INTERNATIONAL ENCYCLOPEDIA OF
PHARMACOLOGY AND THERAPEUTICS

Executive Editor: A. C. SARTORELLI, *New Haven*

Section 115

THE MODULATION OF IMMUNITY

Some Recent and Forthcoming Volumes

INTERNATIONAL ENCYCLOPEDIA OF
PHARMACOLOGY AND THERAPEUTICS

Section 115

THE MODULATION OF IMMUNITY

EDITOR

MALCOLM S. MITCHELL

University of Southern California School of Medicine
Los Angeles, USA

PERGAMON PRESS

OXFORD · NEW YORK · TORONTO · SYDNEY · FRANKFURT

U.K.	Pergamon Press Ltd., Headington Hill Hall, Oxford OX3 0BW, England
U.S.A.	Pergamon Press Inc., Maxwell House, Fairview Park, Elmsford, New York 10523, U.S.A.
CANADA	Pergamon Press Canada Ltd., Suite 104, 150 Consumers Road, Willowdale, Ontario M2J 1P9, Canada
AUSTRALIA	Pergamon Press (Aust.) Pty. Ltd., P.O. Box 544, Potts Point, N.S.W. 2011, Australia
FEDERAL REPUBLIC OF GERMANY	Pergamon Press GmbH, Hammerweg 6, D-6242 Kronberg-Taunus, Federal Republic of Germany

First edition 1985

Library of Congress Cataloging in Publication Data

Main entry under title:
The modulation of immunity.
(International encyclopedia of pharmacology and therapeutics ; section 115)
Includes index.
1. Immune response — Regulation.
2. Immunosuppressive agents. 3. Adjuvants, Immunological. I. Mitchell, Malcolm S. II. Series.
[DNLM: 1. Immunity, Cellular.
2. Antibody Formation. 3. Adjuvants, Immunologic.
QV 4 I58 section 115]
QR186.M63 1985 616.07'9 84–14804

British Library Cataloguing in Publication Data

The modulation of immunity
(International encyclopedia of pharmacology and therapeutics; section 115)
1. Immunology
I. Mitchell, Malcolm S. II. Series
616.07'9 QR181
ISBN 0–08–031977–7

Published as Supplement No. 15 (1985) to the review journal *Pharmacology & Therapeutics*

Printed in Great Britain by A. Wheaton & Co. Ltd., Exeter

PREFACE

This volume devoted to 'The Modulation of Immunity' has attempted by its title and its contents to make two fundamental points. First, the effects that microbial and chemical modulators exert on immunity can best be understood as perturbations of the intrinsic modulations that continually occur within the lymphoid system. Second, the so-called 'immunological adjuvants' or 'immunopotentiators' do not always augment but often decrease the immune response, just as 'immunosuppressive (cytotoxic) agents' are capable of stimulating immunity at certain schedules.

Dosage and scheduling of agents relative to the antigen are critical in determining the outcome of their activity, and even the species and strain of animal must be considered with some agents, but this is exactly what one might expect in the use of any pharmacological agent. It may be of little consolation, but the complexity of the actions of immunological modulators even with defined antigens makes it small wonder that the most appropriate regimens for the use of these agents against tumors have not yet been established. Some agents currently evaluated are probably not being used to their full potential, because they are being given by routes that may permit only their local (inflammatory) effects, while others may prove to have little besides inflammatory actions when tested thoroughly. In addition, the maximal effectiveness of many modulators may depend upon their use with other stimulants of immunity, such as specific antigens with the nonspecific 'adjuvants'.

Regardless of the applications to which extrinsic modulators might be put, it is worth emphasizing that they should be approached as an extension of immunological and other biological regulatory systems. Some modulators currently being tested are in fact biological substances, and it is conceivable that some of the intrinsic mediators released by lymphocytes or macrophages could be used to advantage in the future, particularly if their release is an important mechanism by which extrinsic substances act. In any case, we have chosen first to review the ways in which the immune system regulates itself, to set off the modulators that may impinge upon it, even though many of the mechanisms of action of the latter are incompletely understood. By keeping this framework in mind, not only the mode of action of currently available agents can be determined, but one might predict which new agent might be developed to augment or counteract a specific regulatory step.

The contributors have been invited to review their subjects critically and in many instances have reviewed a good deal of their own work in a broader context than in their shorter original papers. If personal biases have been expressed, that is all to the good I think, since the documentation is ample and the reader can ultimately decide what to believe. We hope that this juxtaposition of 'pure' and 'applied' immunology will help to bridge the gap between two areas of investigations into the immune response, a distinction that many of us have always considered artificial.

M. S. MITCHELL

CONTENTS

LIST OF CONTRIBUTORS xi

Part I: INTRINSIC REGULATION OF THE IMMUNE RESPONSE 1

1. MODULATION OF IMMUNITY BY THYMUS-DERIVED LYMPHOCYTES

SUSAN SOLLIDAY RICH and ROBERT R. RICH, *Baylor College of Medicine, Houston, USA*

1. Introduction 3
2. The Immune System: Cells and Responses 3
3. Facilitative T Cell Regulation of Immune Responses 7
4. Negative T Cell Regulation of Immune Responses 12
5. Genetic Control of Regulatory T Cell Interactions 19
References 23

2. MODULATION OF IMMUNITY BY MACROPHAGES

HOWARD T. HOLDEN, *National Cancer Institute, Bethesda, USA* and RONALD B. HERBERMAN, *Frederick Cancer Center, Maryland, USA*

1. Introduction 35
2. Enhancement of the Immune Response by Macrophages 38
3. Suppression of Immune Responses by Macrophages 51
4. Concluding Remarks 69
References 71

3. MODULATION OF IMMUNITY BY ANTIGENS, ANTIBODIES AND ANTIGEN-ANTIBODY COMPLEXES

NICHOLAS R. STC. SINCLAIR, *The University of Western Ontario, Canada*

1. Introduction 81
2. Cellular Mechanisms in Immune Responses 82
3. Modulation of the Immune Response by Antibody 102
4. Modulation of the Immune Response by Antigen 126
5. Conclusions 135
References 138

4. MODULATION OF IMMUNITY BY SOLUBLE MEDIATORS

BYRON H. WAKSMAN, *National Multiple Sclerosis Society, New York, USA*

1. Introduction 159
2. Classification of MK, LK and other Cytokines 159
3. Biological Role of MK, LK and other Cytokines 163
4. Relation of *in vitro* Observations to *in vivo* Events 165
5. The Central Role of the Macrophage 168
6. Purification and Characterization of MK, LK and other Cytokines 169
7. Target Cell Receptors and Specificity for Soluble Mediators 172
8. Identity of Cells Producing Different Mediators 175
9. Mechanism(s) of Mediator Production and Release 177
10. Action of Cytokines on Target Cell Functions 180
11. Nomenclatural Problems 186
12. Problems for the Future 187
References 188

Part II: EXTRINSIC IMMUNOMODULATION: THE PERTURBATION OF INTRINSIC REGULATION 209

A. Microbes

5. VIRUSES AND THE IMMUNE RESPONSE

STEVEN SPECTER and HERMAN FRIEDMAN, *University of South Florida, Tampa, USA*

1. Introduction 211
2. Historical Background 211
3. Current Concept of Immunity as Related to Virus-induced Immunosuppression 212
4. Mechanisms of Virus-induced Immunosuppression 214
5. Suppression of Humoral Immunity by Oncogenic Viruses 215
6. Effects of Oncogenic Viruses on Cellular Immunity 220
7. Effect of Viruses on Macrophage Functions 224
8. Conclusions 232
9. Summary 233
References 234

6. MODULATION OF IMMUNITY AND HOST RESISTANCE BY MICRO-ORGANISMS

JOHN B. HIBBS, JR., JACK S. REMINGTON and CARLETON C. STEWART, *Veterans Administration Hospital and University of Utah, USA; Palo Alto Medical Research Foundation and Stanford University, USA; Los Alamos National Laboratory, Los Alamos, USA*

1. Introduction 241
2. The Host Response to Intracellular Micro-organisms Results in Increased Nonspecific Resistance to Taxonomically and Antigenically Unrelated Intracellular Micro-organisms 242
3. The Macrophage is the Effector Cell in Expression of Increased Nonspecific Resistance to Intracellular Micro-organisms—the Concept of Acquired Cellular Immunity 243
4. The Host Response to Intracellular Infection Results in Increased Resistance to Neoplasia 245
5. The Macrophage is the Effector Cell in Expression of Increased Nonspecific Resistance to Neoplastic Cells 249
6. The Host Response to Intracellular Infection Results in a Suppressed Response to Specific Immunologic Stimuli 256
7. The Macrophage is an Effector Cell Capable of Suppressing Immunologic Responses 262
8. Does Macrophage Activation Induced by Soluble Lymphocyte Products (Lymphokines) Result in Acquisition of an Increased Potential for Expression of Immunosuppressive as well as Tumoricidal Effect by Activated Macrophages? 263
9. There are a Number of Biochemical Mechanisms that Potentially could have a Role in Producing Immunosuppression Induced by Administration of Microbial Agents 265
10. Conclusion 266
References 267

7. MODULATION OF IMMUNITY BY BACILLUS CALMETTE-GUÉRIN (BCG)

MALCOLM S. MITCHELL, *University of Southern California, Los Angeles, USA* and RICHARD I. MURAHATA, *Armour-Dial Research Laboratory, Arizona, USA*

1. Introduction 275
2. Effects on Specific Types of Lymphoid Cell 281
3. Fractions of BCG 288
4. Clinical Immunotherapy with BCG 291
5. Conclusions and Projections 294
References 295

8. METHANOL EXTRACTION RESIDUE: EFFECTS AND MECHANISMS OF ACTION

SHLOMO BEN-EFRAIM, *Tel-Aviv University, Israel*

1. Introduction 303
2. Effects of MER on States of Resistance and Immunological Reactivity 305
3. Mode of Action Studies 321
4. Concluding Remarks 329
References 331

9. IMMUNOBIOLOGY OF *CORYNEBACTERIUM PARVUM*

JACOB ZIGHELBOIM, *University of California, Los Angeles, USA* and DAVID BERD, *Thomas Jefferson University, Philadelphia, USA*

1. Introduction 339
2. Morphologic Alterations Following *C. parvum* 340
3. Modulation of Reticuloendothelial Function 342
4. Resistance to Infectious Agents 342
5. Antitumor Activity 343
6. Antitumor Effects in Man 345
7. Modulation of the Immune Response 346
8. Delayed Hypersensitivity 347
9. Mechanism of Action 348
10. Effects on Macrophages 348
11. Lymphocytes—B Cells 351
12. Lymphocytes—T Cells 352
13. NK Cells 354
14. Concluding Remarks 354

References 354

B. Chemical Agents

10. MODULATION OF THE IMMUNE RESPONSE BY CHEMOTHERAPY

DONALD P. BRAUN and JULES E. HARRIS, *Rush Presbyterian–St Luke's Medical Center, Chicago, USA*

1. Introduction 359
2. Drugs Effects on Afferent Immune Responses 359
3. Drug Effects on Central Immune Responses 365
4. Drug Effects on Efferent Immune Response 379
5. Conclusions 383

References 384

11. MODULATION OF IMMUNITY BY LEVAMISOLE AND DTC

GÉRARD RENOUX, *Faculté de Médecine, Tours, France*

1. Introduction 393
2. Chemistry, Pharmacology and Metabolism of Levamisole 394
3. Experimental Immunomodulation Studies with Levamisole 395
4. Clinical Use of Levamisole 399
5. Chemistry, Metabolism and Pharmacology of Sodium Diethyldithiocarbamate, DTC 400
6. Experimental Immunomodulation Studies with DTC 402
7. Mechanisms of Action of DTC 404
8. Influences of DTC on Immune Parameters in Man 405
9. General Conclusions 406

References 407

12. THE INFLUENCE OF SYNTHETIC HOMORIBOPOLYNUCLEOTIDE COMPLEXES ON THE IMMUNE RESPONSE

ROBERT E. CONE, *University of Connecticut School of Medicine, Farmington, USA*

1. Introduction 411
2. Historical 411
3. Augmentation of Humoral Immune Response 412
4. Cell Mediated Immunity 414
5. Immune Defense 416
6. Tumor Immunity 417
7. Immunosuppressive Effects of Polynucleotide Adjuvants 418
8. Cellular Sites of Action of Polynucleotide Adjuvants 419
9. Mode of Action of Polynucleotide Adjuvants 421
10. Future Prospects 424

References 425

13. THE BIOLOGICAL ACTIVITY OF THE SYNTHETIC POLYANION, PYRAN COPOLYMER (DIVEEMA, MVE, 46015) AND THE HETEROCYCLIC BIS DEAE FLUORENONE DERIVATIVE, TILORONE AND CONGENERS: CLINICAL AND LABORATORY EFFECTS OF THESE AGENTS AS MODULATORS OF HOST RESISTANCE

WILLIAM REGELSON, *Virginia Commonwealth University, Richmond, USA*

1. Introduction 429
2. Synthetic Polyanions 430
3. Pyran Discussion 435
4. Pyran: Adjuvant Action 441
5. Pyran: Summary and Conclusion 443
6. Tilorone and its Analogs 444
7. Anti-tumour Activity 450
8. Effects on Immune and Inflammatory Response 452
9. Clinical Anti-tumour Studies 455
10. Miscellaneous Action 457
11. Related Compounds 458
12. Conclusion: Tilorone and Analogs 459
13. Final Summary: Pyran, Tilorone and their Derivatives 459
References 461

INDEX 473

LIST OF CONTRIBUTORS

BEN-EFRAIM, S.
Department of Human Microbiology, Sackler School of Medicine, Tel-Aviv University, Ramat-Aviv, Tel-Aviv, Israel.

BERD, D.
Department of Medicine, Thomas Jefferson University, Philadelphia, PA 19111, USA.

BRAUN, D. P.
Department of Medicine, Rush Presbyterian–St. Luke's Medical Center, Chicago, IL 60612, USA.

CONE, R. E.
Department of Pathology, University of Connecticut School of Medicine, Farmington, CT 06030, USA.

FRIEDMAN, H.
Department of Microbiology, University of South Florida, Tampa, FL 33612, USA.

HARRIS, J. E.
Department of Medicine, Rush Presbyterian–St. Luke's Medical Center, Chicago, IL 60612, USA.

HERBERMAN, R. B.
Frederick Cancer Center, Frederick, MD 21201, USA.

HIBBS, J. B.
Department of Medicine, VA Hospital, University of Utah School of Medicine, Salt Lake City, UT 84148, USA.

HOLDEN, H. T.
National Cancer Institute, Bethesda, MD 20205, USA.

MITCHELL, M. S.
Departments of Medicine and Microbiology, University of Southern California School of Medicine, Los Angeles, CA 90033, USA.

MURAHATA, R. I.
Armour-Dial Research Laboratory, Scottsdale, AR 85251, USA.

REGELSON, W.
Department of Medicine, Medical College of Virginia, Richmond, VA 23298, USA.

REMINGTON, J. S.
Department of Immunology and Infectious Diseases, Palo Alto Medical Research Foundation, Palo Alto, CA 94301, USA.

RENOUX, G. E.
Laboratory of Immunology, Faculty of Medicine, Tours, France.

RICH, R. R.
Department of Microbiology and Immunology, Baylor College of Medicine, Houston, TX 77030, USA.

RICH, S. S.
Department of Microbiology and Immunology, Baylor College of Medicine, Houston, TX 77030, USA.

SPECTER, S.
Department of Microbiology, University of South Florida, Tampa, FL 33612, USA.

STC. SINCLAIR, N. R.
Department of Microbiology and Immunology, University of Western Ontario, London, Ontario, Canada.

STEWART, C. C.
Department of Experimental Pathology, Los Alamos National Laboratories, Los Alamos, NM 87545, USA.

WAKSMAN, B. H.
National Multiple Sclerosis Society, 205 E 42nd Street, New York, NY 10017, USA.

ZIGHELBOIM, J.
University of California, Los Angeles School of Medicine, Los Angeles, CA 90024, USA.

PART I

INTRINSIC REGULATION OF THE IMMUNE RESPONSE

CHAPTER 1

MODULATION OF IMMUNITY BY THYMUS-DERIVED LYMPHOCYTES

SUSAN SOLLIDAY RICH and ROBERT R. RICH

Department of Microbiology and Immunology; and The Howard Hughes Medical Institute at Baylor College of Medicine, Houston, Texas, USA

1. INTRODUCTION

Antigenic stimulation of the immune system initiates a complex series of interactions between distinct types of immunologically active cells. Culminating these finely integrated interactions is a biologically effective immune response expressed through specific antibody synthesis and directly active effector cells. The nature of the immune response, its magnitude, tempo and specific form, is determined by an array of modulatory processes which are associated with antigen and its presentation, as well as with intrinsic properties of the immune system. Within the immune system multiple pathways of modulation, or regulation, are associated with different types of immunologically active cells and their products. Thus, a broad spectrum of effect is possible. In this review we shall focus upon the regulation of immunocompetent cell functions by the thymus-derived class of lymphocytes (T cells),* as mediated directly or via their products. The unique and potent regulatory functions of T cells in both facilitation and suppression of various types of immune reactivity will be described; when possible we will attempt to identify target cells and mechanisms of effect. Since induction and regulation of immunity involve complex cellular interactions we shall briefly review the roles of different classes of immunologically active cells, as well as phenotypic and functional heterogeneity within each class. Most of the work discussed has been performed with mice; to the extent that observations have been extended to other species, however, the conclusions appear to be general. Throughout it is hoped that the phenomena described will be seen in the broad context of intercellular communication, which in the specialized context of the immune system results in generation and regulation of immune responses.

2. THE IMMUNE SYSTEM: CELLS AND RESPONSES

After activation of antigen-reactive precursor cells by specific antigens, a complex, coordinated series of cellular interactions is initiated. Two distinct types of immune responses evolve, cell-mediated immunity and antibody synthesis. Discovery of two separate pathways for differentiation of antigen-reactive precursor cells led to definition of the roles that each type of cell plays in such responses. Pluripotent hematopoietic stem cells, derived from the

*Abbreviations used in this review: ALS, anti lymphocyte serum; ABA, azobenzenearsonate; B cell, antibody-producing cell precursor; C_H, constant region of immunoglobulin heavy chain; C_L, constant region of immunoglobulin light chain; Con A, concanavalin A; CTL, cytotoxic thymus-derived lymphocyte; CTL_p, precursor of cytotoxic thymus-derived lymphocyte; DTH, delayed-type hypersensitivity; GAT, terpolymer of L-glutamic acid^{60}–L-alanine^{30}–L-tyrosine^{10}; GVH, graft-versus-host; Id, idiotype; Ig, immunoglobulin; Igh, gene complex controlling immunoglobulin heavy chain structure; IL-1, interleukin 1; IL-2, interleukin 2; KLH, keyhold limpet hemocyanin; MHC, major histocompatibility gene complex; MLR, mixed leukocyte reaction; PHA, phytohemagglutinin; SIRS, soluble immune response suppressor; SLE, systemic lupus erythematosus; SRBC, sheep red blood cell; T cell, thymus derived lymphocyte; T_H, helper T cell; TRF, T cell replacing factor; Ts, suppressor T cell; Ts_2, second order suppressor T cell; Ts_3, third order suppressor T cell; TsF, T cell suppressor factor; V_H, variable region of immunoglobulin heavy chain.

bone marrow, differentiate into immunocompetent, antigen-reactive precursors in the primary lymphoid organs. The thymus promotes differentiation of stem cells into thymus-derived (T) lymphocytes, and the ill-defined mammalian analogue of the avian bursa of Fabricius enables development of stem cells into precursors of antibody-producing cells or B lymphocytes (Katz and Benacerraf, 1973; Pierce and Benacerraf, 1976; Warner, 1974; Cantor and Weissman, 1976). Concomitant with the acquisition of immunocompetence, precursor T and B cells become committed to singular antigen-specific responsiveness (Burnet, 1959).

B cells recognize antigen via membrane-integrated immunoglobulin molecules specific for that antigen. They respond by proliferation and differentiation into plasma cells. These cells secrete antibody molecules with antigen-binding properties identical to those of the B cell membrane immunoglobulins (Warner, 1974). The variable region of an antibody molecule, containing the antigen-binding site, is distinguished by a unique set of determinants associated with the primary amino acid sequence forming the binding site structure. The combination of these determinants is termed *idiotype* (Id) (Capra and Kehoe, 1975; Eichmann, 1978); in sufficient concentration they may themselves be recognized as antigenic. In turn, they can stimulate idiotype-specific (i.e. anti-idiotypic) antibodies and T cells that seem likely to be of major importance in the development of circular immunoregulatory networks (Jerne, 1974). A major fraction of antibodies produced to certain antigens may share a predominant or cross-reactive idiotype (Nisonoff *et al.,* 1977; Makela and Karjalainen, 1977). This class of idiotypes has proven invaluable in determining the relationship of B cell and T cell antigen receptors and mechanisms of interaction among and between these cell types. Some stimulated B cells do not proceed to antibody production but differentiate instead to long-lived memory cells with anamnestic response capabilities on re-exposure to the appropriate antigen (Warner, 1974; Pierce and Benacerraf, 1976; Katz, 1977). Alternatively, under certain circumstances, interaction with antigen renders B cells tolerant or unresponsive, and they differentiate neither to memory cells nor to antibody synthesizing cells (Weigle, 1973; Katz and Benacerraf, 1974; Stocker and Nossal, 1976; Metcalf and Klinman, 1976).

T cells are the effectors of cell-mediated immune responses. Antigen recognition is mediated through interaction with antigen-specific membrane receptors (Warner, 1974; Pierce and Benacerraf, 1976; Katz, 1977; Marchalonis, 1980). In contrast to B cell surface immunoglobulin receptors, the T cell receptor for antigen is not classical immunoglobulin, although it may possess the terminal antigen binding portion of the heavy chain of the immunoglobulin molecule. Idiotypic determinants have been identified on T cell antigen receptors (Binz and Wigzell, 1975; Eichmann and Rajewsky, 1975; Eichmann, 1978; Dietz *et al.,* 1980), and sera specific for framework determinants on immunoglobulin heavy chain variable regions (V_H) interfere with certain T cell functions and bind antigen-specific T cell products (Ben Neriah *et al.*, 1980; Puri *et al.*, 1980; Tada *et al.*, 1980). An additional unique property of T cell antigen recognition is the requirement that mature T cells recognize antigen in the context of major histocompatibility gene complex (MHC) encoded 'self' determinants on the surface of antigen presenting or target cells (Zinkernagel and Doherty, 1979; Shearer and Schmitt-Verhulst, 1977; Schwartz *et al.,* 1976). This phenomenon will be discussed in a subsequent section. The nature of the receptor assembly required to accommodate recognition of both foreign and self moieties, i.e. individual antigen and self-MHC specific receptors or a single receptor which encompasses features of both determinants (Zinkernagel and Doherty, 1977), has not been established.

Following antigenic stimulation T cells do not produce antibody molecules but rather mediate other diverse immunological phenomena. Stimulated T cells, like B cells, may proliferate; when the stimulating antigens are foreign histocompatibility antigens, the proliferative response is termed the mixed leukocyte reaction (MLR). T cells also differentiate into cytotoxic T lymphocytes (CTL) which lyse target cells against which they have been sensitized *in vitro* (Wagner *et al.,* 1973). These *in vitro* T cells responses are mediated by distinct T cell subpopulations that collaborate *in vivo* in the development of complex T cell-mediated immune responses such as graft-versus-host (GVH) reactions and homegraft and tumor rejection (Wagner *et al.,* 1973; Cerottini and Brunner, 1974; Cantor and Weissman, 1976;

Engers and MacDonald, 1976). In addition, activated T cells secrete a variety of soluble factors or lymphokines, including macrophage migration inhibition factor, chemotactic factors, lymphotoxin, skin reactive factors, and interferon (Waksman and Namba, 1976; Cohen, 1980; Gresser, 1980). These factors contribute to the inflammatory processes and tissue damage of cell-mediated delayed hypersensitivity reactions and probably play important roles in host-defence mechanisms in various infectious diseases (Lawrence and Landy, 1969; Bloom, 1971; David, 1975; McGregor and Kostiala, 1976). In addition to direct effector functions, T cells subserve critical regulatory functions which ultimately affect all cellular and soluble aspects of the immune system. In this capacity, T cells secrete a number of specific and nonspecific products that mediate both facilitative and suppressive functions; characteristics of such cells and factors will be addressed in detail in this review. Like B cells, T cells may develop into long-lived antigen-specific memory cells (Cantor and Weissman, 1976), or may be rendered tolerant to specific antigenic challenge under appropriate conditions (Weigle, 1973; Katz and Benacerraf, 1974; Basten *et al.,* 1975; Katz, 1977).

Macrophages are associated with both humoral and cell-mediated immune responses and their related B and T effector cells and constitute the third essential cellular component of immune responses. These cells perform crucial accessory functions in the uptake, catabolism and presentation of antigen to both T and B cells, leading to initiation of immune responsiveness and avoidance of tolerance induction (Unanue, 1972; Nelson, 1976; Dresser and Mitchison, 1968; Moller, 1978). Furthermore, by presenting antigen in association with their cell surface histocompatibility antigens, these cells may be critically important in defining the immunogenic moiety to which T cells respond (Pierce *et al.,* 1976; Rosenthal and Shevach, 1976; Miller *et al.,* 1976; Thomas and Shevach, 1976). Finally, there is substantial evidence that macrophages function as secondary nonspecific effector cells in the expression of both antibody and cell-mediated responses (Unanue, 1972; David, 1975; Nelson, 1976; Unanue *et al.,* 1976).

2.1 T Cell Subpopulations

Characterization of T and B cell responses to antigens and definition of the cellular requirements for cell-mediated and humoral immunity has additionally revealed phenotypic and functional heterogeneity which defines subpopulations within the class of mouse T lymphocytes. One scheme of T cell classification, essentially related to stages of differentiation, is based on membrane alloantigens, lifespan, migration patterns and less definitively, on functional properties (Stobo and Paul, 1973; Kappler *et al.,* 1974; Araneo *et al.,* 1975; Cantor and Weissmann, 1976; Cantor *et al.,* 1975).

The most immature T cell population is resident in thymus, displays abundant Thy-l (previously termed θ, an alloantigen found on all murine T cells) and little major histocompatibility complex (MHC)-coded alloantigens. These cells are highly susceptible to treatment with corticosteroids. They are generally poorly responsive to antigenic stimulation; they do, however, exhibit good proliferative responses to the T cell-specific mitogen concanavalin A (Con A), but not to another T cell mitogen, phytohemagglutinin (PHA). Inferential evidence suggests that these thymocytes differentiate independently of antigenic stimulation to a second relatively immature subpopulation which is found among peripheral T cells and corticosteroid-resistant thymocytes. Such cells display intermediate amounts of Thy-1 and MHC antigens. These cells migrate preferentially to the spleen, do not recirculate extensively through the blood and lymphatic systems, are short-lived, and demonstrate good proliferative responses to both PHA and Con A. Additional characteristics are relative radiosensitivity and insensitivity to small doses of antilymphocyte serum (ALS) or thoracic duct drainage. They are depleted within 2 to 3 weeks after adult thymectomy, indicating dependence on continuing thymic influence. The final functional T cell subset which differentiates independently of the previous short-lived peripheral T cell subpopulation, is more mature, longer-lived, migrates preferentially to lymph nodes and recirculates in peripheral blood and lymphatic vessels. Cell-surface alloantigens reflect reduced Thy-1 and increased MHC-coded antigens. These cells are depleted after treatment with ALS or thoracic duct drainage, but are relatively unaffected by adult thymectomy and respond more vigorously to PHA than to Con A.

The most fruitful approach to distinction among subsets of T cells has been through characterization of Ly (Lymphocyte) surface alloantigens, Ly-1, Ly-2 and Ly-3 (Boyse *et al.*, 1968, 1971: Klein, 1975). Like Thy-1, these antigens are displayed on surfaces of thymocytes and peripheral T cells, but not on B cells. T cells may be divided into three subclasses bearing Ly-1, 2 and 3 (Ly-123$^+$), Ly-1 (Ly-1$^+$) or Ly-2 and 3 together (Ly-23$^+$) antigens. Most thymocytes are Ly-123$^+$. Among peripheral T cells the three classes are present in decreasing proportions, i.e. Ly-123$^+$, approximately 50 per cent of splenic T cells; Ly-1$^+$ (approximately 30 per cent) and Ly-23$^+$ (5–10 per cent). Current evidence suggests that immature T cells bear all three Ly alloantigens, and may differentiate before antigenic stimulation into cells bearing either Ly-1 or both Ly-2 and Ly-3 alloantigens (Cantor and Boyse, 1975a, b; Huber *et al.*, 1976a). While Ly-23 antigens are absent from mature Ly-1$^+$ cells, the Ly-1 antigen is found on all populations; Ly-1$^+$ cells express high levels of the antigen while Ly-23$^+$ cells possess levels detectable only by sensitive flow microfluorometric analyses (Nakayama *et al.*, 1979; Ledbetter and Herzenberg, 1979).

Unequivocal assignment of specific T cell functions to subclasses designated according to specific phenotypic or differentiative criteria has not yet been clearly established. However, the Ly system has been most useful in this regard. Generally, T cells expressing Ly-1 but lacking Ly-23 antigens include effector cells for delayed hypersensitivity responses (Vadas *et al.*, 1976; Huber *et al.*, 1976b) as well as cells that mediate proliferative responses to alloantigens in MLR (Cantor and Boyse, 1975b). In contrast, CTL are Ly-23$^+$ (Cantor and Boyse, 1975a, b; Cantor and Weissman, 1976; Kisielow *et al.*, 1975; Shiku *et al.*, 1975). Interestingly, recent reports document blocking of alloantigen-primed Ly-23$^+$ T cell cytotoxicity by conventional (Shinohara and Sachs, 1979; Nakayama *et al.*, 1980), or monoclonal (Sarmiento *et al.*, 1980; Hollander *et al.*, 1980) anti-Ly-2 reagents. Thus it has been speculated that the molecule bearing Ly-23 is sterically associated with or directly active in CTL receptor interactions.

Classification of regulatory T cells, to be discussed in subsequent sections, reveals complexity regarding both assignment of Ly phenotype and placement of these cells within a differentiation pathway. Generally, mature peripheral T cells of Ly 1$^+$ 23$^-$ phenotype mediate helper or amplifier activity in both humoral and cell-mediated immune responses (Cantor and Boyse, 1975a, b; Kisielow *et al.*, 1975; Feldman *et al.*, 1975a; Jandinski *et al.*, 1976; Cantor *et al.*, 1976; Huber *et al.*, 1976a; Herzenberg *et al.*, 1976a), while Ly-23$^+$ cells are responsible for effector suppressor activities (Feldmann *et al.*, 1975; Jandinski *et al.*, 1976; Cantor *et al.*, 1976; Vadas *et al.*, 1976; Herzenberg *et al.*, 1976a; Tada *et al.*, 1977; Germain and Benacerraf, 1981; Rich, R. and Rich, S., unpublished observation). Although the most populous peripheral Ly-123$^+$ subset has been difficult to define functionally, in addition to serving as antecedents of Ly-1$^+$ and Ly-23$^+$ T cells, it appears to function as an important intermediary in multicellular suppressor cell pathways (Feldmann and Kontiainen, 1976; Eardley *et al.*, 1978; McDougal *et al.*, 1979; Taniguichi and Takuhisa, 1980). The preceding information suggests a relatively consistent association of Ly phenotype and T cell function. An alternate and interesting view has recently been formulated which suggests that Ly phenotypes correlate more directly with the particular class of self or allogeneic MHC-encoded determinant recognized by T cells, regardless of their functions, than with the T cell function *per se* (Swain, 1980). The MHC antigens and their roles in the immune response will be described in a subsequent section. Additional studies using well characterized T cell lines and hybrids should clarify these associations between function and surface phenotype.

While this review is based primarily on work from the murine system, it is pertinant to note recent important accomplishments in phenotypic definition of functional human T cell subsets. Largely through the use of the new technology for identification of cell surface antigens with monoclonal antibodies (Kohler and Milstein, 1976; Scharff *et al.*, 1981) it has become apparent that subpopulations of human T cells with distant effector and regulatory activites can also be identified. A large number of differentiation antigens have been identified using these techniques. Several series of monoclonal antibodies have been studied in considerable detail (Reinherz and Schlossman, 1980; Evans *et al.*, 1981). They define molecules on subpopulations of human T cells that appear to be functional and, perhaps in at least some cases, molecular analogues of the murine Thy-1 and Ly molecules. Thus, the large majority of human peripheral blood T cells, but not B cells or other leukocytes, express determinants recognized by monoclonal antibodies designated OKT-3 and Leu-1. A subpopulation of such T cells with helper activities for both T and B cell responses have generally been characterized as OKT-4$^+$ or Leu-3a$^+$. In contrast, T cells expressing the antigenic determinants OKT-5, OKT-8, Leu-2a and Leu-2b have been identified as suppressors of a number of immune responses and, like their Ly-23$^+$ analogues in the mouse, as effectors of *in vitro* T cell-mediated cytotoxicity.

2.2 Regulatory Activities of T Cells

The observations of Claman *et al.* (1966), rapidly confirmed and extended by Miller and Mitchell (1969), Mitchison (1971b) and others, revealed that the humoral immune response is not a unicellular process but rather a product of complex cellular interactions (reviewed Pierce and Benacerraf, 1976; Katz, 1977). Such studies demonstrated facilitative or helper functions of T cells in antibody responses by B cells to complex multi-determinant antigens such as hapten-protein conjugates or heterologous erythrocytes. The concept of positive regulatory function of helper T lymphocytes (T_H) was extended by documentation of cooperative or amplifying interactions among subsets of T cells in the development of cell-mediated immune responses, such as GVH reactions (Cantor and Weissman, 1976) or CTL generation (Wagner *et al.,* 1973; Cantor and Boyse, 1975b). Thus T cells can function in a cooperative fashion to promote or amplify the responses of B cells and other T cells.

It has been more recently appreciated that the opposite regulatory effect, namely suppression or inhibition of immune responsiveness, is also mediated by T cells, designated suppressor T cells (Ts). As with positive regulation, negative T cell regulation influences the nature and magnitude of both T cell-mediated and B cell-mediated immune responses (Gershon, 1974; Pierce and Kapp, 1976; Germain and Benacerraf, 1981).

Consequently it is evident that T lymphocytes play a unique and powerful role as central cellular modulators of the diverse and complex antigen-driven reactions which culminate in an immune response. As suggested previously, opposite regulatory influences appear to reflect activities of separate and distinct subpopulations of T cells. In succeeding sections each of these regulatory phenomena will be described with reference to the type of immune response affected. We will attempt to identify target cells and mechanisms of induction of regulatory effect, insofar as these mechanisms may be understood at this time. In addition, genetic restraints which affect regulatory cell interactions will be discussed.

3. FACILITATIVE T CELL REGULATION OF IMMUNE RESPONSES

3.1 T Cell Facilitation of Antibody Synthesis

Descriptions of the ability of T lymphocytes to modulate B lymphocyte function rest on experimental models of two general types. The first, termed adoptive transfer, is an experimental system in which lymphoid cells, frequently enriched for a particular lymphocyte class or antigenic reactivity, are tested for immune reactivity after transfer to syngeneic recipients which have been rendered immunologically unresponsive (usually through whole-body irradiation). The measured reactivity is considered a functional assessment of the activity of the transferred cells. The second system is based on induction of antibody formation *in vitro* wherein appropriately selected heterogeneous lymphocyte populations, or combinations of purified cell fractions, are cultured with antigen under defined conditions. These culture systems, described by Mishell and Dutton (1967) and Marbrook (1967), allow considerable manipulation of the constituents of an immune response.

Using adoptive transfer, Claman *et al.* (1966) first showed that T cells and B cells act synergistically in reconstitution of immune responsiveness to heterologous erythrocytes. Subsequently, elegant studies of Miller and Mitchell (1968) and Mitchell and Miller (1968) revealed that at least two functionally distinct lymphoid cell classes must interact to effect antibody production *in vivo,* but that only one of these, the B cell, is the specific precursor of antibody-forming cells. The T cell is stimulated by antigens to divide and interacts with antigen-stimulated B cells to facilitate their differentiation to antibody-synthesizing plasma cells. Initial insights into the structural basis of T cell-B cell interaction were provided during this same period by experiements using defined antigens which consisted of a small molecule, by itself nonimmunogenic, coupled to a larger molecule, usually a heterologous protein (Mitchison, 1969, 1971a, b; Katz *et al.,* 1970; Paul *et al.,* 1970). The small molecule, termed the 'hapten,' is the antibody-binding group against which antibody responses are elicited. Haptens are conjugated to the larger molecule, the 'carrier,' which provides a poorly understood but immunologically-specific matrix required for development of a hapten-specific antibody response. Experiments using hapten-carrier antigen systems demonstrated that development of secondary IgG anti-hapten responses to hapten-carrier conjugates required interactions between two populations of primed cells, one of which was hapten-specific and the other carrier-specific. Raff (1970) subsequently demonstrated that carrier specificity was expressed by T cells and hapten specificity by B cells.

In addition to antigen-specific helper cells which interact with determinants on the carrier molecule, distinct populations of T_H have been identified which (1) are functionally *hapten* specific (Cosenza *et al.,* 1977; Eichmann, 1978); (2) express idiotypic determinants associated with that hapten binding specificity (Krawinkel *et al.,* 1977; Hammerling *et al.,* 1976); and (3) express fine specificity markers which are also associated with the V_H region on hapten binding antibody molecules (Krawinkel *et al.,* 1977). Moreover, anti-idiotypic antibodies related to certain hapten-binding specificities have been used to induce (Eichmann and Rajewsky, 1975; Julius *et al.,* 1978) or to block (Julius *et al.,* 1978; Eichman, 1977) hapten-specific T_H activity. It should be noted that hapten specific T_H have been identified utilizing a special class of antigens, such as phosphorylcholine or Group A streptococcal carbohydrate, in which the antigen includes many repeating determinants, thus permitting close approximation of T_H and B cells which both recognize the same group of haptenic determinants. In addition to providing critical, albeit indirect, evidence supporting utilization of immunoglobulin variable region gene products as T cell antigen binding receptors, these data also indicate that T cells, like B cells, are able to recognize haptenic determinants, and in some instances hapten-specific, idiotype bearing T_H are requisite to production of idotype positive, anti-hapten antibody (Hetzelberger and Eichmann, 1978; Cosenza *et al.,* 1977).

During the past several years there has been increasing evidence that one important mechanism of antigen-specific regulation is provided by the synthesis of circular or mirror-like regulatory networks that result from the development of immune responses to the antigen-specific products of the immune response itself (Jerne, 1974; Rowley *et al.,* 1973; Bona and Hiernaux, 1981). Accordingly, a variety of experimental findings have corroborated the existence of two major types of helper T cells participating in antibody responses characterized by a major population of antibody molecules bearing a common idiotype. The first type of T_H interacts directly with determinants of the antigen as just described; the second, an immunoglobulin-recognizing T_H, reacts with the idiotype of the B cell immunoglobulin receptor. Evidence for the second class of T_H derived initially from experiments demonstrating by regression analysis that two interacting sets of T cells, one of which was immunoglobulin reactive, were limiting for collaboration with B cells in response to hapten-derivatized syngeneic myeloma proteins (Janeway *et al.,* 1977). More recently, a role for T_H cells recognizing idiotype (anti-Id T_H) has been inferred by experiments demonstrating that T_H which had been negatively selected by adsorption to plates coated with idiotype-bearing immunoglobulin no longer supported production of Id^+ antibodies, while the Id^- portion of this response was unaffected (Woodland and Cantor, 1978; Sercarz and Metzger, 1980). It is possible that antigen and antigen-specific T_H provide an early stimulus to unprimed B cells, including those bearing the idiotype of interest; accumulation of Id^+ B cells or secreted Id^+ antibodies may then secondarily stimulate anti-idiotypic T_H which enhance the total antigen-specific antibody response through selective expansion of Id^+ B cell clones (Bottomly and Mosier, 1979; Sercarz and Metzger, 1980).

In addition to the directly or operationally antigen-specific helper effects of antigen or idiotype primed T_H cells detailed above, there exist additional avenues for facilitation of B cell responses by activated T cells. Stimulation by exposure to allogeneic cells or Con A allows these cells to promote B cell proliferation and defferentiation in antibody responses to a variety of antigens (Dutton *et al.*, 1971; Schimpel and Wecker, 1971, 1972; Katz *et al.*, 1971; Katz and Benacerraf, 1972; Wecker *et al.*, 1974). Thus the requirement for interaction with carrier-primed T cells may be abrogated by concomitant nonspecific T cell activation (Katz, 1977).

An increasingly comprehensive view of T cell help is based on systematic analyses of soluble products produced by activated T cells. Essentially three general classes of factors have been described. Antigen specific stimulation of T_H cells in the presence of adherent cells generates factors that provide antigen-specific helper activity to purified primed B cells; such an antigen-specific T cell factor has been produced by cloned T cell hybrids and exhibits both antigen binding and V_H characteristics, suggesting it may represent a shed T_H cell antigen receptor (Eshhar *et al.*, 1980). A second soluble T cell product, termed interleukin 2 (IL-2), has been identified in supernates of T cells stimulated by mitogens, conventional antigens or allogeneic lymphocytes (Aarden, 1979) and in supernates of T cell hybridomas (Harwell *et al.*, 1980; Stull and Gillis, 1981). Murine IL-2, a 30,000–35,000 dalton protein, provides a proliferative signal to other T cells, but not B cells, via a specific receptor which is expressed after antigen activation of the target T cells (Smith *et al.*, 1980). This interaction is neither genetically restricted by MHC antigens *(vide infra)* nor antigen specific. Finally, a third T cell factor, T cell replacing factor (TRF) is produced in cultures of antigen or mitogen-stimulated T cells and acts only when added late in cultures of B cells with antigen (Askonas *et al.*, 1974; Schimpl and Wecker, 1975; Schimpl *et al.*, 1980). TRF is antigen non-specific, MHC non-restricted, and appears to interact directly with proliferating B cells to trigger immunoglobulin synthesis or secretion (Schimpl *et al.*, 1980). A cloned T cell product with similar properties has recently been described (Nabel *et al.*, 1981). Both IL-2 (Wagner and Rollinghoff, 1978) and TRF (Pickel *et al.*, 1976) appear to be products of activated Ly-1^+ T cells. However, it is not known if the various specific and nonspecific helper factors are products of distinct T cell subpopulations.

To postulate mechanisms whereby this complex array of helper T cells and factors provide positive regulation of B cell responses it is important to recognize the quantitative nature of T cell regulatory effects. First, there is a class of antigens (thymus-independent antigens) which do not require T cell participation to promote antibody synthesis (Basten and Howard, 1973). These antigens share interesing common structural properties; many are carbohydrates and most are large polymers which exhibit identical, repeating subunits. T-independent antibody responses are generally characterized by predominance of IgM antibody production and lack of memory B cell development (Katz, 1977). Second, using selected antigen concentrations even thymus-dependent antigens may elicit substantial antibody responses of the IgM class in the absence of T cells (Katz and Benacerraf, 1972; Davie and Paul, 1974). Consequently T cells may enhance antibody sythesis through promotion of IgG as well as other isotype production and differentiation of memory B cells, rather than provide an absolute on or off signal.

Several theories have been proposed to explain the facilitative roles of T cells in B cell immune responses. It is probable that multiple antigen-specific as well as non-specific mechanisms are operative under differing circumstances. One proposal, put forth by Mitchison (Mitchison, 1969; Mitchison *et al.*, 1971a, b) and modified by Feldman and Basten (1972), suggest that T cells concentrate antigen via their carrier-specific receptors and thus present a focus of haptenic determinants, which are present on the carrier molecules, to hapten-reactive B cells. It is suggested that the local concentration of haptenic molecules promotes initial B cell triggering. This proposal postulates that antigen provides a direct bridge between carrier-specific helper T cells and hapten-specific B cells (Mitchison *et al.*, 1970). An extension of the above proposal has incorporated the requirement for an additional signal to the B cell to promote proliferation and differentiation to antibody synthesis (Bretscher and Cohen, 1970; Bretscher, 1975). The initial signal depends upon a particular density or organization of antigens, while the other provides a distinct proliferative and/or differentiative signal. Thus carrier or hapten specific T_H can be brought into close physical approximation to hapten-reactive B cells via antigen bridges, while idiotype-specific T_H may interact directly with B cell surface immunoglobulin receptors. Soluble products from activated T_H might then provide the necessary second signal to antigen activated B cells, as well as expand the initial population of helper T cells. Finally, it should be recognized that this discussion of multiple pathways of T cell potentiation of B cell responsiveness does not reflect an emerging heterogeneity of B cell subpopulations, with the potential differential responsiveness to T cell stimulatory signals which may characterize certain B cell subsets (Janossy and Greaves, 1975; Scher *et al.,* 1976; Gronowicz and Coutinho, 1975; Gorczynski and Feldmann, 1975; McDevitt *et al.,* 1976; Ahmed *et al.,* 1977).

3.2 T Cell Facilitation of Cell-mediated Immune Responses

Helper or amplifier T cell interactions with precursors of effector T cells have been described in numerous models of T cell-mediated immune functions. Synergistic interactions between T cells were initially described for GVH reactions (Cantor and Asofsky, 1970, 1972; Cantor and Weissman, 1976). Two T cell subclasses, differentiated on the basis of homing patterns, density of Thy-1 alloantigen, susceptibility to ALS treatment and anatomic location interacted synergistically to produce good GVH reactions when tested together, whereas meager responses were obtained from each population tested independently. Amplifier T cell activity has also been identified in the generation of cytotoxic lymphocytes *in vitro* (Wagner *et al.,* 1973; Bach *et al.,* 1973; Schendel *et al.,* 1973; Eijsvoogel *et al.,* 1973; Cantor and Boyse, 1975a, b). Wagner (1973) described a population of short-lived T cells, found mainly in the thymes and spleen, which was unable to generate cytotoxic lymphocytes independently. However, these cells effected significant enhancement of the differentiation of cytotoxic T cell precusors found mainly among long-lived recirculating T cells in lymph nodes. Concurrent observations by Bach *et al.* (1976), demonstrated that helper T cells respond primarily to differences encoded by the I region of the major histocompatibility complex on the allogeneic stimulating cell while T effector cell precursors are stimulated by target antigens coded by peripheral regions of the complex (see subsequent section on genetic control). Ly phenotype of helper (Ly-1^+) and cytotoxic precursor cells (Ly-23^+) (Cantor and Boyse, 1975a, b) further verified a discrete T cell subset, which amplified activities of antigen-triggered cytotoxic T cell precursors, according to a two signal-two cell model (Bach *et al.,* 1976). This model postulates that Ly-23^+ cytotoxic T cell precursors must be stimulated independently by alloantigen, perhaps to initiate a differentiative process, in order to render them receptive to helper effects of antigen-activated Ly-1^+ cells. Such helper effects might be mediated either directly or via soluble factors.

The initial alloantigen-induced recognitive and proliferative phases in generation of cytotoxic lymphocyte activity, the MLR, also involve synergistic interactions between T cell subpopulations. Several laboratories (Cohen and Howe, 1973; Tittor and Walford, 1974; Jacobsson and Blomgren, 1974) reported that while neither peripheral T cells, localized in lymph node or peripheral blood, nor thymocytes proliferated significantly in response to allogeneic stimuli, mixtures of the two T cell populations generated responses which significantly exceeded a calculated additive response. The bulk of the proliferative activity could be assigned to the peripheral lymph node T cells, while thymocytes appeared to amplify their response (Howe and Cohen, 1975a, b).

It is generally acknowledged that delayed-type hypersensitivity (DTH) reactions require interactions of both activated T cells and macrophages which are attracted to and retained at the site of antigen deposition. While few studies have addressed the issue, it appears that T-T cell interactions also contribute to this T cell-mediated response. Strassmann *et al.,* (1980) have demonstrated that (T,G)-A--L primed Ly 1^+ 23^- T cells effectively transfer DTH reactivity to recipient animals; the same cells failed to transfer reactivity to recipients which were congenitally athymic (nude), neonatally thymectomized, or irradiated and reconstituted with B cells only. Unprimed Ly-123$^+$ radiosensitive T cells were found to be the requisite synergyzing partner for full DTH expression.

Recent analyses of the alloantigen-induced CTL system, utilizing both conventionally prepared and long-term cloned lines of T cells, have corraborated and extended early interpretations of T cell interactions. Wagner and Rollinghoff (1978) verified that alloantigen-activated Ly-1$^+$23$^-$ T cells mediate helper activity by production of soluble factors, now recognized as interleukin 2. The most striking requirement for effective IL-2 interaction with CTL precursors (CTLp) is a previous alloantigen-mediated triggering event in the CTLp population; unprimed CTLp require the concurrent presence of antigen (McDonald *et al.*, 1980), while previously primed CTLp are induced to proliferate by IL-2 in the absence of additional antigen (Wagner and Rollinghoff, 1978). IL-2 plus antigen also promotes differentiation of thymic or peripheral Ly-123$^+$ CTLp to mature Ly-123$^+$ cytotoxic effector cells (Wagner *et al.*, 1980; Hardt *et al.*, 1980; Goronzy *et al.*, 1981). In addition to directly stimulating CTLp development, IL-2 also induces proliferation of additional Ly-1$^+$ T_H (Wagner *et al.*, 1980). CTL systems specific for hapten or virus-modified self determinants similarly demonstrate such IL-2-mediated events (Wagner *et al.*, 1980). Thus significant IL-2-induced expansion of both T_H and CTL populations contribute to the final profile of T cell-mediated lysis.

Enrichment of functional subsets of alloreactive T cells by continuous *in vitro* stimulation, together with use of T cell growth factors (IL-2) has allowed development of clones of T cells mediating a wide variety of regulatory and effector functions (rev. Moller, 1981), and has provided powerful tools in delineating regulatory T cell interactions. CTL amplifier clones, directly or through secretion of soluble growth factors, presumably IL-2, induce the proliferation of cytolytic T cell clones of a variety of MHC or modified-self specificities (Glasebrook and Fitch, 1980; Guimezanes and Schmitt-Verhulst, 1981; von Boehmer and Haas, 1981). Proliferation of *primed* cloned CTL is absolutely IL-2 dependent, but not antigen dependent (rev. Moller, 1981). Interaction of IL-2 with an IL-2-specific receptor, induced by antigen triggering of the CTL, has been suggested by observations that resting T cells are not stimulated by IL-2 to proliferate in the absence of antigen or mitogen triggering (Larsson and Coutinho, 1979; Smith *et al.*, 1980). Moreover, activated but not resting T cells specifically absorb IL-2 activity for CTL proliferation and bind radiolabelled IL-2 (Smith *et al.*, 1980). In this regard, it is of interest that the immunosuppressive drug cyclosporin A reportedly interferes with activated T cell proliferation by blocking expression of the IL-2 receptor (Larsson, 1980). In contrast to cloned CTL, helper T cell clones require continuing antigenic stimulation; the secreted IL-2, however, has neither antigen specificity nor strain restricted properties in interactions with antigen specific CTL (Glasebrook and Fitch, 1980; Guimezanes and Schmitt-Verhulst, 1981; von Boehmer, 1980). Some amplifier clones bear the anticipated Ly$^+$2$^-$ phenotype while others are Ly negative by flow cytofluorometry (Glasebrook and Fitch, 1980). Thus the original predictions of a two signal triggering model in helper T cell-cytotoxic T cell interactions have been persuasively supported by clonal analysis. Receptor binding of antigen by (Ly-1$^+$) T helper cells, in concert with signals from adherent antigen-presenting cells (to be discussed in a later section) lead to secretion of IL-2; independent antigen triggering of Ly-23$^+$ or Ly-123$^+$ CTL precursors induces the expression of an IL-2 specific receptor (Fig. 1). This receptor apparently persists in the primed CTL population since further antigen is not required to maintain IL-2 sensitivity. Binding of IL-2 to its receptor then triggers proliferation of the primed CTL. Although the frequent use of unpurified or partially purified IL-2 preparations may mask additional important signal molecules, the above model appears to be generally valid.

3.3 T Cell Facilitation of Macrophage Effector Functions

Macrophages have important functions, critical to initiation of immune responses, in uptake, catabolism and presentation of antigen to T and B cells. In this role they are capable of regulating activities of surrounding cells. In addition, macrophages function as nonspecific effector cells of immunological processes. In each of these capabilities the functions of macro-

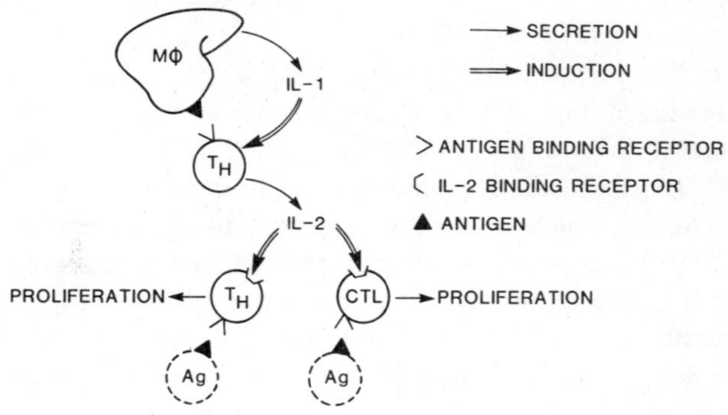

FIG. 1. Model of T cell interactions in CTL generation. Binding of macrophage (M/Ø)-presented antigen together with macrophage-produced interleukin 1 (IL-1) induces helper T cells to secrete interleukin 2 (IL-2). Independent antigen triggering of CTL precursors, as well as of other T_H, promotes expression of IL-2 specific receptors on these cells. Binding of IL-2 to these receptors then induces proliferation of the primed T cells. Antigen presentation to T_H and CTL in IL-2 receptor expression may involve cell types in addition to macrophages.

phages are significantly affected by regulatory influences of T lymphocytes. Antigen handling and presentation by macrophages may be enhanced by helper T cells through concentrated binding of free T cell receptors with attached antigen (Feldmann and Basten, 1972; Feldmann, 1972). In addition, many subclasses of T cells require recognition of conventional antigens in the context of MHC antigens on the macrophage cell surface (to be reviewed in a subsequent section); T cells mediating help or delayed type hypersensitivity reactions are particularly dependent on recognition of Ia antigens, encoded within the I region of the MHC (Miller, 1980). It is now apparent that activated T cells (Beller *et al.*, 1980) or the soluble products of such cells (Steinman *et al.*, 1980) enhance Ia expression on certain macrophage subpopulations. In addition, macrophage participation in antigen presentation and cell interactions also involves the secretion of lympho-stimulatory molecules by macrophages (Unanue *et al.*, 1976). One of the better defined of these molecules, interleukin 1 (IL-1, previously termed lymphocyte activating factor) is a 12,000 to 16,000 dalton single polypeptide molecule which, along with antigen, stimulates the production of IL-2 by helper T cells (rev. Watson, 1981). Interestingly, IL-1 production can be induced in macrophages by T cells in the presence of mitogens or macrophage-bound antigens (Mizel *et al.*, 1978). Thus an effective functional synergy follows binding of macrophage-bound antigen by T cells with the appropriate antigen-specific receptors.

As nonspecific agents of cell-mediated immune functions, phagocytes act as the effector arm of that reaction, while activated T lymphocytes provide the specific recognition. Numerous biological activities have been attributed to soluble factors, or lymphokines, produced by activated T lymphocytes, particularly in models of delayed type hypersensitivity responses, including chemotaxis, immobilization, and activation of phagocytic cells to effect increased destruction of invading agents (Cohen, 1980).

4. NEGATIVE T CELL REGULATION OF IMMUNE RESPONSES

A variety of experiments in which depletion of T cells resulted in enhanced immune responses, or in which addition of thymocytes or selected T cell populations led to reduced responses, suggested that T lymphocytes, in addition to promoting immunity, were also capable of suppressing immune responses of both B and T effector cells (Katz, 1977; Gershon, 1974). Numerous immune phenomena such as antigenic competition, tolerance and autoimmunity have subsequently been associated with suppressor T cell (Ts) activities. Antigenic competition, in which induction of an immune response to one antigen nonspecifically interferes with development of a response to an unrelated antigen, has been ascribed to activation of Ts by the initial antigenic exposure (Taussig, 1973; Gershon, 1974; Pross and Eidinger, 1974; Liacopoulos and Ben-Efraim, 1975). Immunological tolerance in either T or B cell populations may be effected through direct functional inactivation of potentially responsive lymphocytes by antigen or by elimination of specifically reactive clones of cells. On the other hand, suppressor T cells may play a crucial role in some forms of tolerance, both in induction and maintenance (Katz and Benacerraf, 1974; Gershon, 1974; Pierce and Kapp, 1976). A particularly provocative activity of suppressor T cells has been demonstrated in prevention of autoimmune responses. In experimental animal disease models (Allison, 1974a, b; Talal and Steinberg, 1974; Steinberg *et al.*, 1975; Talal, 1976) and perhaps in certain human diseases (Waldmann *et al.*, 1974; Siegel *et al.*, 1976; Abdou *et al.*, 1976; Hoffmann *et al.*, 1977), compromise of normal suppressor T cell function results in occurrence or acceleration of autoimmune disease, implying a regulatory surveillance function of Ts in a biologically balanced system.

Suppressor T cells are of considerable importance as homeostatic regulators of immune responses initiated under normal circumstances; exaggerated suppressor cell activity may be expressed in special situations of antigen or mitogen stimulation. Recent data suggest multiple targets of Ts effect. In following sections, various phenomena attributed to Ts activity will be described in an effort to develop general concepts from diverse experimental models.

4.1 T Cell Suppression of Antibody Synthesis

Suppressor T cell activity in antibody synthesis was initially identified by experimental manipulations such as adult thymectomy or ALS treatment which indiscriminately reduced T cells and consequently increased antibody responses. After administration of ALS, responses to some T-independent antigens such as pneumococcal polysaccharide (Baker *et al.*, 1970a, b, 1974) and polyvinylpyrollidone (Kerbel and Eidinger, 1971, 1972) are markedly enhanced. Adult thymectomy, which decreases Ly-123$^+$ cells in the spleen, enhances responses to some T-independent antigens (Andersson and Blomgren, 1971; Kerbel and Eidinger, 1972; Howard *et al.*, 1973; Gershon, 1974; Rotter and Trainin, 1974), as well as enhancing helper T cell activity for primary responses to T-dependent antigens (Kappler *et al.*, 1974). In other experiments thymocytes were added to normal heterogeneous lymphocyte populations *in vivo* or *in vitro*, leading to antibody responses which were decreased in comparison with that of the normal population alone (Droege, 1971; Droege *et al.*, 1972; Schimpl and Wecker, 1971; Gershon, 1974; Rotter and Trainin, 1974; Cantor and Weissman, 1976). Such experiments suggested that the thymus maintains a suppressor precursor population both locally and secondarily seeded to the spleen, which is a critical regulator of humoral immune responses.

Evidence of naturally occurring suppressor activity also derives from investigations in which normal spleen cells or spleen-seeking cells inhibit responses of other normal peripheral lymphoid populations. Mosier and co-workers (Mosier and Cohen, 1975; Mosier and Johnson, 1975) have demonstrated that the failure of spleen cells from young animals to respond to heterologous erythrocytes *in vitro* is at least partially due to the enhanced activity of suppressor T cells in young spleen. In addition, spleen T cells from young mice suppress antibody responses of adult spleen cells. These findings have obvious implications for the role of suppressor T cells in the maintenance of self-tolerance and the relative ease of tolerance induction in neonatal animals.

Deliberate activation to enhance suppressor cell activity has greatly facilitated investigation of inductive and effector mechanisms in regulation of antibody synthesis. Suppressor cells have been activated both with nonspecific T cell mitogens, e.g. Con A, or with specific antigens, usually presented in relatively high doses or in nonimmunogenic forms. Antigen-specific suppressor cell activity has been described for a wide range of antigens including heterologous erythrocytes (Eardley and Gershon, 1975, 1976), complex proteins (Tada *et al.*, 1975; Basten *et al.*, 1974; Ishizaka and Adachi, 1976; Kontiainen and Feldmann, 1976), synthetic polypeptides (Kapp, 1974a, b) and allotypic (Herzenberg *et al.*, 1976b) and idiotypic (Eichmann, 1975) determinants on immunoglobulin molecules. In such systems suppressor cell effects are specific; antibody responses to unrelated antigens are unaffected. In most responses to hapten-carrier conjugates, suppressor T cell activity is stimulated by, and subsequently expressed specifically against, carrier determinants of the antigenic complex (Okumura and Tada, 1971, 1973). Additionally, antigen-activated suppressors of antibody synthesis may selectively inhibit IgG antibody responses with little effect on IgM production (Tada and Takemori, 1974; Basten *et al.*, 1975; Feldmann, 1974), and may cause decreased average avidity of antibodies produced (Takemori and Tada, 1974). Conversely, loss of suppressor T cell function may lead to disproportionate synthesis of IgG compared with IgM synthesis (Talal, 1976). Due to the central role of helper T cells with regard to both carrier specificity and IgG production, the above evidence strongly suggests that helper T cells are important targets of antigen-specific suppressor T cell activity in antibody synthesis.

Careful analyses of several antigen-specific suppressor systems have suggested that suppression may result from a series of T cell interactions rather than a single Ts-T_H effector cell interaction (Germain and Benacerraf, 1981). Two well-studied systems provide relevant models. A single immunization of mice of certain MHC genotypes with the terpolymer L-glutamic acid^{60}-L-alanine^{30}-L-tyrosine^{10} (GAT) triggers a population of Ts cells; disruption of these cells yields a soluble factor that also suppressed GAT responses (Kapp *et al.*, 1976). This T suppressor cell factor (TsF) binds GAT, shares idiotypic determinants with anti-GAT antibodies, expressed MHC determinants but not Ig constant region markers, is approximately 50,000 mw, and interacts with its target irrespective of the MHC or Igh phenotype of the target cell (rev. Germain and Benacerraf, 1981). The target of GAT-TsF is not a T_H or B cell but rather a second suppressor T cell (Ts_2) found in a nonprimed T cell population (Germain *et al.*, 1978). The activated Ts_2 then suppresses the primary antibody response through interaction with an uncharacterized target. A similar but distinct series of interactions underlies suppression of secondary responses to the protein keyhold limpet hemocyanin (KLH). Multiple exposures to high doses of KLH stimulate splenic and thymic KLH-specific Ts; as above those cells produce a 50,000 mw suppressor factor which has MHC and immunoglobulin V_H, but not C_H or C_L, determinants (Tada *et al.*, 1980). In contrast to the above model, however, KLH-TsF is highly MHC-restricted. That is, suppression is observed only when the cell producing the KLH-TsF and its target cells are of the same MHC phenotype (Taniguchi *et al.*, 1976). Moreover, the target cell is a primed T cell which, upon stimulation with KLH-TsF, acquires suppressive capability and acts directly on T_H without either MHC or Igh restriction (Taniguchi and Takuhisa, 1980). Such data from several systems, including suppression of both humoral and cell-mediated responses, have been integrated to propose a consistent suppressor pathway which generally accounts for the various suppressor T cells, factors and their interactions (Germain and Benacerraf, 1981). Three distinct T suppressor cells, binding either antigen or idiotypic determinants found on receptors for that antigen, act sequentially via soluble mediators; the final Ts_3 cell suppresses in an antigen-nonspecific fashion and without either MHC or Igh restriction. A clear role for anti-idiotypic Ts has been defined in certain of the antibody systems characterized by predominant or cross-reactive idiotypes. Injection of anti-idotypic antibody (Eichmann, 1975; Owen *et al.*, 1977a, b) or syngeneic cells coupled with idiotype-bearing antibody (Dohi and Nisonoff, 1979) both result in selective inhibition of the Id^+ component of a primary response. Ts and TsF with anti-idiotype binding specificity have been associated with such patterns of suppression (Owen *et al.*, 1977a, b; Hirai and Nisonoff, 1980). Anti-idiotypic Ts may then trigger or be triggered by antigen-specific, idiotype-positive Ts within the sequence of the previously described suppressor pathways.

Since a particular antigen activates only the relatively few T cells that possess membrane receptors specific for that antigen, a nonspecific T cell mitogen, Con A has been used to activate large numbers of T cells for antigen-nonspecific suppressor activity. Mitogenic concentrations of Con A added directly to immuno-competent cells and antigen (T-dependent and T-independent), either *in vivo* or *in vitro,* profoundly suppressed primary and secondary IgM and IgG responses (Rich and Pierce, 1973a; Pierce *et al.*, 1975a; Dutton 1972, 1973, 1975). In contrast, *in vivo* generation of memory cells was unimpaired (Rich, 1975). Furthermore, incubation of spleen or lymph node cells with Con A for 48 hr activated a subpopulation of T lymphocytes which, when added in small numbers to cultures of normal cells and antigen, markedly inhibited antibody synthesis. The activity of Con A-activated suppressor cells in antibody synthesis was largely reproduced by a soluble factor secreted by such cells, termed soluble immune response suppressor (SIRS) (Rich and Pierce, 1974; Pierce *et al.*, 1975a, b; Tadakuma *et al.*, 1976). Kinetic analyses of responses suppressed by either Con A-activated T cells or SIRS revealed normal initiation of antibody responses followed by abrupt premature termination (Rich and Pierce, 1973b, 1974). Further studies suggested that the immediate target of SIRS activity is the macrophage (Tadakuma and Pierce, 1976). It has been suggested that SIRS induces macrophages to release an additional soluble inhibitor of cell proliferation which secondarily acts on B cells, accounting for the delayed suppression of antibody responses (Tadakuma and Pierce, 1976). Recent biochemical analyses have indicated that SIRS may be a peroxidase-like molecule that is converted by macrophages to an oxidizing agent; suppression may then be mediated by oxidation of a component required for cell division (Aune and Pierce, 1981). Ly phenotyping has demonstrated that the Con A-activated suppressor of antibody synthesis is a T cell of the Ly-23^+ subclass (Jandinski *et al.*, 1976). This mitogen-stimulated suppressor cell model has thus proven fruitful in dissection of complex regulatory interactions, and may be important to understanding and treating human diseases marked by regulatory cell dysfunction.

4.2 T Cell Suppression of Cell-mediated Immune Responses

Although impeded by less precisely quantitative assay systems, identification of suppressor T cell activity in T cell-mediated immune responses, including generation of cytotoxic T lymphocytes, MLR, GVH, and delayed hypersensitivity, has similarly been achieved. The experiments described below demonstrate negative regulatory effects of suppressor T cells on both the differentiative and effector processes of other subpopulations of T cells.

In cell-mediated immune systems where T lymphocytes with potential suppressor activity are not overtly presensitized, a regulatory role of suppressor T cells may often be inferred. For example, adult thymectomy leads to a decrease of Ly-123^+, cells in the spleen, and results in increased MLR responsiveness (Mosier and Cantor, 1971) and enhanced generation of cytotoxic lymphocytes *in vitro* (Simpson and Cantor, 1975). These experiments suggest that LY-123^+ spleen cells may themselves have regulatory functions, or serve as necessary targets of suppressor activity; in either case removal would interfere with physiologic regulation, allowing enhanced responses to occur.

Antigen-specific suppression mediated by antigen-sensitized T cells is apparent in many models of T cell-mediated immune function, including contact sensitivity (Zembala and Asherson, 1973; Claman *et al.*, 1980; Sunday *et al.*, 1981), delayed-type hypersensitivity (Green *et al.*, 1980; Weinberger *et al.*, 1979; Lieu and Howard, 1980), T cell immunity to syngeneic tumors (Greene, 1980; Fujimoto *et al.*, 1978), cytolytic T cell responses to alloantigens (Truitt *et al.*, 1977) and alloantigen-induced T cell proliferation (Rich and Rich, 1974; Chaouat and Voisin, 1974; Brondz *et al.*, 1980). As with Ts-mediated suppression of humoral immune responses, there is clear evidence that several of the suppressor systems operate via multi-cellular pathways (Fig. 2). Suppression of DTH responses to the hapten azobenzenearsonate (ABA) has been studied extensively and provides the most complete and representative suppressor pathway analysis (rev. Germain and Bencerraf, 1981). Hapten-derivatized syngeneic cells injected intravenously trigger Ts_1, which are antigen binding and share the major cross-reactive idiotype of ABA-binding antibodies. Those cells release an antigen-binding, idiotype positive, genetically-nonrestricted factor, that triggers a second Ts_2 cell characterized by a receptor which binds idiotypic determinants, rather than antigen. Factors released by the second-order suppressor cell, similarly anti-idiotypic, trigger antigen-activated idiotype-positive Ts_3 in a MHC-restricted fashion to finally effect suppression on an unknown target. As in regulation of humoral responses, the final suppressor-target interaction may be mediated by molecules which are entirely antigen nonspecific. Suppression of ongoing immune responses can be achieved by Ts_2 cells or factors, whereas Ts_1 are only effective as afferent regulators given at the time of antigen priming (Dietz *et al.*, 1981). While other suppressor systems are essentially similar in interaction pathway, the intermediary suppressor cell (Ts_2) may express antigen-specific rather than idiotype-specific receptors (Moorhead,

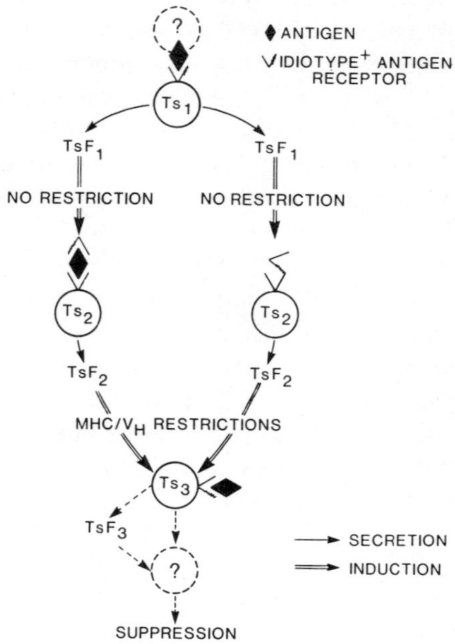

FIG. 2. Model of multicellular cell pathway. The first order suppressor T cell (Ts_1) binds antigen, presented in an unknown fashion, by an idiotype-positive antigen receptor. Activated Ts_1 releases an antigen-binding, idiotype-positive factor which interacts with a second order Ts (Ts_2) expressing an anti-idiotype receptor. The soluble anti-idiotypic factor (TsF_2) produced by this cell triggers idiotype positive Ts_3 in an MHC and V_H restricted fashion. Alternatively, in some systems the Ts_2 cell may be triggered by TsF_1 via an antigen bridge; antigen-binding TsF_2 produced by Ts_2 then similarly activates Ts_3 with MHC restriction. Ts_3, which must be antigen primed before activation by TsF_2, may itself produce a factor, TsF_3, that interacts with an unknown target, in some cases probably a T_H, to mediate suppression. (Adopted from Germain and Benacerraf, 1981.)

1979). Thus either antigen or idiotype can theoretically serve to focus and coordinate such suppressor interactions.

Early studies in a contact sensitivity system demonstrated in addition that normal macrophages incubated with an antigen-specific suppressor factor were armed to perform secondary, nonspecific suppressor activities (Asherson and Zembala, 1974); in such a case macrophages might passively display T cell-derived suppressor products or secondarily produce their own suppressive molecules. There exist a number of reports of antigen-activated suppressor cells which also mediate nonspecific suppression if the original sensitizing antigen is present to elicit suppressor function (Bash and Waksman, 1975; Gelfand and Paul, 1975; Rich, S. and Rich, R., 1975; Schendel *et al.,* 1973; Hirano and Nordin, 1976a, b; Truitt *et al.,* 1977). Consequently it appears that both antigen specific and nonspecific effector functions may accompany the pathway initiated by a specific antigen-T suppressor cell interaction.

Studies of MLR regulation from our laboratory have focused primarily on antigenic and genetic specificity characteristics of splenic suppressor T cells activated *in vivo* by injection of allogeneic cells (Rich, S. and Rich, R., 1974, 1975). Although specific reexposure to the sensitizing alloantigen is required for optimal elicitation of suppressor activity, the suppressor effect *per se* appears to be nonspecific with respect to the stimulator cell in MLR. In contrast, the interaction between the suppressor and the responding cell population in MLR is specific and is controlled by genes encoded in the major histocompatibility gene complex (Rich, S. and Rich, R., 1975, 1976a, b; Rich, S. *et al.* 1977). Alloantigen-activated MLR suppressor cells secrete a soluble product which has been studied to clarify such interactions and to identify the target of suppressor cell activity (Rich, S. and Rich, R., 1975, 1976a, b). Initial attempts to identify a target cell rested on the capacity of various lymphoid cell populations to remove MLR suppressor factor (MLR-TsF) activity by adsorption; only activated T cells were effective adsorbants while resting T cells or activated or resting B cells were ineffective (Rich, S. and Rich, R., 1976b). Thus the function of MLR-TsF may depend on its interaction with a receptor which is expressed only after activation of the susceptible target cell. Additionally, recent studies have demonstrated that MLR-TsF has the capacity to trigger a second order suppressor cell, suggesting a multicellular suppressor pathway in this system as well (Beckwith and Rich, 1981). Recent experiments have also addressed the relationship of binding and functional specificity of MLR-TsF. The majority of suppressor molecules, derived from Ts which are antigen-specific in their triggering requirements (Dennison *et al.*, 1981), appear to be similarly alloantigen-specific and exist mainly in complexes with shed stimulator cell alloantigens. Such complexes suppress MLR in an antigen nonspecific fashion; in contrast noncomplexed MLR-TsF is strictly antigen specific (Rich, S. *et al.*, 1981). Thus the antigen binding specificity only partially establishes the true functional spectrum of an activated suppressor T cell and its products.

Alloantigen-activated suppressor T cells also profoundly suppress the *in vitro* generation of syngeneic cytotoxic lymphocytes (Truitt *et al*, 1977). As in MLR, specificity of suppressor activity elicitation contrasts with nonspecificity of subsequent effect. Soluble factors (CTL-TsF) distinct from those that suppress alloantigen-driven MLR proliferation, mediate CTL suppression and appear to trigger a second order suppressor cell (Truitt *et al.*, 1978, 1979). Interestingly the additional cell in this case is not another T cell but an adherent cell, probably a macrophage. CTL-TsF interacts early, and reversibly with the adherent target, which then effects suppression during the final 48 to 72 h of primary CTL generation (Truitt *et al.*, 1979).

Finally, nonspecific suppression of T cell-mediated immune responses may be achieved by mitogen-activated suppressor T cells (Peavy and Pierce, 1974; Rich, R. and Rich, S., 1975; Shou *et al.*, 1976). Peavy and Pierce (1974) have shown that splenic T cells activated *in vitro* by Con A inhibit differentiation in MLR of syngeneic normal T cells into cytotoxic cells. It is noteworthy that although antibody synthesis (Rich and Pierce, 1973b), and MLR responses (Rich, R. and Rich, S., 1975) and CTL generation (Peavy and Pierce, 1974) are inhibited by Con A-activated T cells, the soluble suppressor elaborated by such cells (SIRS) only suppresses antibody synthesis and does not affect proliferation in MLR or CTL generation (Pierce *et al.*, 1975b; Pierce and Kapp, 1976). It is possible that suppressive regulation by Con A-activated cells may be effected via several functional pathways, e.g. with direct suppressor T cell-responder T cell interaction in MLR and CTL generation, and indirect macrophage-mediated suppression of B cell proliferation (Pierce *et al.*, 1975b). In fact, an additional possibility is raised by experiments of Kastner and Rich (1978) demonstrating that Con A-induced suppressors of CTL generation may act, at least to a significant degree, by direct elimination of allogeneic stimulator cells. Thus the mechanisms of apparent suppressor function of Con A-activated Ts on antibody synthesis and CTL generation may be quite different.

In summary, it has become apparent that there are multiple steps within the generation of a T cell-mediated immune response which require collaborative interactions of discrete subpopulations of T cells. Similarly there may be numerous mechanisms whereby T cells regulate the final magnitude or tempo of such responses. Antigen or idiotype focused suppressor pathways are initiated and integrated with exquisite specificity, while secondary mechanisms allow localized nonspecific extension of the activated regulatory systems.

4.3 Suppressor T Cell Dysfunction and Disease

Disorders of intrinsic suppressor T cell function may play significant roles in the pathogenesis of diseases of autoimmunity and immunodeficiency. Early support for this concept was provided by evidence from several experimental models of autoimmune disease. For example, Allison (1974 a, b) demonstrated active T cell inhibition of autoantibody synthesis in experimental autoimmune thyroiditis. If normal regulatory T cell function was compromised, the autoimmune disease developed or was intensified. Recent data have further supported this hypothesis and have distinguished between naturally occurring Ts, important in the physiological prevention of anti-thyroglobulin antibody responses, and induced Ts, that inhibit responses stimulated by elevated serum levels of native thyroglobulin (Rose *et al.*, 1981).

The most widely studied abnormalities of Ts function in experimental autoimmunity have been those in New Zealand mice. New Zealand Black (NZB) mice develop a spontaneous hemolytic anemia, whereas the F_1 hybrid with New Zealand white (NZB × NZW) develops a syndrome resembling human syngeneic lupus erythematosus (SLE). There is now substantial evidence for suppressor T cell dysfunction in these animals, although the role of the abnormalities in the pathogenesis of clinical disease has remained controversial (Talal and Steinberg, 1974; Steinberg *et al.*, 1981). It is clear, however, that these mice show a premature loss of Ts functions and hyperactivity of B cell functions which precede appearance of disease. These include a marked deficiency in the numbers of Ly-123^+ feedback suppressors recovered from the spleens of young NZB mice (Cantor *et al.*, 1978), as well as the refractoriness of NZB CTL precursors to a soluble suppressor of *in vitro* CTL differentiation (Huston *et al.*, 1979). Additionally, in (NZB × NZW) F_1 mice neonatal thymectomy accelerates the onset of disease; infusion of thymectomized animals with thymocytes from young animals prevents acceleration, whereas thymocytes from older animals are ineffective. This age-dependent loss of suppressor T cell function affects both humoral and cell-mediated responses. Additionally, it has demonstrated that older mice (18 weeks) are incapable of producing SIRS or some other spontaneously released low molecular weight suppressor factor (Krakauer *et al.*, 1976; Raney and Steinberg, 1976). Nonetheless, immunoglobulin synthesis by cultured B cells from these mice is suppressed when they are treated with SIRS from Con A-activated normal cells (Krakauer *et al.*, 1976). A possible role of such suppressor cell factors in pathogenesis is suggested by reports that treatment of young disease-prone mice with regular injections of SIRS (Waldmann *et al.*, 1977) or the low molecular weight suppressor factor (Steinberg *et al.*, 1978) can retard the development of autoimmunity, even after autoantibody production has started. Thus therapeutic replacement of suppressor T cell functions with the soluble products of such cells may eventually find clinical applicability. These observations of autoimmune disease associated with loss of suppressor T cells, coupled with demonstrations of strong suppressor activity in both neonatal animals (Mosier and Johnson, 1975; Mosier and Cohen, 1975) and humans (Miyawaki *et al.*, 1979; Tosato *et al.*, 1980) and with the generalized loss of T cell functions in aging animals (Makinodan and Adler, 1975; Gerbase-DeLima *et al.*, 1975) coincident with increased autoimmunity (Allison, 1974a, b; Stutman, 1974; Burnet, 1974; Good and Yunis, 1974) collectively suggest an inherent role of suppressor T cells in the initiation and maintenance of self-tolerance.

Moreover, recent studies in humans with autoimmune and immunodeficiency diseases now provide considerable support for the clinical relevance of experiments in model disease systems. The work of Waldmann *et al.*, (1974, 1976) first demonstrated suppressor T cell dysfunction in a subset of patients with common variable immunodeficiency. Lymphocytes from individuals with this disease do not synthesize normal quantities of immunoglobulin, although they may possess normal numbers of B cells. T cells from some patients with this disease suppress *in vitro* mitogeninduced immunoglobulin synthesis by B cells from normal individuals. Additionally, B cells from patients synthesize immunoglobulin normally in the presence of normal T lymphocytes (Waldmann *et al.*, 1976). Thus it is postulated that inappropriate suppressor T cell activity inhibits normal B cell function, and that in this form of the disease, the defect in immunoglobulin synthesis may be fundamentally related to T cell dysfunction. Similar evidence for suppressor cell-mediated inhibition of *in vitro* immunoglobulin synthesis has also been obtained in several other, phenotypically quite distinct, immunodeficiency syndromes (Siegal *et al.*, 1976; Broom *et al.*, 1976). Thus one might postulate that Ts dysfunction in such diseases may be either a secondary manifestation or a common primary pathogenetic mechanism. Excessive activity or numbers of suppressor T cells have also been reported in several hematological disorders. These include Hodgkin's disease (Twomey *et al.*, 1975; Hillinger and Herzig, 1978), which may also involve subpopulations of suppressor monocytes; infectious mononucleosis (Crawford *et al.*, 1981); and Felty's syndrome (rheumatoid arthritis, splenomegaly and neutropenia). In the latter disease, Ts-mediated inhibition of granulopoiesis has been advanced as an hypothesis to explain the neutropenia (Abdou *et al.*, 1978). Similarly Ts-induced immunoregulatory dysfunction has been suggested as a contributory mechanism in impaired cellular immunity observed in patients with myesthenia gravis (Birnbaum and Tsairis, 1976) and systemic funcal infections (Stobo *et al.*, 1976).

In accord with findings in experimental autoimmune disease, recent data have been consistent with Ts deficiencies in a wide spectrum of clinical diseases in which autoreactive immunological mechanisms have been invoked. This work is now rapidly accelerating, due in large part to the availability of monoclonal antibodies that can be used to define functional subpopulations of human T cells, differentiating 'helper/inducer' T cells from 'cytotoxic/suppressor' T cells (Reinherz and Schlossman, 1980; Evans *et al.*, 1981). Through *in vitro* studies of the control of T cell responses to antigens or mitogens or of T cell functions as regulators of immunoglobulin synthesis, subnormal Ts function has thus been reported in such diverse diseases as SLE (Fauci *et al.*, 1978; Sakane *et al.*, 1978; Sagawa and Abdou, 1979; Morimoto *et al.*, 1980); insulin-dependent diabetes mellitus (Buschard *et al.*, 1980); inflammatory bowel disease (Hodgson *et al.*, 1978a); hepatitis B antigen-negative chronic hepatitis (Hodgson *et al.*, 1978b; Tremolada *et al.*, 1980); primary biliary cirrhosis (Routhier *et al.*, 1980); multiple sclerosis (Bach *et al.*,1980); asbestosis (Gaumer *et al.*,1981); and familial Mediterranean fever (Ilfeld *et al.*, 1981). Finally, as the capacity to dissect human T cell subpopulations becomes more sophisticated, the definition of defects at multiple points within immunoregulatory circuits seems probable. An interesting example is illustrated by recent data suggesting that an apparent defect in suppressor cell function in patients with juvenile rheumatoid arthritis (Strelkauskas *et al.*, 1978) reflects, in fact, deficiency of $OKT4^+$ suppressor inducer cells, rather than $OKT5^+/OKT8^+$ Ts effector cells (Morimoto *et al.*, 1981).

5. GENETIC CONTROL OF REGULATORY T CELL INTERACTIONS

A provocative feature of interactions of both helper and suppressor T cells with their target cells is the expression and role of products of the major histocompatibility gene complex (MHC). The major histocompatibility complex is a small chromosomal segment of multiple tightly-linked genes which control a variety of immunological functions in addition to cell-surface histocompatibility antigens. The traits and functions associated with the MHC are homologous among mammalian species studied and will be described as identified in the mouse (in which it is designated the *H*-2 complex). The *H*-2 complex has been divided into four regions on the basis of antigens or immunologic functions which each region controls (Schreffler and David, 1975; Klein, 1975) (Fig. 3). The peripheral regions, designated *K* and *D*, encode serologically detectable transplantation antigens, termed Class I antigens, which are present on all tissues of the body. These antigens stimulate T cells to graft rejection and

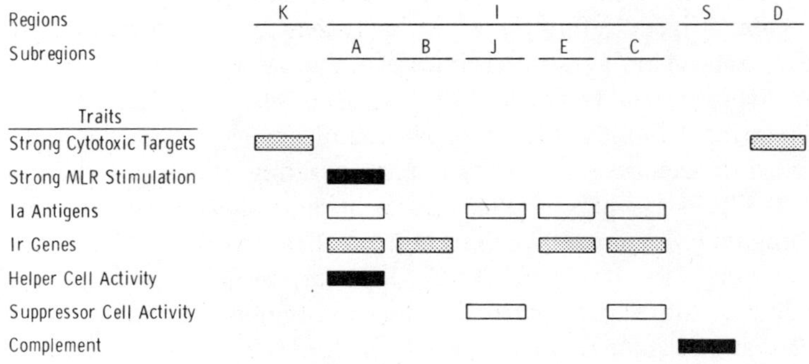

FIG. 3. A map of the genetic subdivisions and associated traits of the mouse major histocompatibility gene complex (H-2).

serve as target antigens of active cytotoxic T cells in these responses. Adjacent to the *D* region is the *S* region which controls serum proteins in the complement sequence, as well as receptors for some of the complement products (Schreffler, 1976; Schreffler *et al.*, 1976). Between the *S* and *K* regions is the *I* region which encodes another family of cell surface alloantigens, the *I* region-associated *(Iα)* antigens, or Class II antigens, represented on lymphocytes, macrophages and epidermal cells (Schreffler and David, 1975). Also mapped to this region are immune response *(Ir)* genes which control immune responsiveness to a number of natural and synthetic antigens (see Benacerraf and Germain, 1978).

The capacity of T cells to regulate immune responses seems to be closely related to their central role in discriminating molecules perceived as self from those recognized as non-self. This capacity is defined largely by the cell surface antigens encoded by the MHC. Although mechanisms are poorly understood, T cells are apparently educated with respect to the identification of self-MHC antigens during the course of their differentiation in the thymus (Zinkernagel *et al.*, 1978). In addition, other autologous molecules encountered by T cells during antenatal or neonatal differentiation (e.g. serum proteins) are also recognized thereafter as self; immune responses against such antigens *per se* after maturation of the immune system are either prevented by deletion of the potentially responsive T cell clones or are actively suppressed by Ts cells. Nevertheless, mature T cells are stimulated by recognition of conventional antigens in the context of self-MHC molecules. In other words, T cell activation requires recognition of both foreign antigens and critical self-MHC determinants (Zinkernagel and Doherty, 1979; Shearer and Schmitt-Verhulst, 1977; Paul and Benacerraf, 1977). The molecular nature of this recognition remains to be established, but experimental data suggest that T lymphocytes are triggered either by recognition of two separate moieties on such antigen-presenting cells as macrophages (i.e. a self-MHC determinants plus an antigenic determinant) or, alternatively, by recognition of a compound antigen comprised of a self-MHC molecule plus the foreign antigen that binds to a single receptor for 'altered-self' (Zinkernagel and Doherty, 1977). Many of the previously described regulatory interactions between subpopulations of T cells or between macrophages and T cells or T cells and B cells apparently also involve self recognition. This is observed experimentally by restrictions on such interactions to cells that are identical with each other for genes encoded within the subregions of the *H-2I* region of the mouse MHC (rev. Miller, 1980). Such interactions are termed 'MHC-restricted' interactions. For example, many helper T cell responses appear to require recognition of self determinants encoded within the *I-A* or *I-E* subregions of the *H-2* complex; both initial antigen priming and subsequent antigen interactions are restricted by this requirement (Katz *et al.*, 1975; Zinkernagel *et al.*, 1978b; Sprent, 1978; Lonai *et al.*, 1981). Moreover, there are recent suggestions that IL-2 production by T_H may also depend upon binding of Ia molecules at the time of antigen triggering (von Boehmer, 1980). In contrast, suppressor T cell restriction, when identified, has been associated with products of the *I-J* or *I-C* subregions (rev. Murphy, 1978; Rich, S. and Rich, R., 1976a, b; Chaouat and Voisin, 1974; Brondz *et al.*, 1980). However, it has been difficult to clearly substantiate a role for antigen presentation to Ts on the surface of an antigen-presenting cell in the context of a particular I region antigen. In fact, Ts appear generally to be primed or restimulated preferentially in the absence of antigen-presenting cells (Ishizaka and Adachi, 1976; Feldmann and Kontianen, 1976; Pierres and Germain, 1978; Dennison *et al.*, 1981), so the mechanistic basis for I-J or I-C restricted Ts interactions is not clear.

MHC-encoded molecules also serve as important differentiative markers on regulatory T cells. Nearly all T cells participating in suppressor pathways express determinants encoded by the *I-J* subregion (Murphy, 1978; Germain and Benacerraf, 1981); some Ts express I-C determinants as well (Rich and David, 1979; Germain and Benacerraf, 1981). Helper T cells have been more difficult to categorize according to I region phenotype. The majority of T_H appear to lack distinguishing Ia molecules (Miller, 1980), but activated T_H bearing determinants encoded within the *I-A* subregion have been reported (Okumura *et al.*, 1976; Tokuhisa *et al.*, 1978), as well as an exceptional example of I-J^+ helper T cells (Tada *et al.*, 1978). It is significant that the Ia molecules identified on regulatory T cells are restricted in expression to T cells alone, and are not identified on B cells (Tada, 1977; Tokuhisa *et al.*, 1978; Rich and David, 1979). Regulatory T cell factors similarly bear Ia determinants; helper T cell factors of both conventional (Tokuhisa *et al.*, 1978; Munro and Taussig, 1975; Mozes and Haimovich, 1979;) and monoclonal (Eshhar *et al.*, 1980; Lonai *et al.*, 1981) preparation bear *I-A* subregion determinants. In contrast, conventional (rev. Murphy, 1978; Germain and Benacerraf, 1981) and monoclonal (Taniguchi *et al.*, 1979, Kapp *et al.*, 1980) suppressor

T cell factors are I-J positive, or I-C positive (Rich and David, 1979; Moorhead, 1979). The function of *I* region-encoded MHC determinants on regulatory T cells and factors is unknown, as is the molecular basis of MHC restrictions within helper or suppressor pathways. However, it is abundantly clear that MHC gene products are critical in differentiative and interactive regulatory communication.

5.1 Induction of Regulatory T Cell Functions

Diverse evidence suggests that helper and suppressor T cells are functionally and phenotypically distinct subpopulations. As previously stated, the most definitive subpopulation characterization is based on Ly alloantigen expression. Primed suppressor T cells are generally Ly-23^+ and helper T cells are Ly-1^+; less differentiated Ly-123^+ T cells are also involved in both types of regulation as precursors, and perhaps also as mediators of fully differentiated T cell function (Shen *et al.,* 1980; Simon and Abenhardt, 1980; Eichmann *et al.,* 1980). MHC-encoded molecules, particularly I–J determinants on suppressor T cells, are also useful surface alloantigens in identification of regulatory subpopulations, although the molecular basis, if any, of such associations with regulatory effector functions has not yet been demonstrated. An additional interesting and largely unexplored area of phenotypic characterization is distinctive cell surface sugars on suppressor and helper T cells. Helper T cells appear to express sugars characterized by sialyl residues while, in contrast, activated Ts may express B-galactosyl residues (Nakano *et al.,* 1980). Similarly, regulatory factors may also be differentially glycosylated (Yodoi, 1980, 1981). The possible role of surface sugars in induction or expression of T cell regulation is currently undetermined.

Preferential organ localization, recirculation patterns and other biological parameters less definitively separate the functionally distinct subsets (Pierce and Kapp, 1976; Cantor and Weissman, 1975). Antigen or mitogen-activated helper and suppressor cells show somewhat different tissue distribution. Active suppressor T cells are found with highest frequency in the spleen and thymus and much lower frequency in lymph nodes; active helper cells are more generally distributed, with relatively higher frequency in lymph nodes. In addition, antigen-activated helper cells develop immunological memory (Katz and Benacerraf, 1972; Cantor and Weissman, 1976; Araneo *et al.,* 1976), whereas some data suggest that priming to suppressor cell activity does not produce a suppressor memory T cell population (Kapp *et al.,* 1975; Benacerraf *et al.,* 1975). A recent report, however, does describe evidence for antigen specific memory Ts for DTH responses by the unusual adoptive transfer method of celomic parabiosis, suggesting a long-lived circulating memory Ts pool (Liew and Howard, 1980).

Although under normal conditions both helper and suppressor populations are present, it is clear that appropriate manipulations will favor the expression of one regulatory activity over the other, perhaps reflecting distinct inductive events associated with each activity. Antigen presentation, dose, physicochemical form, route of injection and adjuvant effects all affect assessment of regulatory phenomena. Suppressor T cell activity is favored by injection with soluble or deaggregated antigens; addition of bacterial products to soluble antigens, insolubilization of antigens and incorporation of antigens into an adjuvant preparation favor the development of helper T cells (Katz and Benacerraf, 1972; Pierce and Kapp, 1976).

A frequent feature of selective generation of suppressor activity is stimulation with supraimmunogenic antigen doses, both *in vivo* and *in vitro* (Eardley and Gershon, 1976; Eardley and Sercarz, 1976; Ishizaka and Adachi, 1976; Kontiainen and Feldmann, 1976; Whisler and Stobo, 1976). In addition, macrophage activity may influence the appearance of suppressor or helper activity. In various *in vitro* systems suppressor cell induction appears to be macrophage independent (Ishizaka and Adachi, 1976; Feldmann and Kontiainen, 1976; Dutton, 1975; Pierres and Germain, 1978), while macrophages may be critical in helper T cell activation (Ishizaka and Adachi, 1976; Feldmann and Kontiainen, 1976; Erb and Feldmann, 1975). This accords with observations that macrophage removal or bypass favors tolerance induction (see Dresser and Mitchison, 1968; Cinader and Fujiwara, 1974; Cowing *et al.,* 1974), which in some cases may involve suppressor cells.

Macrophages supply three important activating principles to T_H cells, i.e., conventional antigen presentation, self Ia antigen presentation, and the soluble factor IL-1. Production of IL-2 by T_H is similarly dependent on these macrophage functions (von Boehmer, 1980). Interruption of these activities, for instance by blocking I–A molecules with specific antiserum (Perry and Greene, 1981), or inactivating antigen-presenting cells by ultra-violet irradiation (Wagner *et al.*, 1980; Greene *et al.*, 1979; Perry and Greene, 1981) or cellular disruption (Wagner *et al.*, 1980), interferes with T_H activation and instead favors Ts induction (Perry and Greene, 1981; Berzofsky and Richman, 1981). At the least, these data suggest that Ts, unlike T_H, do not respond to antigen in the context of I–A subregion determinants on macrophages. Since Ts may be activated in the absence of macrophages, and are easily isolated by adsorption to immobilized antigen in the absence of antigen-presenting cells (Taniguchi and Miller, 1977; Dietz *et al.*, 1980), Ts may be selectively triggered by direct binding of antigen in the absence of macrophage Ia molecules. Thus it is possible that Ts antigen-specific receptors differ qualitatively from those utilized by T_H. Owen has, in fact, described a T cell alloantigen which maps near immunoglobulin allotype genes and is found only on Ts but not T_H or B cells; this determinant is postulated to be a heavy chain constant region marker on a Ts receptor (Owen, 1980; Owen *et al.*, 1981). It should be noted, however, that at least one laboratory has demonstrated triggering of a primed Ts by exposure to antigen-pulsed macrophages only of the proper MHC phenotype (Araneo *et al.*, 1981), so receptor binding activities may vary, perhaps reflecting distinct Ts subclasses within suppressor pathways.

While the above observations fail to provide conclusive evidence for the critical mechanisms of helper and suppressor T cell induction, they do suggest general conclusions. Helper T cells appear to be singularly dependent on macrophage presentation of antigen in the context of Ia antigens, at least for primary antigen interaction. In contrast, suppressor T cells may be triggered by antigen alone, in the absence of macrophage presentation, or perhaps may recognize antigen on the surface of multiple cell types, including other T cells and B cells, in the context of MHC determinants distinct from those recognized by T_H. The inductive requirements involving recognition of receptor idiotypic determinants by both regulatory T cell populations are presently uncharacterized, and may contribute another level of complexity to the above scheme of regulatory cell induction.

5.2 MECHANISMS OF MODULATION OF IMMUNE RESPONSES BY T LYMPHOCYTES

The cellular and molecular foundations of T cell-mediated immune regulation are clearly complex and still poorly understood. Critical questions concerning the ultimate target cell, molecular properties of regulatory molecules and their receptors, and the nature of the susceptible activity of the target cell which is affected, have been only partially answered. However, important advances are being made, particularly with utilization of the monoclonal cell systems and soluble reagents that have been briefly described in this review.

Helper T cell activity appears to derive primarily from their ability to offer proliferative and differentiative signals to other antigen-activated cells within a limited milieu. Once triggered by the combined activities of macrophage-bound antigen and IL-1, T_H generate IL-2 which provides the proliferative signal to other helper T cells and effector T cells that have been activated by antigen to express an IL-2 receptor. Antigen alone fails to trigger proliferation, suggesting that the second, necessary signal is provided by IL-2. The same IL-2 molecule appears to promote proliferation of various T cell subsets, perhaps including Ts (Palacious and Moller, 1981), and IL-2 cross adsorption by functionally distinct T cells suggests expression of a common IL-2 specific receptor (Schreier *et al.*, 1980). Specificity of help derives from the initial antigen interaction with T_H via antigen or idiotype-specific receptors; thereafter T cells activated by any antigenic stimulus are poised for nonspecific IL-2 triggering. Since IL-2 is a T cell-specific molecule, B cell help apparently is provided by distinct T cell replacing factor. Activation of B cells is required before they become susceptible to TRF, which then allows final differentiation to immunoglobulin secretion. Ia molecules have a central role in transmission of helper signals, although the molecular mechanisms of their activities are not clearly understood.

As with helper T cell activity, the molecular mechanisms of suppressor T cell activity are unknown. However, some general observations may be made. A number of studies (Rich and Pierce, 1974; Peavy and Pierce, 1974; Rich, 1975; Dutton, 1975; Gershon, 1974; Thomas *et al.*, 1975; Rich, S. and Rich, R., 1974, 1975) support the conclusion that reduced responsiveness results not from prevention of initial antigenic stimulus itself, but from interference with differentiative and proliferative events subsequent to antigenic stimulation. Some studies suggest that suppressor cells act directly on activated T helper cells to inactivate or ultimately destroy these cells or their products (Herzenberg *et al.*, 1976; Harwell *et al.*, 1977). Recently, a monoclonal sheep red blood cell (SRBC) glycophorin-specific TsF has been developed and partially purified to a 70,000 mw single chain polypeptide (Fresno *et al.*, 1981). Incubation of SRBC-primed Ly-1^+ T_H in this TsF preparation, with the addition of antigen, results in abolition of the capacity of these cells to provide help to B cells in an anti-SRBC antibody response (Fresno *et al.*, 1981). Incubation of B cells in the same TsF had no effect. Consequently, in this system the TsF interacts directly with an activated T_H. The mechanism of inhibition has not yet been identified; TsF could possibly modify antigen presentation by complexing with antigens, such that it prevents subsequent IL-2 production or receptor display in the T_H population; moreover, TsF could compete for IL-2 receptors, blocking the proliferative signal, or interact directly with IL-2, thus modifying its effect. It is interesting that in two systems, monoclonal suppressor products specific for a single determinant on a complex antigen preempt the entire response to that antigen (Taniguchi *et al.*, 1979; Fresno *et al.*, 1981). In this regard it has been demonstrated that the 70,000 mw suppressor molecule breaks down into two subunits upon antigen binding, producing a 25,000 mw piece that retains antigen-binding activity but not suppression, and a 45,000 mw piece that is nonspecifically suppressive (Nabel *et al.*, 1980). Thus occupation of the TsF antigen-binding site may activate a largely nonspecific suppressor effect on nearby cells responding to other determinants of that antigen. Data unequivocally supporting suppressor T cell effects directly on B cells has been more difficult to identify. However, recently two laboratories have reported that idiotype-specific Ts can inhibit the secretion of Id^+ immunoglobulins by myeloma lines (Lynch *et al.*, 1979; Abbas *et al.*, 1980). This direct Ts–B effector cell interaction may also play a role in physiologic processes of suppressive regulation.

In summary, although firm conclusions about underlying mechanisms of regulation of cellular interactions in the immune response are not yet possible, control of an immune response clearly develops through cell–cell interactions which are complex in both induction and expression. The roles of dynamic cell surface determinants and their genetic control are of particular current interest. Finally, the regulatory cell interactions discussed in this review may be of wide general significance; their understanding may be important not only in determining the nature of cooperative and suppressive cell interactions in the immune system, but may be relevant to nonimmunologic cell–cell recognition systems in general.

REFERENCES

AARDEN, L. (1979) Revised nomenclature for antigen-nonspecific T cell proliferation and helper factors. *J. Immunol.* **123:** 2928–2929.

ABBAS, A., BURAKOFF, S., GEFTER, M. and GREENE, M. (1980) T lymphocyte mediated suppression of myeloma function *in vitro*. III. Regulation of antibody production in hybrid myeloma cells by T lymphocytes. *J. exp. Med.* **152:** 969–978.

ABDOU, N. J., NAPOMBEJARA, C., BALENTINE, L. and ABDOU, N. J. (1978) Suppressor cell-mediated neutropenia in Felty's syndrome. *J. Clin. Invest.* **61:** 738–743.

ABDOU, N. J., SAGAWA, A., PASCUAL, E., HEBERT, J. and SADAGHEE, S. (1976) Suppressor T-cell abnormality in idiopathic systemic lupus erythematosus. *Clin. Immunol. Immunopathol.* **6:** 192–199.

AHMED, A., SCHER, I., SHARROW, S. O., SMITH, A. H., PAUL, W. E., SACHS, D. H. and SELL, K. W. (1977) B-lymphocyte heterogeneity: Development and characterization of an alloantiserum which distinguishes B-lymphocyte differentiation alloantigens. *J. exp. Med.* **145:** 101–110.

ALLISON, A. C. (1974a) The role of T and B lymphocytes in self tolerance and autoimmunity. *Contemp. Top. Immunobiol.* **3:** 227–242.

ALLISON, A. C. (1974b) Interactions of T and B lymphocytes in self-tolerance and autoimmunity. In *Immunologic Tolerance: Mechanisms and Potential Therapeutic Applications*, pp. 22–25. KATZ, D. H. and BENACERRAF, B. (eds). Academic Press, New York.

ANDERSSON, B. and BLOMGREN, H. (1971) Evidence for thymus-independent humoral antibody production in mice against polyvinylpyrrolidone and *E. coli* lipopolysaccharide. *Cell. Immunol.* **2:** 411–424.

ARANEO, B. A., MARRACK (HUNTER), P. C. and KAPPLER, J. W. (1975) Functional heterogeneity among T-derived lymphocytes of the mouse. II. Sensitivity of subpopulations to anti-thymocyte serum. *J. Immunol* **114:** 747–751.

ARANEO, B. A., MARRACK, P. C. and KAPPLER, J. W. (1976) Functional heterogeneity among the T-derived lymphocytes of the mouse. VI. Memory T cells stored in the T2 subpopulation. *J. Immunol.* **117:** 2131–2136.

ARANEO, B. A., YOWELL, R., METZGER, D. and SERCARZ, E. (1981) Positive selection of major histocompatibility complex-restricted suppressor T cells bearing the predominant idiotype in the immune response to lysozyme. *Proc. Natl. Acad. Sci. USA* **78:** 499–503.

AUNE, T. and PIERCE, C. (1981) Mechanism of action of macrophage-derived suppressor factor produced by soluble immune response suppressor-treated macrophages. *J. Immunol.* **127:** 368–372.

ASHERSON, G. L. and ZEMBALA, M. (1974) T cell suppression of contact sensitivity in the mouse. III. The role of macrophages and the specific triggering of nonspecific suppression. *Eur. J. Immunol.* **4:** 804–807.

ASKONAS, B., SCHIMPL, A. and WECKLER, E. (1974) The differentiative function of T cell replacing factor in nu/nu spleen cell cultures. *Eur. J. Immunol.* **4:** 164–169.

BACH, F. H., BACH, M. L. and SONDEL, P. M. (1976) Differential functions of major histocompatibility complex antigens in T-lymphocyte activation. *Nature* **259:** 273–281.

BACH, F. H., SEGALL, M., ZIER, K. S., SONDEL, P. M., ALTER, B. J. and BACH, M. L. (1973) Cell mediated immunity: separation of cells involved in recognitive and destructive phases. *Science* **180:** 403–406.

BACH, M. A., PHAN-DINH-TUY, F., TOURNIER, E., CHATENOUD, L., BACH, J. T., MARTIN, C. and DEGOS, J. D. (1980) Deficit of suppressor T cells in active multiple sclerosis. *Lancet* **ii:** 1221–1223.

BAKER, P. J., BARTH, R. F., STASHAK, P. W. and AMSBAUGH, D. F. (1970a) Enhancement of the antibody response to type III pneumococcal polysaccharide in mice treated with anti-lymphocyte serum. *J. Immunol.* **104:** 1313–1315.

BAKER, P. J., STASHAK, P. W., AMSBAUGH, D. F. and PRESCOTT, B. (1974) Regulation of the antibody response to type III pneumococcal polysaccharide. II. Mode of action of thymic-derived suppressor cells. *J. Immunol.* **112:** 404–409.

BAKER, P. J., STASHAK, P. W., AMSBAUGH, D. F., PRESCOTT, B. and BARTH, R. F. (1970b) Evidence for the existence of two functionally distinct types of cells which regulate the antibody response of type III pneumococcal polysaccharide. *J. Immunol.* 1581–1583.

BASH, J. and WAKSMAN, B. (1975) The suppressive effect of immunization on the proliferative responses of rat T cells *in vitro*. *J. Immunol.* **114:** 782–787.

BASTEN, A. and HOWARD, J. G. (1973) Thymus independence. *Contemp. Top. Immunobiol.* **2:** 265–291.

BASTEN, A., MILLER, J. F. A. P. and JOHNSON, P. (1975) T cell-dependent suppression of an anti-hapten antibody response. *Transplant. Rev.* **26:** 130–169.

BASTEN, A., MILLER, J. F. A. P., SPRENT, J. and CHEERS, C. (1974) Cell-to-cell interaction in the immune response. X. T-cell-dependent suppression in tolerant mice. *J. exp. Med.* **140:** 199–217.

BECKWITH, M. and RICH, S. (1981) MLR suppressor factor-target cell interaction: Evidence for a second cell in the suppressor pathway. *Fed. Proc.* **40:** 1062.

BELLER, D., KIELY, J. M. and UNANUE, E. (1980) Regulation of macrophage populations. I. Preferential induction of Ia-rich peritoneal exudates by immunologic stimuli. *J. Immunol.* **124:** 1426–1432.

BENACERRAF, B. and GERMAIN, R. (1978) The immune response genes of the major histocompatibility complex. *Immunol. Rev.* **38:** 70–119.

BENACERRAF, B., KAPP, J. A., DEBRE, P., PIERCE, C. W. and DELACROIX, F. (1975) The stimulation of specific suppressor T cells in genetic non-responder mice by linear random copolymers L-amino acid. *Transplant Rev.* **26:** 21–38.

BEN-NERIAH, Y. B., GIVOL, D., LONAI, P., SIMON, M. and EICHMANN, K. (1980) Allotype-linked genetic control of a polymorphic V_H framework determinant on mouse T-helper cell receptors. *Nature* **285:** 257–259.

BERZOFSKY, J. and RICHMAN, L. (1981) Genetic control of the immune response to myoglobulins. IV. Inhibition of determinant-specific Ir gene-controlled antigen presentation and induction of expression by pretreatment of presenting cells with anti-Ia antibodies. *J. Immunol.* **126:** 1898–1904.

BINZ, H. and WIGZELL, H. (1975) Shared idiotypic determinants on B and T lymphocytes reactive against the same antigenic determinants. I. Demonstration of similar or identical idiotypes on IgG molecules and T-cell receptors with specificity for the same alloantigens. *J. exp. Med.* **142:** 197–211.

BIRNBAUM, G. and TSAIRIS, P. (1976) Suppressor lymphocytes in myesthenia gravis and effect of adult thymectomy. *Ann. N.Y. Acad. Sci.* **274:** 527–535.

BLOOM, B. R. (1971) *In vitro* approaches to the mechanism of cell-mediated immune reactions. *Adv. Immunol.* **13:** 102–208.

BONA, C. and HIERNAUX, J. (1981) Immune response: Idiotype-antiidiotype network. *CRC Critical Rev. Immunol.* **2:** 33–81.

BOTTOMLY, K. and MOSIER, D. (1979) Mice whose B cells cannot produce the T15 idiotype also lack an antigen specific helper T cell required for T15 expression. *J. exp. Med.* **150:** 1399–1409.

BOYSE, E. A., ITAKURA, K., STOCKERT, E., IRITANI, C. and MIVRA, M. (1971) Ly-C: A third locus specifying alloantigens expressed only on thymocytes and lymphocytes. *Transplantation* **II:** 351–352.

BOYSE, E. A., MIYAZAWA, M., AOKI, T. and OLD, L. J. (1968) Ly-A and Ly-B: Two systems of lymphocyte isoantigens in the mouse. *Proc. R. Soc. B* **170:** 175–193.

BRETSCHER, P. A. (1975) The two signal model for B cell induction. *Transplant. Rev.* **23:** 37–48.

BRETSCHER, P. and COHN, M. (1970) A theory of non-self discrimination. *Science* **169:** 1042–1049.

BRONDZ, B., KARAULOV, ABRONINA, I. and BLANDOVA, Z. (1980) Biological, immunological and genetic characterization of specific suppressor T cells and their receptors immune to antigens of the H-2 complex. *Molec. Immunol.* **17:** 833–849.

BROOM, B. C., DE LA CONCHA, J. G., WEBSTER, A. D. B., JANOSSY, G. J. and ASHERSON, G. L. (1976) Intracellular immunoglobulin production *in vitro* by lymphocytes from patients with hypogammaglobulinemic and their effect on normal lymphocytes. *Clin. exp. Immunol.* **23:** 73–77.

BURNET, F. M. (1959) *The Clonal Selection Theory of Acquired Immunity*. Cambridge University Press, London.
BURNET, F. M. (1974) Autoimmunity and aging. *Prog. Immunol. II.* **5:** 27–36.
BUSCHARD, K., MADSBAD, S. and RYGAARD, J. (1980) Depressed suppressor cell activity in patients with newly diagnosed insulin-dependent diabetes mellitus. *Clin. exp. Immunol.* **41:** 25–32.
CANTOR, H. and ASOFSKY, R. (1970) Synergy among lymphoid cells mediating the graft-vs. host (GVH) response. II. Synergy and GVH reactions produced by BALB/c lymphoid cells of differing anatomic origin. *J. exp. Med.* **131:** 235–246.
CANTOR, H. and ASOFSKY, R. (1972) Synergy among lymphoid cells mediating the graft-vs-host response. III. Evidence for interaction between two types of thymus derived cells. *J. exp. Med.* **135:** 764–779.
CANTOR, H. and BOYSE, E. A. (1975a) Functional subclasses of T lymphocytes bearing different Ly antigens. I. The generation of functionally distinct T-cell subclasses is a differentiative process independent of antigen. *J. exp. Med.* **141:** 1376–1389.
CANTOR, H. and BOYSE, E. A. (1975b) Functional subclasses of T lymphocytes bearing different Ly antigens. II. Cooperation between subclasses of Ly^+ cells in the generation of killer activity. *J. exp. Med.* **141:** 1390–1399.
CANTOR, H., MCVAY-BOUDREAU, L., HUGENBERGER, J., NAIDORF, K., SHEN, F. W. and GERSHON, R. K. (1978) Immunoregulatory circuits among T-cell sets. II. Physiologic role of feedback inhibition *in vivo:* Absence in NZB mice. *J. exp. Med.* **147:** 1116–1125.
CANTOR, H., SHEN, F. W. and BOYSE, E. A. (1976) Separation of helper T cells from suppressor T cells expressing different Ly components. II. Activation by antigen: after immunization, antigen-specific suppressor and helper activities are mediated by distinct T-cell subclasses. *J. exp. Med.* **143:** 1391–1401.
CANTOR, H., SIMPSON, E., SATO, V. L., FATHMAN, C. G. and HERZENBERG, L. A. (1975) Characterization of subpopulations of T lymphocytes. I. Separation and functional studies of peripheral T-cells binding different amounts of fluorescent anti-Thy-1.2 (Theta) antibody using a fluorescence-activated cell sorter (FACS). *Cell. Immunol.* **15:** 180–196.
CANTOR, H. and WEISSMAN, I. (1976) Development and function of subpopulations of thymocytes and T lymphocytes. *Prog. Allergy* **20:** 2–64.
CAPRA, J. D. and KEHOE, J. M. (1975) Hypervariable regions, idiotypy, and the antibody-combining site. *Adv. Immunol.* **20:** 1–40.
CEROTTINI, J. C. and BRUNNER, K. T. (1974) Cell-mediated cytotoxicity, allograft rejection, and tumor immunity. *Adv. Immunol.* **18:** 67–132.
CHAOUAT, G. and VOISIN, G. (1974) Regulatory T cell subpopulations in pregnancy. I. Evidence for suppressive activity of the early phase of MLR. *J. Immunol.* **122:** 1383–1388.
CINADER, B. and FUJIWARA, M. (1974) The role of accessory and thymus-derived cells in resistance to tolerance induction. In: *Immunological Tolerance: Mechanisms and Potential Therapeutic Applications,* pp. 67–86. KATZ, D. H. and BENACERRAF, B. (eds.). Academic Press, New York.
CLAMAN, H. N., CHAPERON, E. A. and TRIPLETT, R. F. (1966) Thymus-marrow cell combinations. Synergism in antibody production. *Proc. Soc. exp. Biol. Med.* **122:** 1167–1171.
CLAMAN, H., MILLER, S., SY, M. S. and MOORHEAD, J. (1980) Suppressive mechanisms involving sensitization and tolerance in contact allergy. *Immunol. Rev.* **50:** 105–132.
CLAMAN, H. N., PHANUPHAK, P. and MOOREHEAD, J. W. (1974) Tolerance to contact sensitivity—a role for suppressor T cells? In: *Immunological Tolerance: Mechanisms and Possible Therapeutic Applications,* pp. 123–128. KATZ, D. H. and BENACERRAF, B. (eds.). Academic Press, New York.
COHEN, L. and HOWE, M. L. (1973) Synergism between subpopulations of thymus-derived cells mediating the proliferative and effector phases of the mixed lymphocyte reaction. *Proc. Natl. Acad. Sci.* **70:** 2707–2710.
COHEN, S. (1980) Lymphokines in delayed hypersensitivity. *Prog. Immunol.* **4:** 860–879.
COSENZA, H., JULIUS, M. and AUGUSTIN, A. (1977) Idiotypes as variable region markers: Analogies between receptors on phosphorylcholine-specific T and B lymphocytes. *Immunol. Rev.* **34:** 3–33.
COWING, C., LUKIC, M. and LESKOWITZ, S. (1974) The cellular basis for establishing tolerance or immunity to bovine γ-globulin in mice. In: *Immunological Tolerance: Mechanisms and Potential Therapeutic Applications,* pp. 61–66. KATZ, D. H. and BENACERRAF, B. (eds.). Academic Press, New York.
CRAWFORD, D. H., BRICKNELL, P., TIDMAN, N., MCCONNELL, I., HOFFBRAND, A. V. and JANOSSY, G. (1981) Increased numbers of cells with suppressor T cell phenotype in the peripheral blood of patients with infectious mononucleosis. *Clin. exp. Immunol.* **43:** 291–297.
DAVID, J. R. (1975) Macrophage activation by lymphocyte mediators. *Fed. Proc.* **34:** 1730–1736.
DAVIE, J. M. and PAUL, W. E. (1974) Role of T lymphocytes in the humoral immune response. I. Proliferation of B lymphocytes in thymus-deprived mice. *J. Immunol.* **113:** 1483–1445.
DAVIES, A. J. S. (1969) The thymus and the cellular basis of immunity. *Transplant. Rev.* **1:** 43–91.
DENNISON, D., RICH, S. and RICH, R. (1981) Cellular and antigenic requirements for production of mixed leukocyte reaction suppressor factor. Submitted for publication.
DIETZ, M., SY, M. S., BENACERRAF, B., NISONOFF, A., GREENE, M. and GERMAIN, R. (1981) Antigen and receptor-driven regulatory mechanisms. VII. H-2 restricted anti-idiotype suppressor factor from efferent suppressor T cells. *J. exp. Med.* **153:** 450–463.
DIETZ, M., SY, M-S., GREENE, M. I., NISONOFF, A., BENACERRAF, B. AND GERMAIN, R. (1980) Antigen and receptor-driven regulatory mechanisms. VI. Demonstration of cross-reactive idiotypic determinants on azobenzenearsonate-specific antigen-binding suppressor T cells producing soluble suppressor factor(s). *J. Immunol.* **125:** 2374–2379.
DOHI, Y. and NISONOFF, A. (1979) Suppression of idiotype and generation of suppressor T cells with idiotype-conjugated thymocytes. *J. exp. Med.* **150:** 929–918.
DRESSER, D. W. and MITCHISON, N. A. (1968) The mechanism of immunological paralysis. *Adv. Immunol.* **8:** 129–181.
DROEGE, W. (1971) Amplifying and suppressive effects of thymus cells. *Nature* **234:** 549–551.
DROEGE, W., MALCHOW, D. and STROMINGER, J. L. (1972) Cellular heterogeneity in the thymus. I. Electrophoretic analysis of lymphoid cell populations from chickens. *Eur. J. Immunol.* **2:** 156–161.

DUTTON, R. W. (1972) Inhibitory and stimulatory effects of concanavalin A on the response of mouse spleen cell suspensions to antigen. I. Characterization of the inhibitory cell activity. *J. exp. Med.* **136:** 1445–1460.

DUTTON, R. W. (1973) Inhibitory and stimulatory effects of concanavalin A on the response of mouse spleen cell suspensions to antigen. II. Evidence for separate stimulatory and inhibitory cells. *J. exp. Med.* **138:** 1496–1505.

DUTTON, R. W. (1975) Suppressor T cells. *Transplant. Rev.* **26:** 39–55.

DUTTON, R. W., FALKOFF, R., HURST, J. A., HOFFMAN, M., KAPPLER, J. W., KETTMAN, J. R., LESLEY, J. S. and VANN, D. (1971) Is there evidence for a non-antigen specific diffusable chemical mediator in the initiation of the immune response? *Prog. Immunol.* **1:** 355–368.

EARDLEY, D. D. and GERSHON, R. K. (1975) Feedback inhibitors of suppressor T-cell activity. *J. exp. Med.* **142:** 524–529.

EARDLEY, D. D. and GERSHON, R. K. (1976) Induction of specific suppressor T cells *in vitro. J. Immunol.* **117:** 313–318.

EARDLEY, D. and SERCARZ, E. E. (1976) Modulation of help and suppression in a hapten-carrier system. *J. Immunol.* **116:** 600–605.

EARDLEY, D. D., HUGENBERGER, J., MCVAY-BOUDREAU, L., SHEN, F. W., GERSHON, R. K. and CANTOR, H. (1978). Immunoregulatory circuits among T cell sets. I. T helper cells induce other T cell sets to exert feedback inhibition. *J. exp. Med.* **147:** 1106–1115.

EICHMANN, K. (1975) Idiotype suppression. II. Amplification of a suppressor T cell with anti-idiotypic activity. *Eur. J. Immunol.* **5:** 511–517.

EICHMANN, K. (1977) Heavy chain variable region idiotypes on helper T cells. In: *The Immune System: Genetics and Regulation,* pp. 127–138. SERCARZ, E., HERZENBERG, H. and FOX, F. (eds.). Academic Press, New York.

EICHMANN, K. (1978) Expression and function of idiotypes on haplotypes. *Adv. Immunol.* **26:** 195–254.

EICHMANN, K. and RAJEWSKY, K. (1975) Induction of T and B cell immunity by anti-idiotypic antibody. *Eur. J. Immunol.* **5:** 661–666.

EICHMANN, K., FALK, I., MELCHERS, I. and SIMON, M. (1980) Quantitative studies on T cell diversity. I. Determination of the precursor frequencies for two types of streptococcus A-specific helper cells in nonimmume, polyclonally activated splenic T cells. *J. exp. Med.* **152:** 477–492.

EIJSVOOGEL, V. P., DUBOIS, M. J., MEINESZ, A., BIERHORST-EIJLANDER, A., ZEYLEMAKER, W. P. and SCHELLEKENS, P. T. L. A. (1973) The specificity and activation mechanism of cell-mediated lympholysis (CMI) in man. *Transplant. Proc.* **5:** 1675–1678.

ENGERS, H. D. and MACDONALD, H. R. (1976) Generation of cytolytic T lymphocytes *in vitro. Contemp. Top. Immunobiol.* **5:** 145–190.

ERB, P. and FELDMANN, M. (1975) The role of macrophages in the generation of T-helper cells. II. The genetic control of the macrophage-T-cell interaction for helper cell induction with soluble antigens. *J. exp. Med.* **142:** 460–472.

ESHHAR, Z., APTE, R., LÖWY, I., BEN-NERIAH, Y., GIVOL, D. and MOZES, E. (1980) T cell hybridomas bearing heavy chain variable region determinants producing (T,G)-A—L-specific helper factors. *Nature* **286:** 270–272.

EVANS, R. L., WALL, D. W., PLATSOUCAS, C. D., SIEGAL, F. P., FIKRIG, S. M., TESTA, C. M. and GOOD, R. A. (1981) Thymus-dependent membrane antigens in man: Inhibition of cell-mediated lympholysis by monoclonal antibodies to T_{H2} antigen. *Proc. Natl. Acad. Sci. USA* **78:** 544–548.

FAUCI, A. S., STEINBERG, A. D., HAYNES, B. F. and WHALEN, G. (1978) Immunoregulatory aberrations in systematic lupus erythematosus. *J. Immunol.* **121:** 1473–1479.

FELDMANN, M. (1972) Cell interactions in the immune response *in vitro.* V. Specific collaboration via complexes of antigen and thymus-derived cell immunoglobulin. *J. exp. Med.* **136:** 737–760.

FELDMANN, M. (1974) T cell suppression *in vitro.* I. Role in regulation of antibody response. *Eur. J. Immunol.* **4:** 660–666.

FELDMANN, M. (1976) Lymphoid cell interactions in Japan. *Nature* **269:** 12–14.

FELDMANN, M. and BASTEN, A. (1972) Cell interactions in the immune response *in vitro.* III. Specific collaboration across a cell impermeable membrane. *J. exp. Med.* **136:** 49–67.

FELDMANN, M., BEVERLEY, P. C. L., DUNKLEY, M. and KONTIAINEN, S. (1975) Different Ly antigen phenotypes of *in vitro* induced helper and suppressor cells. *Nature* **258:** 614–616.

FELDMANN, M. and KONTIAINEN, S. (1976) Suppressor cell induction *in vitro.* II. Cellular requirements of suppressor cell induction. *Eur. J. Immunol.* **6:** 302–305.

FRESNO, M., MCVAY-BOUDREAU, L., NABEL, G. and CANTOR, H. (1981) Antigen specific T lymphocyte clones. II. Purification and biological characterization of an antigen-specific suppressive protein synthesized by cloned T cells. *J. exp. Med.* **153:** 1260–1274.

FUJIMOTO, S., MATSUZAWA, T., NAKAGAWA, K. and TADA, T. (1978) Cellular interaction between cytotoxic and suppressor T cells against syngeneic tumors in the mouse. *Cell Immunol.* **38:** 378–387.

GAUMER, H. R., DOLL, N. J., KAIMAL, J., SCHUYLER, M. and SALVAGGIO, J. E. (1981) Diminished suppressor cell function in patients with asbestosis. *Clin. exp. Immunol.* **44:** 108–116.

GELFAND, M. C. and PAUL, W. E. (1975) Prolongation of allograft survival in mice by administration of anti-Thy-1-serum. I. Mediation by *in vivo* activation of regulatory T cells. *J. Immunol.* **115:** 1–4.

GERBASE-DELIMA, M., MEREDITH, P. and WALFORD, R. L. (1975) Age related changes, including synergy and suppression in the mixed lymphocyte reaction in long-lived mice. *Fedn. Proc.* **34:** 159–161.

GERMAIN, R. and BENACERRAF, B. (1981) A single major pathway of T lymphocyte interactions in antigen-specific immune suppression. *Scand. J. Immunol.* **13:** 1–10.

GERMAIN, R., THEZE, J., KAPP, J. and BENACERRAF, B. (1978) Antigen-specific T cell mediated suppression. I. Induction of L-glutamic acid^{60}-L-alanine^{30}-L-tyrosine^{10} specific suppressor T cells *in vitro* requires both antigen-specific T cell suppressor factor and antigen. *J. exp. Med.* **147:** 123–136.

GERSHON, R. K. (1974) T cell control of antibody production. *Contemp. Top. Immunobiol.* **3:** 1–40.

GLASEBROOK, A. and FITCH, F. (1980) Alloreactive cloned T cell lines. I. Interactions between cloned amplifier and cytotytic T cell lines. *J. exp. Med.* **151:** 876–895.

GOOD, R. A. and YUNIS, E. (1974) Association of autoimmunity, immunodeficiency and aging in man, rabbits and mice. *Fedn. Proc.* **33:** 2040–2050.

GORCZYNSKI, R. M. and FELDMANN, M. (1975) B-cell heterogeneity: difference in the size of B lymphocytes responding to T-dependent and T-independent antigens. *Cell. Immunol.* **18:** 88–97.

GRONOWICZ, E. and COUTINHO, A. (1975) Functional analysis of B-cell heterogeneity. *Transplant. Rev.* **24:** 3–40.

GORONZY, J., SCHAEFER, U., EICHMANN, K. and SIMON, M. (1981) Qualitative studies on T cell diversity. II. Determination of the frequencies and Lyt phenotypes of two types of precursor cells for alloreactive cytotoxic T cells in polyclonally and specifically activated splenic T cells. *J. exp. Med.* **153:** 857–870.

GREENE, M. (1980) The genetic cellular basis of regulation of the immune response to tumor antigens. *Cont. Topics Immunobiol.* **11:** 81–116.

GREENE, M., SY, M., KRIPKE, M. and BENACERRAF, B. (1979) Impairment of antigen-presenting cell function by ultraviolet radiation. *Proc. Natl. Acad. Sci. USA* **76:** 6591–6595.

GREENE, M., SY, M. S., NISONOFF, A. and BENACERRAF, B. (1980) The genetic and cellular basis of antigen and receptor stimulated regulation. *Molec. Immunol.* **17:** 857–866.

GRESSER, S. (1980) Interferon and the immune system. *Prog. Immunol.* **4:** 710–719.

GUIMEZANES, A. AND SCHMITT-VERHULST, A. M. (1981) I. Region restricted long-term cultured T cells with helper function for thymic cytotoxic precursor cells. *J. Immunol.* **126:** 563–569.

HAMMERLING, G., BLACK, S. J., BEREK, C., EICHMANN, K. and RAJEWSKY, K. (1976) Idiotypic analysis of lymphocytes *in vitro*. II. Genetic control of T helper cell responsiveness to anti-idiotypic antibody. *J. exp. Med.* **143:** 861–869.

HARDT, C., PFIZENMAIER, K., RÖLLINGHOFF, KLEIN, J. and WAGNER, H. (1980) Alloreactive and H-2 restricted Lyt 23 cytotoxic T lymphocytes derive from a common pool of antecedent Lyt 123 precursors. *J. exp. Med.* **152:** 1413–1418.

HARWELL, L., MARRACK, P. and KAPPLER, J. W. (1977) Suppressor T-cell inactivation of a helper T-cell factor. *Nature* **265:** 57–59.

HARWELL, L., SKIDMORE, B., MARRACK, P. and KAPPLER, J. (1980) Concanavalin A-inducible interleukin-2-producing T cell hybridomas. *J. exp. Med.* **152:** 893–904.

HERZENBERG, L. A., OKUMURA, K., CANTOR, H., SATO, V. L., SHEN, F. W., BOYSE, E. A. and HERZENBERG, L. A. (1976) T-cell regulation of antibody responses: demonstration of allotype-specific helper T cells and their specific removal by suppressor T cells. *J. exp. Med.* **144:** 330–344.

HETZELBERGER, D. and EICHMANN, K. (1978) Recognition of idiotypes in lymphocyte interactions. I. Idiotypic in the cooperation between T and B lymphocytes. *Eur. J. Immunol.* **8:** 846–852.

HILLINGER, S. M. and HERZIG, G. P. (1978) Impaired cell-mediated immunity in Hodgkin's disease mediated by suppressor lymphocytes and monocytes. *J. Clin. Invest.* **61:** 1620–1627.

HIRAI, Y. and NISONOFF, A. (1980) Selective suppression of the major idiotypic component of an antihapten response by soluble T cell-derived factors with idiotypic or anti-idiotypic receptors. *J. exp. Med.* **151:** 1213–1231.

HIRANO, T. and NORDIN, A. A. (1976a) Cell-mediated immune response *in vitro*. I. The development of suppressor cells and cytotoxic lymphocytes in mixed lymphocyte cultures. *J. Immunol.* **116:** 1115–1122.

HIRANO, T. and NORDIN, A. A. (1976b) Cell-mediated immune response *in vitro*. II. The mechanism(s) involved in the suppression of the development of cytotoxic lymphocytes. *J. Immunol.* **117:** 2226–2232.

HODGSON, H. J. F., WANDS, J. R. and ISSELBACHER, K. J. (1978a) Decreased suppressor cell activity in inflammatory bowel disease. *Clin. exp. Immunol.* **32:** 451–458.

HODGSON, H. J. F., WANDS, J. R. and ISSELBACHER, K. J. (1978b) Alteration in suppressor cell activity in chronic active hepatitis. *Proc. Natl. Acad. Sci. USA* **75:** 1549–1553.

HOFFMAN, R., ZEMIANI, E. D., LUTTON, J. D., ZALUSKY, R. and WASSERMAN, L. R. (1977) Suppression of erythroid-colony formation by lymphocytes from patients with aplastic anemia. *New Engl. J. Med.* **296:** 10–13.

HOLLANDER, N., PILLEMER, E. and WEISSMAN, I. (1980) Blocking effect of Lyt-2 antibodies on T cell functions. *J. exp. Med.* **152:** 674–687.

HOWARD, J. G., CHRISTIE, G. H. and SCOTT, M. (1973) Biological effects of *Corynebacterium parvum*. IV. Adjuvant and inhibitory activities on B lymphocytes. *Cell. Immunol.* **7:** 290–301.

HOWE, M. L. and COHEN, L. (1975a) Lymphoid cell subpopulations. I. Synergy between lymph node cells and thymocytes in response to alloantigens and mitogens. *J. Immunol.* **115:** 1227–1232.

HOWE, M. L. and COHEN, L. (1975b) Lymphoid cell subpopulations. II. Characterization of cell populations responsible for synergy in the mixed lymphocyte interaction. *J. Immunol.* **115:** 1233–1238.

HUBER, B., CANTOR, H., SHEN, F. W. and BOYSE, E. A.(1976a) Independent differentiative pathways of Ly 1 and Ly 23 subclasses of T cells. Experimental production of mice deprived of selected T-cell subclasses. *J. exp. Med.* **144:** 1128–1133.

HUBER, B., DEVINSKY, D., GERSHON, R. K. and CANTOR, H. (1976b) Cell-mediated immunity: delayed-type hypersensitivity and cytotoxic responses are mediated by different T-cell subclasses. *J. exp. Med.* **143:** 1534–1539.

HUSTON, D. P., RICH, R. R., STEINBERG, A. D. and TRUITT, G. A. (1979) Regulation of cytotoxic lymphocyte responses in New Zealand mice by alloantigen-activated spleen cells. *J. Immunol.* **122:** 1476–1481.

ILFELD, D. N., WEIL, S. and KUPERMAN, O. (1981) Suppressor cell function in a family with familial Mediterranean fever. *Clin. exp. Immunol.* **43:** 357–361.

ISHIZAKA, K. and ADACHI, T. (1976) Generation of specific helper cells and suppressor cells *in vitro* for the IgE and IgG antibody response. *J. Immunol.* **117:** 40–47.

JACOBSSON, H. and BLOMGREN, H. (1974) Enhancement of the mixed lymphocyte response in the mouse by the addition of thymocytes. *Cell. Immunol.* **10:** 294–309.

JANEWAY, C., MURGITA, R., WEINBAUM, F., ASOFSKY, R. and WIGZELL, H. (1977) Evidence for an immunoglobulin-dependent antigen-specific helper T cell. *Proc. Natl. Acad. Sci. USA* **74:** 4582–4586.

JANDINSKI, J., CANTOR, H., TADAKUMA, T., PEAVY, D. L. and PIERCE, C. W. (1976) Separation of helper T cells from suppressor T cells expressing different Ly components. I. Polyclonal activation: Suppressor and helper activities are inherent properties of distinct T-cell subclasses. *J. exp. Med.* **143:** 1382–1390.

JANOSSY, G. and GREAVES, M. (1975) Functional analysis of murine and human B lymphcyte subsets. *Transplant. Rev.* **24:** 177–236.

JERNE, N. (1974) Towards a network theory of the immune system. *Ann. Immunol. (Inst. Pasteur)* **125c:** 373–389.

JULIUS, M., COSENZA, H. and Augustin, A. (1978) Evidence for the endogenous production of T cell receptors bearing idiotypic determinants. *Eur. J. Immunol.* **8:** 484–491.

KAPP, J., ARANEO, B. and CLEVINGER, B. (1980) Suppression of antibody and T cell proliferative responses to L-glutamic acid^{60}-L-alanine^{30}-L-tyrosine^{10} by a specific monoclonal T cell factor. *J. exp. Med.* **152:** 235–290.

KAPP, J. A., PIERCE, C. W. and BENACERRAF, B. (1974a) Genetic control of immune responses *in vitro.* III. Tolerogeneic properties of the terpolymer L-glutamic acid^{60}-L-alanine^{30}-L-tyrosine^{10} (GAT) for spleen cells from nonresponder (H-2^{s} and H-2^{q}) mice. *J. exp. Med.* **140:** 172–184.

KAPP, J. A., PIERCE, C. W. and BENACERRAF, B. (1975) Role of suppressor T cells in an IR gene controlled immune response. In: *Suppressor Cells in Immunity,* pp. 84–92. SINGHAL, S. K. and SINCLAIR, N. R. (eds.). University of Western Ontario Press, London, Ontario.

KAPP, J. A., PIERCE, C. W., DE BA CROIX and BENACERRAF, B. (1976) Immunosuppressive factor(s) extracted from lymphoid cells of nonresponder mice primed with L-glutamic acid^{60}-L-alanine^{30}-L-tyrosine^{10} (GAT). I. Activity and antigen specificity. *J. Immunol.* **116:** 305–309.

KAPP, J. A., PIERCE, C. W., SCHLOSSMAN, S. and BENACERRAF, B. (1974b) Genetic control of immune responses *in vitro.* V. Stimulation of suppressor T cells in nonresponder mice by the terpolymer L-glutamic acid^{60}-L-alanine^{30}- L-tyrosine^{10} (GAT). *J. exp. Med.* **140:** 648–649.

KAPPLER, J. W., HUNTER (MARRACK), P. C., JACOBS, D. and LORD, E. (1974) Functional heterogeneity among the T-derived lymphocytes of the mouse. I. Analysis by adult thymectomy. *J. Immunol.* **113:** 27–38.

KASTNER, D. and RICH, R. (1978) Regulation of alloantigen induced cytotoxic responses by concanavalin A-activated lymphoid cells: Suppression by antigen elimination. *J. Immunol.* **121:** 1782–1737.

KATZ, D. H. (1977) *Lymphocyte Differentiation, Recognition and Regulation,* pp. 631–675. Academic Press, New York.

KATZ, D. H. and BENACERRAF, B. (1972) The regulatory influence of activated T cells on B cell responses to antigen. *Adv. Immunol.* **15:** 1–94.

KATZ, D. H. and BENACERRAF, B. (eds.) (1974) *Immunological tolerance: Mechanisms and Potential Therapeutic Applications.* Academic Press, New York.

KATZ, D. H., GRAVES, M., DORF, M. E., DIMUZIO, H. and BENACERRAF, B. (1975) Cell interactions between histoincompatiole T and B lymphocytes. VIII. Cooperative responses between lymphocytes are controlled by genes in the I region of the H-2 complex. *J. exp. Med.* **141:** 263–267.

KATZ, D. H., PAUL, W. E., GOIDL, E. A. and BENACERRAF, B. (1970) Carrier functions in anti-hapten immune responses. I. Enhancement of primary and secondary anti-hapten antibody responses by carrier preimmunization. *J. exp. Med.* **132:** 261–282.

KATZ, D. H., PAUL, W. E., GOIDL, E. H. and BENACERRAF, B. (1971) Carrier function in anti-hapten antibody responses. III. Stimulation of antibody synthesis and facilitation of hapten-specific secondary antibody responses by graft-versus-host reactions. *J. exp. Med.* **133:** 169–186.

KERBEL, R. S. and EIDINGER, D. (1971) Variable effects of antilymphocyte serum on humoral antibody formation. Role of thymus-dependency of antigen. *J. Immunol.* **106:** 917–926.

KERBEL, R. S. and EIDINGER, D. (1972) Enhanced immune responsiveness to a thymus independent antigen. Evidence for a short-lived subpopulation of inhibitory thymus-derived lymphocytes. *Eur. J. Immunol.* **2:** 114–118.

KISIELOW, P., HIRST, J., SHIKU, BEVERLY, P. C. L., HOFFMAN, M. K., BOYSE, E. A. and OETTGEN, H. F. (1975) Ly antigens: markers for functionally distinct subsets of thymus-derived lymphocytes of the mouse. *Nature* **253:** 219–220.

KLEIN, J. (1975) *Biology of the Mouse Histocompatibility-2 Complex.* Springer-Verlag, New York.

KÖHLER, G. and MILSTEIN, C. (1976) Derivation of specific antibody-producing tissue culture and tumor lines by cell fusion. *Eur. J. Immunol.* **6:** 511–519.

KONTIAINEN, S. and FELDMAN, M. (1976) Suppressor cell induction *in vitro.* I. Kinetics of induction of antigen-specific suppressor cells. *Eur. J. Immunol.* **6:** 296–301.

KRAKAUER, R. S., WALDMANN, T. A. and STROBER, W. (1976) Loss of suppressor T cells in adult NZB/NZW mice. *J. exp. Med.* **144:** 662–673.

KRAWINKEL, U., CRAMER, M., IMANISHI-KARI, T., JACK, R. S., RAJEWSKY, K. and MÄKELÄ, O. (1977) Isolated hapten-binding receptors of sensitized lymphocytes. I. Receptors from nylon wool-enriched mouse T lymphocytes lack seriological markers of immunoglobulin constant domains but express heavy chain variable portions. *Eur. J. Immunol.* **8:** 566–573.

LARSSON, E. L. (1980) Cyclosporin A and dexamethasone suppress T cell responses by selectively acting at distinct sites of the triggering process. *J. Immunol.* **124:** 2828–2833.

LARSSON, E. L. and CONTINHO, A. (1979) The role of mitogenic lectins in T cell triggering. *Nature* **280:** 239–241.

LAWRENCE, S. H. and LANDY, M. L. (eds.) (1969) *Mediators of Cellular Immunity.* Academic Press, New York.

LEDBETTER, J. and HERZENBERG, L. (1979) Xenogeneic monoclonal antibodies to mouse lymphoid differentiation antigens. *Immun. Rev.* **47:** 63–90.

LIACOPOULOS, P. and BEN-EFRAIM, S. (1975) Antigenic competition. *Prog. Allergy* **18:** 97–204.

LIEW, F. and HOWARD, J. (1980) Regulation of delayed type hypersensitivity V. Suppressor cell memory in antigen-specific suppression of delayed-type hypersensitivity to sheep erythrocytes. *Eur. J. Immunol.* **10:** 937–943.

LONAI, P., PURI, J. and HAMMERLING, G. (1981) H-2 restricted antigen binding by a hydridoma clone that produces antigen-specific helper factors. *Proc. Natl. Acad. Sci. USA* **78:** 549–553.

LYNCH, R., ROHNER, J., ADERMATL, B., GEBEL, H., AUTRY, J. and HOOVER, R. (1979) Immunoregulation of murine myeloma cell growth and differentiation: A monoclonal model of B cell differentiation. *Imm. Rev.* **48:** 45–80.

MÄKELÄ, O. and KARJALAINEN, K. (1977) Inherited immunoglobulin idiotypes of the mouse. *Immunol. Rev.* **34:** 119–138.

MAKINODAN, T. and ADLER, W. H. (1975) Effects of ageing on the differentiation and proliferation potentials of cells of the immune system. *Fed. Proc.* **34:** 153–158.

MARBROOK, J. (1967) Primary immune response in cultures of spleen cells. *Lancet ii:* 1279–1281.

MARCHALONIS, J. (eds.) (1980) The molecular biology of T cell receptors: A symposium. *Molec. Immunol.* **17:** 795–1010.

McDevitt, H. O., Delovitch, T. L., Press, J. L. and Murphy, D. B. (1976) Genetic and functional analysis of the Ia antigens, their possible role in regulating the immune response. *Transplant. Rev.* **30:** 197–235.
McDonald, H., Cerottini, J., Ryser, J., Marijanski, J., Taswell, C., Widmer, M. and Brunner, K. (1980) Quantitation and cloning of cytolytic T lymphocytes and their precursors. *Immunol. Rev.* **51:** 93–123.
McDougal, J. S., Shen, F. W. and Elster, P. (1979) Generation of T helper cells in vitro. V. Antigen-specific Ly 1^+ T cells mediate the helper effect and induce feedback suppression. *J. Immunol.* **122:** 437–442.
McGregor, D. O. and Kostiala, A. A. I. (1976) Role of lymphocytes in cellular resistance to infection. *Contemp. Top. Immunobiol.* **5:** 237–266.
Metcalf, E. S. and Klinman, N. R. (1976) *In vitro* tolerance induction of neonatal murine B cells. *J. exp. Med.* **143:** 1327–1340.
Miller, J. F. A. P. (1980) MHC restrictions in cellular cooperation. *Prog. Immunol.* **4:** 359–374.
Miller, J. F. A. P. and Mitchell, G. F. (1968) Cell to cell interaction in the immune response. I. Hemolysin-forming cells in neonatally thymectomized mice reconstituted with thymus or thoracic duct lymphocyte. *J. exp. Med.* **128:** 801–820.
Miller, J. F. A. P. and Mitchell, G. F. (1969) Thymus and antigen-reactive cells. *Transplant. Rev.* **1:** 3–42.
Miller, J. F. A. P., Vadas, M., Whitlaw, A. and Gamble, J. (1976) Role of major histocompatibility complex gene products in delayed-type hypersensitivity. *PNAS* **73:** 2486–2490.
Mishell, R. I. and Dutton, R. W. (1967) Immunization of normal mouse spleen cell suspensions *in vitro*. *Science* **153:** 1004–1006.
Mitchell, G. F. and Miller, J. F. A. P. (1968) Cell to cell interaction in the immune response. II. The source of hemolysin-forming cells in irradiated mice given bone marrow and thymus or thoracic dust lymphocytes. *J. exp. Med.* **128:** 821–837.
Mitchison, N. A. (1969) Cell populations involved in immune responses. In: *Immunological Tolerance,* pp. 149–151. Landy, M. and Braun, W. (eds.), Academic Press, New York.
Mitchison, N. A. (1971a) Carrier effects in secondary responses to hapten protein conjugates. I. Measurement of the effect with transferred cells and objection to the local environment hypothesis. *Eur. J. Immunol.* **1:** 10–17.
Mitchison, N. A. (1971b) Carrier effects on the secondary immune response. II. Cellular cooperation. *Eur. J. Immunol.* **1:** 18–27.
Mitchison, N. A., Rajewsky, K. and Taylor, R. B. (1970) Cooperation of antigenic determinants and of cells in the induction of antibodies. In: *Developmental Aspects of Antibody Formation and Structure,* pp. 547–561. Sterzl, J. and Riha, I. (eds.). Academic Press, New York.
Miyawaki, T., Seki, H., Kubo, M. and Taniguki, N. (1979) Suppressor activity of T lymphocytes from infants assessed by coculture with unfractionated adult lymphocytes in the pokeweed-mitogen system. *J. Immunol.* **123:** 1092–1096.
Mizel, S., Oppenheim, J. and Rosenstreich, D. (1978) Characterization of lymphocyte-activity factor (LAF) produced by the macrophage cell line $P388D_1$. I. Enhancement of LAF production by activated T lymphocytes. *J. Immunol.* **120:** 1497–1503.
Möller, G. (1978) Role of macrophages in the immune response. *Immunol. Rev.* **40:** 1–255.
Möller, G. (1981) T cell clones. *Immunol. Rev.* **54:** 1–266.
Moorhead, J. (1979) Soluble factors in tolerance and contact sensitivity to 2,4-dinitrofluorobenzene in mice. III. Histocompatibility antigens associated with the hapten dinitrophenol serve as target molecules on 2,4-dinitrofluorobenzene immune T cells for soluble suppressor factor. *J. exp. Med.* **150:** 1432–1447.
Morimoto, C., Reinherz, E. L., Borel, Y., Mantzouranis, E., Steinberg, A. D. and Schlossman, S. F. (1981) Autoantibody to an immunoregulatory inducer population in patients with juvenile rheumatoid arthritis. *J. Clin. Invest.* **67:** 753–761.
Morimoto, C., Reinherz, E. L., Schlossman, S. F., Schur, P. H., Mills, J. A. and Steinberg, A. D. (1980) Alterations in immunoregulatory T cell subsets in active systemic lupus erythematosus. *J. Clin. Invest.* **66:** 1171–1174.
Mosier, D. and Cantor, H. (1971) Functional maturation of mouse thymic lymphocytes. *Eur. J. Immunol.* **1:** 459–461.
Mosier, D. E. and Cohen, P. L. (1975) Ontogeny of mouse function. *Fedn. Proc.* **34:** 137–140.
Mosier, D. E. and Johnson, B. M. (1975) Ontogeny of mouse lymphocyte functions. II. Development of the ability to produce antibody is modulated by T lymphocytes. *J. exp. Med.* **139:** 1354–1359.
Mozes, E. and Haimovitch, J. (1979) Antigen specific T cell helper factor cross reacts idiotypically with antibodies of the same specificity. *Nature* **278:** 56–57.
Munro, A. J. and Taussig, M. J. (1975) Two genes in the major histocompatibility complex control immune response. *Nature* **256:** 103–106.
Murphy, D. (1978) The I-J subregion of the murine H-2 gene complex. *Springer Seminars in Immunopathol.* **1:** 111–131.
Nabel, G., Fresno, M., McVay-Boudreau, Chessman, D., Bucala, R. and Cantor, H. (1980) Generation and preparation of thymus-dependent lymphocytes in continuous culture. *Prog. Immunol.* **4:** 315–337.
Nabel, G., Greenberger, J., Sakakeeny, M. and Cantor, H. (1981) Multiple biologic activities of a cloned inducer T cell population. *Proc. Natl. Acad. Sci. USA* **78:** 1157–1161.
Nakano, T., Imai, Y., Naiki, M. and Osawa, T. (1980) Characterization of mouse helper and suppressor T cell subsets separated by lectins. *J. Immunol.* **125:** 1928–1932.
Nakayama, E., Dippold, W., Shiku, H., Oettgen, H. and Old, L. (1980) Alloantigen-induced T-cell proliferation: Lyt phenotype of responding cells and blocking proliferation by Lyt antisera. *Proc. Natl. Acad. Sci. USA* **77:** 2890–2894.
Nakayama, E., Shiku, H., Stockert, E., Oettgen, H. and Old, L. (1979) Cytotoxic T cells:Lyt phenotype and blocking of killing activity by Lyt antisera. *Proc. Natl. Acad. Sci. USA* **76:** 1977–1981.
Nelson, D. S. (ed.) (1976) *Immunobiology of the Macrophage*. Academic Press, New York.
Nisonoff, A., Ju, S. T. and Owen, F. (1977) Studies of structure and immunosuppression of a cross-reactive idiotype in strain A mice. *Immunol. Rev.* **34:** 89–118.

OKUMURA, K., HERZENBERG, L. A., MURPHY, D. B., McDEVITT, H. O. and HERZENBERG, L. A. (1976) Selective expression of H-2 (I-region) loci controlling determinants on helper and suppressor T lymphocytes. *J. exp. Med.* **144:** 685–698.

OKUMURA, K. and TADA, T. (1971) Regulation of homocytotropic antibody formation in the rat. VI. Inhibitory effect of thymocytes on the homocytotropic antibody response. *J. Immunol.* **107:** 1682–1689.

OKUMURA, K. and TADA, T. (1973) Suppression of hapten-specific antibody response by carrier specific T cells. *Nature New Biol.* **245:** 180–182.

OWEN, F. (1980) A mature T lymphocyte marker closely linked to Igh-1 that is expressed on the precursor for the suppressor T cell regulating a primary response to SRBC. *J. Immunol.* **124:** 1411–1417.

OWEN, F., JU, S. T. and NISONOFF, A. (1977a) Presence on idiotype-specific suppressor T cells of receptors that interact with molecules bearing the idiotype. *J. exp. Med.* **137:** 1559–1566.

OWEN, F., JU, S. T. and NISONOFF, A. (1977b) Binding to idiotype determinants of a large population of T cells in idiotypically suppressed mice. *Proc. Natl. Acad. Sci. USA* **74:** 2084–2088.

OWEN, F., RIBLET, R. and TAYLOR, B. (1981) The T suppressor cell alloantigen T_{su}d maps near immunoglobulin allotype genes and may be a heavy chain constant-region marker on a T cell receptor. *J. exp. Med.* **153:** 801–810.

PALACIOS, R. and MÖLLER, G. (1981) T cell growth factor abrogates concanavalin A-induced suppressor cell function. *J. exp. Med.* **153:** 1360–1365.

PAUL, W. E. and BENACERRAF, B. (1977) Functional specificity of thymus-dependent lymphocytes. *Science* **195:** 1293–1300.

PAUL, W. E., KATZ, D. H., GOIDL, E. A. and BENACERRAF, B. (1970) Carrier function in anti-hapten immune responses. II. Specific properties of carrier cells capable of enhancing antihapten antibody responses. *J. exp. Med.* **132:** 283–299.

PEAVY, D. L. and PIERCE, C. W. (1974) Cell-mediated immune responses *in vitro*. I. Suppression of the generation of cytotoxic lymphocytes by concanavalin A-activated spleen cells. *J. exp. Med.* **140:** 356–369.

PERRY, L. and GREENE, M. (1981) T cell subset interactions in the regulation of syngeneic tumor immunity. *Fed. Proc.* **40:** 39–44.

PICKEL, K., HAMMERLING, U. and HOFFMAN, M. (1976) Ly phenotype of T cells releasing T cell replacing factor. *Nature* **264:** 72–72.

PIERCE, C. W. and BENACERRAF, B. (1976) Cellular basis of immune responses. In: *Textbook of Immunopathology,* pp. 3–14. MIESCHER, P. A. and MULLER-EBERHARD, H. J. (eds). Greene and Stratton, New York.

PIERCE, C. W. and KAPP, J. A. (1976) Regulation of immune responses by suppressor T cells. *Contemp. Top. Immunobiol.* **5:** 91–143.

PIERCE, C. W., KAPP, J. A. and BENACERRAF, B. (1976) Regulation by the *H-2* complex of macrophage-lymphoid cell interactions in secondary antibody responses *in vitro. J. exp. Med.* **144:** 371–381.

PIERCE, C. W., PEAVY, D. L. and TADAKUMA, T. (1975a) Suppressor T cells as regulators of lymphocyte functions. *Ann. N.Y. Acad. Sci.* **256:** 365–374.

PIERCE, C. W., TADAKUMA, T., KUHNER, A. L. and DAVID, J. R. (1975b) Characterization of a soluble immune responses suppressor (SIRS) produced by concanavalin A-activated spleen cells. In: *The Role of Mitogens in Immunobiology,* pp. 583–595. OPPENHEIM, J. J. and ROSENSTREICH, D. L. (eds.). Academic Press, New York.

PIERRES, M. and GERMAIN, R. (1978) Antigen-specific T cell-mediated suppression. IV. Role of macrophages in generation of L-glutamic acid^{60}-L-alanine^{30}-L-tyrosine^{10} (GAT)-specific suppressor T cells in responder mouse strains. *J. Immunol.* **121:** 1306–1314.

PROSS, H. F. and EIDINGER, D. (1974) Antigenic competition: A review of nonspecific antigen-induced suppression. *Adv. Immunol.* **18:** 133–168.

PURI, J., BEN-NERIAH, Y., GIVOL, D. and LONAI, P. (1980) Antibodies to immunoglobulin heavy chain variable regions protect helper cells from specific suicide by radiolabelled antigen. *Eur. J. Immunol.* **10:** 281–284.

RAFF, M. C. (1970) Role of thymus-derived lymphocytes in the secondary humoral response in mice. *Nature, Lond.* **226:** 1257–1258.

RANNEY, D. F. and STEINBERG, A. D. (1976) Differences in the age-dependent releas a low molecular weight suppressor (LWMS) and stimulation by normal and NZB/W lymphoid organs. *J. Immunol.* **117:** 1219–1225.

REINHERZ, E. L. and SCHLOSSMAN, S. F. (1980)The differentiation and function of human T lymphocytes. *Cell* **19:** 821–827.

RICH, R. (1975) Antibody synthesis and immunological memory in concanavalin A-treated mice. *Clin. Immunol. Immunopath.* **3:** 482–491.

RICH, R. R. and PIERCE, C. W. (1973a) Biological expressions of lymphocyte activation. I. Effect of phytomitogens on antibody synthesis *in vitro. J. exp. Med.* **137:** 205–223.

RICH, R. and PIERCE, C. W. (1973b) Biological expressions of lymphocyte activation. II. Generation of a population of thymus-derived suppressor lymphocytes. *J. exp. Med.* **137:** 649–659.

RICH, R. R. and PIERCE, C. W. (1974) Biological expressions of lymphocyte activation. III. Suppression of plaque-forminc cell responses *in vitro* by supernatant fluids from concanavalin A-activated spleen cell cultures. *J. Immunol.* **112:** 1360–1368.

RICH, R. and RICH, S. (1975) Biological expressions of lymphocyte activation. IV. Concanavalin A-activated suppressor cells in mouse mixed lymphocyte reactions. *J. Immunol.* **114:** 1112–1115.

RICH, S. and DAVID, C. (1979) Regulatory mechanisms in cell-mediated immune responses. VIII. Differential expression of I region determinants by suppressor cells and their targets in suppression of mixed leukocyte reactions. *J.exp. Med.* **150:** 1108–1121.

RICH, S and RICH, R. (1974) Regulatory mechanisms in cell-mediated immune responses. I. Regulation of mixed lymphocyte reactions by alloantigen-activated thymus-derived lymphocytes. *J. exp. Med.* **140:** 1588–1603.

RICH, S. and RICH, R. (1975) Regulatory mechanisms in cell-mediated immune responses. II. A genetically restricted suppressor of mixed lymphocyte reactions released by alloantigen-activated spleen cells. *J. exp. Med.* **142,** 1391–1401.

RICH, S. and RICH, R. (1976a) Regulatory mechanisms in cell-mediated immune responses. III. I-region control of suppressor cell interactions with mixed lymphocyte reactions. *J. exp. Med.* **143:** 672–677.

RICH, S. and RICH, R. (1976b) Regulatory mechanisms in cell-mediated immune responses. IV. Expression of a receptor for MLR suppressor factor on activated T lymphocytes. *J. exp. Med.* **144:** 1214–1226.

RICH, S., BECKWITH, M., DENNISON, D. and RICH, R. (1981) Antigenic and cellular interactions in MLR-TsF suppression. *Fed. Proc.* **40:** 1167.

RICH, S., ORSON, F. M. and RICH, R. (1977) *H-2* and non *H-2* gene control of T cell suppression of MLR. In: *Proceedings of the Third IR Gene Workshop,* MCDEVITT, H. O. (ed.). Academic Press, New York. (In press).

ROSE, N. R., KONG, Y. M., OKAYASU, I., GIRALDO, A. A., BEISEL, K. AND SUNDICK, R. S. (1981) T cell regulation in autoimmune thyroiditis. *Immunolog. Rev.* **55:** 299–314.

ROSENTHAL, A. and SHEVACH, E. (1976) The function of macrophages in T-lymphocyte antigen recognition. *Contemp. Top. Immunobiol.* **5:** 47–90.

ROTTER, V. and TRAININ, N. (1974) Thymus cell population exerting a regulatory function in the immune response of mice to polyvinylpyrrolidone. *Cell. Immunol.* **13:** 76–86.

ROUTHIER, G., EPSTEIN, O., JANOSSY, G., THOMAS, H. C., SHERLOCK, S., KUNG, P. C. and GOLDSTEIN, G. (1980) Effects of cyclosporin A on suppressor and inducer T lymphocytes in primary biliary cirrhosis. *Lancet ii:* 1223–1225.

ROWLEY, D., FITCH, F., STUART, F., KÖHLER, H. and COSENZA, H. (1973) Specific suppression of immune responses. *Science (Wash. D.C.)* **181:** 1133–1141.

SAGAWA, A. and ABDOU, N. J. (1979) Suppressor-cell antibody in systemic lupus erythematosus. *J. Clin. Invest.* **63:** 536–539.

SAKANE, T., STEINBERG, A. D. and GREEN, I. (1978) Studies of immune functions of patients with systemic lupus erythematosus. I. (1978) Studies of immune functions of patients with systemic lupus erythematosus. I. Dysfunction of suppressor T-cell activity related to impaired generation of rather than response to suppressor cells. *Arth. Rheum.* **21:** 657–664.

SARMIENTO, M., GLASEBROOK, A. and FITCH, F. (1980) IgG or IgM monoclonal antibodies reactive with different determinants on the molecular complex bearing Lyt 2 antigen block T cell-mediated cytolysis in the absence of complement. *J. Immunol.* **125:** 2665–2672.

SCHARFF, M. D., ROBERTS, S. and THAMMANA, P. (1981) Hybridomas as a source of antibodies. *Hosp. Pract.* **16:** 61–66.

SCHENDEL, D. J., ALTER, B. J. and BACH, F. H. (1973) The involvement of LD- and SD-region differences in MLR and CML: A three-cell experiment. *Transplant. Proc.* **5:** 1651–1655.

SCHER, I., SHARROW, S. O., WISTAR, R., JR., ASOFSKY, R. and PAUL, W. E. (1976) B-lymphocyte heterogeneity: ontogenetic development and organ distribution of B-lymphocyte populations defined by their density of surface immunoglobulin. *J. exp. Med.* **144:** 494–506.

SCHIMPL, A., HÜBNER, L., WONG, C. and WECKER, E. (1980) Non-antigen-specific T cell factors. *Prog. Immunol.* **4:** 403–412.

SCHIMPL, A. and WECKER, E. (1971) Reconstitution of a thymus cell-deprived immune system by syngeneic and allogeneic thymocytes *in vitro*. *Eur. J. Immunol.* **1:** 304–306.

SCHIMPL, A. and WECKER, E. (1972) Replacement of T cell function by a T cell product. *Nature New Biol.* **237:** 15–17.

SCHIMPL, A. and WECKER, E. (1975) A third signal in B cell activation given by TRF. *Transplant. Rev.* **23:** 176–188.

SCHREFFLER, D. C. (1976) The S region of the mouse major histocompatibility complex (H-2): Genetic variation and functional role in complement system. *Transplant. Rev.* **32:** 140–167.

SCHREFFLER, D. C. and DAVID, C. S. (1975) The *H-2* major histocompatibility complex and the I immune response region: genetic variation, function and organization. *Adv. Immunol.* **20:** 125–195.

SCHREFFLER, D. C., MEO, T. and DAVID, C. S. (1976) Genetic resolution of the products and functions of I and S region genes of the mouse *H-2* complex. In: *The Role of Products of the Histocompatibility Gene Complex in Immune Responses,* pp. 3–27. KATZ, D. H. and BENACERRAF, B. (eds.). Academic Press, New York.

SCHREIER, M., ISCOVE, N., TEES, R., CLARDEN, L., VON BOEHMER, H. (1980) Clones of killer and helper T cells: Growth requirements, specificity and retention of function in long term culture. *Immunol. Rev.* **51:** 315–336.

SCHWARTZ, R., DORF, M. E., BENACERRAF, B. AND PAUL, W. E. (1976) The requirement for two complementing Ir-GLØ immune response genes in the T lymphocyte proliferative response to poly-($Glu^{53}Lys^{36}Phe^{11}$). *J. exp. Med.* **143:** 897–905.

SERCARZ, E. and METZGER, D. (1980) Epitope-specific and idiotype-specific cellular interactions in a model protein antigen system. *Springer Semin. Immunopathol.* **3:** 145–170.

SHEARER, G. M. and SCHMITT-VERHULST, A. M. (1977) Major histocompatibility complex restricted cell-mediated immunity. *Adv. Immunol.* **25:** 55–91.

SHEN, F., MCDOUGAL, J., BOND, J. and CORT, S. (1980) Development and communicative interrelations of Ly-123 and Ly 1 cell sets. *J. exp. Med.* **151:** 566–572.

SHIKU, H., KISIELOW, P., BEAN, M. A., TAKAHASHI, T., BOYSE, E. A., OETTGEN, H. F. and OLD, L. J. (1975) Expression of T-cell differentiation antigens of effector cells in cell-mediated cytotoxicity *in vitro*. Evidence for functional heterogeneity related to the surface phenotype of T-cells. *J. exp. Med.* **141:** 227–241.

SHINOHARA, H. and SACHS, D. (1979) Mouse alloantibodies capable of blocking cytotoxic T-cell function. *J. exp. Med.* **150:** 432–444.

SHOU, L., SCHWARTZ, S. A. and GOOD, R. A. (1976) Suppressor cell activity after concanavalin A treatment of lymphocytes from normal donors. *J. exp. Med.* **143:** 1100–1110.

SIEGAL, F. P., SIEGAL, M. and GOOD, R. A. (1976) Suppression of B-cell differentiation by leukocytes from hypogammaglobulinemia patients. *J. Clin. Invest.* **58:** 109–122.

SIMPSON, E. and CANTOR, H. (1975) Regulation of the immune response by subclasses of T lymphocytes. II. The effect of adult thymectomy upon humoral and cellular responses in mice. *Eur. J. Immunol.* **5:** 337–343.

SIMON, M. and ABERHARDT, B. (1980) Generation of effector cells from T cell subsets. II. Ly^{+} 123 T cells contain the precursors for all primary cytotoxic effector cells and for cells involved in the regulation of cytotoxic responses. *Eur. J. Immunol.* **18:** 334–341.

SMITH, K., BAKER, P., GILLIS, S. and RUSSETTI, F. (1980) Functional and molecular characteristics of T cell growth factor. *Molec. Immunol.* **17:** 579–589.

SPRENT, J. (1978) Restricted helper function of F_1 hybrid T cells positively selected to heterologous erythrocytes in irradiated parental strain mice. II. Evidence for restrictions affecting helper cell induction and T-B collaboration, both mapping to the K-end of the H-2 complex. *J. exp. Med.* **147:** 1159–1174.

STEINBERG, A. D., GERBER, N. L., GERSHWIN, N. E., MORTON, R., GOODMAN, D., CHUSED, T. M., HARDIN, J. A. and BARTHOLD, D. R. (1975) Role of suppressor T cells in autoimmunity in New Zealand mice. In: *Suppressor Cells in Immunity,* pp. 174–180. SINGHAL, S. K. and SINCLAIR, N. R. (eds.), University of Western Ontario Press, London, Ontario.

STEINBERG, A. D., HUSTON, D. P., TAUROG, J. D., COWDERY, J. S. and RAVECHE, E. S. (1981) The cellular and genetic basis of murine lupus. *Immunolog. Rev.* **55:** 121–154.

STEINBERG, A. D., KRAKAUER, R., REINERTSEN, J. L., KLASSEN, L. W., ILFELD, D., REEVES, J. P., WILLIAMS, G. W. and ANTONOUYCH, T. (1978) Therapeutic studies in NZB/NZW mice VI. Age-dependent effects of concanavalin A stimulated spleen cell supernate. *Arth. Rheum.* **21:** 204–209.

STEINMAN, R., NAGUEIRA, N., WITMAN, M., TYDINGS, J. and MELVAN, I. (1980) Lymphokine enhances the expression and synthesis of Ia antigens on cultured mouse peritoneal macrophages. *J. exp. Med.* **152:** 1248–1261.

STOBO, J. D. and PAUL, W. E. (1973) Functional heterogeneity of murine lymphoid cells. III. Differential responsiveness of T cells to phytohemagglutinin and concanavalin A as a probe for T cell subsets. *J. Immunol.* **110:** 362–375.

STOBO, J. D., PAUL, S., LAN, R. E. and HERMANS, P. E. (1976) Suppressor thymus-derived lymphocytes in fungal infections. *J. Clin. Invest.* **57:** 319–328.

STOCKER, J. and NOSSAL, G. J. V. (1976) Pathways to immunological tolerance: An approach through the study of maturing B lymphocytes. *Contemp. Top. Immunobiol.* **5:** 191–210.

STRASSMANN, G., ESHHAR, Z. and MOZES, E. (1980) Genetic regulation of delayed-type hypersensitivity responses to poly (L-Tyr, L-Glo)-poly (DL-ALA)-POLY (L-Lys). II. Evidence for a T-T cell collaboration in delayed-type hypersensitivity responses and for a T cell defect at the efferent phase in nonresponder H-2^k mice. *J. exp. Med.* **151:** 628–636.

STRELKAUSKAS, A. J., CALLERY, R. T., MCDOWELL, J., BOREL, Y. and SCHLOSSMAN, S. F. (1978) Direct evidence for loss of human suppressor cells during active autoimmune disease. *Proc. Natl. Acad. Sci. USA* **75:** 5150–5154.

STULL, D. and GILLIS, S. (1981) Constitutive production of interleukin 2 by a T cell hybridoma. *J. Immunol.* **126:** 1680–1683.

STUTMAN, O. (1974) Cell-mediated immunity and aging. *Fedn. Proc.* **33:** 2028–2032.

SUNDAY, M., BENACERRAF, B. and DORF, M. (1981) Hapten specific T cell responses to 4-hydroxy-3-nitrophenyl acetyl. VIII. Suppressor cell pathways in cutaneous sensitivity responses. *J. exp. Med.* **153:** 811–822.

SWAIN, S. (1980) Association of Ly phenotypes, T cell function and MHC recognition. *Fed. Proc.* **39:** 3110–3113.

TADA, T. (1977) Regulation of the antibody response by T cell products determined by different I subregions. *In Regulation of the Immune System,* pp. 345–361. SERCARZ, E. and HERZENBERG, L. A. (eds.). Academic Press, Inc., New York.

TADA, T., HAYAKAWA, K., OKUMURA, K. and TANIGUCHI, M. (1980) Coexistence of variable region of immunoglobulin heavy chain and I region gene products on antigen-specific suppressor T cells and suppressor T cell factor. *Molec. Immunol.* **17:** 867–875.

TADA, T. and TAKEMORI, T. (1974) Selective roles of thymus-derived lymphocytes in the antibody response. I. Differential suppressive effect of carrier-primed T cells on hapten-specific IgM and IgG antibody responses. *J. exp. Med.* **140:** 239–252.

TADA, T., TAKEMORI, T., OKUMURA, K., NONAKA, M. and TOKUHISA, T. (1978). Two distinct types of helper T cells involved in the secondary antibody response: Independent and synergistic effects of Ia^- and Ia^+ helper T cells. *J. exp. Med.* **147:** 446–458.

TADA, T., TANIGUCHI, M. and OKUMURA, K. (1977) Regulation of antibody response by antigen-specific T cell factors bearing I region determinants. *Prog. Immunol.* **3:** 369–377.

TADA, T., TANIGUCHI, M. and TAKEMORI, T. (1975) Properties of primed suppressor T cells and their products. *Transplant. Rev.* **26:** 106–129.

TADAKUMA, T., KUHNER, A. L., RICH, R. R., DAVID, J. R. and PIERCE, C. W. (1976) Biological expressions of lymphocyte activation. V. Characterization of a soluble immune response suppressor (SIRS) produced by concanavalin A-activated spleen cells. *J. Immunol.* **117:** 323–330.

TADAKUMA, T. and PIERCE, C. W. (1976) Site of action of a soluble immune response suppressor (SIRS) produced by concanavalin A-activated spleen cells. *J. Immunol.* **117:** 967–972.

TAKEMORI, T. and TADA, T. (1974) Selective role of thymus-derived lymphocytes in the antibody response. II. Preferential suppression of high-affinity antibody-forming cells by carrier-primed suppressor T cells. *J. exp. Med.* **140:** 253–266.

TALAL, N. (1976) Disordered immunologic regulation and autoimmunity. *Transplant. Rev.* **31:** 240–263.

TALAL, N. and STEINBERG, A. D. (1974) The pathogenesis of autoimmunity in New Zealand black mice. *Curr. Top. Microbiol. Immunol.* **64:** 79–104.

TANIGUCHI, M. and MILLER, J. (1977) Enrichment of specific suppressor cells and characterization of their surface markers. *J. exp. Med.* **146:** 1450–1454.

TANIGUCHI, M., SAITO, T. and TADA, T. (1979) Antigen-specific suppressive factor produced by a transplantable I-J bearing T cell hybridoma. *Nature* **278:** 555–558.

TANIGUCHI, M., TADA, T. and TOKUHISA, T. (1976) Properties of antigen-specific suppressive T cell factor in the regulation of antibody. *J. exp. Med.* **144:** 20–31.

TANIGUCHI, M. and TAKUHISA, T. (1980) Cellular consequences in the suppression of antibody response by the antigen-specific T cell factor. *J. exp. Med.* **151:** 517–527.

TAUSSIG, M. J. (1973) Antigenic competition. *Curr. Top. Microbiol. Immun.* **60:** 125–174.

THOMAS, D. W., ROBERTS, W. K. and TALMAGE, D. W. (1975) Regulation of immune response: Production of soluble suppressor by immune spleen cells *in vitro. J. Immunol.* **114:** 1616–1622.

THOMAS, D. W. and SHEVACH, E. M. (1976) Nature of the antigenic complex recognized by T lymphocytes. I. Analysis with an *in vitro* primary response to soluble protein antigens. *J. exp. Med.* **144:** 1263–1273.

TITTOR, W. and WALFORD, R. L. (1974) Synergistic response between thymus and lymph node cells in the mixed lymphocyte culture. *Nature* **247:** 371–373.

TOKUHISA, T., TANIGUCHI, M., OKUMURA, K. and TADA, T. (1978) An antigen-specific I region gene product that augments the antibody response. *J. Immunol.* **120:** 414–421.

TOSATO, G., MAGRATH, I. T., KOSKI, I. R., DOOLEY, N. J. and BLAESE, R. M. (1980). *J. Clin. Invest.* **66:** 383–388.

TREMOLADA, F., FATTOVICH, G., PANEBIANCO, G., ONGARO, G. and REALDI, G. (1980) Suppressor cell activity in viral and non-viral chronic active hepatitis. *Clin. exp. Immunol.* **40:** 89–95.

TRUITT, G., DENNISON, D., RICH, R. and RICH, S. (1979) Interaction between T cells and non-T cells in suppression of cytotoxic lymphocyte responses. *J. Immunol.* **123:** 745–750.

TRUITT, G., RICH, R. and RICH, S. (1978) Suppression of cytotoxic lymphocyte responses *in vitro* by soluble products of alloantigen-activated spleen cells. *J. Immunol.* **121:** 1045–1051.

TRUITT, G. A., RICH, R. and RICH, S. (1977) Suppression of cytotoxic lymphocyte generation *in vitro* by alloantigen-activated spleen cells. *J. Immunol.* (In press)

TWOMEY, J. J., LAUGHTER, A. H., FARROW, S. and DOUGLASS, C. C. (1975) Hodgkin's disease: An immunodepleting and immunosuppressive disorder. *J. Clin. Invest.* **56:** 467–475.

UNANUE, E. R. (1972) The regulatory role of macrophages in antigenic stimulation. *Adv. Immunol.* **15:** 95–166.

UNANUE, E. R., BELLER, D. I., CALDERON, J., KIELY, J. M. and STADECKER, M. J. (1976) Regulation of immunity and inflammation by mediators from macrophages. *Am. J. Path.* **85:** 65–478.

VADAS, M. A., MILLER, J. F. A. P., MCKENZIE, I. F. C., CHISM, S. E., SHEN, F. W., BOYSE, E. A., GAMBLE, J. R. and WHITELAW, A. M. (1976) Ly and Ia antigen phenotypes of T cells involved in delayed-type hypersensitivity and in suppression. *J. exp. Med.* **144:** 10–19.

VON BOEHMER, H. (1980) Expression of receptor diversity in T lymphocytes. *Prog. Immunol.* **4:** 113–121.

VON BOEHMER, H. and HAAS, W. (1981) H-2 restricted cytolytic and noncytolytic T cell clones: Isolation, specificity and functional analysis. *Immunol. Rev.* **54:** 27–56.

WAGNER, H. and ROLLINGHOFF, M. (1978) T-T cell interactions during *in vitro* cytotoxic allograft responses. I. Soluble products from activated Ly 1^+ T cells trigger autonomously antigen-primed Ly 23^+ T cells to cell proliferation and cytolytic activity. *J. exp. Med.* **148:** 1523–1538.

WAGNER, H., RÖLLINGHOFF, M., PFIZENMAIER, K., HARDT, C. and JOHNSCHER, G. (1980) T-T cell interactions during *in vitro* cytotoxic T lymphocyte CTL responses. II. Helper factor from activated Lyt 1^+ T cells is rate limiting (i) in T cell responses to nonimmunogenic alloantigen, (ii) in thymocyte responses to allogeneic stimulator cells, and (iii) recruits allo- or H-2-restricted CTL precursors from the Lyt 123^+ T subset. *J. Immunol.* **124:** 1058–1067.

WAGNER, H., ROLLINGHOFF, M. and NOSSAL, G. J. V. (1973) T-cell-mediated immune responses induced *in vitro:* A probe for allograft and tumor immunity. *Transplant. Rev.* **17:** 3–36.

WAKSMAN, B. and NAMBA, Y. (1976) On soluble mediators of immunologic regulation. *Cell. Immunol.* **21:** 161–176.

WALDMANN, T. A., BRODER, S., BLAESE, R. M., DURM, M., BLACKMAN, M. and STROBER, W. (1974) Role of suppressor T cells in pathogenesis of common variable hypogammaglobulinemia. *Lancet ii:* 609–613.

WALDMANN, T. A., BRODER, S., KRAKAUER, R., DURM, M., GOLDMAN, C., MEADE, B. and STROBER, W. (1977) Dysfunction of suppressor mechanisms associated with immunodeficiency and autoimmunity. In: *Regulatory Mechanisms in Lymphocyte Activation.* LUCAS, D. O. (ed.). Academic Press, New York.

WALDMANN, T. A., BRODER, S., KRAKAUER, R., MACDERMOTT, R. P., DURM, M., GOLDMAN, C. and MEADE, B. (1976) The role of suppressor cells in the pathogenesis of common variable hypogammaglobulinemia and the immunodeficiency associated with myeloma. *Fed. Proc.* **35:** 2067–2072.

WARNER, N. L. (1974) Membrane immunoglobulins and antigen receptors on B and T lymphocytes. *Adv. Immunol.* **19:** 67–216.

WATSON, J. (1981) Lymphokines and the induction of immune responses. *Transplant.* **31:** 313–317.

WECKER, E., SCHIMPL, A., HUNIG, T. and KUHN, L. (1974) A T cell produced mediator substance active in the humoral immune response. *Ann. N.Y. Acad. Sci.* **249:** 258–263.

WEIGLE, W. O. (1973) Immunological unresponsiveness. *Adv. Immunol.* **16:** 61–122.

WEINBERGER, J., GERMAIN, R., JU, S. I., GREENE, M., BENACERRAF, B. and DORF, M. (1979) Hapten specific T cell responses to 4-hydroxy-3-nitrophenyl acetyl. II. Demonstration of idiotypic determinants on suppressor T cells. *J. exp. Med.* **150:** 761–776.

WHISLER, R. L. and STOBO, J. D. (1976) Heterogeneity of murine regulatory T cells. I. Subpopulations of amplifier and suppressor T cells. *J. exp. Med.* **144:** 398–413.

WIGZELL, H. and BINZ, H. (1980) Lymphocyte receptors. *Prog. Immunol.* **4:** 94–104.

WOODLAND, R. and CANTOR, H. (1978) Idiotype-specific T helper cells are required to induce idiotype-positive B memory cells to secrete antibody. *Eur. J. Immunol.* **8:** 600–606.

YODOI, J., HIRASHIMA, M. and ISHIZAKA, K. (1980) Regulatory role of IgE-binding factors from rat T lymphocytes. II. Glycoprotein nature and source of IgE-potentiating factor. *J. Immunol.* **125:** 1436–1441.

YODOI, J., HIRASHIMA, M. and ISHIZAKA, K. (1981) Lymphocytes bearing Fc receptors for IgE. V. Effect of tunicamycin on the formation of IgE potentiating factor and IgE-suppressive factor by Con A-activated lymphocytes. *J. Immunol.* **126:** 877–882.

ZEMBALA, M. and ASHERSON, G. L. (1973) Depression of the T cell phenomenon of contact sensitivity by T cells from unresponsive mice. *Nature* **244:** 227–228.

ZEMBALA, M. and ASHERSON, G. L. (1974) T cell suppression of contact sensitivity in the mouse. II. The role of soluble suppressor factor and its interaction with macrophages. *Eur. J. Immunol.* **4:** 799–804.

ZINKERNAGEL, R. M., CALLAHAN, G. N., ALTHAGE, A., COOPER, S., KLEIN, P. A. and KLEIN, J. (1978a) On the thymus in the differentiation of 'H-2 self-recognition' by T cells: Evidence for dual recognition? *J. exp. Med.* **147:** 882–911.

ZINKERNAGEL, R., CALLAHAN, G., ALTHAGE, A., COOPER, S., STEILEIN, J. and KLEIN, J. (1978b) The lymphoreticular system in triggering virus plus self-specific cytotoxic T cells: Evidence for T help. *J. exp. Med.* **147:** 897–911.

ZINKERNAGEL, R. and DOHERTY, P. D. (1977) Major transplantation antigens, virus and specificity of surveillance T cells. The 'altered self' hypothesis. *Contemp. Top. Immunobiol.* **7:** 179–220.

ZINKERNAGEL, R. and DOHERTY, P. D. (1979) MHC-restricted cytotoxic T cells: Studies on the biological role of polymorphic major transplantation antigens during T cell restriction specificity, function and responsiveness. *Adv. Immunol.* **27:** 52–177.

Acknowledgements—Research from our laboratory was supported in part by USPHS Research Grants AI-13810, AI-15394 and AI-17048. Robert R. Rich is an Investigator of the Howard Hughes Medical Institute. We gratefully acknowledge the expert assistance of Norma Olivarez in preparation of this manuscript. The literature review for this manuscript was completed in June 1981.

CHAPTER 2

MODULATION OF IMMUNITY BY MACROPHAGES

HOWARD T. HOLDEN* and RONALD B. HERBERMAN**

**National Cancer Institute, Bethesda, USA*
***Frederick Cancer Center, Maryland, USA*

1. INTRODUCTION

The literature concerning the effects of macrophages on the immune response is already large and growing rapidly. Macrophages seem to be involved in almost every phase of the immune response. Not only are they important as effector cells in their own right, but there is now a wealth of information suggesting macrophages may, through a combination of suppressing and enhancing effects, play an important role in regulating the immune response. Evidence obtained both *in vivo* and *in vitro* supports the concept of macrophages as immunoregulatory cells. We shall review here the available *in vivo* and *in vitro* evidence for augmentation and suppression of immune response by macrophages, and will also suggest how macrophages may play a role as effector cells in T cell suppression and antigenic competition.

Many of the *in vitro* experiments, on which important conclusions have been based, have compared the results obtained in assay systems using cell populations depleted of macrophages to those obtained using cell populations containing, or highly enriched for, macrophages. Before discussing the details of these experiments, it is important to note that there are problems with interpreting such data.

There is virtually no way to prepare cell populations completely free of macrophages. None of the available methods have been shown to reduce the proportion of macrophages below 0.1 per cent, and this may not be sufficient to rule out the role of very small numbers of macrophages as auxiliary cells for the induction of immune responses. Most of the macrophage depletion procedures are based on adherent or phagocytic properties of macrophages. Petri dish adherence (Mosier, 1967) allows separation of the cells into two populations which can be tested alone or after recombination. The resultant populations, however, are by no means pure and the degree of depletion of macrophages is not as good as that achieved by other techniques. Passage of lymphoid cells over adherence columns of nylon wool (Julius *et al.*, 1973), rayon cotton (Kirchner *et al.*, 1974b), glass beads (Shortman, 1968), or Sephadex G–10 (Ly and Mishell, 1974) allows rather good depletion of adherent cells. However, since B cells are adherent, albeit less than macrophages, those procedures most effective in depleting adherent cells must of necessity deplete a certain proportion of the B cells. In fact, a procedure based on this principle has been described to obtain a purified population of T cells simply by depleting all of the adherent cells (Julius *et al.*, 1973). Since, however, as many as 80 per cent of the cells are lost when performing such procedures, it is obvious that even some T cells are depleted. In addition to the separation procedures based on the adherent properties of macrophages, incubation of cells with powdered iron to allow phagocytic cells to ingest the iron particles, and then passage of the cells through a strong magnetic field to obtain a population free of phagocytes (iron and magnet technique), has been a useful technique to obtain a phagocyte-depleted population (Kirchner *et al.*, 1974b). However, since the percentage of the cells recovered (50–60 per cent of normal spleen cells) is routinely lower than the percentage of cells which are non-phagocytic, it is clear that even this depletion technique is not entirely selective for macrophages. Another approach to the problem of obtaining purified cell populations has been the use of procedures wherein lymphocytes are allowed to rosette with heterologous erythrocytes and then placed over a Ficoll–Hypaque density gradient which separates the rosette-forming cells (T cells) from the non-rosette-forming cells. The use of such procedures has been reported in guinea pigs (Rosenstreich and Oppenheim, 1976) and humans (West *et al.*, 1976). Combinations of adherence depletion techniques and enrichment techniques such as just described seem likely to yield the purest populations. In addition to the above techniques, several substances and compounds have been reported to be selectively toxic for macrophages. Silica and carrageenan (Allison *et al.*, 1966) have been used *in vivo* and *in vitro* to deplete macrophage activity. Trypan blue (Hibbs, 1974) has been reported to be similarly effective. Finally, there are several reports of the use of 'specific' anti-macrophage sera and complement to kill macrophages (Feldmann and Palmer, 1971; Gorczynski, 1976). Only one allelic form of macrophage surface antigen has been described, Mph-1 (Archer and Davies, 1974), which is similar to the allelic forms of theta and Ly antigens found on mouse T lymphocytes. However, this antiserum has not been widely utilized for studies of macrophage depletion or enrichment. Most of the antisera used for depletion of macrophages from populations or for indentification of macrophages have been heteroantisera which were rendered specific by extensive absorption procedures with cell populations free of macrophages. However, as is apparent from the above discussion, macrophage-free populations are difficult to prepare, and further, if readily available, there would be relatively little need for antimacrophage sera. The difficult problems in this area have been reviewed by Leibovich and Ross (1975). More recently, several monoclonal antibodies have been produced that appear to react specifically with macrophages or subpopulations of macrophages. These have been raised against different antigens on mouse macrophages (Springer, 1982). However, most of the monoclonal antibodies do not react with all macrophages or monocytes and more extensive testing has indicated that several also cross react with small subpopulations of resting or activated lymphocytes (Taniyama and Holden, unpublished observations). Potentially, this type of reagent if sufficiently specific will be very useful for delineating mononuclear phagocytes and for depleting these cells from mixed populations.

Preparation of *pure* macrophage populations is also difficult. In rodents and guinea pigs, a population enriched for macrophages can be obtained by washing out the peritoneal cavity, and many investigators refer to peritoneal exudate cells and macrophages interchangeably. Mice normally have $2–3 \times 10^6$ macrophages resident in the peritoneal cavity which can be washed out. It is important to note, however, that the resultant population is heterogeneous, consisting of about 60 per cent lymphocytes, 35 per cent macrophages, and occasional mast and other cells (Edelson and Cohn, 1976). If irritating agents such as light mineral oil, 10 per cent proteose peptone broth, or thioglycolate are placed in the peritoneal cavity, a sterile peritonitis develops. Initially there is an influx of neutrophils, maximally present about 48 hr after injection of the irritant. By 72–96 hr, most of the neutrophils have disappeared and macrophages make up the majority of the cells in the peritoneal exudate (PEC). Shevach (1976) reported that in guinea pigs, 3 days after i.p. injection of light mineral oil, the PEC consisted of 75 per cent macrophages, 10 per cent neutrophils and 15 per cent lymphocytes. By allowing such PEC to adhere to glass slides for 3 hr and washing off the nonadherent cells, a population consisting largely of macrophages and neutrophils remained (Lipsky and Rosenthal, 1973). Neutrophils, unlike macrophages, do not survive overnight incubation in media at 37° (Edelson and Cohn, 1976). Thus, Lipsky and Rosenthal (1973) reported that after overnight incubation, the adherent PEC remaining on the slides after vigorous washing were 99 per cent pure macrophages. Erb and Feldmann (1975a) used similar adherence techniques to purify PEC from mice. In addition, they treated the adherent PEC with both an anti-T cell and anti-B cell serum and complement followed by irradiation with 200 R. They reported that after thorough washing the macrophages were 99.7 per cent pure. Katz and Unanue (1973) used similar procedures in mice, injecting 1 ml of 10 per cent proteose peptone broth to induce the PEC. After 3 days, $8–15 \times 10^6$ PEC could be obtained which were 85 per cent pure macrophages. When such mice were irradiated with 660 R 24 hr prior to harvesting, only 4×10^6 PEC were recovered but 98 per cent were macrophages. In humans, PEC are obviously not readily available. However, Rode and Gordon (1974) could obtain essentially pure populations of monocytes from human peripheral blood leukocytes (PBL) separated from the red blood cells (RBC) with a Ficoll–Hypaque gradient, by allowing the PBL to adhere to glass Petri dishes for 8 days and vigorously washing off all remaining nonadherent cells. Human peripheral blood monocytes have also been purified by Percoll gradient separation followed by adherence (Kleinerman *et al.*, 1983) or by countercurrent centrifugation elutriation (Stevenson *et al.*, 1983). Both these techniques provide monocytes that are greatly enriched (greater than 95% purity), but as with other methods, there is still a low level of contamination with other types of cells. It should be noted that most of the procedures used to induce macrophages in the peritoneal cavity, or to isolate the macrophages, cause activation and other functional changes. For example, adherence to a surface results in increased protein synthesis and increased enzyme production by macrophages (Bodel *et al.*, 1977).

Whatever procedures are used to prepare macrophage-depleted or -enriched cell populations, it is obvious that the purity of the resultant population must be documented. Several methods are available for identification of macrophages and monocytes, but none are entirely satisfactory. The ingestion of various substances such as latex particles, colloidal carbon and heterologous erythrocytes has been used to identify phagocytic cells. In addition, histochemical staining techniques (Goldstein and Blomgren, 1973), particularly for nonspecific esterase (Yam *et al.*, 1971), are now widely used to identify macrophages. However, it is possible that even these methods may be fallible. Nathan *et al.* (1976) have expressed concern that a population of cells that they have isolated from the peritoneal exudates of mice pretreated with Bacille Calmette–Guerin (BCG) which have strong anti-proliferative effects on tumor cells *in vitro*, although adherent and staining positive for esterase, may be non- or poorly phagocytic under the conditions they used. They have been reluctant to call these cells macrophages and thus raise the question of whether cells other than macrophages and monocytes may stain positive for nonspecific esterase. Confirmatory reports of a discrete population of esterase positive, non-phagocytic cells, however, have not yet appeared. Enumeration of macrophages by any of the procedures is complicated by the fact that in any cell population there are not only mature macrophages and monocytes but also macrophage and monocyte precursors which may not be readily identifiable. These cells, although less adherent (Cline and Sumner, 1972), much less susceptible to anti-macrophage sera and complement (Virolainen *et al.*, 1972), and probably non-phagocytic, can mature during *in vitro* culture and function as macrophages even after the most efficient depletion procedures based on these functional properties. Many of these problems have been extensively discussed in a recent book (Bloom and David, 1976).

Macrophages appear to be a heterogeneous group of cells, both functionally and morphologically. At the present time it is not clear whether the heterogeneity is simply a result of different levels of maturation or whether there are in fact distinct subpopulations of macrophages which can be identified on the basis of certain cell surface or functional characteristics. During maturation from promonocyte through monocyte and immature macrophage to mature macrophage, there are many changes in their functional characteristics. Territo and Cline (1976) have provided evidence that the frequency of cell division decreases as the cells mature, while other characteristics such as phagocytic activity, glass adherence, microbicidal activity, surface receptors for immunoglobulin and the ability to interact with lymphoid cells in various immune reactions, generally increase.

Macrophages or monocytes from different sources display divergent characteristics. Bennet (1966) has shown that when macrophages from different tissue sources were isolated and cultured *in vitro*, their rate of attachment to glass as well as their mitotic rate in culture varied. Based on these features, Bennet described three categories of macrophages: peritoneal and peripheral blood macrophages that attached rapidly and had a low mitotic rate; bone marrow, spleen and liver macrophages that spread slowly and had a high mitotic rate; and alveolar macrophages that spread rapidly and had a high mitotic rate. Nitulescu and Förster (1976) reported that there were antigenic differences between the alveolar and peritoneal macrophages in rats. Walker (1967a) has also discussed the differences in functional activity between macrophages from various sources. He noted that peritoneal macrophages had a higher bactericidal activity than did alveolar macrophages and in addition that they had higher Fc receptor avidity. Furthermore, peritoneal macrophages responded well to chemotactic agents and were very efficient at rendering antigen immunogenic, while alveolar macrophages had low activity in these tests. Similarly, Boumsell and Meltzer (1976) have noted differences in the chemotactic response of blood monocytes and peritoneal macrophages to lymphocyte and complement-derived chemotactic substances with regard to both time-course and dose response. Hence, there is evidence that macrophages from different tissues may vary considerably in their functional characteristics. Whether this is due to stage of maturation or to subpopulation distribution is not clear.

Macrophages from a single tissue source may also be heterogeneous in terms of their surface characteristics and their functional reactivity. Rhodes (1975) found that there was marked variability in the avidity of the Fc receptors among guinea pig peritoneal macrophages. If the macrophages were induced with an inflammatory agent, there was a six-fold increase in the proportion of macrophages with high avidity Fc receptors. Heterogeneity in macrophage function has been noted by a number of investigators and has recently been reviewed by Walker (1976a). Basically, two types of observations suggested there may be functional subclasses of macrophages: (i) only a certain percentage of macrophages performed certain functions under similar conditions (such as phagocytosis of bacteria or erythrocytes), or (ii) macrophage populations which were fractionated based on their density or size, could be identified on the basis of various functional characteristics. Walker (1976b) used a discontinuous Ficoll gradient to fractionate rabbit peritoneal exudate cells into five subpopulations. Several different functional tests were then performed with the cells from each fraction. He found that binding of ^{125}I-T2 antigen was greatest in fraction 1 (least dense) while binding through the Fc receptor was greatest in the denser fractions 3 and 4. In addition, Walker fractionated rat peritoneal exudate cells from animals that had been immunized with a chemically induced tumor (plus BCG) and found that the cytotoxic reactivity of the macrophages resided predominately in two fractions. Similarly, differences in the size of macrophage effector cells were noted by Holden *et al.* (1976) in studies of the growth inhibitory activity of macrophages isolated from murine sarcoma virus-induced tumors. There were two functional subpopulations with different cell sizes (as determined by sedimentation velocity at 1 g).

All of these studies, however, are complicated by the fact that different methods of induction were used for harvesting macrophages and the cells may exhibit various levels of activation. In addition, the process of activation may call in a specific subpopulation of cells or, as suggested recently by Bomford and Olivotto (1975) and Woodruff *et al.* (1975), the activation process may cause macrophage precursors to differentiate into mature cells. Unfortunately at this time there is not enough information on subpopulations of macrophages from any one source to determine whether different functions will regularly be associated with particular macrophage subpopulations.

In all, it is apparent that dogmatic statements concerning the absolute requirement for macrophages, or the lack thereof for various immune responses, require careful documentation to be at all convincing. However, despite the above problems, it has still been possible to extensively study the role of macrophages in enhancing and suppressing immune responses, and evidence has been presented that macrophages play a vital role in regulating the immune response.

2. ENHANCEMENT OF THE IMMUNE RESPONSE BY MACROPHAGES

Macrophages have been shown to enhance almost every phase of the immune response. For many immune responses generated *in vitro*, there appears to be an absolute requirement for macrophages. This, of course, does not prove that macrophages are required *in vivo* or, if they are required, that they perform the same function *in vivo* as they do *in vitro*. When lymphocytes are cultured without macrophages, the viability after 4–5 days under some conditions is lower than when macrophages are present (Chen and Hirsch, 1972; Bevan *et al.*, 1974). In contrast, there is little or no evidence that macrophages enhance the viability of lymphocytes *in vivo*. Thus, it would seem that enhancing effects of macrophages on the immune response *in vitro*, which result *only* from the improvement of lymphocyte viability, may have limited relevance *in vivo*. One way to prevent such problems would be to perform *in vitro* investigations under optimal tissue culture conditions which are not substantially improved by the addition of macrophages. *In vivo* experiments on the role of macrophages in enhancing immune responses also have problems. Observations made *in vivo* occasionally raise as many questions as they answer. Subclinical infections or fluctuations of hormone levels may affect *in vivo* experiments in ways that would be difficult to predict. However, with a combination of *in vivo* observations, and *in vitro* experiments designed to dissect and explain the results obtained *in vivo*, meaningful interpretations may be suggested. In this section we shall discuss the evidence that macrophages can enhance immune response *in vivo* and then we shall discuss the evidence obtained *in vitro* as possible explanations for the *in vivo* findings. Recent concepts regarding the mechanisms of the enhancing effects of macrophages, including some of the current concepts of antigen presentation, will be reviewed.

2.1. Enhancement of the Immune Response *In Vivo*

There is considerable evidence that macrophages can enhance the immune response *in vivo* (Mitchison, 1969; Klaus, 1974; for reviews see Unanue, 1972; Oppenheim and Seeger, 1976). This is supported by many experiments in which injection of soluble protein antigen bound to macrophages (by exposure to live macrophages *in vitro* or *in vivo*) has resulted in stronger immune responses in experimental animals than has injection of equivalent quantities of free soluble antigen. In addition, there is evidence that certain immunodeficient states are a result of an incompetent reticuloendothelial system (Carter and Rector, 1972; Hardy *et al.*, 1973; Blaese, 1975).

Both humoral and cellular responses have been shown to be enhanced by injection of antigens bound to macrophages (Unanue, 1972; Oppenheim and Seeger, 1976). Routinely, macrophages have been washed after exposure to radiolabeled soluble antigen and then injected into the host. The amount of antigen injected with the macrophages has been determined by the radioactivity of the injected cells. With some exceptions (to be discussed below), the response was ten- to a thousand-fold higher on a per microgram basis when the antigen was injected bound to macrophages (Mitchison, 1969; Klaus, 1974). Other cells such as fibroblasts can bind approximately the same amount of soluble antigen as macrophages, but there is general agreement that antigens injected bound to fibroblasts fail to augment strong immune responses (Mitchison, 1969; Klaus, 1974). As has been found with other macrophage functions, the ability to enhance immunogenicity is radioresistant (Unanue, 1972). However, viable macrophages are required. Mitchison (1969) has shown that antigen transferred on dead macrophages was no more immunogenic than antigen injected alone. Also, the ability of the transferred cells to interact with host cells is required. Macrophages in Millipore chambers implanted into the peritoneal cavities of mice did not enhance immunogenicity (reviewed by Unanue, 1972).

Although many soluble antigens are more immunogenic when transferred bound to macrophages, some are as immunogenic when injected alone. The ability of macrophage-bound antigen to enhance immunogenicity has been shown to be inversely related to the ability of macrophages to clear the antigen from the serum *in vivo* (reviewed by Unanue, 1972). Keyhole limpet hemocyanin (KLH) was taken up very well by macrophages *in vivo*. Preincubation with macrophages *in vitro* did not enhance the response to it (Unanue, 1969). Presumably when such antigens are inoculated in soluble form, they are rapidly bound to tissue macrophages and are thus presented to the immune system in the same form as when they are bound to macrophages *in vitro*. On the other hand, human serum albumin (HSA) was phagocytized poorly by murine macrophages *in vivo*, and preincubation of HSA with macrophages *in vitro* increased the resultant antibody response about one thousand fold when compared to equal microgram quantities of free HSA (Mitchison, 1969). In contrast to free soluble antigen, macrophage-bound antigen has not been shown to induce tolerance (Unanue, 1972).

In addition to enhancement of a humoral or cellular immune response to antigen, macrophages can influence the type of response elicited. In guinea pigs, Oppenheim and Seeger (1976) have shown that small doses of tetanus toxoid (0.1 μg), when bound to macrophages and given either intradermally or intracardiacly, induced delayed hypersensitivity type responses to subsequent challenge. In contrast, soluble antigen given in the same dose, schedule and routes resulted in immediate Arthus reactions, indicating high levels of circulating antibody. Further, two sequential injections of macrophage-bound tetanus toxoid resulted only in stronger delayed hypersenstivity. Boosting with tetanus toxoid alone, on the other hand, resulted in high levels of circulating antibody 2 weeks later (Oppenheim and Seeger, 1976). Thus, in some systems the use of macrophage-bound antigen for immunization results not only in an enhanced response but also in a response qualitatively different from that obtained with free soluble antigen.

Finally, many of the immunodeficiencies of newborn animals appear to be associated with the immaturity of the mononuclear phagocytes. Neonatal mice responded very poorly to sheep erythrocytes when compared to adult animals (Argyris, 1968). However, the antibody response could be augmented considerably if the newborn mice were reconstituted with adult peritoneal exudate cells 2 days before immunization. Since mouse spleen cells have been shown to contain antigen sensitive cells 24 hr after birth (Carter and Rector, 1972), the deficiency in neonatal mice would not appear to be in this population of cells. Furthermore, adoptive transfer studies of neonatal and adult mouse spleen cells into X-irradiated recipients also suggested that newborns lacked cells needed to process the antigen, and that these cells were radioresistant, indicating that they might be macrophages (Carter and Rector, 1972). Hardy *et al.* (1973) found that the antibody response in mice to sheep erythrocytes as well as to *Shigella paradysentheria* was not evident until 3–5 days after birth. In exploring the role of the macrophage, they found the PEC from neonatal mice preincubated with *Shigella* antigen were unable to induce an antibody response in adult mice; while the use of PEC from adult mice led to significantly higher titers of antibody in the recipients. From this they concluded that the macrophages from newborn mice were incapable of taking up and processing the *Shigella* antigen sufficiently to induce a detectable antibody response. Blaese (1975) performed studies on the antibody response to several antigens in newborn rats and found that the response of the animal depended on the type of antigen used for immunization. Rats 18 hr old did not respond to sheep or burro erythrocytes, KLH or type III pneumococcal polysaccharide, but responded fairly well to killed *Brucella abortus*. If the sheep erythrocytes given to the neonate were mixed with unfractionated PEC or macrophage-enriched PEC from adults, there was a strong antibody response. Antibody responses to KLH or burro erythrocytes could be induced in neonates in a similar fashion. It is of interest that *Brucella* as well as several other macrophage activators, when injected into newborn rats with the immunogen, were able to substitute for adult macrophages, presumably by activating the resident macrophages. Finally, by inoculating neonates with high doses of antigen it was relatively easy to induce tolerance to that antigen. Blaese (1975) suggested that this was also due to the immaturity of the macrophages in these animals, since the rats did not become tolerant when antigen was injected with adult macrophages. Part of the explanation for the inability of macrophages from young or newborn animals to support immune response may be linked to the lack of expression of Ia antigens on their surfaces. Beller and his colleagues (Beller and Ho, 1982) have been examining the modulation of Ia antigen on macrophages and have found that Ia antigen expression, both *in vitro* and *in vivo*, is labile on macrophages. Macrophages with low expression of Ia cannot function effectively as accessary cells, and macrophages from neonates have been shown to poorly express Ia antigens (Beller, personal communication). However, when such macrophages were stimulated with lymphokine-containing supernatants, they become Ia positive and could function as accessary cells. Apparently, under normal conditions of antigen presentation in neonates, there is a deficiency in the signal to the macrophages to convert them to Ia positive. However, when a macrophage activating agent such as Brucella was injected into newborn rats with the immunogen, the animals mounted an immune response (Blaese, 1972). Such results might be explained by the induction of Ia antigens thereby allowing them to support the host response to antigen.

2.2. Enhancement of the Immune Response *In Vitro*

In vivo experiments such as those described above have shown that macrophages could enhance and, in some cases, qualitatively alter the expression of the immune response. Although demonstrating the significance of macrophages in eliciting various immune responses, such *in vivo* experiments do not allow definition of the mechanisms of action. Unlike experimental models of T cell or B cell deficient animals (e.g. the nude mouse or bursectomized chicken), no model of complete and selective macrophage deficiency is readily available. Macrophages are functionally radioresistant so even in adoptive transfer experiments, resident macrophages may participate in the immune response. Agents which are considered to be selectively toxic for macrophages such as carrageenan, silica (Allison *et al.*, 1966), or trypan blue (Hibbs, 1974) are less than totally effective (Sawicki and Catanzaro, 1975). In addition, in *in vivo* experiments, it is usually difficult to identify the phase in the immune response during which macrophages are required. For example, in the study of Schwartz and Leskowitz (1969), in which simultaneous injection of carrageenan with antigen temporarily suppressed delayed hypersensitivity responses in guinea pigs, one cannot distinguish between the effect of carrageenan on macrophages involved in the afferent or the efferent limb of the response. In contrast, *in vitro* experiments allow more precise dissection of the site of action of macrophages.

2.2.1 *The Macrophage Requirement for the Generation of Antibody-Producing Cells* In Vitro

There are several techniques for generating antibody responses in a totally *in vitro* environment. One of the most commonly used techniques is the Mishell–Dutton culture system (Mishell and Dutton, 1966), followed by a Jerne plaque assay (Jerne and Nordin, 1963). Mosier (1967), using a modification of such a system, was one of the first investigators to show a requirement for two distinct cell types for the *in vitro* primary generation of antibody-forming cells (AFC) in response to sheep erythrocytes (SRBC). After separating murine spleen cells on the basis of adherence to a glass Petri dish, neither the nonadherent nor the adherent fraction could generate antibody-forming cells. However, the recombined fractions responded as well as the unfractionated population. These results have been verified with antibody production to all heterologous RBC tested (Katz and Benacerraf, 1972; Pierce, 1969, 1973; Feldmann and Palmer, 1971; Sjobert *et al.*, 1972; Shortman and Palmer, 1971; Shortman *et al.*, 1970; Cosenza *et al.*, 1971; Mosier, 1968; McIntyre and Pierce, 1973), In addition, the macrophage requirement for AFC production has been demonstrated using hapten–protein conjugates (Feldmann *et al.*, 1974) or synthetic soluble copolymers (Pierce *et al.*, 1974; Kapp *et al.*, 1973) as antigens. IgM, IgG and IgA plaque-forming responses have all been shown to require macrophages *in vitro* (Pierce, 1973). Although early reports suggested that the secondary response was not dependent upon macrophages (Pierce, 1969; Katz and Unanue, 1973), it has now been shown that both primary and secondary responses require adherent and phagocytic cells (reviewed by Oppenheim and Rosenstreich, 1976). Whether other cells without known immunologic effects can substitute for macrophages in these *in vitro* responses is not entirely clear. Katz and Unanue (1973) have reported that DNP–KLH bound to fibroblasts could induce an AFC response comparable to that induced with DNP–KLH bound to macrophages when added to nonadherent DNP–KLH-primed mouse spleen cells in a Mishell–Dutton culture system. Similarly, Möller *et al.* (1976) have recently shown that fibroblasts could reconstitute the primary AFC response of nonadherent mouse spleen cells in a Mishell–Dutton culture system with SRBC. In these cases, however, it is likely that residual macrophages left in the spleen preparations after the macrophage-depletion procedures were responsible for inducing the responses observed and that the fibroblasts simply amplified the response by improving the culture conditions by a nonspecific feeder effect. Be that as it may, in addition to adherent cells and B cells, T cells are required for the generation of AFC to the above antigens *in vitro.* In contrast, another class of antigens which can stimulate AFC *in vitro* in the absence of T cells (T-independent antigens) have until recently been considered macrophage independent (Feldmann *et al.*, 1974; Mosier *et al.*, 1974; Feldmann, 1972a; Lemke *et al.*, 1975). These findings suggested that the primary role of macrophages in enhancing AFC production to T-dependent antigens might be related to the requirement for T cells. However, recent reports (Chused *et al.*, 1976; Lee *et al.*, 1976; Pike and Nossal, 1976), showing that some T-independent antigens do in fact require macrophages, do not support this notion. Polyclonal antibody responses to B cell mitogens such as LPS (Lemke *et al.*, 1975) which are also T-independent, have not (with one exception) been shown to require macrophages *in vitro* (Oppenheim and Rosenstreich, 1976; Rosenstreich and Oppenheim, 1976). The exception is a report by Kragnoff *et al.* (1974) which showed that the LPS-induced proliferative response of B cells from the Peyer's patches of nude mice required either 2-mercaptoethanol or macrophages. However, in this case, T cells were also required, suggesting this situation was unusual if not unique.

2.2.2 *The Requirement for Macrophages for T Cell Responses* In Vitro

Consistent with the enhanced immunogenicity afforded by macrophage-bound antigen in induction of delayed hypersensitivity responses *in vivo* (Oppenheim and Seeger, 1976) are experiments showing that macrophages are required for the generation of T cell responses *in vitro.* T cell proliferative responses in mixed leukocyte culture (MLC) were found to require macrophages in mice (Bevan *et al.*, 1974) and humans (Jones, 1971). Similarly, the *in vitro* generation of cytotoxic effector cells to alloantigens in MLC systems [cell-mediated lympholysis (CML)] has been shown to require macrophages in mice (Wagner *et al.*, 1972). However, whether macrophages function to enhance the immunogenicity of alloantigens is unclear. An alternative explanation for the requirement for macrophages in MLC is that the primary stimulating cell in the MLC is the allogeneic macrophage. This has been observed with MLC in guinea pigs (Greineder and Rosenthal, 1975b), humans (Rode and Gordon, 1974) and rats (Oehler and Herberman, 1977). In these studies, syngeneic macrophages did not reconstitute the MLC responses abrogated by depletion of macrophanges from both stimulating and responding populations.

T cell proliferative responses to nonspecific mitogens have also been shown to require macrophages. Rosenstreich and Oppenheim (1976) have recently reviewed evidence that T cell proliferative responses to Concanavalin A (Con A) and phytohemagglutinin (PHA) in guinea pigs are macrophage dependent. Nonadherent human peripheral blood mononuclear leukocytes (PBL), purified by passage over a column containing glass beads, have a diminished proliferative response to PHA which could be reconstituted with as few as 1 per cent phagocytic cells (Oppenheim *et al.*, 1968). Both Oppenheim *et al.* (1968) and Lohrmann *et al.* (1974) have shown that the dependence of human lymphocytes on monocytes for strong proliferative responses to PHA is much easier to demonstrate when suboptimal concentrations of PHA are used. Our laboratory has recently separated human PBL on the basis of adherence by passage of the cells through Sephadex G–10 columns (Jerrells, Dean and Herberman, unpublished observations) and determined the reactivity to PHA and Con A. We found that populations depleted of adherent cells, with less than 1 per cent esterase positive cells, were essentially unresponsive to Con A, whereas the responses to PHA were diminished less consistently, if at all. Reconstitution of the nonadherent cells with irradiated adherent autologous cells which were enriched for esterase positive cells (monocytes) resulted in enhanced PHA and Con A responses, equal to or even greater than the response of the original untreated population. Similarly, in other experiments, we have observed that human PBL forming rosettes with SRBC (E-RFC), when separated from non-rosetting cells by centrifugation in a Ficoll–Hypaque density gradient, may proliferate little if at all in response to Con A (Dean *et al.*, 1977; West, Dean and Herberman, unpublished observations). As observed with the adherent cell-depleted populations described above, the PHA response was diminished less than the Con A response. Approximately 1 per cent of the cells prepared in this way stained positive for esterase or ingested latex particles, and essentially none of the cells had detectable surface IgM. When such populations were further depleted of cells bearing an Fc receptor by adherence to monolayers of antibody-coated SRBC attached to Petri dishes with poly-l-lysine (West *et al.*, 1977), the nonadherent population (consisting of cells lacking the Fc receptor and esterase) also failed to respond to PHA. When reconstituted with various concentrations of adherent autologous PBL, the response to both mitogens was restored. These observations suggest that human PBL require adherent cells, presumably macrophages, to proliferate in response to Con A and that fewer such cells, or a particular subpopulation of adherent cells bearing an Fc receptor, are needed for responses to PHA. Blaese *et al.* (1977), in studies with human PBL, have provided evidence that different macrophage-dependent *in vitro* responses may have varying requirements for macrophages. By using a series of macrophage depletion techniques, they could show a hierarchy of macrophage dependence for several *in vitro* responses. Monocyte-mediated antibody-dependent cell-mediated cytotoxicity (MMADCC) was the assay system most dependent on macrophages. Since macrophages are the effector cells in this assay, even minimal decreases in the percentage of macrophages were associated with decreased cytotoxicity. As more efficient macrophage depletion techniques were used, the synthesis of immunoglobulin induced by pokeweed mitogen (PWM) was depressed. Only the most efficient means of macrophage depletion caused depression of the proliferative response to soluble antigens (Candida and SK–SD). Although less dependent on macrophages than MMADCC and the PWM response, the proliferative response to soluble antigens was still shown to be macrophage-dependent. In contrast to our findings, these investigators could not demonstrate a macrophage requirement for a proliferative response to PHA even by using a Shortman column (Shortman, 1968), their most effective technique, to deplete the adherent cells. All of these data indicate that the proliferative response of human PBL to optimal concentrations of PHA requires very few macrophages indeed.

T cell proliferation in response to the immunological adjuvant Bacillus Calmette–Guérin (BCG) *in vitro* requires the presence of macrophages (Mokyr and Mitchell, 1975). Mouse thymus cell suspensions, which contain approximately 0.25 per cent macrophages, responded vigorously to BCG, incorporating ^{3}H–thymidine 25–35-fold more than unstimulated controls. When macrophages were depleted to <0.25 per cent (undetectable by Giemsa stain), the response to BCG was abolished. There was no diminution of the response to Con A, indicating viability of the nonadherent thymus cells, and reconstitution of macrophages to 0.5 per cent completely restored the response to BCG. Reduction of macrophages in the spleen from 10 to 0.5 per cent caused no change in two experiments, but significant augmentation of ^{3}H–thymidine incorporation in response to BCG in two others (Mokyr and Mitchell, 1975). Thus, a critical concentration of macrophages 0.25–0.5 per cent was required for the mitogenic effects of BCG on T cells, with higher concentrations tending to cause diminished reactivity of lymphocytes.

T cell proliferative responses induced by sodium periodate or neuraminidase–galactose oxidase (NG) require macrophages in guinea pigs (Greineder and Rosenthal, 1975a). In this system, treatment of either macrophages or T cells alone with these materials resulted in strong proliferative responses when the cells were recombined.

In contrast, purified lymphocytes treated with periodate or NG and also pretreated with mitomycin C to prevent their own proliferation could not induce a T cell proliferative response when added to unfractionated guinea pig lymph node cells. These observations further confirm the requirement for interaction between T cells and macrophages in the generation of proliferative responses to nonspecific stimuli.

Proliferative responses of primed T cells to soluble protein antigens have been shown to require macrophages in several systems. In guinea pigs immunized with ovalbumin (OVA) in complete Freund's adjuvant (CFA), lymph node cells depleted of adherent cells did not proliferate in response to the antigens unless reconstituted with adherent cells (Seeger and Oppenheim, 1970; Walderon *et al.*, 1973; Rosenthal and Shevach, 1973; Paul *et al.*, 1976). In addition, purified macrophages, but not lymphocytes preincubated with purified protein derivative of tuberculin (PPD) or OVA and added to purified lymph node cells from immunized animals, induced strong proliferative responses *in vitro* (Rosenthal and Shevach, 1973; Paul *et al.*, 1976). Similarly, Cline and Swett (1968) have shown that when human PBL from tuberculin-sensitive donors were depleted of adherent cells, no blastogenic response was observed in the presence of PPD. Addition of adherent cells with the characteristics of monocytes to the cultures of purified PBL and PPD resulted in strong proliferative responses. Viable monocytes were required and separation of the responding lymphocytes from the monocytes with cell-impermeable Millipore membranes prevented the enhancing effect. Similar findings using human PBL have been reported by Blaese *et al.* (1972).

Primary T cell proliferative responses to soluble protein antigen *in vitro* have been difficult to demonstrate. However, recently antigen-pulsed macrophages were used to prime purified guinea pig LNC *in vitro* for subsequent proliferative responses upon re-exposure to antigen-pulsed macrophages (Thomas and Shevach, 1976). As will be discussed, these types of experiments have allowed a more detailed understanding of the macrophage–lymphocyte interaction than was previously possible in experiments where T cells were primed *in vivo*.

2.2.2.1. *The requirement for macrophages for the production of lymphokines* in vitro. In addition to the induction of T cell division, antigens and mitogens induce the production by T cells of numerous mediators termed lymphokines. *In vitro* systems have been developed to investigate the events leading to lymphokine production. Thus far, all such *in vitro* systems show that macrophages are required for the production of mediators by T cells.

Migration inhibition factor (MIF) production by guinea pig lymphocytes primed with CFA required macrophages pulsed with PPD (Ohishi and Onoue, 1975). In this case, the macrophage requirement could be replaced by supernatants of macrophages stimulated with lipopolysaccharide (LPS) (Ohishi and Onoue, 1976). Similarly, our laboratory (Landolfo *et al.*, 1978) has recently shown that spleen cells from C57BL/6 mice bearing Moloney sarcoma virus-induced tumors could be induced to produce MIF by culture with 3 M KCl extracts of tumor cells bearing relevant antigens. Spleen cells depleted of macrophages by adherence techniques did not produce MIF when cultured with the 3 M KCl extract. However, when purified macrophages from light mineral oil-induced peritoneal exudates of normal syngeneic mice were added to the ádherent cell-depleted spleen cells in the presence of free antigen, MIF production could again be demonstrated. Further, spleen cells with macrophages which were preincubated with soluble tumor antigens for 2–6 hr and washed to remove all unbound antigen could also produce MIF. More recently, we have shown that only antigen-pulsed spleen cells containing macrophages compatible with the responding cells at the major histocompatibility complex (MHC) could produce MIF (Landolfo *et al.*, 1977). Unlike the findings of Ohishi and Onoue described above for the PPD system in guinea pigs, the macrophage requirement in the MSV tumor system has been shown to require cell–cell contact and could not be replaced by supernatants of LPS-stimulated macrophages (Landolfo, Holden and Herberman, unpublished observations).

In addition to MIF, a number of other mediators are produced by stimulated T cells *in vitro*. Macrophages were required for interferon production by PBL from tuberculin-sensitive human donors in response to PPD *in vitro* (Epstein *et al.*, 1971a). Unprimed human lymphocytes stimulated with PHA produced interferon only in the presence of macrophages (Epstein *et al.*, 1971b). Osteoclast-activating factor (OAF) produced by human PBL in response to PHA required adherent cells (Horton *et al.*, 1974). In guinea pigs, T cell production of macrophage chemotactic factor by primed T cells stimulated with soluble antigen required macrophages (Wahl *et al.*, 1975). In sensitized humans, the production of fibroblast chemotactic factor *in vitro* by PBL stimulated with the sensitizing antigen required the presence of adherent cells (Postlethwaite *et al.*, 1976).

In summary, all immune responses involving triggering of T cells, whether to help B cells respond to T-dependent antigens, to help other T cells to become effector cells, or to mediate effector functions themselves, require at least small numbers of macrophages. In our discussion we have made no effort thus far to distinguish between those macrophage requirements dependent on cellular contact with T cells and the ability of macrophage products to effectively replace the actual adherent cell. Similarly, for most of the systems discussed, we have made no distinction between those T cell responses shown to require macrophages which share some region in the MHC and those in which no genetic restriction has been described. Oppenheim and Rosenstreich (1976) have recently reviewed these issues and have presented evidence suggesting that T cell responses to nonspecific mitogens and cellular antigens, i.e., to alloantigens in MLC or CML or heterologous erythrocyte antigens such as SRBC, do not require the presence of intact and viable macrophages in the culture, but instead only require soluble factors from macrophages such as lymphocyte-activating factor (LAF) (Gery *et al.*, 1972). These factors act, with the cellular antigens or mitogens, as 'second signals' analogous to second signals required for B cell activation to promote T cell triggering and to amplify the response (Rosenstreich and Oppenheim, 1976). Several lines of evidence account for these views. Antibody production to heterologous erythrocytes *in vitro* required T cells and macrophages as well as B cells as previously described. However, Calkins and Golub (1972) have shown that macrophages could provide the helper effect even when separated from macrophage-depleted spleen cells by a cell-impermeable Millipore filter. The antigen (SRBC in this case) and not the macrophages had to be in contact with the responding cells. Further, Chen and Hirsch (1972; and reviewed by Chen and Hirch, 1975) have shown that the requirement for macrophages in a Mishell–Dutton culture system could be replaced entirely with various thiols, of which the most widely used is 2-mercaptoethanol (2–ME). Addition of such agents to lymphoid cells in tissue culture has long been known to enhance the viability of the cells remaining after several days in culture (Fanger *et al.*, 1970; Click *et al.*, 1972). When even small numbers of macrophages were added to nonadherent mouse spleen cells in the absence of 2–ME, the viability was shown to be similarly increased (Pierce and Kapp, 1976). However, Pierce and Kapp (1976) have suggested that rather than replacing macrophages in Mishell–Dutton cultures, 2–ME simply augments the activity of the small number of macrophages left in culture after macrophage depletion procedures. This, of course, may be difficult to directly demonstrate until cell populations can be depleted of macrophages so efficiently that they will not respond to cellular antigens under optimal conditions even in the presence of 2–ME.

T cell responses to cellular alloantigens in MLC and CML have also been shown to be supported by factors from cultures of macrophages (Bach *et al.*, 1970) and by 2–ME in mice (Bevan *et al.*, 1974). As discussed earlier, in guinea pigs, rats and humans, macrophages must be present only in the stimulating cell population as the primary stimulating cells. In this respect, they play a dual role of both presenting the alloantigens to the responding T cells as well as nonspecifically supporting the response (Rosenstreich and Oppenheim, 1976). In addition to T cell responses to alloantigens, T cell proliferative responses to nonspecific mitogens can also be supported by macrophage factors. In the presence of macrophage products, even purified T cells respond well to PHA (Rosenstreich and Oppenheim, 1976). Similarly, the Con A response of T cells requires only macrophage factors. In the situation where macrophage products or thiols such as 2–ME can replace the requirement for macrophages, there is obviously no necessity that the macrophages producing the factors share MHC components with the responding T cells.

In contrast to the T cell responses to cellular antigens and mitogens just discussed, T cell responses to soluble protein antigens have been shown to require the actual presence of viable macrophages in the culture system (for review, see Rosenstreich and Oppenheim, 1976). For these cellular interactions, the MHC does appear to play an important role. This will be discussed in detail in the section on antigen presentation (Section 2.3.2).

2.3. MECHANISMS OF ACTION

The immunogenicity of many soluble protein antigens appears to be correlated with the ability of *in situ* macrophages to take up and process the antigen (discussed above in Section 2.1). Antigens not taken up well *in vivo*, and therefore poorly immunogenic, could be preincubated with macrophages and injected as macrophage-bound antigen. Antigens treated in this way were highly immunogenic and never produced tolerance. B cell tolerance to T-dependent antigens (all soluble protein antigens are T-dependent) has been associated with the prolonged exposure of the B cells to free antigen in the absence of activated helper T cells (for review, see Klaus *et al.*, 1976). One component of the mechanism of increased immunogenicity associated with macrophage-bound antigen may be that antigens administered in this way are less likely to be exposed to B cells in free form than are antigens injected without macrophages. All T cell responses to soluble protein antigens, either production of mediators or proliferative responses, require viable macrophages. In addition to preventing prolonged exposure of B cells to antigens, the evidence suggests that macrophages are also needed to present soluble protein antigens to T cells. With these points in mind, we can first discuss antigen processing by macrophages and then the ability of macrophages to present antigens to T cells. In addition, we will briefly discuss the role of macrophage-produced soluble factors in the activation of the immune response.

2.3.1. *Antigen Processing*

Most antigen picked up by macrophages *in vitro* is endocytosed and rapidly degraded into nonimmunogenic fragments (Unanue, 1972; Ellner and Rosenthale, 1975). However, a small percentage of the antigen associated with the macrophase has been shown to remain in immunogenic form (Unanue and Cerottini, 1970). It is not clear where this antigen is located in the macrophage but it appears that it is slowly released by exocytosis from the cell (Calderon and Unanue, 1974). Some of the immunogenic form of the antigen appears to be expressed on the surface of the cell at some time during the response since in mice, some of the antigen on macrophages has been found to be trypsin-sensitive and could be detected on the cell surface by specific antibodies (Unanue *et al.*, 1969b). Further, when mouse macrophages were preincubated with soluble protein antigens and then exposed to antigen-specific antibody or were trypsinized prior to *in vivo* inoculation, the resulting antibody response was largely abrogated (Unanue, 1972). In guinea pigs the observations are more complex. Walderon *et al.*, (1974) have provided evidence that guinea pig macrophages pulsed with PPD at 4° and then trypsinized while at 4° were no longer immunogenic. In contrast, when guinea pig macrophages were pulsed with PPD at 37°, only a fraction of the immunogenicity was trypsin sensitive. Further, when macrophages were pulsed at 4° and then incubated at 37° before trypsinization, the macrophage-associated immunogenicity became progressively more trypsin resistant. This led these investigators to postulate two steps in antigen processings by macrophages. The first consisted of antigen binding to the macrophage surface, which was trypsin-sensitive and temperature-independent. The second step involved either internalization or sequestration of the immunogenic component in the folds of the membrane rendering it relatively insensitive to trypsinization. Similarly, Ellner and Rosenthal (1975) have shown that antigen taken up by guinea pig macrophages was resistant to trypsin and could not be detected by specific antibody. They have postulated that the macrophage-lymphocyte interaction might induce a return of the antigen to the surface of the macrophage where it would be available for presentation to T cells. Calderon and Unanue (1974) studied the handling of KLH by macrophages and found that a small percentage (3–7 per cent) of the antigen picked up by macrophages *in vitro* was internalized and slowly released into the medium as a smaller molecule than the original antigen, and that part of this fragment was still reactive with anti-KLH antisera. This protein release was associated with live macrophages and was trypsin-resistant. In addition, its release was independent of protein synthesis.

In summary, there is general agreement that the majority of the antigen phagocytized by macrophages is degraded into nonimmunogenic fragments and released. This may play an important role preventing tolerance induction. In addition, a small percentage of the antigen is expressed on the surface of the macrophage where it is highly immunogenic. In mice, the antigen is trypsin-sensitive and detectable by specific antibody. In guinea pigs, the immunogenic fragments are trypsin-resistant and cannot be detected by specific antibody, suggesting they may be sequestered in the membrane. Finally, some of the immunogenic portions of the molecule may be internalized, to be slowly released in an immunogenic form for a variable length of time. The biochemical events involved in these processes are largely unknown.

2.3.2. *Antigen Presentation*

2.3.2.1. *Antigen presentation by macrophages: effects on T cells.* Whereas antigen processing concerns the effects of macrophages on antigens which result in altered and frequently enhanced immunogenicity as compared to the native form, antigen presentation is concerned with the macrophage–lymphocyte interaction which results in antigen-specific triggering of lymphocyte responses. The most recent concepts of antigen presentation by macrophages grew largely out of studies of the genetic control of the immune response. Certain strains of mice (Benacerraf and McDevitt, 1972), guinea pigs (Paul and Benacerraf, 1974) and rats (Kunz and Gill, 1974) have been found to be high or low antibody responders to specific antigens. The ability to mount a strong antibody response to many antigens was linked to the MHC (Benacerraf and McDevitt, 1972; Kunz and Gill, 1974). By use of recombinant strains of mice for genetic mapping, the immune response (Ir) genes have largely been found to be located in the I region of the MHC although in some cases the H–2K region has not yet been ruled out (Shreffler and David, 1975). Ir gene expression, or the ability to generate immune responses to antigens under Ir gene control, was once thought to be primarily a property of T cells (Paul and Benacerraf, 1974). Now, however, macrophages in the guinea pig (Shevach, 1976) and the rat (Tada *et al.*, 1976) and probably B cells, in some cases in mice (Mozes and Shearer, 1971), are thought to express Ir genes. The I region of the MHC also codes for I region-associated (Ia) cell surface antigens found on the membranes of subpopulations of T cells, B cells and macrophages as well as some nonlymphoid cells (Hammerling, 1976). That Ia antigens are important in macrophage–T cell interactions is indicated by the fact that antisera directed toward these Ia antigens have been shown to block T cell proliferative responses to macrophage-bound soluble antigen (Shevach and Rosenthal, 1973; Shevach, 1976). Further, recent evidence has been presented that antisera directed toward Ia antigens coded for in the I–J subregion of the MHC (recently described by Murphy *et al.*, 1976), when preincubated with macrophages but not the macrophage-depleted responding lymphocytes, could block the *in vitro* humoral response to burro red blood cells (BRBC) (Neiderhuber and Shreffler, 1976). Studies of lymphoid cellular interactions have suggested that T cell–B cell collaboration *in vitro* and *in vivo* required identity at various I subregions of the MHC (Katz *et al.*, 1973a, 1976). Similar requirements have been suggested for the ability of macrophages to present antigens to T cells for helper cell induction (Erb and Feldmann, 1975b, 1976) and for induction of antigen-specific T cell proliferative responses (Rosenthal and Shevach, 1973). However, exceptions to this rule have been reported. Pierce *et al.* (1976) and Kapp *et al.* (1973) have shown that completely allogeneic macrophages can prime T cells *in vitro* to become helper cells for antibody-forming cell (AFC) production to GAT (a random terpolymer of L–glutamic acid–L–alanine–L–tryosine). In addition, Heber-Katz and Wilson (1976) have shown rat T cells, 'filtered' through irradiated F_1 hybrid rats to deplete alloreactive cells, could collaborate with allogeneic B cells in a primary *in vitro* anti-SRBC response. These experiments, then, suggest that Ia compatibility may not be required for cellular interactions of unprimed cells.

Similar experiments have been performed *in vivo*. Bechtol *et al.* (1974) have used tetraparental (allophenic) chimeric mice constructed from the fusion of mouse embryos of strains which are high (CWB) and low (C3H) responders to Poly L–(Tyr, Glu)–poly–D, L–Ala–poly–L–Lys (TGAL). These strains are congenic on the C3H background, differing for the Ig allotype and the H–2 complex. The percentage of each parental lymphoid cell type in the adult chimeric mice could be determined by allotype analysis of the serum immunoglobulin. Those mice with a high percentage of the CWB Ig allotype proved to be high responders to TGAL and those with a low percentage of the CWB allotype were poor responders. This suggested that the genetic responsiveness was still associated with the predominant lymphoid cell type in the chimeric mice. However, when high responder chimeric mice were immunized with TGAL, the anti-TGAL response consisted of antibody of both allotypes and the ratio of the CWB allotype to the C3H allotype had not changed from the resting state. This suggested that B cells of both haplotypes responded to CWB T cell help, thus providing evidence that T–B collaboration could occur *in vivo* despite MHC differences. These observations were further supported by the experiments of von Boehmer *et al.* (1975a). They adoptively transferred, into lethally irradiated F_1 mice, SRBC primed T cells from tetraparental bone marrow chimera mice which were depleted of cells from the other parental donor by treatment with alloantisera and complement. The recipients were then inoculated with SRBC and with SRBC-primed B cells depleted of T cells by anit-theta plus complement from the opposite parental strain. These allogeneic, primed T and B cells cooperated well to give a strong anti-SRBC response. Since these investigators (von Boehmer *et al.*, 1975b) had previously demonstrated the lack of alloreactivity between T cells from chimeric mice and cells from mice of one of the parental strains, the observed response was not due to an allogeneic effect. Similarly, Bechtol *et al.* (1976) have provided convincing evidence that the anti-TGAL responses (discussed above) in $C_3H \leftrightarrow CWB$ tetraparental mice were in no way due to an allogeneic effect. These experiments have clearly shown that, at least in some situations, T cells and B cells can collaborate *in vivo* despite I region differences. To provide an explanation for these observations, Pierce *et al.* (1976) have recently pointed out that the Ia identity requirement had been seen in experiments using primed cells in secondary responses, whereas those investigators not observing the Ia identity genetic restriction had tested either primary responses or responses of T cells primed in a chimeric environment (Kapp *et al.*, 1973; Pierce *et al.*, 1976; Heber–Katz and Wilson, 1975). Further, Pierce *et al.* (1976) demonstrated that T cells primed *in vivo* with allogeneic macrophages required macrophages syngeneic to those used for priming, to trigger a secondary response. Moreover, macrophages syngeneic to T cells primed with allogeneic macrophages could not be substituted for allogeneic macrophages for the secondary challenge. These findings are supported by the work of Miller *et al.* (1976a), using an adoptive transfer of delayed hypersensitivity (DTH) system in mice. They have shown that T cells of one parental haplotype, sensitized in a chimeric environment, could adoptively transfer DTH to either of the parents despite total histoincompatibility. Further, T cells from (BALB/c $\times$ CBA)F_1 hybrid mice, sensitized in either BALB/c or CBA nude mice, could transfer DTH reactivity only to the parent syngeneic to the nude mouse in which they were sensitized (Miller *et al.*, 1976a). They previously showed that F_1 cells sensitized in an F_1 environment could transfer DTH reactivity equally well to either parent (Miller *et al.*, 1976b). These experiments support the notion that the original macrophage–T cell interaction is responsible for genetic restrictions observed for macrophage interactions with primed T cells. More direct evidence for this hypothesis has been provided by recent reports of Thomas and Shevach (1976,

1977a, b). They showed that purified lymph node cells of (strain 2 × strain 13)F_1 guinea pigs, primed *in vitro* with OVA-pulsed macrophages from either parent, could be restimulated only with macrophages of the same parent pulsed with the same antigen. In contrast, F_1 LNC primed with F_1 macrophages would respond to either of the parental macrophages in a secondary response (Thomas and Shevach, 1976). These experiments, however, only showed priming of F_1 LNC by macrophages, albeit with interesting genetic restrictions for subsequent T cell restimulation. To examine priming of T cells with totally allogeneic macrophages, they had to pretreat the macrophages with specific anti-Ia antisera to block alloantigen sensitization which would otherwise result in a strong secondary MLC upon reexposure of the allogeneic macrophages to the allosensitized T cells. They found that the antisera, in addition to blocking the Ia determinant on the macrophages, served as an antigen to which the T cells could be sensitized. Once primed, the T cells responded secondarily only to macrophages of the same haplotype which were treated with anti-Ia antisera. Neither macrophages of the proper haplotype without pretreatment with anti-Ia, nor syngeneic macrophages regardless of treatment with anti-Ia stimulated. Therefore, this represents a clear example of T cell priming with histoincompatible macrophages, the secondary response of which was specific not only for the antigen but also for the haplotype of the macrophage used for the initial priming. Further, these investigators found that antisera toward the B.1 MHC determinant (analogous to the H–2 K and D regions in the mouse) also could act as an antigen and that the Ia genetic restriction for secondary stimulation was operative in this case also. On the basis of these data, they have suggested that protein antigens bound to Ia and other MHC molecules on macrophages serve as 'complex antigenic determinants' to which T cells are primed. Moreover, they concluded that Ia antigens must indirectly influence the presentation of antigen bound to other MHC molecules since only anti-B.1 treated macrophages with Ia determinants identical to those of the anti-B.1 treated macrophage used for priming could elicit a secondary proliferative response (Thomas and Shevach, 1977a). In addition, they have shown that TNP-modified macrophages could specifically sensitize allogeneic T cells, but only after the alloreactive clone of T cells was depleted by treatment with BUdR and light during a primary MLC. The reason for this was not obvious, but since not even syngeneic macrophages, modified with TNP, could sensitize T cells during a MLC proliferative response, it was likely that a suppressor mechanism was being generated which was dependent on the proliferation of the alloreactive cells (Thomas and Shevach, 1977b).

Paul *et al.* (1976) have recently shown that guinea pig LNC primed *in vivo* with OVA could be restimulated *in vitro* with antigen-pulsed macrophages from either parent, and if during the proliferative phase of the secondary response induced by such antigen-pulsed macrophages, the responding cells were treated with BUdR and exposed to light, thus eliminating the proliferating clone, the remaining cells could be stimulated only with OVA-pulsed macrophages from the alternate parent. Positive selection experiments showed that if F_1 LNC, primed *in vivo*, were restimulated with OVA-pulsed macrophages of one parent, the responding cells were then hyperresponsive for OVA-pulsed macrophages of that parent but only modestly responsive to OVA-pulsed macrophages of the other parent.

All of these data can be explained by the hypothesis that the original macrophage–T cell MHC relationship established a preference in the secondary response for macrophage MHC antigen which induced the primary response. I, D and K region identity primary sensitization, T cells appear to recognize antigens in complex or association with MHC antigens on macrophages. For secondary stimulation then, the primed T cell requires presentation of antigen in complex or association with the same macrophage MHC antigen which induced the primary response. I, D, and K region identity requirements for secondary T cell stimulation have been demonstrated depending on the antigen used (Miller *et al.*, 1976a; Paul *et al.*, 1976; Thomas and Shevach, 1976; Pierce *et al.*, 1976). In the case of F_1 cells sensitized in an F_1 environment, or parental cells sensitized in a chimeric environment, two clones of antigen-reactive cells may be generated, one for each macrophage haplotype expressed during the sensitization.

In summary, these recent observations indicate that MHC gene products on macrophages play a critical role in the sensitization process of the T cell and that T cell receptors recognize antigen in complex or association with macrophage Ia or other MHC determinants. Paul *et al.* (1976) have postulated that the MHC has evolved as the basis for cellular interactions which are essential for the competence of the immune response. This interesting hypothesis serves to point out the rather central role of macrophages in induction of T cell-dependent immune responses.

2.3.2.2. *Antigen presentation by macrophages: effects on B cells.* In contrast to the recent advances in understanding of the macrophage–T cell interaction, the macrophage–B cell interaction has received little attention. Rather, the T cell–B cell interaction has been stressed (Katz *et al.*, 1973a, b, 1976; reviewed in Katz and Benacerraf, 1972). The demonstration that T-independent B cell antigens were also macrophage independent (Shortman *et al.*, 1970; Mosier *et al.*, 1974; Feldmann, 1972a, b) has suggested that the primary or sole role of macrophages is to sensitize T cells and only through that mechanism could macrophages influence B cell responses. However, recent demonstrations that B cell responses to some T-independent antigens either require or are greatly enhanced by macrophages (Chused *et al.*, 1976; Lee *et al.*, 1976; Pike and Nossal, 1976) suggest that macrophages may play a role in B cell activation and that their effect on B cells in these responses may have been overlooked. There is, in fact, some evidence that activated macrophages produce factors that can stimulate B cells directly to respond to T-dependent antigens in the absence of T cells (Schrader, 1973; Wood and Gaul, 1974; Hoffman *et al.*, 1976a, b; Wood and Cameron, 1975). In addition, there is evidence that T cell helper factors may require macrophages to activate (or provide a second signal for) B cells. Feldmann (1972c) has reported experiments done in double chambered Marbrook vessels in which primed T cells, separated from T cell-depleted spleen cells by a 0.1 μ Nucleopore membrane, could induce specific AFC production by the T cell-depleted spleen cells in the presence of the priming antigen (DNP–KLH). When macrophages were also depleted from the T cell-depleted spleen cells, no specific AFC production could be demonstrated. Reconstitution of the spleen cells with purified anti-theta and complement-treated PEC (macrophages) again resulted in specific AFC production. Further, when primed T cells were cultured in the upper chamber of the Marbrook vessel with DNP–KLH, and purified PEC were cultured alone in the lower chamber, Feldmann (1972c) found that the thoroughly washed PEC could induce a strong antigen-specific AFC response when combined with T cell-depleted spleen cells in a secondary culture devoid of additional antigen. From such experiments, Feldmann (1972c) concluded that macrophages were required to present the antigen–T cell factor complex to B cells. Schrader and Feldmann (1973) arrived at similar conclusions during investigations of antigenic competition. In these experiments, mice which had been primed with fowl gamma globulin (FGG) were injected with donkey RBC (DRBC) i.p. or i.v. 2 days before serving as donors of spleen cells to be used in a Marbrook–Diener culture system to produce AFC to DNP coupled to FGG. They found that the AFC response was very poor when DNP–FGG was used as an antigen, but when DNP was coupled to a thymus-independent antigen such as flagella (FLA), a strong AFC response was observed. This indicated that the B cells were fully competent to produce antibody when triggered by a T-independent antigen and suggested the defect in the response to DNP–FGG was in either the T cells or the macrophages. They found that addition of very small numbers of normal macrophages to the system (0.2 per cent of the responding cells) allowed a normal AFC response, compared to the response of cells from FGG-primed mice not preinjected with DRBC. In addition, the ability to respond to DNP–FGG was restored by trypsinizing the responding cells prior to culture. From these experiments, they concluded that macrophages in the spleens of mice pre-injected with DRBC were unable to present the T cell helper factor to the B cells due to the pre-injection with DRBC *in vivo*. The trypsinization, they concluded, acted to remove a surface inhibitor from the surface of the macrophages.

Further evidence that macrophages alone can enhance B cell antibody production was provided by Opitz *et al.* (1976). They showed that normal mouse spleen cells would generate a polyclonal antibody response in a Mishell–Dutton culture system if cocultivated with high concentrations of mouse PEC for 8 hr before depleting the spleen cells of all phagocytic cells and reculturing them in media containing 2–ME. Control cultures not cultured with high numbers of mouse PEC generated no such response.

In summary then, these observations suggest that macrophages can have significant effects on B cell responses to both T-dependent and T-independent antigens. In view of the recent work describing the mechanisms of antigen presentation to T cells by macrophages (previous section), it seems likely that macrophages may also be involved in the presentation of T cell-dependent helper factors to B cells. Alternatively, primed T cells, upon activation by antigen, may liberate factors which activate macrophages which then provide a second signal to B cells for specific AFC production. Considering the changing concepts of the genetic restrictions (or lack thereof) on T cell–B cell collaboration and macrophage–T cell interactions, it would seem that further investigations are needed on the role of macrophages in the relationship between T cells and B cells as well as their role in stimulating B cells directly.

2.3.3. *Lymphocyte Activation Factor (IL-1)*

In addition to the role of macrophages in the processing and presentation of antigen, it appears that macrophages can also assist in the development of an immune response by providing another signal to the lymphocytes. This is in the form of a soluble factor, initially designated lymphocyte activation factor (LAF) but renamed interleukin 1 (IL-1). IL-1 was first described by Gery and his co-workers (1972) as a factor, produced by adherent human peripheral blood leukocytes, which could stimulate the mitogenic activity of PHA and Con A on murine thymocytes. Subsequently this factor has been identified in a number of mammalian species (for review see Mizel, 1980). Although resting macrophages produce little or no IL-1, activated macrophages produce considerable levels of IL-1. Agents that activate macrophages directly, such as endotoxin and mycobacteria, have been shown to be stimulants of IL-1 production (Oppenhien *et al.,* 1979). In addition, factors produced by lymphocytes in response to antigen stimulation could also induce the production of IL-1 (Moore *et al.,* 1980).

IL-1 has been found to have several effects on lymphocyte populations as reflected in the usual assay for IL-1. Thymocytes can be stimulated directly to proliferate by IL-1 or by IL-1 plus PHA or Con A (Gery *et al.,* 1972). IL-1 can also modestly increase the proliferative response of peripheral T cells to lectins and antigens. Thus IL-1 can act either directly as a mitogen or as a second signal to promote T lymphocyte proliferation. IL-1 can also promote the *in vitro* antibody responses of B lymphocytes (Wood and Gaul, 1974).

3. SUPPRESSION OF IMMUNE RESPONSES BY MACROPHAGES

In the previous sections we have discussed evidence that macrophages can enhance immune responses *in vivo* and *in vitro.* Various mechanisms were discussed, both in terms of the effect of macrophages on the antigen itself and the requirement for macrophages of various lymphocyte responses to antigens and mitogens. In most cases, normal macrophages in very low concentrations were used to demonstrate these enhancing effects.

In this section, we shall concentrate on suppressive effects of macrophages on the immune response. In contrast to the enhancing effects, the suppressive effects have usually been seen with greater concentrations of macrophages or with highly activated macrophages. First, we shall describe a series of basic observations made in our laboratory and in others which provide a framework on which a more general concept of immunosuppression resulting from the inhibition of lymphocyte proliferation by cells of the reticuloendothelial system (RES) can be constructed. What is known about the mechanism of macrophage-mediated cytostatic effects will be reviewed. We suggest that 'activation' of macrophages is a relative term and that the degree of suppression is related not only to the activation state of the macrophages but also to the number of macrophages in the proximity of an expanding clone of lymphocytes. We shall discuss various ways in which macrophages can become activated and thereby become more suppressive. An important recent finding which will be emphasized is that T cells can generate suppressor macrophages via a factor isolated from Con A-induced suppressor T cells. Therefore, suppressor T cells may exert their effects indirectly through activation of suppressor macrophages.

We shall then discuss the evidence that suppressor macrophages *in vitro* and an activated reticuloendothelial system (RES) *in vivo* can be shown to have similar effects on lymphocyte responsiveness. A number of examples of suppressed immune responses associated with an activated RES will be discussed, along with evidence that in many cases the cell which mediates the suppressor effect is probably an activated macrophage. Finally, we shall discuss the observations that macrophages, usually considered to be nonspecific in their effects, may in fact be able to distinguish between neoplastic and non-neoplastic cells.

3.1. Basic Observations

Our laboratory has recently investigated a number of cases of suppressed immune responses *in vitro* and, in many instances, has identified the responsible agent as a macrophage (Kirchner *et al.*, 1974a, b, c, 1975a, b; Oehler *et al.*, 1977a, b; Fernbach *et al.*, 1976a, b; Glaser *et al.*, 1976; reviewed in Kirchner *et al.*, 1976). Many of the original observations were made by Kirchner *et al.* (1974a, b, 1975a). It was initially observed that spleen cells from C57BL/6 mice bearing tumors induced by inoculation with Moloney sarcoma virus (MSV) responded poorly if at all to T cell mitogens such as PHA and Con A and frequently had a depressed response to the B cell mitogen LPS (Kirchner *et al.*, 1974a, b). There were several possible explanations for such findings. If T cells, and occasionally B cells, migrated from the spleen during the growth of the tumor, the lack of cells even potentially capable of responding to mitogens when cultured *in vitro* could account for the defect. However, purification of the lymphocytes by passing the spleen cells from MSV tumor-bearing mice (MSV spleen cells) over a rayon adherence column [a technique by which cells capable of ingesting latex particles were largely depleted but the ratio or surface immunoglobulin (Ig) positive to Ig negative cells was essentially unchanged (Kirchner *et al.*, 1974a)] reconstituted the proliferative response to the mitogens (Kirchner *et al.*, 1974a, b). Therefore, cells capable of responding to the mitogens were present in the spleen. Thus two possible explanations remained: either the potentially responsive cells were diluted by an influx of cells which would not respond to mitogens (Smith and Konda, 1973), or a population of adherent cells was present which somehow prevented the potentially responsive cells from proliferating. To test whether a suppressive effect was playing a role in the failure of the MSV spleens to respond to mitogens, spleen cells from MSV tumor-bearing mice were mixed with spleen cells from normal mice and the mixture was incubated with PHA. Virtually no proliferative response was observed in the cell mixture, demonstrating the role of suppressor cells (Kirchner *et al.*, 1974b). To characterize the cell or cells responsible for the suppressive effect, a number of subpopulations of cells from MSV spleens were tested for their suppressive effects on the proliferative response of normal spleen cells to PHA. Pretreatment of the MSV spleen cells with anti-theta and complement to remove T cells had no effect or actually increased the suppressive effects (Kirchner *et al.*, 1974b, 1975a). In contrast, depletion of adherent cells by passage over a rayon column, or of phagocytic cells by pretreatment with iron powder and magnet, totally abrogated the suppressive effect (Kirchner *et al.*, 1974b). In addition, pretreatment of the cells with carrageenan, which is specifically toxic for macrophages and not for lymphocytes (Lake *et al.*, 1971), largely abrogated the suppression (Kirchner *et al.*, 1975a). Further, the suppressor activity was resistant to 2500 r X-irradiation (Kirchner *et al.*, 1975a). These data indicated that the MSV spleen cells contained a subpopulation of radioresistant, phagocytic, carrageenan-sensitive, non–T cells, and thus probably macrophages or monocytes, which could suppress the proliferative response of lymphocytes to mitogens (reviewed in Kirchner *et al.*, 1976). Subsequent reports concerning studies of tumor-bearing rats (Glaser *et al.*, 1975; Veit and Feldman, 1976b), humans (Broder *et al.*, 1975) and mice (Pope *et al.*, 1976) confirmed that suppressed responses to mitogens could be due to the presence of a population of suppressor macrophages. In addition to the suppression of mitogen responses, macrophage-mediated suppressive effects have been demonstrated in a variety of other *in vitro* reactions. Fernbach *et al.* (1976b) found that MSV spleen cells responded poorly to alloantigens in MLC and CML. When mixed with normal mouse spleen cells, irradiated MSV spleen cells were strongly suppressive compared to the effect of adding equal numbers of irradiated normal spleen cells. When MSV spleen cells were pretreated with carrageenan or when the phagocytes were depleted with iron and magnet, the suppressive effect was no longer seen. In addition, the cells were found to be adherent and radioresistant. As expected, treatment with anti-theta and complement had no effect. Addition of peritoneal exudate cells (PEC), induced with thioglycolate and purified by Petri dish adherence so that greater than 95 per cent of the cells were macrophages morphologically, also resulted in suppression of the MLC and the CML (Fernbach *et al.*, 1976a). Berlinger *et al.* (1976) have shown that depressed MLC responses of PBL from some cancer patients could be restored by passing the PBL over a Sephadex G–10 column which in their hands selectively depleted monocytes. Kirchner *et al.* (1975a) found that the T cell proliferative response of spleen cells from tumor-bearing mice to tumor-associated antigens in a mixed lymphocyte-tumor interaction (MLTI) was greatly improved by depletion of adherent or phagocytic cells. Similarly, Glaser *et al.* (1975) showed that spleen cells taken from rats bearing progressively growing tumors were largely unresponsive to tumor-associated antigens in a MLTI. After depletion of adherent or phagocytic cells, positive responses were detected. We recently confirmed and extended these observations, and have shown that the suppressor cells in tumor-bearing rats were resistant to treatment with a specific heterologous anti-rat thymocyte serum and complement (ATS and C) as well as to a heterologous anti-rat immunoglubulin serum and complement (Oehler *et al.*, 1977a). These data indicated that the suppressor cells in spleens of tumor-bearing rats which inhibit specific lymphoproliferative responses to tumor cells *in vitro* were macrophages. In rats, however, we found that normal spleen cells added to MLTI cultures as third parties were also suppressive, albeit not as suppressive as spleen cells taken from tumor-bearing donors. Extensive characterization procedures showed suppressor cells in the spleens of non-tumor-bearing rats similarly were macrophages. These experiments indicated that the suppressive nature of macrophages may not necessarily represent a pathologic state but rather reflect a normal regulatory mechanism which is intensified in some pathological conditions.

Injection of mice with agents such as heat-killed *Corynebacterium parvum* (*C. parvum*) results in a strong stimulation of the reticuloendothelial system (RES) (Halpern *et al.*, 1963; Halpern, 1975). Splenic macrophages from mice treated with *C. parvum*, strongly supress the lymphoproliferative responses to PHA, Con A and LPS, and, if given in a high enough dose, to pokeweed mitogen (PWM) (Scott, 1972; Kirchner *et al.*, 1975c; reviewed in Kirchner *et al.*, 1976). Mitchell *et al.* (1973) have shown similar effects after treatment of mice with Bacillus Calmette–Guerin (BCG).

Natural killer (NK) cells, a population of effectors that have spontaneous cytolytic activity against tumor cells (Herberman and Holden, 1979), are also subject to the regulatory activity of cells that appear to be macrophages. Adherent macrophages isolated from murine sarcoma virus (MSV)-induced tumors could suppress the effector phase of NK cells (Gerson *et al.*, 1981). In addition adherent cells isolated from spleens of animals inoculated with pyran copolymer could also suppress NK activity when mixed with the effector cells and assayed for cytolytic activity in a 4-hour isotope release assay against YAC-1 tumor targets (Santoni *et al.*, 1980a, b). In the latter studies, higher ratios of macrophages to spleen cells were employed (1:1) than are usually used to demonstrate suppression of other types of functions. Macrophages or macrophage-like cells seem to be responsible for the depression of NK activity induced by hydrocortisone (Hochman and Cudkowicz, 1978), i-carageenan (Hochman *et al.*, 1981) and *Corynebacterium parvum* (Santoni *et al.*, 1983). NK cell activity can also be suppressed by a preincubation with macrophages (Brunda *et al.*, 1982). Under these circumstances, spleen cell suspensions containing natural killer cells are incubated overnight with macrophages that have been isolated from the peritoneal cavity of mice that have not been inoculated with an activating or phlogistic agent (resident macrophages). These macrophages could reduce the spontaneous NK activity or inhibit the augmentation of NK activity by interferon treatment. Macrophages from animals that had been inoculated with *C. parvum* (which activates the macrophages) were much less efficient in their suppressor activity. This was in marked contrast to the ability of pyran activated macrophages to suppress the effector phase of the response. Hence, macrophages at different stages of activation appear to have markedly different abilities to suppress NK activity at different stages of the development of the cytolytic activity.

In contrast to the inhibitory effects of suppressor macrophages on proliferative responses and on the generation of cytotoxic lymphocytes which require proliferation (Cantor and Jandinski, 1974; Peavy and Pierce, 1975), cytotoxicity by previously-generated effector cells seems not to be affected. Primary T cell-mediated cytotoxicity to tumor-associated antigens (Kirchner *et al.*, 1974b), PHA-induced T cell-mediated cytotoxicity (Kirchner *et al.*, 1975a) and antibody-dependent cell-mediated cytotoxicity (Poplack *et al.*, 1976; reviewed in Kirchner *et al.*, 1976) appear to be unaffected by suppressor macrophages. Initially it appeared that only immune responses that required proliferation were sensitive to suppression by macrophages. However, several recent observations indicate that other phases of the immune response, that do not require proliferation, can also be suppressed by macrophages. Klimpel and Henny (1978) demonstrated that the generation of secondary cytotoxic responses could take place in the absence of proliferation and that this response could be inhibited by macrophages activated *in vivo* by Bacillus Calmette Guerin. Studies on the *in vitro* generation of cytotoxicity to methyl-cholanthrene-induced tumors gave similar types of information (Garrigues *et al.*, 1982). Suppressor macrophages added at any time during the first four days of a five day mixed lymphocyte culture could suppress the generation of cytotoxic effector cells. Thus suppressor cells added before and after lymphocyte proliferation could inhibit the generation of the response. Suppressor macrophages have been shown to also inhibit the production of lymphokines, a function that is independent of proliferation. Landolfo *et al.* (1977) demonstrated that spleen cells from mice bearing murine sarcoma virus-induced tumors, at peak tumor size, were deficient in their ability to produce MIF but could have that response restored by removing the macrophages. Subsequently, Varesio *et al.* (1980) showed that activated macrophages, when added to cells that had been stimulated to produce lymphokines, suppressed their response (Varesio *et al.*, 1980a, b, c). Subsequent studies have shown that suppression by macrophages of lymphokine production was seen only when the suppressor cells were added during the first 6 hours of culture (Varesio and Holden, 1980; Varesio *et al.*, 1981). During this period critical protein synthesis steps appear to take place in the lymphocytes that are required for the development of lymphokine synthesis and for the full expression of the proliferative response (Varesio *et al.*, 1980d, e). Suppressor macrophages have been shown to inhibit protein synthesis in responding lymphocytes and therefore appear to interfere with the development of the response by inhibiting this phase of macromolecular synthesis of the lymphocyte (Varesio *et al.*, 1981). Keller (1974a) has emphasized the need for macrophages to be activated to mediate the suppressor effect. His data show that on a per cell basis, peptone broth-induced rat peritoneal macrophages are more suppressive than non-induced peritoneal macrophages. However, in sufficient concentrations, 'resting' or non-induced macrophages also inhibited lymphocyte proliferation (Keller, 1974a). Our laboratory has provided further evidence, in both mice (Fernbach *et al.*, 1976a) and rats (Oehler *et al.*, 1977b), that by simply increasing the concentration of PEC in MLC–CML cultures, lymphoproliferative responses and the resultant generation of cytotoxic effector cells were inhibited without affecting the viability of the cells in the suppressed cultures. Further, the distinction between 'activated' and 'resting' macrophages is complicated by the fact that many substances including lymphocyte mediators (reviewed by David, 1975), with which circulating macrophages must to a variable degree be in contact *in vivo*, activate macrophages. Therefore, it may be better to think of relative degrees of activation rather than of an all or none phenomenon. This would account for both Keller's (1974a) findings that activated macrophages were more suppressive than resting (less activated) macrophages and our observations that increased numbers of peritoneal macrophages added to CML cultures as third parties [5–8 per cent in rats (Oehler *et al.*, 1977b) and greater than 10 per cent in mice (Fernbach *et al.*, 1976a)] were strongly suppressive. In contrast, addition of a thirty fold greater number of X-irradiated thymocytes to rat CML cultures as third parties had no suppressive effect, suggesting that cell crowding was not the cause of suppression by higher numbers of macrophages (Oehler *et al.*, 1977b). Thus, it would appear that macrophages, either low numbers of strongly activated cells or higher numbers of minimally activated cells, can suppress lymphocyte proliferation and in that way inhibit or abrogate the expansion of a clone of sensitized lymphocytes.

3.2. Mechanisms of Action

3.2.1. *Assay Systems*

Much of the information concerning the mechanisms of macrophage-mediated suppression has come from the work of Keller (1974a, b, 1976; Keller *et al.*, 1975) who measured the rate of proliferation of antigen- or mitogen-triggered lymphocytes in Petri dishes containing various concentrations of purified macrophages obtained from rat peritoneal exudates. Basically, Keller demonstrated that high macrophage to lymphocyte ratios (10:1) completely inhibited proliferation of the lymphocytes (Keller, 1975). The effect was nonspecific in that the proliferation of syngeneic, allogeneic, and xenogeneic lymphocytes could be suppressed. Moreover, use of malignant lymphoma cells as targets of suppression has provided a consistent and simpler assay system for analysis of the mechanism of the macrophage-mediated suppression (Keller, 1974a), since these cells did not need to be stimulated to proliferate.

Support for the use of rapidly dividing tumor cells as indicator cells for suppressor macrophage activity has recently been provided by our laboratory (Oehler *et al.*, 1977a). We have directly compared the ability of macrophages to suppress the proliferation rate of lymphoma lines maintained *in vitro* to their ability to suppress specific lymphoproliferative responses of immune rate splenic T cells to tumor-associated antigens in a mixed lymphocyte–tumor interaction (MLTI). Under the proper conditions, results obtained in one assay could be used to predict results obtained in the other. This indicated that the cytostatic mechanism was similarly effective on rapidly proliferating lymphoid cells regardless of the stimulus (Oehler *et al.*, 1977a).

3.2.2. *Metabolic Requirements for Macrophage-Induced Suppression*

Keller (1974b) has evaluated the effects of various agents and treatments to determine the metabolic requirements for macrophage-induced suppression. The suppressive effect was sensitive only to protein synthesis inhibitors and inhibitors of glycolysis (Keller, 1974b). When various parameters of macrophage activity were monitored, such as cellular adherence, pinocytosis, bactericidal capacity, glucose oxidation, production of RNase and DNase, and others, only alterations in the rate of protein synthesis correlated with the cytostatic effects observed (Keller, 1975). Pretreatment of macrophage monolayers with inhibitors of DNA synthesis such as mitomycin C and X-irradiation had no effect on their cytostatic activity. In addition, the suppressor activity was resistant to treatment with a variety of enzymes including trypsin, neuraminidase and pronase. Inhibitors of pinocytosis or phagocytosis had no effect. Moreover, careful microscopic examination of the experimental cultures showed no relationship of increased phagocytic activity to the degree of suppression. Thus, although the mechanisms by which macrophages inhibit lymphoproliferative responses are unknown, the available evidence suggests that the ability to suppress can be correlated with the rate of protein synthesis and not with various other parameters of macrophage activation. This could be interpreted to suggest that only a subpopulation of macrophages, characterized by its increased rate of protein synthesis, is suppressive or that only macrophages which have been activated to undergo increased protein synthesis are suppressive. However, until these findings are confirmed in other laboratories, it may be premature to speculate on the mechanisms by which suppressor macrophages mediate their effects.

3.2.3. *Suppressor Effects of Macrophages Mediated by Soluble Factors*

Although there are a number of reports describing suppressor effects of macrophages which require cell–cell contact (Sjöberg and Britton, 1972; Sjöberg, 1971; Eggers and Wunderlich, 1975; Kirchner *et al.*, 1975a; reviewed in Kirchner *et al.*, 1976), macrophages also appear to mediate suppressor effects through the effects of soluble factors (for review see *Modulation of Immunity by Soluble Mediators* by Byron H. Waksman, in this series). Suppressor factors produced by or dependent on macrophages have been described by a number of investigators. Calderon *et al.* (1974) have described a factor recovered from cultures of mouse peritoneal exudate cells which inhibited ^{3}H–TdR incorporation by, and proliferation of, tumor cells and mitogen-stimulated lymphocytes *in vitro*. It was of low molecular weight and resistant to trypsin digestion. Further, it could be absorbed by tumor cells cultured *in vitro*. Similarly, Waldman and Gottlieb (1973) have described a low molecular weight factor isolated from rat PEC which inhibited proliferation of antigen-stimulated and resting rat lymphocytes. Krakauer *et al.* (1976) have demonstrated a soluble suppressor factor which inhibited immunoglobulin production of PWM-stimulated mouse spleen cells. This factor was apparently produced by macrophages in the ascitic fluid of hypogammaglobulinemic mice bearing plasmacytomas. Similarly, Kolb *et al.* (1977) have demonstrated a suppressor factor apparently originating from macrophages of mice bearing large plasmacytomas which inhibited the PFC response to SRBC in Mishell–Dutton cultures.

Several other defined products of macrophages have been suggested as mediators of macrophage-induced suppression. Goodwin *et al.* (1977) demonstrated that prostaglandins produced by macrophages could suppress proliferation of human peripheral blood lymphocytes. Grimm *et al.* (1978) also demonstrated the *C. parvum* activated, macrophage-mediated suppression could be partially accounted for by the production of prostaglandin by these cells. More recently, Metzger *et al.* (1980) found that macrophages appear to mediate their suppressive effect not only by the production of prostaglandin but also through the release of hydrogen peroxide. Another immunoregulatory mediator, interferon, may also play a role in macrophage-mediated suppression. Neuman and Sorg (1977) have suggested that the interferon produced by macrophages may be one of the mediators of macrophage suppression. In summary there appear to be several mediators that could be involved in the suppression by macrophages. At the present time it is unclear which of these substances is the predominant mediator of suppression or whether suppression may be a composite of the effects of several of these mediators.

Caution must be exercised, however, in evaluating the effects of soluble factors produced from lymphoid cells in tissue culture. When only one parameter such as ^{3}H–TdR incorporation is used as a measure of suppression, the possibility that breakdown products of dying cells are present in the culture which compete with radiolabeled DNA precursors and thus inhibit ^{3}H–TdR incorporation without inhibiting cell proliferation must be ruled out. One group (Opitz *et al.*, 1975a), in fact, has performed a series of biochemical characterizations on a soluble factor which they had previously shown to suppress ^{3}H–TdR incorporation of PHA-stimulated mouse lymphocytes (Opitz *et al.*, 1975b) and conclusively demonstrated that it was thymidine. There are several ways to avoid such tissue culture artifacts. One way is to use a second assay system independent of ^{3}H–TdR incorporation to demonstrate the suppressive effect. Fernbach *et al.* (1976a) showed that macrophages suppressed the generation of cytotoxic effector cells and the appearance of blast cells as well as the incorporation of ^{3}H–TdR by mouse T cells in MLC. In this study, by observing the effects of various concentrations of macrophages on the MLC, they noted that

^{3}H TdR incorporation was inhibited at a slightly lower concentration of macrophages than was the generation of lymphoblasts or the generation of cytotoxic effector cells. It seems likely that the slightly disparate findings were a result of the presence of cell breakdown products in the media. This effect, however, was minor compared to the effect of greater numbers of macrophages which totally suppressed all three parameters of the response generated in the MLC.

In addition to using alternate assay systems, one can measure the incorporation of other labeled protein or nucleic acid precursors such as tritiated uridine, valine or leucine. Opitz *et al.* (1975a) showed that the incorporation of these precursors was not inhibited by supernatants from cultures containing cell breakdown products which artifactually inhibited ^{3}H–TdR incorporation. Similarly, Fernbach *et al.* (1976a) have suggested that the use of low specific activity ^{3}H–TdR (300 mCi/mM instead of 6 Ci/mM) minimized the effect of artifactual ^{3}H–TdR incorporation inhibition. Perhaps the easiest way to avoid such artifacts is to wash the cells immediately before addition of ^{3}H–TdR, thus removing any cell breakdown products which may have accumulated during the culture period.

Thus, in light of the findings of Opitz *et al.* (1975a), who identified their low molecular weight suppressor factor as thymidine, it seems mandatory that any soluble suppressor substance which inhibits ^{3}H–TdR incorporation of proliferating cells *in vitro* must be shown to actually inhibit cellular proliferation to be seriously considered as a factor which may have immunosuppressive activity *in vivo*.

3.2.4. *Macrophage Activation as a Result of Interaction with Exogenous Agents or with Lymphocytes and Their Mediators*

As previously discussed, macrophages which are in states of increased activation, usually associated with increased rates of protein synthesis, are more suppressive on a per cell basis than less activated macrophages. A number of agents are known to stimulate the reticuloendothelial system (RES) which results in the appearance of highly activated macrophages in the organs of the lymphoid system and particularly in the spleen. Similar effects on the activation of macrophages by such agents have been observed *in vitro*. First, we will discuss exogenous agents which activate macrophages and the little that is known about the mechanisms involved. Then we will discuss possible mechanisms by which suppressor macrophage activity may be enhanced or regulated by interaction with lymphocytes or their mediators during the induction of an immune response.

Several agents capable of activating macrophages are known. Bacterial products can activate macrophages. Shilo (1959) has reviewed evidence that in the case of gram negative bacteria, the lipopolysaccharide component of the cell wall, and particularly the lipid A component, is a potent macrophage activator. Other macrophage activators include certain organisms such as *C. parvum* (Halpern *et al.*, 1964), *Listeria monocytogenes*, BCG, *Mycobacterium tuberculosis* (reviewed by McGregor and Logie, 1975) and double-stranded RNA (reviewed by Allison and Davies, 1975). The actual mechanism of macrophage activation by these agents is unknown. *C. parvum* has been extensively studied to learn why it is such a powerful RES stimulant. Prévot (1975) has suggested that a component of the bacterial cell wall is responsible for the intense RES activation and has tentatively named it 'reticulostimulin'. Efforts to purify reticulostimulin, however, have largely resulted in abrogation of the macrophage-activating effect (Adlam *et al.*, 1975) and thus have been unsuccessful. In addition to microbial agents such as *C. parvum*, most soluble adjuvants are known to stimulate reticuloendothelial proliferation and to activate macrophages (Unanue *et al.*, 1969a). Spitznagel and Allison (1970) have correlated the ability of various substances to labilize lysosomes in macrophages with their adjuvant effects. They found that retinol (vitamin A alcohol) and LPS were particularly active in this respect. Despite the large number of empirical observations that the administration of various agents such as those mentioned above results in RES activation, very little is known about the actual mechanisms involved. It seems likely that a greater understanding of the mechanisms of this important aspect of the immune response will enable such agents to be used as one of the means of intervening in and regulating the immune response in the future.

In addition to interaction with exogenous agents, macrophage–lymphocyte interactions also have been shown to result in activation of macrophages. Similar to the requirement for macrophages for the sensitization phase of most immune responses (discussed earlier in this review), macrophages have also been shown to be required to mediate the effector phase of the response in collaboration with sensitized lymphocytes in some cases. McGregor and Koster (1971) have shown that lasting immunity to *Listeria monocytogenes* in rats can be adoptively transferred with thoracic duct lymphocytes, but cannot be mediated without an intact macrophage system. Conversely, purified macrophages from immune animals could not transfer lasting immunity even to intact animals. These results suggest that certain immune effector functions require an interaction between immune T cells and macrophages which neither cell alone can carry out regardless of the immune status. Nathan *et al.* (1973) have studied mediators from T lymphocytes which affect macrophages. They found macrophage migration inhibition factor (MIF) to be particularly active in increasing macrophage adherence, phagocytosis, and glucose carbon 1 oxidative hexose monophosphate shunt pathway metabolism. Moreover, they found that interaction of macrophages with MIF also results in increased protein synthesis. Two to three days of exposure to the lymphokine *in vitro* was required before the effects became detectable in their system (Nathan *et al.*, 1971). In a recent review of the effect of lymphocyte mediators on macrophages, David (1975) has confirmed and extended the reports of Nathan *et al.* (1973). He discussed evidence that, in addition to the metabolic and morphologic effects on macrophages attributed to MIF by Nathan *et al.* (1973), MIF also decreased lysosomal enzymes, increased the cytoplasmic enzyme lactic dehydrogenase, as well as membrane adenylate cyclase, and increased glucosamine incorporation. More importantly, bacteriostasis to *Listeria monocytogenes* and tumoricidal activity have been shown to be strongly enhanced.

Recently Taramelli and her colleagues have examined the signals required for the induction of suppressor macrophages *in vitro*. Blomgren *et al.* (1976) reported that macrophages could be induced to be suppressive for Con A-stimulated lymphocytes after they were treated with a lymphokine supernatant. Similarly, Proteose peptone-elicited macrophages, after treatment overnight with lymphokines, developed the ability to suppress the production of lymphokines (Taramelli *et al.*, 1981). However, not all agents that could activate macrophages to become tumoricidal induced suppressor macrophages. Interferon, poly I:C and endotoxin were found to induce tumoricidal macrophages without concomitantly engendering suppression of lymphokine production. This would suggest that there are different mechanisms involved at either the induction or effector phase of these responses or that different subpopulations of cells are involved.

Thus, there is ample evidence that macrophages can be activated by interaction with a number of agents including lymphocyte mediators, the best studied of which is MIF. As a result of interaction with MIF, various parameters of macrophage activation such as the rate of protein synthesis were found to be increased. As we have discussed, the rate of macrophage protein synthesis correlated quite well with the suppressor activity of macrophages. Therefore, it is obvious that a number of agents, including products of activated lymphocytes (at least MIF), are capable of augmenting suppressor macrophage activity.

3.3. *The Relationship of Suppressor T Cells to Suppressor Macrophages*

Recent reports of suppressor cells other than macrophages include the specific suppressor T cells of Tada and Taniguchi (1976) and the allotype suppressor T cells described by Herzenberg *et al.* (1976). In addition, Dutton (1972) has shown that Con A-stimulated T cells can nonspecifically block anti-SRBC responses in Mishell–Dutton culture systems *in vitro*. Similarly, Peavy and Pierce (1974) have used Con A-stimulated T cells to nonspecifically suppress the generation of cytotoxic effector cells to alloantigens in MLC–CML reactions. The mechanism of action in both cases is thought to be a suppression of the proliferative event required for the expression of the effector function (Dutton, 1972; Peavy and Pierce, 1974). However, just because an element of the suppressor cycle is a T lymphocyte does not mean that the macrophages are not an integral part of the observed suppression. Gershon (1974), in an exhaustive review of suppressor T cells, has allowed that the role of macrophages in the actual inhibition of proliferation resulting from suppressor T cell activity is uncertain. A good example of the contribution of macrophages to T cell-mediated suppression has been elucidated by Pierce and his collaborators. Rich and Pierce (1974) first described a suppressor factor that was isolated from supernatants of Con A-stimulated spleen cells. The factor has been termed 'SIRS' for soluble immune response suppressor. This factor nonspecifically inhibits IgG and IgM plaque-forming cell responses, cytotoxic T cell responses and proliferative responses to a variety of antigens and is produced by Lyt 2^+ T lymphocytes (Peavy and Pierce, 1974; Rich and Pierce, 1974; Jandinski *et al.*, 1976; Pierce and Kapp, 1976). Characterization of SIRS reveals that it is a glycoprotein with a molecular weight of 45,000–55,000 (Tadakuma *et al.*, 1976a). Thus far, SIRS has been indistinguishable from MIF (Tadakuma *et al.*, 1976b). SIRS appears to be distinct from immunoglobulins in that it does not bind to immunoabsorbant columns coated with anti-mouse IgG or IgM (Tadakuma *et al.*, 1976a). Tadakuma *et al.* (1976b) demonstrated that SIRS does not act directly on B or T cells, but requires macrophages to mediate its effect. Subsequently it was shown that SIRS appears to be converted to a macrophage-derived suppressor factor (MØ SF) by macrophage H_2O_2 (Aune and Pierce, 1981a, b). Thus macrophages are involved in the final generation of the suppressor factor.

Folch and Waksman (1974) have shown that normal rat spleens contain suppressor cells which can suppress the proliferative response in mixed leukocyte cultures. The effector cells mediating the suppression were adherent, but cells from donors having undergone adult thymectomy, irradiation and bone marrow reconstitution were inactive. They concluded that the suppressor cell was an adherent suppressor T cell. We have recently confirmed that normal rat spleens contain adherent cells which suppress MLC and CML reactivity (Oehler *et al.*, 1977b). However, we have also shown that the suppressor cells are phagocytic and *resistant* to treatment with a specific anti-T cell serum and complement. Our data indicate that the final effector cell mediating the suppression is a macrophage. To reconcile our findings with those of Folch and Waksman (1974), we have suggested that the activated macrophages in normal rat spleens are a reflection of, and dependent on, T cell activity *in vivo* (Oehler *et al.*, 1977c). The early findings of McGregor and Koster (1971) showing a macrophage requirement for the adoptive transfer by immune thoracic duct lymphocytes of immunity to *Listeria monocytogenes* may be explained in a similar manner. In this case, the immune T cells may have led to the gradual development of activated macrophages with anti-microbial activity.

3.4. Evidence That Suppressor Macrophages Can Suppress Immune Responses *In Vivo*

3.4.1. *Introductory Remarks*

Most of the clear-cut evidence that macrophages can act as suppressor cells comes from *in vitro* observations. It is rather difficult to directly relate such *in vitro* findings to the role of these cells in regulating the immune response *in vivo*. Part of this reflects the general problem of determining the *in vivo* role of *in vitro* phenomena. A classical approach in this direction has been to examine the effects of adoptive transfer of cells with a particular function *in vitro*. However, adoptive transfer of suppressor macrophages seems unlikely to confer a suppressed state on the recipient for at least two reasons. Firstly, highly activated macrophages undoubtedly do not stay highly activated long after transfer. Nathan *et al.* (1973) showed that macrophages activated by lymphocyte mediators *in vitro* remained activated only 24–48 hr after removal of the activating agent. Secondly, adoptively transferred, strongly activated macrophages might lodge at the site of inoculation or some other unwanted location and not migrate into the same lymphoid microenvironment as the lymphocytes engaged in the immune response or even into the appropriate lymphoid organs. Local adoptive transfer of macrophages, either admixed with responding lymphocytes or inoculated into the site of the immune response (e.g. draining lymph node), would be expected to overcome these problems. However, little evidence along these lines has been reported. The main approach which has been made to evaluate the *in vivo* role of macrophages is to administer agents which can stimulate the reticulo-endothelial system (RES) and cause the activation and migration of macrophages into the lymphoid and circulatory systems. In addition, various pathological conditions, both experimentally induced and naturally occurring which are associated with RES stimulation, present opportunities to observe the effect of strongly activated macrophages in high cell densities in the proximity of lymphocytes during the generation of an immune response *in vivo*. There are a number of studies showing a depressed immune response in the presence of either a high macrophage cell density or a highly activated RES. Based in part on the *in vitro* evidence discussed above, one might predict that immune responses requiring the generation of an expanding clone of antigen-sensitized lymphocytes would be suppressed if sufficient suppressor macrophage activity were present during the proliferative phase of the response. Interpretation of such studies, however, is complicated by the fact that the stimulating agents have *in vivo* effects other than activation of macrophages, and also that macrophages are involved at many levels of the immune response, both in initiating immune responses, i.e. antigen presentation, antigen processing, prevention of tolerance, and frequently in the final effector phases of the immune response, i.e. delayed hypersensitivity (Scott, 1974), tumor (Remington *et al.*, 1975; Hibbs *et al.*, 1972; Evans and Alexander, 1972) and tissue graft rejection (Evans and Grant, 1972), and protection from certain infectious agents (Gadebusch, 1972). It has been possible to design experiments to take advantage of the fact that macrophage participation in various phases of an immune response to an antigenic challenge do not necessarily occur simultaneously. Shortly after antigenic challenge, macrophages aid in sensitizing lymphocytes. Then, after a lag period which varies from 24–28 hr to several days, depending on the antigen, the lymphoproliferative phase begins, followed by the appearance of the effector phase of the immune response, i.e. antibody production, cytotoxic T cell appearance, memory cell distribution and/or macrophage activation. Thus, the lymphoproliferative phase occurs some time after antigen inoculation and continues through the time of the appearance of the effector aspect of the response. To demonstrate suppressive effects of macrophage activation, the optimal time of most intense macrophage activation should be during the proliferative phase, i.e. some time after antigen inoculation and before the appearance of effector cells (plasma cells or cytotoxic T cells). Similar to the kinetics of the immune response, the length of time between injection of a stimulating agent and the appearance of maximal macrophage activation must be taken into account. The kinetics of the appearance of suppressor macrophages in the spleen of experimental animals differs slightly with the particular activating agent used, the dose and the route of administration.

Thus the most convincing evidence that suppressor macrophages can inhibit the generation of an immune response *in vivo* would come from experiments in which suppressor macrophages and few proliferating lymphocytes have been shown to be in lymphoid organs at the time when one would expect the lymphoproliferative phase of the immune response to be occurring. Ideally, one might then find that upon removal of inactivation of suppressor macrophages, fully immunocompetent lymphocytes remain. In addition, *in vivo* administration of agents which inactivate macrophages without interfering with their numerous enhancing effects would be expected to reverse the immunosuppression. Such evidence would point to suppressor macrophages as the main or only cause for the suppressed immune response observed *in vivo*.

In the sections to follow, we shall review the available evidence for *in vivo* suppression of immune responses by macrophages. In addition, evidence will be reviewed regarding the possibility that some forms of antigenic competition may be due to the appearance of splenic suppressor macrophages.

3.4.2. *Suppression Directly Related to Macrophage Concentration* In Vivo

A simple but still somewhat artificial way to observe the effects of local adoptive transfer of high macrophage concentrations on antigen-triggered lymphocytes *in vivo* would be to place antigen-primed lymphocytes in a small Millipore chamber with the antigen and a large number of macrophages, and implant the chamber into the peritoneal cavity of a lethally irradiated histocompatible mouse. Measurement of the resultant serum and chamber antibody levels and comparison with levels generated in mice in which similar chambers were implanted without high numbers of macrophages would give some indication of the effect of the extra macrophages.

Using such an experimental design, Perkins and Makinodan (1965) placed SRBC-primed mouse spleen cells in 0.1 μm Milliport chambers with SRBC and various numbers of peritoneal exudate cells and implanted them in irradiated mice. As controls, they implanted chambers to which they added either unprimed mouse spleen cells in numbers equal to the primed responding cells plus SRBC or primed responding cells plus SRBC alone. After 9 days, they measured the hemolysin titer in both the chamber fluid and the serum. The antibody titers from mice bearing chambers containing primed spleen cells plus SRBC were very similar to those with primed spleen cells, SRBC and equal numbers of unprimed spleen cells. In contrast, the chamber fluid or sera from mice bearing chambers containing additional PEC sufficient to make up 20–30 per cent of the primed responding cell had markedly depressed titers. No concentration of PEC produced enhanced antibody production and high numbers of PEC completely suppressed the response. To reduce the artificiality of the approach with Millipore chambers, similar experiments were designed in which mice were injected intraperitoneally with glycogen to increase the number and the level of activation of the peritoneal macrophages, or only with saline. Both groups were challenged with SRBC i.p. and the serum hemolysin titers measured every other day for 10 days. At all time points tested, mice pretreated with glycogen had lower serum antibody levels compared to the saline-injected controls. The objective of these experiments was to obtain *in vivo* data to support the notion that macrophages enhanced the SRBC response, but the results which were in the opposite direction indicated that high cell densities of macrophages in the environment of lymphocytes which were stimulated to proliferate and produce antibody could suppress antibody production *in vivo*. Hoffman (1970), using an *in vitro* Mishell–Dutton culture system, obtained similar results and, in addition, provided evidence that the suppressive effect of the high concentration of macrophages was mediated through an inhibition of the proliferative phase of the response. He found that the optimal macrophage concentration for an *in vitro* SRBC response was 2 per cent of the responding spleen cells. Adding purified peritoneal macrophages to a final concentration of 20 per cent of the responding spleen cell population resulted in profound inhibition of the response. Moreover, analysis of the cells in the suppressed cultures revealed greatly decreased blastogenesis and plasma cell formation. He postulated that the high concentration of macrophages inhibited the proliferation of antigen-sensitive cells, thereby preventing a clonal expansion of cells destined to produce antibody. Alternatively, since T cells are also required to provide a helper factor for the production of antibody to heterologous erythrocytes, both *in vitro* and *in vivo* (reviewed in Oppenheim and Rosenstreich, 1976; Katz and Benacerraf, 1972), the suppressive effect of macrophages could have been mediated through inhibition of the T cell response. However, there is little if any evidence that macrophages can suppress the production and release of factors *per se*. So this alternative seems unlikely. Moreover, evidence has been presented that suppressor macrophages can inhibit LPS-induced B cell proliferative responses in mice (Kirchner *et al.*, 1974b) and rats (Yoshinaga *et al.*, 1972). Since LPS induces B cell proliferation directly without the aid of accessory cells (Lipsky and Rosenthal, 1976; reviewed by Oppenheim and Rosenstreich, 1976), it would appear that macrophages are capable of suppressing B cell proliferation directly. Thus, it is likely that the suppression by high concentrations of macrophages of antibody production in the above cases was due to inhibition of proliferation of the antigen-sensitized clone of B cells.

3.4.3. *Suppression of Antibody Production* In Vivo *by a Macrophage-Activating Agent*

Lipopolysaccharide has been shown to activate macrophages (see Section 3.2.4) and *in vivo* inoculation of this material has been shown to inhibit immune responsiveness (Bradley and Watson, 1964; Franzl and McMaster, 1968). As predicted above, the demonstration of LPS-induced suppression is very dependent on the time of administration of LPS in relation to antigen inoculation. It seems necessary for the LPS to come in contact with macrophages which are closely associated with lymphoid cells prior to exposure to antigen. In other words, if LPS and the antigen (SRBC) were given by the same route, the LPS had to be given 24–48 hr prior to the antigen. Only relatively large doses of LPS induced suppression when given i.p. 24 hr before antigen inoculation into the same area. If LPS was given i.v. 24 hr before antigen i.p., five-fold less endotoxin could totally abrogate the anti-SRBC response (Franzl and McMaster, 1968). Similarly, Bradley and Watson (1964) have shown that a relatively large dose of LPS given to mice at the time of injection of actinophage MSP8 simply delayed the production of neutralizing antibody, whereas daily injections of LPS suppressed the antibody production indefinitely despite continued presence of the phage in the tissues of the animal. Further, hyperimmunized mice with high levels of circulating antibody could be suppressed with daily LPS administration. When the LPS was stopped, the antibody production resumed as indicated by the prompt appearance of high serum levels of neutralizing antibody. The results of these studies indicate that antibody production in mice can be suppressed by an agent which activates macrophages. However, it is possible that the inhibitory effects of LPS are independent of macrophages, since as noted above, LPS can have direct effects on B cells.

3.4.4. *The Suppressive Effect of* C. parvum *on the Generation of Resistance to Tumor Cells*

C. parvum is a powerful RES-activating agent (Halpern *et al.*, 1963) which can induce splenic suppressor macrophages in mice (Kirchner *et al.*, 1975c; Scott, 1972). Similarly, *C. parvum* injection has been shown to suppress some immune responses requiring proliferation *in vivo*. Immunization procedures which normally conferred a significant amount of protection from tumor challenge were much less effective if instituted 4–5 days after *C. parvum* injection (Smith and Scott, 1972; Woodruff *et al.*, 1976). The studies of Scott (1972) demonstrated the temporal relationship between *C. parvum* injection and the appearance of suppressor macrophages. Intravenous inoculation of *C. parvum* produced maximal suppression of responsiveness of spleen cells to PHA at day 7, with some persisting inhibition through day 28. This suppression was shown to be mediated by macrophages. Considering this time course for the appearance of suppressor cells in the spleen after *C. parvum* injection, one might predict that immune responses generated in the spleen and dependent upon the rapid expansion of an antigen-sensitized clone of lymphocytes would be suppressed if the proliferative response occurred about 7 days after *C. parvum* injection. Thereafter (for at least 2 weeks) moderate suppression might be observed. Smith and Scott (1972) investigated the protective effects of *C. parvum* injection on challenge of CBA mice with R–1 leukemia cells (a radiation-induced syngeneic leukemia). Inoculation of unimmunized mice with as few as ten tumor cells i.p. resulted in the death of all recipients with 10–15 days. When mice were immunized with a single dose of 1×10^5 heavily irradiated R–1 cells 7 days prior to the inoculation of 100 R–1 cells i.p., 50 per cent of the mice survived. When *C. parvum* was given 7 days before the immunizing dose of irradiated R–1 cells, 90 per cent of the mice died within 20 days of the injection of non-irradiated R–1 cells. Similarly, Woodruff *et al.* (1976) have reported that in CBA mice, protection against a syngeneic chemically induced fibrosarcoma by immunization with irradiated tumor cells was decreased by pretreatment with *C. parvum* 5 days before the immunizing dose. Recent studies in our laboratory by Kirchner *et al.* (1975b) have provided insight into possible mechanisms operative in the experiments described above. C56BL/6 mice injected with Moloney sarcoma virus developed a tumor at the site of inoculation which reached maximum size 14 days after inoculation and regressed completely by 21 days (MSV mouse tumor system). Spleen cells taken from donors after tumor regression could be stimulated to become cytotoxic *in vitro* by cocultivation with mitomycin C-treated RBL–5 tumor cells, shown to contain relevant antigens (Herberman *et al.*, 1974). To test the effect of *C. parvum* inoculation in this system, mice were given *C. parvum* i.p. 23 days after virus infection, and 7 days later primed spleen cells from these mice were cultured *in vitro* with RBL–5 to generate cytotoxic effector cells. The cytotoxicity generated with such cells was much lower than that generated with spleen cells from immune mice not treated with *C. parvum*. This effect of *C. parvum* appeared to be mediated by suppressor macrophages, since mixture of immune spleen cells with spleen cells from mice inoculated 8–10 days earlier with *C. parvum* resulted in a marked suppression of generation of cytotoxicity. The suppression by the spleen cells from *C. parvum*-treated mice was dependent on the presence of macrophages but not T cells. Bernstein *et al.* (1977) have recently shown that the generation of cytotoxic effector cells from non-cytotoxic primed rat spleen cells required the proliferation of a clone of lymphocytes during cocultivation with mitomycin-treated (C58NT)D tumor cells. Similarly, our laboratory has provided evidence that a proliferative response is also required for the generation of cytotoxic effector cells *in vitro* from non-cytotoxic primed cells in the MSV mouse tumor system (Stiller, Holden and Herberman, unpublished observations). Thus it seems likely that the suppressed cytotoxic response generated *in vitro* by *C. parvum*-pretreated MSV immune mice was due to the inhibition of the required lymphoproliferative response by the *C. parvum*-induced suppressor macrophages. These observations by no means prove that the interference with tumor resistance (Smith and Scott, 1972; Woodruff *et al.*, 1976) was caused by the inhibition of a proliferative response required to generate an immune state, but the similarities between the *in vivo* observations and the *in vitro* findings are striking. An important issue is whether the increased numbers of activated macrophages found in the spleens of animals treated with *C. parvum* (or other RES stimulants) can inhibit lymphoproliferative responses sufficiently to suppress *in vivo* generation of cytotoxic effector cells. Evidence that spleens of *C. parvum*-treated mice can inhibit the proliferation of antigen-stimulated lymphoid cells *in vivo* has been provided by Howard *et al.* (1967). They treated F_1 hybrid mice with i.v. *C. parvum* 4 days before i.v. injection of 10^8 viable parental lymphoid cells, thus initiating a graft versus host (GVH) reaction in the environment of a highly stimulated reticuloendothelial system. The pretreatment with *C. parvum* protected the majority of the mice from the uniformly fatal GVH reaction which occurred in the untreated control mice. Evidence for the mechanism of action of the protective effect was obtained by examining the spleens of representative mice from each group for proliferating lymphocytes. Twelve days after GVH initiation, the percentage of donor cells in mitosis was 85–90 per cent in the untreated F_1 hybrid recipients. In contrast, only 0–5 per cent of the proliferating cells were of donor origin in the mice pretreated with *C. parvum*. These data show that *C. parvum* induced an environment in the spleens of mice which suppressed rapidly-proliferating alloantigen-stimulated parental lymphoid cells *in vivo*. It remains to be directly demonstrated that macrophages were in fact responsible for the anti-proliferative effect.

C. parvum and other potent RES stimulators are frequently used as immunotherapeutic agents to increase resistance against tumor growth. However, the observations discussed above indicate that, under some circumstances, these agents may actually interfere with effective anti-tumor immunity and that these immunosuppressive effects may be mediated by suppressor macrophages.

3.4.5. *The Possible Role of Suppressor Macrophages in Antigenic Competition*

The interference with the immune response to an antigen by prior inoculation with high doses of a non-cross-reactive second antigen has been termed antigenic competition. Antigenic competition has been extensively studied and the subject has been thoroughly reviewed recently (Pross and Eidinger, 1974). As suggested by Pross and Eidinger (1974), it seems likely that numerous mechanisms of action are responsible for the various phenomena grouped under the heading of antigenic competition. Since some instances of antigenic competition can actually be shown to be suppressive phenomena and the suppression is at least associated with an inhibition of proliferative response, suppressor macrophages should be considered as one type of mediator of these effects.

Several lines of evidence suggest that some forms of antigenic competition may actually be mediated through a suppressor mechanism rather than direct competition between antigens for responding cells. Sjöberg and Britton (1972) have shown that spleen cells from mice heavily preimmunized with SRBC suppressed the PFU response of normal mouse spleen cells to horse red blood cells (HRBC) when cocultivated in Mishell–Dutton culture systems in the presence of SRBC. Similarly, Thomas *et al.* (1975) have shown that when spleen cells from mice immunized with ovalbumin (OVA) were added with OVA to Mishell–Dutton cultures with SRBC-primed spleen cells the SRBC-specific PFU response was suppressed compared to cultures in which either the OVA or the OVA immune spleen cells were omitted. Further, Thomas *et al.* (1975) reported that in suppressed cultures, ^{3}H–TdR incorporation was depressed compared to nonsuppressed control cultures, indicating that the mechanism of the suppressor effect involved the proliferation rate of the responding cells. Möller (1971a) has presented evidence that DNA synthesis in the spleen of mice subjected to antigenic competition is reduced compared to normal controls. When mice were preimmunized by two injections of HRBC and then irradiated with 900 r before receiving normal spleen cells in adoptive transfer, the rate of DNA synthesis in the spleen as determined by ^{125}IUdR incorporation *in vivo* was suppressed by 40–50 per cent when compared to unimmunized but otherwise similarly treated control mice. Whether T cells or B cells were preferentially suppressed in these systems was not tested. However, there is evidence that the suppressive effect can be observed on either population. Although it is generally accepted that the induction of antigenic competition requires injection of a T-dependent antigen (reviewed in Pross and Eidinger, 1974), the antibody response to T-independent antigens was shown to be susceptible to suppression (Sjöberg and Britton, 1972), suggesting that B cells could be suppressed directly. On the other hand, Bash *et al.* (1976) have shown that spleen cells from rats injected 24 hr earlier with large doses of OVA i.v. responded poorly to PHA compared to normal controls, and when mixed with normal spleen cells, these cells were highly suppressive. The experiments showed that the suppressive effect on proliferation *in vitro* could also affect T cells. The apparent lack of specificity of the suppressor effect is consistent with the nonspecific nature of suppressor macrophage activity (reviewed by Kirchner *et al.*, 1976). Bash *et al.* (1976) have shown that the suppressor cell activated by injection of large doses of OVA is adherent and somewhat sensitive to carrageenan [a specific macrophage toxin (Lake *et al.*, 1971)]. However, since low doses of cyclophosphamide given i.p. at the time of antigen administration *in vivo* also abrogated the suppressor effect, the authors concluded that T cells and macrophages acted synergistically to be suppressive. Thomas *et al.* (1975) have shown that the suppression of AFC production *in vitro* by OVA immune mouse spleen cells cultured in the presence of OVA was mediated by a soluble suppressor factor produced by T cells. The characteristics of the factor are not unlike those of 'SIRS', another soluble suppressor described by Rich and Pierce (1974) and characterized by Tadakuma *et al.* (1976). SIRS, as discussed above (Section 3.3), is a product of Con A-stimulated T cells which can nonspecifically suppress AFC production to heterologous erythrocytes *in vitro*. The mechanism of action has to some extent been elucidated in that the target cell has been shown to be a macrophage in the responding cell population (Tadakuma *et al.*, 1976). Thus, the role of suppressor macrophages in the experiments reported by Thomas *et al.* (1975) would seem to require further investigation.

In summary, although the mechanisms for antigenic competition are largely unknown and may be quite heterogeneous, in the instances in which suppression of proliferation is associated with the depressed response, it seems likely that suppressor macrophages activated by antigen-stimulated T cells or their products play a role.

3.4.6. *The Role of Macrophages in Immunosuppression Associated with Graft Versus Host Disease*

In mice, antibody responses to SRBC have been shown to be greatly suppressed *in vivo* after induction of chronic GVH disease (Blanden, 1969; Möller, 1971b). Blanden (1969) also has shown that in mice undergoing mild chronic GVH, immunization with KLH in complete Freund's adjuvant was virtually ineffective, as indicated by a greatly depressed immediate hypersensitivity reaction upon challenge with antigen. Similarly, PFU responses generated *in vivo* to T-independent antigens have also been shown to be suppressed in mice undergoing chronic GVH. In contrast to the decreased humoral response to the various types of antigens (cellular, soluble, T-dependent and T-independent), the resistance of such mice to infection with *Listeria monocytogenes* was significantly increased (Blanden, 1969). Such increased resistance has frequently been associated with elevated levels of macrophage activity (McGregor and Koster, 1971). As discussed earlier, states of increased macrophage activation *in vivo* have occasionally been associated with immunosuppressive effects. One might therefore predict that normal syngeneic lymphoid cells adoptively transferred into irradiated animals undergoing chronic GVH disease would be immunosuppressed. Möller (1971b) has shown that this is indeed the case. He found that both primed and normal spleen cells when adoptively transferred into irradiated F_1 mice undergoing chronic GVH disease had strongly suppressed antibody responses to i.v. SRBC when compared to irradiated and adoptively transferred but otherwise normal F_1 control recipients. Byfield *et al.* (1973) showed that viable parental T cells were required in the cells injected to induce GVH disease-related suppression of the response to SIII. However, certain aspects of their findings led them to postulate that macrophages, perhaps activated in response to the alloantigen-stimulated parental T cells, in fact directly mediated the suppressor effect. This was supported by the findings of Sjöberg (1971, 1972). He has shown that spleens taken from F_1 hybrid donors 1 week after induction of GVH disease (GVH spleen cells) were essentially unresponsive to SRBC in Mishell–Dutton cultures. Moreover, when GVH spleen cells were added to normal or primed F_1 or parental spleen cells with SRBC, the response was strongly suppressed compared to F_1 or parental spleen cells cultured with SRBC alone (Sjöberg, 1971). The media from suppressed cultures could support strong anti-SRBC responses of normal spleen cells, indicating the suppression was not due to media exhaustion or a stable soluble factor. Pretreatment of the GVH spleen cells with anti-theta and complement before mixing with normal cells did not abrogate the suppressor activity. Depletion of phagocytes from the GVH spleen cells with iron and magnet treatment did abrogate the suppressor effect, indicating that the suppressor cell was a macrophage (Sjöberg, 1972). Thus, taken together, the findings of Byfield *et al.* (1973) and Sjöberg (1971, 1972) provided further evidence that in some cases, suppressor macrophages can be generated in response to activated T cells.

In addition to the suppressed humoral responses observed in chronic GVH disease, cellular reactions have also been shown to be suppressed. Lapp and Möller (1969) have shown that skin grafts from allogeneic mice survived significantly longer when grafted to unrelated F_1 hybrid recipients undergoing GVH disease. Both primary and secondary set rejection times could be delayed. However, the mechanism for this immune suppression has not been extensively studied.

Chronic GVH disease then appears to be another example of a situation in which suppressed immune responses can be demonstrated *in vivo* and in which the suppression of the responses *in vitro* can be shown to be mediated by macrophages. Further, as in the case of antigenic competition, it seems likely that the suppressor macrophages are T cell-dependent.

3.4.7. *The Role of Macrophages in Immunosuppression Associated with Cancer and Other Pathological Conditions*

Cancer, miliary tuberculosis, sarcoidosis, lepromatous leprosy and severe viral illnesses are among those diseases associated with depressed humoral and cellular responsiveness (Hersh *et al.*, 1973; Smith, 1972; Turk and Waters, 1971). Patients with advanced cancer have long been known to have suppressed delayed hypersensitivity responses when skin tested with tuberculin (Renaud, 1926), mumps (Logan, 1956; Lamb *et al.*, 1962) and other microbial antigens (Logan, 1956; Lamb *et al.*, 1962; Solowey and Rappaport, 1965). In addition, there is evidence that some cancer patients have a delayed rejection of allogeneic grafts of skin and tumor cells (Gardner and Preston, 1962). Lee *et al.* (1970) were able to demonstrate significant impairment of the ability of non-lymphoid cancer patients to generate serum levels of antibody to flagellin from *Salmonella adelaide* when compared to the response of age-matched, hospitalized patients with diseases thought not to have immunosuppressive effects. Whether such depressed cellular and humoral immune responses precede and perhaps play an etiologic role in these conditions, or are a result of them is uncertain. In the case of cancer patients, however, the demonstration of an anergic state is frequently associated with a poor prognosis (reviewed by Hersh *et al.*, 1973). Thus, insight into the mechanisms resulting in such disease-related immunosuppression could be helpful in developing a more sophisticated approach to the medical management of this group of patients.

Patients with multiple myeloma frequently have suppressed serum levels of normal immunoglobulin, respond poorly to antigenic stimulation, and are highly susceptible to infection (Fahey *et al.*, 1963; Broder *et al.*, 1975). Broder *et al.* (1975) have shown that PBL from multiple myeloma patients cultured *in vitro* with pokeweed mitogen (PWM) synthesized significantly less immunoglobulin than PBL from normal volunteers under similar conditions. In addition, in many cases, PBL from multiple myeloma patients, when added to normal PBL, suppressed their immunoglobulin synthesis in response to PWM. When phagocytic mononuclear cells were depleted from the PBL of the multiple myeloma patients, the ability to suppress normal PBL immunoglobulin synthesis in response to PWM was largely abrogated. Moreover, the response of PBLs of a myeloma patient to PWM was greatly improved by removal of phagocytic cells. PWM induces a blastogenic response in both T cells and B cells (reviewed by Oppenheim and Rosenstreich, 1976) and X-irradiation of human B cells prior to culture with PWM prevents the appearance of immunoglobulin in the media (T. Waldmann, personal communication). These findings suggest that monocytes in the PBL of some myeloma patients can suppress the proliferation and immunoglobulin production of human B cells *in vitro*. Similarly, in a rodent plasmacytoma model (Krakauer *et al.*, 1976), ascitic fluid from tumor-bearing hypogammaglobulinemic mice was found to contain a low molecular weight trypsin-sensitive factor which suppressed PWM-induced immunoglobulin synthesis by normal mouse spleen cells or human PBL. When the ascites from such mice was depleted of phagocytic cells, the suppressor factor could no longer be demonstrated. Similarly, Kolb *et al.* (1977) have found that macrophages in the spleens taken from hypogammaglobulinemic mice bearing large plasmacytomas suppressed the PFC response of normal spleen cells to SRBC in a Mishell–Dutton culture system when added in as third parties. These studies taken together provide evidence that in both mice and humans suppressor macrophages and/or their products can suppress the production of immunoglobulin by B cells from normal or tumor-bearing individuals *in vitro*. These findings are consistent with the findings of Kirchner *et al.* (1976) and others (Yoshinaga *et al.*, 1972) that in animal systems, B cell mitogen-induced proliferative responses can be suppressed by suppressor macrophages.

Allogeneic skin graft survival was prolonged on some patients bearing malignant neoplasms (Gardner and Preston, 1962). A number of *in vitro* observations of suppressed MLC responses using cells from cancer patients have provided evidence that suppressor macrophages may be involved in this form of immunosuppression also. Berlinger *et al.* (1976) have compared MLC reactivity of PBL from patients with solid, non-lymphoid malignancies to the reactivity of PBL from normal donors. They were able to identify a group of cancer patients in whom MLC reactivity was consistently depressed compared to normal controls. When the PBL with suppressed responsiveness were passed through a Sephadex G–10 column which selectively depleted monocytes, the MLC reactivity was improved in all cases which were suppressed. When PBL from normal donors were similarly filtered, no such effect was seen. Our laboratory (Jerrells, Dean and Herberman, unpublished observations) has confirmed that the lymphoproliferative responses of some cancer patients to mitogens or to allogeneic PBL could be significantly increased by passage of their PBL over Sephadex G–10 columns. Furthermore, the addition of mitomycin C-treated PBL from these patients to cultures of normal PBL could significantly inhibit proliferative responses to T cell mitogens. However, this mechanism does not appear to account for the depressed lymphoproliferative responses of all such patients, since in some cases, the responses remained depressed after removal of adherent cells. Twomey *et al.* (1975) have shown that PBL from patients with Hodgkin's disease stimulated normal PBL poorly in MLCs. When adherent cells were depleted from the patients' cells used as stimulators, strong MLC responses were observed. They could show that the suppressor cell was radioresistant and required protein synthesis to be suppressive, but their failure to show the cell was phagocytic using a 'modified technique' led them to postulate that the suppressor cell was a lymphocyte similar to that observed in normal rat spleen cells by Folch and Waksman (1974). As discussed earlier, recent evidence suggests that the cells described by Folch and Waksman were actually T cell-dependent suppressor macrophages. Thus it is possible that the findings of Twomey *et al.* (1975) may also support the notion that suppressor macrophages from PBL of cancer patients can suppress the proliferative phase of the response to alloantigens *in vitro*.

Studies in experimental animal tumor systems have provided a firm basis for the role of suppressor macrophages in the immunodepression of tumor-bearing individuals. Our laboratory (Fernbach *et al.*, 1976b) has shown that spleen cells from mice bearing MSV-induced tumors responded poorly in MLC and CML reactions. As described earlier, these depressed responses were shown to be mediated by suppressor macrophages. Veit and Feldman (1976a) have studied a rat tumor model in which they found suppressed MLC responsiveness with spleen cells from tumor-bearing rats. Extensive cell characterization procedures identified the suppressor cells as macrophages (Veit and Feldman, 1976b). Eggers and Wunderlich (1975) have provided evidence that spleen cells from mice bearing a methylcholanthrene-induced tumor also contained suppressor macrophages which suppressed the *in vitro* generation of cytotoxic effector cells to alloantigens. In contrast, Fujimoto *et al.* (1976a) have reported that when mice bearing methylcholanthrene-induced tumors served as donors of thymocytes to be adoptively transferred to syngeneic mice just prior to tumor inoculation, the rate of eventual tumor regression was slowed. Since thymocytes treated with anti-theta and complement had no such effect, Fujimoto *et al.* (1976b) concluded that the suppressor cells were T cells. However, since survival rates of the 'suppressed' and the nonsuppressed groups were identical, despite significant ($p < 0.001$) differences in the rate of tumor regression, it is difficult to draw firm conclusions from these experiments. Further, since all of the experiments were performed *in vivo*, the mechanism of the enhanced tumor growth, i.e. whether mediated through suppressor macrophages and acting on the immune response to the tumor or by direct enhancement of the growth of the tumor, would seem to be an open question.

Thus, suppressed T cell responses to alloantigens have been demonstrated in a variety of tumor systems. In mice, rats and humans, suppressed MLC responses have been shown to be due to cells which have been characterized as monocytes or macrophages by a number of criteria. Spontaneously occurring tumors as well as tumors induced by virus infection and carcinogen inoculation have been shown to induce suppressor monocytes or macrophages in the PBL of humans or spleen of mice and rats which can suppress reactivity to alloantigens. Therefore, these *in vitro* findings provide at least one possible explanation for the observations that allogeneic skin graft survival is prolonged in cancer patients. It would seem that further investigations designed to clearly define the role of suppressor macrophages in suppression of immune responses to alloantigens *in vivo* are indicated.

In addition to cancer, certain infectious diseases are known to be associated with suppression of immune responses. Generally, the degree of immunosuppression has correlated with the severity of the disease. The cause and effect relationship between the phenomena is an important question to be answered. Leprosy, a human disease caused by infection with *Mycobacterium leprae*, has provided insight into the correlation of immunosuppression with the severity of disease. Turk and Waters (1971) studied histological sections of lymph nodes taken from patients with leprosy varying in severity from *tuberculoid* leprosy (with the best prognosis), through *borderline* leprosy (an intermediate stage), to *lepromatous* leprosy (disseminated disease). *Tuberculoid* leprosy was associated either with a completely normal appearing lymph node or with nodes demonstrating a lymphocytosis of the paracortical areas [generally considered to be thymus-dependent (Parrot and Desousa, 1971)]. Occasionally, lymphoblasts were noted in the paracortical areas, indicating the presence of ongoing lymphoproliferative responses. These patients responded well to intradermal lepromin testing and could be sensitized to dinitrochlorobenzene (DNCB). Lymph nodes from patients with leprosy of intermediate severity showed an infiltration of the paracortical regions with epithelioid-like cells which remained distinctly separate from the lymphocytes. These patients responded to intradermal lepromin albeit poorly, but could be sensitized to DNCB. In *lepromatous* leprosy, paracortical areas of lymph nodes were heavily infiltrated with foamy histiocytes and the germinal centers manifested a hyperplastic plasmacytosis. These patients had a negative lepromin test and usually could not be sensitized to DNCB. Thus, this study provides *in vivo* morphological evidence for an association between severity of immunosuppression and macrophage infiltration of lymphoid tissues.

3.5. THE DIFFERENTIAL EFFECT OF MACROPHAGES ON NORMAL VERSUS NEOPLASTIC CELLS

Keller compared the effects of activated macrophages on normal versus neoplastic cells and found that, although both cell types undergo inhibition of proliferation, only neoplastic cells were killed (Keller, 1974a, 1976). Evidence supporting the notion that only neoplastic cells are killed by macrophages, thus establishing the concept of nonspecific but 'selective' macrophage-mediated cytotoxicity, has been provided by several laboratories (Currie and Basham, 1975; Cleveland *et al.*, 1974; Hibbs, 1973; Holterman *et al.*, 1973; Hibbs *et al.*, 1973; Piessens *et al.*, 1975). All of these studies, however, measured target cell lysis rather than target cell proliferation. Our laboratory (Kirchner *et al.*, 1974a, b, 1975) has noted on several occasions that the suppressive effect of macrophages on lymphocytes was not observed unless the lymphocytes were proliferating rapidly (i.e. stimulated by mitogens, tumor antigens, or alloantigens, etc.). One might therefore speculate that some property of transformed cells which is shared by proliferating lymphocytes but not by resting lymphocytes provides the basis by which macrophages exert their cytolytic and/or cytostatic effect. Evidence suggesting that rapidly proliferating cells are more susceptible to lysis by macrophages than resting cells has been provided by Holterman *et al.* (1975). They have shown that rat embryo fibroblasts are susceptible to cytolytic effects only during early passages in tissue culture, when their proliferation rate is high. They hypothesized that neoplastic cells may have certain membrane properties in common with rapidly proliferating embryonic cells of early passage *in vitro* which are subsequently lost through the process of differentiation. Fox *et al.* (1971) have provided evidence that mild proteolytic treatment of normal mouse fibroblasts maintained *in vitro* (3T3) resulted in the appearance of certain agglutinin receptors on the surface of the cell membrane which could always be demonstrated on the membrane of polyoma virus transformed mouse fibroblasts (Py3T3). The expression of the agglutinin receptors on the 3T3 cells was associated with an increased rate of proliferation and a loss of contact inhibition. The effect was transient, however, and when the proliferation rate returned to normal, the agglutinin receptors were no longer demonstrable. Although these studies were done with fibroblasts and not with lymphoid cells, they at least support the notion that rapidly proliferating cells may express receptors or membrane properties normally expressed 'selectively' on continually proliferating (transformed) cells. Shinitzky and Inbar (1974) have provided evidence that the microviscosity of the surface membrane lipid layer of normal lymphocytes and malignant lymphoma cells can be associated with the growth characteristics of the cells, and that by altering the microviscosity of the membrane with lecithin–cholesterol (1:1) liposomes, one can predictably modify the growth characteristics of the cells. These observations further emphasize the possibility that normal cells may transiently acquire membrane characteristics of transformed cells during blastogenesis. Thus, if the mechanism by which macrophages lyse transformed cells is the same as that mediating cytostasis of both cell types, the ability of lymphocytes to cover or fail to express some membrane property when their proliferation is inhibited could account for the findings that macrophages have cytostatic effects on both cell types but lyse only cells which are transformed. Another entirely possible explanation for the findings is that the effector cells involved in the cytolysis are not macrophages at all but instead are natural killer (NK) cells as recently described by Herberman *et al.* (1975). Recently Herberman *et al.* (1977) have shown that many agents with well-known RES activating effects strongly boost NK cell activity when administered to mice, and that the broad specificity of the cytolytic activity is directed primarily toward tumor cells. Similarly, Wolf *et al.* (1976) observed that i.p. injection of BCG caused the appearance of increased cytolytic activity by PEC and that most, if not all, of this activity was mediated by NK cells. Our laboratory is currently investigating the possibility that at least some of the selective cytolytic effects of PEC previously attributed to macrophages may be mediated by highly active NK cells.

4. CONCLUDING REMARKS

In this review we have discussed some of the evidence that macrophages provide both enhancing and suppressive effects on immune responses. The enhancing effects of macrophages might be grouped into three broad categories: prevention of tolerance, antigen presentation and enhancing factor production. In the case of subcellular protein antigens, macrophages phagocytize and break down much of the antigen, thus helping to prevent a prolonged interaction of B cells with high concentrations of free soluble antigen, in the absence of a second signal to produce antibody, which would be likely to result in a state of B cell tolerance. Some of the antigen, however, is not broken down by macrophages, but instead is expressed on the cell surface in a highly immunogenic form. Recent evidence suggests that one form taken by such antigen is that of a complex with the MHC antigens on the surface of the macrophage. As such, at least T cells can be primed or triggered with the resultant generation of helper T cells to provide a second signal to B cells for antibody production and/or a clone of highly reactive memory T cells which are then available to mediate a vigorous secondary response when presented with the same antigen in complex with the same MHC determinant on the surface of a macrophage. In addition to presentation of soluble antigens to T cells, there is a wealth of information suggesting that macrophages produce factors which can enhance the response of T cells to mitogens as well as to cellular antigens such as alloantigens in MLC or antigens on the surface of heterologous erythrocytes. More detailed discussion of these factors can be found elsewhere in this series. Less is known about the macrophage–B cell interaction. There are a number of reports showing that macrophages can stimulate B cells directly to proliferate and produce antibody. In addition, there is some evidence that macrophages may play a vital role in mediating T cell–B cell collaboration. Further investigations are needed to clarify these issues.

On the other hand, we have presented evidence that macrophages, if in sufficient quantity or if sufficiently activated, can suppress immune responses which are dependent or independent of proliferation. Suppression of T cell responses by suppressor macrophages *in vitro* could be correlated with evidence obtained *in vivo*, indicating that when macrophages were strongly activated during the time when a lymphocyte response should have occurred, the resultant immune state was frequently depressed. Similarly, since suppressor macrophages could also suppress B cell proliferative responses *in vitro,* it is not surprising that antibody responses requiring B cell proliferation were frequently suppressed in cases where the RES was highly activated such as in chronic graft versus host disease, some cases of antigenic competition and in the presence of a rapidly growing malignant tumor.

The suppressive effect of macrophages would seem to be important for several reasons. We have discussed evidence that suppressor macrophages could be induced by lymphocyte mediators. The best studied mediator apparently capable of inducing suppressor macrophages is MIF. In fact, as discussed, it seems likely that many if not all suppressor T cells may liberate factors which mediate the suppressor effect through macrophages. This then would appear to represent a mechanism by which a clonal expansion of sensitized lymphocytes could be slowed or stopped by a product of lymphocyte activation. Since 2 or 3 days are required to activate macrophages with lymphocyte mediators (see Section 3.2.4.), such a mechanism would not prevent the appearance of a significant number of effector cells and memory cells but could serve to limit their continued, excessive production. Such negative feedback systems have been described for many regulatory mechanisms in mammalian physiology. As we have discussed, suppressor macrophages have little or no suppressor effect on cytotoxic T cells or other effector cells which do not proliferate. Thus, established immune responses would not be affected through this mechanism.

In addition, macrophages can be activated to become suppressive by agents which may operate through mechanisms independent of lymphocytes. Agents or conditions which activate the RES, including the growth of many tumors, have frequently resulted in the appearance of splenic suppressor macrophages. Although in this review we have concentrated on reports of immunosuppression associated with administration of RES activators (*C. parvum* and BCG), in fact, these agents are generally thought of as immunopotentiators. However, a problem with the use of such agents is that the immunopotentiating effects are seen inconsistently and, frequently, immunosuppression is seen instead. The effects of these agents on the immune response *in vivo* are undoubtedly complex. When used correctly, RES stimulators may eventually prove very useful for immunotherapy. However, when immunosuppression occurs instead of immunopotentiation, it seems likely that suppressor macrophages play a role in the suppression. In the case of RES activation in response to tumor growth, an interesting situation arises. Although perhaps an appropriate response to the tumor, if the RES activation cannot control the growing neoplasm by direct cytostatic effects on the tumor cells, it is entirely possible that the resulting abundance of suppressor macrophages may play a role in the immunosuppressed state frequently observed in cancer patients. There are undoubtedly many ways in which tumors can cause immunosuppression. One way, however, might be through a mechanism by which tumor cells or tumor cell products lead to an activated RES which suppresses immune responses requiring lymphocyte proliferation. In this case, however, unlike the response of local macrophages to mediators from sensitized, activated, proliferating lymphocytes, the RES stimulus from the tumor might be more diffuse, involving a significant proportion of the lymphoid cells. One would predict that this would result in a prolonged, nonspecific state of immunosuppression.

Finally, we have briefly discussed the apparently reproducible observations that, although the cytostatic effects of macrophages on rapidly dividing lymphocytes and transformed cells seem highly correlative, the 'lytic effects of macrophages' are directed selectively toward cells that are neoplastic. Assuming that macrophages are indeed the effector cells, we have suggested that the basic recognition process leading to the cytostatic and the cytolytic events are similar, and that the selective lysis of neoplastic cells reflects the inability of tumor cells to modulate certain surface receptors shared by normal lymphocytes only during blastogenesis.

In summary, macrophages seem to be involved in almost every phase of the immune response. They can both enhance and suppress lymphocyte responses, and most lymphocyte responses require the presence of macrophages for any of a number of reasons to mount any response at all. The observations that suppressor T cells may mediate some if not all of their suppressor effects through suppressor macrophages help to explain what appeared to be a dual suppressor mechanism triggered by similar stimuli but mediated by different effector cells. The evidence discussed in this review supports the concept that macrophages play a central role in regulating some aspects of the immune response. Hopefully, further investigations of the immunobiology of macrophages will enable careful therapeutic intervention via this natural regulatory mechanism.

Acknowledgments—The authors wish to gratefully acknowledge many stimulating discussions with Dr. Holger Kirchner concerning the suppressive effects of macrophages. In addition, we thank Drs Santo Landolfo, Angela Santoni, and James Braatz for knowledgeable suggestions and helpful comments.
Finally, one of us thanks Laurie for being patient and understanding.

REFERENCES

ADLAM, C., REID, D. E. and TORKINGTON, P. (1975) The nature of the active principle of *Corynebacterium parvum*. In: *Corynebacterium Parvum; Applications in Experimental and Clinical Oncology* pp. 35–39, HALPERN, B. (ed.). Plenum Press, New York, London.

ALLISON, A. C. and DAVIES, P. (1975) Increased biochemical and biological activities of mononuclear phagocytes exposed to various stimuli, with special reference to secretion of lysosomal enzymes. In: *Mononuclear Phagocytes in Immunity, Infection and Pathology* pp. 487–506, FURTH, R. V. (ed.). Blackwell Scientific Publications, Oxford, London.

ALLISON, A. C., HAMMINGTON, J. S. and BIRBECK, M. (1966) An examination of the cytotoxic effects of silica on macrophages. *J. exp. Med.* **124**: 141–153.

ARGYRIS, B. F. (1968) Role of macrophages in immunological maturation *J. exp. Med.* **128**: 459–468.

BACH, F. H., ALTER, B. J., SOLLIDAY, S., ZOSCHKE, D. C. and JANIS, M. (1970) Lymphocyte reactivity *in vitro*. II. Soluble reconstituting factor permitting response of purified lymphocytes. *Cell. Immun.* **1**: 219–225.

BASH, J. A., SINGER, A. M. and WAKSMAN, B. H. (1976) The suppressive effect on the proliferative responses of rat T cells *in vitro*. II. Abrogation of antigen-induced suppression by selective cytotoxic agents. *J. Immun.* **116**: 1350–1353.

BECHTOL, K. B., FREED, J. H., HERZENBERG, L. A. and MCDEVITT, H. (1974) Genetic control of the antibody response to poly–L (Tyr, Glu)–poly–D, L–Ala—poly–L–Lys in C3H–CWB tetraparental mice. *J. exp. Med.* **140**:1660–1675.

BECHTOL, K. B. and MCDEVITT, H. O. (1976) Antibody response of C3H↔(CKB × CWB)F_1 tetraparental mice to poly–L (Tyr, Glu)–poly–D, L–Ala—poly–L–Lys immunization. *J. exp. Med.* **144**: 123–144.

BENACERRAF, B. and MCDEVITT, H. O. (1972) Histocompatibility-linked immune response genes. *Science* **175**: 272–274.

BENNET, B. (1966) Isolation and cultivation *in vitro* of macrophages from various sources in the mouse. *Am. J. Path.* **48**: 165–181.

BERLINGER, N. T., LOPEZ, C. and GOOD, R. A. (1976) Facilitation or attenuation of mixed leukocyte culture responsiveness by adherent cells. *Nature* **260**: 145–146.

BERNSTEIN, I., COHEN, E. and WRIGHT, P. (1977) Relationship of cellular proliferation and the generation of cytotoxic cells in an *in vitro* secondary immune response to syngeneic rat lymphoma cells. *J. Immun.* **118**: 1090–1094.

BEVAN, M., EPSTEIN, R. and COHN, M. (1974) The effect of 2–mercaptoethanol on murine mixed lymphocyte cultures. *J. exp. Med.* **139**: 1025–1030.

BLAESE, M. R. (1975) Macrophages and the development of immunocompetence. In: *The Phagocytic Cell in Host Resistance*, 1975 pp. 309–317, BELLANTI, J. A. and DAYTON, D. H. (eds.). Raven Press, New York.

BLAESE, M. R., LAWRENCE, C. E. and POPLACK, D. G. (1977) A critique of techniques of macrophage–monocyte depletion in studies of human peripheral blood mononuclear leukocyte (MNL) function. In: *Proceedings of the Eleventh Leukocyte Culture Conference*, 1977 LUCAS, D. (ed.). Academic Press, New York (in press).

BLAESE, M. R., OPPENHEIM, J. J., SEEGER, R. C. and WALDMAN, T. A. (1972) Lymphocyte–macrophage interaction in antigen induced *in vitro* lymphocyte transformation in patients with the Wiskott–Aldrich syndrome and other diseases with anergy. *Cell. Immun.* **4**: 228–242.

BLANDEN, R. V. (1969) Increased antibacterial resistance and immunodepression during graft-versus-host reactions in mice. *Transplantation* **7**: 484–497.

BLOOM, B. R. and DAVID, J. R. (eds.) (1976) In Vitro *Methods in Cell-Mediated and Tumor Immunity* Academic Press, New York.

BODEL, P. T., NICHOLS, B. A. and BAINTON, D. F. (1977) Appearance of peroxidase reactivity within the rough endoplasmic reticulum of blood monocytes after surface adherence. *J. exp. Med.* **145**: 264–274.

BOMFORD, R. and OLIVOTTO, M. (1975) Inhibition by *Corynebacterium parvum* of lung-nodule formation by intravenously injected fibrosarcoma cells. In: Corynebacterium parvum: *Application in Experimental and Clinical Oncology* pp. 268–275, HALPERN, B. (ed.). Plenum Press, New York.

BOUMSELL, L. and MELTZER, M. S. (1975) Mouse mononuclear cell chemotaxis. I. Differential response of monocytes and macrophages. *J. Immun.* **115**: 1746–1748.

BRADLEY, S. G. and WATSON, D. W. (1964) Suppression by endotoxin of the immune response to actinophage in the mouse (29640). *Proc. Soc. exp. Biol. Med.* **117**: 570–574.

BRODER, S., HUMPHREY, R., DUR, M., BLACKMAN, MEADE, B., GOLDMAN, C., STROBER, W. and WALDMANN, T. (1975) Impaired synthesis of polyclonal (non-paraprotein) immunoglobulins by circulating lymphocytes from patients with multiple myeloma. *New Engl. J. Med.* **293**: 887–892.

BYFIELD, P., CHRISTIE, G. H. and HOWARD, J. G. (1973) Alternative potentiating and inhibitory effects of GVH reaction on formation of antibodies against a thymus-independent polysaccharide (SIII). *J. Immun.* **111**: 72–81.

CALDERON, J., KIELY, J.-M., LEFKO, J. L. and UNANUE, E. R. (1975) The modulation of lymphocyte functions by molecules secreted by macrophages. I. Description and partial biochemical analysis. *J. exp. Med.* **142**: 151–164.

CALDERON, J. and UNANUE, E. (1974) The release of antigen molecules from macrophages: characterization of the phenomena. *J. Immun.* **122**: 1804–1814.

CALDERON, J., WILLIAMS, R. T. and UNANUE, E. R. (1974) An inhibitor of cell proliferation released by cultures of macrophages. *Proc. natn. Acad. Sci. USA* **71**: 4273–4277.

CALKINS, C. E. and GOLUB, E. S. (1972) Direct demonstration of lymphocyte–macrophage cooperation in the absence of physical contact between the two cell types. *Cell. Immun.* **5**: 579–586.

CANTOR, H. and JANDINSKI, J. (1974) The relationship of cell division to the generation of cytotoxic activity in mixed lymphocyte culture. *J. exp. Med.* **140**: 1712–1716

CARTER, B. G. and RECTOR, E. S. (1972) The generation of antigen-sensitive cells in the newborn mouse. *J. Immun.* **109**: 1345–1351.

CHEN, C. and HIRSCH, J. G. (1975) The effects of certain thiols on mouse lymphoid cell survival and on antibody production *in vitro*. In: *Mononuclear Phagocytes in Immunity, Infection and Pathology* pp. 765–774, VAN FURTH, R. (ed.). Blackwell Scientific Publications, London.

CHEN, C. and HIRSCH, J. (1972) The effects of mercaptoethanol and of peritoneal macrophages on the antibody-forming capacity of nonadherent mouse spleen cells *in vitro*. *J. exp. Med.* **136**: 604–617.

CHUSED, T. M., KASSAN, S. S. and MOSIER, D. E. (1976) Macrophage requirement for the *in vitro* response to TNP Ficoll: a thymic independent antigen. *J. Immun.* **116**: 1579–1581.

CLEVELAND, R. P., MELTZER, M. S. and ZBAR, B. (1974) Tumor cytotoxicity *in vitro* by macrophages from mice infected with *Mycobacterium bovis* strain BCG. *J. natn. Cancer Inst.* **52**: 1887–1895.

CLICK, R. E., BENCK, L. and ALTER, B. J. (1972) Immune responses *in vitro*. I. Culture conditions for antibody synthesis. *Cell. Immun.* **3**: 264–276.

CLINE, M. J. and SUMNER, M. A. (1972) Bone marrow macrophage precursors. I. Some functional characteristics of the early cells of the mouse macrophage series. *Blood* **40**: 62–64.

CLINE, M. J. and SWETT, V. C. (1968) The interaction of human monocytes and lymphocytes. *J. exp. Med.* **128**: 1309–1325.

COSENZA, H., LESERMAN, L. and ROWLEY, D. (1971) The third cell type required for the immune response of spleen cells *in vitro*. *J. Immun.* **107**: 414–421.

CURRIE, G. A. and BASHAM, C. (1975) Activated macrophages release a factor which lyses malignant cells but not normal cells. *J. exp. Med.* **142**: 1600–1605.

DAVID, J. R. (1975) Macrophage activation by lymphocyte mediators. *Fedn Proc.* **34**: 1730–1742.

DEAN, J. H., KIBRITE, A., JERRELLS, T. R. and HERBERMAN, R. B. (1977) Technical considerations for the separation of human peripheral blood lymphocyte subpopulations by rosetting with sheep erythrocyte. In: *Proceedings of the Eleventh Leukocyte Culture Conference*, pp. 583–586, LUCAS, D. (ed.). Academic Press, New York.

DUTTON, R. W. (1972) Inhibitory and stimulatory effects of Concanavalin A on the response of mouse spleen cell suspensions to antigen. *J. exp. Med.* **136**: 1445–1460

EDELSON, P. J. and COHN, Z. A. (1976) Purification and culture of monocytes and macrophages. In: In Vitro *Methods in Cell-Mediated and Tumor Immunity* BLOOM, R. and DAVID, J. (eds.). Academic Press, New York.

EGGERS, A. E. and WUNDERLICH, J. R. (1975) Suppressor cells in tumor-bearing mice capable of nonspecific blocking of *in vitro* immunization against transplant antigens. *J. Immun.* **114**: 1554–1556.

ELLNER, J. J. and ROSENTHAL, A. S. (1975) Quantitative and immunologic aspects of the handling of 2,4-dinitrophenyl guinea pig albumin in macrophages. *J. Immun.* **114**: 1563–1569.

EPSTEIN, L. B., CLINE, M. J. and MERIGAN, T. C. (1971a) PPD-stimulated interferon: *in vitro* macrophage–lymphocyte interaction in the production of a mediator of cellular immunity. *Cell. Immun.* **2**: 602–613.

EPSTEIN, L. B., CLINE, M. J. and MERIGAN, T. C. (1971b) The interaction of human macrophages and lymphocytes in the PHA-stimulated production of interferon. *J. natn. Cancer Inst.* **50**: 744–746.

ERB, P. and FELDMANN, M. (1975a) The role of macrophages in the generation of T-helper cells. III. Influence of macrophage-derived factors in helper cell induction. *Eur. J. Immun.* **5**: 759–766.

ERB, P. and FELDMANN, M. (1975b) The role of macrophages in the generation of T-helper cells. II. The genetic control of the macrophage–T cell interaction for helper cell induction with soluble antigens. *J. exp. Med.* **142**: 460–472.

ERB, P., FELDMANN, M. and HOGG, N. (1976) The role of macrophages in the generation of T-helper cells. IV. Nature of genetically related factor derived from macrophages incubated with soluble antigens. *Eur. J. Immun.* **6**: 365–372.

ESTEROFF, T., GALINAUD, P., DORMONT, J., WALLON, C. and TCHERNIA, G. (1976) The xenogeneic effect—evidence for coparticipation of human monocytes and T lymphocytes in the restoration of nude mouse *in vitro* response to sheep red blood cells. *Eur. J. Immun.* **6**: 683–687.

EVANS, R. and ALEXANDER, P. (1972) Role of macrophages in tumor immunity. I. Cooperation between macrophages and lymphoid cells in syngeneic tumor immunity. *Immunology* **23**: 615–626.

EVANS, R. and GRANT, C. K. (1972) Role of macrophages in tumor immunity. III. Cooperation between macrophages and lymphoid factors in an *in vitro* allograft situation. *Immunology* **22**: 667–675.

FAHEY, J. L., SCOOGIN, R., UTZ, J. and SZWED, C. (1963) Infection, antibody response and gamma globulin components in multiple myeloma and macroglobulinemia. *Am. J. Med.* **35**: 698.

FANGER, M. W., HART, D. A., WELLS, J. V. and NISONOFF, A. (1970) Enhancement by reducing agents of the transformation of human and rabbit peripheral lymphocytes. *J. Immun.* **105**: 1043–1045.

FELDMANN, M. (1972a) Induction of immunity and tolerance *in vitro* by hapten protein conjugates. II. Carrier independence of the response to dinitrophenylated polymerized flagellin. *Eur. J. Immun.* **2**: 130–137.

FELDMANN, M. (1972b) Cell interactions in the immune response *in vitro*. II. The requirement for macrophages in lymphoid cell collaboration. *J. exp. Med.* **135**: 1049–1058.

FELDMANN, M. (1972c) Cell interactions in the immune response *in vitro*. V. Specific collaboration via complexes of antigen and thymus-derived cell immunoglobulin. *J. exp. Med.* **136**: 737–760.

FELDMANN, M. and BASTEN, A. (1972) Cell interactions in the immune response *in vitro*. IV. Comparison of the effects of antigen-specific and allogeneic thymus-derived cell factors. *J. exp. Med.* **136**: 722–736.

FELDMANN, M., GREAVES, M. F., PARKER, D. C. and RITTENBERG, M. B. (1974) Direct triggering of B lymphocytes by insolubilized antigen. *Eur. J. Immun.* **4**: 591–597.

FELDMANN, M. and PALMER, J. (1971) The requirement for macrophages in the secondary immune response to antigens of small and large size *in vitro*. *Immunology* **21**: 685–699.

FERNBACH, B. R., KIRCHNER, H. and HERBERMAN, R. B. (1976a) Inhibition of the mixed lymphocyte culture by peritoneal exudate cells. *Cell. Immun.* **22**: 399–403.

FERNBACH, B. R., KIRCHNER, H., BONNARD, G. D. and HERBERMAN, R. B. (1976b) Suppression of mixed lymphocyte responses in mice bearing primary tumors induced by murine sarcoma virus. *Transplantation* **21**: 381–386.

FOLCH, H. and WAKSMAN, B. H. (1974) The spleen suppressor cell. II. Suppression of the mixed lymphocyte reaction by thymus-dependent adherent cells. *J. Immun.* **113**: 140–144.

FOX, T. O., SHEPPARD, J. R. and BURGER, M. M. (1971) Cyclic membrane changes in animal cells: Transformed cells permanently display a surface architecture detected in normal cells only during mitosis. *Proc. natn. Acad. Sci. USA* **68**: 244–247.

FRANZL, R. E. and MCMASTER, P. D. (1968) The primary immune response in mice. I. The enhancement and suppression of hemolysin production by a bacterial endotoxin. *J. exp. Med.* **127**: 1087–1107.

FUJIMOTO, S., GREENE, M. L. and SEHON, A. H. (1976a) Regulation of the immune response to tumor antigens. I. Immunosuppressor cells in tumor-bearing hosts. *J. Immun.* **116**: 791–799.

FUJIMOTO, S., GREENE, M. L. and SEHON, A. H. (1976b) Regulation of the immune response to tumor antigens. II. The nature of immunosuppressor cells in tumor-bearing hosts. *J. Immun.* **116**: 800–806.

GADEBUSCH, H. H. (1972) Mechanisms of native and acquired resistance to infection with *Cryptococcus neoformans*. In: *Macrophages and Cellular Immunity* pp. 3–11, LASKIN, A. I. and LECHEVALIER, H. (eds.). CRC Press, Cleveland.

GARDNER, R. J. and PRESTON, F. W. (1962) Prolonged skin homograft survival in advanced cancer and cirrhosis and the liver. *Surgery Gynec. Obstet.* **115**: 399–402.

GERSHON, R. K. (1974) T cell control of antibody production. In: *Contemporary Topics in Immunobiology* Vol. 3, pp. 1–40, COOPER, M. D. and WARNER, N. L. (eds.). Plenum Press, New York, London.

GERY, I., GERSHON, R. K. and WAKSMAN, B. H. (1972) Potentiation of the T-lymphocyte response to mitogens. I. The responding cell. *J. exp. Med.* **136**: 128–142.

GLASER, M., KIRCHNER, H. and HERBERMAN, R. B. (1975) Inhibition of *in vitro* lymphoproliferative responses to tumor associated antigens by suppressor cells from rats bearing progressively growing Gross leukemia virus-induced tumors. *Int. J. Cancer* **16**: 384–393.

GLASER, M., KIRCHNER, H., HOLDEN, H. T. and HERBERMAN, R. B. (1976) Inhibition of cell-mediated cytotoxicity against tumor-associated antigens by suppressor cells from tumor-bearing mice. *J. natn. Cancer Inst.* **56**: 865–867.

GOLDSTEIN, P. and BLOMGREN, H. (1973) Further evidence for autonomy of T cells mediating specific *in vitro* cytotoxicity: Efficiency of very small amounts of highly purified T cells. *Cell. Immun.* **9**: 127–141.

GORCZYNSKI, R. M. (1976) Control of the immune response: role of macrophages in regulation of antibody– and cell-mediated immune responses. *Scand. J. Immun.* **5**: 1031–1047.

GREINEDER, D. and ROSENTHAL, A. (1975a) The requirement for macrophage–lymphocyte interaction in T-lymphocyte proliferation induced by generation of aldehydes on cell membranes. *J. Immun.* **115**: 932–938.

GREINEDER, D. K. and ROSENTHAL, A. S. (1975b) Macrophage activation of allogeneic lymphocyte proliferation in the guinea pig mixed leukocyte culture. *J. Immun.* **114**: 1541–1547.

HALPERN, B. N. (ed.) (1975) Corynebacterium parvum: *Application in Experimental and Clinical Oncology.* Plenum Press, New York.

HALPERN, B. N., PREVOT, A. R., BIOZZI, G., STIFFEL, C., MOUTON, D., MORARD, J. C., BOUTHILLIER, Y. and DECREUSEFOND, C. (1963) Stimulation de l'activité phagocytaire du système réticuloendothélial provoquée par *Corynebacterium parvum*. *J. Reticuloendothel. Soc.* **1**: 77–85.

HAMMERLING, G. J. (1976) Tissue distribution of Ia antigens and their expression on lymphocyte subpopulations. *Transplant Rev.* **30**: 64–82.

HARDY, B., GLOBERSON, A. and DANON, D. (1973) Ontogenic development of the reactivity of macrophages to antigenic stimulation. *Cell. Immun.* **9**: 282–288.

HEBER-KATZ, E. and WILSON, D. B. (1975) Collaboration of allogeneic T and B lymphocytes in the primary antibody response to sheep erythrocytes *in vitro*. *J. exp. Med.* **142**: 928–935.

HERBERMAN, R. B., AOKI, T., NUNN, M., LAVRIN, D. H., SOARES, N., GAZDAR, A., HOLDEN, H. and CHANG, K. S. S. (1974) Specificity of ^{51}Cr-release cytotoxicity by lymphocytes immune to murine sarcoma virus. *J. natn. Cancer Inst.* **53**: 1103–1111.

HERBERMAN, R. B., NUNN, M. E., HOLDEN, H. T. and LAVRIN, D. H. (1975) Natural cytotoxic reactivity of mouse lymphoid cells against syngeneic and allogeneic tumor. II. Characterization of effector cells. *Int. J. Cancer* **16**: 230–239.

HERBERMAN, R. B., NUNN, M. E., HOLDEN, H. T., STAAL, S. and DJEU, J. Y. (1977) Augmentation of natural cytotoxic reactivity of mouse lymphoid cells against syngeneic and allogeneic target cells. *Int. J. Cancer* **19**: 555–564.

HERSH, E. M., GUTTERMAN, J. U. and MAVLIGIT, G. (1973) Immunological deficiency cancer. In: *Immunotherapy of Cancer in Man* pp. 3–18. Charles C. Thomas, Springfield, IL.

HERZENBERG, L. A., OKUMURA, K., CANTOR H., SATO, V. L., SHEN, F., BOYSE, E. A. and HERZENBERG, L. A. (1976) T-cell regulation of antibody responses: Demonstration of allotype-specific helper T cells and their specific removal by suppressor T cells. *J. exp. Med.* **144**: 330–344.

HIBBS, J. B. (1973) Macrophage nonimmunologic recognition: target cell factors related to contact inhibition. *Science* **180**: 868–870.

HIBBS, J. B. (1974) Heterocytolysis by macrophages activated by Bacillus Calmette–Guerin: Lysosome exocytosis into tumor cells. *Science* **184**: 468–471.

HIBBS, J. B., LAMBERT, L. H. and REMINGTON, J. S. (1972) Possible role of macrophage mediated nonspecific cytotoxicity in tumor resistance. *Nature New Biol.* **235**: 48–50.

HOFFMAN, M. (1970) Peritoneal macrophages in the immune response to SRBC *in vitro. Immunology* **18**: 791–797.

HOFFMAN, M. K., GREEN, S., OLD, L. J. and OETTGEN, H. F. (1976a) Serum containing endotoxin-induced tumour necrosis factor substitutes for helper T cells. *Nature* **263**: 416–417.

HOFFMAN, M. K., HAMMERLING, U., SIMON, M. and OETTGEN, H. F. (1976b) Macrophage requirements of CR− and CR+B lymphocytes for antibody production *in vitro. J. Immun.* **116**: 1447–1451.

HOLDEN, H. T., HASKILL, J. S., KIRCHNER, and HERBERMAN, R. B. (1976) Two functionally distinct anti-tumor effector cells isolated from primary murine sarcoma virus-induced tumors. *J. Immun.* **117**: 440–446.

HOLTERMANN, O. A., KLEIN, E. and CASALE, G. P. (1973) Selective cytotoxicity of peritoneal leucocytes for neoplastic cells. *Cell. Immun.* **9**: 339–352.

HOLTERMANN, O. A., LISAFELD, B. A., KLEIN, E. and KLOSTERGAARD, J. (1975) Cytocidal and cytostatic effects of activated peritoneal leukocytes. *Nature* **257**: 228–229.

HORTON, J. E., OPPENHEIM J. J., MERGENHAGEN, S. E. and RAISZ, L. G. (1974) Macrophage–lymphocyte synergy in the production of osteoclast activating factor. *J. Immun.* **113**: 1278–1287.

HOWARD, J. G., BIOZZI, G., STIFFEL, C., MOUTON, D. and LIACOPOULOS, P. (1967) An analysis of the inhibitory effect of *Corynebacterium parvum* on graft-versus-host disease. *Transplantation* **5**: 1510–1524.

JERNE, N. K. and NORDIN, A. A. (1963) Plaque formation in agar by single antibody-producing cells. *Science* **140**: 405.

JONES, A. L. (1971) Effect of column purification on response of lymphocytes in mixed leukocyte cultures (MLC) and to blastogenic media derived from MLCS. *Clin. exp. Immun.* **8**: 927–939.

JULIUS, M. H., SIMPSON, E. and HERZENBERG, L. A. (1973) A rapid method of the isolation of functional thymus-derived lymphocytes. *Eur. J. Immun.* **3**: 345–347.

KAGNOFF, M. F., BILLINGS, P. and COHN, M. (1974) Functional characteristics of Peyer's patch lymphoid cells. II. Lipopolysaccharide is thymus dependent. *J. exp. Med.* **139**: 407–413.

KAPP, J., PIERCE, W. and BENACERRAF, B. (1973) Genetic control of immune responses *in vitro*. II. Cellular requirements for the development of primary plaque-forming cell responses to the random terpolymer L–glutamic acid^{60} –L–alanine^{30} –L–tyrosine^{10} (GAT) by mouse spleen cells *in vitro. J. exp. Med.* **138**: 1121–1132.

KATZ, D. H. and BENACERRAF, B. (1972) The regulatory influence of activated T-cells on B-cells responses to antigens. *Adv. Immun.* **15**: 2–85.

KATZ, D. H., CHIORAZZI, N., MCDONALD, J. and KATZ, L. R. (1976) Cell interactions between histoincompatible T and B lymphocytes. IX. The failure of histocompatible cells is not due to suppression and cannot be circumvented by carrier-priming T cells with allogeneic macrophages. *J. Immun.* **117**: 1853–1859.

KATZ, D., HAMAOKA, T. and BENACERRAF, B. (1973a) Cell interactions between histoincompatible T and B lymphocytes. II. Failure of physiologic cooperative interactions between T and B lymphocytes from allogeneic donor strains in humoral response to hapten-protein conjugates. *J. exp. Med.* **137**: 1405–1418.

KATZ, D. H., HAMAOKA, T., DORF, M. E. and BENACERRAF, B. (1973b) Cell interactions between histoincompatible T and B lymphocytes. The H–2 gene complex determines successful physiologic lymphocyte interactions. *Proc. natn. Acad. Sci. USA* **70**: 2624–2628.

KATZ, D. H. and UNANUE, E. R. (1973) Critical role of determinant presentation in the induction of specific responses in immuno–competent lymphocytes. *J. exp. Med.* **137**: 967–990.

KELLER, R. (1974a) Modulation of cell proliferation by macrophages: A possible function apart from cytotoxic tumour rejection. *Br. J. Cancer* **30**: 401–415.

KELLER, R. (1974b) Mechanisms by which activated normal macrophages destroy syngeneic rat tumor cells *in vitro. Immunology* **27**: 285–298.

KELLER, R. (1975) Major changes in lymphocyte proliferation evoked by activated macrophages. *Cell. Immun.* **17**: 542–551.

KELLER, R. (1976) Susceptibility of normal and transformed cell lines to cytostatic and cytocidal effects exerted by macrophages. *J. natn. Cancer Inst.* **56**: 369–374.

KELLER, R., KEIST, R. and IVATT, R. J. (1974) Functional and biochemical parameters of activation related to macrophage cytostatic effects on tumor cells. *Int. J. Cancer* **14**: 675–683.

KIRCHNER, H., HERBERMAN, R. B., GLASER, M. and LAVRIN, D. H. (1974b) Suppression of *in vitro* lymphocyte stimulation in mice bearing primary Moloney sarcoma virus-induced tumors. *Cell. Immun.* **13**: 32–40.

KIRCHNER, H., CHUSED, T. M., HERBERMAN, R. B., HOLDEN, H. T. and LAVRIN, D. H. (1974b) Evidence of suppressor cell activity in spleens of mice bearing primary tumors induced by Moloney sarcoma virus. *J. exp. Med.* **139**: 1473–1487.

KIRCHNER, H., FERNBACH, B. R. and HERBERMAN, R. B. (1976) Macrophages suppressing T and B cell mitogen responses and the mixed leukocyte reaction. In: *Mitogens in Immunology* pp. 495–507, OPPENHEIM, J. J. and ROSENSTREICH, D. L. (eds.). Academic Press, New York.

KIRCHNER, H., MUCHMORE, A. V., CHUSED, T. M., HOLDEN, H. T. and HERBERMAN, R. B. (1975a) Inhibition of proliferation of lymphoma cells and T lymphocytes by suppressor cell from spleens of tumor-bearing mice. *J. Immun.* **144**: 206–210.

KIRCHNER, H., GLASER, M. and HERBERMAN, R. B. (1975b) Suppression of cell-mediated tumour immunity by Corynebacterium parvum. *Nature* **257**: 396–398.

KIRCHNER, H., HOLDEN H. T. and HERBERMAN, R. B. (1975c) Splenic suppressor macrophages induced in mice by injection of *Corynebacterium parvum*. *J. Immun.* **115**: 1212–1216.

KLAUS, G. G. B. (1974) Generation of thymus-derived helper cells by macrophage-associated antigen. *Cell. Immun.* **10**: 483–488.

KLAUS, G. G. B., HOWARD, J. G. and FELDMANN, M. (1976) Mechanisms of B cell tolerance. *Br. med. J.* **32**: 141–146.

KOLB, J–P., ARRIAN, S. and ZOLLA–PAZNER, S. (1977) Suppression of the humoral immune response by plasmacytomas: mediation by adherent mononuclear cells. *J. Immun.* **118**: 702–709.

KRAKAUER, R. S., STROBER, W. and WALDMANN, T. A. (1976) Hypogammaglobulinemia in experimental myeloma: the role of suppressor mononuclear phagocytes. *Clin. Res.* **24**: 337a.

KUNZ, H. W., GILL, T. J., III and BORLAND, B. (1974) The genetic linkage of the immune response to poly (Glu52Lys33Tyr15) to the major histocompatibility locus in inbred rate. *J. Immunogenetics* **1**: 277–287.

LAKE, W. W., BICE, D., SCHWARTZ, J. and SALVAGGIO, J. (1971) Suppression of *in vitro* antigen-induced lymphocyte transformation by carrageenan, a macrophage-toxic agent. *J. Immun.* **107**: 1741–1745.

LAMB, D., PILNEY, F., KELLY, W. D. and GOOD, R. A. (1962) A comparative study of the incidence of anergy in patients with carcinoma, leukemia, Hodgkin's disease and other lymphomas. *J. Immun.* **89**: 555–558.

LANDOLFO, S., HERBERMAN, R. B. and HOLDEN, H. T. (1977) Stimulation of mouse migration inhibitory factor (MIF) production from MSV-immune lymphocytes by soluble tumor associated antigen: requirement for histocompatible macrophages. *J. Immun.* **118**: 1244–1248.

LANDOLFO, S., HERBERMAN, R. B. and HOLDEN, H. T. (1978) Cellular immunity to murine sarcoma virus-induced tumors as measured by macrophage migration inhibition assorp. *J. natn. Cancer Inst.* (in press).

LAPP, W. S. and MOLLER, G. (1969) Prolonged survival of H–2 incompatible skin allografts on F_1 animals treated with parental lymphoid cells. *Immunology* **17**: 339–334.

LEE, A. K. Y., ROWLEY, M. and MACKAY, I. R. (1970) Antibody-producing capacity in human cancer. *Br. J. Cancer* **24**; 454–463.

LEE, K. C., SHIOZAWA, C., SHAW, A. and DIENER, E. (1976) Requirement for accessory cells in the antibody response to T cell-independent antigens *in vitro*. *Eur. J. Immun.* **6**: 63–68.

LEIBOVICH, S. J. and ROSS, R. (1975) Macrophages and anti-macrophage serum. In: *Mononuclear Phagocytes in Immunity, Infection and Pathology* pp. 151–160, VAN FURTH, R. (ed.). Blackwell Scientific Publications, London.

LEMKE, H., COUTINHO, A., OPITZ, H. and GRONOWICZ, E. (1975) Macrophages suppress direct B cell activation by lipopolysaccharide. *Scand. J. Immun.* **4**: 707–720.

LIPSKY, P. and ROSENTHAL, A. (1973) Macrophage–lymphocyte interaction. I. Characteristics of the antigen-independent binding of guinea pig thymocytes and lymphocytes to syngeneic macrophages. *J. exp. Med.* **138**: 900–921.

LIPSKY, P. E. and ROSENTHAL, A. S. (1976) The induction and regulation of guinea pig B–lymphocyte proliferation *in vitro*. *J. Immun.* **117**: 1594–1602.

LOGAN, J. (1956) The delayed type of allergic reaction in cancer altered response to tuberculin and mumps virus. *N. Z. med. J.* **55**: 408–410.

LOHRMANN, P. H., NOVIKOVS, L. and GRAW, R. G. (1974) Cellular interactions in the proliferative response of human T and B lymphocytes to phytomitogens and allogeneic lymphocytes. *J. exp. Med.* **139**: 1553–1567.

LY, I. A. and MISHELL, R. I. (1974) Separation of mouse spleen cells by passage through columns of Sephadex G–10. *J. Immun. Meth.* **5**: 239–247.

MCGREGOR, D. D. and KOSTER, F. T. (1971) The mediator of cellular immunity. IV. Cooperation between lymphocytes and mononuclear phagocytes. *Cell. Immun.* **2**: 317–325.

MCGREGOR, D. D. and LOGIE, P. S. (1975) Macrophocyte–lymphocyte interactions in infection immunity. In: *Mononuclear Phagocytes in Immunity, Infection, and Pathology* pp. 631–661, FURTH, R. V. (ed.). Blackwell Scientific Publications, Oxford, London.

MCINTYRE, J. and PIERCE, C. (1973) Immune responses *in vitro*. IX. Role of cell clusters. *J. Immun.* **111**: 1562–1537.

MILLER, J. F. A. P., VADAS, M. A., WHITELAW, A. and GAMBLE, J. (1976a) Role of major histocompatibility complex gene products in delayed-type hypersensitivity. *Proc. natn. acad. Sci. USA.* **73**: 2486–2490.

MILLER, J. F. A. P., VADAS, M. A., WHITELAW, A. and GAMBLE, J. (1976b) H–2 linked Ir gene regulation of delayed-type hypersensitivity in mice. In: *The Role of Products of the Histocompatibility Gene Complex in Immune Responses* pp. 403–415, KATZ, D. and BENACERRAF, B. (eds.). Academic Press, New York.

MISHELL, R. I. and DUTTON, R. W. (1966) Immunization of normal mouse spleen cell suspensions *in vitro*. *Science* **153**: 1004–1005.

MITCHELL, M. S., KIRKPATRICK, D., MOKYR, M. B. and GERY, I. (1973) On the mode of action of BCG. *Nature New Biol.* **243**: 216–217.

MITCHISON, N. A. (1969) The immunogenic capacity of antigen taken up by peritoneal exudate cells. *Immunology* **16**: 1–14.

MOKYR, M. B. and MITCHELL, M. S. (1975) Activation of lymphoid cells by BCG *in vitro*. *Cell. Immun.* **15**: 264–273.

MOLLER, G. (1971a) Induction of antigenic competition with thymus-dependent antigens: Effect on DNA synthesis in spleen cells. *J. Immun.* **106**: 1566–1571.

MÖLLER, G. (1971b) Suppressive effect of graft versus host reaction on the immune response to heterologous red cells. *Immunology* **20**: 597–609.

MÖLLER, G., LEMKE, H. and OPITZ, H.–G. (1976) The role of adherent cells in the immune response. *Scand. J. Immun.* **5**: 2969–280.

MOSIER, D. E. (1967) A requirement for two cell types for antibody formation *in vitro*. *Science* **158**: 1573–1575.

MOSIER, D. E. (1968) Cell interactions in the primary immune response *in vitro*: a requirement for specific cell clusters. *J. Immun.* **129**: 351–362.

MOSIER, D. E., JOHNSON, B. M., PAUL, W. E. and MCMASTER, P. R. B. (1974) Cellular requirements for the primary *in vitro* antibody response to DNP–Ficoll. *J. exp. Med.* **139**: 1354–1360.

MOZES, E. and SHEARER, G. M. (1971) Contribution of bone marrow cells and lack of expression of thymocytes in genetic controls of immune responses for two immunopotent regions with Poly–(Phe, Glu) Poly Pro–Poly–Lys in inbred mouse strains. *J. exp. Med.* **134**: 141–161.

MURPHY, D. B., HERZENBERG, L. A., OKUMURA, K., HERZENBERG, L. A. and MCDEVITT, H. O. (1976) A new *I* subregion (*I–J*) marked by a locus (*Ja–4*) controlling surface. Determinants of suppressor T lymphocytes. *J. exp. Med.* **144**: 699–712.

NATHAN, C. F., HILL, V. M. and TERRY, W. T. (1976) Isolation of a subpopulation of adherent peritoneal cells with anti-tumor activity. *Nature* **260**: 146–148.

NATHAN, C. F., KARNOVSKY, M. L. and DAVID, J. R. (1971) Alterations of macrophage functions by mediators from lymphocytes. *J. exp. Med.* **133**: 1356–1376.

NATHAN, C. F., REMOLD, H. G. and DAVID, J. R. (1973) Characterization of a lymphocyte factor which alters macrophage functions. *J. exp. Med.* **137**: 275–290.

NIEDERHUBER, J. E. and SHREFFLER, D. C. (1977) Anti-Ia serum blocking of macrophage function in the *in vitro* humoral response. *Transplant. Proc.* **9**: 875–879.

NITULESCU, G. and FÖRSTER, O. (1976) Antigenic differences between rat alveolar and peritoneal macrophages. *Adv. exp. Med. Biol.* **73A**: 53–58.

OEHLER, J. R. and HERBERMAN, R. B. (1977) Interaction of T cells with allogeneic macrophages in mixed leukocyte cultures in rats. *J. Immun.* **19**: 1785–1789.

OEHLER, J. R., CAMPBELL, D. A. and HERBERMAN, R. B. (1977a) *In vitro* inhibition of lymphoproliferative responses to tumor associated antigens and of lymphoma cell proliferation by rat splenic macrophages. *Cell. Immun.* **28**: 355–370.

OEHLER, J. R., HERBERMAN, R. B., CAMPBELL, D. A. and DJEU, J. Y. (1977b) Inhibition of rat mixed lymphocyte cultures by suppressor macrophages. *Cell. Immun.* **29**: 238–250.

OEHLER, J. R., CAMPBELL, D. A. and HERBERMAN, R. B. (1977c) Adherent suppressor cells in normal rat spleen. *Proceedings of the Eleventh Leukocyte Culture Conference* pp. 797–799, Academic Press, New York.

OHISHI, M. and ONOUE, K. (1975) Functional activation of immune lymphocytes by antigenic stimulation in cell-mediated immunity. I. Requirement for macrophages in antigen-induced MIF production by guinea pig immune lymphocytes *in vitro*. *Cell. Immun.* **18**: 220–232.

OHISHI, M. and ONOUE, K. (1976) Functional activation of immune lymphocytes by antigenic stimulation in cell-mediated immunity. II. Analysis of the macrophage-replacing activity of the LPS-stimulated macrophage culture supernatant in the antigenic activation of purified immune lymphocytes. *Cell. Immun.* **26**: 295–307.

OPITZ, H.-G., NIETHAMMER, D., JACKSON, R. C., LEMKE, H., HUGET, R. and FLAD, H. D. (1975a) Biochemical characterization of a factor released by macrophages. *Cell. Immun.* **18**: 70–75.

OPITZ, H. G., NEITHAMMER, D., LEMKE, H., FLAD, H. D. and HUGET, R. (1975b) Inhibition of ^{3}H–thymidine incorporation of lymphocytes by a soluble factor from macrophages. *Cell. Immun.* **16**: 379–388.

OPITZ, H. G., OPITZ, U., LEMKE, HUGET, R. and FLAD, H. D. (1976) Polyclonal stimulation of lymphocytes by macrophages. *Eur. J. Immun.* **6**: 457–461.

OPPENHEIM, J., LEVENTHAL, B. and HERSH, E. (1968) The transformation of column-purified lymphocytes with nonspecific and specific antigenic stimuli. *J. Immun.* **101**: 262–270.

OPPENHEIM, J. J. and ROSENSTREICH, D. L. (1976) Signals regulating *in vitro* activation of lymphocytes. *Prog. Allergy* **20**: 65–159.

OPPENHEIM, J. J. and SEEGER, R. C. (1976) The role of macrophages in the induction of cell-mediated immunity *in vitro*. In: *Immunobiology of the Macrophage* pp. 111–130, NELSON, D. S. (ed.). Academic Press, New York.

PARROT, D. M. V. and DESOUSA, M. (1971) Thymus-dependent and thymus-independent populations: Origin, migratory patterns and lifespan. *Clin. exp. Immun.* **8**: 663–684.

PAUL, W. E. and BENACERRAF, B. (1974) Antigen recognition. In: *Mechanisms of Cell-Mediated Immunity* pp. 61–97, MCCLUSKEY, R. T. and COHEN, S. (eds.). John Wiley, New York.

PAUL, W. E., SHEVACH, E. M., THOMAS, D. W., PICKERAL, S. F. and ROSENTHAL, A. S. (1977) Genetic restriction in T–lymphocyte activation by antigen-pulsed peritoneal exudate cells. *Cold Spring Harb. Symp. quant. Biol.* **41**: 571–578.

PEAVY, D. L. and PIERCE, C. W. (1974) Cell-mediated immune response *in vitro*. I. Suppression of the generation of cytotoxic lymphocytes by Concanavalin A and Concanavalin A-activated spleen cells. *J. exp. Med.* **140**: 356–369.

PEAVY, D. L. and PIERCE, C. W. (1975) cell-mediated immune response *in vitro*. III. Elimination of specific cytotoxic lymphocyte responses by ^{3}H–thymidine suicide. *J. Immun.* **115**: 1521–1524.

PERKINS, E. H. and MAKINODAN, T. (1965) The suppressive role of mouse peritoneal phagocytes in agglutinin response. *J. Immun.* **94**: 765–777.

PIERCE, C. W. (1969) Immune responses *in vitro*. I. Cellular requirements for the immune response by non-primed and primed spleen cells *in vitro*. *J. exp. Med.* **130**: 345–350.

PIERCE, C. W. (1973) Immune responses *in vitro*. IV. Cell interactions in the development of primary IgM, and IgA plaque-forming cell responses *in vitro*. *Cell. Immun.* **9**: 453–464.

PIERCE, C. W. and KAPP, J. A. (1976) The role of macrophages in antibody responses *in vitro*. In: *Immunobiology of the Macrophage* pp. 1–33, NELSON, D. S. (ed.). Academic Press, New York.

PIERCE, C., KAPP, J. and BENACERRAF, B. (1976) Regulation by the H–2 gene complex of macrophage–lymphoid cell interactions in secondary antibody responses *in vitro*. *J. exp. Med.* **144**: 371–381.

PIERCE, C., KAPP, J., WOOD, D. and BENACERRAF, B. (1974) Immune responses *in vitro*. X. Functions of macrophages. *J. Immun.* **112**: 1181–1189.

PIESSENS, W. F., CHURCHILL, W. H. and DAVID, J. R. (1975) Macrophages activated *in vitro* with lymphocyte mediators kill neoplastic but not normal cells. *J. Immun.* **114**: 293–299.

PIKE, B. L. and NOSSAL, G. J. V. (1976) Requirement for persistent extracellular antigen in cultures of antigen-binding B lymphocytes. *J. exp. Med.* **144**: 568–572.

PLATA, F., CEROTTINI, J. C. and BRUNNER, K. T. (1975) Primary and secondary *in vitro* generation of cytolytic T lymphocytes in the murine sarcoma virus system. *Eur. J. Immun.* **5**: 227–233.

POPE, B. L., WHITNEY, R. B., LEVY, J. G. and KILBURN, D. G. (1976) Suppressor cells in the spleens of tumor-bearing mice: Enrichment by centrifugation on Hypaque–Ficoll and characterization of the suppressor population. *J. Immun.* **116**: 1342–1346.

POPLACK, D. G., BONNARD, G. D., HOLIMAN, B. J. and BLAESE, R. M. (1976) Monocyte-medicated antibody-dependent cellular toxicity: a clinical test of monocyte function. *Blood* **48**: 809–816.

POSTLETHWAITE, A. E., SNYDERMAN, R. and KAND, A. H. (1976) The chemotactic attraction of human fibroblasts to a lymphocyte-derived factor. *J. exp. Med.* **144**: 1188–1203.

PRÉVOT, A. R. (1975) Bacteriological aspect of anaerobic *Corynebacteria* in relation to RES stimulation. In: Corynebacterium Parvum; *Applications in Experimental and Clinical Oncology* pp. 3–10, HALPERN, B. (ed.). Plenum Press, New York.

PROSS, H. F. and EIDINGER, D. (1974) Antigenic competition: a review of nonspecific antigen-induced suppression. *Adv. Immun.* **18**: 133–168.

REMINGTON, J. S., KRAHENBUHL, J. L. and HIBBS, J. B., JR. (1975) A role for the macrophage in resistance to tumor development and tumor destruction. In: *Mononuclear Phagocytes in Immunity, Infection and Pathology* pp. 869–893, VAN FURTH, R. (ed.). Blackwell Scientific Publications, Oxford.

RENAUD, M. (1926) La cuti réaction à la tuberculine chez les cancereaux. *Bull. Mém. Soc. Méd. Paris* **50**: 1441–1442.

RHODES, J. (1975) Macrophage heterogeneity in receptor activity: the activation of macrophage Fc receptor function *in vivo* and *in vitro*. *J. Immun.* **114**: 976–981.

RICH, R. R. and PIERCE, C. W. (1974) Biological expressions of lymphocyte activation. *J. Immun.* **112**: 1360–1368.

RODE, H. N. and GORDON, J. (1974) Macrophages in the mixed leukocyte culture reaction (MLC). *Cell. Immun.* **13**: 87–94.

ROSENSTREICH, D. L. and OPPENHEIM, J. J. (1976) The role of macrophages in the activation of T and B lymphocytes *in vitro*. In: *Immunobiology of the Macrophage* pp. 162–197, NELSON, D. S. (ed.). Academic Press, London.

ROSENTHAL, A. and SHEVACH, E. (1973) Function of macrophages in antigen recognition by guinea pig T lymphocytes. I. Requirement for histocompatible macrophages and lymphocytes. *J. Immun.* **138**: 1194–1212.

SAWICKI, J. E. and CATANZARO, P. J. (1975) Selective macrophage cytotoxicity of carrageenan *in vivo*. *Int. Archs Allergy appl. Immun.* **49**: 709–714.

SCHRADER, J. W. (1973) Mechanism of activation of the bone marrow-derived lymphocyte. *J. exp. Med.* **138**: 1466–1480.

SCHRADER, J. W. and FELDMANN, M. (1973) The mechanism of antigenic competition. I. The macrophage as a site of a reversible block of T–B lymphocyte collaboration. *Eur. J. Immun.* **3**: 711–717.

SCHWARTZ, H. J. and LESKOWITZ, S. (1969) The effect of carrageenan on delayed hypersensitivity reactions. *J. Immun.* **103**: 87–91.

SCOTT, M. T. (1972) Biological effects of the adjuvant *Corynebacterium parvum*. I. Inhibition of PHA, mixed lymphocyte and GVH reactivity. *Cell. Immun.* **5**: 459–468.

SCOTT, M. T. (1972) Biological effects of the adjuvant *Corynebacterium parvum*. II. Evidence for macrophage–T-cell interaction. *Cell. Immun.* **5**: 469–479.

SCOTT, M. T. (1974) Depression of delayed-type hypersensitivity by *Corynebacterium parvum*: mandatory role of the spleen. *Cell. Immun.* **13**: 251–263.

SEEGER, R. and OPPENHEIM, J. (1970) Synergistic interaction of macrophages and lymphocytes in antigen-induced transformation of lymphocytes. *J. exp. Med.* **132**: 44–65.

SHEVACH, E. M. (1976) The function of macrophages in antigen recognition by guinea pig T-lymphocytes. III. Genetic analysis of the antigens mediating macrophage–T lymphocyte interaction. *J. Immun.* **116**: 1482–1489.

SHEVACH, E. M. and ROSENTHAL, A. S. (1973) The function of macrophages in antigen recognition by guinea pig T-lymphocytes. II. Role of the macrophage in the regulation of genetic control of the immune response. *J. exp. Med.* **138**: 1213–1229.

SHILO, M. (1959) Nonspecific resistance to infections. *Ann. Rev. Microbiol.* **13**: 255–278.

SHINITZKY, M. and INBAR, M. (1974) Difference in microviscosity induced by different cholesterol levels in the surface membrane lipid layer of normal lymphocytes and malignant lymphoma cells. *J. molec. Biol.* **85**: 603–615.

SHORTMAN, K. (1968) The separation of different cell classes from lymphoid organs. II. The purification and analysis of lymphocyte populations by equilibrium density gradient centrifugation. *Aust. J. exp. Biol. med. Sci.* **46**: 375–396.

SHORTMAN, K., DIENER, E., RUSSEL, P. and ARMSTRONG, W. D. (1970) The role of nonlymphoid accessory cells in the immune response to different antigens. *J. exp. Med.* **131**: 461–482.

SHORTMAN, K. and PALMER, J. (1971) The requirement for macrophages in the *in vitro* immune response. *Cell. Immun.* **2**: 399–410.

SHREFFLER, D. C. and DAVID, C. S. (1975) The H-2 major histocompatibility complex and the I immune response region: genetic variation, function, and organization. *Adv. Immunol.* **20**: 125–190.

SJÖBERG, O. (1971) Antigenic competition *in vitro* of spleen cells subjected to a graft-versus-host reaction *Immunology* **21**: 351–361.

SJÖBERG, O. (1972) Effect of allogeneic cell interaction on the primary immune response *in vitro*. *Clin. exp. Immun.* **12**: 365–375.

SJÖBERG, O., ANDERSON, J. and MOLLER, G. (1972) Requirement for adherent cells in the primary and secondary immune response *in vitro*. *Eur. J. Immun.*

SJÖBERG, O. and BRITTON, S. (1972) Antigenic competition *in vitro* between heterologous erythrocytes. *Eur. J. Immun.* **2**: 282–288.

SMITH, R. T. (1972) Possibilities and problems of immunologic intervention in cancer. *New Engl. J. Med.* **287**: 439–450.

SMITH, R. T. and KONDA. S. (1973) The stimulatory effects of bearing primary methylcholanthrene-induced tumors upon the murine lymphoreticular system. *Int. J. Cancer* **12**: 577–588.

SMITH, S. E. and SCOTT, M. T. (1972) Biological effects of *Corynebacterium parvum*. III. Amplification of resistance and impairment of active immunity to murine tumours. *Br. J. Cancer* **26**: 361–367.

SOLOWEY, A. C. and RAPAPORT, F. T. (1965) Immunologic responses in cancer patients. *Surgery Gynec. Obstet.* **121**: 756–760.

SOUTHAM, C. M., BRUNSCHWIG, A. and DIXON, Q. (1962) In: *Biological Interactions in Normal and Neoplastic Growth* p. 723, BRENNAN, M. J. and SIMPSON, W. L. (eds.). Little and Brown, Boston.

SPITZNAGEL, J. K. and ALLISON, A. C. (1970) Mode of action of adjuvants: retinol and other lysosome-labilizing agents as adjuvants. *J. Immun.* **104**: 119–127.

TADA, N., ITAKURA K., and AIZAWA, M. (1976) Immune response gene (Ir–SRBC) exerts its effects via macrophages in inbred rats. *J. Immunogenetics* **3**: 49–60.

TADA, T. and TANIGUCHI, M. (1976) Characterization of the antigen-specific suppressive T cell factor with special reference to the expression of region genes. In: *The Role of Products of the Histocompatibility Gene complex in Immune Responses* pp. 513–541, KATZ, D. H. and BENACERRAF, B. (eds.). Academic Press, New York.

TADAKUMA, T., KUHNER, A. L., RICH, R. R., DAVID, J. R. and PIERCE, C. W. (1976a) Biological expressions of lymphocyte activation. V. Characterization of a soluble immune response suppressor (SIRS) produced by Concanavalin A–activated spleen cells. *J. Immun.* **117**: 323–330.

TADAKUMA, T. and PIERCE, C. W. (1976b) Site of action of a soluble immune response suppressor (SIRS) produced by Concanavalin A–activated spleen cells. *J. Immun.* **117**: 967–972.

TERRITO, M. and CLINE, M. J. (1976) Macrophages and their disorders in man. In: *Immunobiology of the Macrophage* pp. 593–616, NELSON, D. S. (ed). Academic Press, New York.

THOMAS, D. W., ROBERTS, W. K. and TALMAGE, D. W. (1975) Regulation of the immune response: production of a soluble suppressor by immune spleen cells *in vitro*. *J. Immun.* **114**: 1616–1622.

THOMAS, D. W. and SHEVACH, E. (1976) Nature of the antigenic complex recognized by T–lymphocytes. I. Analysis with an *in vitro* primary response to soluble protein antigens. *J. exp. Med.* **144**: 1263–1273.

THOMAS, D. W. and SHEVACH, E. M. (1977a) Nature of the antigenic complex recognized by T-lymphocytes. II. T cell activation by direct modification of macrophage histocompatibility antigens. *J. exp. Med.* **145**: 907–915.

THOMAS, D. W. and SHEVACH, E. M. (1977b) Nature of the antigenic complex recognized by T-lymphocytes. III. Specific sensitization by antigens associated with allogeneic macrophages. *Proc. natn. Acad. Sci. USA* **74**: 2104–2110.

TURK, J. L. and WATERS, F. R. (1971) Immunological significance of changes in lymph nodes across the leprosy spectrum. *Clin. exp. Immun.* **8**: 363–376.

TWOMEY, J. J., LAUGHTER, A., FARROW, S. and DOUGLASS, C. C. (1975) Hodgkin's disease. An immunodepleting and immunosuppressive disorder. *J. clin. Invest.* **56**: 467–475.

UNANUE, E. R. (1969) The immune response of mice to keyhole limpet hemocyanin bound to macrophages. *J. Immun.* **102**: 893–898.

UNANUE, E. R. (1972) The regulatory role of macrophages in antigen stimulation. *Adv. Immun.* **15**: 95–157.

UNANUE, E. R., ASKONAS, B. A. and ALLISON, A. (1969a) A role of macrophages in the stimulation of immune responses by adjuvants. *J. Immun.* **103**: 71.

UNANUE, E. R., CEROTTINI, J.–C. and BEDROD, M. (1969b) The persistence of antigen on the surface of macrophages. *Nature* **222**: 1193–1194.

VEIT, B. C. and FELDMANN, J. D. (1976a) Altered lymphocyte functions in rats bearing syngeneic Moloney sarcoma tumors. I. Mitogen responses, mixed lymphocyte reactions (MLR) and mixed lymphocyte-tumor reactions (MLTR). *J. Immun.* **117**: 646–654.

VETT, B. C. and FELDMANN, J. D. (1975b) Altered lymphocyte functions in rats bearing syngeneic Moloney sarcoma tumors. II. Suppressor cells. *J. Immun.* **117**: 655–660.

VIROLAINEN, M. LAHTI, A. and HÄYRY, P. (1972) Differentiation of macrophage antigen(s) in mouse bone marrow and buffy coat cultures. In: *Experimental Medicine and Biology* Vol. 15. Plenum Press, New York.

VON BOEHMER, H., HUDSON, L. and SPRINT, J. (1975a) Collaboration of histoincompatible T and B lymphocytes using cells from tetraparental bone marrow chimeras. *J. exp. Med.* **142**: 989–997.

VON BOEHMER, H., SPRENT, J. and NABHOLZ, M. (1975b) Tolerance to histocompatibility determinants in tetraparental bone marrow chimeras. *J. exp. med.* **141**: 322–334.

WAGNER, H., FELDMANN, M., BOYLE, W. and SCHRADER, J. W. (1972) Cell-mediated immune response *in vitro*. III. The requirement for macrophages in cytotoxic reactions against cell-bound and subcellular alloantigens. *J. exp. Med.* **136**: 331–343.

WAHL, S. M., WILTON, J. M., ROSENSTREICH, D. L. and OPPENHEIM, J. J. (1975) The role of macrophages in the production of lymphokines by T and B lymphocytes. *J. Immun.* **114**: 1296–1301.

WALDMAN, S. R. and GOTTLIEB, A. A. (1973) Macrophage regulation of DNA synthesis in lymphoid cells: effects of a soluble factor from macrophages. *Cell. Immun.* **9**: 142–146.

WALDRON, J., HORN R. and ROSENTHAL, A. (1973) Antigen-induced proliferation of guinea pig lymphocytes *in vitro*. Obligatory role of macrophages in the recognition of antigen by immune T-lymphocytes. *J. Immun.* **111**: 58–64.

WALDRON, J., HORN, R. and ROSENTHAL, A. (1974) Antigen-induced proliferation of guinea pig lymphocytes *in vitro*: functional aspects of antigen handling by macrophages. *J. Immun.* **112**: 746–755.

WALKER, W. S. (1976a) Functional heterogeneity of macrophages. In: *Immunobiology of the Macrophage* NELSON, D. S. (ed.). Academic Press, New York.

WALKER, W. S. (1976b) Functional heterogeneity of macrophages in the induction and expression of acquired immunity. *J. Reticuloendothelial Soc.* **20**: 57–65.

WEST, W. H., CANNON, G. B., KAY, H. D., BONNARD, G. B. and HERBERMAN, R. B. (1977) Natural cytotoxic reactivity of human lymphocytes against a myeloid cell line: characterization of effector cells. *J. Immun.* **118**: 355–361.

WEST, W. H., SIENKNECHT, C. W., TOWNES, A. S. and HERBERMAN, R. B. (1976) Performance of a rosette assay between lymphocytes and sheep erythrocytes at elevated temperatures to study patients with cancer and other diseases. *Clin. Immun. Immunopath.* **5**: 60–66.

WOLFE, S. A., TRACY, D. E. and HENNEY, C. S. (1976) Induction of 'natural killer' cells by BCG. *Nature* **262**: 584–586.

WOOD, D. D. and CAMERON, P. M. (1975) Studies on the mechanism of stimulation of the humoral response of murine spleen cultures by culture fluids from human monocytes. *J. Immun.* **114**: 1094–1100.

WOOD, D. D. and GAUL, S. L. (1974) Enhancement of the humoral response of T cell-depleted murine spleens by a factor derived from human monocytes *in vitro*. *J. Immun.* **113**: 925–933.

WOODRUFF, M. F. A., GHAFFAR, A., DUNBAR, N. and WHITEHEAD, V. L. (1976) Effect of *C. parvum* on immunization with irradiated tumour cells. *Br. J. Cancer* **33**: 491–495.

WOODRUFF, M. F. A., GHAFFAR, A. and WHITEHEAD, V. L. (1976) Modification of the effect of *C. parvum* on macrophage activity and tumor growth by X-irradiation. *Int. J. Cancer* **17**: 652–658.

YAM, L. T., LI, C. Y. and CROSBY, W. H. (1971) Cytochemical identification of monocytes and granulocytes. *Am. J. clin. Pathol.* **55**: 283–290.

YOSHINAGA, M., YOSHINAGA, A. and WAKSMAN, B. (1972) Regulation of lymphocyte responses *in vitro*. I. Regulatory effect of macrophages and thymus-dependent (T) cells on the response of thymus-independent (B) lymphocytes to endotoxin. *J. exp. Med.* **136**: 956–961.

CHAPTER 3

MODULATION OF IMMUNITY BY ANTIGENS, ANTIBODIES AND ANTIGEN-ANTIBODY COMPLEXES

NICHOLAS R. STC. SINCLAIR

Department of Microbiology and Immunology, The University of Western Ontario, London, Ontario, Canada

1. INTRODUCTION

The immune response has often been described in terms of the simple reflex arc of neurophysiology. Implicit in this analogy is that a spatial and temporal separation can be made between afferent, central and efferent portions of the immune response. However, in many immune responses, the antigen remains in the system not only for further triggering events but may also interact with various immune products. End-products which by definition should occur at the end of the immune response, would not seem to influence the early stages of this response. However, the lateness in arrival of end-products is more an illusion than reality. Antibody, even IgG antibody, can be detected at very early stages of an immune response (Yuan *et al.*, 1970) and various effector and regulator cells make their appearance early in many responses (Sercarz *et al.*, 1975). Therefore, rather than a division of immune responses into compartmentalized steps such as an afferent limb, a central response and an efferent limb, one must consider that the immune response will also have to deal with the presence of antibody during the early stages, of antigen at later stages, and of cells attempting, almost from the very beginning, to suppress as well as generate various immune responses. The progress of an immune response is not the consequence of an immune stimulus on a system capable of responding in a predetermined fashion, as with the simple reflex analogy so often invoked, but as a more complex system in which interactions of stimulating signals with end-products serve to modify the immune response in ways which have been established as appropriate according to evolutionary criteria.

Although not entirely separable, a distinction should be made between triggering events and regulatory phenomena. Triggering events involve the impingement of antigen in an immunogenic form on a cell capable of responding to the antigen, with the production of a clone of cells that produce antibody or express specific cytotoxicity. Regulatory phenomena or modulation involve an interaction between the antigenic trigger and end-products of that immune response which in turn leads to an alteration in the immune response. Although receptors for antigen could perhaps be considered 'end-products', it is nevertheless convenient to describe the consequences of interaction between immunogenic antigen and antigen-receptors as 'triggering', whereas modulation is the interaction of antigen with commonly accepted end-products, such as antibody or cytotoxic cells. The question becomes how early do end-products appear in an immune response and how early can they, on interaction with antigen, lead to the modulation of an immune response. The earlier end-products make their appearance in an immune response the more likely it is that characteristics displayed in an immune response (such as cell cooperative events and the general structure of lymphoid tissue) would have as their basis various modulating or regulatory activities as well as activities related to triggering.

The major concern of this review is an understanding of the mechanisms by which antibody, antigen–antibody complexes and antigen modulate immune responses. This gives some insight to how these forms of modulation may be altered, particularly with the use of pharmacologic agents. As an example, a major point is made with respect to the centrality of the Fc portion of antibodies and Fc-receptors on immunocompetent cells in regulation of immune responses. If pharmacologic agents can be found that react with Fc-receptors, either to block or activate them, it is likely that these pharmacologic agents will play an important role in augmenting or suppressing various immune responses. Since pharmacologic intervention depends upon an understanding of the complexities of the components and interactions of the immune response, it would not be justifiable to simplify unduly. My aim, therefore, has been to present these complexities without losing sight of the underlying principles.

This review on modulation of the immune response by antibody and antigen will begin with a description of the various components of this response. The approach taken will be to assemble the established facts in a way which will allow for the construction of a working model in which regulatory events are seen as an integral part of the immune response rather than a control process which is secondary to the immune mechanism *per se.*

2. CELLULAR MECHANISMS IN IMMUNE RESPONSES

2.1. Antibody Responses

Cellular events that occur in a humoral immune response can be summarized as follows: immunogenic antigen interacts with cells containing receptors for that antigen, (Moller, 1970; Singhal and Wigzell, 1971; Warner, 1974; Klinman and Press, 1975) and two types of specific cells are activated, B and T lymphocytes (Claman and Chaperon, 1969; Davies, 1969; Miller and Mitchell, 1969; Taylor, 1969; Mitchison, 1971a, b). Many of the interactions occurring between B and T cells involve the mediation of an A cell which has both phagocytic and cell-surface-display potentialities (Unanue, 1972), the latter being the most closely associated with immunogenicity (Unanue and Askonas, 1968; Unanue and Cerottini, 1970). B lymphocytes undergo activation, proliferation, and develop into lymphoblastoid then plasmablastoid cells which eventually become mature plasma cells. IgM antibody is synthesized and secreted predominantly during the blast-like stages of plasma cell differentiation, whilst IgG antibody synthesis is highest during the later plasmablast and plasmacyte stages (Janossy and Greaves, 1975). The syntheses of antibodies of IgA and IgE classes is also dependent on the activation of B cells (Dwyer *et al.*, 1976; Chiorazzi *et al.*, 1976), IgE antibody being synthesized somewhat earlier and IgA somewhat later in immune responses (Taylor *et al.*, 1973; Orgel *et al.*, 1975). Helper T lymphocytes are involved in plasma cell differentiation as well as in other cooperative cellular events during the activation of an immune response. However, some B cell activations do not require the presence of T cells or T cell factors (Basten and Howard, 1972).

Although there is still confusion concerning the chemical nature of antigen-specific receptors on T cells, there appears to be little doubt concerning the immunoglobulin nature of antigen-receptors on B cells; these immunoglobulins house the specific antigen-binding activity (Warner, 1974). Some immunoglobulin antigen-receptors may be similar to antibodies formed as a result of the immune response (Vitetta and Uhr, 1972) but most represent unusual forms of immunoglobulins on the surface of B cells, such as 8S IgM (Vitetta *et al.*, 1971) and IgD (Rowe *et al.*, 1973; Melcher *et al.*, 1972; Abney and Parkhouse, 1974). It has been suggested that B cells which respond to thymus-independent antigens do not bear IgD on their surface while cells responsive to T cell-dependent antigens display surface IgD (Cambier *et al.*, 1977). More direct evidence on the relationship between surface IgD and resistance to tolerance induction comes from experiments in which B cells were treated with anti-δ antibody (Scott *et al.*, 1977; Vitetta *et al.*, 1977) in which the susceptibility of B cells to tolerance induction could be raised by treating cells with this antibody or by treating newborns with anti-δ antibody which prevents the development of IgD-bearing cells.

Antibodies directed against μ-chains were unable to induce sensitivity to tolerance induction. Following removal of the surface IgD, either with papain or anti-δ antibodies, the surface IgD regenerates and this regeneration reconfers resistance to tolerance induction. Therefore, 'B cell maturation' giving tolerance resistance is not a cellular maturation process but one in which B cells may be in various stages of cell-surface-receptor expression; this expression determines the reactivity of the B cells particularly with respect to their sensitivity to tolerance induction.

The debate concerning the structural basis for T cell antigen-receptors has been long and contradictory. T cells recognize antigen in roughly the same way as antibody; this conclusion has been deduced from the observation that crossreactions and specificity of the two forms of antigen-recognition appear to be similar (Rajewsky and Mohr, 1974). Furthermore, anti-idiotypic antibodies prepared against the antigen-binding (idiotypic) sites on T cell receptors react with the antigen-binding regions of normal immunoglobulins as well as with those on B and T cell antigen-receptors (Rajewsky and Eichmann, 1977). The structure on T cell antigen-receptors recognized by anti-idiotypic antibody is the variable of the immunoglobulin heavy chain series (Binz and Wigzell, 1975a, b, c; Black *et al.*, 1975, 1976, Hammerling *et al.*, 1976); that is, T cell idiotypes are inherited with the Ig-1 gene complex which codes for heavy chains, the ability of anti-idiotypic antibody to stimulate helper cell activity amongst cells harvested from different strains of mice depends upon the alleles present at the Ig-1 locus and not on the make-up of the H-2 complex and, lastly, antibodies which recognize the light chain idiotypes are ineffective in stimulating helper T cell activity, whereas antibodies recognizing the heavy chain idiotype are effective in helper cell activation. That T cells display the heavy chain idiotype but not the light chain idiotype is a further argument against these particular T cell antigen-receptors being passively absorbed. Although T cells produce antigen-specific factors expressing Ia-antigens, it seems likely that antigen-receptors on T cells which allow T cells to bind to antigen-coated columns possess heavy chain variable regions, detectable with anti-idiotypic sera, but do not possess constant regions of the known immunoglobulin heavy chains or Ia antigens. Since these particular antigen-receptors have molecular weights in the range of 150,000, they must be incorporated into polypeptides for which the constant region has not yet been defined (Rajewsky and Eichmann, 1977). Since both idiotype-containing T cell receptors and Ia-bearing antigen-specific T cell factors can recognize antigen specifically, both molecules must have variable regions which allow for such antigen-specific binding. These two molecules may come together to form a complete antigen-receptor on T cells or may exist independently as two T cell antigen-receptors.

The binding of immunogenic antigen to antigen-receptors triggers specific B and T cells into activity. The mechanisms by which immunogen attachment to antigen-receptors activates B and T cells are, in all likelihood, considerably different. The nature of this triggering event is as yet unknown, however, many contributions to this particular field indicate that triggering involves more than a simple binding process (Bretscher and Cohen, 1968; Schrader, 1974a, b; Bretscher, 1975; Klinman and Press, 1975). Events such as crosslinking, capping and loss of receptors followed by receptor reformation may be repeated many times and serve to activate immunocompetent cells (Diener and Paetkau, 1972; Raff *et al.*, 1973; Barton and Diener, 1975; De Luca *et al.*, 1975; Ault and Unanue, 1974; Ault *et al.*, 1974; Nossal and Layton, 1976). These changes in antigen-receptor distribution are associated with cellular alterations such as the development of an uropod, translational movement and increased metabolic activity (reviewed by Schreiner and Unanue, 1976). An initial round of capping, patching and endocytosis of receptors is not sufficient for either the induction or inactivation (tolerance) of an immune response. It seems that antigen in high doses, sufficient to cause tolerance induction, induces the loss of antigen-receptors through endocytosis and shedding whereas antigen concentrations which are immunogenic allow for the capping of only a portion of the antigen-receptors (Nossal and Layton, 1976). These latter results are in contrast to those involving receptor redistribution with anti-immunoglobulin antibody; in these latter studies there was no way of assessing immunogenicity (Schreiner and Unanue, 1976) while in the experiments performed by Nossal and Layton (1976) a correlation between immunogenicity and receptor behavior has been made. Hapten-specific B cells may require continuous or periodic contact with antigen to mature into an overtly antibody-forming state (Nossal and Pike, 1976; Pike and Nossal, 1976). Other signals, unrelated to antigen-binding but possibly directed by it, may provide additional stimuli for cell proliferation and differentiation. In the process of antigen-recognition by immunocompetent cells, most notably T cells, membrane components on cells displaying the captured foreign antigen are recognized along with the foreign antigen itself (Rosenthal and Shevach, 1973; Thomas and Shevach, 1976; Vadas *et al.*, 1976). The activation of unprimed and primed T cells (Thomas and Shevach, 1976) and unprimed B cells (Pierce and Klinman, 1976) to full antibody production may require a more complex form of associated or dual recognition involving major histocompatibility complex (MHC) antigens, whereas the induction of antibody-formation by primed B cells appears to be a simple antigen determinant recognition (Pierce and Klinman, 1976).

B cells from young mice possess mainly monomeric IgM surface immunoglobulin whereas adult animals display both IgM and the murine homologue of human IgD on the surface of the same cell (Goding and Layton, 1976). These two classes of surface immunoglobulin cap independently with specific antisera directed against either of them but when exposed to antigen they will cocap indicating that they both bind antigen (Goding and Layton, 1976). From studies carried out on leukemic B lymphocytes (Salsano *et al.*, 1974; Fu *et al.*, 1974, 1975), the monomeric IgM and IgD surface immunoglobulin appear to contain the same variable regions. Not only do B cells express more than one class of immunoglobulin antigen-receptor with the same antigen-binding region, they also appear to be able to synthesize and secrete antibody expressing the same variable region but belonging to different classes of immunoglobulin (Sledge *et al.*, 1976). Different immunoglobulin classes of antibody are formed sequentially rather than simultaneously. These results would lead one to believe that single B cells 'switch' in their synthesis from IgM to IgG antibody production. There would also appear to be a switch between IgG and IgA synthesis (Sledge *et al.*, 1976).

Two questions that have been raised on a number of occasions are whether the IgM to IgG switch occurs prior to or after exposure to antigen, and whether cells destined to switch from IgM to IgG or even to IgA production are marked by differences in their antigen-receptors prior to contact with antigen (Cooper *et al.*, 1972). In a population of non-primed cells, the cells synthesizing IgG progress through an initial period of IgM antibody production, whereas cells primed against antigen synthesize IgG antibody without a prior period of IgM production (Press and Klinman, 1973). In the latter case, the switch from IgM to IgG production occurred consequent to antigenic stimulation during the production of a primary response. However, it would also appear that cells destined to switch sooner to IgG antibody secretion possess on their surface larger quantities of immunoglobulin (Lafleur *et al.*, 1973; Osmond and Nossal, 1974) having high avidity for antigen (Lafleur and Mitchell, 1975). Some experiments suggest that animals not previously immunized with a particular antigen appear to possess different precursors for IgG and IgM antibody-secreting cells (Miller and Cudkowicz, 1971; Shearer *et al.*, 1969; Cooper *et al.*, 1972) whereas other investigations indicate that IgM and IgG antibody-secreting cells stem from a common precursor cell population (Pierce *et al.*, 1972; L'age-Stehr and Herzenberg, 1970; Bussard *et al.*, 1970).

T lymphocytes, activated by immunogen, appear to aid in B cell differentiation at various stages during plasma cell production. Although there are some indications for a T lymphocyte requirement early in B cell activation, there are even clearer indications that T lymphocytes are required somewhat later in B cell differentiation particularly when IgM-producing lymphoblast-plasmablast cells differentiate towards plasma cells and begin the formation of IgG antibody (Isakovic *et al.*, 1965; Basch,

1966; Sinclair, 1967b; Miller *et al.*, 1967; Taylor and Wortis, 1968; Gershon and Kondo, 1970; Mitchell *et al.*, 1972a; Ness *et al.*, 1976). During the switch from IgM to IgG antibody production, the constant portion of the heavy chains of these two immunoglobulins is changed from μ-type to γ-type whereas the variable portions of the heavy chain and the total light chain are conserved, allowing for the conservation of the antigen-binding activity of the secreted antibody (Gearhart *et al.*, 1975).

In terms of the hapten-carrier model, B cells react to hapten and produce anti-hapten antibodies, whereas T cells that cooperate in the production of anti-hapten antibody are activated mainly by the carrier portion of the molecule (Mitchison, 1971a, b). However, antibodies are also produced against that portion of the immunogen which the T cell recognizes as carrier. This fact is often overlooked in considering T and B cooperation but must especially be taken into account when discussing model experiments for antibody-feedback.

In antibody-mediated immune responses that depend upon T cell activities for their elicitation, three types of T cells may be involved in various aspects of T–B cell cooperation. The major cell type involved is the Ly-1 population of T cells, which has a marked ability to cooperate with B cells in the production of both IgM and IgG antibody (Cantor and Boyse, 1975a). The Ly-1 population of T cells is a recirculating, long-lived population which displays a low concentration of cell surface theta-antigen and is sensitive to antithymocyte antibody. A second population expressing Ly-2,3 antigens, which is also long-lived, low in theta-antigen, and sensitive to antithymocyte serum has no helper role in the induction of antibody-mediated immune responses but possesses a suppressive activity (Cantor and Boyse, 1975a; Herzenberg *et al.*, 1976). A third T cell population produced by the thymus, appears to be insensitive to antithymocyte serum, has high concentrations of theta-antigen on their surface and expresses the Ly-1,2,3 antigens. This rapidly turning over population of Ly-1,2,3 T cells is important in the production of both helper and suppressor activities and in the induction of expression of priming in antibody-mediated T cell-dependent immune responses (Simpson and Cantor, 1975). Removal of both Ly-1 and Ly-1,2,3 T cell populations with antithymocyte serum and adult thymectomy depresses both primary antibody immune responses and priming (Simpson and Cantor, 1975). A wide range of antibody-mediated, T cell-dependent responses has not yet been studied, so that the division of function amongst the three T cell populations should be considered suggestive rather than established.

In allotype-suppressed mice in which a suppressor T cell removes the ability of helper T cells to respond and cooperate in the formation of circulating antibody (Herzenberg *et al.*, 1976), memory B cells develop in response to an injection of antigen to the same extent and with the same avidity as in nonsuppressed mice. However, when allotype-suppressed mice are boosted they are unable to initiate production of higher avidity antibodies as occurred in the nonsuppressed mice. This freezing of avidity at a lower level in allotype suppressed mice (Okumura *et al.*, 1976b) is in agreement with work previously published by Gershon and Paul (1971) which indicate that the increase in avidity of antibody produced is a notably T cell-dependent step. Therefore, helper T cells are required for expression of B cell antibody-forming potentiality rather than for initial triggering of B cells by antigen (Lipsky and Rosenthal, 1976). Production of antibody itself appears to be the most sensitive step requiring T cell help. In the absence of helper T cells, B cell differentiation may cease when the developing plasma cells attempt to shift from IgM to IgG antibody production.

A number of factors, generated by T cells, have antigen specificity with respect to binding and stimulatory capacity; some have protein components (Ia-antigens) coded for by the I-region of the MHC. These are non-immunoglobulin factors and appear to be involved in the stimulation of B cells probably through the mediation of the macrophages (Taussig and Munroe, 1974; Moses *et al.*, 1975; Taussig *et al.*, 1975; Munroe and Taussig, 1975; Erb and Feldmann, 1975). Antigen-specific factors of a similar nature specifically suppress antibody-mediated immune responses, most likely by interfering with helper T cells (Tada *et al.*, 1975; Tada *et al.*, 1976; Herzenberg *et al.*, 1976; Murphy *et al.*, 1976). Other T-cell factors, which nonspecifically stimulate immune responses at later steps in antibody-forming cell production, are elaborated in response to stimuli such as adjuvant or allogeneic cells (Katz and Benacerraf, 1975; Schimpl and Wecker, 1973). Activation of T cells may lead to the production of factors that inhibit nonspecifically certain B and T cell responses (Rich and Pierce, 1974; Rich and Rich, 1976). Therefore, various T cell factors may either stimulate or suppress B cell responses in either a specific or a non-specific manner.

Once B cells begin the formation of massive amounts of antibody for export; it becomes increasingly difficult to identify surface-bound antigen-receptors (Warner, 1974). Whether these receptors actually disappear or are submerged in the antibody product is still open to question.

2.2. Cell-Mediated Immune Responses

Cell-mediated immune responses are responsible for certain forms of reactivity against foreign allografts or cells whose surface has been modified by various chemicals, viral or bacterial (intracellular) parasites. The reactivity is generally expressed as a cytotoxic attack against antigens on the surface of allogeneic or modified syngeneic target cells. The two major cell-types involved in the expression of cell-mediated immunity are T cells and macrophages. As with antibody responses, cell-mediated immune responses involve cell–cell cooperation which takes place within subsets of T cells as well as between T cells and macrophages. The major category of T cell required for the induction of *in vitro* cell-mediated cytotoxicity is a class of recirculating, long-lived T cells bearing the Ly-2,3 antigens (Cantor and Boyse, 1975a, b). This cell expresses a low concentration of theta-antigen (Cantor *et al.*, 1975) has Ia-antigen on both precursor and cytotoxic cells (Plate, 1976) and is sensitive to antithymocyte serum (Cantor and Simpson, 1975; Cantor *et al.*, 1975). Two other populations of T cells regulate the cytotoxic cell response of the Ly-2,3 cell. One of these is the long-lived, low theta-antigen, Ly-1 T cell subpopulation (Cantor and Boyse, 1975b) and the other is a short-lived Ly-1,2,3 population (Simpson and Cantor, 1975) expressing a large amount of theta-antigen (Cantor *et al.*, 1975). Both the Ly-1,2,3 and the Ly-1 populations augment low level *in vitro* cytotoxic cell responses while suppressing high level cytotoxicity production (Simpson and Cantor, 1975; Cantor and Boyse, 1975b). Thymus cells display the same ability to augment suboptimal responses induced by limiting concentrations of lymphnode cells (Wagner, 1973).

T cells may also be subdivided according to their content of Fc-receptors (Stout and Herzenberg, 1975a, b). Stout *et al.* (1976) reported on synergism occurring between an Fc-receptor-positive and an Fc-receptor-negative T cell population obtained from nylon wool columns. The Fc-receptor-negative T cell population, which lacked Ly-1 antigen, appeared to be functioning as a precytotoxic cell population. The Fc-receptor-positive cell population, which lacked the Ly-2 antigen, augmented the response of the former precytotoxic T cell population. However, we have not been able to repeat these observations (Lee and Sinclair, unpublished data), finding precursor activity in the Fc-receptor-negative population and no amplifier activity in the Fc-receptor-positive fractions.

Another model for T–T cell collaboration has been developed in which T cells, exposed to antigen or syngeneic macrophages which had taken up antigen, become sensitized initiator T lymphocytes (ITL) and recruit into regional lymph nodes a second population, termed recruited T lymphocytes (RTL) (Cohen and Levnat, 1976). Recruitment is not inhibited by irradiating the ITL but is markedly reduced by irradiating the RTL. Whereas ITL are found predominantly in spleen and thymus, RTL are present in greatest concentrations in lymphnode, to a lesser extent in spleen and not in thymus. RTL pass through nylon wool (Julius *et al.*, 1973) and histamine (Weinstein *et al.*, 1973) columns, but ITL attach to both of these columns as do Ly-1,2,3 T cells (Segal *et al.*, 1974). Recruitment of RTL to draining lymphnodes decrease the concentration of RTL in other lymphoid tissues and leads to a loss of graft-versus-host (GVH) reactive lymphocytes, suggesting a correlation between GVH reactive lymphocytes and RTL. Whereas both the ITL and the effector cells generated display specificity for the inciting alloantigen, the RTL recognizes syngeneic ITL as well as the sensitizing alloantigen. Neither the ITL or RTL proliferate and transform into effector cells; therefore, a 'third' T lymphocyte population which has not come in direct contact with free alloantigen must be activated to become effector cells. The ITL, which contact antigen directly are inactivated with respect to any further proliferative event yet are able to pick up antigen in a trypsin-resistant form, migrate to lymphnodes and trigger other cells to respond to the foreign antigen. Binding of alloantigen to the ITL and the activity of the RTL allows contact of alloantigen with a 'third' T cell population in lymphnodes so that activation rather than inactivation occurs. Because of their immaturity and ability to adhere to nylon wool and histamine columns, the ITL resemble Ly-1,2,3-positive cells. The RTL resemble the Ly-1 positive in many characteristics and functions whereas the 'third' population are, because they are the direct precursors of cytotoxic cells, likely to be Ly-2,3-positive. Memory is associated with the development of cells with ITL activity in lymphnodes, beginning with the lymphnode which is primarily stimulated and then spreading to other lymphnodes. The RTL population do not show any great degree of memory; neither does the related GVH reaction (Ford and Simonsen, 1971). If the RTL recognize a structure on ITL as well as foreign antigen, this structure may also be recognized on allogeneic lymphoid cells during a GVH reaction; this nonimmunologic recognition may explain the large numbers of cells capable of giving a GVH reaction against one allogeneic target (Nisbet and Simonsen, 1967; Lafferty and Jones, 1969; Wilson *et al.*, 1972), their lack of priming (Ford and Simonsen, 1971) and their more active response against allogeneic differences compared to xenogeneic differences (Lafferty and Jones, 1969). In summary, the generation of cytotoxic effector cells is accomplished in regional lymphnodes in which the foreign antigen is excluded in a free form, sequestered as it is on the surface of ITL, which stimulates RTL and precytotoxic cells through the dual binding of foreign antigen and MHC products. Since direct exposure to soluble alloantigens does not sensitize (Cohen and Livnat, 1976), this elaborate system may be required to overcome tolerance induction due to direct exposure to antigen which may itself operate in preventing the production of autoreactive cells (Cohen and Wekerle, 1973). Further information on the effect of alloantigens on distribution of reactive lymphocytes may be found in a review by Hay and Morris (1976).

T cells displaying cytotoxic potentiality appear to be restricted in other capacities in that they do not cooperate with B cells in the formation of antibody (Dennert and Lennox, 1972, 1973; Dennert and Tucker, 1972; Dennert, 1976; Cantor and Boyse, 1977), they do not generate a good GVH reaction (Sprent and Miller, 1971), they are not identical to cells proliferating in response to lymphocyte-defined antigens in mixed lymphocyte cultures (Wagner, 1972; Bach *et al.*, 1973; Festenstein, 1973; Eijsvoogel *et al.*, 1972, 1973, 1976) and they may not be involved in the generation of delayed-type hypersensitivity reactions (Dennert and Hatlen, 1975; Miller *et al.*, 1976b). On the other hand, they do demonstrate cytotoxicity and the ability to cause rejection of allogeneic and syngeneic grafts (Sprent and Miller, 1971; Cerottini *et al.*, 1972; Rouse *et al.*, 1972; Rollinghoff and Wagner, 1973). Cytotoxic T lymphocytes can be sensitized against a variety of xenogeneic (Beverley and Simpson, 1972) allogeneic (Cerottini and Brunner, 1974) modified syngeneic (Zinkernagel and Dougherty, 1977; Shearer *et al.*, 1977), or even 'unmodified' syngeneic (Cohen *et al.*, 1971) cells. Hapten-coupled erythrocytes appear to lack the ability to stimulate an antihapten cytotoxic cell response so that nucleated cells may be required as stimulators (Dennert, 1976). Although proliferation of the cytotoxic T lymphocyte lineage is necessary (Cantor and Jandinski, 1974), this proliferation does not have to be expressed against lymphocyte-defined antigens or be demonstrable through increased uptake of DNA precursors (Mawas *et al.*, 1975; Abbasi *et al.*, 1973; Nabholz *et al.*, 1974, 1975; Dennert and

Hatlen, 1975; Long *et al.*, 1976). These latter findings would suggest that the mixed lymphocyte reaction is not an obligatory, even though augmentory, step in the production of killer cells. Although it is usual for killer cells to be demonstrated as cytotoxic against serologically-defined antigens of the MHC (Trinchieri *et al.*, 1972; Alter *et al.*, 1973; Eijsvoogel *et al.*, 1973), they can also be demonstrated to be cytotoxic against lymphocyte-defined regions of the MHC (Klein *et al.*, 1974; Wagner *et al.*, 1975a, b). Therefore, the distinction often made between lymphocyte and serologically-defined antigens of the MHC is more quantitative than qualitative. Hapten-coupled cells syngeneic with stimulator cells were the best competitive inhibitors, indicating that the site recognized by cytotoxic cells was larger than the hapten itself (Shearer *et al.*, 1977; Dennert and Hatlen, 1974; Moller, 1974). Since it is by no means certain that the target recognized by effector cells is the same as that detected by the usual restricted antiallogeneic antisera, it has been suggested that the term cytolytically-defined (CD) be used to describe the usual target for cytotoxic T lymphocytes (Bach *et al.*, 1977). Also, MHC antigens which give rise to cell-mediated cytotoxicity *in vitro* may be coded for by genes close to but not identical with the serologically-defined loci while the relative requirement for a lymphocyte-defined locus difference may relate to a closely linked genetic system required for the *in vitro* evocation of a cell-mediated immune response (Long *et al.*, 1976). Reviews on the specificity of cytotoxic T cells have recently appeared (Moller, 1976; Forman, 1976).

Although differences in the H-2I region or the H-2K and H-2D regions can induce the production of cytotoxic cells capable of killing target cells of the same H-2 type as the stimulator cells, the effector cell production in the presence of both an H-2I and H-2K or H-2D difference was much larger than the sum of the anti-H-2I and anti-H-2D or K responses (Wagner, 1973; Nabholz *et al.*, 1974). This would suggest that a form of synergy exists between responses directed against lymphocyte- and serologically-defined antigens. It is of interest that, while I–B and I–C regions of the H-2I locus stimulate mixed lymphocyte reactions, they do not incite either cytotoxic cell production *in vitro* or graft rejection but nevertheless will mediate a synergistic effect with respect to the generation of cytotoxic lymphocytes reactive to the H-2K and H-2D region encoded antigens (Rollinghoff and Wagner, 1975). This latter result favors the concept that T–T cell synergism occurs and that the synergism takes place between at least two separable populations of T cells recognizing two independent antigen systems.

In an *in vitro* allogeneic immune response, responding lymphoblasts take up alloantigens derived from the stimulator cells (Nagy *et al.*, 1976 a, b). When responder cells are activated against H-2K and H-2I differences, two populations of lymphoblasts are found. One population takes up the allogeneic stimulator H-2K antigens; this cell expresses Ly-2 antigen. Another responder lymphoblast takes up the allogeneic H-2I region antigens; these lymphoblasts express Ly-1 antigens. Therefore it would appear that Ly-1 cells have a capacity to recognize and bind allogeneic Ia-antigens encoded by the H-2I region while the Ly-2,3 population has binding specificity for the H-2K antigens (in these particular experiments the H-2D antigens were not studied). There are minor populations, that is, Ly-2,3 lymphoblasts binding Ia-antigens and Ly-1 cells binding H-2K antigens. The presence of cells of the Ly-2,3 type capable of binding H-2I region antigens explains the presence of H-2I region-directed cytotoxic cells in some systems (Klein *et al.*, 1974; Wagner *et al.*, 1975a, b). The presence of allogeneic H-2K antigens on cells possessing Ly-1 antigen may represent that population of cells which can be stimulated, albeit weakly, in a lymphoblastic response against H-2K differences (Nabholz *et al.*, 1974).

In conclusion, there is good reason to think that there are cell–cell collaborative events between at least two populations of T cells, one of which is an Ly-1 population recognizing predominantly H-2I region differences and a second population possessing Ly-2,3 antigens recognizing predominantly the H-2D and H-2K region differences, giving rise to cytotoxic cells specific for the H-2K and H-2D antigens. However, animals differing in only the H-2I region will reciprocally reject skin grafts (Hauptfeld *et al.*, 1973, 1974) so that the H-2I difference may often, rather than rarely, excite an effector cell response. The requirement for cooperating T cell populations may relate to immunologic triggering phenomena, or, as is favored in this review, to overcome inactivation occasioned by direct exposure of T-cells to antigen.

2.3. Receptors for the Fc Portions of Antibody—Cellular Distribution and Association with Other Cell Surface Components

A number of antibodies may become attached through their Fc portions to cells involved in immune responses (macrophages, B and T lymphocytes, other undefined lymphocytes and monocytes). These forms of attachment may influence or regulate the immune response in various ways. Antibodies may be either cytophilic (able to attach to cells in the absence of antigen) or opsonic (binding to antigen first, then to cells). In both cases, it is the Fc portions of antibodies which bind to cellular receptors, which are consequently termed Fc-receptors (Paraskevas *et al.*, 1972a, b).

Since some of the mechanisms proposed for antibody-feedback involve signals emitted from the Fc portion of antibody and since these signals are likely to be received by Fc-receptors present on the surface of immunocomponent cells, it is necessary that a review of the cellular distribution and associations of Fc-receptors with other cell surface entities be included in the description of the immune system. At the outset, it should be stated that the work carried out to date on the distribution and functional interactions of Fc-receptors on lymphoid cells is far from complete. Nevertheless sufficient information is now available to formulate a reasonable overview of this particular subject and to point out areas where information is required.

A number of authoritative reviews have been published recently on the subject of Fc-receptors on the surface of cells involved in the immune response (Warner, 1974; Kerbel and Davies, 1974; Sachs and Dickler, 1975; Dickler, 1976; Schirrmacher and Festenstein, 1976), attesting to the interest and curiosity which these Fc-receptors have aroused. A limited review will be presented herein and will be directed towards the presentation of information concerning these receptors which bear upon the regulatory function proposed for them (Sinclair and Chan, 1971; Sinclair *et al.*, 1976a; Sinclair, 1978).

Receptors for the Fc portions of immunoglobulin were first described on macrophages (Boyden and Sorkin, 1960). Macrophage cytophilic antibody in mice is mainly of the IgG_1 class (Tizard, 1969, 1972) whereas opsonic antibodies appear to be mainly IgG_2 (Berken and Benacerraf, 1968) and possibly only IgG_{2a} (Cline *et al.*, 1972). However, there is a considerable amount of controversy since, with bacterial opsonization, IgM can act efficiently (Rowley and Turner, 1966) and erythrocyte–antibody complexes can be inhibited from opsonization by IgG_1 and IgG_{2b} proteins but not IgG_{2a} myeloma proteins (Shevach *et al.*, 1972). The Fc portion of cytophilic antibody is required for binding (Berken and Benacerraf, 1966; LoBuglio *et al.*, 1967), particularly the CH_3 region of cytophilic immunoglobulin (Yasmeen *et al.*, 1973).

B cells have receptors for the Fc portion of antibody. These receptors may be visualized with the use of antigen–antibody complexes, aggregated immunoglobulin or antibody-coated erythrocytes. Lymphocytes are able to bind immunoglobulin in immune complexes, but not usually free immunoglobulin (Uhr, 1965; Paraskevas *et al.*, 1972a, b; Basten *et al.*, 1972a, b; Dickler and Kunkel, 1972). There is a requirement for the Fc portion in this form of binding (Cline *et al.*, 1972). The Fc-receptor is distinguishable from the receptor for complement (Eden *et al.*, 1973). The lymphocyte that combines with aggregated immunoglobulin through the Fc portion is primarily the B lymphocyte (Basten *et al.*, 1972a; de Jesus *et al.*, 1972; Paraskevas *et al.*, 1972a, b; Dickler *et al.*, 1973; Brain and Marston, 1973; Lay *et al.*, 1971; Frøland, 1972; Jondal *et al.*, 1972); however, these results did not rule out the presence of Fc-receptors on T cells. Plasma cells appear to have a poor representation of Fc-receptors (Basten *et al.*, 1972b; Cline *et al.*, 1972; Warner *et al.*, 1975), especially when secreting immunoglobulin (Ramasamy *et al.*, 1974). The major class of immunoglobulin binding to

Fc-receptors appears to be IgG (Cline *et al.*, 1972; Basten *et al.*, 1972b; Paraskevas *et al.*, 1972a, b; Dickler and Kunkel, 1972) although some evidence for IgM binding has been presented (Basten *et al.*, 1972b). The relative binding efficiency of the various subclasses of murine IgG to B lymphocytes appears to be different in the diverse experimental systems studied. Claims for preferential binding of either IgG_1 (Basten *et al.*, 1972b) or IgG_{2a} (Anderson and Grey, 1974; Soteriades-Vlachos *et al.*, 1974; Gyöngyössy *et al.*, 1975) have been made, while another study found no difference between the two (Cline *et al.*, 1972). Some differential binding of human IgG subclasses has been observed (Lawrence *et al.*, 1975). Even if differences have been observed, the various subclasses of IgG appear to be binding to the same Fc-receptor (Basten *et al.*, 1972b; Anderson and Grey, 1974; Soteriades-Vlachos *et al.*, 1974; Lawrence *et al.*, 1975). Except for possible binding by IgM, there is no evidence that other classes of secreted immunoglobulin bind to B lymphocytes.

The cell surface characteristics of various lymphoid and plasmacytoid tumor cell lines have been studied with the assumption that tumor cells represent cells transformed at some stage in the differentiation pathway and that malignant transformation would freeze the characteristics at that stage (Warner *et al.*, 1975). Very few T lymphomas possess Fc-receptors (three out of twenty-nine) and of these no association can be made between the presence of Fc-receptors and any T cell characteristics studied or source of the tumor. With the B cell tumors, there appears to be a progression in Fc-receptor development. Some B cell tumors possess very weak Fc-receptor activity, contain low amounts of surface immunoglobulins and do not secrete immunoglobulin; these tumors represent a very early stage in B cell development. Other B cell tumors possess few Fc-receptors, have surface immunoglobulin and still do not secrete immunoglobulin; these tumors represent a slightly later stage in B cell development. Still other B cell lymphomas have high concentrations of surface immunoglobulin and Fc-receptors; these tumors produce immunoglobulin for export at a rate much higher than the former two B cell tumor categories but lower than that of plasma cell tumors. These cells could be activated B cells on their way towards plasma cell development or possibly memory B cells. Lastly, plasma cell tumors generally express less Fc-receptor activity, with the exception of one which produces only L chains and not intact IgA as it did in earlier transplant generations (Cline *et al.*, 1972). If one can interpret these series of B cell lymphomas in terms of the normal differentiation process of the B cell towards the functioning plasma cell, one would suggest that Fc-receptor activity is not expressed in stem cells (Basten *et al.*, 1972b), reaches a height of activity in mature B cells and becomes less demonstrable as immunoglobulin synthesis increases (Cline *et al.*, 1972). One of the most notable tumors is a B cell lymphoma which secretes both L and H_γ chains and has a high proportion of cells with Fc-receptors. This cell may be either a memory B cell or a B cell recently activated by antigen. If the latter is the case, then this would suggest that recently activated B cells form IgG antibody and this raises the possibility of early feedback-inhibition by this class of antibody through an Fc-dependent mechanism.

An argument has been made for cell surface association between Fc-receptors and Ia-antigens coded for by the I-region of the MHC (H-2I) in mice (Dickler and Sachs, 1974), however, the following strongly suggest that the two molecules are distinct, even if frequently associated: (1) non-concordance in tissue and cell distribution; (2) the labile nature of Fc-receptors in response to antibody attachment to many cell surface antigens; (3) independent capping; (4) difference in sensitivity to trypsin; and (5) difference in molecular size (Schirrmacher and Festenstein, 1976; Halloran *et al.*, 1975). On effector cells cytotoxic to antibody-coated target cells (Möller, 1965; MacLennan, 1972; Perlmann *et al.*, 1972; Cerottini and Brunner, 1974), Fc-receptors and Ia-antigens are not associated (Schirrmacher and Halloran, 1975; Dickler, 1976; Solheim *et al.*, 1976). On the other hand, there appears to be an association between some of the H-2I determinants on T cells and Fc-receptors (McDevitt *et al.*, 1976; Dickler *et al.*, 1976; Stout *et al.*, 1977). Therefore, the association between Fc-receptors and Ia-antigens, although not complete, is pronounced especially on lymphocytes which are intimately involved in immune responses, B and T cells.

Cell surface immunoglobulins possess mainly μ (8S IgM) or δ (IgD) heavy chains. In cocapping experiments it appears that anti-μ chain antibody would influence the distribution of Fc-receptors whereas anti-δ chain antibody did not; this suggests that μ chain-containing (IgM) antigen-receptors are more closely linked to Fc-receptors than are δ-chain-containing (IgD) antigen-receptors (Forni and Pernis, 1975). The association between IgM antigen-receptors and Fc-receptors may not be a simple physical one since there was a lack of a reciprocal effect, that is, no redistribution of immunoglobulins followed capping of Fc-receptors (see, however, the experiments of Unanue and Abbas (1975) described below). The cocapping of Fc-receptors with IgM antigen-receptors suggests that a more pronounced Fc-dependent regulation of immune activation would take place with respect to the IgM-bearing cells than the IgD-bearing cells, the end result of which would be that IgM responses may be more affected by immunoregulatory IgG antibody than the cells having only IgD antibody on their surface and destined for IgG antibody synthesis. These latter cells would presumably be a form of stabilized IgG memory B cells and this would coincide with the fact that IgG secondary responses are much more difficult to inhibit with antibody than are primary immune responses (Uhr and Möller, 1968).

The capping of some surface immunoglobulins cocaps Fc-receptors (Unanue and Abbas, 1975; Abbas and Unanue, 1975) but does not influence the distribution of H-2K, H-2D or Ia-antigens on B lymphocytes. The separate surface behavior of Ia-antigens and Fc-receptors in capping with anti-immunoglobulin indicates that these cell surface molecules are separate entities. Capping of Ia (H-2I) antigens does not influence the distribution of H-2K or H-2D molecules. Also, the capping of Fc-receptors has no effect on the distribution of cell surface immunoglobulin. The non-reciprocal relationship between Fc-receptor and surface immunoglobulin capping may be altered by previously binding Fab anti-Ig antibody to the surface immunoglobulins, then capping Fc-receptors with antigen–antibody complexes; under these conditions, the Fab anti-Ig antibody moves into the Fc-receptor cap. This suggests that membrane immunoglobulin, altered by the binding of anti-Ig antibody or similarly by antigen, becomes attached to and can then cocap with Fc-receptors. If such an association occurs, this would no doubt be of great importance in initial antigen-triggering at the B-cell surface and would suggest an early function for the Fc-receptor in influencing B cell activation.

There is an interesting maturation relationship in mice which has been observed when both Fc-receptor and immunoglobulin-bearing cells were measured (Forni and Pernis, 1975). The presence of immunoglobulin on the surface of Fc-receptor-bearing cells increases with age. This suggests that either Fc-receptor-bearing cells take up immunoglobulin produced by the fetal cells but would not take up passive IgG antibodies derived from the mother, or that the population of Fc-receptor-positive immunoglobulin-bearing B cells increases with time to represent the majority of the Fc-receptor-bearing cells. Reciprocally, immunoglobulin-bearing cells do not appear to have many Fc-receptors in young mice whereas, in adult mice, most of the immunoglobulin-bearing cells have Fc-receptors. This may be evidence that, as the B cells mature, they display Fc-receptors as was suggested from the analysis of B-cell tumors (Warner *et al.*, 1975). In humans, the majority of IgM- and IgD-bearing cells do not contain Fc-receptors when the cells are derived from cord blood of newborns but most adult peripheral blood lymphocytes bearing these immunoglobulins have Fc-receptors. These results also indicate that Fc-receptor activity may be associated with B cell maturation (Warner *et al.*, 1975). Unlike the situation in mice, the majority of human Fc-receptor-positive lymphocytes are negative for surface immunoglobulin in both neonates and adults, indicating that the majority of Fc-receptor-positive cells are not B cells even though most mature B cells have Fc-receptors.

Only a small proportion of Fc-receptor-containing cells from human peripheral blood have stable surface immunoglobulin and can be considered to be B cells

(Kumagai *et al.*, 1975). When a population of non-T cells (not forming rosettes with sheep erythrocytes) was treated with neuraminidase and then rosetted with sheep erythrocytes a second time, those cells not displaying surface immunoglobulin but containing Fc-receptors formed rosettes with sheep erythrocytes whereas cells with stable surface immunoglobulin did not form rosettes with sheep erythrocytes even after neuraminidase treatment (Abo *et al.*, 1976). Two possibilities for the derivation of these cells were considered; they were either a pre-B cell population which, on further maturation, would become fully-fledged B cells with surface immunoglobulin and Fc-receptors or, by virtue of their ability to form sheep erythrocyte rosettes after neuraminidase treatment, they were in reality a subpopulation of T cells. In individuals with active autoimmune disease, the number of Fc-receptor-containing cells and the number of cells with a stable surface immunoglobulin marker were approximately equal, indicating that the population of surface immunoglobulin-positive, Fc-receptor-positive cells had increased markedly. On remission of the autoimmune disease, the percentage of cells with a stable surface immunoglobulin decreased with little or no change in the Fc-receptor-containing population thus demonstrating that a population of surface immunoglobulin-negative, Fc-receptor-positive cells reemerged. If the surface immunoglobulin-negative, Fc-receptor-positive cell were a precursor cell for the surface immunoglobulin-positive, Fc-receptor-positive B cell, then active autoimmune disease may be associated with a larger population of mature, rather than immature, B cells compared to both normal individuals and individuals whose disease is inactive. If the surface immunoglobulin-negative, Fc-receptor-positive cell, which under certain conditions will rosette with sheep erythrocytes, were a form of T cell then it would appear that heightened B cell activity in autoimmune disease is associated with the loss of this population. Such an association may be the cause (loss of a suppressor T cell population) or the result (exhaustion of a T helper population) of the autoimmune process.

The presence of Fc-receptors on the surface of T cells has been substantiated in a number of studies (Yoshida and Andersson, 1972; van Boxel and Rosenstreich, 1974; Anderson and Grey, 1974; Soteriades-Vlachos *et al.*, 1974; Fridman and Golstein, 1974; Santana and Turk, 1975). Approximately 20 per cent of peripheral T cells and 10 per cent of thymus cells display measurable amounts of Fc-receptors (Stout and Herzenberg, 1975a). Although earlier work had suggested that Fc-receptors appear during T cell activation, there is no conclusive evidence that Fc-receptor-bearing T cells represent a larger (lymphoblast) population. When T cells are separated into those possessing detectable Fc-receptors and those without detectable Fc-receptors, the Fc-receptor-negative population contains cells capable of demonstrating helper activity. About 25 per cent of activated T cells possess Fc-receptors (Fridman and Golstein, 1974; Fridman *et al.*, 1975). These receptors were lost on incubation of T cells at 37°C for 3 hr or more. Concomitant with the loss of Fc-receptors, an Fc-binding material appeared in the culture fluid. This material was immunosuppressive when added to a Dutton and Mishell (1967) system for the production of an IgM PFC response against sheep erythrocytes.

On labeling with antigen–antibody complexes, less than 0.5 per cent of thymic lymphocytes and 20–55 per cent of splenic lymphocytes are positive at low concentrations of antigen–antibody complexes (Dickler *et al.*, 1976). In the spleen, these labeled cells correspond to Ig-bearing lymphocytes. With high concentrations of complexes, 10–20 per cent of thymocytes and 65–80 per cent of splenic lymphocytes are labeled. The additional labeling at high concentrations of antigen–antibody complexes involves T lymphocytes. About half of this T lymphocyte labeling may be inhibited by either intact or $F(ab')_2$ antibodies directed against Ia-antigens. These results demonstrate the existence of a population of T cells whose Ia-antigens and Fc-receptor surface components are linked, whereas, in another T cell population, these two components are independent of each other. A more detailed discussion of this phenomenon will be given in Section 2.4.

Human peripheral blood lymphocytes contain a minority population which binds both uncoated sheep erythrocytes and IgG antibody-coated erythrocytes, suggesting that there are circulating T lymphocytes, which have Fc-receptors for IgG (Ferrarini *et al.*, 1975; Chiao and Good, 1976). These Fc-receptor-bearing T cells are detected when the assay is carried out in the presence of agammaglobulinemic serum of either human or fetal calf origin. This would suggest that the Fc-receptors on T cells are able to take up immunoglobulins in serum supplements and, to demonstrate Fc-receptors on T cells, immunoglobulins must be eliminated from the serum supplement. Human T cells also appear to have a receptor for IgM immunoglobulin; this receptor was detected when T cells were incubated in the absence of IgM-containing serum and were demonstrated as cells capable of forming rosettes with IgM antibody-coated erythrocytes (Moretta *et al.*, 1975). There are three distinct populations of T cells, one displaying an Fc-receptor for IgM, another binding IgG and a third population possessing no detectable Fc-receptors (Moretta *et al.*, 1976a). The T cell subset with receptors for IgM cooperates in B cell activation to mitogens while the IgG-Fc-receptor T cells are suppressive (Moretta *et al.*, 1976b).

Peripheral blood lymphocytes and thymus cells from agammaglobulinemic birds (made so by treatment with anti-IgM antibody and bursectomy) could passively take up antibody onto their surface (Webb and Cooper, 1973). The antibody used was IgM suggesting that T cells are able to take up IgM antibody either as the free immunoglobulin or as IgM antibody associated in antigen–antibody complexes. Thoracic duct lymphocytes, obtained from rats, contain two populations of lymphocytes which can be separated on the basis of their surface immunoglobulin content (Hunt and Williams, 1974). One population contains a high surface immunoglobulin concentration which is formed endogenously; these cells are B cells. Another population (T lymphocytes) has a low concentration of surface immunoglobulin. The class of antibody found on the surface of the latter cells, is of the IgM type. The endogenous nature of the immunoglobulin found on the surface of cells with a high density of immunoglobulin (B cells) and the exogenous nature of immunoglobulin on T cells was determined by performing an adoptive transfer into rats bearing a different immunoglobulin allotype and demonstrating that thoracic duct lymphocytes (harvested 20–30 hr later) bore the donor allotype on the heavily labeled cells and the recipient allotype on cells demonstrating a low concentration of surface immunoglobulins. Such a difference with respect to allotype suggests that cells with limited numbers of immunoglobulins on their surface obtain them passively, whereas cells with a high concentration of immunoglobulins on their surface synthesize them endogenously. These results are in contradistinction to others which suggest that T cells are capable of forming an IgM like antigen-receptor (Cone *et al.*, 1972; Marchalonis and Cone, 1973), however, these latter studies do not distinguish between endogenously formed and passively acquired immunoglobulins. It is possible that immunoglobulins may be acquired on the surface of T cells with specificity for antigen; this would occur when antigen, coupled to IgM antibody, binds to T cells (Hudson and Sprent, 1976). Following the formation of an immunologically specific complex of the T cell antigen-receptor, antigen and IgM antibody, the IgM antibody may attach to Fc-receptors specific for IgM thus allowing the T cells to take up antibody with specificity for the antigen recognized by the T cell (Playfair, 1974).

The above results suggest that T cells have a rather well-developed ability to bind IgM antibody, presumably through an Fc-receptor specific for IgM antibody. So far, there has been no direct demonstration of a requirement for the Fc portion of IgM antibody. Since small amounts of native IgM could block IgM EA-rosette formation, it is likely that no aggregation phenomenon is required for the attachment of IgM to T cells. This could explain the reason why these receptors on T cells are normally blocked. The presence of a population of T cells which take up IgM antibodies may also explain the relatively poor ability of IgM antibody to induce suppression (Henry and Jerne, 1968). Low responder strain animals may be deficient in T cells specific for antigen and containing Fc-receptors for IgM immunoglobulin; these animals are sensitive to IgM antibody-feedback (Ordal *et al.*, 1976).

Approximately 20 per cent of lymphocytes with T cell markers contain detectable Fc-receptors when the T cells were derived from thymus, normal spleen or the peritoneal cavity (Basten *et al.*, 1975c). Although mouse thymus cells have receptors for aggregated human gammaglobulin they did not appear to possess receptors for aggregated mouse gammaglobulin of either the IgG_1, IgG_{2a} or IgG_{2b} subclasses; this suggests that the appearance of receptors for isologous species immunoglobulin (as distinct from heterologous immunoglubulin) may take place in the process of maturation of T cells. In keeping with the lack of Fc-receptors on thymus cells, Revillard *et al.* (1975) were unable to detect EA-E-RFC in human thymus, that is, cells which would rosette in assays for both T cells and Fc-receptor-bearing cells. In this case, the antibody used was heterologous, suggesting that the difference between isologous and heterologous antibody in detecting Fc-receptor-bearing thymus cells (Basten *et al.*, 1975c) may only be visible when using aggregated immunoglobulin preparations and not immunoglobulin-coated erythrocytes. Activated T cell populations also contain about 20 per cent Fc-receptor-bearing cells. Circulating T cells, obtained from the thoracic ducts of heavily irradiated F_1 mice injected with parental thymus cells, lacked Fc-receptors. The absence of Fc-receptors is not due to the occupation of these receptors by immunoglobulin since incubation removes passively-absorbed immunoglobulin without inducing the expression of Fc-receptors. However, this experiment is not totally convincing since Fc-receptors are known to detach themselves from T cells with *in vitro* incubation (Fridman and Golstein, 1974; Fridman *et al.*, 1975). Although circulating T cells harvested from an F_1 mouse injected with parental thymus cells do not possess Fc-receptors (Basten *et al.*, 1975c) it would be incorrect to conclude that this indicates that activated *helper* T cells are Fc-receptor negative. These activated T cells may be near the end of their proliferative potentiality (Sprent and Miller, 1972, 1976) and may lack Fc-receptors, as do highly differentiated plasma cells (Basten *et al.*, 1972b; Warner *et al.*, 1975). A most interesting observation (Basten *et al.*, 1975c) was that Fc-receptors were expressed on peritoneal T cells, which are from a population with a high concentration of macrophages. This may suggest a relation between the function of macrophages and the appearance of Fc-receptors on T cells. T cells may only gain Fc-receptors during the time in which they are in contact with macrophages. Presumably this would involve some collaborative event in the generation of an immune response and may provide an explanation for the observation, made by Stout and Herzenberg (1975a), that cells active as helpers in T–B cell collaboration were Fc-receptor-negative; these cells may only express Fc-receptors during B–T cell collaboration which requires the presence of macrophages (Feldmann and Nossal, 1972).

When mouse thymic lymphocytes are activated against H-2 antigens by adoptive transfer into irradiated H-2 incompatible mice, thoracic duct lymphocytes of donor origin demonstrate both IgM and IgG on their cell surfaces (Hudson and Sprent, 1976). If immunoglobulin-bearing lymphocytes are removed from the initial thymus cell suspension, no IgM-coating of activated T cells (thoracic duct lymphocytes) occurs indicating that IgM antibody is produced by contaminating B cells in the thymus cell preparation. Nevertheless, the IgG-coating remains suggesting that it is passively acquired. Such surface IgG was only demonstrated in thoracic duct lymphocytes taken 5–6 d after adoptive transfer indicating that Fc-receptors for IgG do not develop until this time. T cells, activated against M-locus determinants which do not induce an antibody response, did not demonstrate any acquisition of IgM but did display IgG_1 and IgG_{2a} (not IgG_{2b}), again only at 5–6 d after adoptive transfer. Anti-H-2 activated thoracic duct lymphocytes, obtained from recipients given B cell-depleted thymus cells, could take up both IgM and IgG. The IgM must be directed against the H-2 determinant to which the donor thoracic duct lymphocytes are activated, whereas the IgG may be non-specific. Therefore, specific anti-recipient IgM antibody must be bound to recipient H-2 antigens either before or during attachment to donor thoracic duct lymphocytes specific for recipient antigens. Whether an Fc-receptor for IgM (Ferrarini *et al.*, 1975; Moretta *et al.*, 1976a; Webb and Cooper,

1973) is involved in this process is not known. On the other hand, the non-specific binding of IgG_1 (and IgG_{2a}) probably occurs through an Fc-receptor attachment, which is somewhat surprising since previous reports indicate that such thoracic duct lymphocytes do not possess Fc-receptors (Krammer *et al.*, 1975; Basten *et al.*, 1975c). Circulating T cells may, therefore, possess Fc-receptors but some modification in methodology is required to demonstrate their presence.

Whereas Fc-receptor-positive T cells respond with cell proliferation to Concanavalin A, the Fc-receptor-negative population does not do so (Stout and Herzenberg, 1975b). Concanavalin A has been shown to induce the production of suppressor cells and factors (Rich and Pierce, 1973; Dutton, 1973). Again, the existence of a suppressor cell population bearing an Fc-receptor does not exclude an Fc-receptor in cooperative events between B and T cells; results such as this may be interpreted as suggesting that an inapproprópriate expression of an Fc-receptor may be involved in suppressor cell activity. The rationale behind the inappropriateness would be that a T cell expressing an Fc-receptor would more likely gather to its surface either immunoglobulin or antigen–antibody complexes which disturb B cell activity or T–B cell collaboration. The same receptors may be of use if expressed at the correct time, freeing B cells of antigen–antibody complexes.

There appears to be no relationship between complement- and Fc-receptors (Eden *et al.*, 1973). If complement-receptors play any role in the immune response, they may help in the induction of the thymus-independent IgM synthesis. Depletion of complement-receptor lymphocytes (CRL) inhibits the production of IgM antibody while limiting IgG responses only slightly (Mason, 1976a, b). Furthermore, cells mediating IgG memory and possessing membrane-bound IgG are found amongst both complement-receptor-positive and complement-receptor-negative cell fractions. On the other hand, IgM positive cells, which make up over 80 per cent of the total Ig-positive cell population, all contain complement-receptors. These results suggest that the production of IgM antibody from cells bearing IgM antigen-receptors requires a complement-receptor. IgM antibody synthesis requires fewer T cells and, although a number of exceptions exist, antigens which are 'T cell independent' activate complement via the alternate pathway (Coutinho *et al.*, 1974). These results would appear to discount the hypothesis that complement-receptors were required in the induction of the switch from IgM to IgG antibody synthesis (Dukor and Hartman, 1973).

In analyzing the cellular distribution of Fc-receptors it is clear that these receptors display a rather dynamic activity in their appearance and disappearance from cells of various types. These changes in distribution can be associated with a differentiation pathway, such as in B cell to plasma cell differentiation; however, their placement within the T cell lineage has yet to be understood in terms of either the function of T cells or in terms of the T cell pathway for differentiation. It is possible that no simple statement may be forthcoming concerning the presence or absence of Fc-receptors on various T cell lines, but that the appearance or disappearance of Fc-receptors from T cells may represent a change associated with cellular activities taking place over a rather short time span rather than as a consequence of long term differentiation processes. This is suggested from work in which Fc-receptors on T cells are shed rather rapidly into culture medium (Fridman and Golstein, 1974; Neauport-Sautes *et al.*, 1975) indicating that T cell Fc-receptors are labile and may undergo rapid changes in association with alterations in T cell activity.

2.4. Cooperative Events Occurring in the Generation of an Immune Response: Influence of MHC Antigens

Initially, it was observed that various strains of mice which differ genetically at the MHC respond well or poorly to a number of antigens, such as synthetic aminoacid oligopolymers or more complex proteins given in low concentration. While not all genetically determined immune responses were associated with the MHC, a sufficient number of immune response genes were mapped in this region to excite interest and experimentation. These immune response genes were located between the two genetic loci which coded for the classical, serologically-defined antigens of the mouse MHC. Besides possessing genetic loci important in immune responsiveness to certain antigens, this region also houses genes which determine lymphocytic alloantigens recognizable in a mixed lymphocyte culture (MLC). Three major discoveries have been made with respect to the function of the gene products of this particular region, now designated as the H-2I region. Firstly, cell–cell cooperation in immune responses often involves the requirement for some form of compatibility with respect to the H-2I region (or its counterpart in other species). Secondly, antisera directed against products of the H-2I region detect antigens that are found on immunocompetent cells and these antisera can alter the function of these cells. Thirdly, H-2I encoded Ia-antigens are found on various specific and non-specific factors produced by both T and B cells which are capable of altering the activities of other T cells or B cells. Receptors for these Ia-antigen-containing factors are associated with other Ia-antigens, therefore, regulating signals and their receptors appear to be made up of proteins encoded for by the I region of the MHC.

Already, the H-2I region has been extensively subdivided (Shreffler and David, 1975; Shreffler *et al.*, 1976). It is presently comprised of A, B, J, E and C subregions and specialized immunologic functions have been assigned to cells bearing Ia-antigens encoded for by various H-2I subregions (Tada *et al.*, 1976; Okumura *et al.*, 1976a; Murphy *et al.*, 1976; Neiderhuber and Frelinger, 1976). Some of these functions are discussed in the following paragraphs.

Cooperative interaction between B and T cells involves more than simple antigen recognition. The experiments of Katz *et al.* (1973a, b, c, 1975) suggest that cooperation between B and T cells requires a syngeneic MHC recognition. To demonstrate a cooperative event, the interacting murine cells must share a common H-2I region background (Katz and Benacerraf, 1975). Some form of syngeneic recognition event occurs on the surface of cells undergoing a cooperative interaction in the generation of immune responses. However, rather than an interaction of syngeneic determinants separate from the recognition of antigen, there may be an initial recognition of antigen on the MHC background of the cooperating cells. When the production of primed B and T cells occurs under conditions in which allogeneic T and B cells are allowed to interact from the beginning, these cells will cooperate when stimulated with antigen for the second time (Bechtol *et al.*, 1974a, b: von Boehmer *et al.*, 1975; Heber-Katz and Wilson, 1975; Pierce and Klinman, 1975; von Boehmer and Sprent, 1976). These results indicate that requirement may not be one of syngeneic interaction but of antigenic recognition by T cells on the background of whatever MHC antigens were present on the initially interacting cell types. Therefore, this initial recognition (associative recognition) seems to restrict subsequent cell–cell collaboration.

In all studies wherein primary exposure to antigen occurred in the presence of histoincompatible cells, there had been ample time for the generation of new surface cell-interaction molecules because the B and T cells were produced from stem cells (Katz *et al.*, 1976). Moreover, T cells obtained from tetraparental or semiallogeneic bone marrow chimeras could synergize with B cells from the allogeneic but tolerated strain even when primed in the absence of cells from this strain (Waldmann *et al.*, 1976).

T cell populations may be depleted of their ability to recognize and respond to foreign MHC antigens by injecting these cells into animals possessing these MHC antigens and obtaining thoracic duct lymphocytes from them 18–40 hr after injection (Sprent and von Boehmer, 1976). These cells, primed against an antigen are unable to synergize with the tolerated allogeneic B cells also primed against the same antigen. Neither a B anti-T nor a T anti-B allogeneic reaction appeared to be responsible for this lack of cell synergism. If, on the other hand, T cells are not simply 'filtered' through an allogeneic host but are obtained from F_1 irradiation chimeras receiving T cell-depleted bone marrow (stem cell source) from both parental types, then these T cells will cooperate across an allogeneic barrier with antigen-primed B cells (von

Boehmer and Sprent, 1976). Although allogeneic T and B cells show no cooperation in the 'filtering' experiment mentioned previously, there appears to be no syngeneic preference for cooperation when both allogeneic and syngeneic B cells are present. This latter observation suggests that cooperation can indeed take place across an allogeneic barrier but that T cells must be activated by syngeneic (?B) cells in order to do so. B cells may begin the process by activating T cells through the presentation of antigen on MHC antigens to the surface of the T cells. Once activated, 'filtered' T cells, not possessing reactivity against allogeneic B cells, may now collaborate with these allogeneic B cells. This latter collaboration may be required for removing otherwise tolerogenic antigen (Mitchell, 1975) or feedback-inhibitory antigen–antibody complexes (Chan and Sinclair, 1971), and may not have as stringent a requirement for syngeneic interactions as that between T cells and B cells or macrophages in the original activation of T lymphocytes.

A recent observation (Cantor and Boyse, 1977) has re-opened the question of an allogeneic reactivity disturbing the ability of MHC histoincompatible B and T cells to cooperate. Although the total population of allogeneic T cells could not cooperate with a given B cell population, the Ly-1 fraction of these allogeneic T cells can do so, giving a response which is even higher than that obtained when syngeneic Ly-1 T cells are employed as helper cells. This suggests that the Ly-2,3 T cell population engages in some alloreaction which directly affects the responding B cells either through an alloaggressive response or through the induction of suppressor cells that inhibit the specific response.

There is direct evidence that T cells recognize antigen against a cell-surface background. Antigen associated with peritoneal exudate cells (macrophages) was able to prime nonsensitized, T lymphocyte-rich lymphnode cell population *in vitro* (Thomas and Shevach, 1976). When these antigen-primed T lymphocytes were added to a layer of antigen-containing macrophages obtained from peritoneal exudate cells, these T cells proliferated in response to the second antigen exposure. There was a two-fold requirement with respect to first and second exposure to antigen. Firstly, the two exposures must be to the same antigen, if a maximum proliferative response were to occur indicating immunologic specificity in an anamnestic (secondary) immune response. Secondly, the exposure to a particular antigen on both occasions must be on macrophages from the same I-region genetic background. In these experiments, strains 2 and 13 guinea pigs were used; these strains differ in the I-region but not in the classical serologically-defined regions (Rosenthal and Shevach, 1976; Schwartz, B. D. *et al.*, 1976). If F_1 lymphocytes were used as the responding cell population, a maximum response would occur when the same parental strain macrophages were used for antigen-stimulation on the first and second exposures. However, if the antigen was attached to macrophages from one parental strain on the first exposure and to the other parental strain on the second exposure, little or no response was obtained. These results demonstrate that T cells recognize the antigen and surrounding cellular antigens of macrophages in the process of their activation and reactivation. A similar restriction in ability of primed F_1 cells to recognize antigen on one parental type when priming occurred in the other parental strain has been observed in the adoptive transfer of delayed-type hypersensitivity of fowl gammaglobulin (Miller *et al.*, 1976a); this restriction appeared to operate because of histocompatibility requirements for macrophage-T cell interactions (Miller *et al.*, 1975, 1976a, b).

Nevertheless, other data suggest that F_1 cells may become restricted in a parental environment even when stimulated by antigen for the first time in the F_1 environment (Bevan, 1975); the prior development in the parental environment may have allowed the F_1 cells to gain recognition structures only to that parent. A second receptor was employed later to bind foreign antigen. This duality in recognition suggests dual receptors, one for foreign antigen and the other for MHC antigens on syngeneic cells, unmodified by the foreign antigen.

In an experimental system in which there was no genetic restriction with respect to the ability of antigen-ladened macrophages to stimulate *primary* responses, such a restriction emerged during the induction of secondary responses (Pierce *et al.*, 1976a). In these secondary responses, there was a requirement for a macrophage–antigen complex made up of macrophages which were syngeneic to the macrophages used to induce the primary response. The restriction has been assigned to a macrophage-T cell interaction and not to a MHC restriction required for T–B cell collaboration (Pierce *et al.*, 1976b). These results again suggest that primed T cells are more fastidious in their MHC requirements for activation than either unprimed T or B cells.

If T cells recognize antigen on the surface of another cell type, then it should be possible to demonstrate that these cell-types are required for the binding of antigen to T cells. The propensity of T cells to be damaged (to 'commit suicide') by highly radioactive antigen occurs only in the presence of primed B cells (Basten *et al.*, 1975a). Also, a most efficient way of activating T cells to carrier is to expose them to antigen bound to Ig determinants (antigen-receptors) on carrier-primed B cells (Miller, 1975). T cell activation is enhanced in the presence of antibody and this enhancement involves the presence of B cells (Miller *et al.*, 1971; Kappler and Marrack, 1977) or macrophages (Cohen and Paul, 1974). T cells may also bind to antigen-laden macrophages through a macrophage-receptor for T cells (Lipsky and Rosenthal, 1973). These results suggest that T cells require cell-cooperation, even for binding antigen, a highly inefficient behavior for a cell population thought to be responsible for 'antigen-focusing'.

Carrier-priming of mice to be used as non-irradiated recipients leads to a heightened antihapten response to hapten-homologous carrier immunization by transferred B cells (Pierce and Klinman, 1976). With transfer of B cells from animals not preimmunized with hapten-carrier, carrier-priming of recipients gave an increased IgM antibody response when donor and recipient were allogeneic, whereas, when donor and recipient were syngeneic, there was an increased production of both IgM and IgG_1 antibody. When the donated B cells came from hapten-carrier-primed animals, the production of both IgM and IgG_1 anti-hapten antibodies increased with carrier-priming in either allogeneic or syngeneic systems. These results suggest that the MHC requirement for stimulation of nonprimed B cells to give an IgG_1 response is higher than that for IgM responses and the IgG_1 responses emanating from hapten-carrier primed B cell populations no longer require H-2I identify with cooperating cells. These results seem to be at variance with previously described work in which priming tended to confer genetic restriction rather than alleviate it. In this system, however, macrophages and T cells, resident in the carrier-primed non-irradiated recipients are syngeneic to each other and interaction between these two histocompatible cell-types may take place irrespective of the B cell derivation. Whereas MHC requirements for macrophage–T cell interaction are increased on priming, later cooperation events between T and B cells becomes less sensitive to allogeneic differences following priming.

Whereas a requirement exists for macrophage presentation of antigen to T cells for efficient T cell activation and proliferation, induction of proliferation in the B cell population occurs most readily when the B cells are exposed to free antigen rather than antigen associated with macrophages (Lipsky and Rosenthal, 1976). Although macrophage-associated antigen did not induce efficient B cell activation, neither did it induce B cell tolerance. These results indicate that the major role of macrophages in the immune response may be the activation of T cells, rather than as an intermediary cell-type in T–B cell collaboration. In this study, the B cell response analysed was that of cell proliferation rather than the generation of antibody which may require additional cell-interaction mechanisms to achieve an optimal level and are not evident in the initial proliferative response of B cells to antigen. Furthermore, priming of a B cell population in this study does not involve a change in either B cell numbers or in the capacity of the B cell population to proliferate in response to antigen. Priming of B cells leads to changes in the ability of B cells to undergo later steps in differentiation, particularly the ability to form IgG antibodies.

If MHC restriction in cell–cell cooperation relates to signals associated with Ia-regions, it should be possible to demonstrate that reactions of anti-Ia antibody with Ia-antigens can alter various immune responses. Indeed anti-Ia antisera in the absence of complement, have been shown to inhibit primary and secondary *in vitro* antibody responses to heterologous erythrocytes (Frelinger *et al.*, 1975) and to LPS (Niederhuber *et al.*, 1975). On further dissection of the specificity of Ia antisera that block the production of immunoglobulins by a B cell population, it was noted that antibodies directed against I-A and I-B encoded Ia-antigens would block both IgM and IgG synthesis; I-A and I-B encoded Ia-antigens have been implicated in cell collaboration (Katz *et al.*, 1975) and for interaction between macrophages and lymphocytes (Erb and Feldmann, 1975). Antibodies directed against I-C encoded Ia-antigens block only the synthesis of IgG antibody (Niederhuber and Frelinger, 1976). Blockade by anti-Ia antisera recognizing antigens coded for by the I-C region specifically inhibits later T–B cell collaboration events rather than other forms of cell collaboration (Erb and Feldmann, 1976); hence, IgG synthesis is depressed while IgM antibody synthesis remains normal. Also, the attachment of anti H-2I-C antibody may have induced a state sensitive to inhibition by Ly-2,3 suppressor cells (Cantor and Boyse, 1977); this experiment should be repeated in the absence of the Ly-2,3 T cell population.

Cytotoxicity caused by some anti-Ia antibodies in the presence of complement destroyed the ability of B cells to produce IgG but did not affect the exclusively IgM antibody forming cells (Press *et al.*, 1975, 1976). Cells producing IgM antibody and switching to IgG production were also removed following the treatment with anti-Ia antibodies plus complement. These results indicate the presence of Ia-antigens on the surface of B cells is associated with B cell production of IgG antibody. Using human cells, an antiserum equivalent to murine anti-Ia antibodies inhibits the production of immunoglobulins in culture (Chess *et al.*, 1976; Breard *et al.*, 1977).

Anti-Ia antibody in the absence of complement inhibits B cell activities (Niederhuber and Frelinger, 1976). In contrast, anti-Ia antibodies in the absence of complement could not block a MLC when these antibodies were directed towards the responder cell population, whereas they could do so when directed towards a stimulator population (Meo *et al.*, 1975; Niederhuber and Frelinger, 1976). In the presence of complement, the response of T cells to Con A is inhibited by anti-Ia serum whereas the response to PHA is unaffected (Niederhuber *et al.*, 1976); the T cell subset inhibitible by anti-Ia sera and complement appears to be that T cell subset (Rich and Pierce, 1974) responsible for Con A-induced suppressive activity. The Ia-antigens that are expressed on Con A responsive cells are assignable to the I-J region of the H-2I complex, again linking Con A activation and suppressor cell activity by their mutual expression of such Ia antigens (Frelinger *et al.*, 1976). Helper T cell activities are either resistant (Hämmerling, 1976; McDevitt *et al.*, 1976) or only partially sensitive (Okumura *et al.*, 1976a) to anti-Ia antibody and complement.

T cells, which express much lower concentrations of Ia-antigens on their surface, are mainly responsible for the secretion of Ia-antigens (Parish *et al.*, 1976). The secretion of Ia-antigen could be prevented by exposing T cells to anti-Ly-1 antisera and antisera directed against T cell antigens indicating that the subclass of T cells that secretes Ia-antigen is the Ly-1 population and not the Ly-2,3 population (McKenzie and Parish, 1976). The T cells secreting Ia-antigens do not appear to contain any surface-bound Ia-antigen. Therefore, it would appear to be that one characteristic of T cells is their ability to synthesize and secrete large quantities of Ia-antigen which may find itself in the various T cell factors that augment or suppress immune responses. On the other hand, B cells appear to have the ability to display surface Ia-antigens and to bind Ia-containing factors released from other cells. This does not seem to be an exclusive characteristic of B cells since helper T cells can bind Ia-antigens derived from suppressor T cells in the process of becoming inhibited by these suppressor cell factors (Tada *et al.*, 1976; Okumura *et al.*, 1976a; Murphy *et al.*, 1976). With respect to the possible acquisition by B cells of Ia-antigens derived from T cells, it would be interesting to determine whether or not the Ia-antigen content on B cells in tetraparental bone marrow chimeras (von Boehmer and Sprent, 1976) is endogenously produced or passively acquired from T cells.

In attempting to unravel the mystery of B–T cell surface interactions between Fc-receptors, antigen-receptors and Ia-antigens, Basten *et al.*, (1975a) analyzed the ability of highly radioactive antigen and aggregated gammaglobulin to destroy T or B cells. Thymus absorbed anti-H-2 Fab antibody (? anti-Ia antibody) prevented irradiation damage of B cells upon exposure to highly radioactive, aggregated gammaglobulin. These results are in keeping with those of Dickler and Sachs (1974) and suggest that Fc-receptors and Ia-antigens on the B cell surface bear a close spatial relationship to each other. The anti-H-2 (Ia) antibody would not prevent irradiation damage of specific antigen-binding B cells when these B cells were exposed to highly radioactive antigen. Therefore, there may be an association on B cells between Ia-antigens and Fc-receptors but not between Ia-antigens and antigen-receptors. T cells could not be damaged by direct exposure to highly radioactive antigen; they could, however, be damaged by exposure to radioactive antigen if it was presented on the surface of a non-T cell population. Also, in contradistinction to B cells, irradiation damage of T cells by highly radioactive antigen could be prevented by treating the T cells with anti-H-2 (Ia) Fab antibodies indicating that antigen-receptors and H-2 (Ia) antigens on T cells may be closely associated (Crone *et al.*, 1972; Hammerling and McDevitt, 1974; Wekerle *et al.*, 1975). T cells may bind antigen firmly only with the help of exogenously-derived antibody (Playfair, 1974). Antigen presented by B cells or macrophages may be associated with antibody. T cells, therefore, would bind to antigen through specific nonimmunoglobulin antigen-receptors but also to antibody associated with the presented antigen through Fc-receptor-Fc portion linkage. This linkage may be inhibited by anti-H-2 (Ia) antisera. Fc-receptors on T cells appear to be linked to Ia-antigens (McDevitt *et al.*, 1976; Dickler *et al.*, 1976; Stout *et al.*, 1977). The inhibitory effect of anti-Ia antibody on aggregated immunoglobulin binding by T cells (McDevitt *et al.*, 1976; Dickler, 1976; Stout *et al.*, 1977) and on the binding of cell-presented antigen to T cells (Basten *et al.*, 1975a) at least raises the possibility that antigen-attachment to T cells involves Fc-receptors on T cells and this in turn raises the possibility that antigen-recognition by T cells may involve the concomitant recognition of antigen and antigen-associated antibody. It is reasonable to suggest that the non-T cell type which is required for the presentation of antigen to activate T cells has acquired (macrophage) or produces (B cell) antibody, that T cells initially interact with antigen–antibody complex via specific antigen-receptors, that T cells take up antigen–antibody complexes from the surface of other cells through additional binding between the Fc portion of antibody and Fc-receptors on T cells, and that this attachment may be interfered with by anti-Ia antibodies, which bind to Ia determinants closely associated with Fc-receptors on T cells. Such a mechanism for antigen–antibody binding by T cells may represent a basic mechanism for T cell helper activity.

Approximately 50 per cent of Fc-receptor-bearing T cells are inhibited in their binding of antigen–antibody complexes by antibodies directed against Ia-antigens coded for by the I-A region of the H-2I complex, 30 per cent by binding of antibody to Ia-antigens derived from the I-C region and another 20–30 per cent which are inhibited by antibodies directed against antigen unassociated with the H-2I system (Stout *et al.*, 1977). Some of these antigens may be coded for by the H-2D and H-2K regions and some by non-H-2 genetic loci (Dickler *et al.*, 1975). Within the H-2I region, antibodies directed against I-A and I-C encoded Ia-antigens appear to be the most inhibitory towards the binding of immune complexes whereas antibodies directed against Ia-antigens coded for by the I-J and I-E regions show no such interference. Since Ia-antigens emanating from the I-J region appear to mark suppressor cells (Okumura *et al.*, 1976a; Murphy *et al.*, 1976; Tada *et al.*, 1976), this would suggest that an unique association between Ia-antigens and Fc-receptors does not occur on the surface of suppressor T cells.

Another example of a possible preemption of Fc portions of heterologous antibody (rabbit anti-human T cell) has been described recently (Evans *et al.*, 1977). Absorbed rabbit anti-human T cell serum plus complement has the capacity to inhibit the MLC and the production of lymphocyte mitogenic factors. This serum did not alter lymphocyte responses to soluble antigens, suggesting that the Fc portion of antibody is made unavailable on those cells which exert a helper function and thus is unavailable for complement-mediated cytotoxicity. Since the heterologous antibody was prepared against normal peripheral T cells, there is no reason for suspecting that it detects a differentiation antigen on one T cell line as opposed to another; the difference in effect that this antisera has on two subsets of T cells may therefore relate to a difference in the handling of the Fc portion of antibody during its attachment to the cell surface of the various T cell subsets.

The above results point out the central importance which the products of H-2I region may have in the generation of an immune response. Associations between the Ia antigens, antigen-receptors of both immunoglobulin and non-immunoglobulin types, and Fc-receptors on the surface of immunocompetent B and T cells have been uncovered and implicated in various aspects of the immune response; these associations must play a central role in determining whether or not an immune response will take place and the degree to which it may be modulated.

Since Ia-antigen containing factors may be implicated in forms of modulation of the immune response by antigen and/or antibody, an account of these factors will be given. T cells obtained from antigen-primed animals produce antigen-specific T cell factors when incubated *in vitro* with antigen. Activity of those T cell factors can be demonstrated by injecting them with antigen and B cells into irradiated animals and measuring the subsequent responses (Taussig and Monroe, 1974; Moses *et al.*, 1975; Taussig *et al.*, 1975: Munroe and Taussig, 1975). Their activity is antigen-specific and they bind to the specific antigen. No immunoglobulin is demonstrable in these specific T cell factors. The molecular weight is approximately 50,000 (measured by gel filtration). Genetic determinants responsible for reactivity against some aminoacid oligopolymers have been mapped in the I-region of the H-2 complex and T cell factors can be removed by absorption with anti-Ia serum. These factors are not produced in certain strains of low responder animals but are produced in other low responder strains to the antigen in question. T cell factors interact with B cells, probably through an ‘acceptor’ for these factors. The acceptors for Ia-containing T cell factors are found on B cells (bone marrow cells and purified peripheral B cells) but not on thymocytes. They are found on a rather large majority of B cells, indicating their non-specific nature. The B cell acceptor for T cell factor is blocked by anti-Ia sera indicating that it also may contain Ia-antigen. Some low responder strains for a particular antigen do not express acceptor sites for the antigen-specific T cell factor. Genetic evidence has come forward to indicate that T cells may require a two gene complementing system for activity (Schwartz, R. H. *et al.*, 1976) implying that a factor produced by one T cell may be accepted by another T cell.

A series of suppressive factors produced by T cells appear to be quite similar in nature to the stimulatory factor discussed above (Tada *et al.*, 1975; Kapp *et al.*, 1976; Herzenberg *et al.*, 1976). These factors are also non-immunoglobulin proteins with molecular weights ranging between 35,000 and 55,000. These factors, which are not effective across an H-2 barrier, express Ia-antigens and are recognized as T cell surface-antigen. These suppressive T cell factors appear to have as their target helper T cells rather than B cells, as is the case for some of the augmentary T cell factors. In mice, one part of the H-2I region (I-J) appears to be involved in suppressor factor production while these factors attach to ‘acceptors’ which have their genetic basis in other parts (I-A, I-B) of the H-2I region (Tada *et al.*, 1976; Murphy *et al.*, 1976). Certain strains of mice lack the ability to emit the factor while others lack the ability to receive the suppressive signal (Taniguchi *et al.*, 1976). Tumors appear to stimulate production of similar factors (Fujimoto *et al.*, 1975, 1976).

Although some non-specific factors which are induced in allogeneic reactions have

Ia-antigen (Armerding *et al.*, 1974) others do not (Schimpl and Wecker, 1978). The latter group of Ia-negative T cell-replacing factors (TRF) is produced by Thy-1-positive, Fc-receptor-negative, Ly-1-positive T cells. These factors react with proliferating B cells to allow these cells to mature into antibody-forming plasma cells. The molecular weights of the factors are heterogeneous, ranging from 25,000 to 35,000 daltons. Recent data (Schimpl and Wecker, 1978) indicate that TRF has the ability to bind to Fc-receptors. These receptors may be present either on B cells, and hence TRF may activate B cells into maturation following such binding, or free in solution having been secreted from T cells (Fridman and Goldstein, 1975); the latter would induce a relative deficiency of TRF and hence may explain the suppressive activity of immunoglobulin binding factor (IBF). TRF may serve two basic functions. Firstly, it may stimulate B cells into a final maturation pathway leading to the production of IgG antibody. The second possibility, one that is in line with the mechanism to be proposed concerning antibody-feedback, is that TRF interacts with Fc-receptors on B cells preventing Fc-dependent inactivation of B cells by antigen–antibody complexes. The demonstration that TRF interacts with Fc-receptors on B cells and is involved in a late maturation step in T cell activity provides molecular evidence which is consistent with the view, elaborated upon below, that T cells are involved in controlling Fc-dependent antibody-feedback.

Although many of the soluble factors active in modifying immune responses emanate from T cells or from macrophages, recent evidence indicates that B cells may be an ultimate source of factors produced in some allogeneic reactions which allow other B cells to progress to IgG antibody synthesis (Delovitch and McDevitt, 1977).

Given this outline of cellular events in an immune response, we can now consider forms of modulation by antibody, antigen and antigen–antibody complexes. Because my primary interest lies in antibody-feedback, and because it provides a convenient starting point in building a framework for modulation, immunoregulatory effects of specific antibody will be discussed first. My task in this regard has been made simpler by the appearance of a review by Fitch (1975) which covers many of the recent observations made since the summary of this field by Uhr and Moller (1968). Whereas Fitch's publication is predominantly factual, the present one will have a more speculative nature. In this way, it is hoped that these two reviews will be mutually complementary.

The sections on specific modulation have been divided into that induced by antibody and that by antigen. Regulation by antigen–antibody complexes has not been given a separate section since the formation of such complexes is considered central to control by antigen or antibody.

3. MODULATION OF THE IMMUNE RESPONSE BY ANTIBODY

The presence of specific antibody, either endogenously produced or passively administered, may suppress or augment various immune responses. This dual effect of antibody has attracted a great deal of attention from immunologists because it raises the possibility of specifically altering immune responses in either an upward or downward direction. Furthermore, any influence that antibody may have on the generation of immune responses provides insight into the mechanisms by which these immune responses are generated. Just as the use of various agents have helped in the assigning of cellular activities to various stages of the immune response (Dutton and Mishell, 1967; MacDonald *et al.*, 1975), the effects that antibody has on the immune system help in the definition of cellular activities associated with this system. Since antibody is one of the major products of the immune system and since end-product control is a common event in various biosynthetic pathways, the concept that antibody may regulate its own level must be seriously considered. Cellular pathways involved in such modulation and those moderating this sort of control may be the *raison d'être* of many of the cellular events taking place in an immune response.

3.1. Antigen-Binding vs Antigen-Masking

For a population of immunoglobulins to suppress, this population must have the capacity to bind antigen (Uhr and Moller, 1968). The requirement for complete coverage of antigen (antigen-masking) to allow for feedback-suppression by antibody has been investigated in two forms of experiments. These are the quantitation of antibody needed to induce suppression in relation to the ability of suppressive amounts of antibody to cover all antigenic determinants contained in the antigen administered, and the analysis of the requirements for specificity of antibody to cause suppression.

In many cases of antibody-mediated immunosuppression, coverage of antigen by antibody appears to be far from complete. Small amounts of antibody, administered or accumulated prior to the injection of antigen, induce a measurable degree of suppression (Haughton and Nash, 1969; Ryder and Schwartz, 1969; Solomon *et al.*, 1972). Under conditions in which there is a deficiency in *T* cells, amounts of hyperimmune serum in the vicinity of 10^{-6} cm^3 (about 10^3 times less than that which could be detected by the usual hemagglutinin or hemolysin techniques) is able to suppress the plaque-forming cell response to sheep erythrocytes in irradiated, adoptively-transferred animals (Sinclair *et al.*, 1976a). In some cases in which large amounts of Rh-positive erythrocytes had been administered accidently to Rh-negative individuals, the use of small amounts of anti-Rh-positive antibody to attain immunosuppression with respect to anti-Rh-positive antibody production has been successful (Mollison, 1972). Minute quantities (0.1–0.5 μl) of anti-donor antibodies have led to noticeable graft survival *in vivo* as well as blocked *in vitro* destruction of target cells (Gorer and Kaliss, 1959; Hutchin *et al.*, 1967; Kaliss 1969; Amos *et al.*, 1970; Linscott, 1970; Feldman, J. D., 1972), and enhanced allografts have the ability to take up further administered antiallograft antibody (French, 1973; Carpenter *et al.*, 1976). It should be pointed out, however, that in a number of model systems for antibody-feedback, particularly those involving suppression of cell-mediated immune responses, the amount of hyperimmune serum which must be given is considerably larger (Kaliss 1969) and, in one *in vitro* study, the suppression by antibody likely involves a simple antigen-masking process (Sinclair *et al.*, 1975a). This may be a reflection of the different immune specificities studied, or a system in which there are additional factors, such as marked T cell activation, which limit the mechanisms and thereby decrease the efficiency with which antibody inhibits (Lees and Sinclair, 1975).

Even in systems in which the amount of antibody was sufficient to bind to all the antigenic determinants present in the immunizing dose of antigen, the thermodynamic advantage of immunocompetent cells, with their multiple antigen-binding sites, could allow these cells to compete effectively with circulating antibody for antigen; when the level of circulating antibody is lowered, but is still in very great excess over antigen, an immune response can be triggered by antigen remaining in various depots (Graf and Uhr, 1969; Bystryn *et al.*, 1970, 1971). However, some earlier work on the necessity to bind all antigenic determinants to produce immunosuppression indicated that antigenic determinants were occupied under conditions wherein the antigen did not trigger the immune response and, when free determinants appeared, an immune response arose (Uhr and Baumann, 1961; Dixon *et al.*, 1967).

A number of recent observations have been made in experimental allograft models for graft enhancement which suggest that forms of reactivity against donor antigens are expressed; this is evidence that complete masking of alloantigen cannot account for prolonged graft survival. Enhancement in one renal allograft model (Carpenter *et al.*, 1976) is associated with a delay but not the absence of cell-mediated immunity, with depression of humoral responses responsible for this form of allograft rejection and, as late affects, with immune complex damage, decreased levels of cellular cytotoxicity and the presence of serum blocking factors which prevent cytotoxic attack. Since small amounts of antibody are able to induce enhancement, complete coverage of antigenic determinants on the enhanced allograft is not necessary. The enhanced state was attained in animals which respond immunologically to the engrafted allogeneic antigens, suggesting that the host's ability to recognize the foreign graft was not completely inhibited.

The complex relationship between production of cytotoxic cells and the phenomenon of renal allograft enhancement has been particularly well worked out recently (Stuart *et al.*, 1976b). In the rat strain combinations used (Lewis and Brown Norway), semi-allogeneic (F_1) kidneys were rejected between 5 and 10 d following grafting in unmodified parental hosts. During the same time period, antidonor cell-mediated cytotoxicity was detected using either a chromium-release assay (a measurement of target cell death usually within 4–24 hr) or a microcytotoxicity assay (a measurement of the ability of cytotoxic cells to kill or induce detachment of target cells from tissue culture surfaces within 40–48 hr). A combination of allogeneic lymphocytes and antibody directed against the allogeneic cells caused an immunologically specific enhancement of renal allografts. In animals receiving the renal allograft directly after treatment with alloantigen and antibody, the production of cytotoxic cells, as measured by the chromium-release method, was somewhat lower but not appreciably delayed; the production of cytotoxic cells, as measured by a microcytotoxicity assay, was neither delayed nor reduced. However, when the transplantation of the renal allograft was carried out 10 d after exposure to antigen and antibody (with this timing, the allografted kidney demonstrated a better survival), there was little or no production of cytotoxic cells as measured by chromium-release or by the microcytotoxicity assay. The latter protocol for treatment with alloantigen and antibody, giving the best allograft srvival, was associated with the appearance of anti-idiotypic antibody (antibody directed against the combining site of the antiallograft antibody) as well as with the abssence of cytotoxic cells in two *in vitro* assay systems. Despite the lack of production of cytotoxic cells, lymphoid cells from animals with enhanced kidney allografts are able to induce a marked, although somewhat weakened GVH reaction against animals bearing the antigens of the kidney donor and, also, animals with enhanced renal allografts reject skin grafts from the donor strain in only a lightly delayed fashion. The conclusion to be drawn from these experiments is that graft enhancement may occur in the absence of a suppressed cytotoxic cell response, although better graft survival may be attained when the production of cytotoxic cells has been markedly suppressed. These results point up the complexity of mechanisms operating in the enhancement phenomenon and suggest that enhancement is not coincident with the lack of recognition (Batchelor and Welsh, 1976; Calne, 1976) nor, consequently, with total antigen-masking by graft enhancing (that is, immunosuppressive) antibody.

Some satisfactory experimental studies show that, for an immune response against a particular antigenic determinant on a given immunogen to be eliminated, antibody must be directed towards that particular antigen determinant; these studies are relatively few. An example of determinant-specific immunosuppression is that which occurs in immune responses to chicken erythrocyte antigens where antibody to one particular erythrocyte antigen does not suppress the immune response to a second antigen present on the same erythrocyte (McBride and Schierman, 1971). In another experimental model, immune responses to two separate areas of the immunogen may be controlled separately with respect to antibody-feedback (Pincus *et al.*, 1971). It should be stressed that immune responses to antigenic determinants, not covered by antibody, were not unaffected; they were often increased, indicating that complex immunoregulatory events are taking place (McBride and Schierman, 1971; Pincus *et al.*, 1971, 1973).

Immunologic responses against various H-2 antigens were studied in the progress of immunologic enhancement of a tumor allograft (Moller, 1963). There were some examples of determinant-specific antibody-feedback, but there were also examples in which antibodies directed against one H-2 antigenic determinant inhibited the antibody response against another H-2 antigenic determinant. Conjoint suppression occurred even when the two antigenic determinants studied were on the different ends of the H-2 complex and would not be explicable in terms of a cocapping phenomenon.

Another often-quoted publication is that of Brody *et al.* (1967) in which there was an independent immunosuppression of immune responses directed against two unrelated haptens present on either the same or on separate carrier molecules. However, this work is subject to an alternative interpretation since a form of molecular rather than determinant specificity was also observed in this system. This molecular specificity was observed with respect to antigenic competition (Pross and Eidinger, 1974) and release from antigenic competition seen in this particular study through the agency of antibody (Brody *et al.*, 1967). When antibody against one of the haptenic determinants was included in an immunization procedure, release from antigenic competition occurred with respect to the antibody response against the second haptenic determinant, provided that the two haptens were on separate carrier molecules. This indicates that release from antigenic compeition does not occur when a hapten-carrier is presented to the immune system coupled directly with a second antibody-coated hapten. Thus a form of particle, rather than determinant-specific regulation, appears likely even in this experiment which has been cited as proof for determinant-specific suppression.

Many more studies indicate that antibody directed against one antigenic determinant on an immunogen can suppress an immune response to another antigenic determinant. Some of these immunogens are cellular in nature, such as erythrocytes (Greenbury and Moore, 1969; Stern *et al.*, 1956) or lymphoid cells (Milton, 1976). In the latter study, a C57B1 anti-DBA/2 antibody inhibited the cytotoxic antibody response of CBA mice, immunized with (C57B1 × DBA/2) F_1 cells, against both DBA/2 and C57B1 cells, whereas, on immunization with a mixture of C57B1 and DBA/2 cells only the anti-DBA/2 response was inhibited. Other studies, involving the use of soluble proteins as immunogens, indicate that suppression by antibody is molecule rather than determinant-specific. Guinea pig antibodies, directed against either the Fab or Fc portions of human gammaglobulin (HGG), inhibited the ability of guinea pigs to respond to HGG with the production of either anti-Fab or anti-Fc antibody (Henney and Ishizaka, 1968). In this study, the anti-Fab antibody was shown not to cover the Fc portions of HGG nor did the anti-Fc antibody cover the Fab portions of HGG. In a further study, Henney and Ishizaka (1970) investigated the antibody-inhibition of dinitrophenylated human gammaglobulin (DNP-HGG) in which the antibody was directed against either the DNP (hapten) or the Fc portion of HGG (carrier). Antibody directed against either the DNP or the Fc portion of HGG inhibited both anti-DNP and anti-HGG antibody formation. However the antibody was ineffective in preventing a delayed-type hypersensitivity reaction, suggesting in retrospect that antibodies do not easily interfere with the activation of T cells and also indicating that antigen has not been completely removed. It is of interest that, following primary immunization with hapten–carrier and antihapten antibody, suppression of the antihapten antibody response may be broken by a second injection of hapten–carrier immunogen but not by hapten on a heterologous carrier. This indicates, also in retrospect, that an increase in T cell activity can relieve an antibody suppressed state.

In an immune response, initiated by antigen coupled by antibody through an Fc-dependent attachment to a macrophage population (Hamaoka and Kitagawa, 1971), a number of properties of antibody-feedback can be analyzed particularly with respect to specificity of suppression (Hamaoka *et al.*, 1971a). Hapten–carrier complexes can be coupled to macrophages using anticarrier antibody and this complex stimulates an antihapten response in a primed cell population provided that this population is primed to the hapten–homologous carrier (Hamaoka *et al.*, 1971b). If passive antibody is administered to animals receiving primed cells and antigen-antibody-coated macrophages, the resulting 10 d antibody titer is markedly suppressed. A complex made up of one carrier and two haptens (DNP and benzyl-penicilloyl (BPO)), coupled to macrophages with anticarrier antibody, stimulates a mixture of DNP-carrier-primed and BPO-carrier-primed cells to produce the two antihapten antibodies. Passively administered antibody, directed against either hapten, specifically suppresses the response to that hapten without affecting the antibody response to either the other hapten or the carrier. However, antibody against the carrier inhibits antibody responses to both haptens as well as the carrier. In this system, as compared to others (Yamashita *et al.*, 1976a, b), there is no evidence of hapten-primed T cells so that all anti-hapten responses involved interaction with a carrier-primed T cell population. It would be interesting to know if anticarrier antibody would or would not inhibit an antihapten response in those systems where hapten-primed T cells are found and are sufficient for the generation of antihapten immune responses (Yamashita *et al.*, 1976a, b). Suppresion demonstrating molecule rather than determinant specificity with respect to antibody-feedback may interfere with a B–T cell collaborative event (Hoffmann *et al.*, 1974). When B–T cell collaborative events can take place without recourse to the carrier antigenic specificities, such as in systems when hapten-primed T cells are present, only determinant-specific immunosuppression by anti-carrier antibody may be demonstrated. Anti-hapten antibody might now show molecular, rather than determinant, specificity in immunosuppression.

Work on the role of anti-Ia antibody in immunologic enhancement has given new insights into the question concerning particle vs determinant specificity of antibody required for immunosuppression in allograft enhancement. Allo-antisera raised against donor tissue may enhance the survival of donor tissue, such as heart allografts in rats, even when the alloantisera have had anti-SD (serologically-defined) antigen activity removed by adsorption with donor erythrocytes (Davies and Alkins, 1974) or with donor platelets (Davies, 1976). The absorbed antiserum behaved like the restricted antiserum described by David *et al.* (1973) which is now recognized as defining Ia-antigens encoded for by the I-region of the MHC. These anti-Ia antibodies must be directed against the stimulator rather than the responder tissue to be active in *in vitro* immunosuppression (Meo *et al.*, 1975; Staines *et al.*, 1975). In organ grafts, which consist primarily of parenchymal cells not possessing Ia antigens, the graft enhancing anti-Ia antibodies may act on passenger leukocytes which carry Ia-antigens and usually serve to stimulate the *in vivo* MLC required for sensitization of the recipient and triggering of the antigraft immune response (Davies and Staines, 1976). However, anti-Ia serum shows an equal ability, compared to unabsorbed anti-H-2 sera, to give enhancement of skin allografts, a tissue rich in Ia-antigens (Staines *et al.*, 1975; Davies and Staines, 1976). Although the degree of enhancement of skin allografts was not as permanent as that which occurred with various organ grafts (Zimmerman and Feldman, 1969, 1970; Davies and Staines, 1976), particularly kidney and heart, nevertheless, anti-Ia antisera were able to block for a time the rejection of allografts in which the parenchymal cells of the allograft bear Ia-antigens. A study involving the ability to demonstrate tumor enhancement in Ia-antigen positive and negative tumor cell lines from the same histologic background would help in deciding whether or not the binding of anti-Ia antibodies to engrafted tissue works through the simple elimination of passenger leukocytes bearing Ia-antigens or whether anti-Ia antibodies can, by masking only a portion of the allogeneic tumor cell surface, induce a form of enhancement which does not require the coverage of all antigenic determinants. It should also be pointed out that, although the MLC-Ia-antigen system is a requirement for production of cytotoxic cells *in vitro* (Eijsvoogel *et al.*, 1972, 1973, 1976) this requirement is not complete either *in vitro* where cytotoxic cells can be generated in the apparent absence of an Ia difference (Egorov, 1974; Abbasi *et al.*, 1973; Nabholz *et al.*, 1975; see, however, Peck *et al.*, 1976) and where tissue can be rejected *in vivo* between individuals identical at the MHC (Najarian and Simmons, 1972). In view of the fact that rejection phenomena can occur without an Ia-antigen difference, the binding of anti-Ia antibodies to Ia-antigens may not in fact operate through a peripheral masking mechanism of either the afferent or efferent type (Davies and Staines, 1976). It is of extreme interest to determine the completeness or incompleteness of coverage of Ia-antigens present in allografts undergoing either short-term or long-term enhancement as has been done previously for the MHC antigens generally (French, 1973). Another argument against either antigen-masking or removal of passenger leucocytes in grafts enhanced with anti-Ia antibodies is that these grafts are rejected when placed in a second, non-suppressed, animal syngeneic to the primary host.

Another example of the suppressive activity associated with anti-Ia antibody comes from the study of a rat renal graft enhancement model. Rejecting Lewis X Brown Norway F_1 kidneys in a Lewis rat host demonstrated both a heavy lymphocytic infiltration and evidence of antibody and complement-induced vasculitis (Strom *et al.*, 1975; Carpenter *et al.*, 1976). In animals in whom the survival of the kidney had been prolonged (enhanced) by the use of Lewis anti-Brown Norway antibody, the lymphocytic cellular infiltrate remained the same but the vascular damage was markedly decreased. This indicates that much of the graft damage was due to the production of antibodies which disturbed the vascular supply to the graft and that this aspect of the antigraft response was inhibited by enhancing antibody. Antibody, active in enhancement, appears to be directed against the Ia-like antigens of the rat (Soulillou *et al.*, 1976). This antibody, prepared by absorbing out serologically-defined antigens with erythrocytes and platelets (which do not contain Ia-like antigens), gives an antibody preparation (anti-Ia) which is potent in graft enhancement, is capable of specifically inhibiting the MLC and inhibits EA-rosette formation by a mechanism not requiring the Fc portion of the antibody. This inhibition of EA-rosettes by intact or $F(ab')_2$ antibody indicates that anti-Ia antibody was bound to and/or inhibited Fc-receptors. The marked ability of anti-Ia-like antibody to inhibit the production of graft-damaging IgG antibody may therefore reflect an interference with a collaborative T response which recognizes the Ia like portion of the rat MHC antigens. If, as would seem likely, the graft-damaging antibodies are directed against the SD (non-Ia-like) antigen systems in the rat, these results may be thought of as a form of particle- or molecular-specific immunosuppression by antibody.

Although a number of investigators have reported that anti-Ia antibodies are required for allograft enhancement whereas antibodies directed against non-Ia antigens of the MHC are ineffective in producing enhancement (Davies and Staines, 1976; Carpenter *et al.*, 1976; Soulillou *et al.*, 1976), other investigators have reported contrary findings in the sense that antibodies absorbed to erythrocytes (i.e. those directed against the SD antigens of the MHC) are the ones which are active in allograft enhancement (Jeekel and van Dongen, 1977; Duc *et al.*, 1977). Perhaps, the immunodominance of the alloantigens recognized in host–graft models differs from system to system. In other words, the relationship between enhancing activity of an antibody preparation and its immunologic specificity may vary depending upon the strength of that particular antigenic specificity within any given graft rejection process. If graft enhancing antibody inhibits immune responses through the generation of antigen–antibody complexes, those antigens which can most readily be detached from the cell surface should produce the most effective enhancing agents. The ability of various MHC antigens to detach may differ from one system to another and this may also account for the different observations made.

All studies involving the differential effect of antibody directed against one cellular determinant on the immune response to another cellular determinant assume that antibody-binding to one determinant on a cell surface does not alter an antigenically unrelated determinant on the same cell surface. This is not always the case, a good example being the lability of Fc-receptors due to the binding of antibody to various unrelated antigenic determinants (Schirrmacher and Festenstein, 1976). The influence that such rearrangements may have on antigenically non-related determinants are of importance in discussing the matter of specificity in antibody-feedback. Also, the rearrangements of various cell surface constituents in an immunogenic target may influence the metabolism of the target in such a way so as to alter its immunogenicity. Such considerations which relate to the properties of immunogenic cells *per se* rather than to the details of immunologic regulation should be kept in mind when assessing results purporting to show particle ('molecular') rather than determinant specificity. A similar note of caution must also be raised with respect to particle-specific suppression when the antigens are soluble; the suppressive antibody may simply remove the antigen and studies must be carried out to ensure that the immunogen is available for other forms of immune response as has been done in some investigations (Henney and Ishizaka, 1970).

3.2. Ability of Antibody Derived from Various Classes of Immunoglobulin to Alter Immune Responses

A number of experiments indicate that the class of antibody plays an important role in its ability to inhibit. Indeed, IgM antibody was found to augment suboptimal immune responses whereas IgG antibody uniformly suppressed (Henry and Jerne, 1968). The augmentation by IgM antibody is related to the ability of IgM antibody to induce localization of immunogen in the spleen (Dennert, 1971). Further work (Wason, 1973) has indicated that IgM antibody may exert two effects: (1) augmentation of immune responses, when given prior to antigen, by diverting antigen through sites suitable for immune responses, such as spleen; and (2) suppression of immune responses, when IgM antibody is given after antigen; IgM antibody, given at this time, leads to degradation of the limited amount of remaining antigen.

Some novel observations have been made in genetic low-responder mouse strains (Ordal and Grumet, 1973) in which the inhibitory activity of antibody-containing plasma could be removed with antibodies directed against μ-chains (Ordal *et al.*, 1976). An unique aspect of this particular system was the length of time, after administration of IgM antibody and antigen, during which the animals remained unresponsive to a second injection of antigen. The administration of passive IgM antibody gave a level of deficiency beyond that which could be explained on the basis of prior exposure of these low responder mice to antigen. The combined re-exposure to antigen and the induction of a GVH reaction allowed the breakage of this form of IgM antibody-induced suppression with the production of an IgM response only (whereas a GVH reaction would allow the production of an IgG response in previously primed animals, not suppressed by antibody). These results demonstrate that in some systems IgM antibody is capable of a rather marked degree of inhibition by mechanisms which appear to be more complicated than the simple masking and removal of antigen. This suppression probably involves the establishment of some active form of regulatory feedback. At present it is not known whether IgM antibody-mediated suppression would occur in responder mice; it may be that the hallmark of non-responder mice is the inability to control IgM feedback-inhibition which does not normally occur with this particular immunoglobulin class because of effective handling of IgM antibody by cooperating T cells (Cooper and Lawton, 1975; Moretta *et al.*, 1976b).

3.3. Ability of Various Subclasses of IgG Antibody to Alter Immune Responses

Most authors would agree that there are differences in the abilities of various subclasses of IgG to induce antibody-mediated immunosuppression, however they disagree as to which subclass is the most suppressive. Some favor IgG_1 (Voisin *et al.*, 1969; Murgita and Vas, 1972; Gordon and Murgita, 1975) others IgG_2 (Irvin *et al.*, 1967; Takasugi and Hildemann, 1969a,b; Zimmerman and Feldman, 1969, 1970; Eustace and Irvin, 1973; Fuller and Winn, 1973; Mitchell *et al.*, 1975) while other studies suggest both subclasses of IgG are suppressive (Takasugi and Klein, 1971; Duc *et al.*, 1975). The differences in results obtained reflect, in part, differences in experimental systems. It does not seem unreasonable to assume that most types of antigen-binding immunoglobulins may be suppressive, that the mechanisms of suppression within each subclass of immunoglobulin may differ, and that the efficacy with which each subclass suppresses may vary from one experimental system to another. Some examples from the recent literature will be described and discussed in the next few paragraphs.

The IgG_1 subclass of antibody, which is responsible for the passive cutaneous anaphylaxis reaction (Ovary, 1958), is associated with a pronounced degree of feedback-inhibition of antibody formation (Voisin *et al.*, 1969; Murgita and Vas, 1972; Gordon and Murgita, 1975). IgG_1 antibodies have been shown to be the subclass most dependent on T cell function (Taylor and Wortis, 1968; Torrigiani, 1972). B cells in mice possess Fc-receptors for aggregated immunoglobulin and a major proportion of these receptors are specific for the IgG_1 subclass of antibody (Basten *et al.*, 1972b). These findings can be accommodated within the concept that such IgG_1 antibody-mediated feedback operates on the surface of B cells through the binding of Fc-portions of exogenous or endogeneous IgG_1 antibody to Fc-receptors when antigen in these antigen–antibody complexes bind to antigen-receptors on B cells, hence the high T cell requirement.

The degree of complexity of results obtained may be transmitted to the reader by summarizing the observations made by Vuagnat *et al.* (1973a, b). *Anticarrier* IgG_1 antibody inhibits both IgG_1 and IgG_2 antihapten antibody production, whereas *anti-hapten* IgG_1 antibody permanently inhibits only antihapten IgG_2 antibody production. The production of antihapten IgG_1 antibody is only delayed, and eventually exceeds levels in immunized controls following secondary stimulation with the hapten-carrier complex. *Anticarrier* IgG_2 antibody inhibits antihapten IgG_2 antibody responses while causing only a slight delay in IgG_1 antihapten responses. *Antihapten* IgG_2 antibody suppresses both IgG_1 and IgG_2 antihapten immune responses, producing a priming defect with respect to IgG_2 antibody production. Antihapten IgG_2 antibody formation is inhibited by either IgG_1 or IgG_2 antibodies specific for carrier or hapten. The effects of passive antibody on IgG_1 production are even more complicated in that antihapten IgG_1 or IgG_2 antibody inhibits, at least initially, the primary antihapten IgG_1 response while anticarrier IgG_2 does not inhibit this response as did anticarrier IgG_1. IgG_2 priming is suppressed by IgG_1 and IgG_2 anti-carrier antibodies but only by IgG_2 type of antihapten antibody. Priming with respect to IgG_1 is weak, can not be inhibited and is augmented by antihapten IgG_1 antibody. The most obvious conclusion to be reached is that suppression by the various immunoglobulin subclasses of antibody is dependent on the response studied and that there is no subclass of IgG antibody which suppresses all varieties of immune responses. Also, without defining minimal concentrations of antibody needed for inhibition, it is difficult to decide on the relative efficacy of the various antibody preparations in suppressing immune responses. A claim was made that the difference between the two subclasses of IgG antibody represented a difference in the Fc portion of antibody. However, the authors studied $F(ab')_2$ antihapten antibody and this antibody fragment appeared to induce more immunosuppression than did intact antibody (Vuagnat *et al.*, 1973a); because of the use of a single high dose of suppressive antibodies, a defect in the ability of $F(ab')_2$ antibody to suppress may have been obscured (see below).

In another study from Voisin's laboratory (Duc *et al.*, 1975), it has been found that the anti-tumor IgG_2 antibody was capable of inducing tumor enhancement. However, the dose level required for such enhancement was much *lower* than that normally used. Only on dilution of the IgG_2 antibody was tumor enhancement visible. The authors attributed this finding to the concept that the complement-fixing IgG_2 antibody destroyed tumors at high concentrations, whereas, at low doses of IgG_2 antibody, the tumor-enhancing effect of this immunoglobulin subclass could be observed. If this were the case, one would have expected unfractionated serum containing high levels of IgG_2 to be equally cytotoxic to the engrafted tumor cells, but this was not the case. The increase in immunosuppression on dilution of enhancing IgG_2 antibody may be a real effect. That is, for IgG_2 antibody to be optimally immunosuppressive so that enhancement of tumor growth occurs, tumor antigens present on tumor cells or solubilized from tumor cells must be covered only to a certain degree; this phenomenon has been described in the regulation of an antibody response against sheep erythrocytes (Sinclair and Chan, 1971; Chan and Sinclair, 1971).

Vuagnat and Vilain (1975) have investigated the ability of antihapten or anticarrier IgG_1 or IgG_2 antibodies derived from guinea pigs to modify the cell-mediated response of syngeneic adoptively transferred cells from rats previously immunized with DNP-human serum albumin (HSA) in Freund's complete adjuvant. Passively administered anti-DNP or anti-HSA IgG_1 antibodies augmented delayed hypersensitivity reactions against DNP-HSA in a dose-dependent fashion. Anti-DNP and anti-HSA IgG_2 antibodies inhibited the expression of delayed hypersensitivity at low doses of antibody whereas, at higher doses of IgG_2 antibody, delayed hypersensitivity reactions were less suppressed.

The clearest distinction between the various IgG subclasses in their ability to inhibit comes from work investigating the feedback-suppression of anti-sheep erythrocyte responses in mice (Murgita and Vas, 1972; Gordon and Murgita, 1975). In these studies IgG_1 was uniformly suppressive whereas IgG_2 demonstrated either a pure augmentory property (Gordon and Murgita, 1975) or augmentation at low doses with suppression at higher concentrations of antibody (Murgita and Vas, 1972). Both augmentation by IgG_2 and the suppression by IgG_1 were dependent upon the presence of the Fc portion of antibody (Gordon and Murgita, 1975). This work clearly shows that there is a difference between various subclasses of IgG antibody in their ability to suppress or augment immune responses and that this difference is assignable to the Fc portion of antibodies. However, a word of warning might be sounded regarding these experiments: when we tested various anti-sheep erythrocyte antibodies kindly provided by Dr Murgita, we noted no difference in the ability of antibody from different IgG subclasses to suppress. In addition we noted that the IgG_1 fraction possessed hemolytic activity whereas the IgG_2 fraction did not (Chan and Sinclair, unpublished observation).

3.4. Requirement for the Fc Portion on Immunoregulatory Antibody

Because of the early observations that various classes and subclasses of antibody possess different abilities to mediate antibody-feedback, we reasoned that the Fc portion of antibody may exert an important function in feedback. Therefore, despite contrary observations (Tao and Uhr, 1966; Rowley and Fitch, 1968; Greenbury and Moore, 1968; Henney and Ishizaka, 1968, Cerottini *et al.*, 1969), we re-examined the difference between intact antibody and its $F(ab')_2$ derivative in causing antibody-feedback. Initial experiments demonstrated that the two forms of antibody differed markedly in their ability to inhibit, the $F(ab')_2$ being much less suppressive than intact antibody (Sinclair *et al.*, 1968; Sinclair, 1969). However, these early experiments did not rule out the possibility that $F(ab')_2$ antibody was a less potent feedback-inhibitor (by a factor of 10^2–10^3-fold) due to its more rapid excretion compared to intact IgG antibody. To rule out such an explanation, intact $F(ab')_2$ antibody were repeatedly injected into animals so that one could compensate for differences between $F(ab')_2$ and intact antibody in rates of excretion (Spiegelberg and Weigle, 1965). Even with adequate compensation, there was a clear difference between the two forms of antibody in their ability to inhibit (Sinclair *et al.*, 1970). The deficiency in inhibitory activity by $F(ab')_2$ antibody compared to intact antibody was also demonstrated in an *in vitro* system in which the two forms of antibody persisted in culture to the same extent (Lees and Sinclair, 1973). The differences in ability of $F(ab')_2$ vs intact IgG antibody to inhibit *in vivo* was not simply quantitative but qualitative since the slopes of inhibition on a log-log plot were significantly different (Sinclair *et al.*, 1970). A final piece of evidence which served to point out the difference between intact IgG and $F(ab')_2$ antibodies with respect to their abilities to inhibit responses was the demonstration that $F(ab')_2$ antibody could interfere with immunosuppression induced by intact antibody (Chan and Sinclair, 1973).

The inability of $F(ab')_2$ antibody to suppress an immune response compared to pronounced suppressive activity assignable to intact IgG antibody has been confirmed by a number of laboratories (Wason and Fitch, 1973; Kappler *et al.*, 1973; Hamaoka *et al.*, 1973; Abrahams *et al.*, 1973; Gordon and Murgita, 1975; Tew *et al.*, 1976). Wason and Fitch (1973) used an *in vitro* system (Mishell and Dutton, 1967) and thereby could state that the observed difference in ability to suppress were not due to excretion

(Sinclair *et al.*, 1970; Lees and Sinclair, 1973). Kappler *et al.* (1971, 1973) could pin-point the suppression as being an interference with B–T cell collaboration (Hoffmann *et al.*, 1974) mediated by the Fc portion of antibody. Hamaoka *et al.* (1973) noted that the Fc-dependency of anticarrier antibody was more pronounced in the suppression of an antihapten response rather than the anticarrier antibody response. Abrahams *et al.* (1973) ascertained that the Fc portion was necessary for antibody to remain on macrophages and inactivate them so that they were no longer immunogenic. Gordon and Murgita (1975) demonstrated that the Fc portion of antibody was necessary for the suppressive activity of one IgG subclass and for the augmentory activity of another. Tew *et al.* (1976) demonstrated that the Fc portion of antibody was necessary even in a system in which antibody production in the late immune response was governed by the level of ambient antibody (Graf and Uhr, 1969; Bystryn *et al.*, 1970, 1971). Tew *et al.* (1976) also gave evidence that $F(ab')_2$ could interfere with intact IgG antibody feedback (Chan and Sinclair, 1973) and that inhibition by antigen-antibody complexes required the presence of the Fc portion on antibody (Sinclair *et al.*, 1974). In another form of suppression, (Mitchell and Mokyr, 1972; Mitchell *et al.*, 1975), where suppressor T cells have been implicated in immunosuppression of macrophages by antigen–antibody complexes (Gershon *et al.*, 1974), the Fc portion of inhibitory antibody was also required (Rao and Mitchell, 1977). $F(ab')_2$ antibody has also been shown to be deficient in an allograft enhancement model (Myburgh and Smit, 1972). A recent report (Nielson *et al.*, 1977) indicates a deficiency in the ability of antiresponder or antistimulator $F(ab')_2$ antibody to inhibit the MLC, although other laboratories have not noted such an Fc-dependency (Horung *et al.*, 1971; Thorsby *et al.*, 1973).

There have been a number of reports, some giving adequate antibody dose-response data, indicating that, in certain systems, there is no demonstrable difference in suppressive activity between $F(ab')_2$ and intact IgG antibody. Immune response studied were to a heterologous protein system in which there is a requirement for Fc portion in an augmentory effect but not in the suppressive activity (Pincus *et al.*, 1971), a hapten–carrier system (Vuagnat *et al.*, 1973a), the T-independent polymerized flagellin system (Feldmann and Diener, 1972), an *in vitro* system for the generation of an allogeneic cytotoxic cell response (Sinclair *et al.*, 1975a), and two tumor enhancement models (Chard, 1968; Kaliss *et al.*, 1976), although in the second tumor enhancement model the production of antiallogeneic antibody was inhibited by passively administered antibody in an Fc-dependent manner.

In the polymerized flagellin system, a T cell independent system, there was no requirement for the presence of the Fc portion of antibody in tolerance-inducing antigen–antibody complexes even when careful dose–response studies were carried out (Feldmann and Diener, 1970, 1972). A strong possibility is that Fc-dependent antibody-mediated immunosuppression may affect predominantly B–T cell collaboration (Hoffmann *et al.*, 1974), a step which would be missing in the T-cell independent response to polymerized flagellin. Another possible explanation for the lack of a requirement for the Fc portion of antibody may center around the observations that polymeric flagellin remains on the surface of B cells for a long time (Nossal and Layton, 1976). Such long-lasting adherence of antigen or antigen–antibody complexes to the surface of B cells may allow antigen-receptors or antibody secreted early to be utilized as a source of immunoglobulin with intact Fc portions for the inactivating signal. In a somewhat analogous situation (Schrader and Feldmann, 1973; Feldmann, 1973), a specific T cell factor ('7S' IgM antibody) was stimulatory when it bound antigen in the presence of macrophages but inhibitory or tolerizing when macrophages were removed. When the Fc portions on cell surface-type IgM antibody are free to bind to Fc-receptors on the B cell surface, immunosuppression may occur. Also inactivation may take place when antigen remains attached to a B cell surface for some time and this would be lessened if antigen were attached to the surface of another cell type (such as macrophages).

In an allogeneic tumor model (Kaliss *et al.*, 1954), the requirement for the Fc portion of antibody in tumor enhancement (Kaliss 1969; Voisin, 1971) was investigated (Kaliss *et al.*, 1976). At high concentrations of $F(ab')_2$ and intact IgG antibody, there was no difference in the degree of enhancement in tumors, whereas the production of antiallogeneic antibody was suppressed by passively administered antibody through a mechanism which was aided by the presence of the Fc portion on inhibiting antibody (Kaliss *et al.*, 1976). In these particular experiments a large dose of antibody was used. In a more recent experiment, in which a number of limiting concentrations of antibody were employed, a difference between $F(ab')_2$ and intact IgG in giving tumor enhancement *in vivo* was observed (Kaliss and Sinclair, unpublished observations). Whether or not the use of more limiting concentrations of antibody explains our present ability to see an effect attributable to the Fc portion, or whether or not other factors, as yet unknown or controlled for, are important in the demonstration of the requirement for the Fc portion is as yet unknown. Again, the difference in results between these two experiments underscores the requirement for extensive antibody dose-response studies in order to see real differences in suppression by the two forms of antibody. This criticism not only holds for our earlier experiments (Kaliss *et al.*, 1976) but also for many others (Tao and Uhr, 1966; Rowley and Fitch, 1968; Greenbery and Moore, 1968; Henney and Ishizaka, 1968; Chard, 1968; Pincus *et al.*, 1971; Vuagnat *et al.*, 1973a).

In a recent review of the work relating to enhancement of rat renal allografts in which antibodies directed against Ia-like antigens and inhibiting both MLC and Fc-receptors, Carpenter *et al.* (1976) suggest that the enhancing antibody in their system may operate through an Fc-dependent mechanism which disturbs B–T collaborative events and, as a direct consequence, the production of graft-damaging IgG antibody is suppressed. They also suggest that there is a complex interplay between the Fc-receptor binding of immunoglobulins on B and T cells and that differential binding of the various subclasses of immunoglobulins to these cells either through Fc-receptors or through complement-receptors may play important, but as yet undefined, roles in the phenomenon of enhancement in this rat model system. However, $F(ab')_2$ antibodies appear to enhance allograft survival in this system (Shaipanich *et al.*, 1973; Strom, personal communication). It is possible that there is a complicating factor in that $F(ab')_2$ antibody may prevent direct graft damage through hyperacute rejection mediated by recipient antigraft antibody (Holter *et al.*, 1973; Habal *et al.*, 1973; Smit and Myburgh, 1974). A critical analysis by extensive dose-response studies has not been carried out. Further work is required to ascertain whether or not anti-Ia-like antibodies induce enhancement (see above) through an Fc-dependent mechanism. It may be that $F(ab')_2$ antibody induces a few days delay in the production of cytotoxic cells, to the same degree as intact antibody; this may contribute to an Fc-independent form of allograft enhancement. However, one would predict that antiallograft antibody, particularly anti-Ia-like antibody (which would be equivalent to anticarrier antibody), would suppress the production of the putative IgG graft-damaging antibody (antihapten equivalent) through a mechanism which would be substantially helped by the presence of Fc portion on enhancing antibody.

3.5. B Cell Inactivation Model for Fc-Dependent Antibody-Feedback

Following the observation that the Fc portion of antibody was necessary for antibody-feedback, we constructed a working hypothesis (Sinclair and Chan, 1971) in which immunocompetent B cells interact with antigen–antibody complexes, the interaction with antigen involves an antigen-receptor while the interaction with antibody takes place via an Fc-receptor. Using this working model, we predicted that, if immunocompetent cells were first stimulated by antigen in the absence of antibody and then antibody was given later, these antigen-triggered cells would be inactivated by antigen–antibody complexes when the level of antibody on the complexes was sufficiently high to form tripartite complexes of immunocompetent cells, antigen and antibody; however, if too much antibody were given less suppression would occur because the antigen would be completely covered by antibody leaving no free antigenic determinants to interact specifically with the antigen-receptors on the responding B cells. In other words, antigen-antibody complexes formed in 'antibody excess' would not be able to interact with specific B cells and, therefore, would not be expected to induce specific suppression of B cells which had been previously activated by antigen in the absence of antibody. Indeed, we found that there was an optimum dose of antibody (added 24 hr after antigen) which led to maximum suppression. Doses of antibody greater than the optimum resulted in lesser suppression (Sinclair and Chan, 1971; Chan and Sinclair, 1971). Such a result would not have been observed if suppression by antibody depended only on the circulating levels of antibody obtained. Two direct confirmations have been published (Vuagnat and Vilain, 1975; Duc *et al.*, 1975) and, in one report (Tew *et al.*, 1976), a decrease in amount of antigen given led in an unexpected increase in a response suppressed by antibody, again suggesting that too much antibody relative to antigen may give suboptimal suppression.

More recently, the same model for antibody-feedback involving Fc-mediated inactivation of B cells has been suggested on the basis of the requirement for the Fc portion of antibody, the differing ability of various subclasses of IgG antibody to immunosuppress (Gordon and Murgita, 1975) and the finding of Fc-receptors on B-cells (Sachs and Dickler, 1975).

Suppression by $F(ab')_2$ antibody occurred only when a much higher antibody dose was given and became more pronounced as the dose was increased. The peculiarities of dose-suppression curves for the two forms of antibody may account for various investigators asserting that there is no difference in suppression by $F(ab')_2$ and intact IgG antibodies. Indeed, at certain concentrations of suppressive antibody, inhibition by $F(ab')_2$ antibody may be greater than that seen with a comparable amount of intact antibody. Such a result would suggest that inhibition of immune responses, mediated through the functioning Fc portion of intact antibody, can only occur when the level of antigen coverage by antibody is within a certain range, and also that the Fc portion of antibody may act as a 'handle' which cells in the lymphoreticular system may use for clearing antibody molecules from the surface of antigen. This latter suggestion is made because high concentrations of $F(ab')_2$ antibody gave more (that is, not the same) suppression than did intact IgG antibody.

3.6. Inactivation of B Cells through Fc-Portion Binding to Fc-Receptors

A number of experimental systems have yielded evidence suggesting an Fc-mediated B cell inactivation. Immobilized antigen–antibody complexes are able to inhibit the mitogenic response of murine spleen cells to lipopolysaccharide (LPS), a B cell mitogen, by a mechanism which is dependent upon the Fc portion of antibody in the immobilized complexes (Ryan *et al.*, 1975a, b; Ryan and Henkart, 1976). This form of inhibition was demonstrated in the absence of T cells, indicating that suppressor T cells are not involved. The authors suggested that inactivation by an Fc-dependent process may provide a central mechanism for immunoregulation by antibody or antigen–antibody complexes, similar to the mechanism proposed by us (Sinclair and Chan, 1971). At first glance, this mechanism would appear to be nonspecific but, if the antigen–antibody complexes are brought to the surface of a B cell in a specific manner through the binding of the antigen component to antigen-receptors on B cells, this inherently nonspecific form of feedback suppression would be made specific.

Prolonged formation of EA rosettes decreases the ability of cells to reform the EA-rosettes or to demonstrate K cell activity (Revillard *et al.*, 1975). Like the effect of immobilized antigen–antibody complexes on B cells, the K cell population may have become inactivated by antibody-coated cells through an Fc-dependent mechanism. The inhibition could not be relieved by incubation at 37° C and extensive washing, therefore, the inactivation was stable under conditions likely to clear the cell surface of adsorbed antigen–antibody complexes. These results suggest that the synthesis of new

Fc-receptors was inhibited or, once removed from the surface, are resynthesized at a very slow rate.

Exposure of B cells to antiimmunoglobulin antibodies prevents their activation by various mitogens (Sidman and Unanue, 1976). The antiimmunoglobulin antibody attaches to surface immunoglobulin (antigen-receptors) and causes their removal from the cell surface. When the Fc portion of the antiimmunoglobulin antibody is removed, the resulting $F(ab')_2$ derivative is 20 times less effective in inhibiting B cell activation by mitogens. Inactivation by intact IgG antiimmunoglobulin antibody persists even after the B cells regenerate their immunoglobulin receptors, indicating that the inactivation of B cells is central in type. The decreased ability of $F(ab')_2$ antiimmunoglobulin antibody to inhibit a B cell mitogenic response is not due to a decrease in the binding of surface immunoglobulins or the subsequent capping and endocytosis of surface immunoglobulin; these events are generated just as readily with $F(ab')_2$ antibody as with intact antiimmunoglobulin antibody. Even when capping is totally prevented by sodium azide and the suppressive antiimmunoglobulin antibody is removed by pronase treatment, the B cells are still inactivated. The authors suggested that the dual binding of antiimmunoglobulin antibodies to the B cell surface through the antiimmunoglobulin $F(ab')_2$ portions and through the Fc portions provides the inactivating signal. They also suggested that the antiimmunoglobulin $F(ab')_2$ portion serves as a focusing mechanism to allow sufficient numbers of Fc portions to interact with Fc-receptors on the B cell surface leading to an Fc-mediated inactivation of B cells. This model, arrived at through a different form of experiment, is equivalent to that proposed by us (Sinclair and Chan, 1971). In other experiments (Andersson *et al.*, 1974; Schuffler and Dray, 1974), the $F(ab')_2$ fragment of antiimmunoglobulin antibody was effective in suppressing actual antibody formation; this suggests that Fc-mediated inactivation of B cells involves the suppression of B cell proliferation whereas B cell differentiation can be inhibited by other mechanisms as well as those operating through an Fc-receptor of the antiimmunoglobulin.

In *in vivo* allotype suppression of rabbits, antibody directed against paternal immunoglobulin allotypes prevents the development of circulating levels of that allotype when injected into newborn animals. The Fc portion of antiallotypic antibody is required for this form of antibody-mediated immunosuppression (Dubiski and Swierezynska, 1971; Shek and Dubiski, 1975). The possible role of complement in ridding the allotype suppressed animal of B cells expressing paternally-derived immunoglobulin allotypes had been raised but ruled out on the basis that B cells are not eliminated, and C5 deficient animals can be allotype suppressed (Cinader and Dubiski, 1976). Complement-mediated inactivation of B cells has been further eliminated by the finding that an antibody fragment lacking the CH3 domain, the Facb fragment, also lacks the ability to give allotype suppression (Connell and Dubiski, 1977); this fragment is fully able to activate complement (Connell and Porter, 1971). Suppressor cells may be generated during allotype suppression in mice (Herzenberg *et al.*, 1975); but these cells have not been studied in rabbits because of the lack of inbred strains. Obviously the requirement for the Fc portion in allotype suppression in mice should be assessed. Despite the later appearance of suppressor cells in some forms of allotype suppression, an early inhibitory event, involving the direct inactivation of B cells through a direct Fc-mediated negative signal on the B cell surface, may take place, and, furthermore, may be involved in the generation of suppressor cells.

Another experimental situation in which the Fc portion of immunoglobulin was required for inactivation of B cells is that of specific antihapten tolerance, induced by immunization with hapten on an isologous immunoglobulin carrier (Havas, 1969; Golan and Borel, 1971). Although both T and B cells are inactivated in this form of tolerance (Borel *et al.*, 1975), it is the B cell population which demonstrates the most profound degree of inactivation (Borel *et al.*, 1975; Schrader, 1975a,b; Chiller *et al.*, 1976; Sehon and Lee, 1976). For the *in vivo* induction of tolerance, there was a strict requirement for the Fc portion of immunoglobulin carrier (Borel, 1976; Sehon and

Lee, 1976), and the most tolerogenic subclasses of murine immunoglobulin (Borel, 1976) appeared to be those which bind most readily to B cell Fc-receptors (Basten *et al.*, 1972b). Although the Fc portion of the carrier immunoglobulin was required for the *in vivo* induction of tolerance, no such requirement appeared to exist for induction of tolerance *in vitro* (Schrader, 1975a) where an inappropriate endogenous formation of IgG antibody *in vitro* may have caused inactivation of B cells through an Fc-dependent mechanism. It is worth stressing that isologous IgG carrier seems to be the most effective physiologic tolerance inducer of all the carrier proteins tested (Golan and Borel, 1971; Havas, 1969) suggesting that haptenated isologous immunoglobulin binds to immunocompetent cells specific for hapten and, because of an additional physiologic Fc-mediated activity (not because of additional antigenicity or avidity considerations), this dual binding may give rise to the pronounced degree of regulation leading to tolerance. Because of this consideration, these experiments are discussed under modulation of immune responses by antibody rather than by antigen. Antigen-binding cells with receptors for antigen occupied by tolerogen have been demonstrated (Borel, 1976) and a correlation exists between tolerogenicity and the ability of hapten-isologous IgG carrier to produce receptor-blockade. However, tolerance is not due to complete blockade of antigen-receptors on the tolerized cells, since unoccupied antigen-receptors can be demonstrated on these cells. Such results indicate that the binding of hapten-isologous IgG carrier to the surface of an immunocompetent cell mediates an Fc-dependent form of central inactivation of that cell.

A similar series of experiments have been reported on the effect of haptenated isologous immunoglobulins on reaginic responses to the hapten, elicited by haptenated ovalbumin in alum (Lee and Sehon, 1976). These authors demonstrated that DNP_8-mouse gammaglobulin inhibits the production of reaginic antibodies to DNP-ovalbumin when given either 3 weeks or 4 hr before the eliciting immunogen. Lee and Sehon (1976) developed a model for the attachment of DNP-isologous mouse gammaglobulin to the surface of the B cell in which an Fc-receptor-Fc portion binding would increase the number of attachments between the tolerogen and the cell. The authors likened this model to that previously described by Diener and Feldmann (1972) in which tolerogenicity was a function of the degree of attachment between tolerogen and the surface of an immunocompetent cell and this, in turn, was related to the number of antigenic sites. Therefore, the model proposed by Lee and Sehon (1976) would not suggest any particular regulatory function in the binding of Fc portions of immunoglobulin to Fc-receptors but simply suggests that this allows a greater opportunity for tolerogenic binding. However, the Fc portions of isologous immunoglobulin ‘carrier’ may provide an unique function which leads to a rapid and pronounced degree of inactivation of the B cells (Sinclair and Chan, 1971) rather than the simple increase in attachment sites. Furthermore, the inactivation model (Diener and Feldmann, 1972) to which Lee and Sehon (1976) liken their results was *not* helped by the presence of the Fc portion (Feldmann and Diener, 1972), indicating that this particular analogy is probably inappropriate.

An interesting extension of work on suppression by haptenated isologous IgG involves the induction of tolerance in NZB/W F_1 mice with the use of nucleosides attached to isologous IgG. NZB/W mice develop an autoimmune disease which resembles human systemic lupus erythematosus. This disease, both in mice and in humans, is characterized by the appearance of anti-DNA antibody which, when coupled to DNA, leads to forms of immune complex vasculitis and renal disease. When NZB/W animals were treated with cortisone and nucleoside IgG-complexes, they showed a distinct decrease in the incidence of the disease and a prolonged life span (Borel *et al.*, 1973, 1977).

Antiidiotypic antibodies induce suppression of antibody production bearing that idiotype through a Fc dependent mechanism (Pawlak *et al.*, 1973; Nisonoff and Bangasser, 1975; Kohler *et al.*, 1977). This form of regulation will be discussed in a later section.

Lastly, antigen–antibody complexes have been shown to inactivate antigen-specific immunocompetent cells tested for activity in an adoptive transfer experiment (Sinclair *et al.*, 1974). Furthermore, antigen–antibody complexes have been shown to inactivate B cells through a mechanism which does not involve the direct participation of T cells and could not be reversed with the later addition of T cell factors (Oberbarnscheidt and Kolsch, 1978). Our previous work indicated that antigen–antibody complexes in activated immunocompetent cells through an Fc-dependent mechanism (Sinclair *et al.*, 1974), however, we could only surmise that the defect resided in the B cells since T cells had already been shown to be rather resistant to antibody-feedback (Kappler *et al.*, 1971) and did not rule out the intermediary role for T cells in this particular experiment.

In summary, these experimental models for B cell inactivation have as a common basis the binding of the Fc-portion of immunoglobulin to Fc-receptors on the B cell surface. In one instance (Ryan and Henkart, 1976), this binding and consequent inactivation had no immunologic specificity. The other models demonstrate degrees of specificity based on the fact that the Fc portions of immunoglobulins are directed towards Fc-receptors on particular B cells because the immunoglobulins are bound to antigen (Sinclair and Chan, 1971; Sinclair *et al.*, 1974, 1976a; Oberbarnscheidt and Kolsch, 1978) or are chemically bound to a specific hapten (Borel, 1976; Lee and Sehon, 1976). In other examples of this model, specificity is provided because the Fc-bearing immunoglobulin has antibody activity directed towards immunoglobulin (Sidman and Unanue, 1976) to allotypic (Cinader and Dubiski, 1976) or to idiotypic determinants (Pawlak *et al.*, 1973). Although Fc-mediated inactivation has no inherent immunologic specificity, it is manifestly incorrect to suggest that this model is incapable of preferentially inactivating immunologically specific B cells (Gorczynski *et al.*, 1974) just as it would be incorrect to suggest that complement-mediated cytotoxicity or opsonization cannot be part of immunologically specific reactions.

3.7. Inactivation of Immunocompetent Cells through an Fc-Dependent Mechanism Involving Various Accessory Factors

Although Fc-dependent feedback suppression by antibody may operate through the interaction of Fc portions of inhibiting antibodies with Fc-receptors on the B cell surface, there are alternative or additional mechanisms that should be considered. One of the more obvious would be that cells, when marked by the presence of antigen–antibody complexes on their surface, become prime candidates for phagocytosis. This is indeed the case where enhancement of kidney allografts is accompanied by phagocytosis of immunocompetent cells (Hutchison and Zola, 1977).

The addition of macrophages to cultures producing antibody-forming cells may decrease such immune responses (Chen and Hirsch, 1972; Gery and Waksman, 1972). Certain levels of heating or treatment with glutaraldehyde destroys the ability of macrophages to inhibit. This inhibition is resistant to treatment with neuraminidase or trypsin (Ptak and Gershon, 1975). Because Fc-receptors of macrophages displayed similar sensitivities and resistances to these agents, it has been suggested that the Fc-receptor function in such macrophages may play a role in this form of immunosuppression, presumably by binding antibody. If antibody were attached to antigen assocated with immunocompetent cells, macrophages may exert a negative influence on these immunocompetent cells possibly by phagocytizing them. These results suggest that macrophages may, under certain conditions, have the opposite effect to that normally ascribed to them (Feldmann, 1972a, b; Diener and Feldmann, 1972; Schrader and Feldmann, 1973; Feldmann, 1973).

Another observation, emerging from clinical renal transplantation is that the presence of antidonor antibody, as detected by an antibody-dependent cell-mediated cytotoxicity (ADCC) assay, was in some cases correlated with prolonged clinical graft survival (Kovithavongs and Dossetor, 1975; Stiller *et al.*, 1976, 1977). It may be that ADCC antibody reacts with donor antigen picked up on the surface of recipient, donor-reactive (precytotoxic) cells and, through the mediation of an ADCC activity, suppresses the activation of these cells. Some of the work indicating the requirement for the Fc portion of antibody for antibody-mediated immunosuppression may eventually find its interpretation in the activation of nonspecific effector cells such as phagocytic or lymphoid killer cells or other cells possessing inhibitory potential.

In experiments dealing with enhancement of allografts, it has been noted that such enhancement-facilitation is most readily demonstrated with the IgG_1 form of alloantibody (Voisin *et al.*, 1969). This antibody has been demonstrated to interact with allogeneic cells which contain chemical mediators and, can further bind via their Fc portions to the Fc-receptors on these chemical mediator-containing cells (Daeron *et al.*, 1975). This dual attachment of allogeneic antibody leads to the release of chemical mediators, a phenomenon referred to as direct allogeneic anaphylactic degranulation (DAAD). The released chemical mediator products have been shown to be immunosuppressive (Voisin, 1976) and may lead to graft enhancement. The interaction between enhancing antibody and a chemical mediator-containing cell through the dual attachment to allogeneic antigens and Fc-receptors represents a model in which Fc-dependent suppression by antigen and antibody operates through another cell type, whereas in the former tripartite model (Sinclair and Chan, 1971, Oberbarnscheidt and Kolsch, 1976) the complex itself is considered to be the direct inactivator of B cells.

The anti-sheep erythrocyte response in mice given a low dose of irradiation (300 rad) displays increased resistance to immunosuppression by intact IgG antibody, compared to non-irradiated controls (Sinclair *et al.*, 1976a). Conversely, the rather poor immunosuppression induced by $F(ab')_2$ anti-sheep erythrocyte antibody is enhanced by the administration of 300 rad γ-irradiation. Therefore, there is a radiation-sensitive step in the Fc-dependent form of feedback-inhibition by intact IgG antibody, suggesting that a radiosensitive cellular response is involved. Since radiation interferes specifically with Fc-mediated antibody feedback, it is likely that the cell involved in this form of inhibition would possess an Fc-receptor. Irradiation does not eliminate Fc-receptor-bearing cells (Gyongyossy *et al.*, 1975) but may alter the capacity of suppressor cells to function in Fc-dependent antibody feedback. Suppressor cells are more sensitive to irradiation than are helper cells (Dutton, 1973; Basten *et al.*, 1975b; McCullagh, 1974). Therefore, this type of suppressor cell may be a T cell which interacts with the Fc portions of antibody attached to antigen on the surface of B cells, following which it may become activated and exert some form of inhibitory influence. Since there appears to be a deficiency in adult thymectomized animals to demonstrate suppressor cell activities (Basten *et al.*, 1975b; Burns *et al.*, 1975; Kanellopoulos-Langevin *et al.*, 1976), the short-lived Ly-1,2,3 T cell, which makes up about 50 per cent of the circulating pool of T cells (Canter and Boyse, 1975a,b) may be a good candidate for this role. If Fc-dependent antibody-feedback were less pronounced in adult thymectomized animals compared to their sham-operated controls, this would indicate that the short-lived Ly-1,2,3 T cell is an effector mechanism in Fc-dependent antibody-feedback. Since the long-lived Ly-2,3 T cell also has suppressive activities (Herzenberg *et al.*, 1976) two forms of suppressor cells activated in antibody-feedback may exist; a short-lived Ly-1,2,3 T cell and a long-lived Ly-2,3 T cell. It will be of interest to see if either of these T cells are called into play by an Fc-dependent form of antibody-feedback and whether this would be different from those called into play by antigen alone, either in a tolerogenic or immunogenic form. A suppressor cell, activated by antibody through an Fc-dependent mechanism would possess receptors for the Fc portion of antibody at least during the time when the activation occurs and possibly when immunocompetent cells are inhibited.

Other indications that feedback suppressive (enhancing) antibody can activate a suppressor cell population comes from a study of the inhibition of the MLC by antibodies directed against the stimulator cell population (Kanellopoulos-Langevin *et al.*, 1976). In these studies, spleen cells obtained from animals which had been thymectomized as adults wer more resistant to the feedback suppressive effects of anti-stimulator antibody than spleen cells obtained from normal or sham-thymectomized animals. The removal of a population of histamine-binding cells also induced resistance in the MLC to antibody-feedback. Cells bearing histamine-receptors have been found to regulate many leukocyte responses (Bourne *et al.*, 1974), antibody responses (Shearer *et al.*, 1972; 1974) and are capable of maintaining tolerance in some systems (Segal *et al.*, 1974). These results suggest that antibody, capable of inhibiting the MLC, did so via a suppressor T cell population activated by a histamine signal elaborated through an Fc-dependent DAAD mechanism.

More direct data indicating that suppressor cells are activated by antigen and antibody (Gershon *et al.*, 1974) come from a system which measures the ability of macrophages to bind via cytophilic antibody to tumor cells through Fc-receptors on the macrophage surface (Mitchell and Mokyr, 1972; Mitchell *et al.*, 1975). Macrophages specifically lose their ability to take up cytophilic antibody and to bind tumor cells in rosettes when derived from animals treated with tumor antigen and anti-tumor antibody. Macrophage-mediated anti-tumor immunity was not inhibited by treatment of adult thymectomized, irradiated and bone marrow reconstituted animals with antigen and antibody, but this inhibition did occur when animals were sham thymectomized prior to irradiation and bone marrow reconstitution. This form of inhibition could be reversed with the use of bone marrow cells, and this reversal was itself inhibited by thymus cells provided that the thymus cells were not activated against allogeneic antigens (Mitchell *et al.*, 1975). These results indicate rather strongly that inhibition of a specific immunologic function by antigen and antibody is mediated by the activation of a suppressor T cell population.

In an *in vitro* system for the generation of cell-mediated immunity detected by a chromium-release assay (Cerottini and Brunner, 1974), anti-stimulator cell antibodies suppress by means of an Fc-independent, antigen-masking process (Sinclair *et al.*, 1975a). Cells activated against stimulator antigen inhibit cytotoxic cell production through a mechanism directed towards the responder cell population and act independently of the concentration of stimulator cell antigen in the system (Sinclair *et al.*, 1975b, 1976b,c). In experiments where both forms of suppression are employed, suppression induced by the combined treatment was four to eight fold greater than that which would be expected on the basis of the suppressive levels produced by each inhibitory agent alone, indicating that a form of synergism between antibody and suppressor cells may occur (Sinclair and Lee, unpublished observations). These results point to the possibility that suppression by antibody may not only operate by inducing suppressor cells but may also utilize suppressor cells in the process of inhibiting immune responses.

Low doses of irradiation enhance the anti-DNP IgE response in animals injected with DNP-ascaris without affecting the IgG antihapten antibody responses to any great extent (Tada *et al.*, 1971; Kind and Macedo-Sobrinho, 1973; Chiorazzi *et al.*, 1976). The augmented IgE immune responses could be reproduced using cyclophosphamide an agent known to inhibit suppressor cell activity (Tanaguchi and Tada, 1971; Polak and Turk, 1974; Askenase *et al.*, 1975; Miller *et al.*, 1976a; Debre *et al.*, 1976). Only occasional instances of augmentation of IgG anti-DNA antibodies have been noted, suggesting that the IgG-forming lineage and the IgE-forming lineage may be separate (Dwyer *et al.*, 1976). In these experiments there was no inverse relationship between IgG and IgE levels, and this was interpreted as indicating that antibody-feedback by IgG antibody on IgE immune responses was not involved in the system, however, a more complex mechanism of antibody-feedback involving the production of suppressor cells or involving an antibody-feedback arc in which suppressor cells play a role has not been ruled out. The dual effect of carrier priming and the presence of a soluble factor which does not withstand adoptive transfer (Strejan *et al.*, 1977), may indicate that the combination of a cellular and noncellular (suppressive IgG antibody against carrier or hapten, or IgE antibody against the carrier) component is required for the regulation of an IgE response.

Data from the Hellströms' laboratory (Tamerius *et al.*, 1976; Nepom *et al.*, 1976) suggest that a blocking factor of molecular weight 56,000 daltons is present in the serum of tumor-bearing mice. This suppressive factor is specific, indicating that the molecule may be either a tumor antigen or an antigen-specific suppressor molecule. The authors suggested that the original interpretation that blocking factors are antigen–antibody complexes with the lower molecular weight component being tumor antigen (Hellström and Helström, 1974) must be reevaluated; the low molecular weight component may be an autonomous suppressive factor (Tada *et al.*, 1975, 1976; Rich and Rich, 1976; Herzenberg *et al.*, 1976) since the factor has been shown to be inhibitory by itself. This again raises the possibility that suppressor cell activation and production of suppressor cell factors occurs following exposure to antigen–antibody complexes.

In allotype suppression in the SJL × BALB/c model, neonatally administered antiallotype antibody inhibits the production of immunoglobulin of that allotype without preventing the B cells from reaching the memory cell stage (Okumura *et al.*, 1976b). Suppression appears to involve the elimination of a population of helper cells which are required for the expression rather than induction of B cell memory (Herzenberg *et al.*, 1976). The results suggest that helper T cells are not only specific for antigen but also demonstrate specificity with respect to allotype. Suppressor cells appear to eliminate this population of allotype-specific helper T cells (Herzenberg *et al.*, 1976). Since the majority of suppressor cells and cytotoxic cells are part of the same T cell subpopulation (the Ly-2,3 population), suppressor T cells may be able to recognize an unique target on allotype specific helper T cells and chronic allotype suppression may result from the stimulation of a population of T cells which express either partial or full cytotoxicity towards the suppressed allotype. Although expressed on the cell surface, the suppressed allotype on B cells would not be available as a target for allotype specific suppressor cells. If the cooperative effect of helper cells is to remove antigen–antibody complexes from B cells thus preventing Fc-mediated inhibition, then in so doing, they would bind and display immunoglobulin with the suppressed allotype. The T cells, now with this immunoglobulin on their surface, may serve as a target for the cytotoxic attack by antiallotype-directed suppressor cytotoxic cells. This form of helper T cell elimination may not be the usual cytotoxic attack in which cell–cell contact is required between effector cell and target, but may be equivalent to a lymphokine-mediated killing. These factors may be analogous to suppressive factors containing I–J encoded determinants (Tada *et al.*, 1976) which interact with an I-region encoded receptor found on T and not B cells (Tanaguchi *et al.*, 1976).

A population of suppressor cells has been identified in the bone marrow (Singhal *et al.*, 1972; Drury and Singhal, 1974). These cells appear to be neither T cells nor macrophages. The Fc-receptor-positive portion of this cell population is suppressive, whereas Fc-receptor-negative cells from the same source augment rather than suppress immune responses (Duwe and Singhal, personal communication). Therefore this cell may be a candidate for the effector cell involved in Fc-dependent antibody-feedback. Since this suppressor cell is radiosensitive, it may be the cell type missing in irradiated animals that are resistant to the Fc-dependent form of antibody-feedback (Sinclair *et al.*, 1976).

The concept that the target for antibody feedback at the level of B–T cell collaboration or on B cells directly would appear to be at odds with the suggestion made by a number of laboratories that suppressor cells have helper T cells as their target (Gershon, 1975; Herzenberg *et al.*, 1976). However, two experimental systems seem to suggest that suppressor cells may operate on B cells directly (Baker *et al.*, 1974; Basten *et al.*, 1975b). With reference to the latter (T-dependent) system, HGG tolerant (suppressor) cells inhibited the anti-DNP plaque-forming cell response of DNP-flagellin-primed B cells in the presence of KLH- and HGG-primed cells (as a source of helper T cells) when exposed to DNP-KLH plus DNP-HGG (Basten *et al.*, 1975b). No such inhibition occurred when the same system was exposed to DNP-KLH and nonhaptenated HGG. Such a result indicates that the HGG-suppressor cells interact with DNP-specific B cells through the DNP-HGG hapten-carrier complex and, since DNP-KLH was not able to stimulate an anti-DNP response in the presence of anti-KLH helper cells, most of the hapten-specific (anti-DNP) B cells must have been inactivated by the anti-HGG suppressor cells. When attempts were made to identify the cell type responsible for suppression, it became clear that two cell types were involved, a T cell and a macrophage (not a B cell) both of which had to be harvested from tolerant animals. The macrophage requirement for suppression could not be interfered with by normal macrophages as in a macrophage-dependent form of Fc-mediated antibody-feedback (Abrahams *et al.*, 1973). This result suggests that the target for suppressor cell activity in this system is the B cell and that the final steps of this process are nonspecific but directed through a hapten–carrier complex. These results are very similar to those described previously which dealt with the suppressive effects of anti-carrier antibody (Henney and Ishizaka, 1970; Hamaoka *et al.*, 1971b, 1973; Vuagnat *et al.*, 1973a, b).

The experiments cited implicating a relationship between inhibition by passively administered antibody and the function of various types suppressive cells are indeed preliminary. Further studies using well-defined systems to work out the various parameters of antibody-feedback are required to increase our understanding of antibody-feedback and of some categories of suppressor cell activity.

3.8. Interference with Antibody-Feedback Mediated by T Cells

A number of observations induced us to look for evidence that helper T cells may function by preventing antibody-feedback. The first of these was that T-cell deficient animals appear to have, as their most obvious defect, a difficulty in switching from IgM to IgG antibody synthesis, the latter immunoglobulin being the most feedback suppressive. Secondly, lethally irradiated, inbred animals given a constant number of bone marrow cells, sheep erythrocytes and a varying number of thymus cells demonstrated a thymus cell dose–response slope which was not a simple straight-line relationship (Chan and Sinclair, 1971). Low doses of thymus cells, augmented the response over that seen with bone marrow and antigen alone, but this antibody response remained IgM in class. At the upper range of thymus cell doses, there was a linear relationship between the number of thymus cells transferred and the level of the anti-sheep erythrocyte response obtained; this response began with the production of IgM antibody and then converted to an IgG antibody response. In the thymus cell dose interval between the permanent IgM response and the response which shifted from IgM to IgG antibody production, *no* antibody response occurred. The suggested that cells shifted to IgG antibody synthesis relatively early in the immune response, terminating all antibody responses in these animals, that is, sufficient number of thymus cells to help in the production of IgG antibody were present but were not sufficient to counteract feedback-suppression by endogenously-produced IgG anti-body.

If a function of T cells is to prevent IgG antibody-feedback, it should be possible to demonstrate that T cells and T cell activities interfere with such IgG antibody-feedback. A number of observations have been made which support this supposition. Firstly, adjuvants, which stimulate T cell activities, interfere with antibody-feedback (Rowley *et al.*, 1969). Secondly, an immune response to burro erythrocytes interferes with the inhibition of an anti-sheep erythrocyte plaque-forming cell response by anti-sheep erythrocyte antibody (Lees and Sinclair, 1973). Burro and sheep erythrocytes cross react at the level of the T cell and T cell-activation by the burro erythrocytes may lessen suppression of an anti-sheep erythrocyte response by anti-sheep erythrocyte antibody. Thirdly, in an adoptive transfer system in which antigen, bone marrow and thymus cells are transferred, the presence of thymus cells interferes with antibody-feedback (Sinclair *et al.*, 1976). This interference occurs even when thymus cells are given late so that they produce little or no augmentation of the control response. Fourthly, in the presence of an allogeneic effect, feedback-suppression by intact antibody is less noticeable (Lees and Sinclair, 1975). An allogeneic effect is mediated through the activity of factors generated by stimulated T cells;

these factors influence B cell proliferation after B-cells have been triggered with specific antigen (Armerding and Katz, 1974; Schimpl and Wecker, 1973). Fifthly, thymus cells, either allogeneic or activated against an unrelated antigen, interfere with tumor antigen–antibody-induced suppression of the macrophage's activity towards tumor antigen (Rao *et al.*, 1977). In summary, thymus cells and the induction of activities ascribable to T cells limit the ability of antibody to feedback-suppress immune responses to antigen. These results raise the possibility that cooperation by T cells may prevent antibody-feedback by endogenously produced IgG antibody.

In the system described previously in which antigen–antibody complexes were shown to inactivate B cells through an Fc-dependent mechanism (Oberbarnscheidt and Kolsch, 1978), investigations were also carried out on the interaction between this antigen–antibody mediated Fc-dependent suppression and T cell activity. T cells were not required for suppression and T cell replacing factor (TRF) given at 48 hr could not overcome the suppressive effects of antigen–antibody complexes given at the initiation of cultures. This latter result helped to determine that the target for the suppressive antibody was likely to be B cells, and that the inactivation did not seem to involve the direct participation of suppressor T cells. However, an experiment designed specifically to investigate the question of whether or not TRF, if added to the cultures prior to exposure to suppressive antigen–antibody complexes, will prevent suppression by these complexes has not yet been carried out. Since there are a number of studies which demonstrate that T cell activities may interfere with antibody feedback (Lees and Sinclair, 1975; Sinclair *et al.*, 1976; Rao *et al.*, 1977), it would seem likely that TRF added prior to antigen–antibody complexes would induce a form of resistance. TRF has been recently shown to bind to Fc-receptors on B cells (Schimpl and Wecker, 1978).

The generation of the primed state (Sinclair, 1967a) and the formation of B memory cells appears to proceed without the requirement for T cell cooperation, while T cells are required to generate cells which actively produce immunoglobulin (Roelants and Askonas, 1972; Diamanstein and Blitstein-Willinger, 1974; Schrader, 1975c). This is also the case in allotype suppression (Okumura *et al.*, 1976b). Therefore, T cell help is required predominantly at the point when antibody is produced.

That T cells cooperate with B cells by preventing antibody-feedback is further supported by some observations on B cell inhibition. B cells, triggered by immunizing quantities of dinitrophenylated polymerized flagellin (DNP-POL), were inhibited from antibody secretion in the presence of dinitrophenylated gelatin (DNP-GEL) (Schrader, 1975d). Despite the fact that secretion of antibody (detectable in a plaque-forming assay) did not occur, B cells reached the point of antibody production and were inhibited at that stage. This was demonstrated by removing the DNP-GEL from the B cell surface with collagenase; shortly thereafter the B cells secreted antibody. These results indicate that triggered B cells are inhibited by contact with antigen when endogenously-produced antibody is secreted, that is, cessation of B cell differentiation occurs at the stage when antibody production begins and suppressive antigen–antibody complexes can be formed on the B cell surface. Experiments reported by Aldo-Benson and Borel (1976) are in apparent disagreement with the work of Schrader (1975d) in which B cells appeared to be stopped at an early stage of B cell activation. However the tolerogen used in this case was DNP-mouse gammaglobulin, therefore, the blockading agent possessed both antigenic determinants and Fc portions of antibody which could bind to Fc-receptors on the B cell surface thus preventing even the early stages of plasma cell activation.

A demonstration of IgG antibody-forming cell susceptibility to an inhibitory influence which could not be observed in cells which preferentially synthesize IgM in the early phases of an immune response comes from experiments in which precursors of antibody-forming cells were fractionated on the basis of their differential ability to bind antigen (Lafleur and Mitchell, 1975). Enrichment for unprimed B cells showing a high avidity for antigen, increases the early IgG response without affecting the IgM immune response a similar degree. Later on in the immune response, IgG antibody production is considerably higher when cells with low avidity for antigen were transferred compared with that obtained with high avidity cells. The early production of IgG antibody is likely inappropriate and led to the termination of the immune response. When the high avidity antigen-binding cells are removed, a prolonged IgM antibody response occurs, and the shift to IgG antibody production is delayed, occurring at a time after antigen had been cleared from the system, such that IgG antibody–antigen complexes were less likely to be formed to mediate feedback-inhibition. In keeping with this concept, near normal levels of IgG antibody could be observed late in primary immune responses to sheep erythrocytes in neonatally thymectomized mice (Sinclair, 1967a) suggesting that the requirement of T lymphocytes for the switch from IgM to IgG antibody synthesis is reduced once the system is cleared of antigen.

Once developing plasma cells have begun the synthesis and secretion of IgG antibody, they may no longer require the help of a T cell population because the antibody product itself would tend to elute antigen away from the plasma cell surface. Furthermore, mature plasma cells do not demonstrate receptors for either antigen or Fc portions of antibody. The observation that recently primed cells lose their requirement for T cells and macrophages (Evans and Ivanyi, 1975) coincident with IgG antibody synthesis (Valentova *et al.*, 1966) supports this possibility.

In summary, T cells can be shown in direct experiments to interfere with feedback-suppression by antibody or antigen-antibody complexes. Many characteristics of the immune response and cellular activities involved in this response indicate that T cells may prevent feedback-suppression by endogenously formed antibody after it has combined with remaining antigen on the surface of B cells.

3.9. Modulation of Immune Response by Antiidiotypic Antibodies

Even when two antibodies come from the same class and subclass and express the same allotypic determinants, they will differ considerably in that region of the molecule that binds antigen. This region has consequently been called the variable region. The variability is due to the existence of different amino acid residues in restricted, hypervariable, portions of the variable region. These structural differences account for the ability of one antibody to bind homologous antigen but not other non-crossreacting antigens. These variable region differences are also perceived by the immune system as different antigenic structures; this form of antigenic diversity is referred to as idiotypy. The analysis of idiotypes have allowed a correspondence to be drawn between the variable regions on antibody modecules and receptors on both B and T cells. T cells appear to express only a portion of the idiotypic determinants which are found on antibody molecules and on B cell antigen-receptors. T cell idiotypes are associated with idiotypic determinants found on the heavy chain of classical immunoglobulins whereas antibody molecules and B cell receptors display both light and heavy chain variable region idiotypes. Studies on the expression of idiotypes have not only helped in the analysis of immunoglobulin and antigen-receptor structure, they have also provided valuable data on regulation of immune responses which antiidiotypic antibody and antiidiotypic cells can engender.

The production of antiidiotypic antibody, which recognizes antibodies or receptors against alloantigens, is most easily accomplished by immunizing an F_1 animal with T cells of one of the parental strains. The injected parental T cells will react against the opposite parental antigens in the F_1 host; these reacting lymphocytes display surface receptors for the opposite parental antigens. Since the F_1 host would not contain receptors that recognize either parent, the receptors for antigen on the injected parental cells directed against the other parental antigens would be recognized as foreign. Autoantiidiotypic antibodies may also be produced spontaneously, suggesting that idiotypes are present in such low concentrations in non-immunized animals that they have not become recognized as self-antigens; hence tolerance to them does not develop. T cells will excite an antiidiotypic response, but B cells will not and their presence in the cell inoculum leads to an overall suppression (Binz and Wigzell, 1977). Production by B cells of classical immunoglobulin molecules possessing a particular idiotype may lead to the inactivation of cells that recognize the idiotype. Against this possibility is the observation that antiidiotypic antibody can be generated against injected immunoglobulins containing the idiotype. In this case, however, the immunogen used to stimulate an antiidiotypic response is a glutaraldehyde-fixed and aggregated material which is given in Freund's complete adjuvant. Such a preparation may have lost its ability to deliver inactivation signals through the Fc portion of the antibody and the presence of Freund's complete adjuvant may induce resistance to antibody feedback by the idiotype-bearing immunoglobulin through the activation of T cells. With the use of B cells, antigen-receptors may be shed and immunoglobulin antibodies may be secreted which can interact with host cells recognizing the idiotype in a way such that inactivation of the antiidiotypic immune response occurs.

The administration of antiidiotypic antibody has been shown to inhibit the antibody responses of that idiotype (Hart *et al.*, 1972; Cozensa and Kohler, 1972a, b; Rowley *et al.*, 1973; Strayer *et al.*, 1974; Eichmann, 1975). When the number of idiotypic specificities of the antibody response are limited (Lee and Kohler, 1974), the inhibition can be demonstrated as a decrease in the total amount of antibody formed.

Repeated immunization of mice with phosphorylcholine, an antigen that induces antibody with a restricted idiotype, leads to the production of antibody against phosphorylcholine as well as antibody directed against an IgA myeloma protein (TEPC-15, T15) which has antiphosophorylcholine activity and contains the major idotype of antibody produced on immunization with phosphorylcholine (Cozensa and Kohler, 1972a,b). Simple administration of T15 does not suppress responses to phosphorylcholine, however, an immune response against T15, which requires a number of injections, suppresses immune responses to phosphorylcholine (Rowley *et al.*, 1976). Conversely, an antibody response against phosphorylcholine inhibits antiidiotypic responses to T15 and this inhibition can be passively transferred. Administration of large, paralytic doses of the phosphorylcholine antigen does not prevent immunization against the idiotype, suggesting that the presence of idiotype-bearing antibody to antigen rather than antigen itself is required for suppression of the antiidiotypic response. Antibody directed against antigen and antibody directed against the idiotype determinants on the initial antibody were mutually regulatory in a primary immune response, while, on succeeding immunization, these two forms of antibody occur together *in vivo* despite the fact that antiphosphorylcholine and anti-T15 idiotype antibody responses are still mutually exclusive *in vitro*. This suggests that mechanisms for overcoming mutual regulation are established in multiply-immunized animals.

Another model system for idiotype suppression involves the production of a class of suppressor cells (Eichmann, 1975). In this system involving an antibody response to a carbohydrate antigen (A-CHO), antibody of the IgG_2 subclass directed against a particular idiotype suppressed the formation of antibody bearing that idiotype; anti-A-CHO antibodies expressing other idiotypic specificities were produced. This form of idiotype specific suppression could be adoptively transferred to sublethally irradiated syngeneic recipients. These recipient mice could not produce the idiotype inhibited in the originally suppressed animal. The suppressor cells were both Thy- and Ia-positive. A lower dose of antiidiotype IgG_2 antibody caused chronic suppression whereas a higher dose of IgG_2 antiidiotypic antibody did not. This result is similar to the demonstration that maximal immune suppression by antibody requires an optimal dose of antibody; if greater than optimal quantities of antibody were administered, a lesser degree of suppression is observed (Sinclair and Chan, 1971; Chan and Sinclair, 1971; Vuagnat and Vilain, 1974; Duc *et al.*, 1975). If IgG_1 antiidiotypic antibody was administered, priming of both B and T cell lines for production of that particular idiotype took place (Eichmann and Rajewsky, 1975; Black *et al.*, 1976). Again, an intermediate dose of IgG_1 antibody induced maximal priming (Rajewsky and Eichmann, 1977). That IgG_1 is an augmentary antibody while IgG_2 is suppressive suggests an Fc portion-based difference in biological activity (Pawlak *et al.*, 1973).

The observation that antiidiotypic antibody may lead to inhibition of specific antibody responses presented the possibility that such an antibody may be an important immunoregulation in other immune responses. Lewis rats can make anti-idiotypic antibody against Lewis anti-Brown Norway (BN) antibody if they are immunized with BN antigen and Lewis anti-BN antibody (McKearn *et al.*, 1974). The highest levels of antiidiotypic antibody are obtained approximately ten days after administration of antigen and antibody (Stuart *et al.*, 1976a). If renal allografts are placed in the recipients when the antiidiotypic antibody was at its height, an optimally functioning renal allograft is obtained. Enhancement of the renal allograft coincides therefore with the production of antiidiotypic antibody, rather than the presence of antigen–antibody complexes, which would be highest at the time antigen and antibody were given. Although enhancement correlates with the appearance of antiidiotypic antibody, such antibody is ineffective in prolonging graft survival when passively administered (Stuart *et al.*, 1976a). Spleen cells from long-term surviving recipients of a renal allograft could induce otherwise untreated Lewis recipients to accept a renal allograft from a Lewis × BN F_1 donor (Stuart *et al.*, 1976b). Such a result suggests that there is a suppressor cell population in animals with enhanced renal allografts which interferes with or controls rejection (Binz and Wigzell, 1977). It would be of interest to determine whether such suppressor cells are antigen-specific and, if so, are they directed against antigen itself or against the idiotype recognizing that antigen.

Antibody may augment immune responses through mechanisms that require the presence of the Fc portion (Pincus *et al.*, 1971; Gordon and Murgita, 1975). The augmentation of immune responses by antibody also requires the presence of a T cell population (McBride and Schiermann, 1973; Janeway *et al.*, 1975). T cells may trap antigen–antibody complexes on their surface, and thereby function in a helper role (Playfair *et al.*, 1974; Playfair, 1974). Chemically-haptenated myeloma protein plus antibody to the hapten could be used to elicit a heightened immune response to the idiotype of the myeloma protein and to the hapten coupled to the myeloma protein (Janeway *et al.*, 1975). This augmentation required the presence of peripheral T cells. The most likely explanation for these results is that the complex of haptenated myeloma protein plus antihapten antibody was absorbed to peripheral T cells by both Fc-portion attachment to Fc-receptors on T cells and by attachment of hapten to specific T cells. Such a binding of the Fc-portions of antibody in antigen–antibody complexes by T cells may make these Fc portions unavailable for binding to B cell Fc-receptors thus preventing Fc-dependent B cell inactivation and at the same time providing an activating signal to T cells with respect to their function in T–B cell collaboration (Sinclair *et al.*, 1976a).

It would have been anticipated that the binding of antigen to antibody would have occupied and thus made unavailable, antigen-binding sites on antibody required as antigen in the production of antiidiotypic antibody. However, complexes may fix to the surface of T cells specific for the antigen, and the Fc portion of antibody may become firmly bound by the Fc-receptors on such T cells. This process may allow for the detachment of antibody from antigen, freeing the antibody's antigen-binding sites which may, on the surface of T cells, become a suitable antigen for stimulation of idiotype-specific B or T cells. One would predict that the production of antiidiotypic antibody would require an intact Fc-portion on the original antibody. Similarly, in the experiments of Stuart *et al.* (1976b), the pronounced enhancement of renal allografts that occurred in association with the production of antiidiotypic activities (cell and/or antibodies) would be expected to show dependence upon the presence of an intact (Fc-bearing) antibody in the original antigen–antibody complex.

In situations where antiidiotypic antibody or cells are regulatory, the requirement for a T cell population in the antiidiotypic response could be viewed as suppressive with respect to the original immune products against which the antiidiotypic activity is directed. This may account for why suppressive and stimulatory Ia-antigen containing factors are so much alike: one stimulates a response against antigen whereas a second stimulates a regulatory response against idiotypes capable of recognizing antigen.

An instructive form of regulation is that seen in patients afflicted with malignant melanoma (Lewis and Phillips, 1972; Bodurtha *et al.*, 1975; Shiku *et al.*, 1976). Antibodies, which are cytotoxic to the melanoma, sometimes disappear prior to the emergence of metastases (Shibata *et al.*, 1976). Four forms of regulation are associated with this loss of antitumor antibodies: (1) antiimmunoglobulin which appears to have antiidiotypic specificities directed against specific binding-sites of antitumor antibodies (Lewis *et al.*, 1971b); (2) various antibodies directed against cytoplasmic antigens which may be in complex form with tumor antigen and may also be responsible for a form of kidney damage associated with malignancy (Lewis *et al.*, 1971a); (3) antibodies against antitumor antibodies which may be directed against nonvariable $F(ab')_2$ determinants (Hartman and Lewis, 1974; Lewis *et al.*, 1976) or against Fc portions (Jerry *et al.*, 1976); and (4) various forms of suppressor cells (Lewis, personal communication). All these results suggest that there may be a hierarchy of immunoregulatory events that involve the production of antibody directed against tumor antigens followed by the production of antibodies directed against these antibodies in either a tumor-specific or more general way. The tumor-specific process would be represented by antiidiotypic activity whereas more general immune complex forms of immunoregulation may involve antibodies directed against altered immunoglobulins. The latter may be directed towards specific reactants in an antitumor immune response because of the pre-existing immunologic specificities. These results, and those of others, suggest that a coordinated series of immunoregulatory mechanisms can activate or secondarily control other forms of immunoregulation. There is a temptation to consider a hierarchy of immunoregulatory mechanisms to be present, beginning with antibody directed against antigen, followed by antibody directed against specific antibody, and leading to suppressor cells which may be activated later. Although this appears to be the sequence in these particular studies, it may be reversed in other systems so that an immunoregulatory grid rather than an undirectional immunoregulatory pathway may exist.

In summary, immunoregulatory processes involving the Fc portion of antibody are powerful in that small amounts of antibody can control immune responses. Only a partial covering of determinants on an immunogenic molecule is required for suppression. Not only does antibody directed against antigen lead to immunoregulatory phenomena, but also antibodies against antigenic determinants found in the combining sites of other antibodies or cells will induce similar regulatory events involving Fc-dependent mechanisms. The interactions between the antigen-binding sites of antibody against antigen and the subsequent antiidiotypic antibodies, followed by succeeding levels of recognition, has suggested to Jerne (1974, 1976) that a branching array of interactions exists: the 'network' or 'web' hypothesis for immunoregulation. Specificity in this form of regulation is mandatory for its biologic importance. The information on the Fc portion of antibody serves to illumine the other aspect of such a regulatory web, its effector mechanisms. As with the understanding of immune reactions such as complement fixation or opsonization, an understanding of immunoregulatory networks would be incomplete without an understanding of the central role of the Fc portion of antibody. The specificity of regulatory antibodies is important but insufficient to explain regulation. Specific antibody elicits and directs the effector mechanisms that actually regulate immunity. Just as complement-induced damage of a cell membrane is primarily directed by the fixation of antibody to these membranes, the regulatory events that take place in an immune response are likely to be impelled by the binding of Fc portions of antibodies to Fc-receptors and of antigen to its adjacent receptors. Specific binding between antigen and antibody begins a chain of humoral and cellular events, which generate the signals that actually cause regulation.

4. MODULATION OF THE IMMUNE RESPONSE BY ANTIGEN

Antigen injected under various conditions may lead to the specific elimination of immune responses (Dresser and Mitchison, 1968; Weigle, 1973; Coutinho and Möller, 1975; Howard and Mitchison, 1975; Brent *et al.*, 1976; Leech and Mitchison, 1976; Klaus *et al.*, 1976; Dresser, 1976). The reduced ability of the lymphoid system to respond as a consequence of exposure to tolerogenic antigen has been demonstrated in most immune responses. The nature of the defect induced by tolerogenic antigen differs from one immune response to another and even within one well-defined immune response. The defect may vary depending upon the conditions under which tolerance was induced. Three major categories of defect that occur in various experimental models for tolerance induction are: (1) irreversible tolerance due to the elimination or inactivation of specific immunocompetent cells; (2) reversible tolerance in which an inhibitory influence need only be removed from the immunocompetent cells to allow them to function; and (3) a peripheral blockade in which the products of an immune response were not visible because they were used up immediately in an immunologic reaction. This latter category is, in reality, not a form of tolerance at all because the immune responsiveness is intact whereas the ability to perceive the products of that immune response have been deranged because of a masking process. The distinction between the first two categories of tolerance is made on the basis of rapidity of reversibility. In the second of these, removal of inhibitory antigen, antibody, or antigen–antibody complexes as well as various types of suppressor cells should allow for the rapid reexpression of immunologic function in immunocompetent cells. Irreversible tolerance by definition cannot be reversed by the simple elimination of an actively suppressing element. Tolerance of this form may wane with time; the emergence of immunocompetence depends upon the production of new immunocompetent cells from primitive lymphoid precursors in the bone marrow.

A number of characteristics may predispose the antigen to induce tolerance. The more immunogenic the antigen is, the less tolerogenic it is likely to be, requiring under these conditions additional immunosuppression of the subject to be tolerized. Certain nonmetabilizable compounds demonstrate a high potentiality for tolerance induction, presumably because of the ease with which antigen-overload may occur. One of the more widely used tolerogens has been the various autologous, isologous or heterologous immunoglobulins; these immunoglobulins may, because of Fc-receptor-binding, have proportionately greater negative effects on lymphoid cells.

When haptens are coupled to carriers suitable for the induction of tolerance, the haptens themselves become active in the induction of antihapten tolerance. Haptens that bind to autologous constituents are able to induce either tolerance or immunity (Claman, 1976; Claman and Moorhead, 1967). There is a correlation between the binding of these reactive haptens to autologous components in the antigenized animal and the ability to influence the immune system either negatively or positively. When these reactive haptens bind to epidermal cells, they tend to elicit a pronounced delayed hypersensitivity reaction. On the other hand, when reactive haptens are given systemically, they apparently bind to other autologous components and are effective in inducing tolerance. One may suggest that binding to epidermal cells would provide a potent stimulus whereas binding to compounds such as autologous immunoglobulins or, indeed, lymphoid cells themselves may make these compounds tolerogenic.

If aggregates are removed from an antigen preparation by either centrifugation (Dresser, 1962) or by *in vitro* filtration (Frei *et al.*, 1965) the remaining deaggregated antigen is effective in inducing tolerance. This maneuver has been found to be successful in producing potent tolerogens with antigens such as solubilized sheep erythrocytes (Anderson *et al.*, 1972) flagellin (Parish and Ada, 1969), polyvinylpyrrolidone (Andersson, 1969) dextran (Kabat and Bezer, 1958) and levan (Miranda *et al.*, 1973). This rule, although general, is not absolute (Howard *et al.*, 1971), suggesting that an alteration in size is not central in the production of highly tolerogenic activity. It would seem, at least in some cases, that removing components which have a high affinity for accessory cells increases tolerogenicity and decreases immunogenicity suggesting that an immunogenic form of antigen antagonizes the induction of tolerance or, at least, its expression. The resistance of primed animals to T cell tolerogens indicates that interference with tolerance induction by an ongoing immune response may be related to the increased ability for antigen to be taken up by various reticuloendothelial cells so that immunogen presentation to competent cells is more efficient while antigen-overload is less likely.

Antigens may be modified chemically to alter their immunogenicity for various immune responses. Procedures such as acetoacetylation decrease the ability of antigen to induce an antibody response while increasing the ability to evoke a delayed hypersensitivity reaction (Parish, 1971a,b, 1973; Parish and Liew, 1972). These results are similar to those in which hapten-autologous carriers are potent tolerogens, particularly of B cells, while allowing the induction of some forms of cell-mediated immune responses. Chemically modified antigens may bind with great avidity to B cells, inactivating them, while serving as a suitable immunogen for T cells which require antigen presentation on another cell surface for their activation. Although this form of mutually exclusive activation with respect to the stimulation of various immune responses is not universal, it occurs with sufficient frequency to be of use in attempting to establish prerequisites for stimulation of various components of the immune system. This is so with regard to the stimulation of antibody responses vs cell-mediated responses, and with respect to the stimulation of IgE vs IgG antibody responses.

Without the coordinated functioning of the immune system either as a consequence of immaturity or immunosuppression, antigens may specifically reduce immune responsiveness. Whether the question of immaturity refers to coordinated cellular events within the architecture of a lymphoid system or whether these questions of immaturity also relate to cells themselves has not been firmly answered. Cells may pass through very sensitive phases in which they are extremely prone to becoming tolerant. This may be a requirement for the generation of a lymphoid system in which the ability to form autoreactive clones is equal to the ability to form clones reactive against foreign antigens (Allison and Denman, 1976).

4.1. Irreversible Tolerance—Clone Elimination or Inactivation

With the initial demonstration of experimental tolerance (Billingham *et al.*, 1956) and even before (Burnet and Fenner, 1949), tolerance was considered or predicted to be consequent to the loss of immunocompetent cells. In some experimental systems such a defect was demonstrated to be present (Gowans *et al.*, 1963; Schwarz, 1968; Wilson and Nowell, 1970; Atkins and Ford, 1972; Brent *et al.*, 1973; Basten *et al.*, 1974; Chiller *et al.*, 1974; Brooks, 1975; Elkins, 1973; von Boehmer and Sprent, 1976). In some of these cases, tolerance was complete with no signs of residual activity. However, under certain experimental conditions, tolerance could be shown to be only partial, in which case residual antigen-reactive cells were detected (Gowans *et al.*, 1963, Heron, 1973; Basten *et al.*, 1974; Bernstein *et al.*, 1975; von Boehmer and Sprent, 1976).

Tolerance of the clonal elimination type often involves the preferential loss of T cells. In some systems, this loss occurs at lower doses of tolerogen, takes place more quickly than inactivation of B cells and recovery from the inactive state is slower than for B cells (Chiller *et al.*, 1970, 1971; Weigle *et al.*, 1973). Experiments in which tolerance was broken with the agency of crossreacting antigens (where antibodies which crossreact to both the tolerance-breaking antigen and the original tolerogen were obtained) can be interpreted as a circumvention of a deficient T cell population (Cinader and Dubert, 1955; Weigle, 1973). An elegant experiment has recently been reported in which animals made tolerant to one protein form a limited array of antibodies on immunization with a crossreactive protein (Cecka *et al.*, 1976). If the tolerance-breaking protein differed from the original tolerogen in a geographically restricted surface area, antibodies formed are totally crossreactive with the original tolerogen. This indicates that this area of difference between the original tolerogen and the crossreacting immunogen is recognized by T cells and, in so doing, is unavailable for recognition by B cells capable of responding to the rest of the molecule which is identical to the original tolerogen. Therefore, a B cell population was available in the tolerant animal but a competent T cell population was lacking. When the tolerance-breaking immunogen differs from the original tolerogen at a number of sites on the surface of the molecule, antibodies formed in the previously tolerant animal are directed against either the tolerance-breaking immunogen alone, or against both it and the tolerogen. No antibodies specific for the original tolerogen but not crossreactive with the tolerance-breaking immunogen were formed. Taken together, these results indicate that the B cell population in the tolerant animal was intact, even if somewhat restricted, that an immune response could be obtained by eliciting a new population of helper T cells, and that the ability of B cells to recognize antigenic determinants may be restricted partly because of steric hindrance by the T cell population or its product. If the original immunogen was administered after tolerance was broken with crossreacting antigen, no immune response occurred against antigenic determinants specific for the original immunogen: the normal complement of T cells against the original immunogen was not restored by immunization with crossreacting antigen. Reexposure to the original immunogen may in fact prevent the breakage of tolerance with crossreacting antigen (Weigle, 1973).

The marked sensitivity of T cells to inactivation by various antigens deserves some comment. T cells are inhibited in two antigen-dose ranges, a low dose range in which T cells are the only population affected and in a high antigen dose range where both T and B cells are inactivated (Dresser and Mitchison, 1968; Leech and Mitchison, 1976; Dresser, 1976). Tolerance to certain self-antigens that are present in the circulation in low concentrations, such as thyroglobulin, involves the loss of T cells, whereas tolerance to self-antigens present in large amounts in circulation extends to both T and B lymphocyte populations (Allison, 1971; Weigle, 1971; Allison and Denman, 1976). Intermediate doses of foreign antigen induce immune responses. Two possible interpretations of these facts can be made. The first is that the development of an immune response obscured, but was otherwise unconnected with, the phenomenon of tolerance induction. The defective ability of immunocompetent cells, particularly T cells to adoptively transfer immune responses when they come from recently immunized animals, may indicate that a concomitant tolerance as well as immunity and activation of immunocompetent cells occurs even during the generation of an immune response (Sprent and Miller, 1974, 1976; Sprent and Lefkovits, 1976). However, this defect in immunocompetence in animals expressing immune responses is restricted to lymphocytes found in certain sites, most notably the thoracic duct, and the defect in T cells was not so profound during the generation of an immune response as that seen in low zone tolerance (Blackstock and Hyde, 1973; Rajewsky and Brenig, 1974; Dresser, 1976). As a second possibility, activation of B cells may prevent T cell tolerance. The direct exposure of soluble antigens to T cells without the intervention of another cell type may lead to inactivation of T cells. T cells are activated most readily by antigen presented on a cell surface, whereas soluble antigens either fail to activate T cells or may even suppress them. Soluble protein antigens most readily elicit high and low zone tolerance. Low doses of such antigens may gain direct access to T cells and induce T cell tolerance. Intermediate doses may activate B cells, causing them to present the antigen on their surface to T cells directly, or to produce a cytophilic antibody by which macrophages might take up and present antigen to T cells. At high doses, soluble antigen may gain direct access to T cells despite the early activation of B cells and the secretion of antibody. This scheme reverses the usual concept of T to B cell collaboration. There is ample evidence that antigen presentation on a cell surface is a requirement for T cell activation. By similar reasoning, since deaggregated (Dresser, 1962) or biologically-filtered proteins (Frei *et al.*, 1965), which have a low avidity for cell surfaces, appear to be highly tolerogenic, direct access of antigen to the surface of the T cell may evoke tolerance. Direct access of antigen to the surface of the T cell may be avoided through an increase in avidity of other lymphoid cell surfaces for antigen, perhaps induced by antigen-aggregation or by a small amount of surface-bound antibody. In the latter case, Fc receptors on lymphoid and nonlymphoid cells may bind antigen–antibody complexes such that the antigen now becomes a suitable immunogen for T cells.

Helper antihapten T cell responses may be generated, provided that the host is tolerant to the carrier (Yamashita *et al.*, 1975, 1976a). When the carrier is isologous, antihapten helper T cells are produced. When animals are made tolerant to a heterologous protein, hapten-specific T cells are produced on immunization with hapten–tolerant-carrier complexes, an immune response which would not have occurred if the animal were non-tolerant towards the heterologous carrier. Stimulating hapten-specific T cells with hapten isologous carrier complexes breaks low zone, but not high zone tolerance. This indicates that helper T cells are missing in low zone tolerance, whereas both B and T cells are lacking in high zone tolerance. Mice possessing hapten-specific helper T cells develop antierythrocyte antibody and anemia when challenged with hapten on isologous mouse erythrocytes (Yamashita *et al.*, 1976b), suggesting that the lack of a response against isologous erythrocytes represents a form of low zone tolerance in which an immunocompetent B cell population directed against autologous erythrocytes may be present. Hapten-specific delayed type hypersensitivity to *p*-azobenzene arsonate, produced with hapten homologous carrier immunization but not with hapten heterologous carrier immunization (Jones and Leskowitz, 1965), may represent an analogous system.

Cell-mediated lympholysis of trinitrophenol or virus modified autologous lymphocytes occurs through effector cell activity directed against modified cell surface components controlled by the H-2K and H-2D serological regions of the murine major histocompatibility complex (Shearer *et al.*, 1975; Doherty and Zinkernagel, 1974; Zinkernagel and Doherty, 1975; Zinkernagel, 1976). It is worth noting that hapten-modified autologous lymphocytes, although they may be able to induce the formation of specific cytotoxic cells, appear to induce a form of tolerance in the absence of FCA with respect to T cell dependent and independent antibody responses (Scott and Long, 1976). In this system, trinitrophenol (TNP)-coupled spleen cells block the *in vitro* production of antibody-forming cells against TNP while simultaneously stimulating a cytotoxic T cell response against TNP-coupled target cells. Also, TNP-coupled lymphoctyes inhibit the production of delayed hypersensitivity reactions *in vitro* (Claman, 1976). It would appear that hapten-modified autologous cells stimulate the Ly-2,3 T cell subset, the T cells responsible for cytotoxic and some suppressor cell activity, while inhibiting the activation of B cells and the Ly-1 T cell subset, responsible for helper effects and the expression of delayed-type hypersensitivity. An exception to this is the hapten-specific induction of delayed-type hypersensitivity by hapten–homologous carrier (Jones and Leskowitz, 1965); it may be that some forms of delayed-type hypersensitivity are mediated by Ly-2,3 T cells (Vadas *et al.*, 1976; Miller *et al.*, 1976b). Although all evidence to date suggests that H-2K and H-2D modifications represent the targets for 'altered-self' syngeneic killing, hapten-modified targets rich in H-2I encoded antigens which are recognized by a minor Ly-2,3 T-cell subset has not been formally investigated (Forman, 1976) so that a rigid compartmentalization of functions amongst the subclasses of T cells may be premature.

In normal mice, hapten-conjugated erythrocytes gave rise to immune responses when the erythrocytes were allogeneic or xenogeneic with respect to the host (Koskimies and Makela, 1976). Conversely, when T cell deficient mice were used, syngeneic, rather than allogeneic or xenogeneic, erythrocytes functioned as a better carrier while semi-allogeneic erythrocytes were intermediate. F_1 to parent immunizations gave responses which were no different than allogeneic erythrocytes conjugates. That responses (IgM) to hapten–syngeneic erythrocyte conjugates by T cell deficient mice were stronger than in normal mice suggests that a suppressor T cell may regulate the immune response to hapten conjugates of syngeneic erythrocytes (Naor *et al.*, 1975). The use of the induction of hapten-specific T helper cells for the investigation of the T cell receptor (Leech and Mitchison, 1976) may be misleading if the limiting factor in the T cell response does not relate to antigen-binding and initial triggering events but to regulatory influences which may be brought to bear on the T cell antihapten response.

Two forms of reactivity against tolerated MHC antigens occur which are still compatible with the clonal deletion hypothesis. Firstly, various forms of antibody derived from nontolerant B cells may be demonstrated in T cell tolerance (Hellström and Hellström, 1974; Voisin *et al.*, 1972; Blair and Lane, 1975) provided that an alternate mechanism to allow expression of B cell immunologic capacity can function. Secondly, T cell responses against gene products of the MHC in mice may be subdivided into those directed predominantly against the H-2D and H-2K products and those directed predominantly against the H-2I region products. A reactivity against the H-2I region can be demonstrated by a mixed lymphocyte reaction in the presence of a clonal deletion of cytotoxic cells directed against H-2D and H-2K antigens. The extent of tolerance differs when irradiated F_1 hosts are repopulated with bone marrow from one, as distinct from both, parental strains (von Boehmer and Sprent, 1976). Tolerance develops in cytotoxic cell responses against H-2K and H-2D antigens in F_1 recipients receiving either one or both parental bone marrow cells. However, cells obtained from F_1 irradiation chimeras produced with T cell-depleted bone marrow cells from one parental strain are reactive against the opposite parental strain in mixed lymphocyte reactions. When irradiated F_1 mice received T cell-depleted bone marrow from *both* parents, cells from these chimeras do not respond in mixed lymphocyte cultures against either parental strain. This result is probably due to the fact that the F_1 background supplies sufficient H-2D and H-2K antigen to tolerize the parental immunocompetent cells but cannot supply a sufficient amount of H-2I antigen to induce tolerance with respect to mixed lymphocyte reactive cells. When bone marrow of both parental cell-types, rich in H-2I encoded Ia-antigens, were given to irradiated F_1 recipients, each parental cell population tolerized the other with respect to H-2I as well as H-2K and H-2D antigens. These results account for the presence of an MLR reactivity in the F_1 animals receiving parental bone marrow from one parent; as yet cytotoxic cells against I-region antigen determinants (Klein *et al.*, 1974; Wagner *et al.*, 1975a,b) have not been specifically studied.

A classification of tolerance may be based on the amount of time which cells from tolerant animals need to respond again when transferred into a tolerogen-free environment (Chiller *et al.*, 1971; Elkins, 1973; Rajewsky and Brenig, 1974; Miyamoto and McCullagh, 1974; Chiller and Weigle, 1975; Silvers *et al.*, 1975; Howard and Mitchison, 1975). When cells from irradiation chimeras, discussed in the preceding paragraph, were transferred to antigen-free, irradiated secondary hosts following elimination of any tolerizing antigen, the cells regained immunologic reactivity against tolerated antigens only after a period of 2 weeks or more (von Boehmer and Sprent, 1976). These results indicate that the tolerant state was not easily reversible and reactivities probably reappeared because prethymic cells had differentiated into T cells expressing the previously missing activity. No suppressor cells were demonstrated. In another system (Sanfilippo *et al.*, 1976), carrier-specific tolerance extended to the bone marrow precursor cells which give rise to mature T cells, so that, in some cases, responses must be regenerated from even more primitive stem cell populations.

In a number of cases, induction of tolerance appears to affect predominantly the function of T cells. B cell suppression is found only at high doses of tolerogen or during the phase of maximum tolerance (Chiller *et al.*, 1971) and when certain antigens are used most notably those which do not demonstrate a good *in vivo* anti-carrier T cell response. Some examples of B cell tolerogens are hapten-syngeneic mouse gammaglobulins (Havas, 1969; Golan and Borel, 1971), dinitrophenol attached to a glutamic acid–lysine oligopolymer (DNP-D-GL) (Katz *et al.*, 1972), levans (Howard *et al.*, 1972) pneumococcal capsular polysaccharide type III (SIII) (Howard *et al.*, 1972),

DNP-lysine SIII (Mitchell *et al.*, 1972b) and hapten–syngeneic erythrocytes (Hamilton and Miller, 1974). In the last study, hapten-specific tolerance was induced in 5–7 d following immunization with hapten-syngeneic mouse erythrocytes and only with respect to antihapten IgG antibody production. Antihapten IgM production was not affected. It is possible that cells destined to form IgG antihapten antibody become coated with hapten-syngeneic erythrocytes and are inactivated through an Fc-mediated mechanism when initial formation of IgG antibody begins. If a considerable proportion of activated cells remain as IgM-producing cells, these would not be tolerized by hapten-syngeneic erythrocytes and would respond normally following challenge with immunogenic hapten. In this system, B cells capable of forming IgG antibody against the haptenic determinant are inactivated. There is no defect in the ability of T cells to function in the presence of an immunogenic carrier and no suppressor cell exists. Even though immunosuppressive complexes were not found in the circulation, this should not be interpreted to mean that immune complexes play no role in the inactivation of B cells, since each B cell could be inactivated by its own product on combination with antigen. Hapten-syngeneic mouse erythrocytes would not induce B cell tolerance when given 3 d after the adoptive transfer of primed spleen cells and antigen, indicating that stimulated B cells had become resistant to tolerogen. The reason for this resistance may be that cells producing sufficient amounts of antibody no longer allow the close approach of hapten-syngeneic mouse erythrocytes to the B cell surface and/or because cells actively synthesizing IgG antibody no longer possessed antigen- or Fc-receptors (Warner, 1974). One possible objection to this concept is that antigen-binding cells, as determined by rosette formation, increase during an immune response and would therefore, appear to be resistant to tolerance induction even though binding antigen (Wilson and Miller, 1971). However, many of these rosette-forming cells are T cells, which do not secrete antibody, (McConnell, 1971; Wilson, 1971). Also, actively antibody-synthesizing cells that do form rosettes attach erythrocytes only tenuously (Greaves *et al.*, 1974). Therefore, there may be insufficient contact between antigen and an actively secreting antibody-forming cell in an immune rosette to allow inactivation of this cell.

In other T independent systems, inactivation of B cells also represents the major cellular effect of a tolerogenic exposure to these particular antigens. With some T independent antigens, there is evidence of a prior activation of B cells and hence B cells are inactivated by the antigen–antibody complexes formed on their surface; this was discussed previously when dealing with suppression by antibody. One particular antigen, levan, has been especially instructive with regard to possible mechanisms of B cell inactivation by T cell-independent antigens (Howard and Mitchison, 1975). Levan is slowly eliminated from the body, induces exclusively an IgM antibody response, has no capacity to induce immunologic memory and displays a high avidity for B cells. In an extensive dose–response analysis, the following results were observed: an increasing antilevan response occurred with antigen doses from 100 pg to 10 μg, beyond this point the primary response decreased. If the animals received a second injection of levan (10 μg) 14 d following the injection of varying doses of levan, no evidence of priming was observed; that is, the second response was the same as the first. With priming doses of 1 μg or larger, a depression occurred after the second exposure. These results indicate that two forms of tolerance induction took place. With priming antigen doses of 1 μg and 10 μg, which gave optimal primary responses, the ability of the animals to respond to a second optimal injection of levan is reduced. This suggested to the authors that some form of exhaustive immunization occurs. An alternative possibility is that levan remained attached to B cells and that 1–10 μg doses of levan, in concert with a good immune response, led to the inactivation of B cells through the mediation of antigen–antibody complexes. At the 1 mg dose level of levan, there was an inactivation of the primary response as well as, presumably, an inability to respond to a second injection of levan. This was described as a direct inactivation by the authors and could be an immediate inactivation of B cells by antigen through a membrane freezing process. However, the possible involvement of endogenously-produced antibody indetectable by the assays used forming immune complexes with the levan, should not be discounted. The latter inactivation would again imply that the synthesis and secretion of antibody could function in tolerance-induction. Sensitivity of this IgM form of antilevan immune response to inactivation by antigen-antibody complexes may resemble that which occurs in low responder animals where inactivation by IgM antibody has been described (Ordal *et al.*, 1976).

The activity of B cell tolerogens depends upon their polymeric structure, a certain minimum size, resistance to metabolic degradation in the body and does not depend upon its inherent immunogenic capacity (Klaus *et al.*, 1976b). Tolerance is induced within hours to days, is independent of T cell activity, can demonstrate dissociation with respect to two antigenic determinants on the same molecule and can be stable or unstable with a period of recovery which is dependent upon the regeneration of new immunocompetent cells from stem cells. IgG antibody-forming precursor B cells appear to be more sensitive to these B cell tolerogens, than those giving rise to IgM antibody-forming cells (Hamilton and Miller, 1965; Klaus and Cross, 1974). Some B cell tolerogens can induce tolerance in immunized mice (Katz *et al.*, 1972; Mitchell *et al.*, 1972b). There is a clear association between the avidity of B cells for antigen and their sensitivity to tolerance induction (Klinman, 1972; Desaymard *et al.*, 1976). All of these results suggest that cells with a higher avidity for antigen, such as would be expected of IgG antibody-forming cell precursors, are more likely to be tolerized because antigen is more likely to remain attached to their cell-surfaces for a sufficient time to allow the molecular events associated with tolerance induction to take place (Klaus, 1975). A simple blockade of plasma cells actively forming antibody is not a likely explanation for B cell tolerance because blockade is more noticeable in IgM antibody-forming cells, rather than IgG-forming cells (Klaus, 1976). Cells forming IgG antibody are more resistant to these tolerogens because their antigen-binding receptors may be no longer available or because of a disappearance of Fc-receptors. On the other hand, *precursors* of IgG antibody-forming cells may possess a larger number of high avidity antigen-receptors and also a larger number of Fc-receptors compared to the precursors of IgM antibody-forming cells and, hence, be prone to B cell tolerance.

The ability to tolerize a B cell population depends upon the avidity of antigen-binding and the hapten-density on the tolerizing antigen (Desaymard, *et al.*, 1976). This appears to be the case when a constant number of mouse spleen cells was exposed to varying concentrations of hapten-substituted tolerizing antigen for four hours and then cultured with hapten-substituted immunogen to provoke an immune response. The antibody-forming cells were counted at the end of the culture period and assessed for their avidity for antigen through the use of a hapten-inhibition assay. IgG antibody-forming cell precursors are generally more susceptible to hapten-substituted tolerogen than are IgM antibody-forming cell precursors. Cells capable of producing antibody of high avidity are more easily tolerized than those cells capable of forming antibody of low avidity. When the tolerizing antigen has a low density of haptens, IgG antibody-forming cell precursors of low avidity were more resistant to tolerance induction than IgM antibody-forming cell precursors expressing the same avidity for antigen. On the other hand, when the tolerizing antigen has a higher density of haptens, IgG antibody-forming cell precursors of roughly the same avidity as IgM antibody-forming cell precursors are more readily tolerized. This suggests that an effective tolerogen for IgG antibody-forming cell precursors may require many haptenic determinants; multiple binding to antigen-receptors on the surface of IgG antibody-forming cell precursors and to the IgG antibody product of these cells induces B cell tolerance consequent to the formation of inhibitory immune complexes on the surface of the B-cell. The resistance of IgG precursor cells to lowly substituted tolerogenic molecules may be because there is sufficient hapten to bind only antigen-receptors on to IgG precursor cells with insufficient amounts available to bind the secreted antibody product. The more prominent production of IgM antihapten antibodies to highly haptenated immunogens (Klaus and Cross, 1974) could be due to inactivation of IgG precursor cells by endogenously produced IgG antibodies binding to the numerous hapten groups, to form an inactivating complex of B cell, antigen and secreted antibody (Sinclair and Chan, 1971). This is equally plausible as an explanation based on a greater potential for activation of IgM precursor cells by multi-determinant antigens.

Tolerant animals can be reconstituted by the adoptive transfer of large numbers of cells primed against the tolerogen. If the tolerant animals receive a low number of cells, they will not be reconstituted and become resistant to a normally reconstituting cell dose (Ramseier and Lindenmann, 1972). Tolerant animals could be immunized by the antigenic specificities present on cells that react to the tolerogen because the tolerant animals lack these particular antigen-receptors. A critical analysis of this work (Brent *et al.*, 1976) suggested that no distinction had been made between the presence of antiidiotypic immune responses causing suppression and the usual forms of antigen–antibody complexes leading to suppression. However, our earlier discussion of the role of antiidiotypic antibodies in the regulation of immune responses, initially triggered by antigen–antibody complexes, again raises the possibility that there may be a cascade of effects beginning with antigen–antibody complexes, through regulation by antiidiotypic antibodies, and proceeding further to the elicitation of regulatory cell types directed against antigen or the idiotypic determinants.

Although certain forms of tolerance clearly involve a clonal deletion mechanism, questions may be raised concerning the mechanisms by which this deletion is accomplished. It has been suggested on a number of occasions that the reversible forms of tolerance lead to, or are part of mechanisms that result in a clonal deletion. Indeed, in a number of studies, particularly in immunologic reactivity to tumor antigens, forms of reversible tolerance may evolve into irreversible tolerance with the loss of immunocompetent cells.

In summary, irreversible tolerance involving clonal elimination is characterized by the following: (1) lymphocytes from tolerant animals cannot be rapidly reactivated on adoptive transfer or by *in vitro* cultures; (2) reactivity reappears slowly (due to the generation of new reactive T and B lymphocytes); (3) there is very little evidence of cellular reactivity in a tolerant animal on exposure to the tolerated antigen in an immunogenic form; (4) immunosuppression does not terminate tolerance; (5) other forms of immunologic reactivity to tolerated antigen are not visible or, if so, are irrelevant to clone elimination; (6) tolerance can be broken by the transfer of normal lymphocytes into these tolerant animals; and (7) tolerance cannot be transferred from tolerant animals to normal animals or to normal lymphocyte populations.

4.2. Reversible Tolerance—Active Suppression

In forms of tolerance of the active suppression type, some element of an immunologically specific nature is present that prevents a normal lymphoid cell population from giving rise to the immune response studied. These inhibitory agents may include antibody, solubilized antigen, various forms of antiidiotypic antibody or cells, and varieties of suppressor cells. These forms of active suppression, are characterized by the following properties: (1) specific nonreactivity is unstable on adoptive transfer when the active suppressor is not transferred; (2) tolerance often lasts a shorter time than in the clone elimination type; (3) the lymphoid system may show signs of partial reactivity to challenge with specific immunogen; (4) some immunosuppressive agents may terminate tolerance; (5) other forms of specific immunologic reactivity are detected which lead to the inactivation of that response; (6) transfer of normal lymphocytes does not abrogate this type of tolerance; and (7) various immunologic products taken from tolerant animals may induce tolerance in otherwise normal animals or normal populations of lymphocytes.

A number of noncellular entities regulate immune responses in some experimental models for immunologic tolerance. Serum antibody (Voisin *et al.*, 1969; 1972), anaphalactic antibody (Voisin, 1976) antigen–antibody complexes (Wright *et al.*, 1973,

1974a,b; Bansal *et al.*, 1973a,b) free antigen (Baldwin *et al.*, 1973; Thompson, 1975; Baldwin and Robbins, 1976) and various suppressor factors (Gershon, 1975; Fugimoto *et al.*, 1975; Hellström and Hellström, 1974) have all been implicated as blocking factors in forms of immunologic tolerance which can be differentiated on the basis of completeness. The question has been raised as to the possibility that there may be a real difference between partial and complete tolerance with respect to the mechanisms involved. It seems reasonable to suggest, as Brent *et al.* (1976) have done, that forms of complete tolerance with respect to alloantigen reactivity involve clonal deletion, whereas examples of partial tolerance may operate through active suppression involving the above mentioned entities.

The possible role that antibody may play in the induction of tolerance has been debated on many occasions. A definite requirement for antibody exists in some experimental models, while in others there seems to be no requirement for circulating antibody or antigen–antibody complexes in the induction of tolerance. Furthermore, in some experimental models for tolerance induction there appears to be no requirement for activation of the immunologic system as would be detected by an increased synthesis of DNA, RNA or protein (Weigle *et al.*, 1974). However, in those systems in which no activation of the immune system could be demonstrated, one cannot conclude that antibody does not play a role in the induction of tolerance. To conclude as much one must make the assumption that antibody, capable of feedback-suppression, is not produced in immunocompetent cells without antigen stimulation. Antigen-binding molecules of an immunoglobulin nature are most certainly produced prior to exposure to antigen and are inserted into the plasma membrane to serve as antigen-receptors and small amounts of immunoglobulin may be secreted by non-stimulated cells. When a B cell interacts with tolerogenic antigen, the signal which leads to inactivation may be mediated through a signal emanating from antibody constitutively formed by B cells. Although it may be difficult to prove the existence or nonexistence of constitutive immunoregulatory antibody *per se*, this concept leads to a testable prediction. Given the fact that one may be able to block Fc-receptors on B cells in a way which allows the B cells to become activated when exposed to antigen, such an Fc-receptor blockade would induce a resistance to inactivation by B cell tolerogens requiring Fc portion-bearing, constitutive antibody to attain suppression.

That antigen may be responsible for a form of reversible inactivation (Baldwin *et al.*, 1973; Thompson, 1975; Baldwin and Robins, 1976) seems to be established with reasonable certainty. The distinction made between the role of antigen in inducing a reversible inactivation vs its activity in inducing clonal deletion should be accentuated. In reversible inactivation, the simple removal of antigen will allow for the immediate expression of immunologic reactivity. On the other hand, in antigen-induced clonal elimination no such rapid reactivation occurs and the re-expression of immunologic reactivity is dependent upon the generation of new immunocompetent cells. The dual role attributed to antigen alerts one to the possibility that these two types of tolerance are not strictly separable but are opposite ends of a continuum of immunologic nonreactivity induced by antigen.

A number of experimental models of antigen-induced hyporesponsiveness (tolerance) have recently yielded evidence of suppressor cell involvement (Gershon and Kondo, 1972; Terman *et al.*, 1973; Gershon, 1974; Pinto *et al.*, 1974; Basten *et al.*, 1974; Silvers, 1974; Baker *et al.*, 1974; Rouse and Warner, 1974; Jirsch *et al.*, 1974; Kilshaw *et al.*, 1975; Droege, 1975; Burns *et al.*, 1975; Droege and Tuneskog, 1974; Zan-Bar *et al.*, 1976; Asherson and Zembala, 1976; Taylor and Basten, 1976). These references on the involvement of suppressor cells in the induction of tolerance are by no means complete; similar observations are continually appearing. Most reports on the induction of suppressor cells in tolerant animals implicate T cells as the active cell type. Therefore, T cells are not only the major target for, but also the mediators of, tolerance induction. These results are similar to those obtained in allotype suppression (Herzenberg *et al.*, 1976) in which inhibition of helper T cell activity in allotype suppressed animals is related to the presence of a suppressor T cell population acting directly on a helper T cell population. The rather pronounced sensitivity of T cells to clonal elimination in the induction of tolerance and the predominant anti-helper T cell attack by suppressor T cells suggests that these two forms of tolerance are not mutually exclusive, but merge one into the other.

In summary, tolerance can be defined operationally as forms of specific hyporesponsiveness induced by antigen. Even though antigen is the starting point in these forms of immunosuppression, the mechanisms by which the hyporesponsive state is reached may involve various products of the immune response such as antibody and effector cells which have suppressive activity.

5. CONCLUSIONS

A number of statements can be made concerning the nature of immune responses and their regulation. These will be listed and consecutively numbered. Beginning with these observations, one may construct a number of hypotheses. By ordering these in a logical sequence, one may be able to create an overview of the immune response and its regulation in which the observations and the hypotheses are clearly differentiated, but at the same time collated in a form that allows for continuity. The purpose of this approach is to reinforce in the reader the facts which seem well established and to place them within a framework suitable for grasping the essence as well as the complexity of immune responses.

(1) B cells are capable of binding antigen and undergoing preliminary steps in activation. (2) B cells may be inactivated or inhibited from further differentiation towards plasma cells at various stages in the differentiation process. (3) B cells display an inordinate sensitivity to suppression by antibody. *Hypothesis*: B cells can be activated by immunogen but may be inactivated or regulated by endogenously- or exogenously-derived antibody.

(4) B cells demonstrate a form of antibody-mediated inactivation which depends upon the Fc portion of antibody. (5) For antibody to be feedback-suppressive it must have the ability to bind antigen. (6) B cells express receptors which bind antigen in a highly specific manner. (7) B cells express Fc-receptors for the binding of Fc portions of antibody. *Hypothesis*: B cells can be inactivated by antibody when the variable region of antibody binds to antigen attached via antigen-receptors to B cells, inhibitory antibody also binds to the B cell surface through the Fc portion and this binding is responsible for the delivery of an inactivating signal.

(8) B cells form antibody constitutively; the amount of antibody formed in the absence of antigenic stimulation may be restricted to antigen-receptor molecules or small amounts of secreted product. (9) Antigen can inactivate B cells at various stages in their differentiation pathway towards antibody-forming plasma cells. *Hypothesis*: Antibody constitutively formed by B cells plays a role in the inactivation of B cells by antigen (B cell tolerogens), no matter at what stage in B cell differentiation these tolerogens inactivate.

(10) B cells are inactivated in some systems by mechanisms that depend upon the avidity of antigen-receptors on the B cells for tolerogen and upon the density of antigen (epitope) on the tolerogen. (11) Low epitope tolerogens preferentially inactivate IgM antibody-forming cell precursors while stimulating IgG antibody-forming precursors. (12) Tolerogens and immunogens with high epitope densities preferentially inactivate IgG antibody-forming cell precursors while stimulating IgM antibody-forming cell precursors. *Hypothesis*: The IgG antibody-forming cell precursors are prone to inactivation when their secreted IgG antibody product binds to multi-determinant immunogen or tolerogen. Immunogens or tolerogens with low epitope densities do not favor the dual binding of B cells and secreted antibody to the same antigenic molecule, hence do not form inactivating complexes.

(13) Thymus cells do not respond to direct antigen contact. (14) Thymus cells are activated most readily by the presentation of antigen on the surface of a histocompatible cell. (15) In many immune responses and in tolerance induction there is evidence that T cells become inactivated; this inactivation is favored by exposure to

intravenously injected soluble antigens. *Hypothesis*: T cells are inactivated by direct contact with antigen.

(16) B cells, as well as macrophages and other T cells, are effective in presenting antigen to T cells in a way which allows for T cell activation. (17) T cell inactivation during an antibody response is less than that which occurs in low zone tolerance. *Hypothesis*: Aside from the presentation of antigen on macrophages or other T cells to a responding T cell population, B cells may also present antigen in a form suitable for T cell activation; this is the major consequence of B-T cell collaboration during the antigen-presentation phase of the immune response.

(18) T cells influence the response of B cells to thymus-dependent antigens at stages beyond the point of initial B cell activation. (19) T cells are involved in the switch from IgM to IgG antibody synthesis. (20) In most systems, IgG antibody demonstrates a more potent feedback-suppression than does IgM antibody. (21) T cells and their activities inhibit Fc-dependent feedback by IgG antibody. *Hypothesis*: In T–B cell collaboration, T cells prevent feedback suppression by antibody (particularly IgG) produced during differentiation of B cells towards plasma cells.

(22) T cells bind antigen which is complexed with antibody. (23) The process of binding is inhibited by antibodies directed against T cell Ia-antigens which are closely linked to T cell Fc-receptors. *Hypothesis*: T cells bind antigen–antibody complexes via both antigen- and Fc-receptors; this form of dual binding activates T cells. By preempting the Fc portions of antibody bound to antigen on B cell surfaces, T cells collaborate with B cells in the process of B cell differentiation towards plasma cells by removing antigen, coated with endogenously-derived antibody, from the B cell surface, thus preventing Fc-dependent antibody-feedback of B cells.

(24) T cells produce factors that bind to Fc-receptors or to Ia antigens on B cells. (25) Some Ia antigens on B cells have a preferential association with Fc-receptors. *Hypothesis*: T cells produce factors that bind to B cell Fc-receptors and this prevents Fc-dependent feedback of B cells by antibody.

(26) Antibodies augment some immune responses to specific antigens. (27) The Fc portion of antibody is important for the expression of this augmentory effect by passive antibody. (28) B cells are sensitive to feedback-suppression by antibody whereas T cells are not sensitive. (29) T cells acquire antigen through a process involving antigen-receptors and Fc-receptors on the T cell surface. *Hypothesis*: The augmentory effects of antibody relate to the greater likelihood of antigen–antibody complexes becoming attached to T cells in a way which allows for adequate activation of T cells and the presentation of antigen to B cells without the concomitant exposure to inactivating Fc-generated signals.

(30) Antiidiotypic antibodies are induced most readily in response to antigen–antibody complexes. (31) Antigen–antibody complexes are taken up on the surface of lymphoid cells. (32) The presence of T cells are required for the induction of antiidiotypic antibody. *Hypothesis*: After dual (that is, antigen- and Fc-receptor) binding of complexes to specific T cells, the antigen-binding sites of antibody become available to stimulate an anti-idiotypic antibody response. The T cell dependency of antiidiotypic immune responses is due to idiotype presentation by T cells with the avoidance of an Fc-attachment to B cells.

(33) Cells that suppress immune responses are found amongst most of the cell populations implicated in immune responses. (34) The most prominent T cell suppressor displays the Ly-2,3 antigens, a class of T cells which houses the cytotoxic cell population. (35) Both cytotoxic cells and suppressor cells display Ia-antigens and may operate through the production of soluble factors as well as direct cell-cell contact with the target cell to effect a cytotoxic attack or suppressive event. (36) The end result of some suppressor activity on a helper cell population is the elimination of the helper cell population. *Hypothesis*: Some suppressor T cells (Ly-2,3) operate by generating a complete or incomplete form of cytotoxicity directed against other T lymphocytes that cooperate in the generation of an antibody-mediated immune response.

(37) Cells are generated in response to specific alloantigen which suppress the *in vitro* production of cytotoxic cells to the given antigen. (38) These antigen-specific suppressor cells, which are inseparable from cytotoxic cells, reduce the activity of the responder cell population both reversibly and irreversibly, even though they are sensitized against the stimulator cell population. (39) Stimulator cell antigen is present on the surface of responding lymphoblasts. *Hypothesis*: Cytotoxic cells can inhibit induction of cytotoxic cells by interacting with potentially responsive cells through a stimulator cell antigen bridge, leading to an inactivation of the responder cell population.

(40) Allogeneic immune responses *in vivo* appear to involve a series of cell-cell communication events in which the antigen is presented to the precytotoxic cell population in a constrained and highly compartmentalized fashion. (41) The cell-type which originally contacts antigen does not become cytotoxic but does transfer the information required for stimulation through a process in which the antigen moiety is recognized along with MHC antigens on the surface of this cell type. (42) Activated cells proliferate in the lymphnodes in response to this antigenic stimulation and are directed mainly against the lymphocyte-defined antigens on both the syngeneic antigen-bearing cell as well as the lymphocyte-defined antigens present on the incoming alloantigen. (43) Precytotoxic cell population recognizes predominantly cytolytically-defined antigens which appear to be linked to the serologically-defined antigens. *Hypothesis*: This form of cell-cooperation in the production of cytotoxic cells has as its basis the prevention of feedback-suppression induced by the direct exposure of antigen to precytotoxic cells; this suppression may be endogenously generated within each cell or may involve interactions between cells with capabilities of expressing cytotoxicity through bridges of specific stimulator antigen.

(44) Induction of immunologic enhancement of allografts by anti-allograft antibody can take place without suppression of cell-mediated immune responses and may involve the suppression of a damaging IgG antibody-mediated immune response. (45) The most potent forms of immunologic enhancement involve the concomitant loss of cytotoxic cell production which, in turn, is coupled to the presence of antiidiotypic reactivity. (46) Antiidiotypic antibody or cells suppress the production of antibody or cells bearing the idiotype. *Hypothesis*: Suppression of cytotoxic T cell production by antibody (or antigen–antibody complexes) involves the elicitation of an antiidiotypic response (antibody or cells) consequent to the exposure of the immune system to antigen-antibody complexes on the surface of T cells. The production of these antiidiotypic entities may control both B and T cell immune responses while antigen-antibody complexes are poor in activating T cells.

(47) Although antigen may be accumulated in lymphnodes and other lymphoid structures, it is restricted in its distribution within these structures and found in areas which do not contain cells differentiating into IgG antibody-forming cells. (48) Antigen may accumulate in a lymphnode consequent to exposure to contact sensitizers or in response to alloantigens or tumor antigens, but these antigens are restricted in their localization and in their mode of exposure on the surface of carrier cells such that, after the initial activation of cytotoxic cell precursors, the generation of cytotoxic cells occurs in areas not noted for their ability to accumulate available antigen. (49) Introduction of solubilized contact allergens or various soluble alloantigens or tumor antigens into a lymphnode leads to a rapid cessation of cytotoxic cell production. *Hypothesis*: The lymphnode serves to allow initial contact or contacts with antigen such that suitable forms of activation of T or B cells can occur and then it keeps these developing cells from further contact with antigen which would lead to their suppression. Once activation of the immunologically specific cells occurs, their maturation into cells, which produce immunologically specific products able to excite pronounced inflammatory reactions following contact with antigen, would take place in the absence of antigen. This separation of synthesis of specific immunologic products from reaction sites allows for undisturbed end product synthesis; when synthesis and reaction sites coincide regulation (inhibition) of the immune response occurs.

The various forms of modulation of the immune response, especially those involving antigen or antibody, are accomplished through a variety of mechanisms. There is considerable interest in finding the most potent and controlable forms of modulation which can be put to use in solving clinical problems. Fc-dependent feedback by antibody is such a form of modulation. So far, it has been shown to operate efficiently on B cells, but T cells may also be susceptible to Fc-dependent inactivation if correct conditions can be obtained. The inactivation of helper T cells by IgG_2 antiidiotypic antibody and by insolubilized immunoglobulin may be examples of T cell sensitivity to Fc-dependent inactivation.

A two signal requirement has been hypothesized for both the induction of immune responses (Bretscher and Cohen, 1970; Bretscher, 1972) and the induction of tolerance (Dresser, 1970, 1976). However, other studies would seem to support a one signal triggering mechanisms relating either to antigen-receptors or to another receptor to which antigens are focused by specific antigen receptors in a rather passive way (Moller, 1975). Hypotheses that suggest that the amount of antigen on the surface of the cell distinguishes between immunity and tolerance (Howard and Mitchison, 1975) again would suggest some form of one signal discrimination. These contrasting concepts of one versus two signals for activation or tolerance induction may be accommodated within the present analysis of the importance of modulating events in immune responses and tolerance induction. For instance, activation of B cells may only require contact with antigen in a way which leads to a perturbation in antigen-receptors. B cell activation may require, at least initially, a number of perturbations. No second signal may be necessary for these initial triggering events. The second signal may be the deletion of a regulatory mechanism or feedback-suppressive effect due to the initial production of highly suppressive antibody or other end products which would provide an intense and overwhelming inactivation signal unless removed by another cellular or subcellular entity. In other words, the second signal could be a mechanism for removal of an inactivating influence generated by responding cells. With respect to T cell inactivation, the continued presence of antigen on the surface of the T cell at the time effector activity is expressed induces T cell inactivation. A second influence (signal) may be the sequestering of antigen so that the T cell does not have antigen incorporated in its membrane at the time it develops effector cell function. Similarily, prevention of B cell inactivation may be accomplished by the removal of antigen prior to the production of sufficient amounts of antibody to form inactivating antigen–antibody complexes. On the other hand, the induction of tolerance of either B or T cell type would result from the expression of these negative signals. The expression of a negative signal would thus be due to the formation of an end product in the continued presence of stimulating antigen. Such an inhibitory event may take place because of the lack of a 'second signal' that interferes with inactivation (a double negative event), rather than a signal that activates directly (a single positive event). These modulatory mechanisms may be required to prevent autoimmune responses and reactions, undesirable aberrations that are well within the capacity of the functioning lymphoid system.

Acknowledgements—The author is indebted to Penny Chan and Rosemary Lees, whose experimental work and discussions have contributed greatly to this review, to Leni Vichos, whose reading and correcting have removed some of the obscurities, and to Judy Verge, Pat Fraser, Rosemary Dishman and Phyllis Hobson for their secretarial assistance in the preparation of this manuscript. Financial support for the author's work reviewed and for the expenses incurred in the writing of this review come from the Medical Research Council of Canada and the National Cancer Institute of Canada.

REFERENCES

Abbas, A. K. and Unanue, E. R. (1975) Interrelationships of surface immunoglobulin and Fc receptors on mouse B lymphocytes. *J. Immunol.* **115**: 1665–1671.

Abbasi, K., Demant, P., Festenstein, H., Holmes, J., Huber, B. and Rychlikova, M. (1973) Mouse mixed lymphocyte reactions and cell-mediated lympholysis: genetic control and relevance to antigenic strength. *Transplant. Proc.* **5**: 1329–1337.

Abney, E. R. and Parkhouse, R. M. E. (1974) Candidate for immunoglobulin D present on murine B lymphocytes. *Nature, Lond.* **2**: 600–602.

ABO, T., YAMAGUCHI, T., SHIMZU, F. and KUMAGAI, K. (1976) Studies of surface immunoglobulins on human B lymphocytes. II. Characterization of a population of lymphocytes lacking surface immunoglobulins but carrying Fc receptor (SIg^-Fc^+ cell). *J. Immunol.* **117**: 1781–1787.

ABRAHAMS, S., PHILLIPS, R. A. and MILLER, R. E. (1973) Inhibition of the immune response by 7S antibody. Mechanism and site of reaction. *J. exp. Med.* **137**: 870–892.

ALDO-BENSON, M. and BOREL, Y. (1976) Loss of carrier-determined tolerance *in vitro* with loss of receptor blockade. *J. Immunol.* **116**: 223–226.

ALLISON, A. C. (1971) Unresponsiveness to self antigens. *Lancet* **ii**: 1401–1403.

ALLISON, A. C. and DENMAN, A. M. (1976) Self-tolerance and autoimmunity. *Br. med. Bull.* **32**: 124–129.

ALTER, B. J., SCHENDEL, D. J., BACH, M. L., BACH, F. H., KLEIN, J. and STIMPFLING, J. H. (1973) Cell-mediated lympholysis. Importance of serologically defined H-2 regions. *J. exp. Med.* **137**: 1303–1309.

AMERDING, D. and KATZ, D. H. (1974) Activation of T and B lymphocytes *in vitro*. II. Biological and biochemical properties of an allogeneic effect factor (AEF) active in triggering specific B lymphocytes. *J. exp. Med.* **140**: 19–37.

AMOS, D. B., COHEN, I. and KLEIN, W. J. (1970) Mechanisms of immunologic enhancement. *Transplant. Proc.* **2**: 68–75.

ANDERSON, C. L. and GREY, H. M. (1974) Receptors for aggregated IgG on mouse lymphocytes. Their presence on thymocytes, thymus-derived, and bone marrow-derived lymphocytes. *J. exp. Med.* **139**: 1175–1188.

ANDERSON, T. H., ROETHLE, J. and AUERBACH, R. (1972) Induction of tolerance to sheep red blood cells. *J. exp. Med.* **136**: 1666–1671.

ANDERSSON, B. (1969) Induction of immunity and immunologic paralysis in mice against polyvinyl pyrrolidone. *J. Immunol.* **102**: 1309–1313.

ANDERSSON, J., BULLOCK, W. W. and MELCHERS, F. (1974) Inhibition of mitogenic stimulation of mouse lymphocytes by anti-mouse immunoglobulin antibodies. I. Mode of action. *Eur. J. Immunol.* **4**: 715–722.

ASHERSON, G. L. and ZEMBALA, M. (1976) Suppressor T cells in cell-mediated immunity. *Br. med. Bull.* **32**: 158–164.

ASKENASE, P. W., HAYDEN, B. J. and GERSHON, R. K. (1975) Augmentation of delayed-type hypersensitivity by doses of cyclophosphamide which do not affect antibody responses. *J. exp. Med.* **141**: 697–702.

ATKINS, R. C. and FORD, W. L. (1972) The effect of lymphocytes and serum from tolerant rats on the graft versus-host activity of normal lymphocytes. *Transplantation* **13**: 442–444.

AULT, K. A. and UNANUE, E. R. (1974) Events after the binding of antigen to lymphocytes. Removal and regeneration of the antigen receptor. *J. exp. Med.* **139**: 1110–1124.

AULT, K. A., UNANUE, E. R., KATZ, D. H. and BENACERRAF, B. (1974) Failure of lymphocytes to reexpress antigen receptors after brief interaction with a tolerogenic D-amino acid copolymer. *Proc. natn. Acad. Sci. U.S.A.* **71**: 3111–3114.

BACH, F. H., SEGALL, M., ZIER, K. S., SONDEL, P. M., ALTER, B. J. and BACH, M. L. (1973) Cell-mediated immunity: separation of cells involved in recognitive and destructive phases. *Science, Wash.* **180**: 403–406.

BACH, F. H., KUPERMAN, O. J., SOLLINGER, H. W., ZARLING, J., SONDEL, P. M., ALTER, B. J. and BACH, M. L. (1977) Cellular immunogenetics and LD–CD collaboration. *Transplant. Proc.* **9**: 859–863.

BAKER, P. J., STASHAK, P. W., AMSBAUGH, D. F. and PRESCOTT, B. (1974) Regulation of the antibody response to type III pneumococcal polysaccharide. II, Mode of action of thymic-derived suppressor cells. *J. Immunol.* **112**: 404–409.

BALDWIN, R. W. and ROBBINS, R. A. (1976) Factors interfering with immunological rejection of tumours. *Br. med. Bull.* **32**: 118–123.

BALDWIN, R. W., PRICE, M. R. and ROBBINS, R. A. (1973) Inhibition of hepatoma immune lymphnode cell cytotoxicity by tumour-bearer serum, and solubilized hepatoma antigen. *Int. J. Cancer* **11**: 527–535.

BANSAL, S. C., HELLSTRÖM, K. E., HELLSTRÖM, I. and SJOGREN, H. O. (1973a) Cell-mediated immunity and blocking serum activity to tolerated allografts in rats. *J. exp. Med.* **137**: 590–602.

BANSAL, S. C., HELLSTRÖM, I., HELLSTRÖM, K. E. and WRIGHT, P. W. (1973b) Cell-mediated immunity and blocking serum activity before and after breakage of allograft tolerance in rats. *Transplantation* **16**: 610–620.

BARTON, M. and DIENER, E. (1975) A new perspective on B cell triggering: control of immune response by organizational changes in the lipid bilayer. *Transplant. Rev.* **23**: 5–22.

BASCH, R. S. (1966) Immunologic competence after thymectomy. *Int. Archs Allergy appl. Immunol.* **30**: 105–119.

BASTEN, A. and HOWARD, J. G. (1972) Thymus independence. *Contemp. Topics Immunobiol.* **2**: 265–291.

BASTEN, A., MILLER, J. F. A. P., SPRENT, J. and CHEERS, C. (1974) Cell-to-cell interaction in the immune response. X. T-cell-dependent suppression in tolerant mice. *J. exp. Med.* **140**: 199–217.

BASTEN, A., MILLER, J. F. A. P., SPRENT, J. and PYE, (1972a) A receptor for antibody on B lymphocytes. I. Method of detection and functional significance. *J. exp. Med.* **135**: 610–626.

BASTEN, A., WARNER, N. L. and MANDEL, T. (1972b) A receptor for antibody on B lymphocytes. II. Immunochemical and electron microscopy characteristics. *J. exp. Med.* **135**: 627–642.

BASTEN, A., MILLER, J. F. A. P. and ABRAHAM, R. (1975a) Relationship between Fc receptors, antigen-binding sites on T and B cells, and H-2 complex-associated determinants. *J. exp. Med.* **141**: 547–560.

BASTEN, A., MILLER, J. F. A. P. and JOHNSON, P. (1975b) T-cell dependent suppression of an anti-hapten antibody response. *Transplant. Rev.* **26**: 130–131.

BASTEN, A., MILLER, J. F. A. P., WARNER, N. L., ABRAHAM, R., CHIA, E. and GAMBLE, J. (1975c) A subpopulation of T cells bearing Fc receptors. *J. Immunol.* **115**: 1159–1165.

BATCHELOR, J. R. and WELSH, K. I. (1976) Mechanisms of enhancement of kidney allograft survival. A form of operational tolerance. *Br. med. Bull.* **32**: 113–117.

BECHTOL, K. B., WEGMANN, T. G., FREED, J. H., GRUMET, F. C., CHESEBRO, B. W., HERZENBERG, L. A. and MCDEVITT, H. O. (1974a) Genetic control of the immune response to (T,G)-A-L in C3H ↔ C57 tetraparental mice. *Cell. Immunol.* **13**: 264–277.

Bechtol, K. B., Freed, J. H., Herzenberg, L. A. and McDevitt, H. O. (1974b) Genetic control of the antibody response to poly-L(Tyr, Glu)-poly-D, L-Ala–poly-L-Lys in C3H ↔ CWB tetraparental mice. *J. exp. Med.* **140**: 1660–1675.

Berken, A. and Benacerraf, B. (1966) Properties of antibodies cytophilic for Macrophages. *J. exp. Med.* **123**: 119–144.

Berken, A. and Benacerraf, B. (1968) Sedimentation properties of antibody cytophilic for macrophages. *J. Immunol.* **100**: 1219–1222.

Bernstein, I. D., Hamilton, B. L., Wright, P. W., Burstein, R. and Hellström, K. E. (1975) Mixed leukocyte culture reactivity in operationally tolerant rats: relationship of lymphocyte-mediated reactivity and serum-blocking activity. *J. Immunol.* **114**: 320–325.

Bevan, M. J. (1975) The major histocompatibility complex determines susceptibility to cytotoxic T cells directed against minor histocompatibility antigens. *J. exp. Med.* **142**: 1349–1364.

Beverley, P. C. L. and Simpson, E. (1972) Cytotoxic activity *in vitro* of thymus-derived lymphocytes sensitized to xenograft antigens. *Nature, New Biol.* **237**: 17–18.

Billingham, R. E., Brent, L. and Medawar, P. B. (1956) Quantitative studies on tissue transplantation immunity. III. Actively acquired tolerance. *Phil. Trans. R. Soc.* **B239**: 357–414.

Binz, H. and Wigzell, H. (1975a) Shared idiotypic determinants on B and T lymphocytes reactive against the same antigenic determinants. I. Demonstration of similar or identical idiotypes on IgG molecules and T-cell receptors with specificity for the same alloantigen. *J. exp. Med.* **142**: 197–211.

Binz, H. and Wigzell, H. (1975b) Shared idiotypic determinants on B and T lymphocytes reactive against the same antigenic determinants. II. Determination of frequency and characteristics of idiotypic T and B lymphocytes in normal rats using direct visualization. *J. exp. Med.* **142**: 1218–1230.

Binz, H. and Wigzell, H. (1975c) Shared idiotypic determinants on B and T lymphocytes reactive against the same antigenic determinants. III. Physical fractionation of specific immunocompetent T lymphocytes by affinity chromatography using antiidiotypic antibodies. *J. exp. Med.* **142**: 1231–1240.

Binz, H. and Wigzell, H. (1977) Antigen-binding, idiotypic T-lymphocyte receptors. *Contemp. Topics Immunobiol.* **7**: 113–177.

Black, S. J., Eichmann, K., Hämmerling, G. J. and Rajewsky, K. (1975) Stimulation and inhibition of T cell helper function by anti-idiotypic antibody. In; *Membrane Receptors of Lymphocytes*, pp. 117–120, Seligmann, M., Preud'homme, J. I. and Kourilsky, F. M. (eds). American Elsevier, New York.

Black, S. J., Hämmerling, G. J., Berek, C., Rajewsky, K. and Eichmann, K. (1976) Idiotypic analysis of lymphocytes *in vitro*. I. Specificity and heterogeneity of B and T lymphocytes reactive with anti-idiotypic antibody. *J. exp. Med.* **143**: 846–860.

Blackstock, R. and Hyde, R. M. (1973) Comparison of the ease of tolerance induction in thymus and bone marrow of three strains of mice. *Cell. Immunol.* **9**: 67–75.

Blair, P. and Lane, M. A. (1975) Non-T cell killing of mammary tumor cells by spleen cells: secretion of antibody and recruitment of cells. *J. Immunol.* **115**: 184–189.

Bodurtha, A. J., Chee, D. O., Laucius, J. F., Mastrangelo, M. J. and Prehn, R. T. (1975) Clinical and immunological significance of human melanoma cytotoxic antibody. *Cancer. Res.* **35**: 189–193.

Borel, Y. (1976) Isologous IgG-induced immunologic tolerance to haptens: A model of self versus non-self recognition. *Transplant. Rev.* **31**: 3–22.

Borel, Y., Lewis, R. M. and Stollar, B. D. (1973) Prevention of murine lupus nephritis by carrier-dependent induction of immunologic tolerance to denatured DNA. *Science, Wash.* **182**: 76–78.

Borel, Y., Reinisch, C. L. and Schlossman, S. F. (1975) T and B cell in hapten-specific carrier-determined tolerance. *J. exp. Med.* **142**: 1254–1262.

Borel, Y., Lewis, R. M., Andre-Schwartz, J., Stollar, B. D. and Diener, E. (1977) Treatment of lupus nephritis in adult (NZB X NZW)F_1 mice by cortisone-facilitated tolerance to nucleic acid antigens.

Bourne, H. R., Lichtenstein, L. M., Melmon, K. L., Henney, C. S., Weinstein, Y. and Shearer, G. M. (1974) Modulation of inflammation and immunity by cyclic AMP. Receptors for vasoactive hormones and mediators of inflammation regulate many leukocyte functions. *Science, N.Y.* **184**: 19–28.

Boyden, S. V. and Sorkin, E. (1960) The adsorption of antigen by spleen cells previously treated with antiserum *in vitro*. *Immunology* **3**: 272–283.

Brain, P. and Marston, R. H. (1973) Rosette formation by human T and B lymphocytes. *Eur. J. Immunol.* **3**: 6–9.

Breard, J. M., Friedman, S. and Chess, L. (1977) Stimulation de lymphocytes B human par des surnageants de cellules T activées par un antigène: le rôle de déterminants semblables aux antigènes Ia. *Ann. Immunol. Inst. Pasteur* **128C**: 145–147.

Brent, L., Hansen, J. A., Kilshaw, P. J. and Thomas, A. V. (1973) Specific unresponsiveness to skin allografts in mice. I. Properties of tissue extracts and their synergistic effect with antilymphocyte serum. *Transplantation* **15**: 160–171.

Brent, L., Brooks, C. G., Medawar, P. B. and Simpson, E. (1976) Transplantation tolerance. *Br. med. Bull.* **32**: 101–106.

Bretscher, P. A. (1975) The two signal model for B cell induction. *Transplant. Rev.* **23**: 37–48.

Bretscher, P. A. and Cohen, M. (1968) Minimal model for the mechanism of antibody induction and paralysis by antigen. *Nature, Lond.* **220**: 444–448.

Brody, N. I., Walker, J. C. and Siskind, G. W. (1967) Studies on the control of antibody synthesis. Interaction of antigenic competition and suppression of antibody formation by passive antibody on the immune response. *J. exp. Med.* **126**: 81–91.

Brooks, C. G. (1975) Neonatally induced transplantation tolerance: *in vitro* evidence supporting a clonal inactivation mechanism. *Eur. J. Immunol.* **5**: 741–747.

Burnet, F. M. and Fenner, F. (1949) *The production of antibodies* (2nd edn). Macmillan, Melbourne, London.

Burns, F. D., Marrack, P. C., Kappler, J. W. and Janeway, C. A. (1975) Functional heterogeneity among the T-derived lymphocytes of the mouse. IV. Nature of spontaneously induced suppressor cells. *J. Immunol.* **114**: 1345–1347.

BUSSARD, A. E., NOSSAL, G. J. V., MAZIE, J. C. and LEWIS, H. (1970) *In vitro* stimulation of antibody formation by peritoneal cells. II. Cell interactions and effects of immunochemical or metabolic inhibitors. *J. exp. Med.* **131**: 917–935.

BYSTRYN, J.-C., GRAF, M. W. and UHR, J. W. (1970). Regulation of antibody formation by serum antibody. II. Removal of specific antibody by means of exchange transfusion. *J. exp. Med.* **132**: 1279–1287.

BYSTRYN, J.-C., SCHENKEIN, I. and UHR, J. W. (1971) A model for the regulation of antibody synthesis by serum antibody. *Prog. Immunol.* **1**: 627–636.

CALNE, R. Y. (1976) Mechanisms in the acceptance of organ grafts. *Br. med. Bull.* **32**: 107–112.

CAMBIER, J. C., VITETTA, E. S., KETTMAN, J. R., WETZEL, G. M. and UHR, J. W. (1977) B-cell tolerance. III. Effect of papain-mediated cleavage of cell surface IgD on tolerance susceptibility of murine B cells. *J. exp. Med.* **146**: 107–117.

CANTOR, H. and BOYSE, E. A. (1975a) Functional subclasses of T lymphocytes bearing different Ly antigens. I. The generation of functionally distinct T-cell subclasses is a differentiative process independent of antigen. *J. exp. Med.* **141**: 1376–1389.

CANTOR, H. and BOYSE, E. A. (1975b) Functional subclasses of T lymphocytes bearing different Ly antigens. II. Cooperation between subclasses of Ly^+ cells in the generation of killer activity. *J. exp. Med.* **141**: 1390–1399.

CANTOR, H. and BOYSE, E. (1977) Regulation of the immune response by T-cell subclasses. *Contemp. Topics Immunobiol.* **7**: 47–67.

CANTOR, and JANDINSKI, (1974) The relationship of cell division to the generation of cytotoxic activity in mixed lymphocyte culture. *J. exp. Med.* **140**: 1712–1716.

CANTOR, H. and SIMPSON, E. (1975) Regulation of the immune response by subclasses of T lymphocytes. I. Interactions between pre-killer T cells and regulatory T cells obtained from peripheral lymphoid tissues of mice. *Eur. J. Immunol.* **5**: 330–336.

CANTOR, H., SIMPSON, E., SATO, V. L., FATHMAN, C. G. and HERZENBERG, L. A. (1975) Characterization of subpopulations of T lymphocytes. I. Separation and functional studies of peripheral T-cells binding different amounts of fluorescent anti-Thy 1.2 (Theta) antibody using a fluorescence-activated cell sorter. *Cell. Immunol.* **15**: 180–196.

CARPENTER, C. B., D'APICE, A. J. F. and ABBAS, A. K. (1976) The role of antibodies in the rejection and enhancement of organ allografts. *Adv. Immunol.* **22**: 1–65.

CECKA, J. M., STRATTON, J. A., MILLER, A. and SERCARZ, E. (1976) Structural aspects of immune recognition of lysozymes. III. T cell specificity restriction and its consequences for antibody specificity. *Eur. J. Immunol.* **6**: 639–646.

CEROTTINI, J.-C. and BRUNNER, K. T. (1974) Cell-mediated cytotoxicity, allograft rejection and tumor immunity. *Adv. Immunol.* **18**: 67–132.

CEROTTINI, J.-C., MACCONAHEY, P. J. and DIXON, F. J. (1969) The immunosuppressive effect of passively administered antibody IgG fragments. *J. Immunol.* **102**: 1008–1015.

CEROTTINI, J.-C., FREEDMAN, L. R. and BRUNNER, K. T. (1972) *In vivo* activity of cytotoxic lymphocytes. *Transplant. Proc.* **4**: 299–301.

CHAN, P. L. and SINCLAIR, N. R. STC. (1971) Regulation of the immune response. V. An analysis of the function of the Fc portion of antibody in suppression of an immune response with respect to interaction with components of the lymphoid system. *Immunology* **21**: 967–981.

CHAN, P. L. and SINCLAIR, N. R. STC. (1973) Regulation of the immune response. VI. Inability of $F(ab')_2$ antibody to terminate established immune responses and its ability to interfere with IgG antibody-mediated immunosuppression. *Immunology* **24**: 289–301.

CHARD, T. (1968) Immunological enhancement by mouse isoantibodies: the importance of complement fixation. *Immunology* **14**: 583–589.

CHEN, C. and HIRSCH, J. G. (1972) The effects of mercaptoethanol and of peritoneal macrophages on the antibody-forming capacity of nonadherent mouse spleen cells *in vitro*. *J. exp. Med.* **136**: 604–617.

CHESS, L., EVANS, R., HUMPHREYS, R. E., STROMINGER, J. L. and SCHLOSSMAN, S. F. (1976) Inhibition of antibody-dependent cellular cytotoxicity and immunoglobulin synthesis by an antiserum prepared against a human B-cell Ia-like molecule. *J. exp. Med.* **144**: 113–122.

CHIAO, J. W. and GOOD, R. A. (1976) Studies of the presence of membrane receptors for complement, IgG, and the sheep erythrocyte rosetting capacity on the same human lymphocytes. *Eur. J. Immunol.* **6**: 157–162.

CHILLER, J. M. and WEIGLE, W. O. (1975) Biography of a tolerant state: cellular parameters of the unresponsive state induced in adult mice to human gamma globulin. *J. reticuloendothel. Soc.* **17**: 180–186.

CHILLER, J. M., HABICHT, G. S. and WEIGLE, W. O. (1970) Cellular sites of immunologic unresponsiveness. *Proc. natn. Acad. Sci. U.S.A.* **65**: 551–556.

CHILLER, J. M., HABICHT, G. S. and WEIGLE, W. O. (1971) Kinetic differences in unresponsiveness of thymus and bone marrow cells. *Science, Wash.* **171**: 813–815.

CHILLER, J. M., LOUIS, J. A., SKIDMORE, B. J. and WEIGLE, W. O. (1974) Cellular parameters of the tolerant state induced to human γ-globulin in mice and of its modulation by bacterial lipopolysaccharides. In: *Immunological Tolerance: Mechanisms and Potential Therapeutic Applications*, pp. 373–390, KATZ, D. H. and BENACERRAF, B. (eds). Proceedings of an International Conference held at Brook Lodge, Augusta, Michigan, 1974. Academic Press, New York.

CHILLER, J. M., PODLESKI, U., EVERLITH, K. and BOREL, Y. (1976) Suppressive capacity of haptenated isologous immunoglobulin on murine antibody responses. *Fedn Proc.* **35**: 433.

CHIORAZZI, N., FOX, D. A. and KATZ, D. H. (1976) Hapten-specific IgE responses in mice. VI. Selective enhancement of IgE antibody production by low doses of X-irradiation and by cyclophosphamide. *J. Immunol.* **117**: 1629–1637.

CINADER, B. and DUBERT, J. M. (1955) Acquired immune tolerance to human albumin and the response to subsequent injections of diazo human albumin. *Br. J. exp. Path.* **36**: 515–529.

Cinader, B. and Dubiski, S. (1976) Suppression of immunoglobulin formation with antibody against immunoglobulin. *Br. med. Bull.* **32**: 171–176.

Claman, H. N. (1976) Tolerance and contact sensitivity to DNFB in mice. V. Induction of tolerance with DNP compounds and with free and membrane-associated DNFB. *J. Immunol.* **116**: 704–709.

Claman, H. N. and Chaperon, E. A. (1969) Immunologic complementation between thymus and marrow cells—a model for the two-cell theory of immunocompetence. *Transplant. Rev.* **1**: 92–113.

Claman, H. N. and Moorhead, J. W. (1976) Tolerance to contact hypersensitivity. *Contemp. Topics Immunobiol.* **5**: 211–236.

Cline, M. J., Sprent, J., Warner, N. L. and Harris, A. W. (1972) Receptors for immunoglobulin on B lymphocytes and cells of a cultured plasma cell tumor. *J. Immunol.* **108**: 1126–1128.

Cohen, B. E. and Paul, W. E. (1974) Macrophage control of time-dependent changes in antigen sensitivity of immune T lymphocyte populations. *J. Immunol.* **112**: 359–369.

Cohen, I. R. and Livnat, S. (1976) The cell-mediated immune response: interactions of initiator and recruited T lymphocytes. *Transplant. Rev.* **29**: 24–58.

Cohen, I. R. and Wekerle, H. (1973) Regulation of autosensitization. The immune activation and specific inhibition of self-recognizing thymus-derived lymphocytes. *J. exp. Med.* **137**: 224–238.

Cohen, I. R., Globerson, A. and Feldman, M. (1971) Autosensitization *in vitro*. *J. exp. Med.* **133**: 834–845.

Cone, R. E., Sprent, J. and Marchalonis, J. J. (1972) Antigen-binding specificity of isolated cell-surface immunoglobulin from thymus cells activated to histocompatibility antigens. *Proc. natn. Acad. Sci. U.S.A.* **69**: 2556–2560.

Connell, G. E. and Dubiski, S. (1977) Allotype suppression in rabbits: The requirement for CH3 domain of anti-allotype antibody. *J. Immunol.* **119**: 540–542.

Connell, G. E. and Porter, R. R. (1971) A new enzymatic fragment (Facb) of rabbit immunoglobulin G. *Biochem. J.* **124**: 53P.

Cooper, M. D. and Lawton, A. R. (1975) Development of T and B cells and their functional interactions. In: *Immunodeficiency in Man and Animals*, pp. 3–5, Bergsma, D., Good, R. A., Finstad, J. and Paul, N. W., (eds). *Birth Defects*: *Original Article Series*, Volume 11. Sinauer Associates, Sunderland, Mass.

Cooper, M. D., Lawton, A. R. and Kinkade, P. W. (1972) A two stage model for development of antibody producing cells. *Clin. exp. Immunol.* **11**: 143–149.

Cosenza, H. and Köhler, H. (1972a) Specific inhibition of plaque formation to phosphorylcholine by antibody against antibody. *Science, Wash.* **176**: 1027–1029.

Cosenza, H. and Köhler, H. (1972b) Specific suppression of the antibody response by antibodies to receptors. *Proc. natn. Acad. Sci. U.S.A.* **69**: 2701–2705.

Coutinho, A. and Moller, G. (1975) Thymus-independent B-cell induction and paralysis. *Adv. Immunol.* **21**: 113–236.

Coutinho, A., Gronowicz, E. and Möller, G. (1974) The role of Ig receptors in antigen-induced activation of B lymphocytes. In: *Progress in Immunology II*, Vol. 2, pp. 167–175. Brent, L. and Holborrow, J. (eds). North-Holland, Amsterdam, Oxford.

Crone, M., Koch, C. and Simonsen, M. (1972) The elusive T cell receptor. *Transplant. Rev.* **10**: 36–56.

Daeron, M., Duc, H. T., Kanellopoulos, J., Le Bouteiller, Ph., Kinsky, R. and Voisin, G. A. (1975) Allogeneic mast cell degranulation induced by histocompatibility antibodies: an *in vitro* model of transplantation anaphylaxis. *Clin. Immunol.* **20**: 133–155.

David, C. S., Shreffler, D. C. and Frelinger, J. A. (1973) New lymphocyte antigen (Lna) controlled by the Ir region of the mouse H-2 complex. *Proc. natn. Acad. Sci. U.S.A.* **70**: 2509–2514.

David, C. S., Niederhuber, J. E., Frelinger, J. A., Dugan, E. P., Meo, T. and Shreffler, D. C. (1976) Murine Ia antigens. Expression on T and B cells and their role in immune response. In: *Proceedings of 10th Lukocyte Culture Conference*, pp. 379–392. Academic Press Inc., New York.

Davies, A. J. S. (1969) The thymus and the cellular basis of immunity. *Transplant. Rev.* **1**: 43–91.

Davies, D. A. L. (1976) The true mechanism of immunologic enhancement, deduced from studies of heart transplants in rats. *Transplant. Proc.* **8**: 37–39.

Davies, D. A. L. and Alkins, B. J. (1974) What abrogates heart transplant rejection in immunological enhancement. *Nature, Lond.* **247**: 294–297.

Davies, D. A. L. and Staines, N. A. (1976) A cardinal role for I-region antigens (Ia) in immunological enhancement, and the clinical implications. *Transplant. Rev.* **30**: 18–39.

de Jesus, D. G., Holborow, E. J. and Brown, J. C. (1972) A defect of B lymphocyte transport of aggregated HGG into germinal centres in NZB and NZB X NZW F_1 hybrid mice. *Clin. exp. Immunol.* **11**: 507–522.

Debré, P. Waltenbaugh, C., Dorf, M. E. and Benacerraf, B. (1976) Genetic control of specific immune suppression. IV. Responsiveness to the random copolymer L-glutamic acid^{50}-L-tyrosine induced in BALB/c mice by cyclophosphamide. *J. exp. Med.* **144**: 277–281.

Delovitch, T. L. and McDevitt, H. O. (1977) *In vitro* analysis of allogeneic lymphocyte interaction. I. Characterization and cellular origin of an Ia-positive helper factor–allogeneic effect factor. *J. exp. Med.* **146**: 1019–1032.

DeLuca, D., Miller, A. and Sercarz, E. (1975) Antigen binding to lymphoid cells from unimmunized mice. IV. Shedding and reappearance of multiple antigen binding Ig receptors of T- and B-lymphocytes. *Cell. Immunol.* **18**: 286–303.

Dennert, G. (1971) The mechanism of antibody-induced stimulation and inhibition of the immune response. *J. Immunol.* **106**: 951–955.

Dennert, G. (1976) Thymus derived killer cells: specificity of function and antigen recognition. *Transplant. Rev.* **29**: 59–88.

Dennert, G. and Hatlen, L. E. (1975) Are contact hypersensitivity cells cytotoxic? *Nature, Lond.* **257**: 486–488.

Dennert, G. and Lennox, E. S. (1972) Cell interactions in humoral and cell-mediated immunity. *Nature New Biol.* **238**: 114–116.

DENNERT, G. and LENNOX, E. S. (1973) Phagocytic cells as effectors in a cell-mediated immunity system. *J. Immunol.* **111**: 1844–1854.

DENNERT, G. and TUCKER, D. F. (1972) Selective priming of T cells by chemically altered cell antigens. *J. exp. Med.* **136**: 656–661.

DESAYMARD, C., PEARCE, B. and FELDMANN, M. (1976) Role of epitope density in the induction of tolerance and immunity with thymus-independent antigens. III. Interaction of epitope density and receptor avidity. *Eur. J. Immunol.* **6**: 646–650.

DIAMANTSTEIN, T. and BLITSTEIN-WILLINGER, E. (1974) T cell-independent development of B memory cells. *Eur. J. Immunol.* **4**: 830–832.

DICKLER, H. B. (1976) Lymphocyte receptors for immunoglobulin. *Adv. Immunol.* **24**: 167–214.

DICKLER, H. B. and KUNKEL, H. G. (1972) Interaction of aggregated γ-globulin with B lymphocytes. *J. exp. Med.* **136**: 191–196.

DICKLER, H. B. and SACHS, D. H. (1974) Evidence for identity or close association of the Fc receptor of B lymphocytes and alloantigens determined by the IR region of the H-2 complex. *K. exp. Med.* **140**: 779–796.

DICKLER, H. B., SIEGAL, F. P. BENTWICH, Z. H. and KUNKEL, H. G. (1973) Lymphocyte binding of aggregated IgG and surface Ig staining in chronic lymphocytic leukaemia. *Clin. exp. Immunol.* **14**: 97–106.

DICKLER, H. B., ARBEIT, R. D., HENKART, P. A. and SACHS, D. H. (1976) Association between Ia antigens and the Fc receptors of certain T lymphocytes. *J. exp. Med.* **144**: 282–287.

DICKLER, H. B., CONE, J. L., KUBICEK, M. T. and SACHS, D. H. (1975) Detection of non-H-2 antigen(s) which, like Ia antigens, are associated with the Fc receptor of B lymphocytes. *J. exp. Med.* **142**: 796–801.

DIENER, E. and FELDMANN, M. (1970) Antibody-mediated suppression of the immune response *in vitro*. II. A new approach to the phenomenon of immunological tolerance. *J. exp. Med.* **132**: 31–43.

DIENER, E. and FELDMANN, M. (1972) Relationship between antigen and antibody-induced suppression of immunity. *Transplant. Rev.* **8**: 76–103.

DIENER, E. and PAETKAU, V. H. (1972) Antigen recognition: early surface-receptor phenomena induced by binding of a tritium-labelled antigen. *Proc. natn. Acad. Sci. U.S.A.* **69**: 2364–2368.

DIXON, F. J., JACOT-GUILLARMOD, H. and MCCONAHEY, P. J. (1967) The effect of passively administered antibody on antibody synthesis. *J. exp. Med.* **125**: 1119–1135.

DOHERTY, P. C. and ZINKERNAGEL, R. M. (1974) T-cell-mediated immunopathology in viral infections. *Transplant. Rev.* **19**: 89–120.

DRESSER, D. W. (1962) Specific inhibition of antibody production. II. Paralysis induced in adult mice by small quantities of protein antigen *Immunology* **5**: 378–388.

DRESSER, D. W. (1976) Tolerance induction as a model for cell differentiation. *Br. med. Bull.* **32**: 147–151.

DRESSER, D. W. and MITCHISON, N. A. (1968) The mechanism of immunological paralysis. *Adv. Immunol.* **8**: 129–181.

DROEGE, W. (1975) Immunosuppressive effect of syngeneic thymus cells on allograft rejection. *Proc. natn. Acad. Sci. U.S.A.* **72**: 2371–2374.

DROEGE, W. and TUNESKOG, M. (1976) Suppressor cells in the embryonic thymus mediate allograft tolerance. *Adv. exp. Med. Biol.* **66**: 571–576.

DRURY, P. J. and SINGHAL, S. K. (1974) Isolation of θ-isoantigen negative, antibody-inhibiting cells from normal mouse bone marrow according to their density and surface-adherent properties. *Int. Archs. Allergy appl. Immunol.* **46**: 707–724.

DUBISKI, S. and SWIERCZYNSKA, Z. (1971) Allotype suppression in rabbits: Operational characterization of the target cells. *Int. Archs. Allergy appl. Immunol.* **40**: 1–18.

DUC, H. T., KINSKY, R. G., KANELLOPOULOS, J. and VOISIN, G. A. (1975) Biologic properties of transplantation immune sera. IV. Influence of the course of immunization, dilution and complexing to antigen on enhancing activity of Ig classes. *J. Immunol.* **115**: 1143–1150.

DUC, H. T., KINSKY, R. G. and VOISIN, G. A. (1977) Sites antigéniques impliqués dans la facilitation des allogreffes tumorales. *Ann. Immunol. Inst. Pasteur* **128C**: 19–20.

DUKOR, P. and HARTMANN, K. U. (1973) Hypothesis: bound C3 as the second signal for B-cell activation. *Cell. Immunol.* **7**: 349–356.

DUTTON, R. W. (1973) Inhibitory and stimulatory effects of concanavalin A on the response of mouse spleen cell suspensions to antigen. II. Evidence for separate stimulatory and inhibitory cells. *J. exp. Med.* **138**: 1496–1505.

DUTTON, R. W. and MISHELL, R. I. (1967) Cellular events in the immune response. The *in vitro* response of normal spleen cells to erythrocyte antigens. *Cold Spring Harb. Symp. quant. Biol.* **32**: 407–414.

DWYER, J. M., ROSENBAUM, J. T. and LEWIS, S. (1976) The effect of anti-mu suppression of γM and γG on the production of γE. *J. exp. Med.* **143**: 781–790.

EDEN, A., BIANCO, C. and NUSSENZWEIG, V. (1973) Mechanism of binding of soluble immune complexes to lymphocytes. *Clin. Immunol.* **7**: 459–473.

EGOROV, I. K. (1974) Genetic control of H-2 alloantigens as inferred from analysis of mutations. *Immunogenetics* **1**: 97–107.

EICHMANN, K. (1974) Idiotype suppression. I. Influence of the dose and of the effector functions of antiidiotypic antibody on the production of an idiotype. *Eur. J. Immunol.* **4**: 296–302.

EICHMANN, K. (1975) Idiotype suppression. II. Amplification of a suppressor T cell with antiidiotypic activity. *Eur. J. Immunol.* **5**: 511–517.

EICHMANN, K. and RAJEWSKY, K. (1975) Induction of T and B cell immunity by antiidiotypic antibody. *Eur. J. Immunol.* **5**: 661–666.

EIJSVOOGEL, V. P., VAN ROOD, J. J., DU TOIT, E. D. and SCHELLEKENS, P. TH. A. (1972) Position of a locus determining mixed lymphocyte reaction distinct from the known HL-A loci. *Eur. J. Immunol.* **2**: 413–418.

Eijsvoogel, V. P., du Bois, R., Melief, C. J. M., Zeylemaker, W. P., Raat-Koning, L. and de Groot-Kooy, L. (1973) Lymphocyte activation and destruction *in vitro* in relation to MLC and HL-A. *Transplant. Proc.* **5**: 1301–1307.

Eijsvoogel, V. P., Schellekens, P. Th. A., Du Bois, M. J. G. J. and Zeijlemaker, W. P. (1976) Human cytotoxic lymphocytes after alloimmunization *in vitro*. *Transplant. Rev.* **29**: 125–145.

Elkins, W. L. (1973) Deficit of specific thymus-dependent lymphocytes in transplantation tolerance in the rat. *J. exp. Med.* **137**: 1097–1102.

Erb, P. and Feldmann, M. (1975) The role of macrophages in the generation of T-helper cells. II. The genetic control of the macrophage–T-cell interaction for helper cell induction with soluble antigens. *J. exp. Med.* **142**: 460–472.

Erb, P., Feldmann, M. and Hogg, N. (1976) The role of macrophages in the generation of T-helper cells. IV. Nature of genetically related factor derived from macrophages incubated with soluble antigens. *Eur. J. Immunol.* **6**: 365–372.

Eustace, J. C. and Irvin, G. L. (1973) Immunological tumor enhancement and *in vitro* cytotoxicity. Further evidence for the involvement of 7S γ_{2a}-immunoglobulin. *Transplantation* **16**: 171–176.

Evans, G. and Ivanyi, J. (1975) Antibody synthesis by chicken spleen cells *in vitro*. I. Requirements of B cells at various stages after immunization for T cells, macrophages and antigen. *Eur. J. Immunol.* **5**: 747–752.

Evans, R. L., Breard, J. M., Lazarus, H., Schlossman, S. F. and Chess, L. (1977) Detection, isolation and functional characterization of two human T-cell subclasses bearing unique differentiation antigens *J. exp. Med.* **145**: 221–233.

Feldman, J. D. (1972) Immunological enhancement: a study of blocking antibodies. *Adv. Immunol.* **15**: 167–214.

Feldmann, M. (1972a) Cell interactions in the immune response *in vitro*. II. The requirement for macrophages in lymphoid cell collaboration. *J. exp. Med.* **135**: 1049–1058.

Feldmann, M. (1972b) Cell interactions in the immune response *in vitro*. V. Specific collaboration via complexes of antigen and thymus-derived cell immunoglobulin. *J. exp. Med.* **136**: 737–760.

Feldmann, M. (1973) Induction of B cell tolerance by antigen specific T cell factor. *Nature New Biol.* **242**: 82–84.

Feldmann, M. and Diener, E. (1970) Antibody-mediated suppression of the immune response *in vitro*. I. Evidence for a central effect. *J. exp. Med.* **131**: 247–274.

Feldmann, M. and Diener, E. (1972) Antibody-mediated suppression of the immune response *in vitro*. IV. The effect of antibody fragments. *J. Immunol.* **108**: 93–101.

Feldmann, M. and Nossal, G. J. V. (1972) Tolerance, enhancement and the regulation of interactions between T cells, B cells and macrophages. *Transplant. Rev.* **13**: 3–34.

Ferrerini, M., Moretta, L., Abrile, R. and Durante, M. L. (1975) Receptors for IgG molecules on human lymphocytes forming spontaneous rosettes with sheep red cells. *Eur. J. Immunol.* **5**: 70–72.

Festenstein, H. (1973) Immunogenetic and biological aspects of *in vitro* lymphocyte allotransformation (MLR) in the mouse. *Transplant. Rev.* **15**: 62–88.

Fitch, F. W. (1975) Selective suppression of immune responses. *Prog. Allergy* **19**: 195–244.

Ford, W. L. and Simonsen, M. (1971) The factor of immunization in the rat. The effect of allogeneic immunization on graft-versus-host activity. *J. exp. Med.* **133**: 938–949.

Forman, J. (1976) The specificity of thymus-derived T-cells in cell-mediated cytotoxic reactions. *Transplant. Rev.* **29**: 146–163.

Forni, L. and Pernis, B. (1975) Interactions between Fc-receptors and membrane immunoglobulins on B lymphocytes. In: *Membrane Receptors of Lymphocytes*, pp. 193–201, Seligmann, M., Preud'homme, J. L. and Kourilsky, F. M. (eds). Proceedings of the International Symposium on Membrane Receptors of Lymphocytes held in Paris, 1975 (INSERM Symposium 1). American Elsevier, New York.

Frei, P. C., Benacerraf, B. and Thorbecke, G. J. (1965) Phagocytosis of the antigen, a crucial step in the induction of the primary response. *Proc. natn. Acad. Sci. U.S.A.* **53**: 20–23.

Frelinger, J. A., Niederhuber, J. E. and Shreffler, D. C. (1975) Inhibition of immune responses *in vitro* by specific antiserums to Ia-antigens. *Science, Wash.* **188**: 268–270.

Frelinger, J. A., Niederhuber, J. E. and Shreffler, D. C. (1976) Effects of anti-Ia sera on mitogenic responses. III. Mapping the genes controlling the expression of Ia determinants on concanavalin A-reactive cells to the I-J subregion of the H-2 gene complex. *J. exp. Med.* **144**: 1141–1146.

French, M. E. (1973) Antibody turnover by enhanced rat kidneys. *Transplant. Proc.* **5**: 621–623.

Fridman, W. H. and Golstein, P. (1974) Immunoglobulin-binding factor present on the produced by thymus-processed lymphocytes (T cells). *Cell. Immunol.* **11**: 442–455.

Fridman, W. H., Neauport-Sautes, C., Guimezanes, A. and Gisler, R. H. (1975) Relation between Fc receptors of activated T cells, immunoglobulin binding factor (IBF) and suppression of *in vitro* antibody synthesis. In: *Membrane Receptors of Lymphocytes*, pp. 217–225, Seligmann, M., Preud'homme, J. L. and Kourilsky, F. M. (eds). Proceedings of the International Symposium on Membrane Receptors of Lymphocytes held in Paris, 1975 (INSERM Symposium 1). American Elsevier, New York.

Frøland, S. S. (1972) Binding of sheep erythrocytes to human lymphocytes. A probable marker of T lymphocytes. *Scand. J. Immunol.* **1**: 269–280.

Fu, S. M., Winchester, R. J., Feizi, T., Walzer, P. D. and Kunkel, H. G. (1974) Idiotypic specificity of surface immunoglobulin and maturation of leukemic bone-marrow-derived lymphocytes. *Proc. natn. Acad. Sci. U.S.A.* **71**: 4487–4490.

Fu, S. M., Winchester, R. J. and Kunkel, H. G. (1975) Similar idiotypic specificity for the membrane IgD and IgM of human B lymphocytes. *J. Immunol.* **114**: 250–252.

FUJIMOTO, S., GREENE, M. and SEHON, A. H. (1975) Immunosuppressor T cells and their factors in tumor-bearing hosts. In: *Suppressor Cells in Immunity*, pp. 136–148. SINGHAL, S. K. and SINCLAIR, N. R. STC. (eds). Proceedings of an International Symposium held at London, Ontario, 1975. University of Western Ontario Press, London, Canada.

FUJIMOTO, S., GREENE, M. I. and SEHON, A. H. (1976) Regulation of the immune response to tumor antigens. I. Immunosuppressor cells in tumor-bearing hosts. *J. Immunol.* **116**: 791–799.

FULLER, T. C. and WINN, H. J. (1973) Immunochemical and biological characterization of alloantibody active in immunological enhancement. *Transplant. Proc.* **5**: 585–587.

GEARHART, P., SIGAL, N. and KLINMAN, N. (1975) Production of antibodies of identical idiotype but diverse immunoglobulin classes by cells derived from a single stimulated B cell. *Proc. natn. Acad. Sci. U.S.A.* **72**: 1707–1711.

GERSHON, R. K. (1974) T cell control of antibody production. *Contemp. Topics Immunobiol.* **3**: 1–40.

GERSHON, R. K. (1975) A disquisition of suppressor T cells. *Transplant. Rev.* **26**: 170–185.

GERSHON, R. K. and KONDO, K. (1970) Cell interactions in the induction of tolerance: the role of thymic lymphocytes. *Immunology* **18**: 723–737.

GERSHON, R. K. and PAUL, W. E. (1971) Effect of thymus-derived lymphocytes on amount and affinity of anti-hapten antibody. *J. Immunol.* **106**: 872–874.

GERSHON, R. K., MOKYR, M. B. and MITCHELL, M. S. (1974) Activation of suppressor T-cells by tumor cells and specific antibody. *Nature, Lond.* **250**: 594–596.

GERY, I. and WAKSMAN, B. H. (1972) Potentiation of the T-lymphocyte response to mitogens. II. The cellular source of potentiating mediator(s). *J. exp. Med.* **136**: 143–155.

GODING, J. and LAYTON, J. E. (1976) Antigen-induced co-capping of IgM and IgD-like receptors on murine B cells. *J. exp. Med.* **144**: 852–857.

GOLAN, D. T. and BOREL, Y. (1971) Nonantigenicity and immunologic tolerance: the role of the carrier in the induction of tolerance to the hapten. *J. exp. Med.* **134**: 1046–1061.

GORCZYNSKI, R., KONTIAINEN, S., MITCHISON, N. A. and TIGELAAR, R. E. (1974) Antigen-antibody complexes as blocking factors on the T lymphocyte surface. In: *Cellular Selection and Regulation in the Immune Response*, pp. 143–154, EDELMAN, G. M. (ed.). Society of General Physiologists Series, Vol. 20. Raven Press, New York.

GORDON, J. and MURGITA, R. A. (1975) Suppression and augmentation of the primary *in vitro* immune response by different classes of antibodies. *Cell. Immunol.* **15**: 392–402.

GORER, P. A. and KALISS, N. (1959) The effect of isoantibodies *in vivo* on three different transplantable neoplasms in mice. *Cancer Res.* **19**: 824–830.

GOWANS, J. L., MCGREGOR, D. D. and COWEN, D. M. (1963) The role of small lymphocytes in the rejection of homografts of skin. In: *The Immunologically Competent Cell: Its Nature and Origin*, pp. 20–29, WOLSTENHOLME, G. E. W. and KNIGHT, J. (eds). Ciba Foundation Study Group No. 16. Churchill, London.

GRAF, M. W. and UHR, J. W. (1969) Regulation of antibody formation by serum antibody. I. Removal of specific antibody by means of immunoadsorption. *J. exp. Med.* **130**: 1175–1186.

GREAVES, M. F., OWEN, J. J. T. and RAFF, M. C. (1974) *T and B Lymphocytes: Origins, Properties and Roles in Immune Responses* (1st edn). Excerpta Medica, Amsterdam.

GREENBURY, C. L. and MOORE, D. H. (1968) Nonspecific antibody-induced suppression of the immune response. *Nature, Lond.* **219**: 526–527.

GYÖNGYÖSSY, M. I. C., ARNAIZ-VILLENA, A., SOTERIADES-VLACHOS, C. and PLAYFAIR, J. H. L. (1975) Rosette formation by mouse lymphocytes. IV. Fc and C3 receptors occurring together and separately on T cells and other leucocytes. *Clin. exp. Immunol.* **19**: 485–497.

HABAL, M. B., CARPENTER, C. B., KOBAYASHI, K., BUSH, G. J., MISRA, M. and BIRTCH, A. G. (1973) The protective effect of $F(ab')_2$ and succinylated IgG in the early treatment of hyperacute rejection in the primate. *Transplant. Proc.* **5**: 601–606.

HALLORAN, P., SCHIRRMACHER, V. and DAVID, C. S. (1975) The specificity and significance of the inhibition of Fc receptor binding by anti-H-2 sera. *Immunogenetics* **2**: 349–361.

HAMAOKA, T. and KITAGAWA, M. (1971) Antibody production in mice. II. The mechanism of antigenic stimulation in the secondary immune response. *Immunology* **20**: 119–203.

HAMAOKA, T., TAKATSU, K., MASAKI, H., MATSUOKA, Y. and KITAGAWA, M. (1971a) Antibody production in mice. III. The suppressive effect of antibody on the initiation of secondary immune response. *Immunology* **20**: 871–881.

HAMAOKA, T., TAKATSU, T. and KITAGAWA, M. (1971b) Antibody production in mice. IV. The suppressive effect of anti-hapten and anti-carrier antibodies on the recognition of hapten-carrier conjugates in the secondary response. *Immunology* **21**: 259–271.

HAMAOKA, T., TAKATSU, K. and KITAGAWA, M. (1973) Antibody production in mice. V. The suppressive effect of anti-carrier antibodies on cellular cooperation in the induction of secondary anti-hapten antibody response. *Immunology* **24**: 409–424.

HAMILTON, J. A. and MILLER, J. F. A. P. (1974) Hapten-specific tolerance in mice. I. Induction with hapten-coupled syngeneic erythrocytes. *Eur. J. Immunol.* **4**: 261–268.

HÄMMERLING, G. J. (1976) Tissue distribution of Ia antigens and their expression on lymphocyte subpopulations. *Transplant. Rev.* **30**: 64–82.

HÄMMERLING, G. J. and MCDEVITT, H. O. (1974) Antigen binding T and B lymphocytes. II. Studies on the inhibition of antigen binding to T and B cells by anti-immunoglobulin and anti-H-2 sera. *J. Immunol.* **112**: 1734–1740.

HÄMMERLING, G. J., BLACK, S. J., BEREK, C., EICHMANN, K. and RAJEWSKI, K. (1976) Idiotypic analysis of lymphocytes *in vitro*. II. Genetic control of T-helper cell responsiveness to antiidiotypic antibody. *J. exp. Med.* **143**: 861–869.

HART, D. A., WANG, A.-L., PAWLAK, L. L. and NISONOFF, A. (1972) Suppression of idiotypic specificities in adult mice by administration of anti-idiotypic antibody. *J. exp. Med.* **135**: 1293–1300.

Hartmann, D. P. and Lewis, M. G. (1974) Presence and possible role of anti-IgG antibodies in human malignancy. *Lancet* i: 1318–1320.

Haughton, G. and Nash, D. R. (1969) Specific immunosuppression by minute doses of passive antibody. *Transplant. Proc.* **1**: 616–618.

Hauptfeld, V., Hauptfeld, M. and Klein, J. (1974) Tissue distribution of I region-associated antigens in the mouse. *J. Immunol.* **113**: 181–188.

Hauptfeld, V., Klein, D. and Klein, J. (1973) Serological identification of an Ir-region product. *Science, Wash.* **181**: 167–169.

Havas, H. F. (1969) The effect of the carrier protein on the immune response and the induction of tolerance to the 2,4-dinitrophenol determinant. *Immunology* **17**: 819–829.

Hay, J. B. and Morris, B. (1976) Generation and selection of specific reactive cells by antigen. *Br. med. Bull.* **32**: 135–140.

Heber-Katz, E. and Wilson, D. B. (1975) Collaboration of allogeneic T and B lymphocytes in the primary antibody response to sheep erythrocytes *in vitro*. *J. exp. Med.* **142**: 928–935.

Hellström, K. E. and Hellström, I. (1974) Lymphocyte-mediated cytotoxicity and blocking serum activity to tumor antigens. *Adv. Immunol.* **18**: 209–277.

Henney, C. S. and Ishizaka, K. (1968) Studies on the immunogenicity of antigen–antibody precipitates. I. The suppressive effect of anti-L and anti-H chain antibodies on the immunogenicity of human γG globulin. *J. Immunol.* **101**: 896–904.

Henney, C. S. and Ishizaka, K. (1970) Studies on the immunogenicity of antigen-antibody precipitates. II. The suppressive effect of anti-carrier and anti-hapten antibodies on the immunogenicity of dinitrophenylated human γG globulin. *J. Immunol.* **104**: 1540–1549.

Henry, C. and Jerne, N. K. (1968) Competition of 19S and 7S antigen receptors in the regulation of the primary immune response. *J. exp. Med.* **128**: 133–152.

Heron, I. (1973) Is transplantation tolerance in the rat serum-mediated? *Transplantation* **15**: 534–539.

Herzenberg, L. A., Okumura, K. and Metzler, C. M. (1975) Regulation of immunoglobulin and antibody production by allotype suppressor T cells in mice. *Transplant. Rev.* **27**: 57–83.

Herzenberg, L. A., Okumura, K., Cantor, H., Sato, V. L., Shen, F.-W., Boyse, E. A. and Herzenberg, L. A. (1976) T-cell regulation of antibody responses: demonstration of allotype-specific helper cells and their specific removal by suppressor T cells. *J. exp. Med.* **144**: 330–344.

Hoffmann, M. K., Kappler, J. W., Hirst, J. A. and Oettgen, H. F. (1974) Regulation of the immune response. V. Antibody-mediated inhibition of T and B cell cooperation in the *in vitro* response to red cell antigens. *Eur. J. Immunol.* **4**: 282-286.

Holter, A. R., Neu, M. R., McKearn, T. J., Lynch, A. F. and Stuart, F. P. (1973) Abrogation of hyperacute rejection of renal allografts by pepsin digest fragments of antidonor antibody. *Transplant. Proc.* **5**: 593–596.

Horung, M. O., Layne, E., McDonald, J. C. (1971) The use of human F(ab′)$_2$ fragments as blocking agents in the mixed lymphocyte reaction. *J. Immunol.* **107**: 979–984.

Howard, J. G., Zola, H., Christie, G. H. and Courtenay, B. M. (1971) Studies on immunological paralysis. V. The effect of variation in molecular weight on the immunogenicity, tolerogenicity and antibody-neutralizing activity of type 3 pneumococcal polysaccharide. *Immunology* **21**: 535–546.

Howard, J. G., Christie, G. H. and Courtenay, B. M. (1972) Studies on immunological paralysis. VII. Rapid reversal of Felton's paralysis as evidence for 'tolerant' cells. *Proc. R. Soc.* **B180**: 347–361.

Howard, J. G. and Mitchison, N. A. (1975) Immunological tolerance. *Prog. Allergy* **18**: 43–96.

Hudson, L. and Sprent, J. (1976) Specific adsorption of IgM antibody onto H-2-activated mouse T lymphocytes. *J. exp. Med.* **143**: 444–449.

Hunt, S. V. and Williams, A. F. (1974) The origin of cell surface immunoglobulins of marrow-derived and thymus-derived lymphocytes of the rat. *J. exp. Med.* **139**: 479–496.

Hutchin, P., Amos, D. B. and Prioleau, W. H. (1967) Interactions of humoral antibodies and immune lymphocytes. *Transplantation* **5**: 68–75.

Hutchison, I. V. and Zola, H. (1977) Antigen reactive cell opsonization in passive enhancement of rat kidney allografts. *Transplant. Proc.* **9**: 961–963.

Irvin, G. L., Eustace, J. C. and Fahey, J. L. (1967) Enhancement activity of mouse immunoglobulin classes. *J. Immunol.* **99**: 1085–1091.

Isakovic, K., Smith, S. B. and Waksman, B. H. (1965) Role of the thymus in tolerance. I. Tolerance to bovine gamma globulin in thymectomized, irradiated rats grafted with thymus from tolerant donors. *J. exp. Med.* **122**: 1103–1123.

Janeway, C. A., Koren, H. S. and Paul, W. E. (1975) The role of thymus-derived lymphocytes in an antibody-mediated hapten-specific helper effect. *Eur. J. Immunol.* **5**: 17–22.

Janossy, G. and Greaves, M. (1975) Functional analysis of murine and human B lymphocyte subset. *Transplant. Rev.* **24**: 177–236.

Jeekel, J. and van Dongen, J. (1977) Enhancement of rat renal allograft with antibodies directed against erythrocyte associated antigens (EAA). *Transplant. Proc.* **9**: 969–972.

Jerne, N. K. (1974) Towards a network theory of the immune system. *Ann. Immunol. Inst. Pasteur* **125C**: 373–389.

Jerne, N. K. (1976) The immune system. A web of V-domains. *Harvey Lect.* **70**: 93–110.

Jerry, L. M., Rowden, G., Cano, P. O. Phillips, T. M., Deutsch, G., Capek, A., Hartmann, D. P. and Lewis, M. G. (1976) Immune complexes in human melanoma: a consequence of deranged immune regulation. *Scand. J. Immunol.* **5**: 845–859.

Jirsch, D. W., Kraft, N. and Diener, E. (1974) Tolerance induction to a heterotopic cardiac allograft in the irradiated reconstituted mouse. *Transplantation* **18**: 155–162.

Jondal, M., Holm, G. and Wigzell, H. (1972) Surface markers on human T and B lymphocytes. I. A large population of lymphocytes forming nonimmune rosettes with sheep red blood cells. *J. exp. Med.* **136**: 207–215.

JONES, V. E. and LESKOWITZ, S. (1965) Role of the carrier in development of delayed hypersensitivity to the azophenyl-arsonate group. *Nature, Lond.* **207**: 596–597.

JULIUS, M. H., SIMPSON, E. and HERZENBERG, L. A. (1973) A rapid method for the isolation of functional thymus-derived murine lymphocytes. *Eur. J. Immunol.* **3**: 645–649.

KABAT, E. A. and BEZAR, A. E. (1958) The effect of variation in molecular weight on the antigenicity of dextran in man. *Archs. Biochem.* **78**: 306–318.

KALISS, N. (1969) Immunological enhancement. *Int. Rev. exp. Path.* **8**: 241–276.

KALISS, N., BORGES, P. R. F. and DAY, E. D. (1954) The survival and metastic spread of homografts of mouse tumors in mice pretreated with lyophilized tissue and cortisone. *Cancer Res.* **14**: 210 219.

KALISS, N., SINCLAIR, N. R. STC. and CANTRELL, J. L. (1976) Immunological enhancement of a murine tumor allograft by passive alloantibody IgG and $F(ab')_2$. *Eur. J. Immunol.* **6**: 38–42.

KANELLOPOULOS-LANGEVIN, C., KANELLOPOULOS, J. and VOISIN, G. A. (1976) Role of suppressor cells in antibody-induced inhibition of mixed lymphocyte reactions. *Ann. Immunol. Inst. Pasteur* **217C**: 775–786.

KAPP, J. A., PIERCE, C. W., DE LA CROIX, F. and BENACERRAF, B. (1976) Immunosuppressive factor(s) extracted from lymphoid cells of nonresponder mice primed with L-glutamic acid^{60}-L-alanine^{30}-L-tyrosine^{10} (GAT). I. Activity and antigenic specificity. *J. Immunol.* **116**: 305–309.

KAPPLER, J. W. and MARRACK, P. (1977) The role of H-2 linked genes in helper T-cell function. I. *In vitro* expression in B cells of immune response genes controlling helper T-cell activity. *J. exp. Med.* **146**: 1748–1764.

KAPPLER, J. W., HOFFMANN, M. and DUTTON, R. W. (1971) Regulation of the immune response. I. Differential effect of passively administered antibody on the thymus-derived and bone marrow-derived lymphocytes. *J. exp. Med.* **134**: 577–587.

KAPPLER, J. W., HAVEN, A., VAN DER DHARMARAJAN, U. and HOFFMANN, M. (1973) Regulation of the immune response. IV. Antibody-mediated suppression of the immune response to haptens and heterologous erythrocyte antigens *in vitro. J. Immunol.* **111**: 1228–1235.

KATZ, D. H. and BENACERRAF, B. (1975) The function and interrelationships of T-cell receptors, Ir genes and other histocompatibility gene products. *Transplant. Proc.* **22**: 175–195.

KATZ, D. H., HAMAOKA, T. and BENACERRAF, B. (1972) Immunological tolerance in bone marrow-derived lymphocytes. I. Evidence for an intracellular mechanism of inactivation of hapten-specific precursors of antibody-forming cells. *J. exp. Med.* **136**: 1404–1429.

KATZ, D. H., HAMAOKA, T. and BENACERRAF, B. (1973a) Cell interactions between histoincompatible T and B lymphocytes. II. Failure of physiologic cooperative interactions between T and B lymphocytes from allogeneic donor strains in humoral responses to hapten–protein conjugates. *J. exp. Med.* **137**: 1405–1418.

KATZ, D. H., HAMAOKA, T., DORF, M. E. and BENACERRAF, B. (1973b) Cell interactions between histoincompatible T and B lymphocytes. III. Demonstration that the H-2 gene complex determines successful physiologic lymphocyte interactions. *Proc. natn. Acad. Sci. U.S.A.* **70**: 2624–2628.

KATZ, D. H., HAMAOKA, T., DORF, M. E. and BENACERRAF, B. (1973c) Cell interactions between histoincompatible T and B lymphocytes. IV. Involvement of the immune response (Ir) gene in the control of the lymphocyte interactions in responses controlled by the gene. *J. exp. Med.* **138**: 734–739.

KATZ, D. H., DORF, M. E. and BENACERRAF, B. (1974) Cell interactions between histoincompatible T and B lymphocytes. VI. Cooperative responses between lymphocytes derived from mouse strains differing at genes in the S and D regions of the H-2 complex. *J. exp. Med.* **140**: 290–295.

KATZ, D. H., GREAVES, M., DORF, M. E., DIMUZIO, M. and BENACERRAF, B. (1975) Cell interaction between histoincompatible T and B lymphocytes. VIII. Cooperative responses between lymphocytes are controlled by genes in the I region H-2 complex. *J. exp. Med.* **141**: 263–268.

KATZ, D. H., CHIORAZZI, N., MCDONALD, J. and KATZ, L. R. (1976) Cell interactions between histoincompatible T and B lymphocytes. IX. The failure of histoincompatible cells is not due to suppression and cannot be circumvented by carrier-priming T cells with allogeneic macrophages. *J. Immunol.* **117**: 1853–1859.

KERBEL, R. S. and DAVIES, A. J. S. (1974) The possible biological significance of Fc receptors on mammalian lymphocytes and tumor cells. *Cell* **3**: 105–112.

KILSHAW, P. J., BRENT, L. and PINTO, M. (1975) Suppressor T cells in mice made unresponsive to skin allografts. *Nature, Lond.* **255**: 489–491.

KIND, L. S. and MACEDO-SOBRINHO, B. (1973) Reaginic antibody formation in mice injected with rabbit anti-mouse thymocyte serum. *Int. Archs. Allergy appl. Immunol.* **45**: 780–788.

KLAUS, G. G. B. (1975) B cell tolerance induced by polymeric antigens. II. Effects of tolerance on hapten-binding lymphocyte levels in primary and secondary antibody responses. *Eur. J. Immunol.* **5**: 366–372.

KLAUS, G. G. B. (1976) B cell tolerance induced by polymeric antigens. VI. Kinetics and reversibility of the inhibition of antibody-forming cells by antigen. *Eur. J. Immunol.* **6**: 389–393.

KLAUS, G. G. B. and CROSS, A. M. (1974) The influence of epitope density on the immunological properties of hapten-protein conjugates. I. Characteristics of the immune response to hapten-coupled albumen with varying epitope density. *Cell. Immunol.* **14**: 226–241.

KLAUS, G. G. B., HOWARD, J. G. and FELDMANN, M. (1976a) Mechanisms of B-cell tolerance. *Br. med. Bull.* **32**: 141–146.

KLAUS, G. G. B., PHILLIPS, J. M., HYMPHREY, J. H., DRESSER, D. W. and CROSS, A. M. (1976b) The immunological properties of haptens coupled to thymus independent carrier molecules. IV. The IgG response to dinitrophenylated Ficoll. *Eur. J. Immunol.* **6**: 429–433.

Klein, J., Hauptfeld, V. and Hauptfeld, M. (1974) Involvement of H-2 regions in immune reactions. In: *Progress in Immunology II*, pp. 197–206, Brent, L. and Holborow, J. (eds). North-Holland, Amsterdam, Oxford.

Klinman, N. R. (1972) The mechanism of antigenic stimulation of primary and secondary clonal precursor cells. *J. exp. Med.* **136**: 241–260.

Klinman, N. R. and Press, J. L. (1975) The B cell specificity repertoire: its relationship to definable subpopulations. *Transplant. Rev.* **24**: 41–83.

Kohler, H., Richardson, B. C., Rowley, D. A. and Smyk, S. (1977) Immune response to phosphorylcholine. II. Requirement of the Fc portion and equal effectiveness of IgG subclasses in anti-receptor antibody-induced suppression. *J. Immunol.* **119**: 1979–1986.

Koskimies, S. and Makela, O. (1976) T-cell-deficient mice produce more antihapten antibodies against syngeneic than against allogeneic erythrocyte conjugates. *J. exp. Med.* **144**: 467–475.

Kovithavongs, T. and Dossetor, J. B. (1975) Lymphocyte-dependent antibody crossmatching in kidney transplantation. *Lancet* **ii**: 915–916.

Krammer, P. H., Hudson, L. and Sprent, J. (1975) Fc-receptors, Ia-antigens, and immunoglobulin on normal and activated mouse T lymphocytes. *J. exp. Med.* **142**: 1403–1415.

Kumagai, K., Abo, T., Sekizawa, T. and Sasaki, M. (1975) Studies of surface immunoglobulin on human B lymphocytes. I. Dissociation of cell-bound immunoglobulin with acid pH or at 37°C. *J. Immunol.* **115**: 982–987.

Lafferty, K. J. and Jones, M. A. J. (1969) Reactions of the graft-versus-host (GVH) type. *Aust. J. exp. Biol. med. Sci.* **47**: 17–54.

Lafleur, L. and Mitchell, G. F. (1975) Differences in the immunologic activities of antibody-secreting cell precursors in mouse spleen selected on the basis of antigen-binding capacity. *Eur. J. Immunol.* **5**: 648–652.

Lafleur, L., Miller, R. G. and Phillips, R. A. (1973) Restriction of specificity in the precursors of bone marrow-associated lymphocytes. *J. exp. Med.* **137**: 954–966.

L'age-Stehr, J. and Herzenberg, L. A. (1970) Immunological memory in mice. I. Physical separation and partial characterization of memory cells for different immunoglobulin classes from each other and from antibody-producing cells. *J. exp. Med.* **131**: 1093–1108.

Lawrence, D. A., Weigle, W. O. and Spiegelberg, H. L. (1975) Immunoglobulins cytophilic for human lymphocytes, monocytes, and neutrophils. *J. clin. Invest.* **55**: 368–376.

Lay, W. H., Mendes, N. F., Bianco, C. and Nussenzweig, V. (1971) Binding of sheep red blood cells to a large population of human lymphocytes. *Nature, Lond.* **230**: 531–532.

Lee, W. and Köhler, H. (1974) Decline and spontaneous recovery of the monoclonal response to phosphorylcholine during repeated immunization. *J. Immunol.* **113**: 1644–1646.

Lee, W. Y. and Sehon, A. H. (1976) Suppression of reaginic antibody formation. III. Relationship between immunogenicity and tolerogenicity of hapten–carrier conjugates. *J. Immunol.* **116**: 1711–1718.

Leech, S. H. and Mitchison, N. A. (1976) Break-down of tolerance. *Br. med. Bull.* **32**: 130–134.

Lees, R. K. and Sinclair, N. R. StC. (1973) Regulation of the immune response. VII. *In vitro* immunosuppression by $F(ab')_2$ or intact IgG antibodies. *Immunology* **24**: 735–750.

Lees, R. K. and Sinclair, N. R. StC. (1975) Regulation of the immune response. XI. Resistance to antibody mediated immunosuppression induced by the presence of the allogeneic effect. *Cell. Immunol.* **17**: 525–531.

Lewis, M. G. and Phillips, T. M. (1972) The specificity of surface membrane immunofluorescence in human malignant melanoma. *Int. J. Cancer* **10**: 105–111.

Lewis, M. G., Loughridge, L. W. and Phillips, T. M. (1971a) Immunological studies in nephrotic syndrome associated with extrarenal malignant disease. *Lancet* **ii**: 134–135.

Lewis, M. G., Phillips, T. M., Cook, K. B. and Blake, J. (1971b) Possible explanation for loss of detectable antibody in patients with disseminated malignant melanoma. *Nature, Lond.* **232**: 52–54.

Lewis, M. G., Hartmann, D. P. and Jerry, L. M. (1976) Antibodies and anti-antibodies in human malignancy: an expression of deranged immune recognition. *Ann. N.Y. Acad. Sci.* **276**: 316–327.

Linscott, W. D. (1970) Effects of cell surface antigen density on immunological enhancement. *Nature, Lond.* **228**: 824–827.

Lipsky, P. E. and Rosenthal, A. S. (1973) Macrophage–lymphocyte interaction. I. Characteristics of antigen-independent-binding of guinea pig thymocytes and lymphocytes to syngeneic macrophages. *J. exp. Med.* **138**: 900–924.

Lipsky, P. E. and Rosenthal, A. S. (1976) The induction and regulation of guinea pig B-lymphocyte proliferation *in vitro*. *J. Immunol.* **117**: 1594–1602.

LoBuglio, A. F., Cotran, R. S. and Jandl, J. H. (1967) Red cells coated with immunoglobulin G; binding and sphering by mononuclear cells in man. *Science, Wash.* **158**: 1582–1585.

Long, M. A., Handwerger, B. S., Amos, D. B. and Yunis, E. J. (1976) The genetics of cell-mediated lympholysis. *J. Immunol.* **117**: 2092–2099.

MacDonald, H. R., Sordat, B., Cerottini, J.-C. and Brunner, K. T. (1975) Generation of cytotoxic T lymphocytes *in vitro*. IV. Functional activation of memory cells in the absence of DNA synthesis. *J. exp. Med.* **142**: 622–636.

MacLennan, I. C. M. (1972) Antibody in the induction and inhibition of lymphocyte cytotoxicity. *Transplant. Rev.* **13**: 67–90.

Marchalonis, J. J. and Cone, R. E. (1973) Biochemical and biological characteristics of lymphocyte surface immunoglobulin. *Transplant. Rev.* **14**: 3–49.

Mason, D. W. (1976a) The requirement for C3 receptors on the precursors of 19S and 7S antibody-forming cells. *J. exp. Med.* **143**: 1111–1121.

Mason, D. W. (1976b) The class of surface immunoglobulin on cells carrying IgG memory in rat thoracic duct lymph: the size of the subpopulation mediating IgG memory. *J. exp. Med.* **143**: 1122–1130.

MAWAS, C., SASPORTES, M., CHARMOT, D., CHRISTEN, Y. and DAUSSET, J. (1975) Cell-mediated lympholysis *in vitro*: independence of mixed lymphocyte reactions and T-cell mitogen responses from the *in vitro* generation of cytotoxic effectors in primary immunodeficiency disease. *Clin. exp. Immunol.* **20**: 83–92.

MCBRIDE, R. A. and SCHIERMAN, L. W. (1971) Passive antibody and the immune response. Factors which determine enhancement and suppression. *J. exp. Med.* **134**: 833–845.

MCCONNELL, I. (1971) Antigen receptors on the surface of antibody-secreting cells. *Nature New Biol.* **233**: 177–179.

MCCULLAGH, P. (1974) The role of cellular interaction in differentiating between the occurrence of immunological tolerance and immunity following antigenic challenge. *Eur. J. Immunol.* **4**: 540–545.

MCDEVITT, H. O., DELOVITCH, T. L., PRESS, J. L. and MURPHY, D. B. (1976) Genetic and functional analysis of the Ia antigens: their possible role in regulating the immune response. *Transplant. Rev.* **30**: 197–235.

MCKEARN, T. J., STUART, F. P. and FITCH, F. W. (1974) Antiidiotypic antibody in rat transplantation immunity. I. Production of antiidiotypic antibody in animals repeatedly immunized with alloantigens. *J. Immunol.* **113**: 1876–1882.

MCKENZIE, I. F. C. and PARISH, C. R. (1976) Secretion of Ia antigens by a subpopulation of T cells which are Ly-1, Ly-2, and Ia^-. *J. exp. Med.* **144**: 847–851.

MELCHER, U., VITETTA, E. S., MCWILLIAMS, M., LAMM, M. E., PHILLIPS-QUAGLIATA, J. M. and UHR, J. W. (1974) Cell surface immunoglobulin. X. Identification of an IgD-like molecule on the surface of murine splenocytes. *J. exp. Med.* **140**: 1427–1431.

MEO, T., DAVID, C. S., RIJNBEEK, A. M., NABHOLZ, M., MIGGIANO, V. C. and SCHREFFLER, D. C. (1975) Inhibition of mouse MLR by anti-Ia sera. *Transplant. Proc.* **7**: 127–129.

MILLER, H. C. and CUDKOWICZ, G. (1971) Density gradient separation of marrow cells restricted for antibody class. *Science, Wash.* **171**: 913–915.

MILLER, J. F. A. P. (1975) T-cell regulation of immune responsiveness. *Ann. N.Y. Acad. Sci.* **249**: 9–26.

MILLER, J. F. A. P. and MITCHELL, G. F. (1969) Thymus and antigen-reactive cells. *Transplant. Rev.* **1**: 3–42.

MILLER, J. F. A. P., DUKOR, P., GRANT, G., SINCLAIR, N. R. STC. and SACQUET, E., (1967) The immunological responsiveness of germ-free mice thymectomized at birth. I. Antibody production and skin homograft rejection. *Clin. exp. Immunol.*, **2**: 531–542.

MILLER, J. F. A. P., SPRENT, J., BASTEN, A., WARNER, N. L., BREITNER, J. C. S., ROWLAND, G., HAMILTON, J., SILVER, H. and MARTIN, W. J. (1971) Cell-to-cell interaction in the immune response. VII. Requirement for differentiation of thymus-derived cells. *J. exp. Med.* **134**: 1266–2184.

MILLER, J. F. A. P., VADAS, M. A., WHITELAW, A. and GAMBLE, J. (1975) H-2 gene complex restricts transfer of delayed-type hypersensitivity in mice. *Proc. natn. Acad. Sci. U.S.A.* **72**: 5095–5098.

MILLER, J. F. A. P., VADAS, M. A., WHITELAW, A. and GAMBLE, J. (1976a) H-2 linked Ir gene regulation of delayed-type hypersensitivity in mice. In: *The Role of Products of the Histocompatibility Gene Complex in Immune Responses*, pp. 403–415, KATZ, D. H. and BENACERRAF, B., (eds). Proceedings of an International Conference held at Brook Lodge, Augusta, Michigan, 1975. Academic Press, New York.

MILLER, J. F. A. P., VADAS, M. A., WHITELAW, A. and GAMBLE, J. (1976b) Role of major histocompatibility complex gene products in delayed type hypersensitivity. *Proc. natn. Acad. Sci. U.S.A.* **73**: 2486–2490.

MILTON, J. D. (1976) The specificity of immunosuppression by alloantibody in the mouse. *Transplantation* **22**: 445–448.

MIRANDA, J. J., ZOLA, H. and HOWARD, J. G. (1973) Studies on immunological paralysis. X. Cellular characteristics of the induction and loss of tolerance to levan (poly-fructose). *Immunology* **23**: 843–855.

MISHELL, R. I. and DUTTON, R. W. (1967) Immunization of dissociated spleen cell cultures from normal mice. *J. exp. Med.* **126**: 423–442.

MITCHELL, G. F. (1975) A proposal that one *in vivo* function of T cells is to regulate the availability of antigen for B cells. *Transplant. Rev.* **23**: 119–125.

MITCHELL, G. F., GRUMET, F. C. and MCDEVITT, H. O. (1972a) Genetic control of the immune response. The effect of thymectomy on the primary and secondary antibody response of mice to poly-L(Tyr,Glu)–poly-D,L-Ala–poly-L-Lys. *J. exp. Med.* **135**: 126–135.

MITCHELL, G. F., HUMPHREY, J. H. and WILLIAMSON, A. R. (1972b) Inhibition of secondary anti-hapten responses with the hapten conjugated to type 3 pneumococcal polysaccharide. *Eur. J. Immunol.* **2**: 460–467.

MITCHELL, M. S. and MOKYR, M. B. (1972) Specific inhibition of receptors for cytophilic antibody on macrophages by isoantibody. *Cancer Res.* **32**: 832–838.

MITCHELL, M. S., MOKYR, M. B. and GOLDWATER, D. J. (1975) Analysis and reversal of the inhibition of cytophilic antibody receptors produced by antibody. *Cancer Res.* **35**: 1121–1127.

MITCHISON, N. A. (1971a) The carrier effect in the secondary response to hapten-protein conjugates. I. Measurement of the effect with transferred cells and objections to the local environment hypothesis. *Eur. J. Immunol.* **1**: 10–17.

MITCHISON, N. A. (1971b) The carrier effect in the secondary response to hapten-protein conjugates. II. Cellular cooperation. *Eur. J. Immunol.* **1**: 18–27.

MIYAMOTO, M. and MCCULLAGH, P. (1974) The reappearance of immunologically reactive lymphocytes following termination of homograft tolerance. *Transplantation* **18**: 116–126.

MÖLLER, E. (1965) Contact-induced cytotoxicity by lymphoid cells containing foreign isoantigens. *Science, Wash.* **147**: 873–879.

MÖLLER, E. (1974) Specificity of hapten-reactive T and B mouse lymphocytes. Affinity and avidity of T- and B-cell receptors and anti-hapten antibodies as factors of dose and time after immunization. *Scand. J. Immunol.* **3**: 339–355.

MÖLLER, G. (1963) Studies on the mechanism of immunological enhancement of tumor homografts. I. Specificity of immunological enhancement. *J. natn. Cancer Inst.* **30**: 1153–1175.

MÖLLER, G. (1970) Antigen-binding lymphocyte receptors. *Transplant. Rev.* **5**: 3–166.

MÖLLER, G. (1976) Specificity of effector T lymphocytes. *Transplant. Rev.* **29**: 3–310.

Mollison, P. L. (1972) *Blood Transfusion in Clinical Medicine*, (5th edn). Blackwell Scientific Publ., Oxford.

Moretta, L., Ferrarini, M., Durante, M. L. and Mingari, M. C. (1975) Expression of a receptor for IgM by human T cells *in vitro*. *Eur. J. Immunol.* **5**: 565–569.

Moretta, L., Ferrarini, M., Mingari, M. C., Roretta, A. and Webb, S. R. (1976a) Subpopulations of human T cells identified receptors for immunoglobulins and mitogen responsiveness. *J. Immunol.* **117**: 2171–2174.

Moretta, L., Webb, S. R., Grossi, C. E., Lylyard, P. M. and Cooper, M. D. (1976b) Functional analysis of two subpopulations of human T cells and their distribution in immunodeficient patients. *Clin. Res.* **24**: 448A.

Moses, E., Isac, R. and Taussig, M. J. (1975) Antigen-specific T-cell factors in the genetic control of the immune responses to poly(Tyr,Glu)–polyDLAla–polyLys. Evidence for T- and B-cell defects in SJL mice. *J. exp. Med.* **141**: 703–707.

Mosier, D. E., Johnson, B. M., Paul, W. E. and McMaster, P. R. B. (1974) Cellular requirements for the primary *in vitro* antibody response to DNP-Ficoll. *J. exp. Med.* **139**: 1354–1360.

Munroe, A. J. and Taussig, M. J. (1975) Two genes in the major histocompatibility complex control immune response. *Nature, Lond.* **256**: 103–106.

Murgita, R. A. and Vas, S. I. (1972) Specific antibody-mediated effect on the immune response. Suppression and augmentation of the primary immune response in mice by different classes of antibodies. *Immunology* **22**: 319–331.

Murphy, D. B., Herzenberg, L. A., Okumura, K., Herzenberg, L. A. and McDevitt, H. O. (1976) A new I subregion (I–J) marked by a locus (Ia-4) controlling surface determinants on suppressor T lymphocytes. *J. exp. Med.* **144**: 699–712.

Myburgh, J. A. and Smit, J. A. (1972) Passive and active enhancement in baboon liver allografting. *Transplantation* **14**: 227–235.

Nabholz, M., Vives, J., Young, H. M., Meo, T., Miggiano, V., Rijnbeek, A. and Schreffler, D. C. (1974) Cell-mediated cell lysis *in vitro*: genetic control of killer cell production and target specificities in mouse. *Eur. J. Immunol.* **4**: 378–387.

Nabholz, M., Young, H., Meo, T., Miggiano, U., Rijnbeek, A. and Shreffler, D. C. (1975) Genetic analysis of an H-2 mutant, B6·C–H-2^{ba}, using cell-mediated lympholysis: T- and B-cell dictionaries for histocompatibility determinants are different. *Immunogenetics* **1**: 457–468.

Nagy, Z., Elliott, B. E. and Nabholz, M. (1976a) Specific binding of K- and I-region products of the H-2 complex to activated thymus-derived (T) cells belonging to different Ly subclasses. *J. exp. Med.* **144**: 1545–1553.

Nagy, Z., Elliott, B. E., Nabholz, M., Krammer, P. H. and Pernis, B. (1976b) Specific binding of alloantigens to T cells activated in the mixed lymphocyte reaction. *J. exp. Med.* **143**: 648–659.

Najarian, J. S. and Simmons, R. L. (1972) *Transplantation*, (1st edn). Lea & Febiger, Philadelphia.

Naor, D., Saltaun, R. and Falkenberg, F. (1975) Lack of requirement for thymocytes for efficient antibody formation to trinitrophenylated mouse red cells in mice: role for thymocytes in suppression of the immune response. *Eur. J. Immunol.* **5**: 220–223.

Neauport-Sautes, C., Dupuis, D. and Fridman, W. H. (1975) Specificity of Fc-receptors of activated T cells. Relation with released immunoglobulin-binding factor. *Eur. J. Immunol.* **5**: 849–854.

Nepom, J. T., Hellström, I. and Hellström, K. E. (1976) Purification and partial characterization of a tumor-specific blocking factor from sera of mice with growing chemically induced sarcomas. *J. Immunol.* **117**: 1846–1852.

Ness, D. B., Smith, S., Talcott, J. A. and Grumet, F. C. (1976) T cell requirements for the expression of the lipopolysaccharide adjuvant effect *in vivo*: evidence for a T cell-dependent and a T cell-independent mode of action. *Eur. J. Immunol.* **6**: 650–654.

Niederhuber, J. E. and Frelinger, J. A. (1976) Expression of Ia antigens on T and B cells and their relationship to immune-response functions. *Transplant. Rev.* **30**: 101–121.

Niederhuber, J. E., Frelinger, J. A., Dugan, E., Coutinho, A. and Shreffler, D. C. (1975) Effects of anti-Ia serum on mitogenic responses. I. Inhibition of the proliferative response to B cell mitogen, LPS, by specific anti-Ia sera. *J. Immunol.* **115**: 1672–1676.

Niederhuber, J. E., Frelinger, J. A., Dine, M. S., Shoffner, P., Dugan, E. and Shreffler, D. C. (1976) Effects of anti-Ia sera on mitogenic response. II. Differential expression of the Ia marker on phytohemagglutinin- and concavalin A-reactive T cells. *J. exp. Med.* **143**: 372–381.

Nielsen, H. E., Heron, I. and Koch, C. (1977) Inhibition of the mixed leucocyte reaction by histocompatibility antibodies requires the Fc part. *Transplantation* **23**: 73–77.

Nisbet, N. W. and Simonsen, M. (1967) Primary immune response in grafted cells. Dissociation between proliferation of activity and proliferation of cells. *J. exp. Med.* **125**: 967–981.

Nisonoff, A. and Bangasser, S. A. (1975) Immunological suppression of idiotypic specificities. *Transplant. Rev.* **27**: 100–134.

Nossal, G. J. V. and Layton, J. E. (1976) Antigen-induced aggregation and modulation of receptors on hapten-specific B lymphocytes. *J. exp. Med.* **143**: 511–528.

Nossal, G. J. V. and Pike, B. L. (1976) Single cell studies on the antibody-forming potential of fractionated, hapten-specific B lymphocytes. *Immunology* **30**: 189–202.

Oberbarnscheidt, J. and Kolsch, E. (1978) Direct blockade of antigen reactive B lymphocytes by immune complexes. An "off" signal provided by the linkage of antigen- and Fc-receptors. *Immunology* **35**: 151–157.

Okumura, K., Herzenberg, L. A., Murphy, D. B., McDevitt, H. O. and Herzenberg, L. A. (1976a) Selective expression of H-2 (I-region) loci controlling determinants on helper and suppressor T lymphocytes. *J. exp. Med.* **144**: 685–698.

Okumura, K., Metzler, C. M., Tsu, T. T., Herzenberg, L. A. and Herzenberg, L. A. (1976b) Two stages of B-cell memory development with different T-cell requirements. *J. exp. Med.* **144**: 345–357.

ORDAL, J. C. and GRUMET, F. C. (1973) Suppression of anti-(T,G)-A–L antibody production in nonresponder mice. *Transplant. Proc.* **5**: 175–178.

ORDAL, J. C., SMITH, S., NESS, D., GERSHON, R. K. and GRUMET, F. C. (1976) IgM-mediated, T cell-independent suppression of humoral immunity. *J. Immunol.* **116**: 1182–1187.

ORGEL, H. A., HAMBURGER, R. N., BAZARAL, M., GORRIN, H., GROSLONG, T., LENOIR, M., MILLER, J. R. and WALLACE, W. (1975) Development of IgE and allergy in infancy. *J. Allergy clin. Immunol.* **56**: 296–307.

OSMOND, D. G. and NOSSAL, G. J. V. (1974) Differentiation of lymphocytes in mouse marrow. I. Quantitative radioautographic studies of antiglobulin binding by lymphocytes in bone marrow and lymphoid tissues. *Cell. Immunol.* **13**: 117–131.

OVARY, Z. (1958) Passive cutaneous anaphylaxis in the mouse. *J. Immunol.* **81**: 355–357.

PARASKEVAS, F., LEE, S.-T., ORR, K. B. and ISRAELS, L. G. (1972a) A receptor for Fc on mouse B-lymphocytes. *J. Immunol.* **108**: 1319–1327.

PARASKEVAS, F., ORR, K. B., ANDERSON, E. D., LEE, S.-T. and ISRAELS, L. G. (1972b) The biological significance of Fc receptor on mouse B-lymphocytes. *J. Immunol.* **108**: 1729–1732.

PARISH, C. R. (1971a) Immune response to chemically modified flagellin. I. Induction of antibody tolerance to flagellin by acetoacetylated derivatives of the protein. *J. exp. Med.* **134**: 1–20.

PARISH, C. R. (1971b) Immune response to chemically modified flagellin. II. Evidence for a fundamental relationship between humoral and cell-mediated immunity. *J. exp. Med.* **134**: 21–47.

PARISH, C. R. (1973) Immune response to chemically modified flagellin. IV. Further studies on the relationship between humoral and cell-mediated immunity. *Cell. Immunol.* **6**: 66–79.

PARISH, C. R. and ADA, G. L. (1969) The tolerance inducing properties in rats of bacterial flagellin cleaved at the methionine residues. *Immunology* **17**: 153–164.

PARISH, C. R. and LIEW, F. Y. (1972) Immune response to chemically modified flagellin. III. Enhanced cell-mediated immunity during high and low zone antibody tolerance to flagellin. *J. exp. Med.* **135**: 298–311.

PARISH, C. R., JACKSON, D. C. and MCKENZIE, I. F. C. (1976) Low molecular weight Ia antigens in normal mouse serum. II. Demonstration of their T cell origin. *Immunogenetics* **3**: 129–137.

PAWLAK, L. L., HART, D. A. and NISONOFF, A. (1973) Requirements for prolonged suppression of an idiotypic specificity in adult mice. *J. exp. Med.* **137**: 1442–1458.

PECK, A. B., ALTER, B. J. and LINDAHL, K. F. (1976) Specificity in T cell mediated lympholysis: identical genetic control of the proliferative and effector phases of allogeneic and xenogeneic reactions. *Transplant. Rev.* **29**: 189–221.

PERLMANN, P., PERLMANN, H. and WIGZELL, H. (1972) Lymphocyte mediated cytotoxicity *in vitro*. Induction and inhibition by humoral antibody and nature of effector cells. *Transplant. Rev.* **13**: 91–114.

PIERCE, C. W., SOLLIDAY, S. M. and ASOFSKY, R. (1972) Immune responses *in vitro*. V. Suppression of γM γG, and γA plaque-forming cell responses in cultures of primed mouse spleen cells by class-specific antibody to mouse immunoglobulins. *J. exp. Med.* **135**: 698–710.

PIERCE, C. W., KAPP, J. A. and BENACERRAF, B. (1976a) Regulation by the H-2 gene complex of macrophage-lymphoid cell interactions in secondary antibody responses *in vitro*. *J. exp. Med.* **144**: 371–381.

PIERCE, C. W., KAPP, J. A. and BENACERRAF, B. (1976b) Stimulation of antibody responses *in vitro* by antigen-bearing syngeneic and allogeneic macrophages. In: *The Role of Products of the Histocompatibility Gene Complex in Immune Responses*, pp. 391–401, KATZ, D. H. and BENACERRAF, B. (eds). Proceedings of an International Conference held at Brook Lodge, Augusta, Michigan, 1975. Academic Press, New York.

PIERCE, S. K. and KLINMAN, N. R. (1975) The allogeneic bisection of carrier-specific enhancement of monoclonal B-cell responses. *J. exp. Med.* **142**: 1165–1179.

PIERCE, S. K. and KLINMAN, N. R. (1976) Allogeneic carrier-specific enhancement of hapten-specific secondary B-cell responses. *J. exp. Med.* **144**: 1254–1262.

PIKE, B. L. and NOSSAL, G. J. V. (1976) Requirement for persistant extracellular antigen in cultures of antigen-binding lymphocytes. *J. exp. Med.* **144**: 568–572.

PINCUS, C. S., LAMM, M. E. and NUSSENZWEIG, V. (1971) Regulation of the immune response: suppressive enhancing effects of passively administered antibody. *J. exp. Med.* **133**: 987–1003.

PINCUS, C. S., MILLER, G. and NUSSENZWEIG, V. (1973) Enhancement of an antihapten response by an antiserum to the carrier protein. *J. Immunol.* **110**: 301–304.

PINTO, M., BRENT, L. and THOMAS, A. V. (1974) Specific unresponsiveness to skin allografts in mice. III. Synergistic effects of tissue extracts, Bordetella pertussis and antilymphocyte serum. *Transplantation* **17**: 477–486.

PLATE, J. M. D. (1976) Cellular responses to murine alloantigens of the major histocompatibility complex. The role of cell subpopulations that express different quantities of H-2 associated markers. *Eur. J. Immunol.* **6**: 180–187.

PLAYFAIR, J. H. L. (1974) The role of antibody in T-cell responses. *Clin. exp. Immunol.* **17**: 1–18.

PLAYFAIR, J. H. L., MARSHALL-CLARK, S. and HUDSON, L. (1974) Cooperation by mouse T lymphocytes: the role of antibody in T cell specificity. *Eur. J. Immunol.* **4**: 54–56.

POLAK, L. and TURK, J. L. (1974) Reversal of immunological tolerance by cyclophosphamide through inhibition of suppressor cell activity. *Nature, Lond.* **249**: 654–656.

PRESS, J. L. and KLINMAN, N. R. (1973) Monoclonal production of both IgM and IgG_1 anti-hapten antibody. *J. exp. Med.* **138**: 300–305.

PRESS, J. L., KLINMAN, N. R., HENRY, C., WOFSY, L., DELOVITCH, T. L. and MCDEVITT, H. O. (1975) Ia antigens on B cells: relationship to B cell precursor function and to surface immunoglobulin. In: *Membrane Receptors of Lymphocytes*, pp. 247–258, SELIGMANN, M., PREUD'HOMME, J. L. and KOURILSKY, F. M. (eds). Proceedings of the International Symposium on Membrane Receptors of Lymphocytes held in Paris, 1975 (INSERM Symposium 1). American Elsevier, New York.

Press, J. L., Klinman, N. R. and McDevitt, H. O. (1976) Expression of Ia antigens on hapten-specific B cells. I. Delineation of B-cell subpopulations. *J. exp. Med.* **144**: 414–427.

Pross, H. F. and Eidinger, D. (1974) Antigenic competition: a review of nonspecific antigen-induced suppression. *Adv. Immunol.* **18**: 133–168.

Ptak, W. and Gershon, R. K. (1975) Immunosuppression effected by macrophage surfaces. *J. Immunol.* **115**: 1346–1350.

Raff, M. C., Feldmann, M. and de Petris, S. (1973) Monospecificity of bone marrow-derived lymphocytes. *J. exp. Med.* **137**: 1024–1030.

Rajewsky, K. and Brenig, C. (1974) Paralysis to serum albumins in T and B lymphocytes in mice. Dose dependence, specificity and kinetics of escape. *Eur. J. Immunol.* **4**: 120–125.

Rajewsky, K. and Eichmann, K. (1977) Antigen receptors of T helper cells. *Contemp. Topics Immunobiol.* **7**: 69–112.

Rajewsky, K. and Mohr, R. (1974) Specificity and heterogeneity of helper T cells in the response to serum albumins in mice. *Eur. J. Immunol.* **4**: 111–119.

Ramasamy, R., Munro, A. and Milstein, C. (1974) Possible role for the Fc-receptor on B lymphocytes. *Nature, Lond.* **249**, 573–575.

Ramseier, H. and Lindenmann, J. (1972) Similarity of cellular recognition structures for histocompatibility antigens and of combining sites of corresponding alloantibodies. *Eur. J. Immunol.* **2**: 109–114.

Rao, V. S. and Mitchell, M. S. (1977) Suppression of macrophage-mediated immunity to leukemia L1210 by immune complexes. *Proc. Am. Ass. Cancer Res.* **18**: 63.

Rao, V. S., Mokyr, M. B., Gershon, R. K. and Mitchell, M. S. (1977) Specific T cell-dependent, antigen-antibody mediated suppression of macrophages: abrogation by nonspecifically stimulated T cells. *J. Immunol.* **118**: 2117–2124.

Revillard, J. P., Samarut, C., Cordier, G. and Brochier, J. (1975) Characterization of human lymphocytes bearing Fc receptors with special reference to cytotoxic (K) cells. In: *Membrane Receptors of Lymphocytes*, pp. 171–184, Seligmann, M., Preud'homme, J. L. and Kourilsky, F. M. (eds). Proceedings of the International Symposium on Membrane Receptors of Lymphocytes held in Paris, 1975 (INSERM Symposium 1). American Elsevier, New York.

Rich, R. R. and Pierce, C. W. (1973) Biological expressions of lymphocyte activation. I. Effects of phytomitogens on antibody synthesis *in vitro*. *J. exp. Med.* **137**: 205–223.

Rich, R. R. and Pierce, C. W. (1974) Biological expressions of lymphocyte activation. III. Suppression of plaque-forming cell responses *in vitro* by supernatant fluids from concanavalin A-activated spleen cell cultures. *J. Immunol.* **112**: 1360–1368.

Rich, S. S. and Rich, R. R. (1976) Regulatory mechanisms in cell-mediated immune responses. IV. Expression of a receptor for mixed lymphocyte reaction suppressor factor on activated T lymphocytes. *J. exp. Med.* **144**: 1214–1226.

Roelants, G. E. and Askonas, B. A. (1972) Immunological B memory in thymus deprived mice. *Nature New Biol.* **239**: 63–64.

Rollinghoff, M. and Wagner, H. (1973) *In vitro* induction of tumor specific immunity: requirements for T lymphocytes and tumor growth inhibition *in vivo*. *Eur. J. Immunol.* **3**: 471–476.

Rollinghoff, M. and Wagner, H. (1975) Secondary cytotoxic allograft response *in vitro*. I. Antigenic requirements. *Eur. J. Immunol.* **5**: 875–879.

Rosenthal, A. S. and Shevach, E. M. (1973) Function of macrophages in antigen recognition by guinea pig T lymphocytes. I. Requirement for histocompatible macrophages and lymphocytes. *J. exp. Med.* **138**: 1194–1212.

Rosenthal, A. S. and Shevach, E. M. (1976) The function of macrophages in T-lymphocyte antigen recognition. *Contemp. Topics Immunobiol.* **5**: 47–90.

Rouse, B. T. and Warner, N. L. (1974) The role of suppressor cells in avian allogeneic tolerance: implications for the pathogenesis of Marek's disease. *J. Immunol.* **113**: 904–909.

Rouse, B. T., Rollinghoff, M. and Warner, N. L. (1972) Anti-θ serum-induced suppression of the cellular transfer of tumour-specific immunity to a syngeneic plasma cell tumour. *Nature. New Biol.* **238**: 116–117.

Rowe, D. S., Hug, K., Faulk, W. P., McCormick, J. N. and Gerber, H. (1973) IgD on the surface of peripheral blood lymphocytes on the human newborn. *Nature New Biol.* **242**: 155–156.

Rowley, D. and Turner, K. J. (1966) Number of molecules of antibody required to promote phagocytosis of one bacterium. *Nature, Lond.* **210**: 496–498.

Rowley, D. A. and Fitch, F. W. (1968) Clonal selection and inhibition of the primary antibody response by antibody. In: *Regulation of the Antibody Response*, pp. 127–140, Cinader, B. (ed.). Thomas, Springfield, Illinois.

Rowley, D. A., Fitch, F. W., Axelrad, M. A. and Pierce, C. W. (1969) The immune response suppressed by specific antibody. *Immunology* **16**: 549–559.

Rowley, D. A. Fitch, R. W., Stuart, F. P., Köhler, H. and Cosenza, H. (1973) Specific suppression of immune responses. *Science, Wash.* **181**: 1133–1141.

Rowley, D. A., Köhler, H., Schreiber, H., Kaye, S. T. and Lorbach, I. (1976) Suppression by autogenous complementary idiotypes: the priority of the first response. *J. exp. Med.* **144**: 946–959.

Ryan, J. L. and Henkart, P. A. (1976) Fc receptor-mediated inhibition of murine B-lymphocyte activation. *J. exp. Med.* **144**: 768–775.

Ryan, J. L., Arbeit, R. D., Dickler, H. B. and Henkart, P. A. (1975a) Fc-receptor mediated inhibition of B lymphocyte mitogenesis. In: *Membrane Receptors of Lymphocytes*, pp. 389–392, Seligmann, M., Preud'homme, J. L. and Kourilsky, F. M. (eds). Proceedings of the International Symposium on Membrane Receptors of Lymphocytes held in Paris, 1975 (INSERM Symposium 1). American Elsevier, New York.

RYAN, J. L., ARBEIT, R. D., DICKLER, H. B. and HENKART, P. A. (1975b) Inhibition of lymphocyte mitogenesis by immobilized antigen–antibody complexes. *J. exp. Med.* **142**: 814–826.

RYDER, R. J. W. and SCHWARTZ, R. S. (1969) Immunosuppression by antibody: localization of site of action. *J. Immunol.* **103**: 970–978.

SACHS, D. H. and DICKLER, H. B. (1975) The possible role of I region determined cell surface molecules in the regulation of immune responses. *Transplant. Rev.* **23**: 159–175.

SALSANO, P., FRØLAND, S. S., NATVIG, J. B. and MICHAELSEN, T. E. (1974) Same idiotype of B-lymphocyte membrane IgD and IgM. Formal evidence for monoclonality of chronic lymphocytic leukaemia cells. *Scand. J. Immunol.* **3**: 841–846.

SANFILIPPO, F., COHN, M. L. and SCOTT, D. W. (1976) Effect of carrier-specific tolerance on the generation of helper cell function. *Eur. J. Immunol.* **6**: 742–746.

SANTANA, V. and TURK, J. L. (1975) Binding of aggregated human immunoglobulin to murine thymocytes and T cells through receptors for the Fc region. *Immunology* **28**: 1173–1178.

SCHIMPL, A. and WECKER, E. (1973) Stimulation of IgG antibody response *in vitro* by T cell-replacing factor. *J. exp. Med.* **137**: 547–552.

SCHIMPL, A. and WECKER, E. (1978) Non-antigen-specific mediators in T–B cell cooperation (in press).

SCHIRRMACHER, V. and FESTENSTEIN, H. (1976) Interaction of Fc and C3 receptors of lymphoid cells with antibodies against products of the major histocompatibility complex: association of MHC products with complement receptors. *Transplant. Rev.* **30**: 140–173.

SCHIRRMACHER, V. and HALLORAN, P. (1975) Independence of Fc receptors and Ia antigens on a variety of cells including cytotoxic K cells. In: *Membrane Receptors of Lymphocytes*, pp. 267–280, SELIGMANN, M., PREUD'HOMME, J. L. and KOURILSKY, F. M. (eds). Proceedings of the International Symposium on Membrane Receptors of Lymphocytes held in Paris, 1975 (INSERM Symposium 1). American Elsevier, New York.

SCHRADER, J. W. (1974a) The mechanism of bone marrow-derived (B) lymphocyte activation. I. Early events in antigen-induced triggering in the presence of polymerized flagellin. *Eur. J. Immunol.* **4**: 14–20.

SCHRADER, J. W. (1974b) The mechanism of bone marrow-derived (B) lymphocyte activation. II. A "second signal" for antigen-specific activation provided by flagellin and lipopolysaccharide. *Eur. J. Immunol.* **4**: 20–24.

SCHRADER, J. W. (1975a) The *in vitro* induction of immunological tolerance in the B lymphocyte by oligovalent thymus-dependent antigens. *J. exp. Med.* **141**: 962–973.

SCHRADER, J. W. (1975b) Tolerance induction in B lymphocytes by thymus-dependent antigens. T cells may abrogate B-cell tolerance induction but prevent an antibody response. *J. exp. Med.* **141**: 974–989.

SCHRADER, J. W. (1975c) The role of T cells in IgG production; thymus-dependent antigens induce B cell memory in the absence of T cells. *J. Immunol.* **114**: 1665–1669.

SCHRADER, J. W. (1975d) Effector-cell blockade. II. A demonstration of the reversible masking of an immune response by blockade of antibody-forming cells. *Eur. J. Immunol.* **5**: 808–812.

SCHRADER, J. W. and FELDMANN, M. (1973) The mechanism of antigenic competition. I. The macrophage as a site of a reversible block of T–B lymphocyte collaboration. *Eur. J. Immunol.* **3**: 711–717.

SCHREINER, G. F. and UNANUE, E. R. (1976) Membrane and cytoplasmic changes in B lymphocytes induced by lignand-surface immunoglobulin interaction. *Adv. Immunol.* **24**: 37–165.

SCHUFFLER, C. and DRAY, S. (1974) *In vitro* suppression of immunoglobulin allotype synthesis by Fab and $F(ab')_2$ fragments of anti-allotype antibody. *Cell. Immunol.* **11**: 367–376.

SCHWARTZ, B. D., PAUL, W. E. and SHEVACH, E. M. (1976) Guinea-pig Ia antigens: functional significance and chemical characterization. *Transplant. Rev.* **30**: 174–196.

SCHWARTZ, R. H., DORF, M. E., BENACERRAF, B. and PAUL, W. E. (1976) The requirement for two complementing Ir–GLØ immune response genes in the T-lymphocyte proliferative response to poly-$(Glu^{53}Lys^{36}Phe^{11})$. *J. exp. Med.* **143**: 897–905.

SCHWARZ, M. R. (1968) The mixed lymphocyte reaction: an *in vitro* test for tolerance. *J. exp. Med.* **127**: 879–889.

SCOTT, D. W. and LONG, C. A. (1976) Role of self-carriers in the immune response and tolerance. I. B-cell unresponsiveness and cytotoxic T-cell immunity induced by haptenated syngeneic lymphoid cells. *J. exp. Med.* **144**: 1369–1374.

SCOTT, D. W., LAYTON, J. E. and NOSSAL, G. J. V. (1977) Role of IgD in the immune response and tolerance. I. Anti-δ pretreatment facilitates tolerance induction in adult B cells *in vitro. J. exp. Med.* **146**: 1473–1483.

SEGAL, S., WEINSTEIN, Y., MELMON, K. L. and MCDEVITT, H. O. (1974) Termination of tolerance by removal of a suppressor cell. *Fedn Proc.* **33**: 723A.

SEHON, A. H. and LEE, W. Y. (1976) Abrogation des anticorps réaginiques antihaptènes chez la souriş. *Congrès Francophone International d'Immunologie*, p. 11 (Abstract).

SERCARZ, E. D., CORENZWIT, D. T., EARDLEY, D. D. and MORRIS, K. M. (1975) Suppressive versus helper effects in carrier priming. In: *Suppressor Cells in Immunity*, pp. 19–26, SINGHAL, S. K. and SINCLAIR, N. R. STC. (eds). Proceedings of an International Symposium held May, 1975, London, Ontario. University of Western Ontario Press, London, Canada.

SHAIPANICH, T., WREN, S., VON HAEFEN, U., KOPPENHOFFER, T., BUSCH, G. and WILSON, R. E. (1973) Evaluation of organ specificity in renal allograft enhancement with $(F(ab')_2$ fragments. *Transplant. Proc.* **5**: 581–583.

SHEARER, G. M., CUDKOWICZ, G. and PRIORE, R. L. (1969) Cellular differentiation of the immune system of mice. II. Frequency of unipotent splenic antigen-sensitive units after immunization with sheep erythrocytes. *J. exp. Med.* **129**: 185–199.

SHEARER, G. M., MELMON, K. L., WEINSTEIN, Y. and SELA, M. (1972) Regulation of antibody response by cells expressing histamine receptors. *J. exp. Med.* **136**: 1302–1307.

Shearer, G. M., Weinstein, Y. and Melmon, K. L. (1974) Enhancement of immune response potential of mouse lymphoid cells fractionated over insolubilized conjugated histamine columns. *J. Immunol.* **113**: 597–607.

Shearer, G. M., Rehn, T. G. and Garbarino, C. A. (1975) Cell-mediated lympholysis of trinitrophenyl-modified autologous lymphocytes. Effector cell specificity to modified cell surface components controlled by the H-2K and H-2D serological regions of the murine major histocompatibility complex. *J. exp. Med.* **141**: 1348–1364.

Shearer, G. M., Schmitt-Verhulst, A.-M. and Rehn, T. G. (1977) Significance of the major histocompatibility complex as assessed by T-cell-mediated lympholysis involving syngeneic stimulating cells. *Contemp. Topics Immunobiol.* **7**: 221–243.

Shek, P.-N. and Dubiski, S. (1975) Allotype suppression in rabbits: competition for target cell receptors between isologous and heterologous antibody and between native antibody and antibody fragments. *J. Immunol.* **114**: 621–625.

Shevach, E., Herberman, R., Lieberman, R., Frank, M. M. and Green, I. (1972) Receptors for immunoglobulin on mouse leukemias and lymphomas. *J. Immunol.* **108**: 325–328.

Shibata, H. R., Jerry, L. M., Lewis, M. G., Mansell, P. W. A., Capek, A. and Marquis, G. (1976) Immunotherapy of human malignant melanoma with irradiated tumor cells, oral bacillus Calmette–Guérin and levamisole. *Ann. N.Y. Acad. Sci.* **277**: 355–366.

Shiku, H., Takamashi, T., Oettgen, H. F. and Old, L. J. (1976) Cell surface antigens of human malignant melanoma. II. Serological typing with immune adherance assays and definition of two surface antigens. *J. exp. Med.* **144**: 873–881.

Shreffler, D. C. and David, C. S. (1975) The H-2 major histocompatibility complex and the I immune response region: genetic variation, function, and organization. *Adv. Immunol.* **20**: 125–195.

Shreffler, D. C., Meo, T. and David, C. S. (1976) Genetic resolution of the products and functions of I and S region genes of the mouse H-2 complex. In: *The role of Products of the Histocompatibility Gene Complex in Immune Response*, pp. 3–37, Katz, D. H. and Benacerraf, B. (eds). Proceedings of an International Conference held at Brook Lodge, Augusta, Michigan, 1975. Academic Press, New York.

Shustick, C., Cohen, I. R., Schwartz, R. S., Latha-Griffin, E. and Waksal, S. D. (1976) T lymphocytes with promiscuous cytotoxicity. *Nature, Lond.* **263**: 699–671.

Sidman, C. L. and Unanue, E. R. (1976) Control of B-lymphocyte function. I. Inactivation of mitogenesis by interaction with surface immunoglobulin and Fc-receptor molecules. *J. exp. Med.* **144**: 882–896.

Silvers, W. K. (1974) The influence of removing lymphoid tissue on the persistence of tolerance of skin allografts in mice. *J. Immunol.* **113**: 804–809.

Silvers, W. K., Elkins, W. L. and Quimby, F. W. (1975) Cellular basis of tolerance in neonatally induced mouse chimeras. *J. exp. Med.* **142**: 1312–1315.

Simpson, E. and Cantor, H. (1975) Regulation of the immune response by subclasses of T lymphocytes. II. The effect of adult thymectomy upon humoral and cellular responses in mice. *Eur. J. Immunol.* **5**: 337–343.

Sinclair, N. R. StC. (1967a) A comparison of primary and secondary haemolysin responses to sheep erythrocytes in neonatally thymectomized, sham-thymectomized and normal Swiss mice. A time-course study of total 19*S* and 7*SS* antibody. *Immunology* **12**: 559–564.

Sinclair, N. R. StC. (1967b) Delayed development of primary immunological responsiveness in neonatally thymectomized Swiss albino mice. *Clin. exp. Immunol.* **2**: 701–704.

Sinclair, N. R. StC. (1969) Regulation of the immune response. I. Reduction in ability of specific antibody to inhibit long-lasting IgG immunological priming following removal of the Fc-fragment. *J. exp. Med.* **129**: 1183–1201.

Sinclair, N. R. StC. (1978) Immunoregulation by antibody and antigen-antibody complexes. *Transplant. Proc.* **10**: 349–353.

Sinclair, N. R. StC. and Chan, P. L. (1971) Regulation of the immune response. IV. The role of the Fc-fragment in feedback inhibition by antibody. *Adv. exp. Med. Biol.* **12**: 609–615.

Sinclair, N. R. StC., Lees, R. K. and Elliott, E. V. (1968) Role of the Fc-fragment in the regulation of the primary immune response. *Nature, Lond.* **220**: 1048–1049.

Sinclair, N. R. StC., Lees, R. K., Chan, P. L. and Khan, R. H., (1970) Regulation of the immune response. II. Further studies on differences in ability of $F(ab')_2$ and 7*S* antibodies to inhibit an antibody response. *Immunology* **19**: 105–116.

Sinclair, N. R. StC., Lees, R. K., Abrahams, S., Chan, P. L., Fagan, G. and Stiller, C. R. (1974) Regulation of the immune response. X. Antigen–antibody complex inactivation of cells involved in adoptive transfer. *J. Immunol.* **113**: 1493–1500.

Sinclair, N. R. StC., Lees, R. K., Fagan, G. and Birnbaum (1975a) Regulation of the immune response. VIII. Characteristics of antibody-mediated suppression of an *in vitro* cell-mediated immune response. *Cell. Immunol.* **16**: 330–347.

Sinclair, N. R. StC., Lees, R. K., Missiuna, P. C. and Fung, F. Y. (1975b) *In vitro* generation of cells capable of suppressing *in vitro* cell-mediated immunity. In: *Suppressor Cells in Immunity*, pp. 42–49, Singhal, S. K. and Sinclair, N. R. StC. (eds). Proceedings of an International Symposium held in London, Canada, 1975. University of Western Ontario Press, London, Canada.

Sinclair, N. R. StC., Lees, R. K. and Chan, P. L. (1976a) Interference with antibody-feedback by irradiation, thymus cells, the allogeneic effect, and serum factors. *Adv. exp. Med. Biol.* **66**: 623–633.

Sinclair, N. R. StC., Lees, R. K., Missiuna, P. C. and Vichos, E. E. (1976b) Regulation of the immune response. XII. Targets for suppressor cell activity in an *in vitro* cell-mediated immune response. *Cell. Immunol.* **27**: 163–170.

Sinclair, N. R. StC., Lees, R. K. Wheeler, M. E., Vichos, E. E. and Fung, F-Y. (1976c) Regulation of the immune response. XI. Cell-mediated feedback of an *in vitro* cell-mediated immune response. *Cell Immunol.* **27**: 152–162.

Singhal, S. K. and Wigzell, H. (1971) Cognition and recognition of antigen by cell associated receptors. *Prog. Allergy* **15**: 188–222.

SINGHAL, S. K., KING, S. and DRURY, P. (1972) Antibody-inhibiting activity of bone marrow cells *in vitro*. *Int. Archs. Allergy appl. Immunol.* **43**: 934–940.

SLEDGE, C., FAIR, D. S., BLACK, B. KRUEGER, R. G. and HOOD, L. (1976) Antibody differentiation: apparent sequence identity between variable regions shared by IgA and IgG immunoglobulins. *Proc. natn. Acad. Sci. U.S.A.* **73**: 923–927.

SMIT, J. A. and MYBURGH, J. A. (1974) Enhancement of baboon liver allografts with noncytotoxic preparations of alloimmune IgG. *Transplantation* **18**: 63–70.

SOLHEIM, B. G., THORSBY, E. and MILLER, E. (1976) Inhibition of Fc receptor of human lymphoid cells by antisera-recognizing determinants of the HLA system. *J. exp. Med.* **143**: 1568–1574.

SOLOMON, J. B., RIDDELL, G. S. and WHYTE, D. F. (1972) Specific immunosuppressive delay of the plaque-forming response by trace amounts of antibody of material origin in young rats injected with mouse or sheep erythrocytes. *Immunology* **22**: 219–226.

SOTERIADES-VLACHOS, C., GYÖNGYÖSSY, M. I. C. and PLAYFAIR, J. H. L. (1974) Rosette formation by mouse lymphocytes. III. Receptors for immunoglobulin on normal and activated T cells. *Clin. exp. Immunol.* **18**: 187–192.

SOULILLOU, J.-P., CARPENTER, C. B. D'APICE, A. J. F. and STROM, T. B. (1976) The role of nonclassical, Fc associated, Ag-B antigens (Ia) in rate allograft enhancement. *J. exp. Med.* **143**: 405–421.

SPIEGELBERG, H. L. and WEIGLE, W. O. (1965) The catabolism of homologous and heterologous 7S gamma-globulin fragments. *J. exp. Med.* **121**: 323–333.

SPRENT, J. and LEFKOVITS, I. (1976) Effect of recent antigen priming on adoptive immune responses. IV. Antigen-induced selective recruitment of recirculating lymphocytes to the spleen demonstrable with a microculture system. *J. exp. Med.* **143**: 1289–1298.

SPRENT, J. and MILLER, J. F. A. P. (1971) Activation of thymus cells by histocompatibility antigens. *Nature New Biol.* **234**: 195–198.

SPRENT, J. and MILLER, J. F. A. P. (1972) Interaction of thymus lymphocytes with histoincompatible cells. II. Recirculating lymphocytes derived from antigen-activated thymus cells. *Cell. Immunol.* **3**: 385–404.

SPRENT, J. and MILLER, J. F. A. P. (1974) Effect of recent antigen priming on adoptive immune responses. II. Specific unresponsiveness of circulating lymphocytes from mice primed with heterologous erythrocytes. *J. exp. Med.* **139**: 1–12.

SPRENT, J. and MILLER, J. F. A. P. (1976) Effect of recent antigen priming on adoptive immune responses. III. Antigen-induced selective recruitment of subsets of recirculating lymphocytes reactive to H-2 determinants. *J. exp. Med.* **143**: 585–600.

SPRENT, J. and VON BOEHMER, H. (1976) Helper function of T cells depleted of alloantigen-reactive lymphocytes by filtration through irradiated F_1 hybrid recipients. I. Failure to collaborate with allogeneic B cells in a secondary response to sheep erythrocytes measured *in vivo*. *J. exp. Med.* **144**: 617–626.

STAINES, N. A., GUY, K. and DAVIES, D. A. L. (1975) The dominant role of Ia antibodies in the passive enhancement of H-2 incompatible skin grafts *Eur. J. Immunol.* **5**: 782–789.

STERN, K., DAVIDSON, I. and MASAITIS, L. (1956) Experimental studies on Rh immunization. *Am. J. clin. Path.* **26**: 833–843.

STILLER, C. R., SINCLAIR, N. R. STC., ABRAHAMS, S., MCGIRR, D., SINGH, H., HOWSON, W. T. and ULAN, R. A. (1976) Anti-donor immune responses in prediction of transplant rejection. *New Engl. J. Med.* **294**: 978–982.

STILLER, C. R., DOSSETOR, J. B., CARPENTER, C. B. and MYBURGH, J. A. (1977) Immunologic monitoring of the transplant recipient. *Transplant. Proc.* **9**: 1245–1254.

STOUT, R. D. and HERZENBERG, L. A. (1975a) The Fc receptor on thymus-derived lymphocytes. I. Detection of a subpopulation of murine T lymphocytes bearing the Fc receptor. *J. exp. Med.* **142**: 611–621.

STOUT, R. D. and HERZENBERG, L. A. (1975b) The Fc receptor on thymus-derived lymphocytes. II. Mitogen responsiveness of T lymphocytes bearing the Fc receptor. *J. exp. Med.* **142**: 1041–1051.

STOUT, R. D., WAKSAL, S. D. and HERZENBERG, L. A. (1976) The Fc receptor on thymus-derived lymphocytes. III. Mixed lymphocyte reactivity and cell-mediated lympholytic activity of Fc^- and Fc^+ lymphocytes. *J. exp. Med.* **144**: 54–68.

STOUT, R. D., MURPHY, D. B., MCDEVITT, H. O. and HERZENBERG, L. A. (1977) The Fc receptor on thymus-derived lymphocytes. IV. Inhibition of binding of antigen-antibody complexes to Fc^+ T cells by anti-Ia antisera. *J. exp. Med.* **145**: 187–203.

STRAYER, D. S., COSENZA, H., LEE, W. M. F., ROWLEY, D. A. and KÖHLER, H. (1974) Neonatal tolerance induced by antibody against antigen-specific receptor. *Science, Wash.* **186**: 640–643.

STREJAN, G. H., RABHERU, K., WHITE, R. and SURLAN, D. (1977) Reaginic antibody production to Ascaris suum allergen, ASC-1. II. Influence of type of adjuvant and of carrier priming on the induction of IgE and IgG antibodies to dinitrophenyl conjugates. *Int. Archs. Allergy. appl. Immunol.* **54**: 502–516.

STROM, T. B., CARPENTER, C. B., GAROVOY, M. R., ABBAS, A. K., CARSON, J. M., BEAR, R. A. and SOULILLOU, J. P. (1975) Modification of the rat alloimmune response by enhancing antibodies and the role of blocking factors in the survival of renal grafts. *Transplantation* **20**: 368–380.

STUART, F. P., MCKEARN, T. J. and FITCH, F. W. (1976a) Immunological enhancement of renal allografts by antireceptor antibody. *Surgery* **80**: 130–136.

STUART, F. P., SCOLLARD, D. M., MCKEARN, T. J. and FITCH, F. W. (1976b) Cellular and humoral immunity after allogeneic renal transplantation in the rat. V. Appearance of antiidiotypic antibody and its relationship to cellular immunity after treatment with donor spleen cells and alloantibody. *Transplantation* **22**: 455–466.

TADA, T., TANIGUCHI, M. and OKUMURA, K. (1971) Regulation of homocytotropic antibody formation in the rat. II. Effect of X-irradiation. *J. Immunol.* **106**: 1012–1018.

TADA, T., TANIGUCHI, M. and TAKEMORI, T. (1975) Properties of primed suppressor T cells and their products. *Transplant. Rev.* **26**: 106–129.

TADA, T., TANIGUCHI, M. and DAVID, C. S. (1976) Properties of the antigen-specific suppressive T-cell factor in the regulation of antibody response of the mouse. IV. Special subregion assignment of the gene(s) that codes for the suppressive T-cell factor in the H-2 histocompatibility complex. *J. exp. Med.* **144**: 713–725.

Takasugi, M. and Hildemann, W. H. (1969a) Regulation of immunity toward allogeneic tumors in mice. I. Effect of antiserum fractions on tumor growth. *J. natn. Cancer. Inst.* **43**: 843–856.

Takasugi, M. and Hildemann, W. H. (1969b) Regulation of immunity toward allogeneic tumors in mice. II. Effect of antiserum and antiserum fractions on cellular and humoral response. *J. natn. Cancer. Inst.* **43**: 857–867.

Takasugi, M. and Klein, E. (1971) The role of blocking antibodies in immunological enhancement. *Immunology* **21**: 675–684.

Tamerius, J., Nepom, J., Hellström, I. and Hellström, K. E. (1976) Tumor-associated blocking factors: isolation from sera of tumor-bearing mice. *J. Immunol.* **116**: 724–730.

Taniguchi, M. and Tada, T. (1971) Regulation of homocytotropic antibody formation in the rat. IV. Effects of various immunosuppressive drugs. *J. Immunol.* **107**: 579–585.

Taniguchi, M., Tada, T. and Tokuhisa, T. (1976) Properties of the antigen-specific suppressive T-cell factor in the regulation of antibody response of the mouse. III. Dual gene control of the T-cell-mediated suppression of the antibody response. *J. exp. Med.* **144**: 20–31.

Tao, T. W. and Uhr, J. W. (1966) Capacity of pepsin-digested antibody to inhibit antibody formation. *Nature, Lond.* **212**: 208–209.

Taussig, M. J. and Munroe, A. J. (1974) Removal of specific cooperative T cell factor by anti-H-2 but not by anti-Ig sera. *Nature, Lond.* **251**: 63–65.

Taussig, M. J., Munro, A. J., Campbell, R., David, C. S. and Staines, N. A. (1975) Antigen-specific T-cell factor in cell cooperation. Mapping within the I region of the H-2 complex and ability to cooperate across allogeneic barriers. *J. exp. Med.* **142**: 694–700.

Taylor, B., Norman, A. P., Orge, H. A., Stokes, C. R., Turner, M. W. and Soothill, J. F. (1973) Transient IgA deficiency and pathogenesis of infantile atopy. *Lancet* **ii**: 111–113.

Taylor, R. B. (1969) Cellular cooperation in the antibody response of mice to two serum albumins: specific function of thymus cells. *Transplant. Rev.* **1**: 114–149.

Taylor, R. B. and Basten, A. (1976) Suppressor cells in humoral immunity and tolerance. *Br. med. Bull.* **32**: 152–157.

Taylor, R. B. and Wortis, H. H. (1968) Thymus dependence of antibody response: variation with dose of antigen and class of antibody. *Nature, Lond.* **220**: 927–928.

Terman, D. S., Minden, P. and Crowle, A. J. (1973) Adoptive transfer of neonatally induced tolerance into normal mice. *Cell. Immunol.* **6**: 284–291.

Tew, J. G., Greene, E. J. and Makoski, M. H. (1976) *In vitro* evidence indicating a role for the Fc region of IgG in the mechanism for the long-term maintenance and regulation of antibody levels *in vivo*. *Cell. Immunol.* **26**: 141–152.

Thomas, D. W. and Shevach, E. M. (1976) Nature of the antigenic complex recognized by T lymphocytes. I. Analysis with an *in vitro* primary response to soluble protein antigens. *J. exp. Med.* **144**: 1263–1273.

Thompson, D. M. P. (1975) Soluble tumour-specific antigen and its relationship to tumour growth. *Int. J. Cancer* **15**: 1016–1029.

Thorsby, E., Bondevik, H. and Solheim, B. G. (1973) The inhibitory effect of HL-A antibodies on lymphocyte transformation *in vitro*. *Transplant. Proc.* **5**: 343–348.

Tizard, I. R. (1969) Macrophage cytophilic antibody in mice. *Int. Archs. Allergy appl. Immunol.* **36**: 332–346.

Tizard, I. R. (1972) Elution of macrophage-bound immunoglobulins by temperature changes *in vitro*. *Immunology* **22**: 69–73.

Torrigiani, G. (1972) Quantitative estimation of antibody in the immunoglobulin classes of the mouse. II. Thymic dependence of the different classes. *J. Immunol.* **108**: 161–164.

Trinchieri, G., Bernoco, D., Curtoni, S. E., Miggiano, U. C. and Ceppellini, R. (1972) Cell-mediated lympholysis in man: relevance of HL-A antigens and antibodies. In: *Histocompatibility Testing*, pp. 509–519, Dausset, J. (ed). Munksgaard, Copenhagen.

Uhr, J. W. (1965) Passive sensitization of lymphocytes and macrophages by antigen-antibody complexes. *Proc. natn. Acad. Sci. U.S.A.* **54**: 1599–1606.

Uhr, J. W. and Baumann, J. B. (1961) Antibody formation. I. The suppression of antibody formation by passively administered antibody. *J. exp. Med.* **113**: 935–957.

Uhr, J. W. and Möller, G. (1968) Regulation of effect of antibody on the immune response. *Adv. Immunol.* **8**: 81–127.

Unanue, E. R. (1972) The regulatory role of macrophages in antigenic stimulation. *Adv. Immunol.* **15**: 95–165.

Unanue, E. R. and Abbas, A. K. (1975) Relationship on the B cell surface of immunoglobulin, Fc receptors and histocompatibility antigen. In: *Membrane Receptors of Lymphocytes*, pp. 281–285, Seligmann, M., Preud'homme, J. L. and Kourilsky, F. M. (eds). Proceedings of the International Symposium on Membrane Receptors of Lymphocytes held in Paris, 1975 (INSERM Symposium 1). American Elsevier, New York.

Unanue, E. R. and Askonas, B. A. (1968) Persistence of immunogenicity of antigen after uptake by macrophages. *J. exp. Med.* **127**: 915–926.

Unanue, E. R. and Cerottini, J. C. (1970) The immunogenicity of antigen bound to the plasma membrane of macrophages. *J. exp. Med.* **131**: 711–725.

Vadas, M. A., Miller, J. F. A. P., McKenzie, I. F. C., Chism, S. E., Shen, F-W. Boyse, E. A., Gamble, J. R. and Whitelaw, A. M. (1976) Ly and Ia antigen phenotypes of T cells involved in delayed-type hypersensitivity and in suppression. *J. exp. Med.* **144**: 10–19.

Valentova, V., Cerny, J. and Ivanyi, J. (1966) The characterization of the immunological memory of the IgM type of response in chickens. *Folia Biol. Prague* **12**: 207–211.

van Boxel, J. A. and Rosenstreich, D. L. (1974) Binding of aggregated γ-globulin to activated T lymphocytes in the guinea pig. *J. exp. Med.* **139**: 1002–1012.

VITETTA, E. S. and UHR, J. W. (1972) Cell surface immunoglobulin. V. Release from murine splenic lymphocytes. *J. exp. Med.* **136**: 676–696.

VITETTA, E. S., BAUR, S. and UHR, J. W. (1971) Cell surface immunoglobulin. II. Isolation and characterization of immunoglobulin from mouse splenic lymphocytes. *J. exp. Med.* **134**: 242–264.

VITETTA, E. S., CAMBIER, J. C., LIGLER, F. S., KETTMAN, J. R. and UHR, J. W. (1977) B-cell tolerance. IV. Differential role of surface IgM and IgD in determining tolerance susceptibility of murine B cells. *J. exp. Med.* **146**: 1804–1808.

VOISIN, G. A. (1971) Immunological facilitation, a broadening of the concept of the enhancement phenomenon. *Prog. Allergy* **15**: 328–485.

VOISIN, G. A. (1976) Biological roles of rodent anaphylactic IgG_1 antibodies. *Agents, Actions* **6**: 5–15.

VOISON, G. A., KINSKY, R. G., JANSEN, F. and BERNARD, C. (1969) Biological properties of antibody classes in transplantation immune sera. *Transplantation* **8**: 618–632.

VOISON, G. A., KINSKY, R. G. and DUC, H. T. (1972) Immune status of mice tolerant of living cells. II. Continuous presence and nature of facilitation-enhancing antibodies in tolerant animals. *J. exp. Med.* **135**: 1185–1203.

VON BOEHMER, H. and SPRENT, J. (1976) T cell function in bone marrow chimeras: absence of host-reactive T cells and cooperation of helper T cells across allogeneic barriers. *Transplant. Proc.* **29**: 3–23.

VON BOEHMER, H., HUDSON, L. and SPRENT, J. (1975) Collaboration of histoincompatible T and B lymphocytes using Cells from tetraparental bone marrow chimeras. *J. exp. Med.* **142**: 989–997.

VUAGNAT, P., NEVEU, T. and VOISON, G. A. (1973a) Immunodeviation by passive antibody, an expression of selective immunodepression. I. Action of guinea pig IgG1 and IgG2 anti-hapten antibodies. *Eur. J. Immunol.* **3**: 90–95.

VUAGNAT, P. and VILAIN, C. (1975) Differential effects of antibody classes on the expression of delayed hypersensitivity. *Transplant. Proc.* **7**: 431–433.

VUAGNAT, P., NEVEU, T. and NOISON, G. A. (1973b) Immunodeviation by passive antibody, an expression of selective immunodepression. II. Action of guinea pig IgG1 and IgG2 anti-carrier antibodies. *J. exp. Med.* **137**: 265–274.

WAGNER, H. (1972) The correlation between the proliferative and the cytotoxic responses of mouse lymphocytes to allogeneic cells *in vitro*. *J. Immunol.* **109**: 630–637.

WAGNER, H. (1973) Synergy during *in vitro* cyclotoxic allograft responses. I. Evidence for cell interaction between thymocytes and peripheral T cells. *J. exp. Med.* **138**: 1379–1397.

WAGNER, H., GOTZE, D., PTSCHELINZEW, L. and ROLLINGHOFF, M. (1975a) Induction of cytotoxic T lymphocytes against I-region-coded determinants: *in vitro* evidence for a third histocompatibility locus in the mouse. *J. exp. Med.* **142**: 1477–1487.

WAGNER, H., HÄMMERLING, G. and ROLLINGHOFF, M. (1975b) Enhanced *in vitro* cytotoxic anti-H-2 responses in the presence of Ia antigens. *Immunogenetics* **2**: 257–268.

WALDMANN, H., POPE, H. and MUNROE, A. J. (1976) Cooperation across the histocompatibility barrier: $H\text{-}2^d$ T cells primed to antigen in an $H\text{-}2^d$ environment can cooperate with $H\text{-}2^k$ B cells. *J. exp. Med.* **144**: 1707–1711.

WARNER, N. L. (1974) Membrane immunoglobulin and antigen receptors on B and T lymphocytes. *Adv. Immunol.* **19**: 67–216.

WARNER, N. L., HARRIS, A. W. and GUTMAN, G. A. (1975) Membrane immunoglobulin and Fc receptors of murine T and B cell lymphomas. In: *Membrane Receptors of Lymphocytes*, pp. 203–216, SELIGMANN, M., PREUD'HOMME, J. L. and KOURILSKY, F. M. (eds). Proceedings of the International Symposium on Membrane Receptors of Lymphocytes held in Paris, 1975 (INSERM Symposium 1). American Elsevier, New York.

WASON, W. M. (1973) Regulation of the immune response with antigen specific IgM antibody; a dual role. *J. Immunol.* **110**: 1245–1252.

WASON, W. M. and FITCH, F. W. (1973) Suppression of the antibody response to SRBC with $F(ab')_2$ and IgG *in vitro*. *J. Immunol.* **110**: 1427–1429.

WEBB, S. R. and COOPER, M. D. (1973) T cells can bind antigen via cytophilic IgM antibody made by B cells. *J. Immunol.* **111**: 275–277.

WEIGLE, W. O. (1971) Recent observations and concepts in immunological unresponsiveness and autoimmunity. *Clin. exp. Immunol.* **9**: 437–477.

WEIGLE, W. O. (1973) Immunological unresponsiveness. *Adv. Immunol.* **16**: 61–122.

WEIGLE, W. O., CHILLER, J. M. and HABICHT, G. S. (1973) Effect of immunological unresponsiveness on different cell populations. *Transplant. Rev.* **8**: 3–25.

WEIGLE, W. O., CHILLER, J. M. and LOUIS, J. A. (1974) Tolerance: central unresponsiveness or peripheral inhibition. In: *Progress in Immunology II*, Vol. 3, pp. 187–196, BRENT, L. and HOLOBOROW, J. (eds). Proceedings of the Second International Congress of Immunology, Brighton, U.K., July, 1974. North-Holland, Amsterdam–Oxford.

WEINSTEIN, Y., MELMON, K. L., BOURNE, H. R. and SELA, M. (1973) Specific leukocyte receptor for small endogenous hormones. Detection by cells binding to insolubilized hormone preparations. *J. clin. Invest.* **52**: 1349–1361.

WEKERLE, H., ESHHAR, Z., LONAI, P. and FELDMAN, M. (1975) Thymus-derived rat lymphocyte receptor for cell surface antigen is a nonseriologically defined product of the major histocompatibility gene complex. *Proc. natn. Acad. Sci. U.S.A.* **72**: 1147–1151.

WILSON, D. B. and NOWELL, P. C. (1970) Quantitative studies on the mixed lymphocyte interaction in rats. IV. Immunologic potentiality of the responding cells. *J. exp. Med.* **131**: 391–407.

WILSON, D. B., HOWARD, J. C. and NOWELL, P. C. (1972) Some biological aspects of lymphocytes reactive to strong histocompatibility alloantigens. *Transplant. Rev.* **12**: 3–29.

WILSON, J. D. (1971) The relationships of antibody-forming cells to rossette-forming cells. *Immunology* **21**: 233–235.

WILSON, J. D. and MILLER, J. F. A. P. (1971) T and B. rossette-forming cells. *Eur. J. Immunol.* **1**: 501–503.

Wright, P. W., Hargreaves, R. E., Bansal, S. C., Bernstein, I. D. and Hellström, K. E. (1973) Allograft tolerance: presumptive evidence that serum factors from tolerant animals that block lymphocyte mediated immunity *in vitro* are soluble antigen-antibody complexes. *Proc. natn. Acad. Sci. U.S.A.* **70**: 2539–2543.

Wright, P. W., Bernstein, I. D., Hamilton, B., Gluckman, J. C. and Hellström, K. E. (1974a) Cell-mediated reactivity and serum blocking activity in tolerant rats. Studies on ten rats operationally tolerant to skin allografts using several independent assays. *Transplantation* **18**: 46–55.

Wright, P. W., Hargreaves, R. E., Bernstein, I. D. and Hellström, I. (1974b) Fractionation of sera from operationally tolerant rats by DEAE cellulose chromatography: evidence that serum blocking factors are associated with IgG. *J. Immunol.* **112**: 1267–1270.

Yamashita, U., Takami, T. and Kitagawa, M. (1975) Induction of anti-hapten antibody response by hapten-isologous carrier conjugate. II. Specificity of hapten-reactive helper T cells. *Cell. Immunol.* **18**: 396–410.

Yamashita, U., Takami, T., Hamaoka, T. and Kitagawa, M. (1976a) The role of hapten-reactive T lymphocytes in the induction of autoimmunity in mice. I. Establishment of the experimental conditions for the termination of immunological tolerance to human gamma globulin. *Cell. Immunol.* **25**: 15–31.

Yamashita, U., Takami, T., Hamaoka, T. and Kitagawa, M. (1976b) The role of hapten-reactive T lymphocytes in the induction of autoimmunity mice. II. Termination of self-tolerance to erythrocytes by immunization with hapten-isologous erythrocytes. *Cell. Immunol.* **25**: 32–40.

Yasmeen, D., Ellerson, J. R., Dorrington, K. J. and Painter, R. H. (1973) Evidence for the domain hypothesis: location of the site of cytophilic activity toward guinea pig macrophage in the CH_3 homology region of human immunoglobulin G. *J. Immunol.* **110**: 1706–1709.

Yoshida, T. O. and Andersson, B. (1972) Evidence for a receptor recognizing antigen complexed immunoglobulin on the surface of activated mouse thymus lymphocytes. *Scand. J. Immunol.* **1**: 401–408.

Yuan, L., Garvey, J. S. and Campbell, D. H. (1970) Molecular forms of antigen in the circulation following immunization. *Immunochemistry* **7**: 601–618.

Zan-Bar, I., Nachtigal, D. and Feldman, M. (1976) Studies on suppressor T cells in tolerance. *Adv. exp. Med. Biol.* **66**: 585–592.

Zimmerman, B. and Feldman, J. D. (1969) Enhancing antibody. I. Bioassay for normal skin grafts. *J. Immunol.* **102**: 507–512.

Zimmerman, B. and Feldman, F. D. (1970) Enhancing antibody. III. Site of activity. *J. Immunol.* **104**: 626–632.

Zinkernagel, R. M. (1976) H-2 restriction of virus-specific T-cell-mediated effector functions *in vivo*. II. Adoptive transfer of delayed-type hypersensitivity to murine lymphocytic chromiomeningitis virus is restricted by the K and D region of H-2. *J. exp. Med.* **144**: 776–787.

Zinkernagel, R. M. and Doherty, P. C. (1975) H-2 compatibility requirement for T-cell-mediated lysis of target cells infected with lymphocytic choriomeningitis virus. Different cytotoxic T-cell specificities are associated with structures coded for in H-2K or H-2D. *J. exp. Med.* **141**: 1427–1436.

Zinkernagel, R. M. and Doherty, P. C. (1977) Major transplantation antigens, viruses, and specificity of surveillance T cells. *Contemp. Topics Immunobiol.* **7**: 179–220.

CHAPTER 4

MODULATION OF IMMUNITY BY SOLUBLE MEDIATORS

BYRON H. WAKSMAN

National Multiple Sclerosis Society, New York, USA

1. INTRODUCTION

Most or all immunologically active cells appear to make and release soluble products other than antibody and transfer factor (both discussed elsewhere in the present volume). These affect the outcome of immune reactions, whether to infectious agents, to tissue or tumor antigens, or to autoantigens. They are known as 'cytokines' or more specifically as 'lymphokines' (LK), for products of activated lymphocytes, and 'monokines' (MK), for macrophage products. There is no generally accepted classification of cytokines active in immunity. However a broad distinction may be made between factors whose production is governed by MHC (major histocompatibility complex) genes and those which are not. These may have originated by evolution, on the one hand, from specific recognition factors in the cellular plasma membrane and, on the other, from products of tissue injury.

2. CLASSIFICATION OF MK, LK AND OTHER CYTOKINES

So-called specific factors (specific immunoregulatory MK and LK) possess the ability to bind antigen specifically—indeed some appear to function biologically as a complex with antigen (Table 1). These react only with a restricted range of target lymphocytes bearing the same MHC antigens as the donor. The genes which control production of these factors lie in the I region of MHC, I-A for helper factors (Erb and Feldmann, 1975a, b; Taussig *et al.*, 1975; Taussig and Munro, 1976), and I-J for

TABLE 1. *Specific Mediators, Restricted by MHC*

Factors	MK/LK/Other	References
Helper		
GRF (genetically restricted factor)	MK	Erb and Feldmann, 1975a, b; Erb *et al.*, 1976a, b
'IgT'	LK	Feldmann, 1972; Feldman and Basten, 1972a; Gisler *et al.*, 1973
Helper factor for IgE	LK	Taniguchi and Tada, 1974; Kishimoto and Ishizaka, 1973, 1974, 1975
Antigen-specific T-cell factor	LK	Munro *et al.*, 1974; Marrack and Kappler, 1975; Taussig and Munro, 1976
Antigen-specific TRF	LK	Kirov and Parish, 1976
TF (transfer factor)	LK	Lawrence, 1974; Ascher *et al.*, 1976
Suppressor		
'Ig T'	LK	Feldmann, 1974a, b
Antigen-specific suppressive T-cell factor	LK	Takemori and Tada, 1975; Taniguchi *et al.*, 1976a, b; Tada *et al.*, 1976a; Tada, 1976
IgE suppressor factor	LK	Tada *et al.*, 1973; Okumura and Tada, 1974; Kishimoto and Ishizaka, 1974, 1975
Allotype suppression factor	LK	Jacobson, 1973
Soluble suppressor of contact sensitivity	LK	Zembala and Asherson, 1974; Asherson *et al.*, 1976
Immunosuppressive factor (GAT)	LK	Kapp *et al.*, 1976, 1977
Tumor-specific blocking factor		Nepom *et al.*, 1976
Acting on macrophages		
SMAF (specific macrophage arming factor)	LK	Granger and Weiser, 1964, 1966; Evans and Alexander, 1972; Evans and Grant, 1972; Evans *et al.*, 1972; Grant *et al.*, 1972
Antigen-dependent MIF	LK	Švejcar *et al.*, 1968; Hochová *et al.*, 1975

suppressor factor (Taniguchi *et al.*, 1976b; Tada *et al.*, 1976a, b). The specific receptors on appropriate target cells are governed by genes closely linked with those controlling production of the factor, in each case (Tada *et al.*, 1976a, b). The adaptive value of such linkage during evolution, is apparent. The function of specific helper and suppressor factors is to regulate the immune response. One specific factor is also recognized at present that 'arms' macrophages, rendering them cytotoxic for tumor or other cells bearing the specific antigen; others may yet be found, such as 'antigen-specific MIF'.

Two classes of immunoregulatory molecules are recognized which appear not to have specificity for antigen, though governed by MHC genes (Table 2). AEF and the MLR suppressor factor are released in response to stimulation with I region gene products, and bind to receptors with I region specificity like that governing production of the factor, (I-A and I-C respectively). The second case involves certain complement components, which specifically recognize particular immunoglobulin domains, other components of the complement cascade, or unidentified cell membrane components. These are controlled by the S subregion of the MHC.

Most nonspecific factors do not bind antigen and have not so far been found to show any MHC restrictions. In addition to nonspecific immunoregulatory MK and LK, which act on lymphocytes, (Tables 3a and 3b), there is a large group of lymphokines with the power to mobilize and activate different inflammatory cells, i.e. macrophages, neutrophils, eosinophils and basophils, as well as lymphocytes and fibroblasts, at sites of inflammation (Table 3c). Others promote inflammation by an action on vascular endothelium or on the thermoregulatory center of the brain. Still others stimulate proliferation of these same cells, either at local sites or in their tissue of origin, i.e. bone marrow.

A variety of mediators act directly to kill or inhibit proliferation of target cells (Table 3d). Normal or neoplastic tissues or indeed protozoan or metazoan parasites may serve as targets for these factors.

The factors listed in Tables 1–3 are without exception proteins or glycoproteins or, in some instances, smaller polypeptides. Attention should be called to certain other types of molecules released by macrophages or lymphocytes which may also play a role, particularly in immunoregulation. Among these are: DNA fragments, which have been shown to be released from stimulated lymphocytes and to enhance T-cell functions in particular (Braun and Nakano, 1965; Cone and Johnson, 1972; Hamaoka and Katz, 1973; Rogers *et al.*, 1972; Sarma and Zubroff, 1973; Olsen and Harris, 1974; Rogers, 1976; Hoessli *et al.*, 1977; Mutchnick *et al.*, 1977); RNA with an attached fragment of antigen, released from macrophages (Rittenberg and Nelson, 1960; Fishman, 1961; Friedman *et al.*, 1965; Askonas and Rhodes, 1965; Cohen *et al.*, 1965; Bell and Dray, 1971; Gottlieb and Waldmann, 1972) and prostaglandins (Lykke *et al.*, 1967; Moncada *et al.*, 1973; Williams and Morley, 1973; Webb *et al.*, 1977; Webb and Oppenheim in First International Workshop, 1976); cyclic nucleotides (Whitfield *et al.*,

TABLE 2. *Nonspecific Mediators, Restricted by MHC*

Factors	MK/LK/Other	References
Helper		
AEF (allogeneic effect factor)	LK	Armerding and Katz, 1974; Armerding *et al.*, 1974
Specific autostimulatory factor	LK	Powles *et al.*, 1971
Complement components	MK, other	Havemann *et al.*, 1970; Forsdyke, 1973; Milthorp and Forsdyke, 1973
Suppressor		
MLR suppressor factor	LK	Rich and Rich, 1974, 1975, 1976a, b
Low MW Ia	MK?	McKenzie and Parish, 1976; Parish *et al.*, 1976
Complement components	MK, other	Havemann *et al.*, 1970; Forsdyke, 1973; Milthorp and Forsdyke, 1973

TABLE 3a. *Nonspecific Factors, Unrestricted by MHC*

Factors	MK/LK/Other	References
Helper		
LAF (lymphocyte activating factor)	MK	Bach, *et al.*, 1970; Hoffman and Dutton, 1971; Gery *et al.*, 1971, 1972
NMF (normal macrophage factor)	MK	Erb and Feldmann, 1975a, b
BAF (B-cell activating factor)	MK	Schrader, 1973; Wood and Gaul, 1974; Wood and Cameron, 1975, 1976
TRF (T-cell replacing factor)	MK?	Watson, 1973
MP (mitogenic protein)	MK	Beller, 1977
TDF (thymus differentiation factor)	MK	Beller and Unanue, 1977
Transferrin	MK	Tormey and Mueller, 1972; Haurani *et al.*, 1973
MF (mitogenic or blastogenic factor)	LK	Kasakura and Lowenstein, 1965; Feldmann and Basten, 1972b; Wolstencroft and Dumonde, 1970; Falk *et al.*, 1970, 1972; Doria *et al.*, 1972
NSF (nonspecific factor)	LK	Waldmann and Munro, 1973, 1974; Waldmann 1975; Waldman *et al.*, 1976
TRF (T-cell replacing factor)	LK	Rubin and Coons, 1972a, b; Schimpl and Wecker, 1972; Askonas *et al.*, 1974; Gorczynski *et al.*, 1973b; Marrack and Kappler, 1975, 1976
TDEF (T-cell-derived enhancing factor)	LK	Alevy and Battisto, 1976a, b
TEF (thymus extract factor)	LK	Armerding and Katz, 1975
Complement components	MK, only	Havemann *et al.*, 1970a, b; Forsdyke, 1973a, b, c; Milthorp and Forsdyke, 1973
DSRF (deficient serum restoring factor)	spleen cells	Watson and Thomas, 1972
Fetuin	other	Hsu *et al.*, 1973

TABLE 3b. *Nonspecific Factors, Unrestricted by MHC*

Factors	MK/LK/Other	References
Suppressor		
Inhibitor(s) of DNA synthesis	MK	Waldman and Gottlieb, 1973; Nelson, 1973; Calderon *et al.*, 1974
AIM (antibody inhibitory material)	LK	Ambrose, 1969, 1975
IDS (inhibitor of DNA synthesis)	LK	Smith *et al.*, 1970; Green *et al.*, 1974; Namba and Waksman, 1975a; Thomas *et al.*, 1975a, b
LIF (lymphoblastogenesis inhibition factor)	LK	Han *et al.*, 1975
FIF (feedback inhibition factor)	LK	Dwyer and Kantor, 1973, 1975; Outteridge and Lepper, 1973
SIRS (soluble immune response suppressor)	LK	Rich and Pierce, 1974; Tadakuma *et al.*, 1976
LIFT (lymphocyte inhibiting factor-thymus)	LK	Kiger *et al.*, 1971, 1973; Florentin *et al.*, 1973, 1976
IRA (immunoregulatory α-globulin)	LK, other?	Mowbray, 1963; Kamrin, 1959; Mannick and Schmid, 1967; Carpenter *et al.*, 1971; Cooperband *et al.*, 1972
'Chalones' (extracted, released)	LK	Houck *et al.*, 1971, 1973a, 1976; Garcia-Giralt and Macieira-Coelho, 1974
IF (interferon)	MK, LK, other[a]	Gisler *et al.*, 1974; Blomgren *et al.*, 1974; Brodeur and Merigan, 1974, 1975
AFP (α-fetoprotein, feutin)	other	Mendelsohn *et al.*, 1971; Murgita and Tomasi, 1975a, b; Yachnin, 1975
LDL (low density lipoprotein)	?	Curtiss and Edgington, 1976; Curtiss *et al.*, 1977
CRP (C-reactive protein)	other[a]	Oishi *et al.*, 1973; Mortensen *et al.*, 1975; Mortensen and Gewurz, 1976
Fibrinogen degradation products	?	Girman *et al.*, 1976
NIP (normal immunosuppressive protein)	?	Havemann *et al.*, 1970; Nelken, 1973; Veit and Michael, 1973; Nelson and Schneider, 1974
LMWS (low MW suppressor)	?	Ranney and Steinberg, 1976
HSF (histamine-induced suppressor factor)	other	Rocklin, 1977

[a]Production after viral infection, cell injury.

TABLE 3c. *Nonspecific Factors, Unrestricted by MHC*

Factors	MK/LK/Other	References
Acting on Inflammatory Cells		
MCF (monocyte chemotactic factor)	LK	Ward *et al.*, 1969, 1970; Rühl *et al.*, 1974
MIF (migration inhibitory factor)	LK, other[a]	David, 1966; Bloom and Bennett, 1966; Bennett and Bloom, 1968
MSF (macrophage slowing factor)	LK	Carnegie *et al.*, 1973
MEF (migration enhancement factor)	LK	Weisbart *et al.*, 1974
MAF (macrophage aggregation factor)	LK	Lolekha *et al.*, 1970; Douglas *et al.*, 1972; Gotoff and Vizral, 1972; Galindo *et al.*, 1975
MAF (macrophage activation factor)	LK	Mooney and Waksman, 1970; Patterson and Youmans, 1970; Nathan *et al.*, 1971, 1973; Simon and Sheagren 1971, 1972a, b; Godal *et al.*, 1971; Krahenbuhl and Remington, 1971
MFF (macrophage fusion factor)	LK	Galindo, 1972; Galindo *et al.*, 1974
OAF (osteoclast activation factor)	LK	Horton *et al.*, 1974; Chen *et al.*, 1976
PRS (pyrogen releasing substance)	LK	Atkins *et al.*, 1972
LIF (leukocyte inhibition factor)	LK	Ward *et al.*, 1970; Søberg, 1970; Clausen, 1971, 1972; Rocklin, 1974; Chess *et al.*, 1975; Lomnitzer *et al.*, 1975
Leukotactic factor	LK	Ward *et al.*, 1970
PAR (products of antigenic recognition)	LK	Ramseier, 1969; Warrington *et al.*, 1976
BCF (basophil chemotactic factor)	LK	Boetcher and Leonard, 1973; Ward *et al.*, 1975; Lett-Brown *et al.*, 1976
ECF (eosinophil chemotactic factor)	LK	Torisu *et al.*, 1973; Hirashima *et al.*, 1976
ESP (eosinophil stimulation promoter)	LK	Colley, 1973, 1976
LCF (lymphocyte chemotactic factor)	LK	Ward *et al.*, 1971
Lymphocyte trapping factor	LK	Curtis and de Sousa, 1973
Fibroblast chemotactic factor	LK?	Postlethwaite *et al.*, 1976
Acting on vascular endothelium		
SRF (skin-reactive factor)	LK	Bennett and Bloom, 1968; Schwartz *et al.*, 1970; Pick *et al.*, 1969, 1970a, b; Maillard *et al.*, 1972
TPF (thymic permeability factor)	LK	Lykke *et al.*, 1967
LNPF (LN permeability factor)	LK	Willoughby *et al.*, 1963, 1964; Spector and Willoughby, 1964
LN activating factors	LK	Kelly *et al.*, 1972; Korčaková *et al.*, 1975
AIPF (anaphylactoid inflammation-promoting factor)	LK	Koltai, 1975
Pyrogens	MK, Other	Johanovsky *et al.*, 1962; Hahn *et al.*, 1967; Siegert *et al.*, 1967; Atkins and Bodel, 1972
Growth Stimulating		
MGF (macrophage growth factor)	MK, Other	Moore, 1976; Stanley *et al.*, 1976
MF (mitogenic or blastogenic factor)	LK	Kasakura and Lowenstein, 1965; Wolstencroft and Dumonde, 1970; Falk *et al.*, 1970, 1972; Feldman and Basten, 1972b; Doria *et al.*, 1972
LIAF (lymphocyte-induced angiogenesis factor)	LK	Sidky and Auerbach, 1975
CSF (colony stimulating factor)	MK, LK, Other	Chervenick and Lo Buglio, 1972; Golde and Cline, 1972; Moore *et al.*, 1973; Cerny, 1974
TDF (thymus differentiation factor)	MK	Beller and Unanne, 1977
Thymopoietin, thymosin	Other	Wolstenholme and Knight, eds., 1970; Friedman, ed., 1975

[a]Production after viral infection, cell injury.

1971; Bach and Bach, 1973; Watson *et al.*, 1973; Bourne *et al.*, 1974; Kook and Trainin, 1974; Watson, 1975b); and histamine (Bourne *et al.*, 1974).

I have chosen to limit my list of mediators to those that are either produced by immunologically active cells or act upon them. However these limits are necessarily arbitrary. Thus many hormones of the pituitary, thyroid and adrenal cortex affect lymphoid organ development (Wolstenhome and Knight, eds., 1970), just as hormone(s) produced by the thymus (epithelium) and thymic macrophages affect T-cell maturation at a more intimate level (Friedman, ed., 1975; Armerding and Katz,

TABLE 3d. *Nonspecific Factors, Unrestricted by MHC*

Factors	MK/LK/Other	References
Direct Action		
Lysosomal enzymes	MK	Cohn and Wiener, 1963; Davies and Allison, 1976
CTF (cytotoxic factor(s))	MK	Pincus, 1967a, b, c; Sintek and Pincus, 1970; Pincus *et al.*, 1970, 1971
MTF (macrophage toxic factor)	MK	Heise and Weiser, 1969; Kramer and Granger, 1972
SMC (specific macrophage cytotoxin)	MK	McIvor and Weiser, 1971a, b; Piper and McIvor, 1975; Bell and McIvor, 1976
MCF (macrophage cytolytic factor)	MK	Melsom *et al.*, 1974
ACT (adherent cell toxin)	MK	Walker *et al.*, 1976
Chromosoma breakage factors	MK	Fialkow and Gartler, 1966; Fialkow, 1967; Fialkow *et al.*, 1968
Microbicidal factors		Sharma and Middlebrook, 1977a, b
LT (lymphotoxin)	LK	Ruddle and Waksman, 1968; Granger and Williams 1968; Williams and Granger, 1968; Shacks and Granger, 1971; Rosenau and Tsoukas, 1976
PIF (proliferation inhibitory factor)	LK	Green *et al.*, 1970; Badger *et al.*, 1971, 1973a, b; Jeffes and Granger, 1976
CIF (cloning inhibition factor)	LK	Holzman *et al.*, 1973a, b; Jeffes and Granger, 1976
IDS (inhibitor of DNA synthesis)	LK	Smith *et al.*, 1970; Green *et al.*, 1974; Namba and Waksman, 1975a; Thomas *et al.*, 1975a, b
Transforming factors	LK	Green *et al.*, 1967

1975; Beller and Unanue, 1977). Many of the immunoregulatory (helper and suppressor) factors we have described are clearly members of a larger group of intercellular mediators (local hormones and chalones) governing proliferation and differentiation of particular cell types, the most commonly studied being liver, fibroblasts, epithelium and hematopoietic cells (see for example Bullough and Rytomää, 1965; Lozzio, 1973; Houck, ed., 1976). The term 'chalone' is in common use for factors inhibiting proliferation of cells identical with those which produce them. Nothing will be said here about mediators produced by polymorphonuclear leukocytes, basophils, eosinophils and platelets, which are almost as diverse as those produced by macrophages (Becker and Henson, 1973), including proteins and peptides such as ECF-A, enzymes such as 'chymase' and sulfatase, membrane constituents such as SRSA-A and PAF, and small molecules such as histamine and serotonin.

Ward and his colleagues have described a new class of substances, present in human serum, which inactivate known LK (Berenberg and Ward, 1973; Ward and Talamo, 1973; Ward and Berenberg, 1974; Ward and Rocklin, 1975). The first was CFI (chemotactic factor inactivator), which acted on leukotactic factor and MCF, as well as on chemotactic fragments of human C3, C5, and C567 and on chemotactic factor from *E. coli.* This substance is decreased in sera deficient in α_1-antitrypsin activity and markedly increased in Hodgkin's disease, possibly accounting in part for the anergy characteristic of this disease. A factor inactivating MIF has also been described (Ward and Rocklin, 1975).

3. BIOLOGICAL ROLE OF MK, LK AND OTHER CYTOKINES

The mediators listed in Tables 1–3 may be regarded as providing an intricate network which links all the cell types playing a role in defense and which controls their development and maturation, their movement and their activation in response to 'foreign' stimuli (Waksman and Namba, 1976). At the same time, by way of the system of suppressor cells and their mediators, regulation of these responses is maintained, with damping down of excessive reactions and elimination of those potentially noxious to the host, notably reactions against self-constituents.

Thus, throughout the life of the individual, certain mediators are responsible for the development of the lymphoid system, among them CSF, thymus hormones (Bach and Beaurain, 1976) and yet to be discovered hormones regulating B-cell maturation (Hämmerling *et al.*, 1976). As the system grows, the need to restrict responses to self-antigens results in a series of controls. This restriction may be sweeping and nonspecific in fetal life, mediated by α-fetoprotein (Murgita and Tomasi, 1975; Yachnin, 1975); IRA (Mowbray, 1963) and perhaps other factors. In later development and adult life, a highly specific tolerance for individual self-antigens develops, mediated by specific suppressor cells and their products, the specific suppressor LK (Katz and Benacerraf, eds., 1974). In situations where tissue damage occurs as a consequence of trauma, infection or tumor, release of self-antigens in immunogenic form poses a renewed threat of autoimmunization. Here, local production of such mediators as CRP, fibrinogen degradation products, and IF may effectively suppress the unwanted reactions (Oishi *et al.*, 1973; Mortensen *et al.*, 1975; Girman *et al.*, 1976; Epstein, 1976). Suppression of maternal reactions against the conceptus bearing paternal antigens is another possible role of AFP (Murgita, 1976).

A second level of regulation affects the homing of T- and B-lymphocytes, 'ecotaxis', to the correct regions of spleen, lymph nodes and gut-associated lymphoid tissues (Zatz and Lance, 1970; Parrott and de Sousa, 1971). This homing appears to be governed by recognition units in the lymphocyte surface and vascular endothelium (Gowans and Knight, 1964; Gesner *et al.*, 1969). In antigen- or adjuvant-stimulated organs, there is enhanced local trapping of lymphocytes, particularly those reactive with the antigen used (Taub *et al.*, 1970; Emeson and Thursh, 1971; Zatz and Lance, 1971; Zatz and Gershon, 1974). This effect, produced in part by LN activating factor and possibly other vasoactive mediators, serves to mobilize the maximum number of lymphocytes capable of responding to a given antigen at the site of immunization.

The third level of regulation concerns the immune response itself, with the production of specific antibody of different molecular classes and the various effector cells of cell-mediated immunity within the peripheral lymphoid organs. Here many specific and nonspecific helper mediators play a role in promoting proliferation and differentiation of the T- and B-cells which become the effectors after a first exposure to antigen and, as memory cells, in secondary responses. Nonspecific suppressor mediators such as IDS, SIRS and FIF play a role as well in restricting responses to competing antigens and in regulating the overall level of response.

At the peripheral level, the effector cells of various types of cell-mediated immunity release a battery of factors which act in concert to produce fever and inflammation (Waksman, 1960; Lawrence and Landy, eds., 1969; David and David, 1972; Waksman, 1976). They bring to a site of antigenic challenge both highly activated phagocytic cells capable of destroying bacterial and other pathogens, cells producing interferon which inhibits local viral replication, and cells such as basophils and eosinophils whose products enhance the inflammatory process and may act to damage metazoan parasites (Capron *et al.*, 1976; Askenase, 1977). The specificity of this reaction resides principally in the specificity of the triggering reaction between antigen and circulating effector T-cells of cell-mediated immunity (Yoshida *et al.*, 1973; Müller, ed., 1973). At the same time an antigen-specific mediator similar to MIF and specific macrophage arming factor determine a second order of specificity at the level of the infiltrating macrophages. In cell-mediated responses to certain membrane antigens, the infiltrating cells may be antigen-specific cytotoxic T-cells (killer cells) (Möller, ed., 1973, 1976a). Since viral infections of nonlymphoid cells may result in their producing typical inflammatory cytokines such as MIF (Yoshida *et al.*, 1975a), infiltrative lesions comparable to those of cell-mediated immunity may sometimes be triggered in the absence of a specific immunologic event.

It should be noted that humoral antibodies of appropriate molecular class also play a role, distinct from that of MK and LK, in regulating immune reactions, both in the lymphoid organs and in the periphery. The first studies of MIF showed considerable confusion between MIF itself and cytophilic antibodies or antigen–antibody complexes which could inhibit macrophage migration (see David and David, 1972). A similar confusion was apparent in early studies of 'IgT' (antibody ? LK ?) and specific helper factors (Taniguchi and Tada, 1974). It is now generally accepted that antibodies, in the form of antigen–antibody complexes, can duplicate the effects of soluble mediators on both the infiltrative and target cell killing phases characteristic of cell-mediated immune reactions (Lovchik and Hong, 1977; Waksman, 1976; Askenase, 1977). This is particularly striking in reactions to metazoan parasites (Capron *et al.*, 1975; Butterworth *et al.*, 1975, 1977; Dean *et al.*, 1975; Askenase *et al.*, 1976; review in Capron *et al.*, 1976; Askenase, 1977). Some cell-mediated immune reactions are characterized by massive plasma cell infiltration, mediated presumably by chemotactic and helper types of LK (Flax, 1966). Here local antibody release may contribute to the final effector phase of the reaction.

At all levels of regulation involving cytokines, both specific and nonspecific mediators have been identified which apparently subserve the same biological role. They thus ensure the effective functioning of the system by providing backup mechanisms throughout (Waksman and Namba, 1976). In general, specific mediators governed by I region genes appear to serve as a first level of control and nonspecific mediators as a second, while prostaglandins and/or cyclic nucleotides may provide an additional, more subtle level of control. The fine tuning of control, as it were, depends on the short-range action of some of these or (in the case of prostaglandins) their brief survival at the site, on their target cell specificity (macrophage, T-cell, B-cell) and the function governed (proliferation, differentiation, activation, movement). Thus in cooperation between T- and B-lymphocytes, we see a specific mediator, IgT, acting at the level of the macrophage or dendritic reticulum cell and a nonspecific mediator acting directly on the B-cell (Feldmann, 1972). Other examples abound.

4. RELATION OF *IN VITRO* OBSERVATIONS TO *IN VIVO* EVENTS

Almost all studies of LK and MK have been carried out in cultures of more or less well defined cell populations. We tend to infer that what is observed *in vitro* also occurs *in vivo* and plays a significant role in the evolution of the immune response or of peripheral cell-mediated lesions. Formal proof that this inference is justified requires convincing demonstration of at least some of the following points: (i) that the factor is produced and released *in vivo*, where its role is postulated, and in an effective concentration and at the correct time; (ii) that injection of the factor reproduces the phenomena attributed to it; (iii) that failure of factor production, e.g. in desensitized or immunologically deficient individuals is correlated with failure of the associated phenomena; (iv) that appropriate use of an antibody or pharmacologic agent specific for the factor inhibits its action *in vitro* and results *in vivo* in failure of the associated phenomena.

Additional common-sense considerations may also be brought to bear. For example, MIF and MCF are produced equally by stimulated T- and B-cells (Yoshida *et al.*, 1973; Rocklin *et al.*, 1974). Yet T-cells circulate while B-cells are predominantly sessile in the LN and spleen; thus MIF from T-cells might be expected to play a role in delayed skin reactions, while that from B-cells would not. On the other hand B-cell production of MIF in stimulated lymph nodes might contribute to inflammation within the nodes. Similarly PIF and CIF (dilute LT) do not inhibit proliferation in lymphocytes (Peter *et al.*, 1973; Namba and Waksman, 1976) and thus cannot be regarded as immunoregulatory.

The application of the criteria listed here, while very incomplete, has been most successful thus far with inflammatory and vasoactive LK presumed to play a role in peripheral cell-mediated reactions. MCF and leukotactic factor, but not MIF, have been isolated from extracts of dermal delayed hypersensitivity reactions (Cohen *et al.*, 1973; Hirashima *et al.*, 1976) and local graft-versus-host reactions (Ward and Volkman, 1975); and permeability factors (Willoughby *et al.*, 1964), ECF (Hirashima *et al.*, 1976), IF (Lodmell *et al.*, 1976) and MAF (Mackaness, 1969) have also been demonstrated more or less convincingly. In lymph draining the site of a tuberculin reaction (in sheep), both MF and MIF were reported to be present (Hay *et al.*, 1973). Similarly a MIF-like molecule has been found in joint fluid after local antigenic stimulation and MCF and MIF in peritoneal exudates exposed to antigen and demonstrating the macrophage disappearance reaction (Yoshida and Cohen, 1974b). MIF also appears in serum after i.v. injection of antigen in sensitized animals (Krejči *et al.*, 1968; Yoshida and Cohen, 1974a). Egg granulomas taken intact from *Schistosoma mansoni* infected mice have been shown to release large quantities of ESP (James and Colley, 1975). Similarly the inflamed synovia from joints affected by rheumatoid arthritis produce large quantities of MIF (Ziff *et al.*, 1974).

Conversely, injection of LN extracts (LNPF), crude supernatants (Dumonde *et al.*, 1969), more or less purified SRF (Bennett and Bloom, 1968; Schwartz *et al.*, 1970; Pick *et al.*, 1970a, b; Yoshida and Cohen, 1974b) or MCF (Cohen *et al.*, 1973) in the skin results in inflammation, with permeability changes and mononuclear cell infiltration. ECF_p gives an eosinophil infiltrate (Yoshida and Cohen, 1974b), and IF given intradermally suppresses normal local cellular reactions (Ngan *et al.*, 1976). MCF given i.p. causes a mononuclear exudate to form (Cohen *et al.*, 1973). Endogenous pyrogen, when injected, produces fever (Atkins and Bodel, 1972). No *in vivo* equivalent has been demonstrated for the reported transformation of human or guinea pig lymphocytes by 'immune' RNA into MIF-producing cells (Thor, 1967; Thor and Dray, 1968; Jureziz *et al.*, 1968). However the injection of transfer factor in man (Lawrence, 1974) may be an approximate equivalent of this experimental observation.

The occasional striking discrepancy between effective MIF production by lymphocytes of patients with chronic mucocutaneous candidiasis, when these are exposed to Candida antigens *in vitro*, and the absence of delayed skin reactivity to the same antigen, is well known (e.g. Goldberg *et al.*, 1971). In desensitization experiments, carried out by injecting sensitized rats or guinea pigs with antigen, loss of skin reactivity has commonly been said to parallel loss of the ability of the individual's lymphocytes to produce MIF in response to antigen (Jokipii, 1973). In careful cross desensitization experiments, however (Dwyer and Kantor, 1973 and 1975; Sonozaki *et al.*, 1975), loss of delayed skin reactivity was found to agree with loss of ability to produce MCF, while the macrophage disappearance reaction in the peritoneal cavity paralleled MIF competence, in agreement with the LK isolation experiments described above.

The use of 'monospecific' antisera against LK or MK to study their role *in vivo* is in its infancy. Antibodies against crude rat or guinea pig LN extracts (LNPF) effectively suppress intradermal delayed reactions (Meacock *et al.*, 1968), as well as the reactions elicited by injection of partially purified SRF (Pick *et al.*, 1969). Presumed monospecific rabbit antiserum against guinea pig MIF (Kuratsuji *et al.*, 1976), which also suppresses delayed skin reactions, was found *in vitro* to neutralize MCF, MIF and SRF (but not LT, MF or leukotactic factor) (Yoshida *et al.*, 1975a,b). The same antiserum neutralized human leukotactic factor but not human MIF (Yoshida *et al.*, 1976)! Geczy *et al.* (1976a, b) and Sorg and Geczy (1976) have used an elaborate procedure to obtain antisera monospecific for guinea pig MF and MIF (see below). These sera too, given either systematically or intradermally, wipe out delayed reactions to PHD or dinitrochlorobenzene without affecting nonspecific reactions elicited with histamine or turpentine.

Perhaps the most successful studies which make use of antibodies have been carried out with LT, but these have not as yet led to any significant study of the possible role of this LK *in vivo*. On the one hand, such antibodies have proved useful in establishing the identity of LT and one or more of the macrophage cytotoxins (MIF) (Heise and Weiser, 1969; Kramer and Granger, 1972), the identity of LT obtained by different methods of lymphocyte stimulation (Walker and Lucas, 1974), the probable relationships among different components making up human LT (Walker *et al.*, 1976; Hiserodt *et al.*, 1976b; Lewis *et al.*, 1977) and the possible structural relationship of LT to human immunoglobulin (Amino *et al.*, 1974). On the other hand, the use of antibody has permitted resolution of the controversial question of the possible role of LT in direct cell-mediated lymphocytotoxicity (CML) (see summary in Rosenau and Tsoukas, 1976). Such a role was suspected from the time LT was first described (Ruddle and Waksman, 1968). Evidence from the use of drugs affecting protein synthesis, cyclic nucleotide levels, microtubule and microfilament function, etc. (e.g. Henney *et al.*, 1974) were at best inconclusive. However a highly monospecific rabbit anti-guinea pig LT was without effect (*in vitro*) on the course of CML (M. K. Gately *et al.*, 1975, 1976; Granger, in First International Workshop, 1976). Thus presumably LT plays no role in conventional graft or tumor rejection *in vivo*. However this observation in no way rules out a possible role for LT in cytotoxicity associated with K-cells (antibody-dependent cell-mediated cytotoxicity, ADCC) or mitogenic stimulation. More important, the use of BCG in immunotheraphy of tumors may involve stimulation of a different subclass of T-cells (in mice, cells bearing the Lyl marker) from killer T-cells (Ly23) and opens the possibility that LT may play a role in killing tumor cells in this situation.

An entirely different but equally interesting problem concerns the *in vivo* role of vasoactive amines in relation to LK production and action in producing inflammation. Dvorak, Askenase and others have established that in some species, basophils are an important component of the cellular infiltrate of a variety of cell-mediated lesions (reviewed in Askenase, 1977). Gershon *et al.* (1975) showed that serotonin inhibitors of various sorts, serotonin (5-hydroxytryptamine) being a major product of activated basophils, inhibit the elicitation of delayed skin reactions in intact mice. These authors have emphasized the action of serotonin on vascular endothelium as an important element of the delayed reaction. Since, however, as noted above, serotonin also triggers MCF release and MCF has been shown to be a principal mediator of mononuclear cell infiltration in such reactions, it seems reasonably clear that serotonin must also participate in the evolution of a delayed skin reaction *in vivo* by its action in releasing MCF.

When we turn to immunoregulatory LK and MK, the situation is relatively less satisfactory. Such substances as AFP, complement components, transferrin, NIP and LDL are of course found in normal serum, while CRP is formed at local sites of trauma and can be readily demonstrated there, e.g. by specific immunofluorescence. Undefined circulating suppressor factors have been shown to increase in lepromatous leprosy (Bullock and Fasal, 1971), in graft-versus-host disease (McMaster and Levy, 1975), and after injection in normal animals of antigens, LPS endotoxin, Freund adjuvant or poly A:U (Lee and Paraskevas, 1976a). Cells taken at the appropriate moment of a systematic graft-versus-host reaction are actively producing AEF (Armerding and Katz, 1974; Armerding *et al.*, 1974). On the other hand, 24 hr after systemic injection of a large dose of antigen in rats, their spleen cells can be shown to be actively producing and releasing large amounts of IDS (Waksman and Namba, First International Workshop, 1976; Namba *et al.*, 1977). Thus there is no question about the presence of these mediators in the intact animal. In most experiments involving antigenic stimulation, however, the presence of a soluble mediator *in vivo* has been inferred rather than demonstrated. Examples include competition of antigens injected into opposite sides of the same animal (Radovich and Talmage, 1967; Fauci and Johnson, 1971a, b), competition between reactions to simultaneous tuberculin tests on opposite sides of the same animal (Outteridge and Lepper, 1973), or indeed competition of one delayed reaction with another elicited by a different antigen in the same animal (Kantor *et al.*, 1971; Dwyer and Kantor, 1973, 1975; Sonozaki *et al.*, 1975).

A number of workers have tested the effect of injecting putative mediators on immune responses. Crude supernatants of activated lymphocytes, when injected into lymphatics draining the skin, produce a striking trapping of circulating lymphocytes in the draining LN (Kelly *et al.*, 1972), while similar supernatants given systemically cause trapping in the spleen (Roehm, 1977). Antigen-specific suppressor factors injected into rats or mice inhibit IgE and IgG responses, respectively, against antigens bearing the same carrier protein as that used in the donor (Tada *et al.*, 1973; Takemori and Tada, 1975). Injection of GAT-specific suppressor factor inhibits immune responses to GAT-MBSA in normal nonresponder mice (Kapp *et al.*, 1977). Adoptively transferred contact sensitivity is specifically suppressed by admixture of an antigen-specific suppressor factor with the transferred cells (Zembala and Asherson, 1974). Nonspecific 'chalones', extracted from spleen or thymus and injected into normal animals, effectively inhibit antibody responses, skin graft rejection and graft-versus-host reactions (Kiger, 1971; Kiger *et al.*, 1973; Houck *et al.*, 1973a; Garcia-Giralt and Macieira-Coelho, 1974). NIP from normal serum, if injected in huge doses, is also immunosuppressive (Nelkin, 1973). Repeated injection of SIRS into (NZB × NZW)F_1 mice, starting in early life, is said to delay the development of autoimmune responses (Krakauer *et al.*, 1977).

Antibody to immunoregulatory LK or MK has not been used *in vivo*.

5. THE CENTRAL ROLE OF THE MACROPHAGE

While we normally think of lymphocytes as the cellular protagonists of the immunologic drama, their differentiation and function is governed at almost every level by macrophages acting either by providing sites of attachment of antigen and recognition by lymphocytes (Rosenthal *et al.*, 1976; Paul *et al.*, 1977), or by release of mediators (MK) which affect lymphocyte function (Unanue, 1976; Nelson, ed., 1976). On the other hand, at the peripheral level in reactions of cell-mediated immunity, the macrophage itself becomes the target of various LK and serves as the principal effector cell.

A brief survey of these macrophage functions would include the following (see Tables 1–3). *Systemic*: macrophages synthesize and release transferrin, complement components and interferon. *Bone marrow*: macrophages are major producers of CSF, which controls growth and differentiation of lymphocyte precursors, as well as other hematopoietic cells. *Thymus*: macrophages produce MP and TDF, which may be the principal agents promoting replication of T_1 cells and their transformation to T_2 cells. *GALT*: macrophages may play a role in the amplification and/or IgA switching functions of this system (Waksman and Ozer, 1976). This question remains open for investigation. *Spleen and LN*: macrophages subserve immunization in a number of ways. They provide attachment sites for particular classes of antigenic molecules (Drutz *et al.*, 1967; Rabinovitch and Gary, 1968), and other types of receptor sites for antigen–antibody or antigen–antibody complement complexes (Fc and C3 receptors), as well as recognition sites for lymphocytes reacting with these antigens (governed by I region and/or K/D region genes). They release antigen-specific helper factors such as GRF, and nonspecific factors promote proliferation of T-cells (LAF, NMF) and B-cells (BAF) and differentiation of the latter (TRF). At the same time, they participate in suppression (e.g. in competition of antigens), usually in conjunction with suppressor T-cells which produce SIRS; they themselves may act by producing inhibitor(s) of DNA synthesis or thymidine nucleosides. Since they simultaneously produce factors that stimulate lymphocytes, they thus become participants in a feedback loop that exaggerates the observed suppression. *Sites of peripheral inflammation triggered by specific lymphocytic reactions*: macrophages first participate in the lymphocyte triggering and second serve as targets for a variety of LK leading to their diapedesis (MIF), directed movement (MCF), replication (MGF), aggregation and fusion (MAF, MFF) and activation (MAF, OAF). Antigen-dependent MIF and SMAF contribute to their movement and activation at specific sites containing antigen. Once activated, they become highly phagocytic and release hydrolases, several types of cytotoxic factors (CTF, MTF, SMC, MC, ACT and LT) and complement components (Littman and Ruddy, 1977), as well as plasminogen activor, interferon and pyrogen.

The extreme diversity of these functions and the membrane components and soluble factors which mediate them reflects the probable ancestral role of macrophage-like (ameboid, phagocytic) cells in relation to all the others under discussion. However, the diversity of lymphocytic functions and mediators is nearly as great, while the granulocytes (neutrophil, basophil, eosinophil) clearly have a much more specialized role, as judged by the cytokines which act on them and the products which they release (Becker and Henson, 1973). Their functions appear to be linked to the evolution of different classes of antibody.

6. PURIFICATION AND CHARACTERIZATION OF MK, LK AND OTHER CYTOKINES

The purification and characterization of soluble mediators produced by lymphoid cells are required if discriminating studies are to be carried out either *in vitro* or *in vivo*. For preparation of 'monospecific' antisera, purified preparations are asbolutely essential. Yet such purification is technically difficult because of the complexity of the cell populations used to produce active supernatants, the multiplicity of factors produced even in simplified *in vitro* systems and the extremely low concentration of any particular factor of interest. As noted by Mayer some time ago, a special approach is needed which, in many ways, resembles that followed in studying complement components. A great deal may nevertheless be learned about the properties of a mediator by carrying out standard fractionation procedures and noting in which fractions activity appears, without ever obtaining the active substance itself in pure form.

In general, the best purification studies have attempted to simplify each system investigated by purifying the initial cell population, for example by removal of macrophages, by density centrifugation (e.g. on Ficoll-Hypaque) or velocity sedimentation, by separation of T- and B-cells, etc. (Natvig *et al.*, 1976). To eliminate the need for separation of mediators from serum proteins, cells are cultured in serum-free medium. In some systems, insolubilized antigen or mitogens are used, to stimulate the cells. Active supernatants are obtained and fractionated by any or all the standard techniques of protein chemistry, notably $(NH_4)_2SO_4$ precipitation, gel filtration, ion exchange chromatography, preparative starch or Pevikon block electrophoresis, Amicon or hollow fiber filtration, cesium chloride and sucrose density gradient centrifugation, isoelectric focusing, and polyacrylamide gel electrophoresis (Remold, 1972; Russell *et al.*, 1972b; Yoshida and Cohen, 1974b; Namba and Waksman, 1975a, b; C. L. Gately *et al.*, 1975, 1976; Blyden and Handschumacher, 1977). When feasible, passage through a column bearing the putative cell membrane receptor for the factor, usually oligosaccharide, results in substantial purification; an example here is purification of LIF on a column of α-L-fucose conjugated to sepharose (Bendtzen, 1976). For antigen-specific factors, of course, a column bearing antigen provides a very straightforward means of separating out the factor, as in the use of GAT-Sepharose columns to obtain purified GAT-specific suppressive factor (Theze *et al.*, 1977).

Ingenious methodologies for handling mediators have been developed by several laboratories in the last few years; I will mention one or two recent examples. Yoshida and his collaborators (1975b) prepared an LK-containing supernatant from guinea pig lymphocytes stimulated with antigen and a control supernatant from unstimulated lymphocytes. Control fractions (from Sephadex G-100) were used to immunize rabbits and the resulting antibody, coupled to agarose beads and used in a column procedure, served as a reagent to remove undesired contaminants from the corresponding G-100 fraction of the LK-containing supernatant. The final purified material was now used to immunize rabbits and obtain an LK-specific antiserum (neutralizing MIF, MCF and CRF but not several other LK). The converse procedure was used by Geczy *et al.* (1976a, b). Guinea pig supernants containing MIF, MF, and SRF were used to make a rabbit antiserum. The LK were then purified from crude supernatant by passage through a column to which the antiserum was coupled, and only then used to raise a 'specific' antiserum in a goat.

A particularly useful technique was developed by Sorg and Bloom (1973). These authors mixed an LK-containing supernatant (from guinea pig cells stimulated with antigen or Con A) internally labeled with ^{3}H-leucine and a control (unstimulated) supernatant labeled with ^{14}C-leucine and separated the mixture of the two supernatants on Sephadex G-75 columns and by isoelectric focusing. 14 protein peaks were found which were synthesized *de novo*, i.e. attributable to the stimulation. When antisera 'specific' for different lymphokines were used to precipitate individual peaks, and the precipitates were solubilized and run on SDS-polyacrylamide gels, several of the peaks could be identified with specific LK and assigned molecular weights, among them MIF (45,000) and LT (20,000) (Sorg and Geczy, 1976, and in First International Workshop, 1976).

In spite of these problems, quite a lot is already known about the mediators listed in Tables 1–3. Almost all the factors governed by I region genes have been shown to be relatively heat resistant (80°C) glycoproteins, with molecular weights close to 50,000 (35–60,000). This holds for the following entities: antigen-specific helper factor (Munro *et al.*, 1974; Taussig and Munro, 1976); antigen-specific suppressor factor (Takemori and Tada, 1975; Taniguchi *et al.*, 1976a; Tada, 1976); immunosuppressive factor (GAT) (Kapp *et al.*, 1976, 1977); antigen-specific IgE suppressor (Tada *et al.*, 1973; Okumura and Tada, 1974; Tada, 1976); the Hellström blocking factor (Nepom *et al.*, 1976); and allogeneic effect factor (Armerding and Katz, 1974; Katz and Armerding, 1976). The antigen-specific and GAT-specific factors are not freely released from the cell membrane and must be obtained by physical disruption of the cells, while others are secreted. Active molecules which are smaller have also been reported (Kishimoto and Ishizaka, 1975; Katz and Armerding, 1976). Ia is described as consisting of two noncovalently linked, glycosylated polypeptides weighing 33,000 and 28,000 (Möller, ed., 1976b; Crumpton and Snary, 1977). Its antigenic specificity appears to reside in its oligosaccharide moiety (McKenzie *et al.*, 1977). In some instances, and possibly in all, the active mediator actually consists of Ia complexed with antigen (Kapp *et al.*, 1977; Ramseier and Lindenmann, 1977). One wonders if one or more mediators may not be found some day to be K or D region gene products.

Antigen-specific helper factors for IgM and IgE, on the other hand, appear to be typical immunoglobulin, with a molecular weight of 150,000 (Taniguchi and Tada, 1974; Kishimoto and Ishizaka, 1975). IgT is described as a typical immunoglobulin; with an H-chain similar to μ in size plus an L-chain (Cone *et al.*, 1972). It is very cytophilic for macrophages (Cone *et al.*, 1974) and has H-chain idiotypes indistinguishable from those of conventional immunoglobulins (Binz *et al.*, 1976).

Thymus hormones are all polypeptides of less than 10,000 in molecular weight (Friedman, ed., 1975; Van Bekkum, 1975; Bach and Carnaud, 1976). The various nonspecific soluble helper LK have been ascribed MW from 27,000 (Hunter and Kettman, 1974) to 75,000 (Rubin and Coons, 1972a, b; Rubin *et al.*, 1973) and even 150,000 (Watson, 1973), the most common values being close to 35,000 (Waldmann *et al.*, 1976; Rubin and MacDonald, 1976; Harwell *et al.*, 1977). MF is smaller, 20–30,000 (C. L. Gately *et al.*, 1975; Mills, 1975). Among inhibitory factors, IDS and similar molecules from both human and animal sources appear to be acid glycoproteins, resistant to temperatures of 70–80°C, having a pI as low as 3.0, and with molecular weights varying between 40,000 and 80,000 (Namba and Waksman, 1975b, 1976, 1977; Thomas *et al.*, 1975a; Green *et al.*, 1974; Hersh *et al.*, 1974; Lee and Lucas, 1977). SIRS is closely similar to MIF, is thermostable up to 80°C and is 48–67,000 (Tadakuma *et al.*, 1976). FIF, also stable up to 80°C, is described as 10–45,000 (Yoshida *et al.*, in First International Workshop, 1976). Lymphocytic 'chalone' (extracted) was originally described as 30–50,000 daltons (Houck *et al.*, 1972, 1973b). More recently it was found to be complexed with RNA, the true MW being closer to 5000 (Houck *et al.*, 1977). The molecule was a strongly cationic glycoprotein, very similar to fibroblastic 'chalone' (extracted or released). LMWS, described by Ranney and Steinberg (1976) has a MW of 500–800 and is stable at 100°C. Human lymphocytic cell lines release Fc receptor (MW 100,000) capable of inhibiting antibody production in tissue culture (Molenaar *et al.*, 1977). It would be interesting to know the relationship of this material to IBF.

Complement components and other well-known serum proteins which have been found to have a possible role in regulating immune responses, among them AFP, transferrin, CRP and fibrinogen (Tables 2 and 3) are subjects of a substantial literature, which lies beyond the scope of this review. Less well known entities, such as NMS, DSRF and IRA have proven to be glycoproteins of α-globulin mobility (Veit and Michael, 1973; Watson and Thomas, 1972; Watson and Epstein, 1973; Menzoian *et al.*, 1974), though the active moiety of IRA may be a small peptide (Menzoian *et al.*, 1974). LDL-In is described as having a MW of $2–3 \times 10^6$ daltons, being 75–80 per cent lipid, and showing β mobility (Curtiss and Edgington, 1976; Curtiss *et al.*, 1977).

The factors which act on inflammatory cells seem, on the basis of present knowledge, to fall into a few well-defined categories. At one extreme are large molecules (>100,000 MW) such as MAF (macrophage aggregation factor) (Postlethwaite and Kang, 1976). At the other is a group of small peptides (12,500–15,000) serving as chemotactic factors for macrophages (MCF) (Altman *et al.*, 1975; Foon *et al.*, 1976; Leonard and Meltzer, 1976) and basophils (BCF) (Lett-Brown *et al.*, 1976). The best studied LK, of course, is MIF, a glycoprotein which occupies an intermediate size range but appears to differ from one species to another. Human MIF is described as 23–25,000 (Remold, 1972; Rocklin, 1974, 1975; Lomnitzer *et al.*, 1975), guinea pig MIF as 35–67,000 (Bennett and Bloom, 1968; Remold, 1972; Houck *et al.*, 1973c) and mouse as 48–100,000 (Hochová *et al.*, 1975; Kühner and David, 1976). These molecules also vary somewhat in their other properties from one species to another. MAF could not be distinguished from MIF (Nathan *et al.*, 1973), and SRF is quite similar (about 39,000) (Pick *et al.*, 1969; Maillard *et al.*, 1972). LIF, on the other hand, is a serine esterase with a MW of approximately 68–69,000 (40–80,000) (Rocklin, 1974, 1975; Lomnitzer *et al.*, 1975; Bendtzen, 1976). It is readily inactivated by DFP, phenylmethyl sulfonyl fluoride, soybean trypsin inhibitor and aprotinin (Bendtzen, 1977a). Indeed such substances as BAEE, a typical trypsin substrate, and BNPP (bis-*p*-nitrophenyl phosphate), a phosphodiester, both block LIF action and block its binding of DFP or PMSF (Bendtzen, 1977b). Other proteases derived from neutrophil granules have been shown to act on thymocytes (Nakamura *et al.*, 1976) and B-cells (Vischer *et al.*, 1976).

Lymphotoxin (LT) also shows marked species variability. Guinea pig LT has a MW of 50–60,000 (Remold, 1972; Goguel and Nauciel, 1974a) or 23,000 Remold (1972); its pI is given as 4.8–4.9. The Gatelys describe it as a single homogeneous molecule (M. K. Gately *et al.*, C. L. Gately *et al.*, 1976). Mouse LT is 90–100,000 (Kolb and Granger, 1968; Williams and Granger, 1969) or 41,000 (Trivers *et al.*, 1976) and has a pI of 4.4–4.8, while the rat molecule is larger (55–90,000) and has a pI of 7.2–7.6 (Trivers *et al.*, 1976; Namba and Waksman, 1975c). These vary as well in thermostability. Human LT turns out to be a family of molecules, produced at different times in the cycle of triggered cells and varying in both molecular size and heat stability (Shacks and Granter, 1971; Hiserodt *et al.*, 1976a, b; Hiserodt and Granger, 1976; Lee and Lucas, 1976; Walker *et al.*, 1976). The α form has a MW of 75–85,000 and pI of 7.0. The β form, which predominates in early supernatants, is 45–50,000 and is unstable at 37°C. There is also a γ form of 10–15,000. These do not appear to bear a simple polymeric relationship to one another. It should be added that LT was thought to act as a RNase (Walker *et al.*, 1976), but this finding is in doubt.

Macrophages, in accord with the diversity of their functions, produce an astonishingly diverse battery of mediators. Two large proteins have been described: SMC, trypsin sensitive, with a MW of 200,000 or more (Piper and McIvor, 1975; Bell and McIvor, 1976); and MTF, trypsin resistant, with assigned MW of 150,000 or 47,000, said to be identical with lymphocyte-derived LT (Kramer and Granger, 1972). Intermediate sized glycoproteins include: antigen-specific GRF, with MW 55,000; endogenous pyrogen, with MW 38,000 and pI 5.1 (the corresponding figures for EP from neutrophils are 15,000 and 6.9) (Dinarello *et al.*, 1974), and TDF (MW 35–40,000) (Beller and Unanue, 1977). A variety of small peptides has been described: LAF (mitogenic for thymocytes), 13–21,000, heat resistant at 80–100°C, pI 6.8–7.0 (Knyszinski and Burger, 1971; Gery and Handschumacher, 1974; Calderon and Unanue, 1975; Blyden and Handschumacher, 1977; Lachman and Handschumacher, 1976); variously described 'TRF', <7000 or 15–40,000 (Watson, 1973); and BAF, 18,000 (Wood *et al.*, 1976). Larger LAF molecules have also been described: 30–35,000 (Ulrich, 1976, 1977) and 50–80,000 (Blyden and Handschumacher, 1977; Hacker *et al.*, 1977). (Again, a factor produced by neutrophils, which potentiates T-cell responses to mitogen is given as 19,000 (Nakamura *et al.*, 1976).) Very small (dialyzable) mediators include MCF, which is heat resistant (60°C) but is labile in the presence of serum (Melsom *et al.*, 1974), and CTF, which may be the same and appears to be phospholipid (Pincus *et al.*, 1971). In addition to all these, we must count the lysosomal enzymes (Cohn and Wiener, 1963), as having a possible role at almost any level of macrophage function in the immune response.

The chemistry of TF, described elsewhere in this review and in other recent reviews (Ascher *et al.*, 1976), is far from clear. There is agreement that the MW of active material is <10,000, but this material is variously reported to consist of multiple small polypeptides, oligonucleotides or even pure hypoxanthine!

7. TARGET CELL RECEPTORS AND SPECIFICITY FOR SOLUBLE MEDIATORS

There is a sharp division between mediators governed by I region genes and all others with respect to target cell specificity. The former react only with cells of the same species and I region genotype. In general their action is restricted to a single type of lymphocyte. Thus GRF acts in the generation of helper T-cells (Erb and Feldmann, 1975a, b; Erb *et al.*, 1976a, b), while antigen-specific T-cell factor (Taussig and Munro, 1976) and AEF (Armerding and Katz, 1974) act only on B-cells. Antigen-specific suppressive T-cell factor also acts to suppress generation of helper T-cells (Tada, 1976), while the MLR-suppressor factor acts only on T-cells undergoing blast transformation (Rich and Rich, 1975, 1976a, b). The action of these mediators may be further restricted by the presence of specific receptors only at 'sensitive' periods of the target cell cycle (see below).

On the other hand, the heterogeneous group of nonspecific immunoregulatory mediators, in many instances, acts effectively across strain and species lines but show restrictions determined by their function. Thus thymocytes are targets of thymus hormones (Friedman, ed., 1975), TDF (Beller, 1977), at least one type of LAF (MP?) (Knyszyinski and Burger, 1971; Gery *et al.*, 1971, 1972; Gery and Waksman, 1972; Calderon and Unanue, 1975) and MF (Vischer, 1972). Peripheral T-cells are targets of MF and various helper factors (Vischer, 1972; Geha and Merler, 1974; Jacobson and Blomgren, 1975; Blomgren, 1976b). Cycling T-cells are helped by a second type of LAF (Gery *et al.*, 1971, 1972; Ulrich, 1976, 1977; Kierszenbaum and Waksman, 1977) and inhibited by IF (Blomgren *et al.*, 1974; Brodeur and Merigan, 1974, 1975; Heron *et al.*, 1976), LIFT (Kiger *et al.*, 1973; Florentin *et al.*, 1973, 1976), IDS (Green *et al.*, 1974; Hersh *et al.*, 1974a, b; Namba and Waksman, 1975b), various chalones (Houck *et al.*, 1971; Houck, 1973; Tibbetts *et al.*, 1975), and such serum factors as AFP (Murgita and Wigzell, 1976), CRP (Oishi *et al.*, 1973; Mortensen and Gewurz, 1976) and IRA (Menzoian *et al.*, 1974). B-cells serve as targets for BAF (Wood and Gaul, 1974; Wood and Cameron, 1975), MF (Vischer, 1972; Geha and Merler, 1974; Jacobson and Blomgren, 1975), NSF (Waldmann and Munro, 1974; Waldmann *et al.*, 1976), DSRF (Watson and Epstein, 1973) and cycling B-cells for TRF (Askonas *et al.*, 1974), while they are inhibited by IF (Gisler *et al.*, 1974; Brodeur and Merigan, 1974, 1975) and, when cycling by IDS, or chalones (Green *et al.*, 1974; Hersh *et al.*, 1974a, b; Ranney and Oppenheim, 1973), respectively. Help may be mediated at the macrophage surface by IgT (Feldmann and Basten, 1972a; Feldmann, 1972) and suppression by SIRS or other factors (Tadakuma and Pierce, 1976; Zembala and Asherson, 1974). There are types of chalones (Garcia-Giralt and Macieira-Coelho, 1974; Houck, 1971; Houck *et al.*, 1973) which act on types of cycling cells other than lymphocytes, among them tumor cells.

The inflammatory MK and LK also most frequently act across strain and species lines and show specificity uniquely in terms of the functional type of target cell affected. This has been well established for MIF (Rocklin *et al.*, 1970; Friedrich *et al.*, 1975) and some of the other mediators acting on macrophages (Evans *et al.*, 1972; Fidler *et al.*, 1976; Moore, 1976). It must be presumed to be true as well for LK acting on basophils, eosinophils, vascular endothelium, etc.

In the case of direct action mediators such as MTF (Kramer and Granger, 1972), LT (Williams and Granger, 1968; Shacks and Granger, 1971; Jeffes and Granger, 1976), macrophage IDS (Calderon *et al.*, 1974) and IDS (Namba and Waksman, 1975b; Thomas *et al.*, 1975a), there seems to be little restriction even at the level of cell type. However LT (and its more dilute versions PIF and CIF) does not act on lymphocytes (Namba and Waksman, 1976; Jeffes and Granger, 1976). There may even be mediators which act across phylum lines, e.g. on such protozoan parasites as *Leishmania* spp. (Brun *et al.*, 1976) and on bacteria (Klun *et al.*, 1973).

These observations do little more than provide general clues to the distribution of receptors in target cell membranes, to which different mediators bind and through which they exert their effects. The actual identification and characterization of these receptors may make use of any of several general approaches. In the case of mediators governed by I region genes, the nature of the receptor can be inferred from genetic studies of target cell specificity (Taussig *et al.*, 1975; Taniguchi *et al.*, 1976b; Tada *et al.*, 1976; Tada, 1976). Sometimes such factors can actually be shown to be taken up by target cells, e.g. uptake of antigen-specific T-cell factor by bone marrow cells and B-cells (Taussig and Munro, 1976). Among nonspecific mediators, some may produce a visible effect on target cells, e.g. the agglutination of macrophages by MAF (Fox *et al.*, 1974). Alternatively they may be absorbed from crude or purified supernatant by target cells: examples include uptake of MIF on macrophages (Bartfeld and Atoynatan, 1969; Leu *et al.*, 1972; Pick, 1976), of LT on various target cells (Williams and Granger, 1973), of TDEF-T by thymocytes of TDEF-B by bone marrow cells (Alevy and Battisto, 1976b), and of the MLR suppressor on lymphocytic blasts (Rich and Rich, 1976b). If the mediator has been purified, it can be radiolabeled and its uptake measured (Rosenau and Tsoukas, 1976). Inhibition of uptake may provide an indirect means of characterizing the receptor and binding, whether by purified unlabeled mediator (Rosenau and Tsoukas, 1976), by sugars presumed to be part of the binding site of the receptor molecule (Remold, 1973; Fox *et al.*, 1974; Rocklin, 1976) or by enzymes which destroy the receptor site (Bartfeld and Atoynatan, 1969; Leu *et al.*, 1972; Remold, 1973; Pick, 1976; Rocklin, 1976). Finally, direct binding of putative receptor molecules or their component sugars can be assayed (Bendtzen, 1976).

By the use of these techniques, immunoregulatory mediators, which are I region gene products are found to act on receptor (acceptor) sites governed by the same subregion of I as that which codes for the mediator itself. The antigen-specific T-cell factor controlled by I-A acts on an acceptor site also controlled by I-A (Taussig *et al.*, 1975), and the antigen-specific suppressive T-cell factor controlled by I-J on an acceptor controlled by I-J (Taniguchi *et al.*, 1976b; Tada *et al.*, 1976; Tada, 1976). The same relationship between the mediator and its acceptor appears to hold for nonspecific MK and LK governed by genes in the I region, e.g. AEF (Katz and Armerding, 1976) and the MLR suppressor factor, which acts on a site controlled by I-C (Rich and Rich, 1975, 1976a, b). These receptors may be presumed to be glycoproteins like other Ia (Möller, ed., 1976b). Taussig (1976) has shown that the acceptor site for his helper factor is governed by both H-2 and non-H-2 genes and suggests that the molecule, in accord with the known two chain structure of Ia, has one chain which is an I region gene product and one which is not. Whether their specificity as receptors depends on the sugar moiety which determines their antigenic specificity (Möller, ed., 1976b; McKenzie and Parish, 1976) remains to be determined.

If MIF is taken as an example of a large class of nonspecific mediators, it seems clear that the receptor is a glycoprotein and that it is specificity dependent on sugars. Thus macrophages treated with trypsin (Bartfeld and Atoynatan, 1969; Leu *et al.*, 1972; Pick, 1976) or α-L-fucosidase (Remold, 1973; Rocklin, 1976; Pick, 1976) lose their sensitivity to MIF. Conversely α-L-fucose, and possibly certain other methyl pentoses, inhibit MIF binding (Remold, 1973; Fox *et al.*, 1974; Rocklin, 1976). LIF too appears to bind α-L-fucose (Bendtzen, 1976) or *N*-acetyl-galactosamine (Rocklin, 1976). MIF possesses proteolytic activity (Havemann *et al.*, 1972) as does LIF (Rocklin, 1974, 1975; Lomnitzer *et al.*, 1975; Bendtzen, 1976, 1977a, b) and this seems independent of the receptor binding specificity of these LK. However, for other enzymatically active mediators like those derived from neutrophil or macrophage lysosomes (Nakamura *et al.*, 1976; Vischer *et al.*, 1976; Cohn and Wiener, 1963), it is possible that binding to a 'receptor' site may not be a necessary prerequisite for action of the molecule on its substrate in the target cell membrane.

In a very few well-studied cases, saturation curves of binding or of mediator action permit study of the binding affinity of the receptor sites and estimates of the number of such sites per cell. This has been done for MIF (Leu *et al.*, 1972), IDS (Namba and Waksman, 1975a) and LT (Rosenau and Tsoukas, 1976). The latter authors found two types of binding sites for LT: high affinity sites of limited capacity, easily saturated, and low affinity sites of unlimited capacity, which could not be saturated. Cytotoxicity of LT paralleled binding by high affinity sites, which were estimated as numbering approximately 600 per cell in sensitive L-cells (fibroblasts). Similar cells which showed genetically determined insensitivity to LT (Kramer and Granger, 1975; Namba and Waksman, 1976) had a markedly reduced number of high affinity sites (Rosenau and Tsoukas, 1976). Dose response curves with LT, nevertheless, show single hit kinetics (Namba and Waksman, 1975a), suggesting that action at a single site is sufficient to result in cell lysis. With IDS, no estimate has been made of the actual number of available sites, but extrapolation of dose-response curves obtained with purified IDS suggests that effective action of the mediator requires binding on 20–40 sites per cell in sensitive lymphocyte populations, and more than a hundred sites on less sensitive fibroblasts (Namba and Waksman, 1975b). In this case, sensitivity of the target cell may be related less to the number of receptor sites available than to some other aspect of target cell action (e.g. adenylate cyclase activity in the cell membrane). Binding of IDS has been shown by using lymphocytes in G_1 (Jegasothy *et al.*, 1977) but was demonstrable with difficulty, perhaps because it is of low affinity. Interestingly, MIF binding has also proved very difficult to demonstrate (Leu *et al.*, 1972; Pick, 1976; but see First International Workshop, 1976). The reaction of α-L-fucose with MIF is very easily reversible (Remold, 1973).

In summary, target cell specificity must be concerned either with the number and character of receptor sites or in some instances (as in the lymphocyte–fibroblast comparison made with IDS) on other details of LK action. With such mediators as LT and IDS, the receptor molecule is a cell membrane component common to a wide variety of cells. For most mediators, however, the receptor is limited to cells of a given type, e.g. macrophage, T-lymphocyte, etc. For the genetically restricted factors, it appears to be an Ia. The majority of receptors identified thus far are glycoproteins. In a few instances, a dominant role of oligosaccharides in their specificity has been established. For most, this remains at present no more than an interesting hypothesis.

The receptors for the Fc portion of certain subclasses of IgG on macrophages and lymphocytes, receptors for the Fc of other IgG subclasses and IgE on basophils, mast cells and eosinophils, and the receptors for C3b and C3d on macrophages, B-lymphocytes, and other cells, are all proteins, most probably glycoproteins (Dorrington, 1976; Dickler, 1976; Ishizaka, 1976; Nussenzweig, 1974; Bianco and Nussenzweig, 1977). There may be some ancestral relationship among membrane components which subserve the receptor function. The B-lymphocyte receptor for the Fc portion of IgG consists of a single polypeptide chain plus sialic acid; its MW is 65–70,000. It has no relation to immunoglobulin or to the C3 receptor, but appears somehow associated with cell membrane Ia. The Fc receptor for IgG on T-cells (IBF ?) is MW 150,000, and that for IgE on rat basophils and mast cells 60,000. As an example, the number of such receptors, for IgE on human basophils, is 40–100,000 per cell (Ishizaka, 1976). Binding affinities of 10^6–10^8 M^{-1} are given for macrophages and IgG and 10^9 M^{-1} for basophils. Note that on the macrophage surface, different mediators bind to different receptor sites: IgT presumably to an Fc receptor, SMAF to an Ia, MIF and/or SIRS to another glycoprotein, C3b and C3d to still others.

A particularly interesting point concerns the rather sharply defined cell cycle specificity of certain mediators and its relation to the presence of effective receptors on the target cells. Rich and Rich (1976b) have shown that the receptor for the MLR suppressor factor is not present on resting T-cells but only on blasts resulting from mitogenic or allogenic stimulation. This receptor, as noted above, is an I-C subregion gene product. Similarly IDS, a nonspecific suppressor of DNA synthesis acts on stimulated T-cells (Namba and Waksman, 1975b; Jegasothy *et al.*, 1976) and synchronized fibroblasts (Wagshal *et al.*, 1977) only in late G_1, i.e. precisely the moment when, by raising cAMP, it is possible to inhibit DNA synthesis without producing other undesired effects. The presence of a receptor for IDS in this limited phase of the cell cycle is thus the crucial element determining and limiting the action of the mediator.

8. IDENTITY OF CELLS PRODUCING DIFFERENT MEDIATORS

The various mediators under discussion differ strikingly with respect to the range of cells which produce them. LK which regulate the immune response (both helper and suppressor factors) are apparently made by T-cells exclusively. This includes all the antigen-specific T-cell factors listed in Table 1, i.e. antigen-specific T-cell factor, helper factor for IgE, antigen-specific suppressive T-cell factor, immunosuppressive factor (GAT), IgE suppressor factor, soluble suppressor of contact sensitivity and SMAF, as well as AEF and the MLR suppressor factor (see Tables 1 and 2 for references). It also includes nonspecific helper and suppressor factors such as MF (Oates *et al.*, 1972; Rockin *et al.*, 1974; Jacobsson and Blomgren, 1975), NSF (Waldmann and Munro, 1973, 1974) and TRF (Schimpl and Wecker, 1972; Marrack and Kappler, 1975, 1976). T_1 cells of the thymus cortex and spleen make IDS (Namba *et al.*, 1977), although it appears that T_2 cells, after prolonged cycling, may also make this factor (Thomas *et al.*, 1975a; Namba *et al.*, 1977). In view of the role of T_1 cells (in mice, cells of Lyl+, 23+ phenotype) in feedback helper and suppressor loops, other mediators produced by these cells may soon be identified.

Inflammatory LK are produced, by and large, by both T- and B-cells, among them MIF (Yoshida *et al.*, 1973; Rocklin *et al.*, 1974; Bloom *et al.*, 1975), LIF (Chess *et al.*, 1975), OAF (Chen *et al.*, 1976), MCF (Altman *et al.*, 1975; Chess *et al.*, 1975) and leukotactic factor (Yoshida *et al.*, 1976). Continuous tissue culture lines, both T and B, produce MIF (Granger *et al.*, 1970; Papageogiou *et al.*, 1972; Tubergen *et al.*, 1972; Yoshida *et al.*, 1976). However, since the circulating sensitized cells of cell-mediated immunity are T-cells, LK production by these would appear to be the significant event *in vivo*. It may be anticipated that LK such as SRF, acting on vascular endothelium, will also be found to be produced by both T and B cells. Fibroblasts in culture may also produce MIF (Tubergen *et al.*, 1972), and this mediator is produced even by virus (SV40)-infected cells (Yoshida *et al.*, 1975a). Thus *in vivo* a macrophage infiltrate may be called forth by nonimmunologic means.

Direct action mediators such as IF, which inhibits viral replication (Chess *et al.*, 1975; Epstein, 1976), and LT (Peter *et al.*, 1973; Bloom *et al.*, 1975) are made by both

T- and B-cells and by macrophages as well (MTF) (Heise and Weiser, 1969; Kramer and Granger, 1972). Many lymphocytic cell lines in culture produce LT (Granger *et al.*, 1970; Glade, 1971; Amino *et al.*, 1974). Macrophages alone produce a wide range of additional nonspecific factors, which play a role at every level of immune function, as noted earlier, among them stimulatory substances such as CSF, MP, TDF, LAF, BAF and transferrin, and inhibitors or cytotoxins such as lysosomal enzymes, CTF, MTF, SMC, MCF and ACT (see Table 3 for references) complement components such as factor B (Bentley *et al.*, 1977) and a single antigen-specific immunoregulatory product, GRF (Erb and Feldmann, 1975a, b).

Other cells are involved in the production of particular mediators, i.e. thymus epithelium and thymus hormones such as thymopoietin (Friedman, ed., 1975; van Bekkum, 1975), macrophages, gastrointestinal epithelium, and liver cells and complement components (Stecher *et al.*, 1967; Colten *et al.*, 1968; Strunk *et al.*, 1975; Lai *et al.*, 1975); damaged muscle and CRP (Kushner and Kaplan, 1961), and so on.

It can be seen from this catalog that the range of cells which produce a given mediator corresponds to a larger degree to the range of cells on which it acts and to its *in vivo* role.

The fact that continuous cell lines in culture produce cytokines is highly significant, in view of the possibility that particular MK or LK or antibody against them may some day prove to have therapeutic value in as yet undefined clinical situations. A variety of inflammatory and direct action mediators has been shown to be produced by human lymphocytic cell lines, even lines cultured as long as 8 years, and to resemble closely the products of antigen or mitogen-stimulated normal lymphocytes, among them LT, MIF, MCF, MF, IDS, IF (and enzymes and immunoglobulins) (Granger *et al.*, 1970; Glade, 1971; Papageorgiou *et al.*, 1972). These could be assayed by perfectly standard techniques: LT on L-cells or HeLa, MIF on guinea pig macrophages, etc. Additional factors have been found by subsequent workers, such as LIF and leukotactic factor and it has become clear that both T- and B-cell lines produce most or all of the factors listed (Amino *et al.*, 1974; Han *et al.*, 1975; Yoshida *et al.*, 1976). Many of these can also be obtained from other types of cells in culture, e.g. human embryonic lung fibroblasts, kidney cells and HeLa cells (Granger *et al.*, 1970; Papageorgiou *et al.*, 1972; Tubergen *et al.*, 1972; Yoshida *et al.*, 1976). Yoshida and his co-workers (1975) have shown that African green monkey kidney cells, infected with SV40 virus, produce an MIF_v which is identical by all chemical and immunological criteria with MIF_L produced by sensitized lymphocytes stimulated with antigen.

On the other hand, immunoregulatory mediators are produced by much more restricted classes of continuous cell lines in culture. IDS (or an IDS-like molecule) is apparently produced only by human T-cell blasts (Smith *et al.*, 1970; Green *et al.*, 1974; Hersh *et al.*, 1974a; Takada *et al.*, 1974; Papageorgiou *et al.*, 1974). MF may also be released only by dividing blasts (Smith *et al.*, 1970). LAF-like molecules are obtained only from macrophages in continuous culture (Hacker *et al.*, 1977). In several of these instances an additional stimulus is required to induce mediator formation and/or release. Thus MOLT-4 (a human T-cell blast), when stimulated by rosetting with SRBC, produces an IDS-like molecule (Takada *et al.*, 1974). With CRBC, which do not bind and form rosettes, the MOLT-4 cells are not stimulated and do not produce the mediator. Similarly Rubin and MacDonald (1976) obtained HEF from cell lines mixed to give an MLR in culture. The macrophage lines studied by Hacker *et al.* (1977) produced LAF only upon stimulation with LPS.

No antigen-specific mediators have yet been obtained from continuous cell lines. However an important technical development, which will perhaps make this possible is the hybridization of specific T-cells with continuous lymphocytic cell lines. In one experimental instance, rat T-cells were hybridized with a mouse cell line, and the resulting hybrids shown to produce both rat and mouse MIF (Namba and Waksman, 1975a). MIF and other mediators can also be extracted from cell lines which produce it in large quantity (Papageorgiou *et al.*, 1974; Prystowsky *et al.*, 1975).

9. MECHANISM(S) OF MEDIATOR PRODUCTION AND RELEASE

Lymphocyte 'activation', as the term is used in current immunological literature, refers to at least three distinct events: (i) complexing of a ligand with the corresponding cell membrane receptor and aggregation of the complexes, followed by ingestion of the complexes or alternatively shedding into the ambient medium; (ii) gene stimulation; and (iii) initiation of the cell cycle, with a shift of the cell from G_0 to G_1 and a further shift into S phase (DNA synthesis) at ≥ 16 hr. A substantial literature shows that each of these events can occur independently of the others. It may be supposed, therefore, that they have different signalling requirements. However, the significant details have yet to be worked out.

Of the different mediators discussed here, some appear actually to be ligand–cell membrane complexes released in the first phase of cell activation, others proteins newly synthesized in the second phase, and some are produced only in relation to the later proliferative event itself. However ligands which stimulate blast transformation and entry into the cell cycle are, in general, found also to stimulate LK release.

Those factors which are made up of Ia or a complex of Ia with antigen are only produced after stimulation with antigen and are probably all in the first category. The nonspecific mediators, however, which are unrelated to the MHC and are almost all produced in the second phase of activation, i.e. in G_1, are formed equally well after stimulation of sensitized cells with specific antigen or of normal cells with conventional mitogens, antilymphocyte serum, allogeneic antigen (in mixed lymphocyte culture), or a wide variety of other ligands. This was shown clearly in the early studies of LT by Granger and Williams (Granger and Williams, 1968; Williams and Granger, 1969) and in similar investigations of MIF (Remold *et al.*, 1972), SRF (Maillard *et al.*, 1972), IF (Epstein *et al.*, 1971a, b; Gifford *et al.*, 1971; Falcoff *et al.*, 1972) and many other inflammatory and direct action LK produced by T-cells. B-cells could be effectively triggered by mitogens, antigen–antibody complexes or aggregated immunoglobulin, anti-immunoglobulin antibody, or activated C3 (in the form of EAC) with production of MCF and presumably other LK (Wahl *et al.*, 1974). Even such pharmacologic mediators as serotonin, acting on human peripheral lymphocytes via its specific receptor, could stimulate production of MCF and leukotactic factor (Foon *et al.*, 1976). Histamine acting on normal guinea pig LN cells via a H-2 type of receptor (inhibitable by burinamide) stimulates production of HSF, a suppressor factor (Rocklin, 1977). Such immunoregulatory LK as IDS, produced in the third phase of cell activation, i.e. in close relation to the proliferative event, are also obtained equally well with antigen and mitogen (Namba and Waksman, 1975b, c; Namba *et al.*, 1977).

The existence of broad groups of LK related to the different phases of lymphocyte activation is supported by a variety of evidence showing, on the one hand, that inflammatory and direct action mediator production can be readily dissociated from DNA synthesis and, on the other, that immunoregulatory LK synthesis cannot. Thus Shacks and Granger (1971) showed that LT production is associated with early protein synthesis, starting as early as 2–3 hr after lymphocyte stimulation and showing no correlation with later blast transformation. Similarly MIF (see David and David, 1972), MCF (Foon *et al.*, 1976), OAF (Horton *et al.*, 1974), CIF (Holzman *et al.*, 1973b) and ESP (Colley, 1976) have all been described as being produced within the first 3–8 hr and peaking by 24 hr. Shacks and Granger (1971) further showed that at low levels of lymphocyte stimulation, transformation is induced but not LT production; at high levels, both are observed; at very high levels, LT production increases but transformation is inhibited. Inhibition of DNA synthesis by vinblastine, irradiation (5000 r) or hot thymidine suicide fails to reduce LT release. Similarly, MIF is produced by sensitized LN cells exposed to antigen in the presence of amounts of cytosine arabinoside or vinblastine which completely inhibit DNA synthesis and mitosis (Bloom *et al.*, 1972). MCF and LTF are produced in normal amounts by antigen or mitogen-stimulated human lymphocytes incubated in 95 per cent O_2 or asparaginase, which more or less completely eliminate DNA synthesis (Valentine, 1972; Rühl *et al.*, 1974). On the other hand, LK production is inhibited by inhibitors of protein synthesis (David, 1966). Findings with mitomycin C (Clausen, 1972) are suspect because this agent tends to act as a general cell poison.

Such findings demonstrate separation of the two functions but leave open the question whether they occur in the same or in different cells. However Rocklin (1973) showed that MIF is produced in normal amounts by cells in which the transformable subpopulation has first been eliminated by a triggering with antigen and treatment with BUdR and light and the remaining subpopulation is then restimulated with antigen. This suggests that different cells are actually involved in at least some instances. In continuous cell lines, LK such as MIF are obviously made by cells which are cycling. If these cells are synchronized, e.g. by double thymidine block, LK production is found in late G_1–S and is inhibited if cycling is arrested (Thomas, 1972; Tubergen *et al.*, 1972). Wagshal and Waksman (1977) have found, however, that LT production by normal mitogen-stimulated lymphocytes is actually enhanced if the cells are arrested in late G_1.

The association of immunoregulatory LK production with late protein synthesis, DNA synthesis and mitosis, in contrast to the mediators discussed above, seems fairly unequivocal. An association in time has been clearly shown for such factors as MF (Maini *et al.*, 1971; Vischer, 1972), IDS (Hersh *et al.*, 1974; Namba *et al.*, 1977), IF (Gifford *et al.*, 1971) and AIM (Ambrose, 1969). In addition, production of these factors is inhibited by agents which affect either protein or DNA synthesis. Thus IDS production is ablated by cycloheximide, puromycin, actinomycin D, arabinosyl cytosine, and arabinosyl-6MP (Hersh *et al.*, 1974) and by mitomycin C and BUdR (Namba *et al.*, 1977). MF production is dissociated from MIF production by different antigen dose requirements (Ford *et al.*, 1976). However, there appear to be two types of MF, one of which is produced in association with early protein synthesis (Sjöberg *et al.*, 1972; Hart *et al.*, 1973; Hirschberg *et al.*, 1974; Mills, 1975). SIRS, which is apparently identical with MIF, is of course also produced early (Rich and Pierce, 1974). CSF production too is independent of DNA synthesis and can be separated from it by judicious use of drugs (Ruscetti and Vhervenick, 1975). So-called 'chalones' extracted from resting T- and B-cells (Tibbetts *et al.*, 1975) do not fit the distinction drawn here.

Some mediators have been studied after extraction from the cell rather than release in one ot the three phases of cell 'activation'. This is the case with several of the antigen-specific LK such as the suppressor factors studied by Tada (Takemori and Tada, 1975) and Kapp (Kapp *et al.*, 1976). It is possible that these *are* released under appropriate physiologic conditions and at the correct time in the cell cycle or, alternatively that cell interaction requires cell contact and that the 'factors' in question fulfill their role without leaving the cell. Several 'chalones' have been extracted materials e.g. from rat LN and spleen or calf thymus and spleen (Houck *et al.*, 1971, 1973). The same alternatives apply.

A good deal of effort has been expended in determining whether any one product, made after different types of stimulation, is in fact always the same. Much of the early work, on MIF for example, seemed to show differences related both to the species of origin and to the mode of cell triggering (see Remold, 1972). However the majority of instances, in which an LK produced after antigenic stimulation has been compared with that produced with mitogen or an MLR, have affirmed the identity of the products studies. A partial list of cases would include: LT (Granger and Williams, 1968; Williams and Granger, 1969), PIF (Badger *et al.*, 1973a) and CIF (Holzman *et al.*, 1973a); MIF (Remold *et al.*, 1972), SRF (Maillard *et al.*, 1972) and LIF (Rocklin, 1975); MCF (Wahl *et al.*, 1974; Ward and Volkman, 1975; Koopman *et al.*, 1976) and BCF (Boetcher and Leonard, 1973; Lett-Brown *et al.*, 1976); IF (Epstein *et al.*, 1971a, b), NSF (Waldmann and Munro, 1973, 1974; Waldmann *et al.*, 1976), IBF (Guimezanes *et al.*, 1975) and IDS (Namba and Waksman, 1975b, c; Namba *et al.*, 1977).

The signalling requirements for production of LK may be more complex than simply the binding of ligand, as implied above. For T-cells, a second signal derived from macrophages appears to be a frequent if not an absolute requirement. Yoshinaga and Waksman (1973) established this for production of LT by rat lymphocytes stimulated with antigen or PHA, and a similar requirement was subsequently shown for such other mediators as OAF (Horton *et al.*, 1974), MIF (Ohishi and Onoue, 1975) and antigen-specific TRF (Kirov and Parish, 1976). The role of the macrophage in the triggering of T-cells by antigen appears to involve dual (simultaneous) recognition of Ia in the macrophage surface membrane and of antigen (Shevach, 1976; Paul, in Paul, ed., 1976). With mitogens, the macrophage's role in triggering remains unclear. Yoshinaga and Waksman (1973) did not find a macrophage requirement for Con A triggering of rat cells to produce LT, nor were macrophages needed for LT production by human cells stimulated with PHA (Walker *et al.*, 1976). On the other hand, B-cell stimulation by antigen (for production of MCF) was shown to require a second signal derived from T-cells, whereas stimulation by mitogens apparently did not (Wahl and Rosenstreich, 1976). A detailed study of B-cell triggering and MCF production by C3 (Koopman *et al.*, 1976) established that C3b binds to both C3b and C3d receptor sites, possibly cross-linking these, and is an effective trigger, while C3d, binding only to the C3d receptor, is not.

Crowding has been invoked as a significant requirement for triggering production of immunosuppressive molecules resembling IDS (Green *et al.*, 1974; Hersh *et al.*, 1974a). However it has been shown that this result is simply a consequence of the 'multihit' kinetics of IDS (Namba and Waksman, 1975b), and the consequent requirement for a high concentration of cells before a threshold concentration of product is attained (Namba *et al.*, 1977).

The triggering of macrophages, in view of the diversity of active substances produced by these cells, appears complex, but may involve the same basic events seen in lymphocyte stimulation. At least five separate situations can be distinguished. Simple incubation of these cells without any known 'stimulant' results in release of NSF or NMF (Waldmann, 1975; Erb and Feldmann, 1975a, b), factor(s) which replace macrophages and even T-cells in situations involving particulate antigens. Some experiments on so-called LAF may be concerned with the same mediator(s). Particles and other ligands which induce phagocytosis, such as LPS endotoxin, result in production of LAF (Blyden and Handschumacher, 1977; Unanue *et al.*, 1976). This has been linked to increased levels of cGMP (Diamantstein and Ulmer, 1976), and appears to involve actual triggering of new protein synthesis, starting several hours after the triggering event. Action on macrophages of certain T-cell-derived 'activating' LK also results in LAF production (Unanue *et al.*, 1976), and this fact results in a feedback loop in which T-cells and macrophages stimulate each other to ever higher levels of activity (Gery and Waksman, 1972). Endogenous pyrogen is similarly produced and released from macrophages stimulated by phagocytosis or by 'activating' LK from T-cells (see Atkins *et al.*, 1972). At the same time, but distinct from the above, phagocytosis results in release of preformed lysosomal enzymes (Cohn and Wiener, 1963). Certain ligands which bind surface membrane constituents, without necessarily leading to phagocytosis, cause release of BAF (Wood and Cameron, 1976), perhaps by the capping and shedding mechanism. Finally soluble antigens interacting with the macrophage surface result in release of GRF, which contains both the antigen itself and Ia, coming presumably from preformed cell membrane recognition structures (Erb and Feldmann, 1975a, b). GRF can substitute for the usual recognition event involving macrophage and antigen in stimulating T-cells. Of the various cytotoxic factors produced and/or released by macrophages, some appear to be products of new protein synthesis, e.g. MTF (Kramer and Granger, 1972), and others preformed lysosomal constituents (enzymes) or membrane components (CTF, SMC ?) (Pincus *et al.*, 1971; McIvor and Weiser, 1971a, b). The term 'activation', used in describing the production of both stimulatory and inhibitory mediators, tends to be confusing inasmuch as it may refer to any of the above events.

Of the factors found in serum, some, such as AFP and complement components, are normal constituents characteristic of the level of development of the individual. Others are specifically associated with tissue injury (CRP) or viral infection (IF), and require new protein synthesis. Still others require *in vivo* antigenic stimulation by microorganisms, such as the leprosy bacillus (Bullock and Fasal, 1971; Nelson *et al.*, 1975) or BCG (Salvin *et al.*, 1973, 1975), by tumors (Oishi *et al.*, 1973; North *et al.*, 1976), by systemic graft-versus-host disease (McMaster and Levy, 1975) or by injected antigens (Dwyer and Kantor, 1973, 1975; Lee and Paraskevas, 1976a; Nelson and Gatti, 1976). Release of Ia *in vivo* after immunologic stimulation has been recently demonstrated (Parish *et al.*, 1976). The presence of circulating immunosuppressive mediators has been demonstrated in systemic diseases associated with ongoing immune reactions, such as systemic lupus erythematosus (Horwitz *et al.*, 1977) and sarcoid (Mangi *et al.*, 1974a, b). Actual signalling events involved in production of these substances can only be guessed at on the basis of what is learned from study of comparable *in vitro* models like those discussed above.

10. ACTION OF CYTOKINES ON TARGET CELL FUNCTIONS

In spite of the importance of learning the mechanism of mediator action, our depth of understanding in this area is still pitifully limited. As in the case of cell phenomena associated with production of mediators, a few single themes stand out from what has so far been learned. LT is unique in producting direct damage of the target cell membrane and lysis. Certain mediators, mainly those which act on inflammatory cells, cause enhanced motility, adherence, endocytosis and exocytosis, and directed movement, phenomena associated with membrane activity and possibly homologous with aggregate formation, capping and ingestion or shedding of surface complexes by lymphocytes. Vascular endothelial change leading to increased permeability or to inflammatory cell adherence and diapedesis may be an effect of this type. Another group of mediators, mainly mitogenic and some helper factors, initiate the cell cycle, i.e. cause resting lymphocytes to move from G_0 into G_1. Still others are unable to effect a G_0–G_1 shift but promote movement from G_1 to S. Suppressor factors may act directly on target lymphocytes to arrest the cell cycle, usually in G_1. Two groups of mediators induce phenotypic change, those that stimulate mediator production by noncycling cells—these cannot at the moment be separated from those which initiate the cell cycle by a G_0–G_1 shift—and those that act on cycling cells to induce differentiation. The latter category includes both hormones acting on various precursor cells to induce maturation, and factors such as TRF, which causes cycling B-cells to become plasma cells. Many mediators act via feedback loops involving other cells, and the final pathway of action may be a function of these other cells. However, here too the final target cell effect will be one of those just listed.

In almost every case, the mechanism of action at the biochemical level remains unknown. There is binding to specific target cell receptors (discussed above) with presumably, deformation of the cell membrane. In a few instances, the mediator is a proteolytic enzyme and thus alters the membrane. In others it activates adenylate and/or guanylate cyclase. It appears that in a few cases it merely blocks membrane receptors for metabolically significant molecules.

The two LK whose mechanism of action has been studied most carefully are LT and MIF (Rosenau and Tsoukas, 1976; Pick, 1976). LT lyses a wide variety of cells of different species (Williams and Granger, 1969, 1973). Within a single species, different target cells vary widely in susceptibility to LT, a difference well brought out by use of dilute LT (Williams and Granger, 1973; Goguel and Nauciel, 1974b), and mutant lines of, for example, fibroblasts have been developed which are partially or completely resistant to its action (Namba and Waksman, 1976; Kramer and Granger, 1975). The primary event in LT action on target cells is binding to cell membrane receptors, and the relative resistance of particular target cells has been shown to depend on variation in the relative number of available receptors for LT (Williams and Granger, 1973; Rosenau and Tsoukas, 1976).

Most studies of LT action agree in describing its lytic effect as starting within approximately 12 hr and increasing progressively over a 36–48 hr period (Ruddle and Waksman, 1968a, b, c; Williams and Granger, 1969, 1973; Russell *et al.*, 1972; Goguel and Nauciel, 1974b). However, dilute LT fails to kill, but merely inhibits cell proliferation, presumably via its effect on the cell membrane (Goguel and Nauciel, 1974b; Namba and Waksman, 1976; Jeffes and Granger, 1976; Rosenau and Tsoukas, 1976). It seems likely that a repair mechanism effectively counteracts the lytic effect of dilute LT at the cell surface, and when this mechanism is inhibited, as by the use of actinomycin D, cell lysis is seen earlier and at concentrations of LT which normally would inhibit DNA synthesis but would not kill the cells (Rosenau *et al.*, 1973; Eifel *et al.*, 1975).

LT action clearly results in cell lysis associated with a failure of osmotic regulation (Russell *et al.*, 1972; Rosenau and Tsoukas, 1976), and may in fact be prevented by the osmotic effect of high molecular weight dextran in the ambient medium (Tsoukas and Rosenau, 1977). Cinematographic observation of human LT action on L-cells (mouse) (Russell *et al.*, 1972) shows both slow ballooning over 1–2 hr and a fast (3–5 min) lytic event with cell shrinkage and internal agitation ('popcorn type' cytolysis). At the ultrastructural level, one sees expansion of the cell sap, condensation of mitochondria, ballooning of rough endoplasmic reticulum, and separation of polysomes into individual ribosomes, all characteristic of osmotic lysis. Rosenau and Tsoukas (1976) also describe both a slow ballooning over 30–120 min, leading to cell rupture, and a rapid fragmentation of cells occurring in 2–5 min. Mitosis is inhibited before cytolysis.

LT action bears no relation to the cell cycle, since it is effectively lytic for resting cells (Goguel and Nauciel, 1974b) and cells treated with mitomycin C, which do not synthesize DNA (Peter *et al.*, 1973). However, it does shut down DNA synthesis and mitosis in cycling cells in about 8 hr (Williams and Granger, 1973; Russell *et al.*, 1972; but see Walker and Lucas, 1972). Its action does not require protein synthesis (Goguel and Nauciel, 1974b). There appears to be no change in permeability up to the moment of cell lysis (Walker and Lucas, 1972), but lysis is accompanied by sudden release of ^{51}Cr and of labeled cell proteins (Peter *et al.*, 1973). Rosenau *et al.* (1973) failed to show any effect of LT on glycolysis, oxidative phosphorylation, or the Na–K pump. However there was a striking early decrease in polysomes and increase in RNA synthesis, especially mRNA, attributable to increased RNA polymerase II activity, presumably associated with the repair mechanism mentioned earlier (Rosenau and Tsoukas, 1976). The suggestion that LT is itself an RNase (Lee and Lucas, 1976) has apparently been abandoned (Moy and Rosenau, 1977).

LT action does not involve complement (Gately and Mayer, 1972; Rosenau and Tsoukas, 1976). However its cell membrane action, with the production of osmotic lysis, requires investigation by the techniques in current use to study complement-mediated lysis and lysis by cytotoxic (killer) T-cells. The same methods must be applied in studying the mechanism of action of cytotoxic factors released by macrophages, notably CTF, a phospholipid which lyses rapidly after binding to the target cell membrane (Pincus *et al.*, 1971), and SMC, an antigen-specific complex (?) which is distinct from LT and lyses target cells within 2 hr (Bell and McIvor, 1976).

Studies on MIF have also shown primarily membrane effects (see David and David, 1972; Pick, 1976). It should be noted first that there is complete confusion between MIF and MAF (see below). These may be one and the same substance. If they are in fact different, effects due to one have surely often been attributed to the other. In this discussion they are treated as the same. The effect of MIF (MAF) on target macrophages was described in early studies as increased adherence and spreading (Mooney and Waksman, 1970), increased motility and phagocytosis (Nathan *et al.*, 1971, 1973), and enhanced bacteriostatic and bactericidal activity (Godal *et al.*, 1971).

A change in surface tension characteristics of the membrane, related to the increase in spreading and phagocytosis, can be demonstrated by a decreased contact angle of membrane with a drop of saline (Thrasher *et al.*, 1973). After 2–3 days of exposure to MIF, macrophages show *decreased* phagocytic activity (Remold and Mednis, 1975–1976).

The increased membrane activity produced by MIF (MAF) is accompanied by increased synthesis of TCA-precipitable membrane components (Hammond and Dvorak, 1972), increased incorporation of glucosamine and increased glucose oxidation by way of the hexose monophosphate shunt (Poulter and Turk, 1975a, b; Pick, 1976). There is contradictory evidence as to late (3 day) increases (or decreases) in such lysosomal hydrolases as acid phosphatase, β-glucuronidase and cathepsin D (Poulter and Turk, 1975a, b; Remold and Mednis, 1975–1976). MIF action is mimicked by proteases and inhibited by antiproteases (Havemann *et al.*, 1972). Similarly, Dy *et al.* (1976) report that macrophages treated with pronase become insusceptible to MAF. MIF (MAF) action is also blocked by DFP (Remold, 1974), suggesting involvement of a serine esterase in the membrane event. It is reported that pretreatment of macrophages with puromycin or cycloheximide reduces their sensitivity to active supernatants (Caspary, 1972). Glycocorticoids, hydrocortisone, and dexamethasone also diminish macrophage sensitivity to MIF (MAF) without affecting production of the factor(s) (Weston *et al.*, 1973; Balow and Rosenthal, 1973).

Pick (1976) lists the following suggested mechanisms of MIF action: (i) MIF is a divalent agglutinating agent; (ii) MIF inhibits transport or a metabolic process linked to membrane function; (iii) MIF competes with a component of the medium essential for migration; (iv) MIF induces loss of a glycoprotein coat, which normally prevents aggregation; (v) MIF causes release of an autoaggregating molecule; (vi) MIF causes complexing of a surface glycosyl transferase of one cell with the glycosyl acceptor on another. His own model suggests that entry of Ca^{2+} into the cell, in association with a rise in cGMP, leads to enhanced tubulin polymerization, associated with assembly of microtubules and immunobilization of the cell. Colchicine and vinblastine, which inhibit microtubule assembly, enhance migration of normal macrophages and counteract the inhibitory effect of MIF on migration (Pick and Abraham, 1973). Agents which raise cyclic AMP and thereby act in opposition to elevated cGMP, among them cAMP, dibutyryl cAMP, isoproterenol, theophylline, PGE_1 and PGE_2 (but not $PGF_{2\alpha}$), and epinephrine, all inhibit MIF action effectively (Koopman *et al.*, 1973). The same agents are said themselves to inhibit migration (Pick, 1972). They raise cAMP, however (Higgins *et al.*, 1976), whereas MIF does not (Higgins and David, 1976).

Thus the mode of MIF action at the level of the cell membrane remains unsolved. The antimicrobial mechanisms triggered or enhanced by MIF (MAF) have been clarified by recent work (Sbarra *et al.*, 1972) but are beyond the scope of the present discussion.

The mechanism of action of other inflammatory mediators, which leads to 'activation' and/or directed movement of neutrophils, basophils, eosinophils and lymphocytes, has received little attention as yet. LIF action is blocked by the serine esterase inhibitors DFP and PMSF (Bendtzen, 1976, 1977a), and cAMP or dibutyryl cAMP partially block the effect of LIF on migration (Bendtzen and Palit, 1977). In these respects it closely resembles MIF except for the identity of the target cell. LIF itself seems to possess esterolytic activity (Rocklin, 1974, 1975; Lomnitzer *et al.*, 1975), and its action is inhibited by soybean trypsin inhibitor and by typical trypsin substrates, such as BAEE (benzyl arginine ethyl ester) (Bendtzen, 1977a, b). This activity then may be the basis of its interaction with the cell membrane. Possible enzymatic activity of other mediators of this type has yet to be investigated, as and when sufficient quantities of purified mediator become available to permit testing.

Nonspecific helper factors in general may play any of three roles. This first became clear when Schimpl and Wecker (1972) distinguished a helper LK (TEF) causing lymphocyte proliferation, i.e. a G_0–G_1 shift, from a different factor (TRF) governing phenotypic differentiation of B-cells already in the cycle. Subsequent studies of helper LK with other names fit them into one or the other of these categories, although LK acting only on G_1–S have not been identified. MK with helper function, originally designated collectively as LAF (Gery *et al.*, 1971, 1972; Gery and Waksman, 1972), include factors purely mitogenic for T-cells (G_0–G_1) (Blyden and Handschumacher, 1977; Unanue, 1976) and others which cause differentiation of cycling cells, e.g. the TDF newly described by Beller and Unanue (1977). Recent careful timing studies, however, have brought out the fact that some LAF preparations are nonmitogenic but act to enhance the G_1–S portion of the cycle (Ulrich, 1976, 1977; Kierszenbaum and Waksman, 1977). Transferrin, produced by macrophages, also acts on mitogen-stimulated cells in mid G_1 to stimulate G_1–S (Tormey and Mueller, 1972). Thus factors described as 'helper' or potentiating, i.e. acting in concert with another stimulant but unable to stimulate alone, may act to enhance either G_0–G_1 or G_1–S, whereas mitogenic factors do both. This applies to macrophage factors such as NMF and BAF, acting on both T- and B-cells (Erb and Feldmann, 1975a, b; Schrader, 1973; Wood and Cameron, 1975), and to a variety of serum factors such as fetuin and 'mitogenic' constituents of fetal calf serum also acting on B-cells (Byrd, 1971; Watson and Epstein, 1973; Hsu *et al.*, 1973). Differentiation hormones, such as CSF, may include factors of all three types, which have not yet been separated. Early LK production results from the G_0–G_1 shift and is enhanced by any factors that enhance this process.

The biochemical mechanisms, for all three aspects of triggering, remain hopelessly confused, both with respect to events at the cell membrane (the signal(s)) and within the cell (second messengers and their biochemical targets), but this is an area of intense investigation (Wedner and Parker, 1976). Some effective mitogens (trypsin, periodate) clearly initiate triggering by enzymatic splitting of cell membrane protein(s) or oligosaccharides, perhaps with secondary bridging, deformation of the membrane and delivering of an effective signal to the interior of the cell. Attention has been called to proteolytic enzymes released by neutrophils as possible mediators of T-cell (Nakamura *et al.*, 1976) or B-cell (Vischer *et al.*, 1976) triggering. The physiologic role of these substances is in considerable doubt, but the possibility that other helper mediators act enzymatically should be carefully investigated. Cyclic nucleotides may possibly play a role in mitogenesis by antigen or mitogens (Wedner and Parker, 1976), and theories concerning the cGMP/cAMP ratio as the essential determinant of triggering of B-cells in particular have been put forward (Watson, 1975). However no attempt has yet been made to relate cyclic nucleotides to the action of lymphocytic mediators which are purely mitogenic, e.g. MF (Jones *et al.*, 1973; Jacobsson and Blomgren, 1975), TEF (Schimpl and Wecker, 1972), or act as 'nonspecific' helper factors (Feldmann and Basten, 1972a, b; Gisler *et al.*, 1973). LK that promote diperentiation of B-cells into plasma cells, notably TRF (NSM) and HEF, are most effective if added to antigen-stimulated cells *in vitro* 1–2 days after initial triggering, i.e. after the B-cells have entered the cell cycle (Askonas *et al.*, 1974; Rubin and MacDonald, 1976). It is not at all unlikely that cAMP plays a role here. In any case, the principal role of mitogenic and nonspecific helper factors of both macrophage and lymphocyte origin is to deliver a second signal to the target T-cell or B-cell and thus to enhance the total stimulus to one of the three phases of triggering. In such cases, the factor effectively substitutes for T-cells in appropriate *in vitro* situations.

Many of the antigen-specific helper and suppressor factors act by way of feedback loops involving either macrophages or T-cells carrying both the Ly 1 and Ly 2.3 markers. The loop mechanism provides amplification of LK or MK actions which, because of the specificity imposed by antigen, are presumably limited to a few clones of mediator-producing cells. Thus IgT and perhaps other specific helper factors appear to act at the macrophage surface (Feldmann and Basten, 1972a, b; Gisler *et al.*, 1973). This may be a means of providing for dual recognition by either T- or B-cell, i.e. recognition of the antigen and of membrane constituents of the macrophage (Ia ?), the helper factor merely serving to anchor antigen to the macrophage surface. Alternatively, the final result may simply be mitogenesis. The specific mediator GRF, resulting from interaction of soluble antigen with macrophages and consisting of a complex of antigen with macrophage membrane-derived Ia (Erb and Feldmann, 1975a, b) is the expression of this type of loop in soluble mediator form. The complex is a direct stimulant to helper T-cells bearing the same Ia (genetic control in I-A subregion), presumably via a dual recognition mechanism. Conversely, suppression in contact sensitization systems involves an antigen-specific soluble mediator also acting at the macrophage surface (Zembala and Asherson, 1974). Again dual recognition of antigen and a macrophage membrane component (K/D ?) by another (suppressor ?) cell may be involved, or alternatively, production by the macrophage of nonspecific suppressor factors. DNFB conjugates of purified membranes have been shown to stimulate suppressor T-cells (Miller *et al.*, 1977). Ptak *et al.* (1977) have found that macrophage membrane alone can regulate the action of specific helper or suppressor factors. Tada has described a feedback loop involving a specific suppressor cell of Ly 2.3 phenotype and a second cell of Ly 1.2.3. phenotype (Tada *et al.*, 1976, in First International Workshop), but here too the effector mechanism is obscure. Yonkosky *et al.* (1966a, b) describe a similar complex mechanism in specific allotype suppression. AEF and the MLR suppressor factor, whose production is not clonally restricted, appear to act directly on target lymphocytes or lymphoblasts without loop amplification.

Among nonspecific helper factors MF, which is usually regarded as a direct T- or B-cell mitogen (Vischer, 1972; Geha and Merler, 1974; Jacobsson and Blomgren, 1975), may also act via a feedback loop involving a second type of cell, described as non-T, nonadherent and nonphagocytic (Blomgren, 1976b). Another type of feedback loop, enhancing helper effects, may involve MAF production by lymphocytes and macrophage production of LAF, which is stimulatory to lymphocytes (Gery and Waksman, 1972). Suppression may be produced directly by IDS, which acts directly on the target cell in G_1 to shut off DNA synthesis (see below) and can effectively neutralize the stimulatory action of MF (Namba, unpublished data). However, suppression may also be produced by SIRS acting via an effect on the macrophage (Tadakuma and Pierce, 1976). The final effect is inhibition of clonal expansion of the stimulated B-cell population.

Cyclic nucleotides play an important role in several aspects of mediator action. Hormonal mediators concerned with lymphocyte precursor differentiation act by raising cAMP. This has been established for thymus hormone (thymosin, thymopoietin, thymic factor, thymus humoral factor) converting prothymocytes from the bone marrow, fetal liver or spleen, into thymocytes (acquisition of high levels of surface membrane Thy 1 and other antigens characteristic of cortical thymocytes, notably G_{IX}, Ly 1, Ly 2.3 and Ly 5); immunocompetent thymocytes into competent T-cells (reacquistion of H-2 and of responsiveness to mitogens, allogeneic stimulation, etc.) in the thymus; or T_1 cells into competent T_2 cells in the spleen (Scheid *et al.*, 1973; Bach *et al.*, 1975; Kook and Trainin, 1975). In the same manner, agents that raise cAMP in precursor cells of the B-series, such as LPS endotoxin (or DBcAMP, PGE_1, etc.) move these cells along successive steps in which they acquire surface immunoglobulin, Ia, the C3 receptor and finally PC-1 (Hämmerling *et al.*, 1975, 1976). The physiologic mediator (hormone) that carries out this function in the intact tissue is unknown, but must be presumed to act in the same manner as LPS. A particularly significant point is that this action of elevated cAMP is limited to large or intermediate-sized target cells which are cycling, in both T- and B-cell series. Studies of the precise point in the cycle at which cAMP acts have yet to be carried out. Presumably mediator (hormone) action is made cell cycle specific by provision of a specific receptor for the mediator in the cell membrane only during the correct phase of the cycle. As the thymus hormone and B-precursor cell stimulants are not interchangeable, the receptors are not only cell cycle specific but also specific with respect to the mediators involved. Both presumably are linked to adenylate cyclase in the membrane. A macrophage product TDF is described as carrying out the same differentiative function on thymocytes from thymus cortex to medulla (Beller and Unanue, 1977), and there is suggestive evidence that this mediator may also act by raising cAMP (Oppenheim *et al.*, 1976).

The nonspecific immunoregulatory mediator IDS acts to suppress DNA synthesis in triggered peripheral lymphocytes by raising cAMP at a restricted point in the cell cycle. Jegasothy has shown in mitogen-stimulated lymphocytes, that in the presence of IDS, cAMP rises abruptly to several times the normal level at 16 hr, i.e. in late G_1 (Jegasothy *et al.*, 1976; Jegasothy and Waksman, in First International Workshop). Elevation of cAMP to this level was shown to inhibit DNA synthesis totally, presumably by arresting the cells in G_1. Agents which inhibit phosphodiesterase action (isobutyl methyl xanthine) or enhance it (imidazole) and thus enhance or inhibit cAMP action within the cell, were shown to enhance and inhibit IDS-mediated inhibition of DNA synthesis, respectively. Finally, IDS was shown to activate adenylate cyclase in cell homogenates prepared in late G_1. Essentially identical findings were obtained with IDS acting on synchronized L-cells (Wagshal *et al.*, 1977); mediator action was strictly limited to a brief period in late G_1 but resulted in a sustained rise in cAMP. Again it is clear that a specific receptor for IDS is present on the cell membrane only at the correct moment of the target cell cycle and absorption experiments have borne this out (Jegasothy *et al.*, 1977).

IDS has no action on thymocytes sensitive to thymus hormone action nor on lymphocytes in the earliest phases of triggering by antigen or mitogen, both presumably lacking IDS receptors though highly sensitive to rises in cAMP. Students of tissue-specific, non-cytotoxic chalones have divided them into G_1 factors (S chalones) which inhibit cell entry into S, and G_2 factors (M chalones), which prevent mitosis, both acting by activation of adenylate cyclase (Iversen, in Houck, ed., 1976; Attallah, in Hock, ed., 1976). Thus IDS is a typical S chalone, except for its relative lack of tissue specificity. There seems little basis for believing that IDS acts directly as an inhibitor of DNA polymerase α (Lee and Lucas, 1977), though this may serve as the ultimate target of the elevated cAMP. Also, the proposition that a prostaglandin step intervenes between IDS and adenylate cyclase (Webb and Nowowiejski, in First International Workshop, 1976) requires more study.

Suppressor factors other than IDS, which have been described as regulating lymphocyte proliferation, have been imperfectly studied, from the standpoint of cell cycle specificity. Among these are the extracted 'chalones' studied by Houck *et al.* (1971, 1973) and by Garcia-Giralt and Macieira-Coelho (1974), IRA (Cooperband *et al.*, 1968; Menzoian *et al.*, 1974) and LIFT (Kiger *et al.*, 1973; Florentin *et al.*, 1976). IRA is reported to raise cAMP (Cooperband, personal communication) and to act selectively on DNA synthesis (Phillips *et al.*, 1975). It thus may act similarly to IDS. Attalah and Houck (in Houck, ed., 1976) conclude that lymphocytic 'chalone' simply blocks uptake of substrate molecules for DNA synthesis. Other factors, notably those found in serum, are effective only at very high concentrations and may be suspected either of not having a significant physiological role or possibly of acting simply to coat the target cell and render it inaccessible to antigen. Among these are NIP (Nelken, 1973), serum α-glycoprotein (Milton and Mowbray, 1972), certain complement components (Forsdyke, 1973a, c; Milthorp and Forsdyke, 1973), hyaluronic acid (Darzynkiewicz and Balazs, 1971) and LDL-In (Curtiss and Edgington, 1976; Curtiss *et al.*, 1977). All act only at high dose. Bovine serum α-glycoprotein inhibits lymphocyte binding of PHA or anti-globulin reversibly. LDL-In, on the other hand, inhibits DNA synthesis irreversibly, but only if it acts on target cells prior to mitogenic stimulation.

There are additional mechanisms illustrated by IF, IBF and AFP. IF has been extensively studied in relation to its effect on virus replication, but the mechanism of its effect in suppressing lymphocytic responses (e.g. Johnson *et al.*, 1975) is still unknown. It is reported to suppress the first phase (G_0–G_1) of B-cell activation during primary immunization with SRBC in Marbrook cultures, without affecting clone size, which depends on G_1–S (Finlay *et al.*, 1977). IBF, produced by activated T-cells binds the Fc moiety of IgG and effectively inhibits both IgM and IgG responses to thymus-independent as well as thymus-dependent antigens (Gisler and Fridman, 1976). It acts optimally if added to stimulated cultures as late as 48–72 hr and, in fact, is ineffective if removed before 60 hr. Interestingly AFP has been shown in tissue culture studies to activate a highly efficient nonspecific suppressor T-cell (Murgita *et al.*, 1977). Its presence at high concentration in newborn and young individuals may thus be responsible for the elevated suppressor activity found both in newborn infants (Olding *et al.*, 1974) and in fetal and young mice (Mosier and Johnson, 1975).

Very little has been done so far to investigate the role of LK in either promoting or suppressing the production of other mediators. MF has been shown to stimulate LT production (Gately *et al.*, 1976a). In this its role does not differ significantly from that of antigen or any mitogenic ligand. Conversely, certain immunoregulatory LK, among them Houck's 'chalones' and FIF, have been reported to turn off MIF production (Houck *et al.*, 1971, 1973; Kantor *et al.*, 1977). HSF suppresses MIF production in antigen-triggered lymphocytes (Rocklin, 1977). Mechanism here remains unknown. While elevation of cAMP inhibits production of many LK, notably TRF (Bösing–Schneider and Haug, 1976), MIF (Pick, 1974; Koopman *et al.*, 1973) and others, it is not clear at present that any immunoregulatory LK really acts by this means. Wagshal has shown that IDS, by arresting triggered cells in G_1, actually enhances LT production since this is the phase of the cycle in which it is most actively produced (Wagshal and Waksman, 1977).

There may, on the other hand be direct neutralization of LK by a special class of mediators. Harwell *et al.* (1977) have shown that NSM (TRF) is neutralized by a suppressor factor from Con A-stimulated T-cells. A serum factor which neutralizes leukotactic factor (CFI or chemotactic factor inactivator) has been described by Ward and his colleagues in normal human serum (Berenberg and Ward, 1973; Ward and Talamo, 1973; Ward and Berenberg, 1974). This factor also inactivates MCF, chemotactic fragments of human C3 and C5 and C567, and even *E. coli* chemotactic factor. The same or a similar factor neutralizes MIF (Ward and Rocklin, 1975).

11. NOMENCLATURAL PROBLEMS

It should be apparent from the above discussion that a single mediator may produce more than one *in vitro* phenomenon, particularly if receptors with which it can interact are present on more than one type of target cell. Thus, since each mediator's name is determined primarily by the *in vitro* assay first used to define it, a certain number of mediators will ultimately prove to be the same. At the same time a mediator's role *in vivo* may correspond to no more than one of the *in vitro* assays in current use or even, possibly, to none of them.

LT provides a convenient example of this problem. It was originally described by its ability to reduce actual target cell numbers in culture (Ruddle and Waksman, 1968a, b, c) or the ability of target cells to incorporate radiolabeled amino acids (Williams and Granger 1968; Shacks and Granger, 1971). Other assays have multiplied (Rosenau and Tsoukas, 1976), among them the measurement of isotope release from labeled target cells, use of unusually sensitive target cells (e.g. certain lines of L-cells), use of target cells treated with mitomycin C in order to eliminate inhibition of cell proliferation as a confusing element of the assay (Peter *et al.*, 1973), and finally use of target cells treated with actinomycin D, which are unable to repair all damage produced by LT and thus are much more sensitive to its action (Rosenau *et al.*, 1973; Eifel *et al.*, 1975). Other names were applied to substances which appeared to inhibit cell proliferation or clone formation in culture without killing the target cells, notably PIF and CIF (Badger *et al.*, 1971; Holzman *et al.*, 1973a, b). It later appeared, however, that these were nothing more than dilute LT, since the two types of activity could not be obtained separately by various physical separation techniques, since they paralleled each other perfectly in mediator action on a variety of different target cells, and finally since cytolytic activity could be converted into anti-proliferative activity by simple dilution (Jeffes and Granger, 1975, 1976; Namba and Waksman, 1975c, 1976; Goguel and Nauciel, 1974b). Conversely, PIF (CIF) activity is converted to lytic activity by inhibition of repair mechanisms with actinomycin D.

A second example is provided by MIF. The original explant technique of Rich and

Lewis (1927–1928) has been completely supplanted by George and Vaughan's capillary tube method (1962), and a variety of further methods have appeared more recently (Pick, 1976), among them inhibition of migration into a notch cut in a macrophage monolayer or migration under a layer of agarose of cells placed in a well cut into the agarose. Pick lists other assays of altered macrophage function, with the note that some of these may be due to other mediators than MIF, notably increased adherence, enhanced phagocytic and pinocytic activity, increased glucosamine uptake, increased glucose oxidation via the hexose monophosphate shunt, and increased bacteriostatic or bactericidal activity. In fact many of them are the characteristic findings associated with MAF (macrophage activation factor). MAF was first described in terms of increased adherence and spreading (Waksman and Matoltsy, 1958; Mooney and Waksman, 1970), increased motility and phagocytic activity (Nathan *et al.*, 1971, 1973; Meade *et al.*, 1974), and is considered to produce such additional effects as stimulation of macrophage proliferation and inhibition of intracellular proliferation of microorganisms (*M. lepraemurium*, vole bacillus) (Godal *et al.*, 1976). MIF and MAF have not been effectively separated by the usual methods of protein chemistry, and may actually be the same (Nathan *et al.*, 1973). The immunoregulatory mediator SIRS was also found to be indistinguishable in its physicochemical properties from MIF (Tadakuma *et al.*, 1976) and to act by way of macrophages (Tadakuma and Pierce, 1976). Its action may simply be another manifestation of macrophage activation. Similar problems surround the relationship between MCF and SRF (Yoshida *et al.*, 1975b; de Franco *et al.*, 1977), and between chemotactic factors and lysosomal enzymes (Howell *et al.*, 1976).

Additional examples are found among immunoregulatory LK and MK. MF was simply described as a mitogen for T- and B-cells (Kasakura and Lowenstein, 1965; Maini *et al.*, 1971; Feldmann and Basten, 1972b), but one must wonder about its possible relation to nonspecific helper factors which act on the proliferative phase of the antibody response, TEF (Schimpl and Wecker, 1972), NSF (Waldmann and Munro, 1974; Waldmann, 1975), TDEF (Alevy and Battisto, 1976a), HP-1 (Farrar *et al.*, in First International Workshop, 1976) and BCAF (Wahl and Rosenstreich, in First International Workshop, 1976). TRF (Schimpl and Wecker, 1972) may well be identical with NSM (Marrack and Kappler, 1975, 1976; Marrack *et al.*, in First International Workshop, 1976), HEF (Rubin and MacDonald, 1976) and HP-2 (Farrar *et al.*, in First International Workshop, 1976). NSF, which stimulates both proliferation and differentiation of B-cells, acts like MF and TRF. The type of LAF mitogenic for thymocytes (Gery *et al.*, 1971, 1972) clearly is the same as MP (Beller and Unanue, 1977), while the type of LAF which potentiates peripheral T-cell responses is probably the same as NMF (Erb and Feldmann, 1975a, b). Conversely, IDS plays different roles determined by the mode of assay: regulation of proliferation in stimulated T- and B-lymphocytes (Namba and Waksman, 1975b; Wagshal and Waksman, 1977), inhibition of proliferation in tumor cells and tumor cell lines (Thomas *et al.*, 1975a, b), and inhibition of antibody responses (Thomas *et al.*, 1975a, b). Its possible identity with AIM, FIF, IRA and the various extracted chalones must be carefully investigated.

While the preceding paragraphs stress the multiplicity of effects that may be produced by a single mediator, one should not overlook the point, stressed earlier in this review, that there may be specific and nonspecific mediators producing virtually identical effects, and that antigen–antibody complexes may also do so (Waksman, 1976). The separation of MIF from immune complexes with similar activity has represented a troublesome problem since it was first described (Amos *et al.*, 1967; Heise *et al.*, 1968; Švejcar *et al.*, 1969; Spitler *et al.*, 1969), as has the similarity of SMAF to cytophilic antibody (Granger and Weiser, 1964, 1966; Evans and Alexander, 1972).

12. PROBLEMS FOR THE FUTURE

A tremendous amount of purely phenomenological information about LK and MK has been accumulated since the description of MIF in 1966. The current task of identifying new mediators may be expected to continue for some time. However, greater interest now attaches to the problem of sorting these out, purifying and characterizing each, preparing monospecific antisera, and learning for certain which are the same and which are different. It remains a continuing challenge to determine the exact biological role of each mediator: when and by what cells it is produced, what cells serve as targets, and what cell functions are affected.

With the achievement of these goals, exact biochemical and biophysical investigation of the mechanism of action of each mediator will become possible. The problem is of course quite different for different types of mediator. The mechanism of cell membrane damage, e.g. by LT, must be distinguished from that produced by complement, CML, ADCC and mitogen-stimulated cells. The phenomena of directed movement, endo- and exocytosis, and other aspects of membrane 'activation' have already received a good deal of attention in connection with other ligands (antigen–antibody complexes, activated complement components, etc.) but remain virtually unexplored in the context of mediator action, except for MIF. Here microfilament and microtubule physiology appear to provide the central problems. For those mediators which affect the cell cycle or which lead to differentiation (phenotypic change), different biochemical mechanisms are significant, and the first clue to these is provided by the observations with cyclic nucleotides. The cell's ability to distinguish stimuli which initiate a G_0–G_1 shift, arrest the cell in G_1, move it from G_1 to S, arrest it in G_2 and/or cause it to differentiate, is not matched by our understanding of the different trigger events, to say nothing of the subsequent steps in each biochemical pathway. Even for the single problem of arrest of the cycle, one supposes that IDS, IF, IBF and dilute LT (PIF, CIF) may all act by different pathways. Thus the real challenge of the future lies in study of mediator action at the molecular level.

A final group of problems lies more in the practical sphere, to obtain large amounts of certain mediators (or of specific antibodies against them) for therapeutic use. Here the use of continuous cell lines remains the avenue of greatest promise, but the fulfilment of the promise inherent in this approach also requires full understanding, at the most basic level, of the identity and mechanism of action of individual mediators.

Acknowledgment—The author gratefully acknowledges the support of USPHS grants AI-06112, AI-06455 and AI-13949, and NCI Contract CB-43926, in the preparation of this review and the personal research cited in the text.

[Editor's note: This review was completed in January 1979. Because of its unique incisiveness and comprehensive coverage of the subject, we decided to republish it even though Dr. Waksman was unable to update it for this volume.]

REFERENCES

Reviews and Symposia

General

LAWRENCE, H. S. and LANDY, M. (1969) *Mediators of Cellular Immunity.* Academic Press, New York, London.

STETSON, C. A. (1970) President's symposium on effectors of cellular immunity. *Am. J. Path.* **60**: 435–504.

BECKER, E. L. and HENSON, P. M. (1973) *In vitro* studies of immunologically induced secretion of mediators from cells and related phenomena. *Adv. Immun.* **17**: 93–193.

FIRST INTERNATIONAL WORKSHOP on mechanism of action and characterization of lymphocyte mediators (1976) *Cell. Immun.* **27**: 332–358.

Methods

BLOOM, B. R. and GLADE, P. R. (1971) In vitro *Methods in Cell-Mediated Immunity.* Academic Press, New York.

BLOOM, B. R. *et al.* (1973) *In vitro* methods in cell-mediated immunity: a progress report. *Cell. Immun.* **6**: 331–347.

BLOOM, B. R. and DAVID, J. R. (1976) In vitro *Methods in Cell-Mediated and Tumor Immunity.* Academic Press, New York, San Francisco, London.

Immunoregulatory Factors

LAWRENCE, H. S. (1974) Transfer factor: initiation and augmentation of cell-mediated immunity. In:

Mechanisms of Cell-Mediated Immunity, pp. 289–329, McCluskey, R. T. and Cohen, S., (eds). Wiley, New York.
Paul, W. E. (1976) Cellular and soluble factors in the regulation of lymphocyte activation. *Fedn Proc.* **35**: 2044–2072.
Munro, A. and Bright, S. (1976) Products of the major histocompatibility complex and their relationship to the immune response. *Nature* **264**: 145–152.
Waksman, B. H. and Namba, Y. (1976) On soluble mediators of immunologic regulation. *Cell. Immun.* **21**: 161–176.
Cooperband, S. R., Nimberg, R., Schmid, K. and Mannick, J. A. (1976) Humoral immunosuppressive factors. *Transplant. Proc.* **8**: 225–242.
Houck, J. C. (1976) *Chalones.* North Holland, Amsterdam, Oxford.
Epstein, L. B. (1976) The ability of macrophages to augment *in vitro* mitogen- and antigen-stimulated production of interferon and other mediators of cellular immunity by lymphocytes. In: *Immunobiology of the Macrophage*, pp. 201–234, Nelson, D. S. (ed). Academic Press, New York, San Francisco, London.
Johnson, H. M. and Baron, S. (1976) Regulatory role of interferons in the immune response. *IRCS J. Med. Sci.* **4**: 50–52.
Ascher, M. S., Gottlieb, A. A. and Kirkpatrick, C. H. (1976) *Transfer Factor. Basic Properties and Clinical Applications.* Academic Press, New York, San Francisco, London.
Wedner, H. J. and Parker, C. W. (1976) Lymphocyte activation. *Prog. Allergy* **21**: 195–300.

Thymus Hormones
Friedman, H. (1975) Thymus factors in immunity. *Ann. N.Y. Acad. Sci.* **249**: 1–547.
van Bekkum, D. W. (1975) *The Biological Activity of Thymic Hormones.* Kooijker Ci., Rotterdam.
Bach, J.-F. and Carnaud, C. (1976) Thymic factors. *Prog. Allergy* **21**: 342–408.

Serum Factors
Möller, G. (1974) Tumor-associated embryonic antigens. *Transplant. Rev.* **20**: 1–129.
Cooperband, S. R., Nimberg, R., Schmid, K. and Mannick, J. A. (1976) Humoral immunosuppressive factors. *Transplant. Proc.* **8**: 225–242.
Nelson, D. S. and Gatti, R. S. (1976) Humoral factors influencing lymphocyte transformation. *Prog. Allergy* **21**: 261–341.

Factors Acting on Inflammatory Cells
Bloom, B. R. and Chase, M. W. (1967) Transfer of delayed-type hypersensitivity. A critical review and experimental study in the guinea pig. *Prog. Allergy* **10**: 151–255.
Spector, W. G. and Willoughby, D. A. (1968) Mediators of delayed hypersensitivity reactions. In: *Mechanisms of Inflammation Induced by Immune Reactions*, pp. 281–288, Miescher, P. A. and Grabar, P. (eds), 5th International Symposium on Immunopathology. Grune & Stratton, New York.
Dumonde, D. C. (1970) 'Lymphokines': Molecular mediators of cellular immune responses in animals and man. *Proc. R. Soc. M.* **63**: 899–902.
Bloom, B. R. (1971) *In vitro* approaches to the mechanism of cell-mediated immune reactions. *Adv. Immun.* **13**: 102–208.
David, J. R. and David, R. A. (1972) Cellular hypersensitivity and immunity: Inhibition of macrophage migration and the lymphocyte mediators. *Prog. Allergy* **16**: 300–449.
Pick, E. and Turk, J. L. (1972) The biological activities of soluble lymphocyte products. *Clin. Exp. Immun.* **10**: 1–23.
Remold, H. G. (1972) Purification and characterization of lymphocyte mediators in cellular immunity. *Transplant. Rev.* **10**: 152–176.
Pick, E. (1976) The mechanism of action of macrophage migration inhibitory factor (MIF). A personal view. *Current Titles Immun.* **4**: 565–568; 597–601.
Rocklin, R. E. (1976a) Products of activated lymphocytes. *Clin. Immunobiol.* **3**: 195–220.
Waksman, B. H. (1976) Commentary: Immunoglobulins and lymphokines as mediators of inflammatory cell mobilization and target cell killing. *Cell. Immun.* **27**: 309–315.

Lymphotoxin
Shacks, S. J. and Granger, G. A. (1971) Studies on *in vitro* models of cellular immunity. *J. Reticuloendoth. Soc.* **10**: 28–49.
Rosenau, W. and Tsoukas, C. D. (1976) Lymphotoxin. A review and analysis. *Am. J. Path.* **84**: 580–596.

Pyrogens
Wolstenholme, G. E. W. and Birch, J. (1971) *Ciba Foundation Symposium on Pyrogens and Fever.* Churchill Livingstone, Edinburgh, London.
Atkins, E. and Bodel, P. (1972) Fever. *New Engl. J. Med.* **286**: 27–34.

Articles

Alevy, Y. G. and Battisto, J. R. (1976a) Dextran-triggered T-cells heighten T- and B-cell reactions to mitogens. *Immunology* **30**: 379–390.
Alevy, Y. G. and Battisto, J. R. (1976b) Characterization of dextran-activated T-cell factors. *Immunology* **30**: 391–399.

ALTER, B. J. and BACH, F. H. (1970) Lymphocyte reactivity *in vitro*. I. Cellular reconstitution of purified lymphocyte response. *Cell. Immun.* **1**: 207–218.

ALTMAN, L. C., CHASSY, B. and MACKLER, B. F. (1975) Physiocochemical characterization of chemotactic lymphokines produced by human T and B lymphocytes. *J. Immun.* **115**: 18–21.

AMBROSE, C. T. (1969) Regulation of the secondary antibody response *in vitro*. Enhancement by actinomycin D and inhibition by a macromolecular product of stimulated lymph node cultures. *J. exp. Med.* **130**: 1003–1029.

AMBROSE, C. T. (1975) Regulation of the secondary antibody response *in vitro*. III. Inhibitor-containing cells of antigen-stimulated rabbit lymph node organ cultures. *Annls d'Immun.* **126C**: 3–13.

AMINO, N., LINN, E. S. PYSHER, T. J., MIER, R., MOORE, G. E. and DE GROOT, L. J. (1974) Human lymphotoxin obtained from established lymphoid lines: Purification and characteristics and inhibition by anti-immunoblobulin. *J. Immun.* **113**: 1334–1345.

AMOS, H. E., GURNER, B. W., OLDS, R. J. and COOMBS, R. R. A. (1967) Passive sensitization of tissue cells. II. Ability of cytophilic antibody to render the migration of guinea pig peritoneal exudate cells inhibitable for antigen. *Int. Archs Allergy* **32**: 496–505.

ARMERDING D. and KATZ, D. H. (1974) Activation of T and B lymphocyte *in vitro*. II. Biological and biochemical properties of an allogeneic effect factor (AEF) active in triggering specific B-lymphocytes. *J. exp. Med.* **140**: 19–37.

ARMERDING, D. and KATZ, D. H. (1975) Activation of T. and B lymphocytes *in vitro*, IV. Regulatory influence on specific T cell functions by a thymus extract factor. *J. Immun.* **114**: 1248–1254.

ARMERDING, D., SACHS, D. H. and KATZ, D. H. (1974) Activation of T and B lymphocytes *in vitro*. III. Presence of Ia determinants on allogeneic effect factor. *J. exp. Med.* **140**: 1717–1722.

ASCHER, M. S., GOTTLIEB, A. A. and KIRPATRICK, C. H. (1976) *Transfer Factor. Basic Properties and Clinical Applications*. Academic Press, New York, San Francisco, London.

ASHERSON, G. L. and ZEMBALA, M. (1974) Suppression of contact sensitivity by T cells in the mouse. I. Demonstration that suppressor cells act on the effector stage of contact sensitivity; and their induction following *in vitro* exposure to antigen. *Proc. R. Soc. B.* **187**: 329–348.

ASHERSON, G. L. and ZEMBALA, M. (1974) Suppression of contact sensitivity by T cells in the mouse. I. Demonstration that suppressor cells act on the effector stage of contact sensitivity; and their induction following *in vitro* exposure to antigen. *Proc. R. Soc. B.* **187**: 329–348.

ASHERSON, G. L., ZEMBALA, M., MAYHEW, B. and GOLDSTEIN, A. (1976) Adult thymectomy prevention of the appearance of suppressor T cells which depress contact sensitivity to picryl chloride and reversal of adult thymectomy effect by thymus extract. *Eur. J. Immun.* **6**: 699–703.

ASKENASE, P. W. (1977) The role of basophils, mast cells and vasoamines in hypersensitivity reactions with a delayed time course. *Prog. Allergy* **23** (in press).

ASKENASE, P. W., HAYDEN, B. and HIGASHI, G. I. (1976) Cutaneous basophil hypersensitivity and inhibited macrophage migration in guinea-pigs with schistosomiasis. *Clin. exp. Immun.* **23**: 318–327.

ASKONAS, B. A. and RHODES, J. M. (1965) Immunogenicity of antigen-containing ribonucleic acid preparations from macrophages. *Nature* **205**: 470–474.

ASKONAS, B. A., SCHIMPL, A. and WECKER, E. (1974) The differentiation function of T cell-replacing factor in nu/nu spleen cell cultures. *Eur. J. Immun.* **4**: 164–169.

ATKINS, E., FELDMAN, J. D., FRANCIS, L. and HERSH, E. (1972) Studies on the mechanism of fever accompanying delayed hypersensitivity. The role of the sensitized lymphocyte. *J. exp. Med.* **135**: 1113–1132.

BACH, F. H., ALTER, B. J., SOLLIDAY, S., ZOSCHKE, D. C. and JANIS, M. (1970) Lymphocyte reactivity *in vitro*. II. Soluble reconstituting factor permitting response of purified lymphocytes. *Cell. Immun.* **1**: 219–227.

BACH, M.-A. and BACH, J.-F. (1973) Studies on thymus products. VI. The effects of cyclic nucleotides and prostaglandins on rosette-forming cells. Inter-reactions with thymic factor. *Eur. J. Immun.* **3**: 778–783.

BACH, M.-A. and BEAURAIN, G. (1976) Cyclic AMP and T-cell differentiation. *Annls d'Immun.* **127C**: 967–973.

BACH, M.-A. FOURNIER, C. and BACH, J.-F. (1975) Regulation of θ-antigen expression by agents altering cyclic AMP level and by thymic factor. *Ann. N.Y. Acad. Sci.* **249**: 316–327.

BADGER, A. M., COOPERBAND, S. R. and GREEN, J. A. (1971) Direct observations on the effect of 'proliferation inhibitory factor' on the clonal growth of target cells. *J. Immun.* **107**: 1259–1267.

BADGER, A. M., COOPERBAND, S. R. and GREEN, J. A. (1973a) Culture conditions affecting induction and release of lymphocyte produced proliferation inhibitory factor (PIF). *Cell. Immun.* **8**: 12–27.

BADGER, A. M., COOPERBAND, S. R., MERLUZZI, V. J. and GREEN, J. A. (1973b) Sensitivity of non-human cells to human lymphocyte proliferation inhibitory factor (PIF) *in vitro*. *Clin. Exp. Immun.* **15**: 435–444.

BALOW, J. E. and ROSENTHAL, A. S. (1973) Glucocorticoid suppression of macrophage migration inhibitory factor. *J. Exp. Med.* **137**: 1031–1041.

BANG, F. B. (1975) A search in Asterias and ascidia for the beginnings of vertebrate immune responses. *Ann. N.Y. Acad. Sci.* **266**: 334–342.

BARTFELD, H. and ATOYNATAN, T. (1969) Cytophilic nature of migration inhibitory factor associated with delayed hypersensitivity. *Proc. Soc. exp. Biol. Med.* **130**: 497–501.

BECKER, E. L. and HENSON, P. M. (1973) *In vitro* studies of immunologically induced secretion of mediators from cells and related phenomena. *Adv. Immun.* **17**: 93–193.

BELL, C. and DRAY, S. (1971) Conversion of non-immune rabbit spleen cells by ribonucleic acid of lymphoid cells from an immunized rabbit to produce IgM and IgG antibody of foreign heavy chain allotype. *J. Immun.* **107**: 83–95.

BELL, R. B. and MCIVOR, K. L. (1976) The effects of a macrophage-derived cytotoxin on the growth and metabolism of target cells. *Cell. Immun.* **22**: 19–27.

BELLER, D. I. (1977) Secretion of lymphostimulatory molecules from macrophages. In: *Symposium on Macrophage Functions in Immunity*, UNANUE, E. R. and FRIEDMAN, H. (eds). *Fedn Proc.* (in press).

BELLER, D. I. and UNANUE, E. R. (1977) Thymic maturation *in vitro* by a secretory product from macrophages. *J. Immun.* **118**: 1780–1787.
BENDTZEN, K. (1976a) Some physicochemical properties of human leucocyte migration inhibitory factor (LIF). *Acta Path. Microb. Scand. C* **84**: 471–476.
BENDTZEN, K. (1976b) Affinity chromatography. A new technique for partial purification of human leucocyte migration inhibitory factor. *J. Immun. Meth.* **11**: 147–151.
BENDTZEN, K. (1977a) Human leukocyte migration inhibitory factor (LIF). I. Effect of synthetic and naturally occurring estarase and protese inhibitors. *Scand. J. Immun.* **6**: 125–131.
BENDTZEN, K. (1977b) Human leukocyte migration inhibotory factor (LIF). II. Partial biochemical characterization of the substrate specificities of this lymphokine. *Scand. J. Immun.* **6**: 133–140.
BENDTZEN, K. and PALIT, J. (1977) *In vitro* modulation of human leucocyte migration and migration inhibitory factor (LIF) activity by cyclic 3',5'-AMP and cyclic 3',5'-GMP. *Acta Path. Microb. Scand.* **85**: 78–80.
BENNETT, B. and BLOOM, B. R. (1968) Reactions *in vivo* and *in vitro* produced by a soluble substance associated with delayed-type hypersensitivity. *Proc. natn. Acad. Sci. USA* **59**: 756–762.
BENTLEY, C., HADDING, U., BITTER-SUERMAN, D. and BRODE, V. (1977) Effect of *in vivo* stimulation of mice on the secretion of factor B of the alternative complement pathway by peritoneal macrophages. *Eur. J. Immun.* **7**: 188–190.
BERENBERG, J. L. and WARD, P. A. (1973) Chemotactic factor inactivation in normal human serum. *J. Clin. Invest.* **52**: 1200–1206.
BIANCO, C. and NUSSENZWEIG, V. (1977) Complement receptors. *Contemp. Top. Mol. Immun.* **6**: 145–176.
BINZ, H., WIGZELL, H. and BAZIN, H. (1976) T-cell idiotypes are linked to immunoglobulin heavy chain genes. *Nature* **264**: 639–642.
BLOMGREN, H. (1976a) Evidence for the release of mitogenic factors by both T and B lymphocytes in the human. *Scand. J. Immunol.* **5**: 1173–1178.
BLOMGREN, H. (1976b) DNA synthetic responses of fractionated human lymphocytes exposed to lymphocyte-derived mitogenic factor. *Scand. J. Immun.* **5**: 1179–1184.
BLOMGREN, H., STRANDER, H. and CANTELL, K. (1974) Effect of human leukocyte interferon on the response of lymphocytes to mitogenic stimuli *in vitro*. *Scand. J. Immun.* **3**: 697–705.
BLOOM, B. R. and BENNETT, B. (1966) Mechanism of a reaction *in vitro* associated with delayed-type hypersensitivity. *Science* **153**: 80–82.
BLOOM, B. R., GAFFREY, J. and JIMENEZ, L. (1972) Dissociation of MIF production and cell proliferation. *J. Immunol.* **109**: 1395–1398.
BLOOM, B. R., STONER, G., GUBFNEY, J., SHEVACH, E. and GREEN, I. (1975) Production of migration inhibitory factor and lymphotoxin by non-T cells. *Eur. J. Immun.* **5**: 218–220.
BLYDEN, G. and HANDSCHUMACHER, R. E. (1977) Purification and properties of human lymphocyte activating factor (LAF). *J. Immun.* **118**: 1631–1638.
BOETCHER, D. A. and LEONARD, E. J. (1973) Basophil chemotaxis: augmentation by a factor from stimulated lymphocyte cultures. *Immun. Commun.* **2**: 421–429.
BORYSENKO, M. (1976) Phylogeny of immunity: an overview. *Immunogenetics* **3**: 305–326.
BOSING-SCHNEIDER, R. and HAUG, M. (1976) Role of cyclic AMP on differentiation of T- and B-lymphocytes during the immune induction. *Cell. Immun.* **27**: 121–125.
BOURNE, H. R., LICHTENSTEIN, L. M., MELMON, K. L., HENNEY, C. S., WEINSTEIN, Y. and SHEARER, G. M. (1974) Modulation of inflammation and immunity by cyclic AMP. Receptors for vasoactive hormones and mediators of inflammation regulate many leukocyte functions. *Science* **184**: 19–28.
BRAUN, W. and NAKANO, M. (1965) Influence of oligodeoxyribonucleotides on early events in antibody formation. *Proc. Soc. exp. Biol. Med.* **119**: 701–707.
BRODEUR, B. R. and MERIGAN, T. C. (1974) Suppressive effect of interferon on the humoral immune response to sheep red blood cells in mice. *J. Immun.* **113**: 1319–1325.
BRODEUR, B. R. and MERIGAN, T. C. (1975) Mechanism of the suppressive effect of interferon on antibody synthesis *in vivo*. *J. Immun.* **114**: 1323–1328.
BROOKS, R. F. (1976) Regulation of the fibroblast cell cycle by serum. *Nature* **260**: 248–250.
BRUN, R., BERENS, R. L. and KRASSNER, S. M. (1976) Inhibition of *Leishmania donovani* transformation by hamster spleen homogenates and active human lymphocytes. *Nature* **262**: 689–691.
BULLOCK, W. E., JR and FASAL, P. (1971) Studies of immune mechanisms in leprosy. III. The role of cellular and humoral factors in impairment of the *in vitro* immune response. *J. Immun.* **106**: 888–899.
BULLOUGH, W. S. and RYTÖMAA, T. (1965) Mitotic homeostasis. *Nature* **205**: 573–578.
BUTTERWORTH, A. E., DAVID, J. R., FRANKS, D., MAHMOUD, A. A. F., DAVID, P. H., STURROCK, R. F. and HOUBA, V. (1977) Antibody-dependent eosinophil-mediated damage to ^{51}Cr-labeled schistosomula of *Schistosoma mansoni*: damage by purified eosinophils. *J. exp. Med.* **145**: 136–150.
BUTTERWORTH, A. E., STURROCK, R. F., HOUBA, V., MAHMOUD, A. A. F., SHER, A. and REES, P. H. (1975) Eosinophils as mediators of antibody-dependent damage to schistosomula. *Nature* **256**: 727–729.
BYRD, W. (1971) Restoration of the immune response to sheep erythrocytes by a serum factor. *Nature New Biol.* **231**: 280–282.
CALDERON, J., KIELY, J.-M., LEFKO, J. L. and UNANUE, U. R. (1975) The modulation of lymphocyte functions by molecules secreted by macrophages. *J. exp. Med.* **142**: 151–164.
CALDERON, J., WILLIAMS, R. T. and UNANUE, E. R. (1974) An inhibitor of cell proliferation released by cultures of macrophages. *Proc. natn. Acad. Sci. USA* **71**: 4273–4277.
CAPRON, A., DESSAINT, J.-P., CAPRON, M. and BAZIN, H. (1975) Specific IgE antibodies in immune adherence of normal macrophages to *Schistosoma mansoni* schistosomules. *Nature* **253**: 474–475.
CAPRON, A., DESSAINT, J.-P., JOSEPH, M., ROUSSEAUX, R. and BAZIN, H. (1976) Macrophage cytotoxicity mediated by IgE antibody. *In vitro* study on *S. mansoni* schistosomules. In: *Molecular and Biological Aspects of the Acute Allergic Reaction*, pp. 153–171, JOHANSSON, S. G. O., STRANDBERG, K. and ILVNÄS, B. (eds). Plenum, New York.
CARNEGIE, P. R., CASPARY, E. A., DICKINSON, J. P. and FIELD, E. J. (1973) The macrophage electrophoretic

migration (MEM) test for lymphocyte sensitization. A study of the kinetics. *Clin. Exp. Immun.* **14**: 37–45.

CARPENTER, C. B., BOYLSTON, A. W., II and MERRILL, J. P. (1971) Immunosuppressive alpha globulin from bovine thymus. I. Preparation and assay. *Cell. Immun.* **2**: 425–434.

CASPARY, E. A. (1972) The mechanism of antigen-induced electrophoretic mobility reduction of guinea pig macrophages. *Clin. Exp. Immun.* **11**: 305–309.

CERNY, J. (1974) Stimulation of bone marrow haemopoietic stem cells by a factor from activated T cells. *Nature* **249**: 63–66.

CHEN, P., TRUMMEL, C., HORTON, J., BAKER, J. J. and OPPENHEIM J. J. (1976) Production of osteoclast-activating factor by normal human peripheral blood rosetting and nonrosetting lymphocytes. *Eur. J. Immun.* **6**: 732–736.

CHERVENICK, P. A. and LOBUGLIO, A. F. (1972) Human blood monocytes: Stimulators of granulocyte and mononuclear colony formation *in vitro*. *Science* **178**; 164–166.

CHESS, L., ROCKLIN, R. E., MACDERMOTT, R. P., DAVID, J. R. and SCHLOSSMAN, S. F. (1975) Leukocyte inhibitory factor (LIF): production by purified human T and B lymphocytes. *J. Immun.* **115**: 315–317.

CLAUSEN, J. E. (1971) Tuberculin-induced migration inhibition of human peripheral leucocytes in agarose medium. *Acta aller.* **26**: 56–80.

CLAUSEN, J. E. (1972) Migration inhibitory effect of cell-free supernatants from mixed human lymphocyte cultures. *J. Immun.* **108**: 453–459.

COHEN, E. P., NEWCOMB, R. W. and CROSBY, L. K. (1965) Conversion of nonimmune spleen cells to antibody-forming cells by RNA: strain specificity of the response. *J. Immun.* **95**: 583–590.

COHEN, S., WARD, P. A., YOSHIDA, T. and BUREK, C. L. (1973) Biologic activity of extracts of delayed hypersensitivity skin reaction sites. *Cell. Immun.* **9**: 363–376.

COHN, Z. A. and WIENER, E. (1963) The particulate hydrolases of macrophages. II. Biochemical and morphological response to particle ingestion. *J. exp. Med.* **118**: 1009–1020.

COLLEY, D. G. (1973) Eosinophils and immune mechanisms. I. Eosinophil stimulation promoter (ESP): A lymphokine induced by specific antigen or phytohemagglutinin. *J. Immun.* **110**: 1419–1423.

COLLEY, D. G. (1976) Eosinophils and immune mechanisms. IV. Culture conditions, antigen requirements, production kinetics and immunologic specificity of the lymphokine eosinophil stimulation promoter. *Cell. Immun.* **24**: 328–335.

COLTEN, H. R., GORDON, J. M., RAPP, H. J. and BORSOS, T. (1968) Synthesis of the first component of guinea pig complement by columnar epithelial cells of the small intestine. *J. Immun.* **100**: 788–792.

CONE, R. E., FELDMANN, M., MARCHALONIS, J. J. and NOSSAL, G. J. V. (1974) Cytophilic properties of surface immunoglobulin of thymus-derived lymphocytes. *Immunology* **26**: 49–60.

CONE, R. E. and JOHNSON, A. G. (1972) Regulation of the immune system by synthetic polynucleotides. IV. Amplification of proliferation of thymus-influenced lymphocytes. *Cell. Immun.* **3**: 283–293.

CONE, R. E., SPRENT, J. and MARCHALONIS, J. J. (1972) Antigen-binding specificity of isolated cell-surface immunoglobulin from thymus cells activated to histocompatibility antigens. *Proc. natn. Acad. Sci. USA* **69**: 2556–2560.

COOPER, E. L. (1974) Invertebrate immunology. *Contemp. Topics Immunobiol.* **4**: 1–299.

COOPERBAND, S. R., BADGER, A. M., DAVIS, R. C., SCHMID, K. and MANNICK, J. A. (1972) The effect of immunoregulatory α-globulin (IRA) upon lymphocytes *in vitro*. *J. Immun.* **109**: 154–163.

COOPERBAND, S. R., BONDEVIK, H., SCHMID, K. and MANNICK, J. A. (1968) Transformation of human lymphocytes: inhibition by homologous alpha globulin. *Science* **159**: 1243–1244.

CRUMPTON, M. J. and SNARY, D. (1977) Isolation and structure of human histocompability (HLA) antigens. *Contemp. Topics Mol. Immun.* **6**: 53–82.

CURTIS, A. S. G. and DE SOUSA, M. (1973) Factors influencing adhesion of lymphoid cells. *Nature New Biol.* **244**: 45–47.

CURTISS, L. K., DE HEER, D. H. and EDGINGTON, T. S. (1977) *In vivo* suppression of the primary immune response by a species of low density serum lipoprotein. *J. Immun.* **118**: 648–652.

CURTISS, L. K. and EDGINGTON, T. S. (1976) Regulatory serum lipoproteins: regulation of lymphocyte stimulation by species of low density lipoprotein. *J. Immun.* **116**: 1452–1458.

DARZYNKEWICZ, Z. and BALAZS, E. A. (1971) Effect of connective tissue intercellular matrix on lymphocyte stimulation. I. Suppression of lymphocyte stimulation by hyaluronic acid. *Exp. Cell Res.* **66**: 113–123.

DAVID, J. R. (1966) Delayed hypersensitivity *in vitro*: its mediation by cell-free substances formed by lymphoid cell-antigen interaction. *Proc. natn. Acad. Sci. USA* **56**: 73–77.

DAVIES, P. and ALLISON, A. C. (1976) Secretion of macrophage enzymes in relation to the pathogenesis of chronic inflammation. In: *Immunobiology of the Macrophage*, pp. 428–461, NELSON, D. S. (ed). Academic Press, New York, San Francisco, London.

DEAN, D. A., WISTAR, R. and CHEN, P. (1975) Immune response of guinea pigs to *Schistosoma mansoni*. I. *In vitro* effects of antibody and neutrophils, eosinophils and macrophages on schistosomula. *Am. J. Trop. Med.* **24**: 74–82.

DE FRANCO, M. F., HANSON, J. M., MORLEY, J., WOLSTENCROFT, R. A. and DUMONDE, D. C. (1977) Leucocyte chemotactic activity in the parallel bioassay of guinea pig lymphokines. *Immunology* **32**: 179–190.

DEKARIS, D., SMERDEL, S. and VESELIĆ, B. (1971) Inhibition of macrophage spreading by supernatants of antigen-stimulated sensitized lymphocytes. *Eur. J. Immun.* **1**: 402–404.

DIAMANTSTEIN, T. and ULMER, A. (1976) Two distinct lymphocyte-stimulating soluble factors (LAF) released from murine peritoneal cells. I. The cellular source and the effect of cGMP on their release. *Immunology* **30**: 741–747.

DICKLER, H. B. (1976) Lymphocyte receptors for immunoglobulin. *Adv. Immun.* **24**: 167–214.

DINARELLO, C. A., GOLDIN, N. P. and WOLFF, S. M. (1974) Demonstration and characterization of two distinct human leukocytic pyrogens. *J. exp. Med.* **139**: 1369–1381.

DORIA, G., AGAROSSI, G. and DI PIETRO, S. (1972) Enhancing activity of thymocyte culture cell-free medium on the *in vitro* immune response of spleen cells from neonatally thymectomized mice to sheep RBC. *J. Immun.* **108**: 268–270.

DORRINGTON, K. J. (1976) Properties of the Fc receptor on macrophages. *Immun. Commun.* **5**: 263–280.

DOUGLAS, S. D. LOUIE, J. S. and GOLDBERG, L. S. (1972) Human monocyte aggregation *in vitro*. *Int. Archs Allergy* **43**: 72–79.

DRUTZ, D. J., KOENIG, M. G. and ROGERS, D. E. (1967) Further observations on the mechanism of reticuloendothelial blockade. *J. exp. Med.* **126**: 1087–1098.

DUMONDE, D. C., WOLSTENCROFT, R. A., PANAYI, G. S., MATTHEW, M., MORLEY, J. and HOWSON, W. T. (1969) 'Lymphokines': non-antibody mediators of cellular immunity generated by lymphocyte activation. *Nature* **224**: 38–42.

DWYER, J. M. and KANTOR, F. S. (1973) Regulation of delayed hypersensitivity. Failure to transfer delayed hypersensitivity to desensitized guinea pigs. *J. exp. Med.* **137**: 32–41.

DWYER, J. M. and KANTOR, F. S. (1975) *In vivo* suppression of delayed hypersensitivity: prolongation of desensitization in guinea pigs. *J. exp. Med.* **142**: 588–599.

DY, M., DIMITRIU, A., GOUGEROT, M. A. and HAMBURGER, J. (1976) Nature of macrophage modifications induced by the macrophage activating factor(s) (MAF): Effect of enzymes and temperature. *J. Reticuloendoth. Soc.* **20**: 93–102.

EIFEL, P. J., WALKER, S. M. and LUCAS, Z. J. (1975) Standardization of a sensitive and rapid assay for lymphotoxin. *Cell. Immun.* **15**: 208–221.

EMERSON, E. E. and THURSH, D. R. (1971) Immunologically specific retention of long-lived lymphoid cells in antigenically stimulated lymph nodes. *J. Immun.* **106**: 635–643.

EPSTEIN, L. B., CLINE, M. J. and MERIGAN, T. C. (1971a) The interaction of human macrophages and lymphocytes in the phytohemagglutinin stimulated production of interferon. *J. Clin. Invest.* **50**: 744–753.

EPSTEIN, L. B., CLINE, M. J. and MERIGAN, T. C. (1971b) PPD-stimulated interferon: *in vitro* macrophage-lymphocyte interaction in the production of a mediator of cellular immunity. *Cell. Immun.* **2**: 602–613.

ERB, P. and FELDMANN, M. (1975a) The role of macrophages in the generation of T-helper cells. I. The requirement for macrophages in helper cell induction and characteristics of the macrophage-T cell interaction. *Cell. Immun.* **19**: 356–367.

ERB, P. and FELDMANN, M. (1975b) The role of macrophages in the generation of T-helper cells. III. Influence of macrophage-derived factors in helper cell induction. *Eur. J. Immun.* **5**: 759–766.

ERB, P., FELDMANN, M. and HOGG, N. (1976a) Role of macrophages in the genration of T-helper cells. IV. Nature of genetically related factor derived from macrophages incubated with soluble antigens. *Eur. J. Immun.* **6**: 365–372.

ERB, P., MEIER, B. and FELDMANN, M. (1976b) Two-gene control of T-helper cell induction. *Nature* **263**: 601–604.

EVANS, R. and ALEXANDER, P. (1972) Mechanism of immunologically specific killing of tumour cells by macrophages. *Nature* **236**: 168–170.

EVANS, R. and GRANT, C. K. (1972) Role of macrophages in tumour immunity. III. Cooperation between macrophages and lymphoid factors in an *in vitro* allograft situation. *Immunology* **23**: 677–687.

EVANS, R., GRANT, C. K., COX, H., STEELE, K. and ALEXANDER, P. (1972) Thymus-derived lymphocytes produce an immunologically specific macrophage-arming factor. *J. exp. Med.* **136**: 1318–1322.

FALCOFF, E., FALCOFF, R., CATMOT, L., DE VOMECOURT, A. and SANCEAU, J. (1972) Synthesis of interferon in human lymphocytes stimulated *in vitro* by antilymphocytic serum. *Rev. Eur. Et. Clin. Biol.* **17**: 20–26.

FALK, R. E., FALK, J. A. and HANCOCK, D. J. (1972) Restoration of immunological competence in irradiated, thymectomized rats with bone marrow cells and thymus supernants. In: *Proceedings Sixth Leucocyte Culture Conference*, pp. 359–373, SCHWARZ, M. R. (ed). Academic Press, New York, London.

FALK, R. E. FALK, J. A., MÖLLER, E. and MÖLLER, G. (1970) Lymphocyte-activating factors released *in vitro* by sensitized and nonsensitized human lymphocytes. *Cell. Immun.* **1**: 150–161.

FAUCI, A. S. and JOHNSON, J. S. (1971a) Suppression of antibody synthesis. I. Evidence for a circulating inhibitor of antibody synthesis demonstrated at the cellular level. *J. Immun.* **107**: 1052–1056.

FAUCI, A. S. and JOHNSON, J. S. (1971b) Suppression of antibody synthesis. II. The effect of carrier-specific cells upon haptenic competition. *J. Immun.* **107**: 1057–1062.

FELDMANN, M. (1972) Cell interactions in the immune response *in vitro*. V. Specific collaboration via complexes of antigen and thymus-derived cell immunoglobulin. *J. exp. Med.* **136**: 737–760.

FELDMANN, M. (1974a) T cell suppression *in vitro*. I. Role in regulation of antibody responses. *Eur. J. Immun.* **4**: 660–666.

FELDMANN, M. (1974b) T cell suppression *in vitro*. II. Nature of specific suppressive factor. *Eur. J. Immun.* **4**: 667–674.

FELDMANN, M. and BASTEN, A. (1972a) Cell interactions in the immune response *in vitro*. III. Specific collaboration across a cell impermeable membrane. *J. exp. Med.* **136**: 49–67.

FELDMANN, M. and BASTEN, A. (1972b) Cell interactions in the immune response *in vitro*, IV. Comparison of the effects of antigen-specific and allogeneic thymus-derived cell factors. *J. exp. Med.* **136**: 722–736.

FIALKOW, P. J. (1967) Chromosomal breakage induced by extracts of human allogeneic lymphocytes. *Science* **155**: 1676–1677.

FIALKOW, P. J. and GARTLER, S. M. (1966) Hyperploidy effect of lymphocte extract on fibroblasts *in vitro*. *Nature* **211**: 713–715.

FIALKOW, P. J., HELLSTRÖM, I. and HELLSTRÖM, K. E. (1968) Chromosomal abnormalities induced *in vitro* by extracts of mouse allogeneic lymphocytes. *Exp. Cell Res.* **49**: 223–225.

FIDLER, I., DARNELL, J. H. and BUDMEN, M. B. (1976) *In vitro* activation of mouse macrophages by rat lymphocyte mediators. *J. Immun.* **117**: 666–673.

FINLAY, G. J., BOOTH, R. J. and MARBROOK, J. (1977) Interferon-induced antibody suppression: a selective effect on high density, late responding precursor cells. *Eur. J. Immun.* **7**: 123–126.

FISHMAN, M. (1961) Antibody formation *in vitro*. *J. exp. Med.* **114**: 837–856.

FLAX, M. H. (1966) Experimental allergic thyroiditis. *Meth. Achievem. exp. Path.* **1**: 493–513.

FLORENTIN, I., KIGER, N. and MATHÉ, G. (1973) T lymphocyte specificity of a lymphocyte-inhibiting factor (chalone) extracted from the thymus. *Eur. J. Immun.* **3**: 624–627.

FLORENTIN, I., KIGER, N. and MATHÉ, G. (1976) The lymphocyte inhibiting factor extracted from the thymus (Lift): inhibition of the DNA synthesis *in vitro*. *Cell. Immun.* **23**: 1–10.

FOON, K. A., WAHL, S. M., OPPENHEIM, J. J. and ROSENSTREICH, D. L. (1976) Serotonin-induced production of a monocyte chemotactic factor by human peripheral blood leukocytes. *J. Immun.* **117**: 1545–1552.

FORD, W. H., ASHWORTH, L. A. E. and INDER, S. (1976) Effect of the concentration of inducing agent on the output of lymphokines in the guinea pig. *Eur. J. Immun.* **6**: 135–138.

FORSDYKE, D. R. (1973a) Serum factors affecting the incorporation of ^{3}H-thymidine by lymphocytes stimulated by antigen. I. Serum concentration. *Immunology* **25**: 583–595.

FORSDYKE, D. R. (1973b) Serum factors affecting the incorporation of ^{3}H-thymidine by lymphocytes stimulated by antigen. II. Evidence for a role of complement from studies with heated serum. *Immunology* **25**: 597–612.

FORSDYKE, D. R. (1973c) Serum factors affecting the incorporation of ^{3}H thymidine by lymphocytes stimulated by antigen. III. Evidence for a role of complement from studies with specific complement inhibitors. *Immunology* **25**: 613–619.

FOWLES, R. E., FAJARDO, I. M., LEIBOWITCH, J. L. and DAVID, J. R. (1973) The enhancement of macrophage bacteriostasis by products of activated lymphocytes. *J. exp. Med.* **138**: 952–964.

FOX, R. A., GREGORY, D. S. and FELDMAN, J. D. (1974) Macrophage receptors for migration inhibitory factor (MIF), migration stimulatory factor (MSF) and agglutinating factor. *J. Immun.* **112**: 1867–1872.

FRIEDMAN, H. P., STAVITSKY, A. B. and SOLOMON, J. M. (1965) Induction *in vitro* of antibodies to phage T_2: Antigens in the RNA extract employed. *Science* **149**: 1106–1107.

FRIEDRICH, W., LAZARY, S., GECZY, C. and DE WECK, A. L. (1975) Lymphokines. I. Use of insoluble concanavalin A for the production of migration inhibitory factor in guinea pig lymphocyte cultures. *Int. Archs Allergy* **49**: 504–518.

GALINDO, B. (1972) Antigen-mediated fusion of specifically sensitized rabbit alveolar macrophages. *Infect. Immun.* **5**: 583–594.

GALINDO, B., LAZDINS, J. and CASTILLO, R. (1974) Fusion of normal rabbit alveolar macrophages induced by supernatant fluids from BCG-sensitized lymph node cells after elicitation by antigen. *Infect. Immun.* **9**: 212–216.

GALINDO, B., MYRVIK, Q. N. and LOVE, S. H. (1975) A macrophage agglutinating factor produced during a pulmonary delayed hypersensitivity reaction. *J. Reticuloendoth. Soc.* **18**: 295–304.

GARCIA-GIRALT, E. and MACIEIRA-COELHO, A., (1974) Differential effect of a lymphoid chalone on the target and nontarget cells *in vitro*. In: *Lymphocyte Recognition and Effector Mechanism*, pp. 457–463, LINDAHL-KIESSLING, K. and OSOBA, D. (eds). Academic Press, New York, London.

GATELY, C. L., GATELY, M. K. and MAYER, M. M. (1975) The molecular dimensions of mitogenic factor from guinea pig lymph node cells. *J. Immun.* **114**: 10–16.

GATELY, C. L., GATELY, M. K. and MAYER, M. M. (1976) Separation of lymphocyte mitogen from lymphotoxin and experiments on the production of lymphocoxin by lymphoid cells stimulated with the partially purified mitogen: A possible amplification mechanism of cellular immunity and allergy. *J. Immun.* **116**: 669–675.

GATELY, M. K., GATELY, C. L., HENNEY, C. S. and MAYER, M. M. (1975) Studies on lymphokines: the production of antibody to guinea pig lymphotoxin and its use to distinguish lymphotoxin from migration inhibitory factor and mitogenic factor. *J. Immun.* **115**: 817–826.

GATELY, M. K. and MAYER, M. M. (1972) The effect of antibodies to complement components C2, C3 and C5 on the production and action of lymphotoxin. *J. Immun.* **109**: 728–734.

GATELY, M. K., MAYER, M. M. and HENNEY, C. S. (1976) Effect of anti-lymphotoxin on cell-mediated cytotoxicity. Evidence for the pathways, one involving lymphotoxin and the other requiring intimate contact between the plasma membranes of killer and target cells. *Cell. Immun.* **27**: 82–93.

GECZY, C. L., GECZY, A. F. and DE WECK, A. L. (1976a) Antibodies to guinea pig lymphokines. II. Suppression of delayed hypersensitivity reactions by a 'second generation' goat antibody against guinea pig lymphokines. *J. Immun.* **117**: 66–72.

GECZY, C. L., GECZY, A. F. and DE WECK, A. I. (1976b) Antibodies to guinea pig lymphokines. IV. Suppression of the mixed leukocyte culture reaction by anti-lymphokine globulin. *J. Immun.* **117**: 1824–1831.

GEHA, R. S. and MERLER, E. (1974) Human lymphocyte mitogenic factor: Synthesis by sensitized thymus-derived lymphocytes. Dependence of expression on the presence of antigen. *Cell. Immun.* **10**: 86–104.

GEIGER, B., GALLILY, R. and GERY, I. (1973) The effect of irradiation on the release of lymphocyte activating factor (LAF). *Cell Immun.* **7**: 177–180.

GEORGE, M. and VAUGHAN, J. H. (1962) *In vitro* cell migration as a model for delayed hypersensitivity. *Proc. Soc. exp. Biol. Med.* **111**: 514–521.

GERSHON, R. K., ASKENASE, P. W. and GERSHON, M. D. (1975) Requirement for vasoactive amines for production of delayed-type hypersensitivity skin reactions. *J. exp. Med.* **142**: 732–747.

GERY, I., GERSHON, R. K. and WAKSMAN, B. H. (1971) Potentiation of cultured mouse thymocyte responses by factors released by peripheral leucocytes. *J. Immun.* **107**: 1778–1780.

GERY, I., GERSHON, R. K. and WAKSMAN, B. H. (1972) Potentiation of lymphocyte responses to mitogens. I. The responding cell. *J. exp. Med.* **136**: 128–142.

GERY, I. and HANDSCHUMACHER, R. E. (1974) Potentiation of the T lymphocyte response to mitogens. III. Properties of the mediator(s) from adherent cells. *Cell. Immun.* **11**: 162–169.
GERY, I. and WAKSMAN, B. H. (1972) Potentiation of lymphocyte responses to mitogens. II. The cellular source of potentiating mediators. *J. exp. Med.* **136**: 143–155.
GERY, I. and WIENER, E. (1975) Potentiation of the T lymphocyte response to mitogens. IV. Relationship between LAF production and 'activation' of macrophages. *J. Reticuloendoth. Soc.* **18**: 252–259.
GESNER, B. M., WOODRUFF, J. J. and MCCLUSKEY, R. T. (1969) An autoradiographic study of the effect of neuraminidase or trypsin on transfused lymphocytes. *Am. J. Path.* **57**: 215–230.
GIFFORD, G. E., TIBOR, A. and PEAVY, D. L. (1971) Interferon production in mixed lymphocyte cell cultures. *Infect. Immun.* **3**: 164–166.
GIRMAN, G., PEES, H., SCHWARZE, G. and SCHEURLEN, P. G. (1976) Immunosuppression by micromolecular fibrinogen degradation products in cancer. *Nature* **259**: 399–401.
GISLER, R. H. and FRIDMAN, W. H. (1976) Inhibition of the *in vitro* 19S and 7S antibody response by immunoglobulin-binding factor (IBF) from alloantigen-activated T cells. *Cell. Immun.* **23**: 99–107.
GISLER, R. H., LINDAHL, P. and GRESSER, I. (1974) Effects of interferon on antibody synthesis *in vitro*. *J. Immun.* **113**: 438–444.
GISLER, R. H., STABER, F., RÜDE, E. and DUKOR, P. (1973) Soluble mediators of T–B interaction. *Eur. J. Immun.* **3**: 650–652.
GLADE, P. R. (1971) In: *Immunological Intervention*, pp. 27–30, UHR, J. W. and LANDY, M. (eds). Academic Press, New York, London.
GODAL, T. (1974) The role of immune responses to *Mycobacterium leprae* in host defence and tissue damage in leprosy. *Prog. Immun.* 2, **4**: 161–169.
GODAL, T., REES, R. J. W. and LAMVIK, J. O. (1971) Lymphocyte-mediated modification of blood-derived macrophage function *in vitro*; inhibition of growth of intracellular mycobacteria with lymphokines. *Clin. Exp. Immun.* **8**: 625–637.
GOGUEL, A. F. and NAUCIEL, C. (1974a) Lymphotoxine de cobaye. Mise en évidence et étude de certaines propriétés physicochimiques. *Annls d'Immun.* **125C**: 569–579.
GOGUEL, A. F. and NAUCIEL, C. (1974b) Guinea pig lymphotoxin. II. Study of its mechanism of action, its differentiation from migration inhibitory factor and interferon. *Annals d'Immunol.* **125C**; 789–802.
GOLDBERG, L. S., BLUESTONE, R., BARNETT, E. V. and LANDAU, J. W. (1971) Studies on lymphocyte and monocyte function in chronic mucocutaneous candidiasis. *Clin. Exp. Immun.* **8**: 37–43.
GOLDE, D. W. and CLINE, M. J. (1972) Identification of the colony-stimulating cell in human peripheral blood. *J. Clin. Invest.* **51**: 2981–2983.
GOLDMAN, M. B. and GOLDMAN, J. N. (1976) Relationship of functional levels of early components of complement to the H-2 complex of mice. *J. Immun.* **117**: 1584–1588.
GORCZYNSKI, R. M., MILLER, R. G. and PHILLIPS, R. A. (1973a) Reconstitution of T cell-depleted spleen cell populations by factors derived from T cells. I. Conditions for the production of active T cell supernatants. *J. Immun.* **110**: 968–983.
GORCZYNSKI, R. M., MILLER, R. G. and PHILLIPS, R. A. (1973b) Reconstitution of T cell-depleted spleen cell populations by factors derived from T cells. III. Mechanism of action of T cell-derived factors. *J. Immun.* **111**: 900–913.
GOTOFF, S. P. and VIZRAL, I. F. (1972) The macrophage aggregation assay for delayed hypersensitivity: development of the response, role of the macrophage, and the independence of humoral antibody. *Cell. Immun.* **3**: 53–61.
GOTTLIEB, A. A. and WALDMAN, S. R. (1972) The multiple functions of macrophages in immunity. *Critical Rev. Microbiol.* **Feb.**: 321–352.
GOWANS, J. L. and KNIGHT, E. J. (1964) The route of recirculation of lymphocytes in the rat. *Proc. R. Soc. B.* **159**: 257–282.
GRANGER, G. A., MOORE, G. E., WHITE, J. G., MATZINGER, P., SUNDSMO, J. S., SHUPE, S., KOLB, W. P., KRAMER, J. and GLADE, P. R. (1970) Production of lymphotoxin and migration inhibitory factor by established human lymphocytic cell lines. *J. Immun.* **104**: 1476–1485.
GRANGER, G. A. and WEISER, R. S. (1964) Homograft target cells: specific destruction *in vitro* by contact interaction with immune macrophages. *Science* **145**: 1427–1429.
GRANGER, G. A. and WEISER, R. S. (1966) Homograft target cells: contact destruction *in vitro* by immune macrophages. *Science* **151**: 97–99.
GRANGER, G. A. and WILLIAMS, T. W. (1968) Lymphocyte cytotoxicity *in vitro*: activation and release of a cytotoxic factor. *Nature* **218**: 1253–1254.
GRANT, C. K., CURRIE, G. A. and ALEXANDER, P. (1972) Thymocytes from mice immunized against an allograft render bone-marrow cells specifically cytotoxic. *J. exp. Med.* **135**: 150–164.
GREEN, J. A., COPPERBAND, S. R., RABINOWITZ, L., NAHMIAS, A. J. and KIBRICK, S. (1967) Production of a factor by blood lymphocytes which induces fibroblastoid transformation in epithelial cells. *Fedn Proc.* **26**: 702 (abstract).
GREEN, J. A., COOPERBAND, S. R., RUTSTEIN, J. A. and KIBRICK, S. (1970) Inhibition of target cell proliferation by supernatants from cultures of human peripheral lymphocytes. *J. Immun.* **105**: 48–54.
GREEN, S. S., WISTAR, R., JR and SELL, K. W. (1974) Mitogen-stimulated lymphocyte inhibition by supernatants of crowded lymphocytoblasts. *Transplantation* **18**: 496–502.
GUIMEZANES, A., FRIDMAN, W. H. and KOURILSKY, F. M. (1975) Immunoglobulin binding factor (IBF) produced by slow T cells: Selective interaction with slow migrating rabbit IgG. *Annls Inst. Pasteur* **126C**: 541–551.
HACKER, M., LACHMAN, L. B., BLYDEN, G. and HANDSCHUMACHER, R. E. (1977) Lymphocyte activating factor production by mouse tumor in culture. *Fedn Proc.* **36**: 1300 (abstract).
HAHN, H. H., CHAR, D. C., POSTEL, W. B. and WOOD, W. B., JR (1967) Studies on the pathogenesis of fever. XV. The production of endogenous pyrogen by peritoneal macrophages. *J. exp. Med.* **126**: 385–394.

HAMAOKA, T. and KATZ, D. H. (1973) Mechanism of adjuvant action of poly A:U on antibody responses to hapten-carrier conjugates. *Cell. Immun.* **7**: 246–260.

HÄMMERLING, U., CHIN, A. F., ABBOTT, J., GOLDSTEIN, G., SONENBERG, M. and HOFFMAN, M. K. (1976) The ontogeny of B lymphocytes. III. Opposite signals transmitted to B lymphocyte precursor cells by inducing agents and hormones. *Eur. J. Immun.* **6**: 868–872.

HÄMMERLING, U., CHIN, A. F., ABBOTT, J. and SCHEID, M. P. (1975) The ontogeny of murine B lymphocytes. I. Induction of phenotypic conversion of Ia^- to Ia^+ lymphocytes. *J. Immun.* **115**: 1425–1431.

HAMMOND, M. E. and DVORAK, H. F. (1972) Antigen-induced stimuaation of glucosamine incorporation by guinea pig peritoneal macrophages in delayed hypersensitivity. *J. exp. Med.* **136**: 1518–1532.

HAN, T., PAULY, J. L. and MINOWADA, J. (1975) Disparity in the production of lymphoblastogenesis inhibition factor by cultured human B and T lymphoid cell lines. *Clin. Exp. Immun.* **20**: 73–81.

HANNA, N., KALDERON, R. and NELKEN, D. (1975) Inhibition of T- and B-lymphocyte functions by normal immunosuppressive protein. *Immunology* **29**: 433–443.

HART, D. A., JONES, J. M. and NISONOFF, A. (1973) Mitogenic factor from inbred guinea pigs. I. Isolation of the factor. *Cell. Immun.* **9**: 173–185.

HARWELL, L., KAPPLER, J. W. and MARRACK, P. (1976) Antigen-specific and nonspecific mediators of T cell/B cell cooperation. III. Characterization of the nonspecific mediator(s) from different sources. *J. Immun.* **116**: 1379–1384.

HARWELL, L., MARRACK, P. and KAPPLER, J. W. (1977) Suppressor T-cell inactivation of a helper T-cell factor. *Nature* **265**: 57–59.

HAURANI, F. I., MEYER, A. and O'BRIEN, R. (1973) Production of transferrin by the macrophages. *J. Reticuloendoth. Soc.* **14**: 309–316.

HAVEMANN, K., BÜRGER, S. and DOSCH, H. M. (1970a) Phythämagglutinin (PHA) und Serum Proteine in der Lymphocytenkultur. II. Die Präcipitation von Serumproteine durch PHA. *Z. ges. exp. Med.* **153**: 308–323.

HAVEMANN, K., DOSCH, H. M. and BÜRGER, S. (1970b) Phythamägglutinin (PHA) und Serum Proteine in der Lymphocytenkulture. I. Nachweis von Fördernden und Hemmenden Serum Faktoren. *Z. ges. exp. Med.* **153**: 297–307.

HAVEMANN, K., HORVAT, M., SODOMANN, C.-P., HAVEMANN, K. and BÜRGER, S. (1972) Protease activity as a possible mechanism of migration inhibitory factor. *Eur. J. Immun.* **2**: 97–99.

HAY, J. B., LACHMANN, P. J. and TRNKA, Z. (1973) The appearance of migration inhibition factor and a mitogen in lymph draining tuberculin reactions. *Eur. J. Immun.* **3**: 127–131.

HEISE, E. R., HAN, S. and WEISER, R. S. (1968) *In vitro* studies on the mechanism of macrophage migration inhibition in tuberculin sensitivity. *J. Immun.* **101**: 1004–1015.

HEISE, E. R. and WEISER, R. S. (1969) Factors in delayed sensitivity: Lymphocyte and macrophage cytotoxins in the tuberculin reaction. *J. Immun.* **103**: 570–576.

HENNEY, C. S., GAFFNEY, J. and BLOOM, B. R. (1974) On the relation of products of activated lymphocytes to cell-mediated cytolysis. *J. exp. Med.* **140**: 837–852.

HERON, I., BERG, K. and CANTELL, K. (1976) Regulatory effects of interferon on T cells *in vitro*. *J. Immun.* **117**: 1370–1373.

HERSH, E. M., MCCREDIE, K. B. and FREIREICH, E. J. (1974a) Mechanisms of production of inhibitor of lymphocyte blastogenic response to mitogens by cultured lymphoblastoid cell line cells. *Transplantation* **17**: 221–227.

HERSH, E. M., MCCREDIE, K. B. and FREIREICH, E. J. (1974b) Inhibition of *in vitro* lymphocyte blastogenesis by inhibitor produced by cultured human lymphoblasts. *Clin. Exp. Immun.* **17**: 463–473.

HIGGINS, T. J. and DAVID, J. R. (1976) Effect of isoprotirenol and aminophylline on cyclic AMP levels of guinea pig macrophages. *Cell. Immun.* **27**: 1–10.

HIGGINS, T. J., WINSTON, C. T. and DAVID, J. R. (1976) Effect of migration inhibitory factor (MIF) on cyclic AMP levels of guinea pig macrophages. *Cell. Immun.* **27**: 11–16.

HIRASHIMA, M., HONDA, M. and HAYASHI, H. (1976) The mediation of tissue eosinophils in hypersensitivity reactions. II. Separation of a delayed eosinophil chemotactic factor from macrophage chemotactic factors. *Immunology* **31**: 263–271.

HIRSCHBERG, H., RANKIN, B. and THORSBY, E. (1974) Production of blastogenic factor by mitomycin-treated cells in mixed lymphocyte cultures. *Transplantation* **17**: 323–325.

HISERODT, J. C., FAIR, D. S. and GRANGER, G. A. (1976a) Identification of multiple cytolytic components associated with the β-LT class of lymphotoxin released by mitogen activated human lymphocytes *in vitro*. *J. Immun.* **117**: 1503–1506.

HISERODT, J. C. and GRANGER, G. A. (1976) *In vitro* lymphocyte cytotoxicity. II. Unstable lymphotoxins (β-LT) secreted and inactivated by mitogen-stimulated human lymphocytes. *Cell. Immun.* **26**: 211–216.

HISERODT, J. C., PRIEUR, A.-M. and GRANGER, G. A. (1976b) *In vitro* lymphocyte cytotoxicity. I. Evidence of multiple cytotoxic molecules secreted by mitogen activated human lymphoid cells *in vitro*. *Cell. Immun.* **24**: 277–288.

HOCHOVÁ, B., KREJČÍ, J., PEKÁREK, J., ŠVEJCAR, J. and JOHANOVSKÝ, J. (1975) Further characterization of antigen-dependent migration inhibitory factor in mice. *Immunology* **29**: 231–236.

HOESSLI, D. C., JONES, A. P. and WAKSMAN, B. H. (1977) Potentiation of the T-lymphocyte response to mitogens. IV. Serum-free production and testing of macrophage soluble products. *Cell. Immun.* **30**: 310–320.

HOFFMANN, M. and DUTTON, R. W. (1971) Immune response restoration with macrophage culture supernatants. *Science* **172**: 1047–1048.

HOLZMAN, R. S., LEBOWITZ, A. S., VALENTINE, F. T. and LAWRENCE, H. S. (1973a) Preparation and properties of cloning inhibitory factor. I. Inhibition of HeLa cell cloning by stimulated lymphocytes and their culture supernatants. *Cell. Immun.* **8**: 249–258.

HOLZMAN, R. S., VALENTINE, F. T. and LAWRENCE, H. S. (1973b) Preparation and properties of cloning inhibitory factor. II. Factors affecting its production and assay. *Cell. Immun.* **8**: 259–269.

HORTON, J. E., OPPENHEIM, J. J., MERGENHAGEN, S. E. and RAISZ, L. G. (1974) Macrophage–lymphocyte synergy in the production of the osteoclast activating factor. *J. Immun.* **113**: 1278–1287.

HORWITZ, D. A., GARRETT, M. A. and CRAIG, A. H. (1977) Serum effects on mitogenic reactivity in subjects with systemic lupus erythematosus, rheumatoid arthritis and scleroderma. Technical considerations and lack of correlation with anti-lymphocyte antibodies. *Clin. Exp. Immun.* **27**: 100–110.

HOUCK, J. C., ATTALLAH, A. M. and LILLY, J. R. (1973a) Immunosuppressive properties of the lymphocyte chalone. *Nature* **245**: 148–150.

HOUCK, J. C., IRAUSQUIN, H. and LEIKIN, S. (1971) Lymphocyte DNA synthesis inhibition. *Science* **173**: 1139–1141.

HOUCK, J. C., KANAGALINGHAM, K., HUNT, C., ATTALAH, A. and CHUNG, A. (1977) Lymphocyte and fibroblast chalones: some chemical properties. *Science* **196**: 896–897.

HOUCK, J. C., SHARMA, V. K. and CHENG, R. F. (1973b) Fibroblast chalone and serum mitogen (anti-chalone). *Nature New Biol.* **246**: 111–113.

HOUCK, J. C., WEIL, R. L. and SHARMA, V. K. (1972) Evidence for a fibroblast chalone. *Nature New Biol.* **240**: 210–211.

HOWELL, H. J., FREER, R. S., ZIGMOND, S. H., SCHIFFMAN, E., ASWANIKUMAR, S., CORCORAN, B. and BECKER, E. L. (1976) The structure-activity relations of synthetic peptides as chemotactic factors and inducers of lysosomal enzyme secretion for neutrophils. *J. exp. Med.* **143**: 1154–1169.

HSU, C. C. S., WAITHE, W. I., HATHAWAY, P. and HIRSCHHORN, K. (1973) The effects of foetinin on lymphocytes; lymphocyte-stimulating property. *Clin. Exp. Immun.* **15**: 427–434.

HUNTER, P. and KETTMAN, J. R. (1974) Mode of action of a supernatant activity from T-cell cultures that nonspecifically stimulates the humoral immune response. *Proc. natn. Acad. Sci. USA* **71**: 512–516.

ISAC, R. and MOZES, E. (1977) Antigen-specific T cell factors: a fine analysis of specificity. *J. Immun.* **118**: 584–588.

ISHIZAKA, T. (1976) Functions and development of cell receptors for IgE. In: *Molecular and Biological Aspects of the Acute Allergic Reaction*, pp. 199–215, JOHANSSON, S. G. O., STRANDBERG, K. and UVNÄS, B. (eds). Plenum, New York.

JACOBSON, E. B. (1973) *In vitro* studies of allotype suppression in mice. *Eur. J. Immun.* **3**: 619–624.

JACOBSSON, H. and BLOMGREN, H. (1975) Characterization of mouse spleen cells releasing or responding to mitogenic factor induced by phytomitogens *in vitro*. *J. Immun.* **114**: 1631–1637.

JAMES, S. L. and COLLEY, D. G. (1975) Eosinophils and immune mechanisms: production of the lymphokine eosinophil stimulation promotor (ESP) *in vitro* by isolated intact granulomas. *J. Reticuloendoth. Soc.* **18**: 283–293.

JEFFES, E. W. B., III and GRANGER, G. A. (1975) Relationship of cloning inhibition factor, 'lymphotoxin' factor and proliferation inhibition factor release *in vitro* by mitogen activated human lymphocytes. *J. Immun.* **114**: 64–69.

JEFFES, E. W. B., III and GRANGER, G. A. (1976) Relationship of CIF, LT and PIF released *in vitro* by activated human lymphocytes, II. A further functional comparison of LT and PIF activities on HeLa and L-929 target cells. *J. Immun.* **117**: 174–179.

JEGASOTHY, B. V., PACHNER, A. R. and WAKSMAN, B. H. (1976) Cytokine inhibition of DNA synthesis: effect on cyclic adenosine monophosphate in lymphocytes. *Science* **193**: 1260–1262.

JEGASOTHY, B. V., NAMBA, Y. and WAKSMAN, B. H. (1978) Regulatory substances produced by lymphocytes. VII. IDS (Inhibitor of DNA synthesis) inhibits stimulated lymphocytes proliferation by activating of membrane adenylate cyclase at a restriction point in G_1. *Immunochemistry* (to be published).

JOHANOVSKÝ, J., VRÁNA, M. and STEJSKAL, A. (1962) Characteristics of fever produced by hypersensitivity pyrogen. *Folia Microb.* **7**: 12–25.

JOHNSON, H. M., BUKOVIC, J. A. and BARON, S. (1975) Interferon inhibition of the primary *in vitro* antibody response to a thymus-independent antigen. *Cell. Immun.* **20**: 104–109.

JOKIPII, L. (1973) Migration inhibition of peritoneal exudate cells from sensitized and desensitized rats. *Immunology* **25**: 283–295.

JONES, J. M., HART, D. A. and NISONOFF, A. (1973) Mitogenic factor from inbred guinea pigs. II. Properties of the factor. *Cell. Immun.* **9**: 186–197.

JUREZIZ, R. E., THOR, D. E. and DRAY, S. (1968) Transfer with RNA extracts of the cell migration inhibition correlate of delayed hypersensitivity in the guinea pig. *J. Immun.* **101**: 823–829.

KAMRIN, B. B. (1959) Successful skin homografts in mature non-littermate rats treated with fractions containing alpha-globulins. *Proc. Soc. exp. Biol. Med.* **100**: 58–61.

KANTOR, F. S., HALL, C. B. and LIPSMEYER, E. A. (1971) Regulatory mechanisms in delayed hypersensitivity. In: *Cellular Interactions in the Immune Response*, pp. 213–218, COHEN, S., CUDKOWICZ, G. and MCCLUSKEY, R. T. (eds). Karger, Basel.

KAPP, J. A., PIERCE, C. W. and BENACERRAF, B. (1977) Immunosuppressive factor(s) extracted from lymphoid cells of nonresponder mice primed with L-glutamic acid^{60}-L-alanine^{30}-L-tyrosine^{10} (GAT). II. Cellular source and effect on responder and nonresponder mice. *J. exp. Med.* **145**: 829–838.

KAPP, J. A., PIERCE, C. W., DE LA CROIX, F. and BENACERRAF, B. (1976) Immunosuppressive factor(s) extraced from lymphoid cells of nonresponder mice primed with L-glutamic acid ^{60}L-alanine^{30}-L-tyrosine^{10} (GAT). I. Activity and antigenic specificity. *J. Immunol.* **116**: 305–309.

KASAKURA, S. and LOWENSTEIN, L. (1965) A factor stimulating DNA synthesis derived from the medium of leucocyte cultures. *Nature* **208**: 794–795.

KASAHARA, T. and SHIOIRO-NAKANO, K. (1976) Splenic suppressing factor: purification and characterization of a factor suppressing thymidine incorporation into activated lymphocytes. *J. Immun.* **116**: 1251–1256.

KATZ, D. H. and ARMERDING, D. (1976) The role of histocompatibility gene products in lymphocyte triggering and differentiation. *Fedn. Proc.* **35**: 2053–2060.

KATZ, D. H. and BENACERRAF, B. (eds) (1974) *Immunological Tolerance. Mechanism and Potential Therapeutic Applications.* Academic Press, New York, San Francisco, London.

KELLY, R. H., WOLSTENCROFT, R. A., DUMONDE, D. C. and BALFOUR, B. M. (1972) Role of lymphocyte activation products (LAP) in cell-mediated immunity. II. Effect of lymphocyte activation products on lymph node architecture and evidence for peripheral release of LAP following antigenic stimulation. *Clin. Exp. Immun.* **10**: 49–65.

KIERSZENBAUM, F. and WAKSMAN, B. H. (1977) Mechanisms of action of 'lymphocyte activating factor' (LAF). I. Association of LAF action with early DNA synthesis in PHA-stimulated lymphocytes. *Immunology* **33**: 663–669.

KIGER, N. (1971) Isolation and immunological study of thymic lymphocytic inhibitory factors. *Rev. Eur. Etudes Clin. Biol.* **16**: 566–572.

KIGER, N., FLORENTIN, I. and MATHÉ. G. (1973) Inhibition of graft-versus-host reaction by preincubation of the graft with a thymic extract (lymphocyte chalone). *Transplantation* **16**: 393–397.

KIROV, S. M. and PARISH, C. R. (1976) Carrier-specific B-cells play a role in the production of an antigen-specific T-cell replacing factor. *Scand. J. Immun.* **5**: 1155–1162.

KISHIMOTO, T. and ISHIZAKA, K. (1973) Regulation of antibody response *in vitro*. VII. Enhancing soluble factors for IgG and IgE antibody response. *J. Immun.* **111**: 1194–1205.

KISHIMOTO, T. and ISHIZAKA, K. (1974) Regulation of antibody response *in vitro*. VIII. Multiplicity of soluble factors released from carrier-specific cells. *J. Immun.* **112**: 1685–1697.

KISHIMOTO, T. and ISHIZAKA, K. (1975) Immunologic and physicochemical properties of enhancing soluble factors for IgG and IgE antibody responses. *J. Immun.* **114**: 1177–1184.

KLUN, C. L., NEIBURGER, R. G. and YOUMANS, G. P. (1973) Relationship between mouse migration-inhibitory factor in supernatant fluids from mouse lymphocyte cultures. *J. Reticuloendoth. Soc.* **13**: 310–318.

KNYSZYNSKI, A. and BURGER, M. (1971) Stimulation of DNA synthesis *in vitro* in mouse thymic cells by bone marrow preparation. *Blood* **37**: 231–239.

KOLB, W. P. and GRANGER, G. A. (1968) Lymphocyte *in vitro* cytotoxicity: characterization of human lymphotoxin. *Proc. natn. Acad. Sci. USA.* **61**: 1250–1255.

KOLTAI, M., BLAZSÓ, G., MINKER, E., LONOVICS, J. and OTTLECZ, A. (1975) Anaphylactoid-inflammation-promoting factor. An insulin-induced factor derived from non-sensitized lymphocytes increases anaphylactoid inflammation in rats. *Int. Arcs Allergy* **49**: 358–370.

KONTIAINEN, S. and FELDMANN, M. (1977) Suppressor cell induction *in vitro*. III. Antigen-specific suppression by supernatants of suppressor cells. *Eur. J. Immun.* **7**: 310–314.

KOOK, A. I. and TRAININ, N. (1974) Hormone-like activity of a thymus humoral factor on the induction of immune competence in lymphoid cells. *J. exp. Med.* **139**: 193–207.

KOOK, A. I. and TRAININ, N. (1975) Intracellular events involved in the induction of immune competence in lymphoid cells by a thymus humoral factor. *J. Immun.* **114**: 151–157.

KOOPMAN, W. J., GILLIS, M. H. and DAVID, J. R. (1973) Prevention of MIF activity by agents known to increase cellular cyclic AMP. *J. Immun.* **110**: 1609–1614.

KOOPMAN, W. J., SANDBERG, A. L., WAHL, S. M. and MERGENHAGEN, S. E. (1976) Interaction of soluble C3 fragments with guinea pig lymphocytes. Comparison of effects of C3a, C3b, C3c, C3d on lymphokine production and lymphocyte proliferation. *J. Immun.* **117**: 331–336.

KORCAKOVÁ, L., HAŠKOVÁ, V., SVOBODOVÁ, J., MACUROVÁ, H., SAJDLOVÁ, H., IVAŠKOVÁ, E. and HINZOVA, E. (1975) Mouse lymph node activating factor release during contact of HL-A different blood lymphocytes. *Transplantation* **20**: 273–277.

KRAHENBUHL, J. L. and REMINGTON, J. S. (1971) *In vitro* induction of nonspecific resistance in macrophages by specifically sensitized lymphocytes. *Infect. Immun.* **4**: 337–343.

KRAKAUER, R. S., STROBER, W., RIPPEON, D. L. and WALDMANN, T. A. (1977) Prevention of autoimmunity in experimental lupus erythematosus by soluble immune response suppressor. *Science* **196**: 56–59.

KRAMER, J. J. and GRANGER, G. A. (1972) The *in vitro* induction and release of a cell toxin by immune C57 B1/6 mouse peritoneal macrophages. *Cell. Immun.* **3**: 88–100.

KRAMER, S. L. and GRANGER, G. A. (1975) The role of lymphotoxin in target cell destruction by mitogen-activated human lymphocytes. I. The correlation of target cell sensitivity to lymphotoxin and the intact lymphocyte. Cell. Immun. **15**: 57–68.

KRAMER, S. L. and GRANGER, G. A. (1976) The role of lymphotoxin in target cell destruction induced by mitogen-activated human lymphocytes *in vitro*. II. The correlation of temperature and trypsin-sensitive phases of lymphotoxin-induced and lymphocyte-mediated cytotoxicity. *J. Immun.* **116**: 562–567.

KREJČÍ, J., ŠVEJCAR, J., PEKÁREK, J. and JOHANOVSKÝ, J. (1968) Demonstration of migration inhibiting substances in sera of guinea pigs with delayed type hypersensitivity to ovalbumin influenced with systemic antigen administration. *Z. Immunitstät.* **136**: 259–267.

KUHNER, A. L. and DAVID, J. R. (1976) Partial characterization of murine migration inhibitory factor (MIF). *J. Immun.* **116**: 140–145.

KURATSUJI, T., YOSHIDA, T. and COHEN, S. (1976) Anti-lymphokine antibody. II. Specificity of biological activity. *J. Immun.* **117**: 1985–1991.

KUSHNER, I. and KAPLAN, M. H. (1961) Studies of acute phase protein. I. An immunohistochemical method for the localization of Cx-reaction protein in rabbits. Association with necrosis in local inflammatory lesions. *J. exp. Med.* **114**: 961–974.

LACHMAN, L. B. and HANDSCHUMACHER, R. E. (1976) Electromobility and purification of human lymphocyte activating factor. *Fedn Proc.* **35**: 489 (abstract).

LAI, R. F. M., FAT, A. and VAN FURTH, R. (1975) *In vitro* synthesis of some complement components (C1q, C3 and C4) by lymphoid tissues and circulating leucocytes in man. *Immunology* **28**: 359–368.

LEE, S.-C. and LUCAS, Z. J. (1976) Regulatory factors produced by lymphocytes. I. The occurrence of multiple α-lymphotoxins associated with ribonuclease activity. *J. Immun.* **117**: 283–291.

LEE, S.-C. and LUCAS, Z. J. (1977) Regulatory factors produced by lymphocytes. II. Inhibition of cellular DNA synthesis associated with a factor inhibiting DNA polymerase α activity. *J. Immun.* **118**: 88–97.
LEE, S. T. and PARASKEVAS, F. (1976a) Soluble factors in immune sera of mice. I. Specific and non-specific suppressive activity. *Clin. Exp. Immun.* **24**: 177–184.
LEE, S. R. and PARASKEVAS, F. (1976b) Soluble factors in immune sera of mice. II. Reversible loss of surface immunoglobulin induced *in vitro*. *Clin. Exp. Immun.* **24**: 185–195.
LEFKOVITS, I., QUINTANS, J., MUNRO, A. and WALDMANN, H. (1975) T-cell-dependent mediator and B-cell clones. *Immunology* **28**: 1149–1154.
LEONARD, E. J. and MELTZER, M. S. (1976) Characterization of mouse lymphocyte-derived chemotactic factor. *Cell. Immun.* **26**: 200–210.
LETT-BROWN, M. A., BOETHCER, D. A. and LEONARD, E. J. (1976) Chemotactic responses of normal human basophils to C5a and to lymphocyte-derived chemotactic factor. *J. Immun.* **117**: 246–252.
LEU, R. W., EDDLESTON, A. L. W. F., HADDEN, J. W. and GOOD, R. A. (1972) Mechanism of action of migration inhibitory factor (MIF). I. Evidence for a receptor for MIF present on the peritoneal macrophage but not on the alveolar macrophages. *J. exp. Med.* **136**: 589–603.
LEWIS, J. E., CARMACK, C. E., YAMAMOTO, R. and GRANGER, G. A. (1977) Antibodies against human lymphokines. I. Methods for induction of antibodies capable of neutralizing stable (α) and unstable (β) lymphotoxins released *in vitro* by activated human lymphocytes. *J. Immun. Meth.* **14**: 163–176.
LITTMAN, B. H. and RUDDY, S. (1977) Production of the second component of complement by human monocytes: stimulation by antigen-activated lymphocytes or lymphokines. *J. exp. Med.* **145**: 1344–1352.
LODMELL, D. L., EWALT, L. C. and NOTKINS, A. L. (1976) Inhibition of vaccinia virus replication in skin of tuberculin-sensitized animals challenged with PPD. *J. Immun.* **117**: 1757–1761.
LOLEKHA, S., DRAY, S. and GOTOFF, S. P. (1970) Macrophage aggregation *in vitro*. A correlate of delayed hypersensitivity. *J. Immun.* **104**: 296–304.
LOMNITZER, R., RABSON, A. R. and KORNHOF, H. J. (1975) Production of leucocyte inhibitory factor (LIF) and macrophage inhibitory factor (MIF) by PHA-stimulated lymphocytes. *Clin. Exp. Immun.* **22**: 522–527.
LOVCHIK, J. C. and HONG, R. (1977) Antibody-dependent cell-mediated cytolysis (ADCC). *Prog. Allergy* **22**: 1–45.
LOZZIO, B. B. (1973) Regulators of cell division. A review. I. Endogenous mitotic inhibitors of hematopoietic cells. *Exp. Hematol.* **1**: 309–339.
LYKKE, A. W. J., WILLOUGHBY, D. A. and KOSCHE, E. R. (1967) Thymic permeability factor: its relationship to lymph-node permeability factor and its antagonism by pyridinol carbamate agents. *J. Path. Bact.* **94**: 381–388.
MACKANESS, G. B. (1969) The influence of immunologically committed lymphoid cells on macrophage activity *in vivo*. *J. exp. Med.* **129**: 973–992.
MAILLARD, J. L., PICK, E. and TURK, J. L. (1972) Interactions between 'sensitized lymphocytes' and antigen *in vitro*. V. Vascular permeability induced by skin-reactive factor. *Int. Archs. Allergy* **42**: 50–68.
MAINI, R. N., DUMONDE, D. C., FAUX, J. A., HARGREAVE, F. E. and PEPYS, J. (1971) The production of lymphocyte mitogenic factor and migration-inhibition factor by antigen-stimulated lymphocytes of subjects with grass pollen allergy. *Clin. Exp. Immun.* **9**: 449–465.
MANGI, R. J., DWYER, J. M., GEE, B. and KANTOR, F. S. (1974a) The immunological competence of subjects with sarcoidosis. *Clin. Exp. Immun.* **18**: 505–517.
MANGI, R. J., DWYER, J. M. and KANTOR, F. S. (1974b) The effect of plasma upon lymphocyte response *in vitro*. Demonstration of a humoral inhibitor in patients with sarcoidosis. *Clin. Exp. Immun.* **18**: 519–528.
MANNICK, J. A. and SCHMID, K. (1967) Prolongation of allograft survival by an alpha globulin isolated from normal blood. *Transplantation* **5**: 1231–1238.
MARAMOROSCH, K. and SHOPE, R. E. (eds) (1975) Hemolymph components in invertebrate immunity. In: *Invertebrate Immunity*, pp. 201–289. Academic Press, New York, San Francisco, London.
MARRACK (HUNTER) P. C. and KAPPLER, J. W. (1975) Antigen-specific and nonspecific mediators of T cell/B cell cooperation. I. Evidence for their production by different T cells. *J. Immun.* **114**: 1116–1125.
MARRACK, P. C. and KAPPLER, J. W. (1976) Antigen-specific and nonspecific mediators of T cell/B cell cooperation. II. Two helper T cells distinguished by their antigen sensitivities. *J. Immun.* **116**: 1373–1378.
MCCONNELL, I. and LACHMANN, P. J. (1977) Complement receptors and cell-associated complement components. *Immun. Commun.* **6**: 111–132.
MCIVOR, K. L. and WEISER, R. S. (1971a) Mechanisms of target cell destruction by alloimmune peritoneal macrophages. I. The effect of treatment with sodium fluoride. *Immunology* **20**: 307–313.
MCIVOR, K. L. and WEISER, R. S. (1971b) Mechanisms of target cell destruction by alloimmune peritoneal macrophages. II. Release of a specific cytotoxin from interacting cells. *Immunology* **20**: 315–322..
MCKENZIE, I. F. C., CLARKE, A. and PARISH, C. R. (1977) Ia antigenic specificities are oligosaccharide in Nature: hapten-inhibition studies. *J. exp. Med.* **145**: 1039–1053.
MCKENZIE, I. F. C. and PARISH, C. R. (1976) Secretion of Ia antigens by a subpopulation of T cells which are $Ly\text{-}1^+$, $Ly\text{-}2^-$, and Ia^-. *J. exp. Med.* **144**: 847–851.
MCMASTER, R. and LEVY, J. G. (1975) Immunosuppression of normal lyphoid cells by serum from mice undergoing chronic graft-vs-host disease. *J. Immun.* **115**: 1400–1403.
MEACOCK, S. C. R., HEESOM, N. and WILLOUGHBY, D. A. (1968) Further studies on the suppression of delayed hypersensitivity reactions in the rat and guinea pig by antibody against lymph node abstracts. *Immunology* **15**: 115–122.
MEADE, C. J., LACHMANN, P. J. and BRENNER, S. (1974) A sensitive assay for cellular hypersensitivity based on the uptake of radioactive colloidal gold. *Immunology* **27**: 227–239.
MELSOM, H., KEARY, G., GRUCA, S. and SELJELID, R. (1974) Evidence for a cytolytic factor released by macrophages. *J. exp. Med.* **140**: 1085–1096.MELTZER, M. S. and OPPENHEIM, J. J. (1977) Bidirectional

amplification of macrophage–lymphocyte interactions: enhanced lymphocyte activation factor production by activated mouse peritoneal cells. *J. Immun.* **118**: 77–82.

MENDELSOHN, J., SKINNER, A. and KORNFELD, S. (1971) The rapid induction by phytohemagglutinin of increased α-aminoisobutyric acid uptake by lymphocytes. *J. Clin. Invest.* **50**: 818–826.

MENZOIAN, J. O., GLASGOW, A. H., NIMBERG, R. D., COOPERBAND, S. R., SCHMID, K., SAPORESCHETZ, I. and MANNICK, J. A. (1974) Regulation of T lymphocyte function by immunoregulatory alpha globulin (IRA). *J. Immun.* **113**: 266–273.

MILLER, S. D., SY, M.-S. and CLAMAN, H. N. (1977) The induction of hapten-specific T cell tolerance using hapten-modified lymphoid membranes. II. Relative roles of suppressor T cells and clone inhibition in the tolerant state. *Eur. J. Immun.* **7**: 165–170.

MILLS, J. A. (1975) Characterization of guinea pig mitogenic factor. *J. Immun.* **114**: 45–50.

MILTHORP, P. and FORSDYKE, D. R. (1973) Serum factors affecting the incorporation of (^{3}H) uridine by lymphocytes stimulated by concanavalin A. Studies of the role of complement. *Biochem. J.* **132**: 803–820.

MILTON, J. D. and MOWBRAY, J. F. (1972) Reversible loss of surface receptors on lymphocytes. *Immunology* **23**: 599–608.

MOLENAAR, J. L., VAN GALEN, M., HANNEMA, A. J., ZEIJLEMAKER, W. and PONDMAN, K. W. (1977) Spontaneous release of Fc receptor-like material from human lymphoblastoid cell lines. *Eur. J. Immun.* **7**: 230–236.

MÖLLER, G. (ed) (1973) Effector cells in cell-mediated immunity. *Transplant. Rev.* **17**: 1–171.

MÖLLER, G. (ed) (1976a) Specificity of effector T lymphocytes. *Transplant. Rev.* **29**: 1–310.

MÖLLER, G. (ed) (1976b) Biochemistry and biology of Ia antigens. *Transplant. Rev.* **30**: 1–322.

MONCADA, S., FERREIRA, S. H. and YANE, J. R. (1973) Prostaglandins, aspirin-like drugs and the oedema of inflammation. *Nature* **246**: 217–219.

MOONEY, J. J. and WAKSMAN, B. H. (1970) Activation of normal rabbit macrophage monolayers by supernatants of antigen-stimulated lymphocyte. *J. Immun.* **105**: 1138–1145.

MOORE, M. A. S. (1976) Regulatory role of macrophages in hemopoiesis. *J. Reticuloendoth. Soc.* **20**: 89–91.

MOORE, M. A. S., WILLIAMS, N. and METCALF, D. (1973) *In vitro* colony formation by normal and leukemic human hematopoietic cells: interaction between colony-forming and colony-stimulating cells. *J. natn. Ca. Inst.* **50**: 591–602.

MORTENSEN, R. F., BROWN, D. and GEWURZ, H. (1977) Effects of C-reactive protein on lymphocyte functions. III. Inhibition of antigen-induced lymphocyte stimulation and lymphokine production. *Cell. Immun.* **28**: 59–68.

MORTENSEN, R. F. and GEWURZ, H. (1976) Enects of C-reactive protein on the lymphoid system. II. Inhibition of mixed lymphocyte reactivity and generation of cytotoxic lymphocytes. *J. Immun.* **116**: 1244–1250.

MORTENSEN, R. F., OSMAND, A. P. and GEWURZ, H. (1975) Effects of C-reactive protein on the lymphoid system. I. Binding to thymus-dependent lymphocytes and alteration of their functions. *J. exp. Med.* **141**: 821–839.

MOSIER, D. E. and JOHNSON, B. M. (1975) Ontogeny of mouse lymphocyte function. II. Development of the ability to produce antibody is modulated by T-lymphocytes. *J. exp. Med.* **141**: 216–226.

MOWBRAY, J. F. (1963) Ability of large doses of an alpha$_2$ plasma protein fraction to inhibit antibody production. *Immunology* **6**: 217–225.

MOY, J. and ROSENAU, W. (1977) Evidence that human α-lymphotoxin is not a RNase. *J. Immun.* **118**: 1507–1508.

MUNRO, A. J., TAUSSIG, M. J., CAMPBELL, R., WILLIAMS, H. and LAWSON, Y. (1974) Antigen-specific T-cell factor in cell cooperation: physical properties and mapping in the left hand (K) half of N-2. *J. exp. Med.* **140**: 1579–1586.

MURGITA, R. A. (1976) The immunosuppressive role of alpha-fetoprotein during pregnancy. *Scand. J. Immun.* **5**: 1003–1014.

MURGITA, R. A., GOIDL, E. A., KONTIAINEN, S. and WIGZELL, H. (1977) α-fetoprotein induces suppressor cells *in vitro*. *Nature* **267**: 257–259.

MURGITA, R. A. and TOMASI, T. B., JR (1975a) Suppression of the immune response by α-fetoprotein. I. The effect of mouse α-fetoprotein on the primary and secondary antibody response. *J. exp. Med.* **141**: 269–286.

MURGITA, R. A. and TOMASI, T. B., JR (1975b) Suppression of the immune response by α-fetoprotein. II. The effect of mouse α-fetoprotein on mixed lymphocyte reactivity and mitogen-induced lymphocyte transformation. *J. exp. Med.* **141**: 440–452.

MURGITA, R. A. and WIGZELL, H. (1976) The effects of mouse alpha-fetoprotein on T-cell-dependent and T-cell-independent immune responses *in vitro*. *Scand. J. Immun.* **5**: 1215–1220.

MUTCHNICK, M. G., HAN, I. H. and JOHNSON, A. G. (1977) Mouse thymocyte membrane uptake of polyadenylic-polyuridylic acid complexes. *Proc. Soc. exp. Biol. Med.* **154**: 264–268.

NAKAMURA, S., YOSHINAGA, M. and HAYASHI, H. (1976) Interaction between lymphocytes and inflammatory exudate cells. II. A proteolytic enzyme released by PMN as a possible mediator for enhancement of thymocyte response. *J. Immun.* **117**: 1–6.

NAMBA, Y., JEGASOTHY, B. V. and WAKSMAN, B. H. (1977) Regulatory substances produced by lymphocytes. V. Production of inhibitor of DNA synthesis (IDS) by proliferating T-lymphocytes. *J. Immun.* **118**: 1379–1384.

NAMBA, Y. and WAKSMAN, B. H. (1975a) Analysis of T-cell-specific functions in continuous lymphocytic cell lines. I. Combined expression of thymocyte antigen and MIF production in rat-mouse hybrid lines. *Exp. Cell Res.* **94**: 22–30.

NAMBA, Y. and WAKSMAN, B. H. (1975b) Regulatory substances produced by lymphocytes. I. Inhibitor of DNA synthesis in the rat. *Inflammation* **1**: 5–21.

NAMBA, Y. and WAKSMAN, B. H. (1975c) Regulatory substances produced by lymphocytes. II. Lymphotoxin in the rat. *J. Immun.* **115**: 1018–1022.

NAMBA, Y. and WAKSMAN, B. H. (1976) Regulatory substances produced by lymphocytes. III. Evidence that lymphotoxin and proliferation inhibitory factor are identical and differ from the inhibitor of DNA synthesis. *J. Immun.* **116**: 1140–1144.

NAMBA, Y. and WAKSMAN, B. H. (1977) Regulatory substances produced by lymphocytes. IV. Further characterization of the inhibitor of DNA synthesis. *Immunochemistry* **14**: 143–147.

NATHAN, C. F., KARNOVKSY, M. L. and DAVID, J. R. (1971) Alterations of macrophage functions by mediators from lymphocytes. *J. exp. Med.* **133**: 1356–1376.

NATHAN, C. F., REMOLD, H. G. and DAVID, J. R. (1973) Characterization of a lymphocyte factor which alters macrophage functions. *J. exp. Med.* **137**: 275–290.

NATVIG, J. B., PERLMANN, P. and WIGZELL, H. (eds) (1976) *Lymphocytes, Isolation, Fractionation, and Characterization.* University Park Press, Baltimore, London, Tokyo.

NELKEN, D. (1973) Normal immunosuppressive protein (NIP). *J. Immun.* **110**: 1161–1162.

NELSON, D. S. (1973) Production by stimulated macrophages of factors depressing lymphocyte transformation. *Nature* **246**: 306–307.

NELSON, D. S. (ed) (1976) *Immunobiology of the Macrophages.* Academic Press, New York, San Francisco, London.

NELSON, D. S., PENROSE, J. M., WATERS, M. F. R., PEARSON, J. M. H. and NELSON, M. (1975) Depressive effect of serum from patients with leprosy on mixed lymphocyte reactions. Influence of anti-leprosy treatment. *Clin. Exp. Immun.* **22**: 385–392.

NELSON, D. S. and SHNEIDER, D. N. (1974) Effect of normal mouse serum on mouse lymphocyte transformation *in vitro. Eur. J. Immun.* **4**: 79–86.

NEPOM, J. T., HELLSTRÖM, I. and HELLSTRÖM, K. E. (1976) Purification and partial characterization of a tumor-specific blocking factor from sera of mice with growing chemically induced sarcomas. *J. Immun.* **117**: 1846–1852.

NGAN, J., LEE, S. H. S. and KIND, L. S. (1976) The suppressive effect of interferon on the ability of mouse spleen cells synthesizing IgE to sensitize rat skin for heterologous adoptive cutaneous anaphylaxis. *J. Immun.* **117**: 1063–1066.

NORTH, R. J., KIRSTEIN, D. P. and TUTTLE, R. L. (1976) Subversion of host defense mechanisms by murine tumors. I. A circulating factor that suppresses macrophage-mediated resistance to infection. *J. exp. Med.* **143**: 559–573.

NOVOGRODSKY, A. and GERY, I. (1972) Enhancement of mouse thymus cells response to periodate treatment by a soluble factor. *J. Immun.* **109**: 1278–1281.

NUSSENZWEIG, V. (1974) Receptors for immune complexes on lymphocytes. *Adv. Immun.* **19**: 217–258.

OATES, C. M., BISENDEN, J. F., MAINI, R. N., PAYNE, L. N. and DUMONDE, D. C. (1972) Thymus and bursa dependence of lymphocyte mitogenic factor in the chicken. *Nature New Biol.* **239**: 137–139.

OCCHINO, J. C., GLASGOW, A. H., COOPERBAND, S. R., MANNICK, J. A. and SCHMID, K. (1973) Isolation of an immunosuppressive peptide fraction from human plasma. *J. Immun.* **110**: 685–694.

OHISHI, M. and ONOUE, K. (1975) Functional activation of immune lymphocytes by antigenic stimulation in cell mediated immunity. I. Requirement for macrophages in antigen-induced MIF production by guinea pig immune lymphocytes *in vitro. Cell. Immun.* **18**: 220–232.

OISHI, N., TORIKAWA, C., OCHIAI, H. and HOKAMA, Y. (1973) Relationship of c-reactive protein in autologous plasma of cancer patients and choline phosphate in lymphocyte responses to phytohemagglutinin. *J. Reticuloendoth. Sco.* **14**: 242–249.

OKUMURA, K. and TADA, T. (1974) Regulation of homocytotropic antibody formation in the rat. IX. Further characterization of the antigen-specific inhibitory T cell factor in hapten-specific homocytotropic antibody response. *J. Immun.* **112**: 783–791.

OLDING, L. B., BENIRSCHKE, K. and OLDSTONE, M. B. A. (1974) Inhibition of mitosis of lymphocytes from human adults by lymphocytes from human newborns. *Clin. Immun. Immunopath.* **3**: 79–89.

OLSEN, I. and HARRIS, G. (1974) Uptake and release of DNA by lymphoid tissue and cells. *Immunology* **27**: 973–987.

OPITZ, H. G., NIETHAMMER, D., JACKSON, R. C., LEMKE, H., HUGET, R. and FLAD, H. D. (1975a) Biochemical characterization of a factor released by macrophages. *Cell. Immun.* **18**: 70–75.

OPITZ, H. G., NIETHAMMER, D., LEMKE, H., FLAD, H. D. and HUGET, R. (1975b) Inhibition of ^{3}H-thymidine incorporation of lymphocytes by a soluble factor from macrophages. *Cell. Immun.* **16**: 379–388.

OPPENHEIM, J. J., SHNEYOUR, A. and KOOK, A. I. (1976) Enhancement of DNA synthesis and cAMP content of mouse thymocytes by mediator(s) derived from adherent cells. *J. Immun.* **116**: 1466–1472.

OUTTERIDGE, P. M. and LEPPER, A. W. D. (1973) Immunosuppressive factors released by transforming lymphocytes in the delayed hypersensitivity skin response to tuberculin. *Immunology* **25**: 981–994.

PAPAGEORGIOU, P. S., HENLEY, W. L. and GLADE, P. R. (1972) Production and characterization of migration inhibitory factor(s) (MIF) of established lymphoid and non-lymphoid cell lines. *J. Immun.* **108**: 494–504.

PAPAGEORGIOU, P. S., TIBBETS, L., SOROKIN, C. F. and GLADE, P. R. (1974) Presence of a reversible inhibitor(s) for human lymphoid cell RNA, protein, and DNA synthesis in the extracts of established human lympoid cell lines. *Cell. Immun.* **11**: 354–366.

PARISH, C. R., CHILCOTT, A. B. and MCKENZIE, I. F. C. (1976) Low molecular weight Ia antigens in normal mouse serum. II. Demonstration of their T cell origin. *Immunogenetics* **3**: 129–137.

PARKER, J. W. and METCALF, D. (1974a) Production of colony-stimulating factor in mitogen-stimulated lymphocyte cultures. *J. Immun.* **112**: 502–510.

PARKER, J. W. and METCALF, D. (1974b) Production of colony-stimulating factor in mixed leucocyte cultures. *Immunology* **26**: 1039–1049.

PARROTT, D. M. V. and DE SOUSA, M. (1971) Thymus-dependent and thymus-independent populations: origin, migratory patterns and lifespan. *Clin. Exp. Immun.* **8**: 663–684.

PATTERSON, R. J. and YOUMANS, G. P. (1970) Demonstration in tissue culture of lymphocyte-mediated immunity to tuberculosis. *Inf. Immunity* **1**: 600–603.

PAUL, W. E., SHEVACH, E. M., PICKERAL, S., THOMAS, D. W. and ROSENTHAL, A. S. (1977) Independent populations of primed F_1 guinea pig T lymphocytes respond to antigen-pulsed parental peritoneal exudate cells. *J. exp. Med.* **145**: 618–630.

PETER, J. B., STRATTON, J. A., STEMPEL, K. E., YU, D. and CARDIN, C. (1973) Characteristics of a cytotoxin ('lymphotoxin') produced by stimulation of human lympoid tissue. *J. Immun.* **111**: 770–782.

PHILLIPS, S. M., CARPENTER, C. B. and LAUE, P. (1975) Immunosuppressive globulin from bovine thymus and serum: mode of action upon afferent and efferent arcs of the mouse immune response. *Ann. N.Y. Acad. Sci.* **249**: 236–247.

PICK, E. (1972) Cyclic AMP effects macrophage migration. *Nature New Biol.* **238**: 176–177.

PICK, E. (1974) Soluble lymphocytic mediators. I. Inhibition of macrophage migration inhibitory factor production by drugs. *Immunology* **26**: 649–658.

PICK, E. and ABRAHAMER, H. (1973) Blocking of macrophage migration inhibitory factor action by microtubular disruptive drugs. *Int. Archs Allergy* **44**: 215–220.

PICK, E., BROSTOFF, J., KREJČÍ, J. and TURK, J. L. (1970a) Interaction between 'sensitized lymphocytes' and antigen *in vitro*. II. Mitogen-induced release of skin reactive and macrophage migration inhibitory factors. *Cell. Immun.* **1**: 92–109.

PICK, E., KREJČÍ, J., ČECH, K. and TURK, J. L. (1969) Interaction between 'sensitized lymphocytes' and antigen *in vitro*. I. The release of skin reactive factor. *Immunology* **17**: 741–767.

PICK, E., KREJČÍ, J. and TURK, J. L. (1970b) Release of skin reactive factor from guinea pig lymphocytes by mitogens. *Nature* **225**: 236–238.

PINCUS, W. B. (1967a) Formation of cytotoxic factor by macrophages from normal guinea pigs. *J. Reticuloendoth. Soc.* **4**: 122–139.

PINCUS, W. B. (1967b) Cell-free cytotoxic fluids from tuberculin-treated normal guinea pigs. *J. Reticuloendoth. Soc.* **4**: 140–150.

PINCUS, W. B., SPANIS, C. W. and SINTEK, D. E. (1971) Cytotoxic factor from peritoneal cells: site of action. *J. Reticuloendoth. Soc.* **9**: 552–567.

PINCUS, W. B., WOODS, W. W. and PANG, R. K. (1970) Immune-specific cytotoxic factor formation by small lymphocytes. *J. Reticuloendoth. Soc.* **7**: 220–237.

PIPER, C. E. and MCIVOR, K. L. (1975) Alloimmune peritoneal macrophages as specific effector cells: characterization of specific macrophage cytotoxin. *Cell. Immun.* **17**: 423–430.

POSTLETHWAITE, A. E. and KANG, A. H. (1976) Guinea pig lymphocyte-derived macrophage aggregation factor: its separation from macrophage migration inhibitory factor. *J. Immun.* **117**: 1651–1655.

POSTLETHWAITE, A. E., SNYDERMAN, R. and KANG, A. H. (1976) The chemotactic attraction of human fibroblasts to a lymphocyte-derived factor. *J. Immun.* **144**: 1188–1203.

POULTER, L. W. and TURK, J. L. (1975a) Studies on the effect of soluble lymphocyte products (lymphokines) on macrophage physiology. I. Early changes in enzyme activity and permeability. *Cell. Immum.* **20**: 12–24.

POULTER, L. W. and TURK, J. L. (1975b) Studies on the effect of soluble lymphocyte products (lymphokines) on macrophage physiology. II. Cytochemical changes associated with activation. *Cell. Immun.* **20**: 25–32.

POWLES, R., BLACHIN, L., CURRIE, G. A. and ALEXANDER, P. (1971) Specific autostimulating factor released by lymphocytes. *Nature* **231**: 161–164.

PRENDERGAST, R. A. and LIU, S. H. (1976) Isolation and characterization of sea star factor. *Scand. J. Immun.* **5**: 873–880.

PRYSTOWSKY, M. B., SOROKIN, C. F., CEGLOWSKI, W. S., HIRSCHHORN, K. and GLADE, P. R. (1975) Intracellular localization of the migration inhibitory factor (MIF) in a long-term human lympoid cell line. *Int. Archs Allergy* **48**: 225–235.

PTAK, W., NAIDORF, K. F. and GERSHON, R. K. (1977) Interference with the transmission of T cell derived messages by macrophage membranes. *J. Immun* **119**: 444–449.

RABINOVITCH, M. and GARY, P. P. (1968) Effect of the uptake of staphylococci on the ingestion of glutaraldehyde-treated red cells attached to macrophages. *Exp. Cell Res.* **52**: 363–369.

RADOVICH, J. and TALMAGE, D. W. (1967) Antigenic competition: cellular or humoral. *Science* **158**: 512–514.

RAMSEIER, H. (1969) Quantitative studies on antigenic recognition. I. Immunological and nonimmunological parameters of the response. *J. exp. Med.* **130**: 1279–1294.

RAMSEIER, H. and LINDENMANN, J. (1977a) Studies on the product of antigenic recognition. I. Formation of the product in recognition of alloantigens. *Exp. Cell Biol.* **45**: 60–88.

RAMSEIER, H. and LINDENMANN, J. (1977b) Studies on the product of antigenic recognition. II. Formation of the product in recognition of alloreceptors. *Exp. Cell Biol.* **45**: 89–100.

RAMSEIER, H. and LINDENMANN, J. (1977c) Studies on the product of antigenic recognition. III. Nature of PAR. *Exp. Cell Biol.* **45**: 100–117.

RANNEY, D. F. and OPPENHEIM, J. J. (1973) *In vitro* generation of lymphocytic chalone by rat spleen cells. *Fedn Proc.* **32**: 979 (abstract).

RANNEY, D. F. and STEINBERG, A. D. (1976) Differences in the age-dependent release of a low molecular weight suppressor (LMWS) and stimulators by normal and NZB/W lymphoid organs. *J. Immun.* **117**: 1219–1225.

REMOLD, H. G. (1973) Requirement for α-L-fucose on the macrophage membrane receptor for MIF. *J. exp. Med.* **138**: 1065–1076.

REMOLD, H. G. (1974) The enhancement of MIF activity by inhibition of macrophage associated esterases. *J. Immun.* **112**: 1571–1577.

REMOLD, H. G., DAVID, R. A. and DAVID, J. R. (1972) Characterization of migration inhibitory factor (MIF) from guinea pig lymphocytes stimulated with concanavalin A. *J. Immun.* **109**: 578–586.

REMOLD, H. G. and MEDNIS, A. (1975–1976) Decrease of three lysosomal enzymes in guinea pig macrophages activated by lymphocyte mediators. *Inflammation* **1**: 175–188.

RICH, A. R. (1941) The significance of hypersensitivity in infections. *Physiol. Revs.* **21**: 70–111.

RICH, A. R. and LEWIS, M. R. (1927–1928) Mechanism of allergy in tuberculosis. *Proc. Soc. exp. Biol. Med.* **25**: 596–598.

RICH, R. R. and PIERCE, C. W. (1974) Biological expressions of lymphocyte activation. III. Suppression of plaque-forming cell responses *in vitro* by supernatant fluids from concanavalin A-activated spleen cell cultures. *J. Immun.* **112**: 1360–1368.

RICH, S. S. and RICH, R. R. (1974) Regulatory mechanisms in cell-mediated immune responses. I. Regulation of mixed lymphocyte reactions by alloantigen-activated thymus-derived lymphocytes. *J. exp. Med.* **140**: 1588–1603.

RICH, S. S. and RICH, R. R. (1975) Regulatory mechanisms in cell-mediated immune responses. II. A genetically restricted suppressor of mixed lymphocyte reactions released by alloantigen-activated spleen cells. *J. exp. Med.* **142**: 1391–1402.

RICH, S. S. and RICH, R. R. (1967a) Regulatory mechanisms in cell-mediated immune response. III. I-region control of suppressor cell interaction with responder cells in mixed lymphocyte reactions. *J. exp. Med.* **143**: 672–677.

RICH, S. S. and RICH, R. R. (1976b) Regulatory mechanisms in cell-mediated immune responses. IV. Expression of a receptor for mixed lymphocyte reaction suppressor factor on activated T lymphoytes. *J. exp. Med.* **144**: 1214–1226.

RITTENBERG, M. B. and NELSON, E. L. (1960) Macrophages, nucleic acids, and the induction of antibody formation. *Am. Nat.* **94**: 321–342.

ROCKLIN, R. E. (1973) Production of migration inhibitory factor by non-dividing lymphocytes. *J. Immun.* **110**: 674–678.

ROCKLIN, R. E. (1974) Products of activated lymphocytes: leukocyte inhibitory factor (LIF) distinct from migration inhibitory factor (MIF). *J. Immun.* **112**: 1461–1466.

ROCKLIN, R. E. (1975) Partial characterization of leukocyte inhibitory factor by concanavalin A-stimulated human lymphocytes (LIF Con A). *J. Immun.* **114**: 1161–1165.

ROCKLIN, R. E. (1976b) Role of monosaccharides in the interaction of two lymphocyte mediators with their target cells. *J. Immun.* **116**: 816–820.

ROCKLIN, R. E. (1977) Histamine-induced suppressor factor (HSF): effect on migration inhibitory factor (MIF) production and proliferation. *J. Immun.* **118**: 1734–1738.

ROCKLIN, R. E., MACDERMOTT, R. P., CHESS, L., SCHLOSSMAN, S. F. and DAVID, J. R. (1974) Studies on mediator production by highly purified human T and B lymphocytes. *J. exp. Med.* **140**: 1303–1316.

ROCKLIN, R. E., MEYERS, O. L. and DAVID, J. R. (1970) An *in vitro* assay for cellular hypersensitivity in man. *J. Immun.* **104**: 95–102.

ROEHM, N. (1977) Induction of splenomegaly with stimulated leukocyte supernatants. *Transplantation* **23**: 49–52.

ROGERS, J. C. (1976) Characterization of DNA excreted from phytohemagglutinin-stimulated lymphocytes. *J. exp. Med.* **143**: 1249–1264.

ROGERS, J. C., BOLDT, D., KORNFELD, S., SKINNER, A. and VALERI, C. R. (1972) Excretion of deoxyribonucleic acid by lymphocytes stimulated with phytohemagglutinin or antigen. *Proc. natn. Acad. Sci. USA* **69**: 1685–1689.

ROSENAU, W., GOLDBERG, M. L. and BURKE, G. C. (1973) Early biochemical alterations induced by lymphotoxin in target cells. *J. Immun.* **111**: 1128–1135.

ROSENTHAL, A. S., BLAKE, T. J., ELLNER, J. J., GREINEDER, D. K. and LIPSKY, P. E. (1976) Macrophage function in antigen recognition by T lymphocytes. In: *Immunobiology of the Macrophage*, pp. 131–160, NELSON D. S. (ed). Academic Press, New York, San Francisco, London.

RUBIN, A. S. and COONS, A. H. (1972a) Specific heterologous enhancement of immune responses. III. Partial characterization of supernatant material with enhancing activity. *J. Immun.* **108**: 1597–1604.

RUBIN, A. S. and COONS, A. H. (1972b) Specific heterologous enhancement of immune responses. IV. Specific generation of a thymus-derived enhancing factor. *J. exp. Med.* **136**: 1501–1517.

RUBIN, A. S. and MACDONALD, A. B. (1976) Partial characterization of an immunoenhancing factor from allogeneic human lymphocytic cell lines. *Immunology* **30**: 69–81.

RUBIN, A. S. MACDONALD, A. B. and COONS, A. H. (1973) Specific heterologous enhancement of immune responses. V. Isolation of a soluble enhancing factor from supernatants of specifically stimulated and allogeneically induced lymphoid cells. *J. Immun.* **111**: 1314–1325.

RUDDLE, N. H. and WAKSMAN, B. H. (1968a) Cytotoxicity mediated by soluble antigen and lymphocytes in delayed hypersensitivty. I. Characterization of the phenomenon. *J. exp. Med.* **128**: 1237–1254.

RUDDLE, N. H. and WAKSMAN, B. H. (1968b) Cytotoxicity mediated by soluble antigen and lymphocytes in delayed hypersensitivity. II. Correlation of the *in vitro* response with skin reactivity. *J. exp. Med.* **128**: 1255–1265.

RUDDLE, N. H. and WAKSMAN, B. H. (1968c) Cytotoxicity mediated by soluble antigen and lymphocytes in delayed hypersensitivity. III. Analysis of mechanism. *J. exp. Med.* **128**: 1267–1278.

RÜHL, H., VOGT, W., BOCHERT, G., SCHMIDT, S., MOELLE, R. and SCHAOUA, H. (1974) Effect of L-asparaginase and hydrocortisone on human lymphocyte transformation and production of a mononuclear leucocyte chemotactic factor *in vitro*. *Immunology* **26**: 989–994.

RUPPERT, B. L. and RICHIE, E. R. (1977) Phytohemagglutinin response of murine spleen cells during pregnancy and inhibition of normal phytohemagglutinin response by pregnancy or post-partum serum. *Exp. Hemat.* **5**: 59–68.

RUSCETTI, F. W. and CHERVENICK, P. A. (1975) Regulation of the release of colony stimulating activity from mitogen-stimulated lymphocytes. *J. Immun.* **114**: 1513–1517.

RUSSELL, S. W., ROSENAU, W., GOLDBERG, M. L. and KUNITOMI, G. (1972a) Purification of human lymphotoxin. *J. Immun.* **109**: 784–790.

RUSSELL, S. W., ROSENAU, W. and LEE, J. C. (1972b) Cytolysis induced by human lymphotoxin. *Am. J. Path.* **69**: 103–118.

SALVIN, S. B., RIBI, E., GRANGER, D. L. and YOUNGNER, J. S. (1975) Migration inhibitory factor and Type II interferon in the circulation of mice sensitized with mycobacterial components. *J. Immun.* **114**: 354–359.

SALVIN, S. B., YOUNGNER, J. S. and LEDERER, W. H. (1973) Migration inhibitory factor and interferon in the circulation of mice with delayed hypersensitivity. *Infect. Immunity* **7**: 68–75.

SARMA, D. S. R. and ZUBROFF, J. (1973) Synthesis and fragmentation of DNA in phytohaemagglutinin-stimulated human peripheral blood lymphocytes. *Immun. Commun.* **2**: 277–285.

SAWADA, J.-I., SHIOIRI-NAKANO, K. and OSAWA, T. (1975) Purification and characterization of guinea pig lymphotoxin produced by lymph node cells stimulated by phytohemagglutinin. *Transplantation* **19**: 335–342.

SBARRA, A. J., PAUL, B. B., JACOBS, A. A., STRAUSS, R. R. and MITCHELL, G. W., JR (1972) Role of the phagocyte in host-parasite interactions. XXXVIII. Metabolic activities of the phagocyte as related to antimicrobial action. *J. Reticuloendoth. Soc.* **12**: 109–126.

SCHEID, M. P., HOFFMANN, M. K., KOMURO, K., HÄMMERLING, U., ABBOTT, J., BOYSE, E. A., COHEN, G. H., HOOPER, J. A., SCHULOF, R. S. and GOLDSTEIN, A. L. (1973) Differentiation of T cells induced by preparations from thymus and by nonthymic agents. The determined state of the precursor cell. *J. exp. Med.* **138**: 1027–1032.

SCHIMPL, A. and WECKER, E. (1972) Replacement of T-cell function by a T-cell product. *Nature New Biol.* **237**: 15–17.

SCHRADER, J. W. (1973) Mechanism of activation of the bone marrow-derived lymphocyte. III. A distinction between a macrophage-produced triggering signal and the amplifying effect in triggered B lymphocytes of allogeneic interactions. *J. exp. Med.* **138**: 1466–1480.

SCHWARTZ, H. J., LEON, M. A. and PELLEY, R. P. (1970) Concanavalin A-induced release of skin-reactive factor from lymphoid cells. *J. Immun.* **104**: 265–268.

SHACKS, S. J., CHILLER, J. and GRANGER, G. A. (1973) Studies on *in vitro* models of cellular immunity: The role of T and B cells in the secretion of lymphotoxin. *Cell. Immun.* **7**: 313–321.

SHARMA, S. D. and MIDDLEBROOK, G. (1977a) Partial purification and properties of an antibacterial product of peritoneal exudate cell cultures from BCG-infected guinea pigs. *Infect. Immunity* **15**: 737–744.

SHARMA, S. D. and MIDDLEBROOK, G. (1977b) Antibacterial product of peritoneal exudate cell cultures from guinea pigs infected with mycobacterial, listeriae, and rickettsiae. *Infect. Immunity* **15**: 745–750.

SHEVACH, E. M. (1976) The role of the macrophage in genetic control of the immune response. *Fedn Proc.* **35**: 2048–2052.

SIDKY, Y. A. and AUERBACH, R. (1975) Lymphocyte-induced angiogenesis: a quantitative and sensitive assay of the graft vs. host reaction. *J. exp. Med.* **141**: 1084--1100.

SIEGERT, R., SHU, H. L. and KOHLHAGE, H. (1967) Correlation between fever and interferon titer in rabbits after induction with myxoviruses. *Life Sci.* **6**: 615–620.

SIMON, H. B. and SHEAGREN, J. N. (1971) Cellular immunity *in vitro*. I. Immunologically mediated enhancement of macrophage bactericidal capacity. *J. exp. Med.* **133**: 1377–1389.

SIMON, H. B. and SHEAGREN, J. N. (1972a) Enhancement of macrophage bactericidal capacity by antigenically stimulated immune lymphocytes. *Cell. Immun.* **4**: 163–174.

SIMON, H. B. and SHEAGREN, J. N. (1972b) Migration inhibitory factor and macrophage bactericidal function. *Infect. Immunity* **6**: 101–103.

SINTEK, D. E. and PINCUS, W. B. (1970) Cytotoxic factor from peritoneal cells: purification and characteristics. *J. Reticuloendoth. Soc.* **8**: 508–521.

SJÖBERG, O., ANDERSSON, J. and MÖLLER, G. (1972) Reconstitution of the antibody response *in vitro* of T cell-deprived spleen cells by supernatants from spleen cell cultures. *J. Immun.* **109**: 1379–1385.

SMITH, R. T., BAUSHER, J. A. C. and ADLER, W. H. (1970) Studies of an inhibitor of DNA synthesis and a nonspecific mitogen elaborated by human lymphoblasts. *Am. J. Path.* **60**: 495–504.

SØBORG, M. (1970) *In vitro* demonstration of microbial cellular hypersensitivity in man. *Proc. R. Soc. M* **63**: 903–905.

SONOZAKI, H., PAPERMASTER, V., YOSHIDA, T. and COHEN, S. (1975) Densensitization: effects on cutaneous and peritoneal manifestations of delayed hypersensitivity in relation to lymphokine production. *J. Immun.* **115**: 1657–1661.

SORG, C. and BLOOM, B. R. (1973) Products of activated lymphocytes. I. The use of radiolabeling techniques in the characterization and partial purification of the migration inhibitory factor of the guinea pig. *J. exp. Med.* **137**: 148–170.

SORG, C. and GECZY, C. L. (1976) Antibodies to guinea pig lymphokines. III. Reactions with radiolabeled lymphocyte activation products. *Eur. J. Immun.* **6**: 688–693.

SPECTOR, W. G. and WILLOUGHBY, D. A. (1964) The effect of vascular permeability factors on the emigration of leucocytes. *J. Path. Bact.* **87**: 341–346.

SPITLER, L., HABER, H. and FUDENBERG, H. H. (1969) Inhibition of capillary migration by antigen–antibody complexes. *J. Immun.* **102**: 404–411.

STANLEY, E. R., CIFONE, M., HEARD, P. M. and DEFENDI, V. (1976) Factors regulating macrophage production and growth: identity of colony-stimulating factor and macrophage growth factor. *J. exp. Med.* **143**: 631–647.

STECHER, V. J., MORSE, J. H. and THORBECKE, G. J. (1967) Sites of production of primate serum proteins associated with the complement system. *Proc. Soc. exp. Biol. Med.* **124**: 433–438.

STRUNK, R. C., TASHJIAN, A. H., JR and COLTEN, H. R. (1975) Complement biosynthesis *in vitro* by rat hepatoma cell strains. *J. Immun.* **114**: 331–335.

ŠVEJCAR, J., PEKÁREK, J. and JOHANOVSKÝ, J. (1968) Studies on production of biologically active substances which inhibit cell migration in supernatants and extracts of hypersensitive lymphoid cells incubated with specific antigen *in vitro*. *Immunology* **15**: 1–11.

ŠVEJCAR, J., PEKÁREK, J. and JOHANOVSKÝ, J. (1969) Tissue culture studies on the mechanism of delayed type hypersensitivity. XIII. Passive transfer of the cell migration inhibition capacity by means of a factor released following interaction of lymph node cells from sensitized rabbits with specific antigen. *Zsch. Immunitatsf.* **138**: 342–354.

TADA, T. (1976) T cell-mediated regulation of IgE antibody production. Nobel Symposium on *Molecular and Cellular Aspects of the Acute Allergic Reaction.* March.

TADA, T., OKUMURA, K. and TANIGUCHI, M. (1973) Regulation of homocytotropic antibody formation in the rat. VIII. An antigen-specific T cell factor that regulates anti-hapten homocytotropic antibody response. *J. Immun.* **111**: 952–961.

TADA, T., TANIGUCHI, M. and DAVID, C. S. (1976a) Properties of the antigen-specific suppressive T cell factor in the regulation of antibody response of the mouse. IV. Special subregion assignment of the gene(s) that codes for the suppressive T-cell factor in the H-2 histocompatibility complex. *J. exp. Med.* **144**: 713–725.

TADA, T., TANIGUCHI, M. and TAKEMORI, T. (1976b) The role of receptors for T cell products in antibody formation. *Immun. Commun.* **5**: 717–736.

TADAKUMA, T., KÜHNER, A. L., RICH, R. R., DAVID, J. R. and PIERCE, C. W. (1976) Biological expressions of lymphocyte activation. V. Characterization of a soluble immune response suppressor (SIRS) produced by concanavalin A-activated spleen cells. *J. Immun.* **117**: 323–330.

TADAKUMA, T. and PIERCE, C. W. (1976) Site of action of a soluble immune response suppressor (SIRS) produced by concanavalin A-activated spleen cells. *J. Immun.* **117**: 967–972.

TAKADA, A., TAKADA, Y. and MINOWADA, J. (1974) Immunological functions of human T-lymphoid cell line (MOLT). I. Release of immunosuppressive factors from the mixture of MOLT-4 cells and sheep red blood cells. *J. exp. Med.* **140**: 538–548.

TAKEMORI, T. and TADA, T. (1975) Properties of antigen-specific suppressive T-cell factor in the regulation of antibody response of the mouse. I. *In vivo* activity and immunochemical characterization. *J. exp. Med.* **142**: 1241–1253.

TANIGUCHI, M., HAYAKAWA, K. and TADA, T. (1976a) Properties of antigen-specific suppressive T cell factor in the regulation of antibody response of the mouse. II. *In vitro* activity and evidence for the I region gene product. *J. Immun.* **116**: 542–548.

TANIGUCHI, M. and TADA, T. (1974) Regulation of homocytropic antibody formation in the rat. X. Ig T-like molecule for the induction of homocytotropic antibody response. *J. Immun.* **113**: 1757–1769.

TANIGUCHI, M., TADA, T. and TOKUHISA, T. (1976b) Properties of the antigen-specific suppressive T-cell factor in the regulation of antibody response of the mouse. III. Dual gene control of the t-cell-mediated suppression of the antibody response. *J. exp. Med.* **144**: 20–31.

TAUB, R. N., KRANTZ, A. R. and DRESSER, D. W. (1970) The effect of localized injection of adjuvant material on the draining lymph node. I. Histology. *Immunology* **18**: 171–186.

TAUSSIG, M. J. (1976) I-region products in Cell-interaction. In: *Basel Institute Immunology, Annual Report*, p. 71 (abstract).

TAUSSIG, M. J., FINCH, A. P. and KELUS, A. S. (1976) Antigen-specific helper factors in rabbit lacking both V and C region Ig determinants. *Nature* **264**: 776–778.

TAUSSIG, M. J. and MUNRO, A. J. (1976) Antigen-specific T-cell factor in cell cooperation and genetic control of the immune response. *Fedn Proc.* **35**: 2061–2066.

TAUSSIG, M. J., MUNRO, A. J., CAMPBELL, R., DAVID, C. S. and STAINES, N. A. (1975) Antigen-specific T-cell factor in cell cooperation. Mapping within the I region of the H-2 complex and ability to cooperate across allogeneic barriers. *J. exp. Med.* **142**: 694–700.

THEZE, J., KAPP, J. A. and BENACERRAF, B. (1977) Immunosuppressive factor(s) extracted from lymphoid cells of nonresponder mice primed with L-glutamic acid^{60}-L-alanine^{30}-L-tyrosine^{10} (GAT). III. Immunochemical properties of the GAT-specific suppressive factor. *J. exp. Med.* **145**: 839–856.

THOMAS, D. B. (1972) The restriction of the release of mibration inhibitory factor to certain phases of the cell cycle of murine leukemia, L 1210. *Eur. J. Immun.* **2**: 478–481.

THOMAS, D. W., ROBERTS, W. K. and TALMAGE, D. W. (1975a) Regulation of the immune response: production of a soluble suppressor by immune spleen cells *in vitro*. *J. Immun.* **114**: 1616–1622.

THOMAS, D. W., TALMAGE, D. W. and ROBERTS, W. K. (1975b) Inhibition of tumor cell proliferation: a second role for suppressor cells? *J. Immun.* **115**: 1366–1369.

THOR, D. E. (1967) Delayed hypersensitivity in man: a correlate *in vitro* and transfer by an RNA extract. *Science* **157**: 1567–1569.

THOR, D. E. and DRAY, S. (1968) The cell migration-inhibition correlate of delayed hypersensitivity. Conversion of human nonsensitive lymph node cells to sensitive cells with an RNA extract. *J. Immun.* **101**: 469–480.

THRASHER, S. G., YOSHIDA, T., VAN OSS, C. J., COHEN, S. and ROSE, N. R. (1973) Alteration of macrophage interfacial tension by supernatants of antigen-activated lymphocyte cultures. *J. Immun.* **110**: 321–326.

TIBBETTS, L. M., GLADE, P. R. and PAGAGEORGIOU, P. S. (1975) Presence of a reversible inhibitor for human lymphoid cell DNA synthesis in the extracts of human peripheral lymphocytes. *Cell. Immun.* **18**: 384–395.

TORISU, M. YOSHIDA, T., WARD, P. A. and COHEN, S. (1973) Lymphocyte-derived eosinophil chemotactic factor. II. Studies on the mechanism of activation of the precursor substance by immune complexes. *J. Immun.* **111**: 1450–1458.

TORMEY, D. C. and MUELLER, G. C. (1972) Biological effects of transferrin on human lymphocytes *in vitro*. *Exp. Cell. Res.* **74**: 220–226.

TRIVERS, G., BRAUNGART, D. and LEONARD, E. J. (1976) Mouse lymphotoxin. *J. Immun.* **117**: 130–135.

TSOUKAS, C. D. and ROSENAU, W. (1977) Inhibition of lymphotoxin- and lymphocyte-mediated cytolysis by high molecular weight dextran. *Proc. Soc. exp. Biol. Med.* **154**: 215–218.

TSUCHIMOTO, T., TUBERGEN, D. G. and BLOOM, A. D. (1972) Synthesis of macrophage migration inhibitory factor (MIF) by immunoglobulin-producing lymphocyte lines and their clones. *J. Immun.* **109**: 884–886.

TUBERGEN, D. G., FELDMAN, J. D., POLLOCK, E. M. and LERNER, R. A. (1972) Production of macrophage migration inhibition factor by continuous cell lines. *J. exp. Med.* **135**: 255–266.

ULRICH, F. (1976) Lymphocyte activating factor from alveolar macrophages. *Fedn Proc.* **35**: 280 (abstract).

ULRICH, F. (1977) Studies of lymphocyte activating factor from alveolar macrophages. *J. Reticuloendoth. Soc.* **21**: 33–51.

UNANUE, E. R. (1976) Secretory function of mononuclear phagocytes. *Am. J. Path.* **83**: 396–417.

UNANUE, E. R., KIELY, J.-M. and CALDERON, J. (1976) The modulation of lymphocyte functions by molecules secreted by macrophages. II. Conditions leading to increased secretion. *J. exp. Med.* **144**: 155–166.

VALENTINE, F. T. (1972) The dissociation by 95 per cent oxygen of the production of lymphocyte transforming factor and the proliferation of lymphocytes stimulated with antigen. In: *Proceedings Sixth Leucocyte Culture Conference*, pp. 337–356. SCHWARZ, M. R. (ed). Academic Press, New York, San Francisco, London.

VEIT, B. and MICHAEL, J. G. (1973) Characterization of an immunosuppressive factor present in mouse serum. *J. Immun.* **111**: 341–351.

VISCHER, T. L. (1972) Mitogenic factors produced by lymphocyte activation: effect on T- and B-cells. *J. Immun.* **109**: 401–402.

VISCHER, T. L., BRETZ, U. and BAGGIOLINI, M. (1976) *In vitro* stimulation of lymphocytes by neutral proteinases from human polymorphonuclear leukocyte granules. *J. exp. Med.* **144**: 863–872.

VOISIN, G. A. (1977) A. (1977) Anticorps régulateurs et cellules suppressives: leur interactions dans le cadre de la réaction de facilitation. *Annals Immun.* **128C**: 431–443.

WAGSHAL, A. B., JEGASOTHY, B. V. and WAKSMAN, B. H. (1977a) Cell cycle specificity of inhibitor of DNA synthesis action. *Fedn Proc.* **36**: 1320 (abstract).

WAGSHAL, A. B., JEGASOTHY, B. V. and WAKSMAN, B. H. (1978) Regulatory substances produced by lymphocytes. VI. Cell cycle specificity of inhibitor of DNA synthesis in L cells. *J. exp. Med.* **147**: 171–181.

WAGSHAL, A. B. and WAKSMAN, B. H. (1978) Regulatory substances produced by lymphocytes. VIII. Cell cycle specificity of inhibitor of DNA synthesis (IDS) action in lymphocytes. *J. Immun.* (submitted).

WAHL, S. M., IVERSON, G. M. and OPPENHEIM, J. J. (1974) Induction of guinea pig β-cell lymphokine synthesis by mitogenic and nonmitogenic signals to Fc, Ig and C3 receptors. *J. exp. Med.* **140**: 1631–1645.

WAHL, S. M. and ROSENSTREICH, D. L. (1976) Role of B-lymphocytes in cell-mediated immunity. I. Requirement for T-cells or T-cell products for antigen-induced B-cell activation. *J. exp. Med.* **144**: 1175–1187.

WAKSMAN, B. H. (1960) A comparative histopathological study of delayed hypersensitive reactions. In: *Ciba Foundation Symposium on Cellular Aspects of Immunity*, pp. 280–329, WOLSTENHOLME, G. E. W. and O'CONNOR, M. (eds). Churchill, London.

WAKSMAN, B. H. and MATOLTSY, M. (1958) The effect of tuberculin on peritoneal exudate cells of sensitized guinea pigs in surviving cell culture. *J. Immun.* **81**: 220–234.

WAKSMAN, B. H. and OZER, H. (1976) Specialized amplification elements in the immune system. The role of nodular lymphoid organs in the mucous membranes. *Prog. Allergy* **21**: 1–113.

WALDMANN, H. (1975) T cell-dependent mediator in the immune response. III. The role of non-specific factor (NSF) in the *in vitro* immune response. *Immunology* **28**: 497–507.

WALDMANN, H. and MUNRO, A. (1973) T cell-dependent mediator in the immune response. *Nature* **243**: 356–357.

WALDMANN, H. and MUNRO, A. (1974) T cell-dependent mediator in the immune response. II. Physical and biological properties. *Immunology* **27**: 53–64.

WALDMANN, H., POULTON, P. and DESAYMARD, C. (1976) Antigen non-specific T-cell factor in B-cell activation. Origin, biological properties and failure to show a relationship to H-2. *Immunology* **30**: 723–733.

WALDMANN, S. R. and GOTTLIEB, A. A. (1973) Macrophage regulation of DNA synthesis in lymphoid cells: effects of a soluble factor from macrophages. *Cell. Immun.* **9**: 142–156.

WALKER, S. M., LEE, S.-C. and LUCAS, Z. J. (1976) Cytotoxic activity of lymphocytes. VI. Heterogeneity of cytotoxins in supernants of mitogen-activated lymphocytes. *J. Immun.* **116**: 807–815.

WALKER, S. M. and LUCAS, Z. J. (1972) Cytotoxic activity of lymphocytes. II. Studies on mechanism of lymphotoxin-mediated cytotoxicity. *J. Immun.* **109**: 1233–1244.

WALKER, S. M. and LUCAS, Z. J. (1974) Cytotoxic activity of lymphocytes. IV. Preparation of heterologous antibody to human lymphotoxin. *J. Immun.* **113**: 813–823.

WARD, P. A. and BERENBERG, J. L. (1974) Defective regulation of inflammatory mediators in Hodgkin's disease. Supernormal levels of chemotactic-factor inactivator. *New Engl. J. Med.* **290**: 76–80.

WARD, P. A., DVORAK, H. F., COHEN, S., YOSHIDA, T., DATA, R. and SELVAGGIO, S. S. (1975) Chemotaxis of basophils by lymphocyte-dependent and lymphocyte-independent mechanisms. *J. Immun.* **114**: 1523–1531.

WARD, P. A., OFFEN, C. D. and MONTGOMERY, J. R. (1971) Chemoattractants of leukocytes, with special reference to lymphocytes. *Fedn Proc.* **30**: 1721–1724.

WARD, P. A., REMOLD, H. G. and DAVID, J. R. (1969) Leukotactic factor produced by sensitized lymphocytes. *Science* **163**: 1079–1081.

WARD, P. A., REMOLD, H. G. and DAVID, J. R. (1970) The production by antigen-stimulated lymphocytes of a leukotactic factor distinct from migration inhibitory factor. *Cell. Immun.* **1**: 162–174.

WARD, P. A. and ROCKLIN, R. E. (1975) Regulation of MIF by a factor in human serum. *J. Immun.* **115**: 309–311.
WARD, P. A. and TALAMO, R. C. (1973) Deficiency of the chemotactic factor inactivator in human sera with α_1-anti trypsin deficiency. *J. Clin. Invest.* **52**: 516–519.
WARD, P. A. and VOLKMAN, A. (1975) The elaboration of leukotactic mediators during the interaction between parental-type lymphocytes and F1 hybrid cells. *J. Immun.* **115**: 1394–1399.
WARRINGTON, R. J., BUEHLER, S. K. and ROBERTS, K. B. (1976) Inflammation-inducing factors from human lymphocytes. Correlation with polymorphonuclear leucocyte migration enhancement or inhibition. *Int. Arch. Allergy* **51**: 186–197.
WATSON, J. (1973) The role of humoral factors in the initiation of *in vitro* primary immune responses. III. Characterization of factors that replace thymus-derived cells. *J. Immun.* **111**: 1301–1313.
WATSON, J. (1975a) Cyclic nucleotides as intracellular mediators of B cell activation. *Transplant. Rev.* **23**: 223–249.
WATSON, J. (1975b) The influence of intracellular levels of cyclic nucleotides on cell proliferation and the induction of antibody synthesis. *J. exp. Med.* **141**: 97–111.
WATSON, J. and EPSTEIN, R. (1973) The role of humoral factors in the initiation of *in vitro* primary immune responses. I. Effects of deficient bovine serum. *J. Immun.* **110**: 31–42.
WATSON, J., EPSTEIN, R. and COHN, M. (1973) Cyclic nucleotides as intracellular mediators of the expression of antigen-sensitive cells. *Nature* **246**: 405–409.
WATSON, J. and THOMAR, M. (1972) A factor that can be used to regulate an *in vitro* primary immune response. *Proc. natn. Acad. Sci. USA* **69**: 594–598.
WEBB, D. R., NOWOWIEJSKI, I., DAUPHINEE, M. and TALAL, N. (1977) An induced alteration in splenic prostaglandin and cyclic nucleotide levels in NZB mice. *J. Immun.* **118**: 446–450.
WEISBART, R. H., BLUESTONE, R., GOLDBERG, L. S. and PEARSON, C. M. (1974) Migration enhancement factor: a new lymphokine. *Proc. natn. Acad. Sci. USA* **71**: 875–879.
WEISBART, R. H. ISAACSON, J., BLUESTONE, R. and GOLDBERG, L. S. (1975) Human polymorphonuclease leucocyte migration inhibitory factor. Evidence for antigen dependency. *Immunology* **29**: 223–230.
WESTON, W. L., CLAMAN, H. N. and KRUEGER, G. G. (1973) Site of action of cortisol in cellular immunity. *J. Immun.* **110**: 880–883.
WHITFIELD, J. F., MACMANUS, J. P., YOUDALE, T. and FRANKS, D. J. (1971) The roles of calcium and cyclic AMP in the stimulatory action of parathyroid hormone on thymic lymphocyte proliferation. *J. Cell Phys.* **78**: 355–368.
WILLIAMS, T. W. and GRANGER, G. A. (1968) Lymphocyte *in vitro* cytotoxicity: lymphotoxins of several mammalian species. *Nature* **219**: 1076–1077.
WILLIAMS, T. W. and GRANGER, G. A. (1969) Lymphocyte *in vitro* cytotoxicity: mechanism of lymphotoxin-induced target cell destruction. *J. Immun.* **102**: 911–918.
WILLIAMS, T. W. and GRANGER, G. A. (1973) Lymphocyte *in vitro* cytotoxicity: mechanism of human lymphotoxin-induced target cell destruction. *J. Immun.* **6**: 171–185.
WILLIAMS, T. J. and MORLEY, J. (1973) Prostaglandins as potentiators of increased vascular permeability in inflammation. *Nature* **246**: 215–217.
WILLOUGHBY, D. A., BOUGHTON, B. and SCHILD, H. O. (1963) A factor capable of increasing vascular permeability present in lymph node cells. A possible mediator of the delayed reaction. *Immunology* **6**: 484–498.
WILLOUGHBY, D. A., SPECTOR, W. G. and BOUGHTON, B. (1964) A lymph-node permeability factor in the tuberculin reaction. *J. Path. Bact.* **87**: 353–363.
WOLSTENCROFT, R. A. and DUMONDE, D. C. (1970) *In vitro* studies of cell-mediated immunity. I. Induction of lymphocyte transformation by a soluble 'mitogenic' factor derived from interaction of sensitized guinea pig lymphoid cells with specific antigen. *Immunology* **18**: 599–610.
WOLSTENHOLME, G. E. W. and KNIGHT, J. (eds) (1970) *Hormones and the Immune Response.* Ciba Foundation Study Group, No. 36. Churchill, London.
WOOD, D. D. and CAMERON, P. M. (1975) Studies on the mechanism of stimulation of the humoral response of murine spleen cultures by culture fluids from human monocytes. *J. Immun.* **114**: 1094–1100.
WOOD, D. D. and CAMERON, P. M. (1976) Stimulation of the release of a B cell-activating factor from human monocytes. *Cell. Immun.* **21**: 133–145.
WOOD, D. D., CAMERON, P. M., POE, M. T. and MORRIS, C. A. (1976) Resolution of a factor that enhances the antibody response of T cell-depleted murine splenocytes from several other monocyte products. *Cell. Immun.* **21**: 88–96.
WOOD, D. D. and GAUL, S. L. (1974) Enhancement of the humoral response of T cell-depleted murine spleens by a factor derived from human monocytes *in vitro*. *J. Immun.* **113**: 925–933.
YACHNIN, S. (1975) Fetuin, an inhibitor of lymphocyte transformation. The interaction of fetuin with phytomitogens and a possible role for fetuin in fetal development. *J. exp. Med.* **141**: 242–256.
YONKOSKY, D., BUFFETT, R. F. and BENNETT, M. (1976a) Suppression of antibody responses in allogeneic mice by products of lymphoid tissue. I. Allogeneic suppressive factor (ASF) from spleens repopulated with thymus cells. *J. Immun.* **116**: 1688–1694.
YONKOSKY, D., BUFFETT, R. F. and BENNETT, M. (1976b) Suppression of antibody responses in allogeneic mice by products of lymphoid tissue. II. Lack of antigenic specificity and immunogenetic requirements of allogeneic suppressive factor (ASF). *J. Immun.* **116**: 1695–1703.
YOSHIDA, T., BIGAZZI, P. and COHEN, S. (1975a) Biologic and antigenic similarity of virus-induced migration inhibition factor to conventional lymphocyte-derived migration inhibition factor. *Proc. natn. Acad. Sci. USA* **72**: 1641–1644.
YSHIDA, T., BIGAZZI, P. E. and COHEN, S. (1975b) The production of anti-guinea pig lymphokine antibody. *J. Immun.* **114**: 688–691.

YOSHIDA, T. and COHEN, S. (1974a) Lymphokine activity *in vivo* in relation to circulating monocyte levels and delayed skin reactivity. *J. Immun.* **112**: 1540–1547.

YOSHIDA, T. and COHEN, S. (1974b) *In vivo* manifestations of lymphokine and lymphokine-like activity. In: *Mechanisms of Cell-Mediated Immunity*, pp. 43–60, MCCLUSKEY, R. T. and COHEN, S. (eds). Wiley, New York.

YOSHIDA, T. KURATSUJI, T., TAKADA, A., TAKADA, Y., MINOWADA, J. and COHEN, S. (1976) Lymphokine-like factors produced by human lymphoid cell lines with B or T cell surface markers. *J. Immun.* **117**: 548–554.

YOSHIDA, T., SONOZAKI, H. and COHEN, S. (1973) The production of migration inhibition factor by B and T cells of the guinea pig. *J. exp. Med.* **138**: 784–797.

YOSHINAGA, M. and WAKSMAN, B. H. (1973) Regulation of lymphocyte response *in vitro*. IV. Role of macrophages in rat lymphocyte responses and their inhibition by cytochalasin B. *Ann. Immun.* **124C**: 97–120.

YOUMANS, G. P. (1971) The role of lymphocytes and other factors in antimicrobial cellular immunity. *J. Reticuloendoth. Soc.* **10**: 100–119.

ZATZ, M. M. and GERSHON, R. K. (1974) Thymus dependence of lymphocyte trapping. *J. Immun.* **112**: 101–106.

ZATZ, M. M. and LANCE, E. M. (1970) The distribution of chromium^{51}-labelled lymphoid cells in the mouse. A survey of anatomical compartments. *Cell. Immun.* **1**: 3–17.

ZATZ, M. M. and LANCE, E. M. (1971) The distribution of ^{51}Cr-labeled lymphocytes into antigen stimulated mice. Lymphocyte trapping. *J. exp. Med.* **134**: 224–241.

ZEMBALA, M. and ASHERSON, G. L. (1974) T cell suppression of contact sensitivity in the mouse. II. The role of soluble suppressor factor and its interaction with macrophages. *Eur. J. Immun.* **4**: 799–804.

ZIFF, M., HURD, E. R. and STASTNY, P. (1974) B- and T-lymphocytes in rheumatoid synovitis and the effect of cyclophosphamide. *Proc. R. Soc. Med.* **67**: 536–539.

ZINSSER, H. and TAMIYA, T. (1926) An experimental analysis of bacterial allergy. *J. exp. Med.* **44**: 753–776.

PART II

EXTRINSIC IMMUNOMODULATION: THE PERTURBATION OF INTRINSIC REGULATION

CHAPTER 5

VIRUSES AND THE IMMUNE RESPONSE

STEVEN SPECTER and HERMAN FRIEDMAN
University of South Florida, Tampa, USA

1. INTRODUCTION

Highly complex cellular and humoral events mediate the interaction between infectious microorganisms and the immune defense system. Evolutionary pressures by microbial agents undoubtedly helped to shape the immune response mechanism. In this regard, there is a vast literature concerning the immune responses of normal individuals to infectious microorganisms such as bacteria and viruses (Schwab, 1975; Dent, 1972, 1975; Gross, 1970; Notkins *et al.*, 1970; Woodruff and Woodruff, 1975a). Considerably less is known regarding how these infectious agents affect the immune system, although it is now widely recognized that both specific and nonspecific defense mechanisms, including humoral and cellular immunity, may be altered in an individual infected with a microbe. Not only can a host respond in a positive manner to an infecting microorganism such as a bacterium or a virus, but the infecting agent may also influence the manner in which the host responds. For example, it is now recognized that many microorganisms elaborate substances which either protect the organism from the host immune response mechanism or, even more drastically, may abrogate the immune response entirely (Schwab, 1975). Therefore, it is somewhat surprising that the observations of Von Pirquet (1908), and others at the beginning of the century, showing that infection of an individual by measles virus may alter immune function, went largely unappreciated for many decades.

It is now widely recognized that viruses, in addition to many bacteria, may markedly affect the immune response mechanism in a negative manner. For example, much effort during the past decade or so has increased the knowledge concerning how viruses modulate immune responses of the infected host. Indeed, the topic of effects of viral infection on immunity has been recently reviewed in detail by a number of authors (Dent, 1975; Notkins *et al.*, 1970; Woodruff and Woodruff, 1975a). Similarly, the subject of modulation of immune responsiveness by bacteria and their products has also been recently reviewed (Schwab, 1975). Therefore, the major purpose of the present review is to summarize some of the mechanisms whereby viruses directly or indirectly influence the immune response system, the nature of viruses, both oncogenic and non-oncogenic, that are known to affect immunity and, lastly, some of the mechanisms whereby viruses are known to modulate immune responses, including effects on humoral and cellular immunity.

2. HISTORICAL BACKGROUND

The relationship between infectious agents and depressed immune competence was appreciated both in ancient times as well as in more modern eras of medicine by studying populations and individuals with infections. Nevertheless, it is widely accepted that the observations by Von Pirquet, as well as others, at the beginning of this century first brought attention to the fact that measles infection could be accompanied by marked depression of a preexisting immune status, i.e. cutaneous hypersensitivity to tuberculin (Dent, 1972). Very little progress was made in this area during the subsequent 5–6 decades. The beginning of increased interest concerning the effects of viruses on immunity occurred in the early 1960s when Old and colleagues mentioned in a general review concerning the effects of leukemia virus infection on the reticulo-endothelial system that mice infected with Friend virus failed to produce expected levels of serum antibody to sheep red blood cells (Old *et al.*, 1960).

Other studies with tumor viruses in the early 1960s demonstrated that several parameters of the immune response could be impaired in mice infected with oncogenic viruses. These early studies have been reviewed extensively. In brief, it should be mentioned that in an attempt to relate the thymus to immunologic functions, Dent *et al.* (1965) showed that mice vertically infected with Gross leukemia virus failed to mount a normal allograft response upon challenge with a skin graft or form normal amounts of anti-phage antibody after challenge immunization. Such immunosuppression was thought to be related to the effects of the virus on development of the thymus in the neonatally infected mice. Odaka and colleagues in Japan, in 1966, reported that Friend virus could infect macrophages, both *in vitro* and *in vivo*, and also that mice infected with this virus showed depressed humoral antibody responses, both at the serum and antibody plaque levels (Odaka *et al.*, 1966). Simultaneously, Siegel and Morton reported that mice infected with Rauscher leukemia virus do not produce a normal immune response to bovine serum albumin or sheep erythrocytes at the serum level (Siegel and Morton, 1966a,b, 1967). Salaman and Wedderburn similarly showed that the antibody plaque response to sheep red blood cells was depressed in Friend virus infected mice (Salaman and Wedderburn, 1966). At about the same time, extensive studies by Ceglowski and Friedman showed that Friend virus infection depressed the hemolytic antibody response of mice to sheep red blood cells by affecting precursor B lymphocytes, and that the depressed numbers of antibody-forming cells in mice infected with this virus was related to the dose and time of virus infection (Ceglowski and Friedman, 1967, 1968a,b, 1969a,b,c, 1970). These studies set the stage for extensive studies concerning both oncogenic and non-oncogenic viruses on immune responses.

The implications of such virus-induced modulation of immunity on mechanisms affecting the host-parasite relationship in both experimental animals and man are many. As discussed by Kantzler *et al.* (1974), in studies concerning influenza virus infection, immunosuppression induced by viruses may lead to severe complications. Furthermore, depressed immune functions related to common and rarer viral infections in man may be causally related to secondary bacterial infections. Thus, effects of virus infections, either direct or indirect, on immune competence may result in clinical manifestations of certain symptoms unrelated to the virus effects on target cells *per se* and could affect the balance of an interaction between the host and endogenous latent infection such as those associated with tuberculosis or brucellosis. Furthermore, it is now felt that virus-induced immunosuppression may be somehow associated with tumorigenesis, regardless of whether or not the virus is oncogenic, since transformed tumor cells might more easily 'escape' immune direction due to local or systemic immunosuppression. Finally, one should consider the possibility that 'live' virus vaccines, either directly or because of contamination with passenger viruses which may affect immune mechanisms, could alter immune responsiveness to either the same or other infectious agents, and thus lead to unwanted consequences.

3. CURRENT CONCEPT OF IMMUNITY AS RELATED TO VIRUS-INDUCED IMMUNOSUPPRESSION

The marked complexity of the interaction among cellular and humoral components of the immune system has become widely accepted over the past few years. Nevertheless, our understanding of the mechanisms of cellular and humoral interactions in immunity is still incomplete. It is noteworthy that at the beginning of this century, at the time when Von Pirquet first reported that measles virus infection suppressed tuberculin hypersensitivity, there was a major controversy as to the relative role and function of humoral versus cellular components of the immune response systems. There was a marked debate concerning the importance of antibody and serum factors as compared to cells in protective immunity against microorganisms. Although some controversy still smolders in contemporary immunology, concerning the relative importance of cellular versus humoral factors in immunity, it is now clear that both are essential. It is generally accepted that several distinct populations of lymphocytes are involved in immunity, i.e. thymus derived T-lymphocytes, bursal equivalent or bone marrow derived B-lymphocytes, and mononuclear phagocytic cells (i.e. macrophages). In addition more recent studies have identified at least two other lymphocyte populations which may be involved in anti-viral immunity. These are the cells involved in antibody-dependent cellular cytotoxicity (ADCC) or K cells and cytotoxic cells found in unstimulated animals or man known as natural killer (NK) cells. Mature B-lymphocytes are directly involved in synthesis and secretion of immunoglobulins and are responsible for the humoral components of the specific immune response mechanism. B-lymphocytes are known to depend upon the inductive influence of the bursa of Fabricius in birds and the bursal equivalent or gut-associated lymphoid tissue in mammalian species. The bone marrow and, early in life, the fetal liver are considered the initial sources of stem cells for B-lymphocytes.

T-lymphocytes also are derived from stem cells in the bone marrow. However, these cells mature in the thymus, most likely under the influence of thymus epidermal cells which secrete a factor(s), i.e. hormones. Upon migration from the thymus, the immunocompetent T-cells may interact with antigen in a specific manner but do not synthesize immunoglobulins. These cells, however, may elaborate a wide variety of soluble factors with potent biologic activity (i.e. kinins). T-cells may also interact directly with cellular antigens and cause their destruction. Furthermore, it is now widely accepted that certain T-cells serve as 'helper' or auxiliary cells required for antibody formation by mature B-lymphocytes, especially those secreting IgG antibodies. Other T-lymphocytes may also serve as 'suppressor' cells, influencing B-lymphocytes in a negative manner.

Although a categorization of T- and B-lymphocytes according to their function in cellular or humoral immunity has been attempted during the past decade, a complete understanding of their activities has not yet been achieved. The involvement of T-lymphocytes in the humoral component of the immune response as helper or suppressor cells may be related either to direct interaction of the cells, or to factors released by T-cells that influence other T-cells. Furthermore, subcellular factors (lymphokines) released by T-lymphocytes, as well as humoral antibody secreted by B-cells, are known to influence functional activities of the third important cell class, the macrophage. These monocytic cells, which are highly heterogenous in function as well as anatomical location, appear to serve an important role in initiating, amplifying and terminating immune responses, especially those directed toward cellular or particulate antigens.

Macrophages, also derived from bone marrow stem cells, circulate freely, and readily phagocytize particulate substances, whether antigenic or not. These cells are known to function as accessory cells for many categories of immune responses. Macrophages are generally regarded as constituting the first line of defense of a host against microbial agents. After injection of a particulate substance such as bacteria, foreign erythrocytes or an inanimate particulate antigen, macrophages are thought to 'process' the antigen and present the appropriate immunogenic determinant to the relevant lymphocytes for initiating an immune response. Although the mechanisms involved in such 'processing' and/or 'presentation' of antigen are not clearly understood, this concept of the afferent limb of the immune system is generally well accepted. Macrophages are also thought to contribute to the efferent or effector limb of the immune response mechanism, ingesting antibody-coated microorganisms and/or particulate antigens, resulting in their enzymatic digestion. Macrophages, as indicated earlier, may also respond to T-cell derived factors, resulting in their activation. A number of recent reviews, discussing the role of macrophages, T- and B-lymphocytes in antibody formation and cellular immunity, have summarized how these cells function and interact in a variety of immune responses (Cooper *et al.*, 1967; Cooper and Lawton, 1974; Katz and Benacerraf; 1972).

K cells and NK cells are apparently bone-marrow derived. The morphologic, physiologic and biologic nature of these cells is currently under scrutiny. Several studies have implied that ADCC and natural killing are both carried out by the same cell population (Kay *et al.*, 1977; Herberman and Holden, 1978). Recently, Timonen *et al.* (1981) have reported that both NK and K cells are associated with large granular lymphocytes. While the majority of studies have focused on anti-tumor effects of NK and K cell cytotoxicity studies on virus infected cells have also been performed (Ching and Lopez, 1979; Minato *et al.*, 1980). There has been an intimate association of NK cells and enhanced activity upon interferon stimulation. Thus, some anti-viral effects of interferon may be mediated via the NK cell (Minato *et al.*, 1980).

4. MECHANISMS OF VIRUS-INDUCED IMMUNOSUPPRESSION

As indicated earlier, it is now quite apparent that various parameters of the immune response mechanism may be influenced by virus infection. However, the manner in which viruses affect immunity has not been totally delineated. Several general mechanisms have been suggested, as follows:

(i) Specific antigen-induced immunologic unresponsiveness may occur when the immune response mechanism is so affected that re-exposure to a normal immunizing dose of the same antigen does not result in a detectable immune response—this type of antigen-specific unresponsiveness is generally referred to as immunologic tolerance. Tolerance may involve both T- and B-cells, and may be either finite (i.e. temporary) or permanent. This form of immune suppression has been reviewed in depth recently (Weigle, 1971).

(ii) Nonspecific immunologic unresponsiveness—a generalized impairment of immune function associated with a variety of initiating agents, including irradiation, radiomimetic drugs, etc. Infection with certain microorganisms, including viruses, may result in nonspecific immunosuppression, as evidenced by generalized decreases or at least alterations in an individual's response to a wide variety of antigens. The induction of nonspecific immunosuppression can be divided into four basic categories: (a) antigenic competition; (b) competition between viruses and antigen for a common stem cell; (c) alteration of phagocytic activity; and (d) lymphocyte dysfunction.

In antigenic competition, a virus may serve as a 'foreign antigen' and thus compete with another antigen for immunocompetent cells. This phenomenon obviously is not restricted to systems where one antigen is an infectious agent, but has been demonstrated with many antigens, including non-replicating ones. The mechanism of antigenic competition is not known and it is felt by some investigators that humoral immune factors may be involved, or that antigens may compete with each other for finite numbers of stem cells or even for finite numbers of antigen reactive or phagocytic cells. Such postulated competition for finite numbers of stem cells may be important not only for non-replicating antigens, but also for infectious 'antigens' such as a virus. For example, if a virus preferentially infects a specific stem cell line, then all subsequent immune responses which would normally derive from such stem cells would be impaired. If such an infected stem cell were a B-cell precursor, a virus infection might prevent the maturation of such B-cells into normal antibody-producing cells, thus reducing the subsequent immune response to the relevant antigen.

Altered phagocytosis has been repeatedly demonstrated when macrophages are directly infected by viruses (Allison, 1970; Notkins *et al.*, 1970). Thus, it is presumed that such depression of phagocytosis after virus infection is mirrored by a defect in antigen processing or presentation, resulting in a reduced immune response, not because immunocompetent cells *per se* are affected, but because antigen is not presented to these cells in the proper manner.

Defects in lymphocyte number, function or activity also may occur because of virus infection. Immunological impairment may result when B- or T-lymphocytes *per se* are either directly affected by a virus or by products of other cells which have been infected by the virus. The direct interaction of a virus, or virus-associated factor, with lymphocytes may therefore result in impaired immune responsiveness. Development of suppressor cells, either T-cells, macrophages or other yet unknown cell types may also result as a consequence of virus infection, as well as by stimulation by other agents (Gorczynski, 1974; Kirchner *et al.*, 1974a, 1974b). Such cells may, in turn, depress either humoral or cellular immune responses, or both. Similarly, factors derived from virus-stimulated cells, or cells responding to some component of the virus, may similarly act as a 'suppressor' factor. In the present review, virus-induced suppression and some possible mechanisms of such suppression will be discussed mainly from the viewpoint of different categories of virus and classes of immune responses.

5. SUPPRESSION OF HUMORAL IMMUNITY BY ONCOGENIC VIRUSES

Friend Virus Complex

One of the most thoroughly investigated model systems concerning virus-induced suppression of humoral immunity is based on murine leukemia associated immunosuppression. Initially, much of the work concerning immunosuppression by murine leukemia viruses was based on the immune response of rodents to sheep erythrocytes (SRBC), considered a T-dependent antigen. Old and his colleagues first reported that immunosuppression to erythrocytes occurred in Friend leukemia virus (FLV)-infected mice (Old *et al.*, 1960). This work has been consistently confirmed and expanded in many laboratories (Bennet and Steeves, 1970; Ceglowski and Friedman, 1967; Cerny and Waner, 1975; Odaka *et al.*, 1966; Wedderburn and Salaman, 1968). Immunodepression by FLV is characterized by a decrease in circulating antibody titers to SRBC, as determined by either titration for hemagglutination or hemolytic antibody in the sera of infected mice (Dent, 1972). In addition, decreased numbers of antibody plaque forming cells (PFCs) to SRBC occur in the spleen and other lymphoid organs in FLV-infected mice, as determined by the localized hemolytic plaque assay (Jerne *et al.*, 1963). The decline in humoral immunity is temporally related to the time of virus infection in relation to the time of antigen administration. Greater immunosuppression occurs when the duration between FLV infection of susceptible mouse strains and challenge immunization with SRBC is longest (Ceglowski and Friedman, 1967). However, significant immunodepression is also evident when antigen is administered even on the day of infection with FLV or one day earlier (Ceglowski and Friedman, 1968b).

The relationship between leukemogenesis, as measured by splenomegaly or blood cell dyscrasia, and immunosuppression is imperfect, since suppression occurs even during the first few days after infection, when the spleen is morphologically unaltered (Ceglowski and Friedman, 1969a). Furthermore, splenectomy does not necessarily prevent immunodepression in FLV-infected mice (Salaman and Wedderburn, 1966), and lymph nodes, which are uninvolved in Friend leukemia, may also show an alteration in responsiveness to SRBC (Bennet and Steeves, 1970; Ceglowski and Friedman, 1968a). It has recently been noted that C57BL/6 mice, which are genetically resistant to Friend leukemia, show a transient but nevertheless marked immunosuppression when the virus is injected 1–3 days before antigen (Ceglowski and Friedman, 1969c). This decrease in responsiveness measured by hemolytic plaque-forming cells (PFC) is directly associated with viremia, and clearly separates the leukemogenic from the immunosuppressive properties of the virus infection. In support of the distinction between leukemogenesis and immunosuppression is the observation that treatment of FLV by *in vitro* incubation with Concanavalin A (Con A) inhibits the leukemogenic properties of the virus but does not completely eliminate the immunosuppressive property (Kateley and Friedman, 1976). Con A-treated FLV induces a latent infection in which viremia occurs in mice, as well as moderate immunosuppression, but there is no evidence of splenomegaly for at least several months. This is similar to the situation which occurs with the lymphatic leukemia virus component of the Friend virus complex, which by itself causes only slight splenomegaly but, nevertheless, depresses the humoral antibody response to sheep RBCs in FLV susceptible mice (Ceglowski and Friedman, 1969c; Eckner, 1975).

Depression of immunoresponsiveness to SRBC has been assessed at both the primary and secondary antibody response level. The degree of immunodepression of either primary or secondary antibody responses to SRBC is somewhat controversial, depending upon the laboratory performing the studies (Ceglowski and Friedman, 1967, 1968b, 1969a; Odaka *et al.*, 1966; Wedderburn and Salaman, 1968). Nevertheless, the IgG antibody response appears to be more suppressed than the IgM response after secondary immunization of FLV-infected mice, suggesting that early events in antibody formation may be less affected (Dent, 1972). In addition, depressed immune responses to a wide variety of antigens besides SRBC have been reported for murine leukemia virus-infected animals. For example, depressed immune responses to lipopolysaccharide antigens from *E. coli*, as well as the bacteria themselves, occur in FLV-infected mice. In addition, immune responses to *Salmonella typhimurium*, *Vibrio cholerae*, bacteriophage, influenza, coxsackie viruses, etc., have been reported to be depressed under certain conditions in leukemia virus-infected mice (Evans and Patterson, 1972; Hirano *et al.*, 1969, 1971; Millian and Schaeffer, 1968; Ransom *et al.*, 1969). On the other hand, no suppression of the 'true' primary immune response to vibrios occurs, although secondary antibody-forming responses to these bacteria are completely inhibited. This is attributed to the nature of the 'true' primary immune response to the vibrios (Cerny *et al.*, 1971; Friedman and Ceglowski, 1974). In the case of most bacterial antigens, there is a low level of antibody response, even in unimmunized animals, referred to as 'background'. This response is probably due to cross reactions with environmental antigens. However, no such background antibody response can be detected in mice which have not been immunized with vibrios. Thus it appears that mice exposed to vibrio antigens for the first time respond with a true primary antibody response. Since no lymphoid cells are committed to producing vibriolytic antibody in unimmunized mice, it has been proposed that only antigen-committed cells or possibly memory cells are the primary targets of the virus leading to suppression. Once mice have been 'primed' with vibrio antigens, resulting in an antigen-induced 'background', the committed cells are now susceptible to suppression by leukemia virus infection.

In attempts to determine the relationship between leukemia virus infection of cells and antibody formation, Koo *et al.* examined individual antibody-producing cells from leukemia virus-infected mice by transmission electron microscopy (Chan *et al.*, 1968; Koo *et al.*, 1971a,b). Such studies indicated that individual antibody-forming cells may be infected with virus, thus eliminating the possible cytotoxic effect of virus on antibody-producing lymphocytes *per se*. It had already been shown by cell transfer studies that antibody-producing precursor cells and FLV target cells were not identical (Ceglowski and Friedman, 1970; Friedman, 1975b; Friedman and Ceglowski, 1968). Thus, immunosuppression by infection with FLV in susceptible mice did not appear to be due primarily to a competition for common stem cells. The transfer experiments using FLV-infected splenocytes injected into X-irradiated recipient mice indicated that precursor B-cells may be affected by the virus and that this population of cells could be involved in the dysfunction of the immune response. However, this conclusion was questioned, since Bendinelli and Bainbridge (1968) found that FLV-infected cells did not 'home' in a normal manner into the spleen, as did splenocytes from normal mice. However, Ceglowski and Friedman showed that such inhibition of 'homing' may not be sufficient to account for the marked immunosuppression noted after FLV infection, and that non-responsiveness was more likely due to a defect in the proliferative activity of FLV-infected B-lymphocytes (Ceglowski *et al.*, 1976; Friedman, 1975a; Friedman and Ceglowski, 1974; Chakrabarty *et al.*, 1970).

The establishment of *in vitro* procedures for induction and maintenance of antibody formation by lymphocytes has led to further studies concerning the nature of immunosuppression by FLV (Dracott *et al.*, 1972). Using the culture system first described by Marbrook (1967), Kateley *et al.* demonstrated that FLV-infected splenocytes were immunosuppressed when challenged with SRBC *in vitro* (Kateley *et al.*, 1974b; Kamo *et al.*, 1975). In additional experiments, Kateley *et al.* (1974b), as well as Weislow and Wheelock (1975), independently showed that relatively low numbers of cells (10^5–5×10^5 splenocytes from infected mice) could suppress 5×10^6 normal spleen cells immunized *in vitro* with SRBC. Further studies showed that cell-free homogenates containing FLV were also immunodepressive, suggesting a direct role for the virus in impairing immune responses (Specter *et al.*, 1976a). Using double-chambered Marbrook vessels with normal and FLV-infected splenocytes subdivided by membrane filters, it was also shown that a factor larger than 300,000 molecular weight but small enough to pass through a 0.05μ membrane was capable of suppressing the immune response of normal splenocytes immunized *in vitro* with SRBC (Kateley *et al.*, 1974b). This immunosuppressive activity was prevented by specific isogeneic mouse anti-FLV serum, suggesting further that the virus was the responsible agent. In studies using a virus-free homogenate of FLV-infected splenocytes clarified by centrifugation at $100{,}000\times g$, no suppression of the antibody response to SRBC was noted (unpublished observation), even though this material inhibited cellular immunity. Thus, it appears that the suppression of antibody formation, at least *in vitro*, is mediated by a non-soluble factor which differs, at least in part, from the factor responsible for unresponsiveness of cell mediated immunity (Mascio and Ceglowski, 1975).

An advantage of *in vitro* procedures for studying immunosuppression by leukemia viruses is the ease of separating cell populations, so that different components of the lymphoid system can be examined systematically. Using separated T-cells, B-cells and macrophage-rich populations, Bendinelli *et al.* established that proteose-peptone-induced peritoneal macrophages from normal mice could restore immunological responsiveness to Rowson Parr Virus (RPV)-infected splenocytes immunized *in vitro* with SRBC (Bendinelli and Friedman, 1976; Bendinelli and Nardini, 1973). RPV is a lymphatic leukemia virus component of the Friend complex (Carter *et al.*, 1970). Further studies indicated that neither B- or T-cells, nor glass adherent (macrophages) or non-adherent (lymphocytes) from the spleen could restore immunity *in vitro* (Bendinelli *et al.*, 1975). Specter *et al.* (1976b) demonstrated similar effects *in vitro* for FLV-infected splenocytes, and further indicated that normal resident peritoneal cells were much less effective in overcoming immunosuppression. This implied that immunosuppression was due to dysfunction of virus-stimulated macrophages, but more information must be obtained before any firm conclusions can be drawn.

Other Murine Leukemia Viruses

Several other murine leukemia tumor virus models have been examined with regard to effects on humoral immune responses (Dent, 1972, 1975; Woodruff and Woodruff, 1975a). For example, Rauscher leukemia virus (RLV), much like Friend virus, results in a marked immunosuppression with decreased numbers of antibody producing cells and circulating antibody (Borella, 1969, 1971, 1972; Gelzer and Dietrich, 1968; Hayry *et al.*, 1970; Millian and Schaeffer, 1968; Seidel and Lauenstein, 1969; Siegel and Morton, 1966a,b, 1967, 1976). The 7S (IgG) antibody response appears to be more suppressed than 19S (IgM) antibody formation (Borella, 1969; Siegel and Morton, 1966b). Suppression, however, is not observed for antibody-forming cells in lymph nodes, suggesting that immunologic impairment may be due to an effect only on the target organ where malignancy develops, i.e. the spleen (Dent, 1972). For example, Siegel and Morton (1976) proposed that competition for a common immunoreactive stem cell by the virus causes the decrease of antibody response in RLV-infected mice.

Using the Moloney leukemia virus model, Cremer and associates observed a variety of humoral immune impairments, especially decreased circulating antibody, including that associated with IgM immunoglobulins, as well as a strong suppression of IgG versus IgM immunobulin synthesis. A limited synthesis of IgG and less heterogeneity of the IgG response was noted in the studies with Moloney virus (Cerny and Stiller, 1975; Cremer, 1967; Cremer *et al.*, 1966, 1969, 1973; Cure and Cremer, 1969). On the other hand, the studies by Kirchner *et al.* (1974a,b) indicated that Moloney virus inhibited cellular formation of hemolytic antibody by more than 90 per cent; this suppression appeared to be associated with suppressor cells that were non-reactive with anti-thymocyte serum and complement, implicating macrophages as the responsible cell class. Such suppression could be due to exertion of an immune modulation by cells which had been de-repressed or otherwise affected by the virus.

Impaired antibody formation has been observed in a spontaneous leukemia system occurring in a high percentage (greater than 80 per cent) of inbred AKR mice (Davidson and Stern, 1954; Dore *et al.*, 1969; Gottlieb *et al.*, 1972; Metcalf and Moulds, 1967; Perkins *et al.*, 1969). Although others have indicated that these mice, which are vertically infected with Gross leukemia virus, may respond normally to a variety of antigenic stimuli, studies have indicated that there is an inhibition of the hemolytic antibody plaque response to sheep erythrocytes even before overt signs of leukemia become evident (Metcalf and Moulds, 1967). When compared to C57BL mice, AKR mice showed decreased numbers of plasma cells and reduced gamma globulin levels (Schmid and Hutchison, 1968). The animals were less reactive to anaphylaxis when exposed to horse serum as compared to CFW mice and showed a lower response to pertussis antigen (Hargis and Malkiel, 1970).

Gross virus, which 'normally' infects AKR mice, was considered for some time to be a suppressive virus (Ellman *et al.*, 1970; Gross, 1970). For example, mice neonatally infected with this agent, prior to development of leukemia, show a decreased ability to form neutralizing antibody to bacteriophage (Peterson *et al.*, 1963). More recent studies have shown that Gross leukemia virus-infected spleen cells have a decreased capacity to form antibody, while allogeneic responses are not affected, suggesting that several mechanisms may be involved (Dent, 1975). Thus, it should be noted that many different types of murine leukemia virus can induce a generalized nonspecific depression of humoral immunity, and the circumstances of immunosuppression may be different for each virus. However; in all instances immune depression seems to result from the effect of the virus *per se*, often through suppressor factors elicited in the host or cells initiated as a result of virus infection.

Avian Viruses

Although the avian leukosis virus system has not been as thoroughly studied as the murine leukemia model, a number of reports have indicated deficiency in circulating antibody formation to serum albumin, bacteriophage, *Brucella abortus*, Salmonella vaccine, as well as sheep and human erythrocytes (Dent *et al.*, 1968; Peterson *et al.*, 1966; Purchase *et al.*, 1968). On the other hand, Dent *et al.* (1968) have reported normal responses to several of these antigens, raising some question as to the suppressive activity of the Avian leukosis virus. It should be noted that Cooper recently re-examined some of the mechanisms that may be involved in immunosuppression by the Avian leukosis viruses. The tumor virus induced lymphoid tumors which had characteristics of B-cells, although they appeared to have IgM surface immunoglobulin marker rather than IgG molecules, indicating a possible genetic defect resulting in the absence of natural cell maturation necessary for sequential expression of C region genes from μ to γ to α (Cooper *et al.*, 1974). Similarly, the DNA oncogenic Herpes virus which is known to cause Marek's disease in fowls, has been reported to suppress humoral immunity to bovine serum albumin and several different species of bacteria (Burg *et al.*, 1971; Evans and Patterson, 1971, 1972; Payne, 1970; Purchase *et al.*, 1968). While electrophoretic examination revealed no deficiencies of immunoglobulin synthesis, more susceptible strains of chickens showed lower IgG levels, suggesting a possible genetic deficiency, which might predispose them to the suppressive effects of these viruses (Howard *et al.*, 1967).

Other DNA Viruses

Oncogenic DNA viruses have not been extensively studied in terms of immunomodulation, but some reports do exist. Friedman and Goldner (1970a,b) reported that Adenovirus 12 and SV_{40} virus, which cause tumors when inoculated into newborn hamsters, resulted in a moderate decrease of antibody responses to sheep

RBC, but only in neonatal hamsters. Hamburg *et al.* (1970) further examined this effect and showed that the response to Sendai viruses was decreased in SV_{40}- or Adenovirus 16-infected hamsters. A human strain of Adenoviruses was found to suppress the anti-SRBC response in chickens (Beladi *et al.*, 1973). In more recent studies Friedman and associates indicated that the antibody response to T-independent *E. coli* LPS was moderately depressed in SV_{40}- and Adenovirus 12-infected hamsters, but only during the early neonatal period and after the emergence of the tumors later in life (unpublished observation).

Suppression of Humoral Immunity by Non-Oncogenic Viruses

Among those non-oncogenic viruses which have been studied in terms of effects on humoral immunity, many different DNA and RNA viruses of human and non-human origin may affect antibody formation. The most frequent contaminant of many tissue cell cultures is the lactic dehydrogenase (LDH) virus, which is now known to have marked effects on immune responsiveness, thus often masking the true effects of other viruses (Riley, 1974; Mella and Lang, 1967; Notkins, 1965). LDH virus has been reported to suppress the antibody response to keyhole limpet hemocyanin and to low doses of goat RBCs, while high doses of such erythrocytes result in normal responses in infected animals (Notkins *et al.*, 1966; Oldstone *et al.*, 1974). Thus, it has been postulated by Oldstone that either antigenic competition, or more likely a T-cell defect or dysfunction, may occur in LDH virus-infected animals. Oldstone also found an enhanced response to human immunoglobulin G, indicating that while suppression is nonspecific, it may be antigen-selective, depending on the antigen used (Oldstone *et al.*, 1974). This raises the question of whether too few antigens have been used in other systems in which generalized immunosuppression has been alleged.

Lymphocytic choriomeningitis virus (LCM), known to cause infection not only in animals but also in man, may have immunomodulating effects (Mims and Wainwright, 1968). Bro-Jørgensen recently indicated that both T-dependent and T-independent antigens, including SRBC, *E. coli* LPS, pneumococcal polysaccharides (SSSIII) and polyvinyl pyrrolidone, are affected (Bro-Jørgensen *et al.,* 1975; Bro-Jørgensen and Volkert, 1974). Suppression to SRBC was greater than 90 per cent and lasted for at least 2–4 weeks, while responses to the three T-independent antigens tested were at normal or near normal levels at all times, indicating that the defect may be related mainly to an influence on T-cells (Bro-Jørgensen and Volkert, 1974). Bro-Jørgensen and Volkert (1974) also reported that the number of colony-forming stem cells for lymphocyte precursors was depleted in mice with LCM infection. Thus the populations of immunocompetent precursor cells were markedly diminished. No other morphologic changes, however, were observed with regard to individual antibody forming cells.

Hepatitis virus has been studied with regard to effects on humoral immunity. Human peripheral blood lymphocytes from individuals infected with Hepatitis A virus (i.e. infectious hepatitis) showed markedly reduced B-cell rosette-forming ability, although the numbers of T-cell rosettes were unaffected. There was also a slight decrease in the number of cells with surface IgM. Lymphocytes with other surface Ig markers were normal. Hepatitis B virus, the etiologic agent of serum hepatitis, did not appear to be suppressive, as determined by similar assays (Aiuti *et al.*, 1973). Thus, there appears to be a marked difference in the effects of these two viruses on the immune response system, at least in man.

As indicated earlier, the first association of immunosuppression with a viral disease was made with measles. In more recent studies, measles virus has repeatedly been shown to cause immunosuppression (Joseph and Oldstone, 1975; McFarland, 1974). A defect in the antibody response to the hapten DNP in mice infected with measles virus appeared related to the effects on helper T-cells, although some effects on B-cells were noted (McFarland, 1974). Suppression, however, was transient and directly related to the presence of viral antigen in the spleen. In cell transfer experiments it was found that T-cells were directly involved in immunological impairment, although T-cell numbers were not reduced in infected animals. However, increasing the numbers of T-cells from infected animals overcame the immunological impairment, suggesting that in all probabiltiy, T-cells were affected. Perhaps only those cells directly infected with virus were immunologically impaired (McFarland, 1974). Nevertheless, the mechanism whereby measles virus causes a T-cell defect has not yet been elucidated. Similar effects occur with mouse thymic virus, which depresses antibody responses to T-dependent SRBCs but not to T-independent antigens such as pneumococcal polysaccharide, DNP-ficoll, etc. (Cohen *et al.*, 1975; Morse *et al.*, 1976). Furthermore, the B-cell mitogenic response, although apparently requiring a helper T-cell population, also is not affected.

The relationship between virus infection and alterations of different lymphocyte populations has been studied with a variety of virus models. Lodmell, studying Aleutian disease of minks, reported that the Sapphire strain showed a greater suppression to goat RBCs than Pastel minks (Lodmell *et al.*, 1970, 1973). Such suppression was directly related to susceptibility of the different strains to the virus. In canine distemper infection, a decrease in the number of lymphocytes was related to an increase in absolute antibody titer to antigens in the infected host and development of an autoimmune type of disease (Krakowka *et al.*, 1973, 1975). On the other hand, in equine infectious anemia, normal numbers of lymphocytes were evident despite a decreased immunocompetence of lymphocytes (Banks and Henson, 1973; Williams *et al.*, 1968), suggesting a relationship between the effects on certain lymphocyte populations and immune responsiveness. Furthermore, when rabbit lymphoid cells were infected *in vitro* with Newcastle Disease virus, a decreased antibody response to bovine serum albumin was evident (Medzon and Vas, 1964). This response could be directly related to morphologic alteration of the rabbit spleen cells, the major source of antibody-producing lymphocytes. An apparent toxic effect of the virus was implicated in mice infected with encephalomyocarditis virus which evinced a decreased level of the anti-viral protein interferon (Stringfellow and Glasgow, 1974). This appeared related to production of a species specific factor which inhibited interferon production. The factor appeared to be non-viral and was apparently produced by the host. Other viruses causing depression of interferon levels have also been noted (Cure and Cremer, 1969; Demaeyer-Guignard, 1972; Hirano *et al.*, 1969; Osborn and Meddaris, 1967; Wagner *et al.*, 1963).

6. EFFECTS OF ONCOGENIC VIRUSES ON CELLULAR IMMUNITY

Friend Leukemia Virus

Cell-mediated immunity, including the *in vitro* correlates of such immunity, has been demonstrated in recent years to be markedly affected by FLV, as well as many other oncogenic viruses. Allograft survival has been reported to be prolonged in FLV-infected mice (Friedman *et al.*, 1973; Mortensen *et al.*, 1973a), although the conclusions of Schneider and Dore (1969) differ in this regard as compared to studies from other laboratories. Delayed cutaneous hypersensitivity to tubercle bacilli, as measured by the mouse foot pad swelling assay, also has been shown to be decreased when FLV was given after sensitization but before challenge with PPD (Mortensen *et al.*, 1973a). Such observations, however, differ from observations for humoral immunity in FLV-infected animals, where suppression did not normally occur when the virus was given after challenge immunization. Similar to the findings with humoral immunity, the degree of immunosuppression of cellular immunity depends upon the dose of virus used for infection and the time interval between infection and challenge with antigen. In *in vitro* studies, production of migration inhibition factors (MIF) and lymphocyte-mediated cytotoxicity has been found to be depressed after FLV infection (Ceglowski *et al.*, 1976; Friedman and Ceglowski, 1971a,b; Mascio and

Ceglowski, 1975; Mortensen *et al.*, 1973a,b). Fractionation of spleen cells into adherent and non-adherent populations indicated that the defect in cellular immunity was due to alteration of the non-adherent spleen cell populations (i.e. lymphocyte-rich). The failure of cytotoxicity, along with reduced MIF activity, implicated the T-lymphocyte population as the defective cell type (Mascio and Ceglowski, 1975). A number of studies suggested that the decrease in the number of effector T-cells was mainly responsible for depression in cytolytic activity by splenocytes from FLV-infected animals. This has been supported by results of studies which showed a reduced number of the theta-bearing lymphocytes in the spleen of FLV-infected mice (Friedman and Kateley, 1975; Kateley *et al.*, 1974a). In addition, Ceglowski (1976) recently reported that depressed cytotoxicity of splenocytes from FLV-infected mice could be restored by treating the spleen cells with neuraminidase, an enzyme which affects sialic acid. The ability of this enzyme to apparently strip off 'blocking' or masking substance(s) from the T-cells could account for re-expression of blocked receptors as a result of alteration due to FLV infection. Ceglowski and co-workers also demonstrated a soluble substance which could be separated from splenic extracts of FLV-infected mice (Friedman and Ceglowski, 1971a,b; Mascio and Ceglowski, 1975). This material was free of virus *per se* or virus-antibody complexes, but readily suppressed *in vitro* expression of cellular immunity. This material was resistant to heating at 56°C for 30 min and was also resistant to treatment with nucleases, neuraminidase and anti-virus serum, but was susceptible to inactivation by trypsin digestion (Ceglowski, 1976). It has not yet been determined whether this factor is a product of a suppressor cell population or of the leukemia cells *per se*. The factor was not suppressive, however, for humoral immunity as determined by examining effects of the extracts on PFC formation to sheep RBCs (Specter *et al.*, unpublished observations).

Friend virus has also been reported to enhance the susceptibility of mice to oncogenic and non-oncogenic viruses (Chirigos *et al.*, 1968; Gledhill, 1961), as well as to tumor grafts (Deodhar and Chiang, 1970). Such increased susceptibility seemed to reflect mainly the depression of cellular immunity. Several possibilities have been raised as the mechanisms of impairment of immunity. Infection by FLV may lead to the development of blocking substances (perhaps sialic acid) on the surface of T-cells, preventing expression of receptors needed for immune competence. Alternatively, a suppressor substance may be elicited, possibly by 'blocked' T-cells infected with the virus, preventing a normal immune response. It is also plausible that a suppressive factor may be released from other infected cells, resulting in blockade or inhibition of other T-lymphocytes. Regardless of the mechanism involved, it seems clear that FLV, which was felt for many years to infect exclusively B-lymphocytes, can also affect expression of immune competence by T-cells. Suppression of such cellular immunity in FLV-infected animals does not appear directly related to suppression of humoral immunity, especially since the soluble factor noted in FLV-infected lymphoid cells which depress cellular immunity has been found to have no effect on antibody formation. Furthermore, this soluble factor was not inactivated by anti-FLV serum, whereas soluble extracts from FLV-infected mice which affect antibody formation could readily be neutralized by such anti-FLV serum. More recently Israel and Wainberg (1981) have reported that a soluble factor was produced by mouse macrophages after infection with FLV or other viruses which depressed blastogenic responses to PHA or ConA. This factor was greater than 20,000 molecular weight, sensitive to trypsin and its biosynthesis was inhibited by cycloheximide. The factor does not have any anti-viral activity and its mode of action remains to be determined.

Mice infected with FLV also exhibited a decrease in the ability of their spleen natural killer (NK) cells to kill YAC-1 lymphoma cells in vitro. Peripheral lymph node cells were not depleted in NK activity even 40 days post-infection when spleen NK activity was non-existent. The mechanism of this decrease is not as yet understood. However, FLV infected spleen cells did result in decreased NK activity of normal spleen cells versus YAC-1 target cells. This indicated that infected spleens contain a suppressive component, either infected cells or suppressor host cells (Bendinelli *et al.*, unpublished observations).

OTHER MURINE TUMOR VIRUSES

Chan and co-workers have reported that Moloney virus prolongs allograft rejection responses in mice (Chan *et al.*, 1970). Moreover, Moloney sarcoma virus (MSV) has been shown by Gorczynski (1974) and Kirchner *et al.* (1974b) to suppress cellular immune responses, including mitogenic responses. Although both investigators stress the importance of suppressor cell populations for reduced immune responsiveness, the cell type that may be involved differs. Gorczynski (1974) reported that immunoglobulins are present on the surface of the suppressor cells involved in immune impairment in MSV infected animals; cytolysis with anti-Ig and complement indicated further that such cells may be B-cells. However, no information has been presented as to whether or not these cells may be macrophages with absorbed surface antibody. This is an important point since Kirchner and colleagues have implicated macrophages as the suppressor cell population, based on resistance of suppressor cells to anti-theta serum and complement and the observation that these cells are readily removed by glass absorption and treatment with iron filings (Kirchner *et al.*, 1974a,b). In both cases, however, removal of the suppressor cell population by cell separation procedures resulted in a cell population fully competent to evince cellular immune reactions *in vitro*. Thus no true defect in the effector T-cell population occurred in the MSV-bearing mice. Addition of the separated suppressor cell population to normal mouse splenocytes depressed responsiveness to PHA, indicating that direct suppression by spleen cells occurred, rather than suppression by tumor cells, tumor viruses or tumor cell products (Kirchner *et al.*, 1974a). C57B1/6 mice with MSV induced tumors were reported to also be depressed in NK cell activity (Herberman *et al.*, 1980). However, CBA mice did not show a significant decrease. Unlike the T-cell responses mentioned above, removal of adherent cells (macrophages) did not significantly affect NK cell depression in the C57B1 mice.

Inhibition of graft rejection has also been reported for other C type viruses, including AKR (Doell *et al.*, 1967; Dore *et al.*, 1969), Gross (Dent *et al.*, 1968) and feline leukemia viruses (Perryman *et al.*, 1972). In addition, mammary tumor virus (MTV), a type B virus, has been found to prolong skin grafts (Blair *et al.*, 1971), similar to the radiation leukemia viruses (Peled and Haran-Ghera, 1971). In addition, the *in vivo* delayed hypersensitivity skin test reactions were found depressed after MTV infection (Griswold *et al.*, 1973). As with the Friend virus system, all the above viruses caused little or no depression of the graft versus host (GvH) reaction (Bennet and Steeves, 1970; Dent, 1972), although there have been reports suggesting some decreased GvH reactions (Dore *et al.*, 1969). In the AKR leukemia system, a decrease in lymphocyte populations as shown by fewer circulating lymphocytes, reduced spleen weight and reduction in bone marrow cellularity, has been related to increased skin graft survival time (Schmid and Hutchison, 1968). Decreased lymphocyte numbers have also been observed in Gross virus infected mice (Olson, 1973). Furthermore, this virus appeared to affect the thymus preferentially, especially in neonatal mice. Measurement of PHA-responsiveness *in vitro*, and examinations for theta antigen on lymphocytes have shown that there are fewer immunocompetent cells in AKR mice (Zatz *et al.*, 1973a,b). During the pre-leukemic state, migration inhibition reactions were found to be impaired, further suggesting that an immunologic defect of T-lymphocytes precedes overt signs of leukemia (Ceglowski and Friedman, 1969b; Frey-Wettstein and Hays, 1970). Although leukemic cells *per se* may be directly involved in these alterations, it is important to note that the virus *per se*, or at least virus antibody complexes in the circulation, may be involved in such immunosuppression. *In vitro* studies for cellular immunity based on lymphocyte stimulation with mitogens or specific antigens showed that Rauscher, Moloney and Gross leukemia viruses were immunosuppressive in these systems (Cerny and Stiller, 1975; Hayry *et al.*, 1970; Kirchner *et al.*, 1974a,b; Olson, 1973).

AVIAN VIRUSES

Avian leukosis virus has been shown by several investigators to depress cellular immunity, as measured by allograft rejection; however, little or no effect has been observed for GvH reactions (Dent, 1972, 1975; Purchase *et al.*, 1968). Among the DNA avian viruses, Marek's disease virus reportedly depressed delayed hypersensitivity to intradermal injection of antigen, as well as mitogen-induced blast cell stimulation. No effects on GvH have been observed (Alm *et al.*, 1972; Burg *et al.*, 1971; Theis *et al.*, 1975).

Other Oncogenic Viruses

Fibroma virus has been reported to depress cutaneous hypersensitivity to viral antigens as well as affect macrophage migration inhibition in rabbits with progressively growing tumors induced by the virus *per se*. Upon tumor regression, immunity is restored (Tompkins *et al.*, 1973). Cellular immunity, as assessed by *in vitro* and *in vivo* assays for hypersensitivity to mycobacteria and skin allografts, was shown to be moderately depressed during the latent period of Adenovirus 12 and SV_{40} tumorigenesis. However, after a tumor appeared, these forms of cellular immunity were markedly depressed. Furthermore, cellular immunity measured by *in vitro* assays to SV_{40} and Adenovirus 12 antigens *per se*, were also markedly depressed after appearance of tumors but not during the latent phase.

Non-oncogenic Viruses

In a number of tumor model systems, suppression of cellular immunity has been clearly associated with the virus causing the tumor. However, it should be noted that in several cases, immunosuppression appeared due to a contaminating virus. Similar to the situation for humoral immunity, the most common virus associated with such 'nonspecific' immunosuppression of cellular immunity was the LDH virus. Snodgrass *et al.* (1972) indicated that LDH virus directly affect the thymus, causing cytotoxic depletion of thymic lymphocytes. Also LDH virus has been shown to alter cellular immune reactions and to potentiate tumor growth, both indicative of T-cell defects. Bonnard and his colleagues reported that suppression of cellular immunity in their Moloney Sarcoma system was due to a contaminating virus, the minute virus of mice (Bonnard *et al.*, 1976). This virus reportedly leads to decreased responsiveness via a suppressor population of macrophages (Kirchner *et al.*, 1974a,b). Another virus associated with tumors is the lymphocytic choriomeningitis virus (LCM). This virus induces an autoimmune-like disease, affecting the ability of the infected individual to mount a normal immune response (Mims and Wainwright, 1968; Pincus *et al.*, 1970). LCM infection reportedly also impairs hypersensitivity, although resistance to other virus infections, a function associated with cellular immunity, is variable (Bro-Jørgensen *et al.*, 1974, 1975; Hoterman and Havell, 1970).

The list of non-oncogenic viruses not associated with tumors, but which result in modulation of immunity, is extensive (Table 1). The methods for assessing immunoresponsiveness in relationship to infection by such viruses have varied considerably. The most common assay utilized in recent years has been the response of leukocytes to phytomitogens, such as phytohemagglutinin and concanavalin A. This response measures T-cell blastogenesis, considered an *in vitro* correlate of cellular immunity. Decreases in PHA responsiveness have been observed by Olsen (1973) as a result of infection with Adenovirus, Herpes simplex virus, influenza, mengovirus and Newcastle disease (NDV) virus. On the other hand, Sendai virus and vaccinia virus, as well as LDH and polyoma viruses, have been reported to enhance PHA-responsiveness (Olson, 1973). Willems *et al.* (1969), in a similar study, reported depressed responses with human wart virus, as well as those mentioned by Olson. In addition, polio, Echo, mumps and Vesicular stomitis virus (VSV), Reovirus and Hepatitis A (infectious hepatitis) virus also affect PHA-responsiveness (Willems *et al.*, 1969). The ability of these viruses to depress PHA responses has been associated with replication of the virus in lymphocyte cytoplasm. Several other viruses, including canine distemper virus (Krakowka *et al.*, 1975), equine infectious anemia virus (Banks and Henson, 1973), mouse cytomegalovirus (Howard *et al.*, 1974; Selgrade *et al.*, 1976), mouse thymus virus (Bro-Jørgensen and Volkert, 1974), rinderpest virus (Willems *et al.*, 1969) and rubella virus (Ganguly *et al.*, 1976; Olson *et al.*, 1968; Vesikari and Buimovici-Klein, 1975) have also been found to suppress PHA-responsiveness of normal lymphocytes Loh and Hudson (1981) have implicated infected adherent spleen cells (macrophages) as the cells responsible for depressed blastogenic responses to plant lectins in murine cytomegalovirus infection. A reduction in the number of infections centers resulted in restoration of responsiveness, suggesting that infected cells were directly responsible for suppression. Combined with the studies of Israel and Wainberg (1981), these data indicate that macrophages are intimately involved in suppression of cell mediated immune responses by oncogenic and non-oncogenic viruses.

Other *in vitro* correlates of cellular immunity have also been found altered by viral infection. Leukocyte migration inhibition is often impaired by rubella infection (Ganguly *et al.*, 1976), and infectious mononucleosis (associated with Epstein-Barr virus) patients often evince decreased killing in leukocyte reactions (Twomey, 1974). The classic methodology for measuring cellular immunity, i.e. delayed cutaneous skin hypersensitivity, has been shown to be inhibited by several viruses, including infectious mononucleosis, influenza (Hall and Kantor, 1972; Kaufman *et al.*, 1974b; Twomey, 1974), NDV, rinderpest, rubella and mumps (Bloomfield and Mateer, 1919; Kantzler *et al.*, 1974; Kauffman *et al.*, 1974b, 1976; McGregor *et al.*, 1976; Twomey, 1974; Yamanouchi *et al.*, 1974). A wide variety of antigens has been used for skin testing to indicate that immunosuppression is not virus specific or even antigen specific. With influenza-killed vaccines, as well as virulent virus, depressed skin reactivities have been noted (Kantzler *et al.*, 1974). This supports the earlier concern about the effects of widespread use of such vaccines in man. No T-cell defect, however, has been noted *in vitro* as a correlate with such reduced skin responses, possibly indicating a specific block of inflammation.

Prolonged skin allograft survival is yet another widely noted defect of cellular immunity in virus-infected individuals. NDV has been shown to prolong skin grafts (Woodruff and Woodruff, 1975a,b). On the other hand, canine distemper virus, which causes a prolonged depression of PHA-responsiveness, has no effect on allograft survival (Krakowka *et al.*, 1975). Again, this suggests that *in vitro* correlates of cellular immunity may be misleading as compared to *in vivo* responsiveness of infected hosts. LDH, mentioned earlier as a depressor of cellular immunity, has also been found to depress allograft survival and graft versus host disease (Howard *et al.*, 1974). The mechanism, although not determined, has been suggested by Howard *et al.* to be related to increased macrophage function, since LDH does not infect this cell class.

Perhaps the most likely mechanism for decreased immunocompetence during viral infection is a direct effect of the virus on lymphocytes *per se*. After infection by some of the above named viruses, defects in lymphocyte cellular activity are evident. A generalized lymphocyte depletion is seen in canine distemper (Krakowka *et al.*, 1975) and in NDV infection (Woodruff and Woodruff, 1975b). LDH and NDV are also capable of altering lymphocyte movement *in vivo* (i.e. homing), which may be a reflection of immunocompetence (McGregor *et al.*, 1976; Morgini and Rosenberg, 1976). Other alterations include a decrease in surface immunoglobulins (usually associated with humoral immunity) on lymphocytes in animals with equine infectious anemia, Hepatitis A, as well as occasionally measles (Aiuti *et al.*, 1973; Mella and Lang, 1967; Williams *et al.*, 1968). Rosette formation of B-cells is also inhibited in patients with Hepatitis A and measles (Aiuti *et al.*, 1973). T-cell rosettes have been found to be present in normal numbers in mice infected with several other viruses. In most cases, however, defects in E rosettes (presumably T-cells) and EAC rosettes (considered B-cells), as well as surface immunoglobulins on lymphocyte membranes, are not evident or even possibly slightly elevated in many instances (Aiuti *et al.*, 1973).

7. EFFECT OF VIRUSES ON MACROPHAGE FUNCTIONS

Macrophages are considered critical in controlling an individual's susceptibility to virus infection, as conclusively demonstrated by Mims (1964) in the 1960s. As the initial cell type of the host defense system to encounter a virus, macrophages may obviously be quite important in modulation of the immune responses in virus

TABLE 1. *Modulation of Immunoresponsiveness by Oncogenic and Non-oncogenic Viruses*

Virus	Response tested	Effect	Antigen	Test animal	References
ONCOGENIC					
DNA					
Adenovirus	Antibody production	depressed	SRBC, sendai	Hamster	Friedman and Goldner, 1970a, b; Hamburg *et al.*, 1970
Fibroma	Delayed hypersensitivity	depressed	Fibroma Ag	Newborn rabbit	Tompkins *et al.*, 1973
	Migration inhibition	depressed	Fibroma Ag	Newborn rabbit	
Marek's disease	Antibody production	depressed	BSA, Bact. antigens	Chicken	Burg *et al.*, 1971; Evans and Patterson, 1971, 1972; Payne, 1970; Purchase *et al.*, 1968
	Immunoglobulin levels	depressed		Chicken	Jakowski *et al.*, 1973
		normal		Chicken	Howard *et al.*, 1967
	Lymphocyte stimulation	depressed	PHA	Chicken	Alm *et al.*, 1972; Theis *et al.*, 1975
	Susceptibility-infection	increased	Coccidiodes	Chicken	Biggs *et al.*, 1968
Polyoma	Lymphocyte stimulation	increased	PHA	Mouse	Olson, 1973
SV_{40}	Antibody production	depressed	SRBC	Hamster	Friedman and Goldner, 1970a,b
	Lymphocyte stimulation	normal	PHA	Human	Willems *et al.*, 1969
RNA					
AKR leukemia	Antibody production	depressed	CRBC, SRBC	Mouse	Davidson and Stern, 1954; Dore *et al.*, 1969; Gottlieb *et al.*, 1972; Metcalf and Moulds, 1967; Perkins *et al.*, 1969
	Gamma globulin levels	depressed		Mouse	Schmid and Hutchison, 1968
	Lymphocyte numbers, proliferation, homing	depressed		Mouse	Schmid and Hutchison, 1968; Zatz *et al.*, 1973a,b
	Anaphylactic reaction	depressed	Pertussis Ag, horse serum	Mouse	Hargis and Malkiel, 1970
	Allograft rejection	depressed		Mouse	Dore *et al.*, 1969; Dracott *et al.*, 1972
	Migration inhibition	depressed		Mouse	Ceglowski and Friedman, 1969c; Frey-Wettstein and Hays, 1970
	Lymphocyte stimulation	depressed	PHA	Mouse	Strauss *et al.*, 1972; Zatz *et al.*, 1973a, b
	Interferon production	depressed		Mouse	Demaeyer-Guignard, 1972
Mammary tumor	Antibody response	depressed	SRBC	Mouse	Blair *et al.*, 1971; Griswold *et al.*, 1973
	Delayed hypersensitivity	depressed		Mouse	Griswold *et al.*, 1973
	Allograft rejection	depressed		Mouse	Blair *et al.*, 1971

TABLE 1. *Modulation of Immunoresponsiveness by Oncogenic and Non-oncogenic Viruses (continued)*

Virus	Response tested	Effect	Antigen	Test animal	References
Avian leukosis	Antibody production	depressed	BSA, phage, *Br. abortus*	Chicken	Dent *et al.*, 1968; Peterson *et al.*, 1966; Purchase *et al.*, 1968
	Cellular immunity	normal		Chicken	Dent *et al.*, 1968; Purchase *et al.*, 1968
Feline leukemia	Antibody production	normal		Cat	Perryman *et al.*, 1972
	Allograft rejection	depressed		Cat	Perryman *et al.*, 1972
Friend leukemia	Antibody production	depressed	SRBC, Viral Ag, Bacterial Ag	Mouse	Ceglowski, 1976; Ceglowski *et al.*, 1972; Ceglowski and Friedman, 1967, 1968a, b, 1969a, b, c, 1970, 1975; Ceglowski *et al.*, 1976; Cerny *et al.*, 1971; Cerny and Stiller, 1975; Cerny and Waner, 1975; Flickinger and Gentile, 1970; Hirano *et al.*, 1969, 1971; Millian and Schaeffer, 1968; Notkins *et al.*, 1970; Peterson *et al.*, 1963; Salaman and Wedderburn, 1966; Wedderburn and Salaman, 1968
	Lymphocyte homing and type	depressed		Mouse	Bendinelli and Bainbridge, 1968; Farber *et al.*, 1975
	Delayed hypersensitivity	depressed		Mouse	Mortensen *et al.*, 1973a
	Allograft rejection	depressed		Mouse	Mortensen *et al.*, 1973a
	GvH	normal		Mouse	Bennet and Steeves, 1970
	Migration inhibition	depressed	PPD	Mouse	Mortensen *et al.*, 1973a
	Lymphocyte stimulation	depressed	PHA, Con A	Mouse	Israel and Wainberg, 1981; Mortensen *et al.*, 1973b; Olson, 1973
	Interferon production	depressed		Mouse	Demaeyer-Guignard, 1972; Wheelock *et al.*, 1974
	Phagocytosis	depressed	SRBC, carbon	Mouse	Koo *et al.*, 1971b; Mortensen *et al.*, 1973a; Utermohlen and Zabriskie, 1973; Levy and Wheelock, 1976; Old *et al.*, 1960; Wheelock *et al.*, 1974
	Susceptibility infection	increased	Mouse hepatitis	Mouse	Gledhill, 1961
	Lymphocyte cytotoxicity	depressed		Mouse	Mascio and Ceglowski, 1975; Mortensen *et al.*, 1973b
Gross leukemia	Antibody production	depressed	Bacteriophage	Mouse	Peterson *et al.*, 1963
	Allograft rejection	depressed		Mouse	Dent *et al.*, 1965
	Lymphocyte stimulation	depressed	PHA	Mouse	Olson, 1973

TABLE 1. *Modulation of Immunoresponsiveness by Oncogenic and Non-oncogenic Viruses (continued)*

Virus	Response tested	Effect	Antigen	Test animal	References
Moloney sarcoma	Antibody production	depressed	SRBC, BSA	Mouse	Cerny and Stiller, 1975; Cremer, 1967; Cremer *et al.*, 1966, 1969, 1973; Salaman and Wedderburn, 1966
	Immunoglobulin levels	depressed		Mouse	Cure and Cremer, 1969
	Allograft rejection	depressed		Mouse	Cerny and Stiller, 1975
	Lymphocyte stimulation	depressed	PHA, LPS	Mouse	Cerny and Stiller, 1975; Kirchner *et al.*, 1974a, b
Radiation leukemia	Antibody production	depressed	SRBC	Mouse	Peled and Haran-Ghera, 1974
	Lymphocyte population	altered		Mouse	Haran-Ghera *et al.*, 1976
	Allograft rejection	normal		Mouse	Peled and Haran-Ghera, 1971
Rauscher leukemia	Antibody production	depressed	SRBC, BSA, Viral Ags, Diphth. toxoid	Mouse	Borella, 1969; Ceglowski and Friedman, 1968b; Gelzer and Dietrich, 1968; Millian and Schaeffer, 1968; Schmid and Hutchison, 1968; Schneider and Dore, 1969; Schwab, 1975; Scott and Walker, 1976; Seidel and Lauenstein, 1969; Siegel and Morton, 1966a, b, 1967, 1976; Siegel *et al.*, 1969; Starr and Berkovich, 1964; Turner and Chirigos, 1969
	Lymphocyte stimulation	depressed	PHA, alloAGS	Mouse	Hayry *et al.*, 1970
Rowson-Parr	Antibody production	depressed	SRBC	Mouse	Bendinelli *et al.*, 1975; Bendinelli and Nardini, 1973
	Lymphocyte morphology	altered		Mouse	Bendinelli and Friedman, 1976
Schwartz leukemia	Lymphocyte stimulation	depressed	PHA	Mouse	Olson, 1973
NON-ONCOGENIC DNA					
Adenovirus	Antibody production	depressed	SRBC	Chicken	Beladi *et al.*, 1973
	Lymphocyte stimulation	depressed	PHA	Human	Willems *et al.*, 1969
	Lymphocyte stimulation	normal	PHA	Human, mouse	Olson, 1973; Willems *et al.*, 1969
Ectromelia (mouse pox)	Phagocytosis	depressed		Mouse	Gledhill *et al.*, 1965; Notkins, 1965
Fowl pox	Macrophage killing	increased	Salmonella, viruses	Chicken	Pathak *et al.*, 1974
Hepatitis B	Lymphocyte number	normal		Human	Aiuti *et al.*, 1973
	Lymphocyte stimulation	depressed	PHA	Human	Willems *et al.*, 1969

TABLE 1. *Modulation of Immunoresponsiveness by Oncogenic and Non-oncogenic Viruses (continued)*

Virus	Response tested	Effect	Antigen	Test animal	References
Herpes simplex	Lymphocyte number	decreased		Mouse	Olson, 1973
	Lympyhocyte stimulation	depressed	PHA	Mouse, human	Olson, 1973; Rosenberg *et al.*, 1974; Willems *et al.*, 1969
	Monocyte chemotaxis	depressed		Mouse	Kleinerman *et al.*, 1974
Infectious mononucleosis	Delayed hypersensitivity	depressed		Human	Twomey, 1974
	Lymphocyte number	normal		Human	Aiuti *et al.*, 1973
	Lymphocyte stimulation	depressed	PHA	Human	Pincus *et al.*, 1970; Rubin, 1966
	Mixed lymphocyte reaction	depressed		Human	Twomey, 1974
Minute virus (mouse)	Mixed leukocyte reaction	depressed		Mouse	Bonnard *et al.*, 1976
Mouse cyto-megalovirus	Antibody production	depressed	SRBC, NDV	Mouse	Howard and Najarian, 1974; Osborn *et al.*, 1968; Osborn and Meddaris, 1967
	Allograft rejection	depressed		Mouse	Howard *et al.*, 1967, 1974
	Lymphocyte stimulation	depressed	PHA, LPS, PWM, Con A	Mouse	Howard *et al.*, 1967, 1974; Salaman and Wedderburn, 1966; Selgrade *et al.*, 1976
	Interferon production	depressed		Mouse	Osborn and Meddaris, 1967
Mouse thymic virus	Antibody production	depressed	SSSIII	Mouse	Morse *et al.*, 1976
	Lymphocyte number	depressed		Mouse	Carter *et al.*, 1970
	Lymphocyte stimulation	depressed	PHA, alloAgs	Mouse	Carter *et al.*, 1970
Wart virus	Lymphocyte stimulation	depressed	PHA	Human	Willems *et al.*, 1969
Vaccinia	Lymphocyte stimulation	depressed	PHA, Con A	Mouse, rabbit, human	McLaren *et al.*, 1976; Olson, 1973; Vesikari and Buomovici-Klein, 1975; Willems *et al.*, 1969
Varicella (chicken pox)	Lymphocyte stimulation	depressed	Tuberculin	Human	Notkins *et al.*, 1970
RNA					
Aleutian mink disease	Antibody production	depressed	GRBC, BGG, KLH, Br.abort.	Mink	Kenyon, 1966; Lodmell *et al.*, 1973, 1970; Porter *et al.*, 1974
	Gamma globulin levels	depressed		Mink	Porter and Larsen, 1965
	Lymphocyte stimulation	depressed	PHA, Con A	Mink	Perryman *et al.*, 1975
Canine distemper	Antibody production	increased	Myelin	Dog	Krakowka *et al.*, 1975
	Lymphocyte number	depressed		Dog	Krakowka *et al.*, 1973
	Allograft rejection	normal		Dog	Krakowka *et al.*, 1973
	Lymphocyte stimulation	depressed	PHA	Dog	Krakowka *et al.*, 1973
Dengue	Phagocytosis	depressed	SRBC	Human	Wagner *et al.*, 1963
Echovirus 9	Lymphocyte stimulation	depressed	PHA	Human	Willems *et al.*, 1969

TABLE 1. *Modulation of Immunoresponsiveness by Oncogenic and Non-oncogenic Viruses (continued)*

Virus	Response tested	Effect	Antigen	Test animal	References
Encephalomyo-carditis	Interferon levels	depressed		Mouse	Siegel *et al.*, 1969; Stringfellow and Glasgow, 1974
Equine infectious anemia	Immunoglobulin levels	decreased		Horse	Williams *et al.*, 1968
	Lymphocyte number	normal		Horse	Banks and Henson, 1973
	Lymphocyte stimulation	depressed	PHA	Horse	Banks and Henson, 1973
	Lymphocyte stimulation	normal	PWM	Horse	Banks and Henson, 1973
Hepatitis A	Lymphocyte number	depressed		Human	Aiuti *et al.*, 1973
	Lymphocyte number	normal		Human	Aiuti *et al.*, 1973
	Lymphocyte stimulation	depressed	PHA	Human	Mella and Lang, 1967; Willems *et al.*, 1969
Influenza	Lymphocyte number	increased		Mouse	Scott and Walker, 1976
	Delayed hypersensitivity	depressed	SK–SD, tuberc.	Human	Bloomfield and Mateer, 1919; Kantzler *et al.*, 1974
	Lymphocyte stimulation	depressed	PHA	Human, mouse	Kantzler *et al.*, 1974; Kauffman *et al.*, 1976; Olson, 1973; Willems *et al.*, 1969; Kauffman *et al.*, 1974a, 1976
	Lymphocyte stimulation	normal	PHA	Human	Kauffman *et al.*, 1974a, 1976
Junin	Antibody production	depressed	HuRBC	Guinea pig	Oldstone *et al.*, 1974; Parodi *et al.*, 1967
Lactic dehydrogenase	Antibody production	depressed	KLH, GRBC	Mouse	Oldstone *et al.*, 1974
	Antibody production	increased	GRBC, HuGG	Mouse	Notkins *et al.*, 1966; Oldstone *et al.*, 1974
	Gamma globulin levels	increased		Mouse	Oldstone *et al.*, 1974
	Lymphocyte number	depressed		Mouse	Snodgrass *et al.*, 1972
	Lymphocyte trapping	depressed		Mouse	Morgini and Rosenberg, 1976
	Tolerance induction	depressed		Mouse	Mergenhagen *et al.*, 1967
	Allograft rejection	depressed		Mouse	Howard *et al.*, 1969
	GvH	depressed		Mouse	Howard *et al.*, 1969
	Lymphocyte stimulation	normal or increased	PHA, Con A	Mouse	Morgini and Rosenberg, 1976; Olson, 1973
Lymphocytic chloriomeningitis	Antibody production	depressed	SRBC, HSA, BSA, HuGG	Mouse	Bro-Jørgensen *et al.*, 1975; Bro-Jørgensen and Volkert, 1974; Morgini and Rosenberg, 1976
	Antibody production	normal	T-independent	Mouse	Bro-Jørgensen *et al.*, 1975
	Lymphocyte number	depressed		Mouse	Bro-Jørgensen and Volkert, 1974; Hanoka *et al.*, 1969
	Interferon levels	depressed		Mouse	Hoterman and Havell, 1970
	Tolerance induction	depressed	BGG, HGG	Mouse	Pincus *et al.*, 1970

TABLE 1. *Modulation of Immunoresponsiveness by Oncogenic and Non-oncogenic Viruses (continued)*

Virus	Response tested	Effect	Antigen	Test animal	References
M-P virus	Antibody production	depressed or increased	SRBC	Mouse	Padnos *et al.*, 1969
Measles	Lymphocyte number	depressed		Mouse	Molomut *et al.*, 1965
	Antibody production	depressed	DNP	Mouse	McFarland, 1974
	Lymphocyte number	normal		Human	Aiuti *et al.*, 1973
	Delayed hypersensitivity	depressed	Tuberculin	Human	Von Pirquet, 1908
	Migration inhibition	depressed	Measles Ag	Human	Mellman and Wetton, 1963; Starr and Berkovich, 1964; Utermohlen and Zabriskie, 1973
	Lymphocyte stimulation	depressed	PHA	Human	Allen *et al.*, 1973; Sullivan *et al.*, 1975
Mengovirus	Lymphocyte stimulation	depressed	PHA	Mouse	Olson, 1973
Mumps	Delayed hypersensitivity	depressed		Mouse	Hall and Kantor, 1972
	Lymphocyte stimulation	depressed	PHA	Human	Willems *et al.*, 1969
Newcastle disease	Antibody production	depressed	BSA	Rabbit	Medzon and Vas, 1964
	Delayed hypersensitivity	depressed	Sol.Ags.	Rat	McGregor *et al.*, 1976
	Lymphocyte stimulation	depressed	PHA, PPD	Human, guinea pig	Belehu and Olson, 1971; Willems *et al.*, 1969
Poliovirus	Susceptibility-infection	depressed	Listeria	Rat	McGregor *et al.*, 1976
	Lymphocyte number	depressed		Human	Woodruff and Woodruff, 1975a
	Delayed hypersensitivity	depressed	Tuberculin	Human	Notkins *et al.*, 1970
	Lymphocyte stimulation	depressed	PHA	Human	Willems *et al.*, 1969
	Monocyte chemotaxis	normal			Kleinerman *et al.*, 1974
Reovirus	Lymphocyte stimulation	depressed	PHA	Human	Willems *et al.*, 1969
	Monocyte chemotaxis	normal		Human	Kleinerman *et al.*, 1974
Rinderpest	Antibody production	depressed	SRBC, CRBC	Rabbit	Yamanouchi *et al.*, 1974
	Delayed hypersensitivity	depressed	PPD	Rabbit	Yamanouchi *et al.*, 1974
	Lymphocyte stimulation	depressed	PHA	Rabbit	Yamanouchi *et al.*, 1974
	Phagocytosis	normal		Rabbit	Yamanouchi *et al.*, 1974
Rubella	Delayed hypersensitivity	depressed	SK-SD	Human	Kauffman *et al.*, 1974b
	Migration inhibition	depressed		Human	Ganguly *et al.*, 1976
	Lymphocyte stimulation	depressed	PHA	Human	Ganguly *et al.*, 1976; Olson *et al.*, 1968; Vesikari and Buomovici-Klein, 1975
	CMI versus virus	increased	Rubella	Human	Fuccillo *et al.*, 1974
Sandfly fever	Phagocytosis	depressed		Human	Wagner *et al.*, 1963
Sendai	Lymphocyte stimulation	depressed	PHA	Human, mouse	Olson, 1973; Willems *et al.*, 1969
Sinbis	Lymphocyte stimulation	increased	PHA	Human	Willems *et al.*, 1969

TABLE 1. *Modulation of Immunoresponsiveness by Oncogenic and Non-oncogenic Viruses (continued)*

Virus	Response tested	Effect	Antigen	Test animal	References
Vesicular stomatitis	Lymphocyte stimulation	depressed	PHA	Human	Willems *et al.*, 1969
Venezuelan equine encephalitis	Antibody production	increased	BGG, HuGG	Mouse, guinea pig	Craig *et al.*, 1969; Howard *et al.*, 1969

infections. It has already been discussed that suppressor macrophages may be involved in Moloney virus-induced immunosuppression (Kirchner *et al.*, 1974a,b). Direct suppression of macrophage function by viruses has been demonstrated. For example, Wheelock and co-workers found that macrophages from FLV-infected mice are markedly inhibited in their ability to phagocytize sheep RBCs *in vitro* (Wheelock *et al.*, 1974). Old and colleagues earlier showed that FLV-infected mice evince an inhibited carbon clearance rate, at least soon after infection (Old *et al.*, 1960). Gledhill *et al.* (1965) and Notkins (1965) have reported decreased phagocytic activity in mice infected with LDH, ectromielia (mouse pox), LCM and hepatitis viruses. Wagner *et al.* (1963) reported that human macrophages had a depressed phagocytic activity when infected by Dengue or Sandfly fever viruses. Others have reported enhanced phagocytosis in some virus infections (Levy and Wheelock, 1976), yet phagocytosis does not seem critical in determining the ability of a virus-infected animal to form antibodies, since phagocytic function appears normal in animals which show decreased antibody responsiveness. Reduced interferon levels have also been observed in peritoneal exudate cells, rich in macrophages, after EMC virus infection (Stringfellow and Glasgow, 1974). On the other hand, increased microbicidal activity during fowl pox infection indicates the wide varieties of modulation of functional activities which may occur with macrophages from animals infected with different viruses (Pathak *et al.*, 1974).

Macrophage function may be critical in overcoming immunosuppression, even if not the central defect in virus-infected individuals. For example, Bendinelli *et al.* (1975), utilizing the Rowson-Parr virus system, demonstrated *in vitro* that mouse peritoneal exudate cells induced with sterile protease peptone could restore antibody responsiveness of infected splenocytes immunized *in vitro* with sheep erythrocytes. The active cell population responsible for this restoration was shown to be macrophages. Specter *et al.* (1976b), in similar experiments using the FLV leukemia model, also found that peritoneal exudate cells could partially restore antibody responses to SRBC. However, Ceglowski and Friedman (1975) were unable to restore the antibody response to SRBC in FLV-infected mice *in vivo*. While these experiments suggest an important role for macrophages in explaining immunosuppression in some virus infections, they do not resolve the question of the nature and mechanism of immunosuppression *per se*. In LCM infection, decreased antibody formation is not accompanied by a defect in macrophage function (Mims and Wainwright, 1968). Thus, macrophages may be involved only in minor aspects of the complex cellular and molecular interactions involved in immunodepression induced by virus.

CONCLUSIONS

It is now widely recognized that virus infections may result in a wide variety of effects on the immune response system, including alterations of humoral and cellular immunity, as well as macrophage function. By analyzing the nature of immunosuppression resulting from infection by various viruses, both oncogenic and non-oncogenic, it seems evident that more than one mechanism must be involved. While some enlightening information has been obtained concerning possible mechanisms, very little has been established concerning the manner in which viruses actually modulate the immune responses of a host. Much more information must be obtained before a complete understanding of virus-induced immunosuppression will permit development of rational measures that can deal effectively with these phenomena and their consequences. We speculate here that virus induced immunodepressive effects may be important in establishing decreased resistance to superinfection by microbial organisms whether viral, bacterial, fungal, mycotic or parasitic. Interactions between microbial agents possibly through alteration of immune responsiveness are probably required in the etiology of some diseases, especially tumors (e.g. EBV and ? in Burkitt's lymphoma). Furthermore, viruses may interact with or stimulate hormonal factors or other host substances in the presence of depressed immunity to cause neoplasia (MMTV and mammary adenocarcinoma). However, in both these examples a critical role for decreased immunity remains to be proven.

Early events in the immune response system apparently are most affected by virus infections, since immunosuppression often occurs prior to apperance of illness or even malignant cells when oncogenic viruses are studied. In the case of tumor viruses, it is even possible that depressed immune responsiveness may be a prerequisite for progression of transformed neoplastic cells. Virus-induced suppression of the host's defense mechanism may contribute to establishment of a neoplasm. This view is supported by the many observations of an association between immunosuppression and increased incidence of malignancy.

Since cellular immunity is considered an important component of the immune system for controlling virus infection, it seems important to note that the most apparent effects of viral immunosuppression involve T-cell dysfunction. It is now accepted that T-cell activities also include regulation of many B-cell responses, either by helper or suppressor cells, or factors that either enhance or depress humoral immunity. Decreased antibody formation may thus be related to a defect in certain cell classes, possibly as a direct result of virus replication in immunocompetent cells or precursors. Alternatively, immunomodulation may involve the induction or stimulation of suppressor T-lymphocytes or macrophages by virus infection. This could enhance either T- or B-cell responses, even though these cells may not be directly affected by the virus. Furthermore, impairment or elimination of suppressor cells during infection with a virus may result in enhanced antibody formation, as noted with the LDH system. More importantly, alteration of control mechanisms by suppressor cells could also be the cause of excessive lymphoid cell malignancies in immunosuppressed individuals. In addition to possible direct effects of virus on lymphoid cells involved in immunity or cells controlling immune response, it is possible that completely indirect mechanisms may be involved. Since viruses may rapidly replicate and shed either non-infectious virus or virus-associated antigens into the circulation, it is conceivable that antibody, complexed with virus or virus products, could result in immunoregulatory factors or antigen–antibody complexes which affect the immune system, either directly or indirectly. In addition, those viruses which replicate preferentially in lymphoid cells would be expected to alter the surface antigenicity of such cells, making them now 'foreign' to the immune system of the host. Thus, as suggested for a number of virus infections, both oncogenic and non-oncogenic, an 'autoimmune'-like response against the virus-infected lymphoid cells could develop, which in turn would depress immune responsiveness, both to virus specific and nonspecific antigens. It seems clear that there are a number of possible mechanisms involved in immunomodulation by viruses and virus products. An understanding of those mechanisms, especially of oncogenic viruses, may be necessary to permit development of methods for controlling not only the virus infection, but also its untoward consequences. Prevention of the malignancies caused by viruses, perhaps in man as well as animals, may be aided by understanding how to control immunomodulation. While altered immunologic functions have been recorded with a plethora of viruses, little is known concerning the role of immune suppression in the primary virus infection. Whether this dysfunction participates in the pathogenesis of various viruses remains to be studied. Since several virus infections (e.g. lymphocytic choriomeningitis virus, hepatitis viruses, dengue hemorrhagic fever) are dependent upon immunologic processes for pathogenesis, immunodepression may moderate formation of immune complexes, etc., which could precipitate more severe disease.

SUMMARY

The nature and mechanisms by which virus infection depresses the immune response are the focus of much attention in experimental and clinical immunology, virology and oncology. It has been widely recognized since early studies with measles virus that infection with certain viruses may depress immunoresponsiveness in a nonspecific manner. However, such virus-induced immunomodulation, especially immunosuppression, is not completely understood. It seems evident that a wide variety of viruses, both oncogenic and non-oncogenic, may affect the immune response system in either a negative or positive manner. *In vivo* infections may alter the expected humoral or cellular immune response, or both, although some viruses affect neither type of response. *In vitro* model systems have been quite useful in recent years for examining the possible mechanisms whereby viruses affect immune responsiveness. Certain viruses appear to preferentially affect B-lymphocytes and their precursors, whereas others affect T-lymphocyte number, function and activity. On the other hand, some viruses preferentially affect macrophages, and thus indirectly modulate the immune response of T- or B-cells. Although the oncogenic RNA viruses, especially those which cause murine leukemia, have been studied in greatest detail for their mechanism of immunosuppression, a wide variety of non-oncogenic RNA and DNA viruses also modulate immune responses, especially *in vitro*. The blastogenic response of lymphoid cells to PHA has been used as a model system in which to investigate how viruses affect T-lymphocytes, while the immune response *in vitro* to sheep erythrocytes, measured by hemolytic plaque formation, has also provided valuable information concerning the effects of viruses on B-cells and their precursors. The influence of virus infections on macrophage function, both *in vivo* and *in vitro*, including phagocytic activity and antigen uptake, has provided information concerning the role of macrophages in virus-induced immunosuppression. However, it is evident that much more information is needed, concerning not only the actual cellular and subcellular mechanisms of virus-induced immunomodulation, but also the significance of such effects on the normal immune expression of an individual, in relation to susceptibility to microbial infection and tumorigenesis.

REFERENCES

AIUTI, F., CIARLA, M. V., D'ASERO, C., D'AMELIO, R. and GAROFALO, J. A. (1973) Surface markers on lymphocytes of patients with infectious diseases. *Inf. Immun.* **8**: 110–117.

ALLEN, J., OPPENHEIM, J., BRODY, J. B. and MILLER, J. (1973) Labile inhibitor of lymphocyte transformation in plasma from a patient with subacute sclerosing panencephalitis. *Inf. Immun.* **8**: 80–82.

ALLISON, A. C. (1970) On the role of macrophages in some pathologic processes. In: *Mononuclear Phagocytes*, pp. 422–444, VAN FURTH, R. (ed). Davis, Philadelphia.

ALM, G. V., SICCARDI, F. J. and PETERSON, R. D. A. (1972) Impairment of the lymphocyte response to phytohemagglutinin in chickens with Marek's disease. *Acta path. microbiol. Scand.* **80**: 109–114.

BANKS, K. L. and HENSON, J. B. (1973) Quantitation of immunoglobulin bearing lymphocytes and lymphocyte response to mitogens in horses persistently infected by Equine infectious anemia virus. *Inf. Immun.* **8**: 679–682.

BELEHU, A. and OLSON, G. B. (1971) Viral-induced unresponsiveness of tuberculin-sensitized guinea pig lymphocytes. *Proc. Soc. exp. Biol. Med.* **136**: 824–829.

BELADI, I., PUSZTAI, R., MUCSI, I., BAKAY, M. and BAJSZAI, G. (1973) Effect of human Adenoviruses on the response of chickens to sheep erythrocytes. *Inf. Immun.* **7**: 22–28.

BENDINELLI, M. and BAINBRIDGE, D. R. (1968) The effect of Friend virus infection on the distribution of infected lymphoid cells. *Rep. Br. Emp. Cancer Campn* **45**: 137.

BENDINELLI, M. and FRIEDMAN, H. (1976) Lymphocyte surface markers and Ig capping responses of spleen and lymph node cells in Rowson-Parr virus infected mice. *Inf. Immun.* **14**: 613–617.

BENDINELLI, M., KAPLAN, G. S. and FRIEDMAN, H. (1975) Reversal of leukemia virus induced immunosuppression *in vitro*: role of peritoneal exudate macrophages. *J. natn. Cancer Inst.* **55**: 1425–1432.

BENDINELLI, M. and NARDINI, L. (1973) Immunodepression by Rowson-Parr virus in mice. II. Effect of Rowson-Parr virus infection on the antibody response to sheep red blood cells *in vivo* and *in vitro*. *Inf. Immun.* **7**: 160–166.

BENNET, M. and STEEVES, R. A. (1970) Immunocompetent cell functions in mice infected with Friend leukemia virus. *J. natn. Cancer Inst.* **44**: 1107–1109.

BIGGS, P. M., LONG, P. L., KENZY, S. G. and ROOTES, D. G. (1968) Relationship between Marek's disease and coccidiosis. II. The eeffect of Marek's disease on the susceptibility of chickens to coccidiodal infection. *Vet. Res.* **83**: 284–289.

BLAIR, P. B., KRIPKA, M. L., LAPPE, M. A., BONHAG, R. S. and YOUNG, L. (1971) Immunologic deficiency associated with mammary tumor virus (MTV) infection in mice: hemagglutinin response and allograft survival. *J. Immun.* **106**: 364–370.

BLOOMFIELD, A. L. and MATEER, J. G. (1919) Changes to skin sensitivieness to tuberculin during epidemic influenza. *Am. Rev. Tuberc. pulm. Dis.* **3**: 166–168.

BONNARD, G. D., MANDERS, E. K., CAMPBELL, M. J., JR, HERBERMAN, R. B. and COLLINS, M. J., JR (1976) Immunosuppressive activity of a subline of the mouse EL-4 lymphoma. Evidence for minute virus of mice causing the inhibition. *J. exp. Med.* **143**: 187–205.

BORELLA, L. (1969) The suppressive effect of Rauscher leukemia virus on the secondary antibody response of spleen cells cultured in cell-impermeable diffusion chambers. *J. Immun.* **103**: 185–195.

BORELLA, L. (1971) The immunosuppressive effects of Rauscher leukemia virus upon spleen cells cultured in cell-impermeable diffusion chambers. II. Effects upon IgM and IgG immunologic memory and on response to phytohemagglutinin and stimulation with allogeneic cells. *J. Immun.* **107**: 464–475.

BORELLA, L. (1972) The immunosuppressive effect of Raucher leukemia virus (RLV) upon spleen cell cultures in cell-impermeable diffusion chambers. III. Inhibition of RLV-induced cell pathways by antigenic stimulation with hemocyanin. *J. Immun.* **108**: 45–53.

BRO-JØRGENSEN, K., GUTTLER, F., JØRGENSEN, P. and VOLKERT, M. (1975) T-lymphocyte function as the principal target of Lymphocytic choriomeningitis virus-induced immunosuppression. *Inf. Immun.* **11**: 622–629.

BRO-JØRGENSEN, K. and VOLKERT, M. (1974) Defects in the immune system of mice infected with Lymphocytic choriomeningitis virus. *Inf. Immun.* **9**: 605–614.

BURG, R. W., FELDBUSH, T., MORRIS, C. A. and MAAG, T. A. (1971) Depression of thymus and bursa-dependent immune systems of chicks with Marek's disease. *Avian Dis.* **15**: 662–671.

CARTER, R. L., CHESTERMAN, F. C., ROWSON, K. E. K., SALAMAN, M. H. and WEDDERBURN, N. (1970) A new virus of minimal pathogenicity associated with Friend virus. II. Histological changes and immunodepressive effect. *Int. J. Cancer* **5**: 103–110.

CEGLOWSKI, W. S. (1976) Effect of leukemia virus infections on antibody formation and cellular immunity. *Ann. N.Y. Acad. Sci.* **276**: 411–416.

CEGLOWSKI, W. S., CAMPBELL, B. P. and FRIEDMAN, H. (1972) Immunosuppression by leukemia viruses. XI. Effect of Friend leukemia virus on humoral immune competence of leukemic resistant C57Bl/6 mice. *J. Immun.* **114**: 231–236.

CEGLOWSKI, W. S. and FRIEDMAN, H. (1967) Suppression of the primary antibody plaque response of mice following infection with Friend disease virus. *Proc. Soc. exp. Biol. Med.* **126**: 662–666.

CEGLOWSKI, W. S. and FRIEDMAN, H. (1968a) Immunosuppressive effects of Friend and Rauscher leukemia disease viruses on cellular and humoral antibody formation. *J. natn. Cancer Inst.* **40**: 983–995.

CEGLOWSKI, W. S. and FRIEDMAN, H. (1968b) Immunosuppression by leukemia viruses. I. Effect of Friend disease virus on cellular and humoral hemolysin response of mice to a primary immunization with sheep erythrocytes. *J. Immun.* **101**: 594–604.

CEGLOWSKI, W. S. and FRIEDMAN, H. (1969a) Immunosuppression by leukemia viruses. II. Cytokinetics of appearance of hemolysin-forming cells in infected mice during the anamnestic response to sheep erythrocytes. *J. Immun.* **102**: 338–346.

CEGLOWSKI, W. S. and FRIEDMAN, H. (1969b) Immunosuppression by leukemia viruses. III. Adoptive transfer of antibody-forming cells to Friend disease virus infected mice. *J. Immun.* **103**: 460–466.

CEGLOWSKI, W. S. and FRIEDMAN, H. (1969c) Murine virus leukemogenesis. Relationship between susceptibility and immunodepression. *Nature* **224**: 1318–1319.

CEGLOWSKI, W. S. and FRIEDMAN, H. (1970) Immunosuppression by leukemia viruses. IV. Effect of Friend leukemia virus on antibody precursors as assessed by cell transfer studies. *J. Immun.* **105**: 1406–1415.

CEGLOWKSI, W. S. and FRIEDMAN, H. (1975) Failure of peritoneal exudate macrophages to reverse immunologic impairment induced by Friend leukemia virus. *Proc. Soc. exp. Biol. Med.* **148**: 808–811.

CEGLOWKSI, W. S., LABADIE, G. U. and MASCIO, A. A. (1976) Effects of leukemia viruses on cellular immune responses. In: *Tumor Virus Infections and Immunity*, pp. 165–173, CROWELL, R. L., FRIEDMAN, H. and PRIER, J. (eds). University Park Press, Baltimore.

CERNY, J., MCALACK, R. F., CEGLOWSKI, W. S. and FRIEDMAN, H. (1971) Divergence between immunosuppression and immunocompetence during virus-induced leukemia. *Proc. natn. Acad. Sci. U.S.A.* **68**: 1862–1865.

CERNY, J. and STILLER, R. A. (1975) Immunosuppression by spleen cells from Moloney leukemia: comparison of the suppressive effect on antibody response and on mitogen induced response. *J. Immun.* **115**: 943–949.

CERNY, J. and WANER, E. B. (1975) Specific susceptibility of sensitized (memory) B cells to suppression and antigenic alteration by murine leukemia virus. *J. Immun.* **114**: 571–580.

CHAKRABARTY, A. K., FRIEDMAN, H. and CEGLOWSKI, W. S. (1970) Biochemical aspects of leukemia virus-induced immunosuppression. Effect of Friend disease virus on spleen nucleases and nucleic acids. *Cancer Res.* **30**: 617–624.

CHAN, G., RANCOURT, M. W., CEGLOWSKI, W. S. and FRIEDMAN, H. (1968) Leukemia virus suppression of antibody-forming cells: ultrastructure of infected spleens. *Science* **159**: 437–439.

CHAN, S. P., HOOK, W. A., TURNER, N. and CHIRIGOS, M. A. (1970) Immunosuppression by murine sarcoma virus (Moloney). *Inf. Immun.* **1**: 288–292.

CHING, C. and LOPEZ, C. (1979) Natural killing of herpes simplex virus type 1-infected target cells: Normal human responses and influence of antiviral antibody. *Infect. Immun.* **26**: 49–56.

CHIRIGOS, M. A., PERK, K., TURNER, W., BURKA, B. and GOMEZ, M. (1968) Increased oncogenicity of the murine sarcoma virus (Moloney) by coinfection with murine leukemia virus. *Cancer Res.* **28**: 1055–1063.

COOPER, M. D., GABRIELSEN, A. E. and GOOD, R. A. (1967) Role of the thymus and other central lymphoid tissues in immunological disease. *Ann. Rev. Med.* **18**: 113–138.

COOPER, M. D. and LAWTON, A. R., III (1974) The development of the immune system. *Sci. Am.* **231**: 58–70.

COOPER, M. D., PURCHASE, H. G., BOCKMAN, D. E. and Gathings, W. E. (1974) Studies on the nature of the abnormality of B-cell differentiation in avain lymphoid leukosis. Production of heterogeneous IgM by tumor cells. *J. Immun.* **113**: 1210–1222.

COHEN, P. L., CROSS, S. S. and MOSIER, D. E. (1975) Immunologic effects of neonatal infection with mouse thymic virus. *J. Immun.* **115**: 706–710.

CRAIG, C. P., REYNOLDS, S. L., AIRHART, J. W. and STAAB, E. V. (1969) Alteration in immune responses by attenuated Venezuelan equine encephalitis vaccine. I. Adjuvant effect of VEE virus infection in guinea pigs. *J. Immun.* **102**: 1220–1227.

CREMER, N. E. (1967) Selective immunoglobulin deficiencies in rats infected with Moloney virus. *J. Immun.* **99**: 71–81.

CREMER, N. E., TAYLOR, D. O. N. and LENNETTE, E. H. (1966) Antibody formation, latency and leukemia: infection with Moloney virus. *J. Immun.* **96**: 495–508.

CREMER, N. E., TAYLOR, D. O. N. and LENNETTE, E. H. (1969) Localization of immunoglobulin and viral antigen in rats infected with Moloney virus. *J. natn. Cancer Inst.* **42**: 695–705.
CREMER, N. E., TAYLOR, D. O. N., LENNETTE, E. H. and HAGENS, S. J. (1973) IgM production in rats infected with Moloney leukemia virus. *J. natn. Cancer Inst.* **51**: 905–915.
CURE, S. F. and CREMER, N. E. (1969) Decreased rate of synthesis of immunoglobulin (IgG) in rats infected with Moloney leukemia virus. *J. Immun.* **102**: 1345–1353.
DAVIDSON, I. and STERN, K. (1954) Heterhemoantibodies in inbred strains of mice. II. Immune agglutinins and hemolysins for sheep and chicken red cells. *J. Immun.* **72**: 216–223.
DEMAEYER-GUIGNARD, J. (1972) Mouse leukemia: depression of serum interferon production. *Science* **177**: 797–799.
DENT, P. B. (1972) Immunodepression by oncogenic viruses. *Prog. med. Virol.* **14**: 1–35.
DENT, P. B. (1975) Immunodepression by oncogenic viruses. In: *The Immune System and Infectious Diseases*, 4th Int. Convoc. Immunol., Buffalo, N.Y., pp. 95–107. Karger, Basel.
DENT, P. B., COOPER, M. D., PAYNE, L. N., SOLOMON, J. J., BURMESTER, B. R. and GOOD, R. A. (1968) Pathogenesis of avian lymphoid leukosis. II. Immunologic activity during lymphogenesis. *J. natn. Cancer Inst.* **41**: 391–401.
DENT, P. B., PETERSON, R. D. A. and GOOD, R. A. (1965) A defect in cellular immunity during the incubation period of passage A leukemia in C_3H mice. *Proc. Soc. exp. Biol. Med.* **119**: 869–871.
DEODHAR, S. D. and CHIANG, T. (1970) Immunosuppression with Friend virus in allogeneic murine tumor system. *Fedn Proc.* **29**: 560.
DOELL, R. G., DEVAUX ST. CYR, C. and GRABAR, P. (1967) Immune reaction prior to development of thymic lymphoma in C57BL mice. *Int. J. Cancer* **2**: 103–108.
DORE, J. F., SCHNEIDER, M. and MATHE, G. (1969) Reactions immunitaires chez les souris AKR leucemique ou preleucemique. *Revue fr. Etud. clin. biol.* **14**: 1003–1007.
DRACOTT, B. N., WEDDERBURN, N. and SALAMAN, M. H. (1972) *In vitro* immune responses of spleen cells from Friend virus infected mice. *J. gen. Virol.* **14**: 77–86.
ECKNER, R. J. (1975) Continuous replication of Friend virus complex (spleen focus forming virus-lymphatic leukemia inducing virus) in mouse embryo fibroblasts. Retention of leukemogenicity and loss of immunosuppressive properties. *J. exp. Med.* **142**: 936–948.
ELLMAN, L., GREEN, I. and MARTEN, W. J. (1970) Histocompatibility genes, immune responsiveness and leukemia. *Lancet* **i**: 1104–1106.
EVANS, D. L. and PATTERSON, L. T. (1971) Correlation of immunologic responsiveness with lymphocyte changes in chickens infected with Marek's disease. *Inf. Immun.* **4**: 567–574.
EVANS, D. L. and PATTERSON, L. T. (1972) Changes in serum proteins associated with the immunosuppressive effects of acute leukosis (Marek's disease). *J. Ret. End. Soc.* **11**: 325–342.
FARBER, P., SPECTER, S. and FRIEDMAN, H. (1975) Leukemia virus induced immunosuppression. Scanning electron microscopy of infected spleen cells. *Science* **160**: 467–471.
FLICKINGER, J. T. and GENTILE, J. M. (1970) Effects of Friend leukemia virus on the immune response of mice to bacterial antigens. *Can. J. Microbiol.* **16**: 741–745.
FREY-WETTSTEIN and HAYS, E. F. (1970) Immune response in preleukemic mice. *Inf. Immun.* **2**: 398–403.
FRIEDMAN, H. (1975a) Effects of Friend leukemia virus on cells of the immune system. In: *Immunological Parameters of Host-Tumor Relationships*, Vol. 3, pp. 238–251, WEISS, D. (ed). Academic Press, N.Y.
FRIEDMAN, H. (1975b) Immunosuppression by murine leukemia viruses. In: *Viruses and Immunity*, pp. 27–47, KOPROWSKI, H. (ed). Academic Press, New York.
FRIEDMAN, H. and CEGLOWSKI, W. S. (1968) Cellular basis for the immunosuppressive properties of a leukemogenic virus. *Nature* **218**: 1232–1234.
FRIEDMAN, H. and CEGLOWSKI, W. S. (1971a) Defect in cellular immunity of leukemia virus infected mice assessed by a macrophage migration inhibition assay. *Proc. Soc. exp. Biol. Med.* **136**: 154–158.
FRIEDMAN, H. and CEGLOWSKI, W. S. (1971b) Immunosuppression by leukemia viruses. VIII. Rapid depression of an *in vitro* leukocyte migration after infection of mice with Friend leukemia virus. *J. Immun.* **107**: 1673–1679.
FRIEDMAN, H. and CEGLOWSKI, W. S. (1974) Virus tumorigenesis and immunity: influence of immunostimulation and immunodepression. In: *The Role of Immunologic Factors in Viral and Oncogenic Processes*, pp. 187–210, BEERS, R. F., TILGHMAN, R. C. and BASSET, E. G. (eds). Johns Hopkins University Press, Baltimore.
FRIEDMAN, H. and KATELEY, J. R. (1975). Lymphocyte surface receptors and leukemia virus-induced immunosuppression. *Am. J. clin. Path.* **63**: 735–747.
FRIEDMAN, H. and GOLDNER, H. (1970a) Effect of a DNA tumor virus on antibody forming cells in neonatally infected hamsters. *Nature* **225**: 455–456.
FRIEDMAN, H. and GOLDNER, H. (1970b) Relationship between immunologic maturity and viral oncogenesis in hamsters. *J. natn. Cancer Inst.* **44**: 809–817.
FRIEDMAN, H., MELNICK, H., MILLS, L. and CEGLOWSKI, W. S. (1973) Depressed allograft immunity in leukemia virus infected mice. *Transp. Proc.* **5**: 981–986.
FUCCILLO, D. A., STEELE, R. W., HENSEN, S. A., VINCENT, M. M., HARDY, J. B. and BELLANTI, J. A. (1974) Impaired cellular immunity to Rubella virus in congenital rubella. *Inf. Immun.* **9**: 81–84.
GANGULY, R., CUSUMANO, C. L. and WALDMAN, R. H. (1976) Suppression of cell-mediated immunity after infection with attenuated rubella virus. *Inf. Immun.* **13**: 464–469.
GELZER, J. and DIETRICH, F. M. (1968) Haemagglutinin production in tumor-bearing and leukemic mice. *Int. J. Cancer* **31**: 51–60.
GLEDHILL, A. W. (1961) Enhancement of the pathogenicity of mouse hepatitis virus (MHV) by prior infection of mice with certain leukemia agents. *Br. J. Cancer* **15**: 531–538.
GLEDHILL, A. W., BILBEY, D. L. J. and NIVEN, J. S. F. (1965) Effects of certain murine pathogens on phagocytic activity. *Br. J. exp. Path.* **46**: 433–442.
GORCZYNSKI, R. M. (1974) Immunity to murine sarcoma virus induced tumors. II. Suppression of T-cell mediated immunity by cells from progressor animals. *J. Immun.* **112**: 1826–1838.

GOTTLIEB, C. F., PERKINS, E. H. and MAKINODAN, T. (1972) Genetic regulation of the thymus dependent humoral immune response in leukemia prone AKR (H-2^k) and non-leukemia C_3H (H-2^k) mice. Description of the genetic control of the immune response at the level of proliferation. *J. Immun.* **109**: 974–981.

GRISWOLD, D. E., HEPPNER, G. H. and CALABRESI, P. (1973) Alteration of immunocompetence by mammary tumor virus. *J. natn. Cancer Inst.* **50**: 1035–1038.

GROSS, L. (1970) *Oncogenic Viruses* (2nd edn). Pergamon Press, London.

HALL, C. B. and KANTOR, F. S. (1972) Depression of established delayed hypersensitivity by Mumps virus. *J. Immun.* **108**: 81–85.

HAMBURG, V. P., SCHERBAKONA, O. E. and SVET-MOLDOVSKY, G. J. (1970) Suppression of antibody formation against Sendai virus in the SV_{40} and Adenovirus 16 infected hamsters. *Experientia* **26**: 532–534.

HANAOKA, M., ZUZUKI, S. and HOTCHIN, J. (1969) Thymus dependent lymphocytes: destruction by lymphocytic choriomeningitis virus. *Science* **163**: 1216–1219.

HARAN-GHERA, N., CHAZAN, R. and BEN-YAAKOV, M. (1976) Spontaneous and induced changes in thymus pattern. In: *Immune Reactivity of Lymphocytes*, pp. 135–140, FELDMAN, M. and GLOBERSON, A. (eds). Plenum Press, New York.

HARGIS, B. J. and MALKIEL, S. (1970) The immunocapacity of the AKR mouse. *Fedn Proc.* **29**: 825.

HAYRY, P., RAGO, D. and DEFENDI, V. (1970) Inhibition of phytohemagglutinin and alloantigen induced lymphocyte stimulation by Rauscher leukemia virus. *J. natn. Cancer Inst.* **44**: 1311–1319.

HERBERMAN, R. B. and HOLDEN, H. T. (1978) Natural cell mediated immunity. *Adv. Cancer Res.* **27:** 305.

HERBERMAN, R. B., HOLDEN, H. T., VARESIO, L., TANIYAMA, T., PUCCETTI, P., KIRCHNER, H., GERSON, J., WHITE, S., KEISARI, Y. and HASKILL, J. S. (1980) Immunologic reactivity of lymphoid cells in tumors. *Contemp. Topics in Immunobiol.* **10:** 61–78.

HIRANO, S., CEGLOWSKI, W. S., ALLEN, J. L. and FRIEDMAN, H. (1969) Effect of Friend leukemia virus on antibody forming cells to a bacterial somatic antigen. *J. natn. Cancer Inst.* **43**: 1337–1345.

HIRANO, S., FRIEDMAN, H. and CEGLOWSKI, W. S. (1971) Immunosuppression by leukemia viruses. VII. Stimulatory effects of Friend leukemia virus on pre-existing antibody forming cells to sheep erythrocytes and *E. coli* in non-immunized mice. *J. Immun.* **107**: 1400–1409.

HOTERMAN, O. A. and HAVELL, E. A. (1970) Reduced interferon response in mice congenitally infected with Lymphocytic choriomeningitis virus. *J. gen. Virol.* **9**: 101–103.

HOWARD, E. B., JANNKI, C., VICKERS, J. and KENYON, A. J. (1967) Elevated γ-globulin levels in Marek's disease (neural lymphatosis) of domestic fowl. *Cornell Vet.* **57**: 183–194.

HOWARD, R. J., CRAIG, C. P., TREVINO, G. S., DOUGHERTY, S. F. and MERGENHAGEN, S. E. (1969) Enhanced humoral immunity in mice infected with attenuated Venezuelan equine encephalitis virus. *J. Immun.* **103**: 699–707.

HOWARD, R. J., MILLER, J. and NAJARIAN, J. S. (1974) Cytomegalovirus induced immune suppression. II. Cellular immunity. *Clin. Exp. Immun.* **18**: 119–126.

HOWARD, R. J. and NAJARIAN, J. S. (1974) Cytomegalovirus induced immune suppression. I. Humoral immunity. *Clin. Exp. Immun.* **18**: 109–111.

HOWARD, R. J., NOTKINS, A. L. and MERGENHAGEN, S. E. (1969) Inhibition of cellular immune reactions in mice infected with Lactic dehydrogenase virus. *Nature* **221**: 873–874.

ISRAEL, E. and WAINBERG, M. A. (1981) Viral inhibition of lymphocyte mitogenesis. The role of macrophages as primary targets of virus-cell interactions. *J. Ret. Endo. Soc.* **29:** 105–116.

JAKOWSKI, R. M., FREDRICKSON, T. N. and LUGINBUHL, R. E. (1973) Immunoglobulin response in experimental infection with cell-free and cell-associated Marek's disease virus. *J. Immun.* **111**: 238–248.

JERNE, N. K., NORDIN, A. A. and HENRY, C. (1963) The agar plaque technique for recognizing antibody producing cells. In: *Cell Bound Antibodies*, pp. 109–131, AMOS, B. and KOPROWSKI, H. (eds). Wistar Institute Press, Philadelphia.

JOSEPH, B. S. and OLDSTONE, M. B. A. (1975) Immunologic injury in Measles virus infection. II. Suppression of immune injury through antigenic modulation. *J. exp. Med.* **142**: 864–876.

KAMO, I., KATELEY, J. R., KAPLAN, G. and FRIEDMAN, H. (1975) Immunosuppression *in vitro* induced by leukemia virus infected splenocytes. *Proc. Soc. exp. Biol. Med.* **148**: 383–386.

KANTZLER, G. B., LAUTERIA, S. F., CUSUMANO, C. L., LEE, J. D., GANGULY and WALDMAN, R. H. (1974) Immunosuppression during Influenza virus infection. *Inf. Immun.* **10**: 996–1002.

KATELEY, J. R. and FRIEDMAN, H. (1976) Impairment of B lymphocyte functions in Concanavalin A-treated Friend virus infected mice. *Ann. N. Y. Acad. Sci.* **276:** 466–478.

KATELEY, J. R., HOLDERBACH, J. and FRIEDMAN, H. (1974a) Leukemia virus induced alteration of lymphocyte Ig surface receptors and the 'capping' response of mouse spleen and lymph node cells. *J. natn. Cancer Inst.* **53**: 1135–1141.

KATELEY, J. R., KAMO, I., KAPLAN, G. and FRIEDMAN, H. (1974b) Suppressive effect of leukemia virus-infected lymphoid cells on *in vitro* immunization of normal splenocytes. *J. natn. Cancer Inst.* **53**: 1371–1378.

KATZ, D. H. and BENACERRAF, B. (1972) The regulatory influence of activated T cells on B cell responses to antigen. *Adv. Immun.* **15**: 1–94.

KAY, H. D., BONNARD, G. D., WEST, W. H. and HERBERMAN, R. B. (1977) A functional comparison of human Fc-receptor bearing lymphocytes active in natural cytotoxicity and antibody dependent cellular cytotoxicity. *J. Immunol.* **118:** 2058–206.

KAUFFMAN, C. A., LINNEMANN, C. C., JR, SCHIFF, G. M. and PHAIR, J. P. (1976) Effect of viral and bacterial pneumonias on cell mediated immunity in humans. *Inf. Immun.* **13**: 78–83.

KAUFFMAN, C. A., LINNEMANN, C. C., JR, TAN, J. S., SCHIFF, G. M. and PHAIR, J. P. (1974a) Cell-mediated immunity in humans during viral infection: dermal hypersensitivity and *in vitro* lymphocyte proliferation during mild viral respiratory infections. *Inf. Immun.* **10**: 757–761.

KAUFFMAN, C. A., PHAIR, J. P., LINNEMANN, C. C., JR and SCHIFF, G. M. (1974b) Cell-mediated immunity in humans during viral infection. I. Effect of Rubella on dermal hypersensitivity, phytohemagglutinin response, and T lymphocyte numbers. *Inf. Immun.* **10**: 212–215.

KENYON, A. J. (1966) Immunologic deficiency in Aleutian mink disease. *Am. J. vet. Res.* **27**: 1780–1782.
KIRCHNER, H., CHUSED, T. M., HERBERMAN, R. B., HOLDEN, H. T. and LARVIN, H. (1974a) Evidence of suppressor cell activity in spleens of mice bearing primary tumors induced by Moloney sarcoma virus. *J. exp. Med.* **139**: 1473–1487.
KIRCHNER, H., HERBERMAN, R. B., GLASER, M. and LARVIN, H. (1974b) Suppression of *in vitro* lymphocyte stimulation in mice bearing primary Moloney sarcoma virus-induced tumors. *Cell. Immun.* **13**: 32–40.
KLEINERMAN, E. S., SNYDERMAN, R. and DANIELS, C. A. (1974) Depression of human monocyte chemotaxis by Herpes simplex and Influenza viruses. *J. Immun.* **113**: 1562–1567.
KOO, G. C., CEGLOWSKI, W. S. and FRIEDMAN, H. (1971a) Immunosuppression by leukemia viruses. V. Ultrastructural studies of antibody forming spleens of mice infected with Friend leukemia virus. *J. Immun.* **106**: 799–814.
KOO, G. C., CEGLOWSKI, W. S., HIGGINS, M. and FRIEDMAN, H. (1971b) Immunosuppression by leukemia viruses. VI. Ultrastructure of individual antibody-forming cells in the spleens of Friend leukemia virus-infected mice. *J. Immun.* **106**: 815–830.
KRAKOWKA, S., COCKERELL, G. and KOESTNER, A. (1975) Effects of Canine distemper virus infection on lymphoid function *in vitro* and *in vivo*. *Inf. Immun.* **11**: 1069–1078.
KRAKOWKA, S., MCCULLOUGH, B., KOESTNER, A. and OLSEN, R. (1973) Myelin-specific autoantibodies associated with central nervous system demyelination in Canine distemper virus. *Inf. Immun.* **8**: 819–827.
Letter to the Editor (1974) Erroneous interpretation of valid experimental observations through interference by the LDH virus. *J. natn. Cancer Inst.* **52**: 1673–1676.
LEVY, M. H. and WHEELOCK, E. F. (1976) The role of macrophages in suppression of established Friend virus leukemia. *J. Ret. End. Soc.* **20**: 243–254.
LODMELL, D. L., BERGMAN, R. K. and HADLOW, W. J. (1973) Antibody-forming cells and hemolysin responses of Pastel and Sapphire mink inoculated with Aleutian disease virus. *Inf. Immun.* **8**: 769–774.
LODMELL, D. L., MUNOZ, J. J., HADLOW, W. J. and WHITFORD, H. W. (1970) Hemagglutinin antibody response of normal and Aleutian disease-affected mink to keyhole limpet hemocyanin. *J. Immun.* **104**: 878–888.
LOH, L. and HUDSON, J. B. (1981) Murine cytomegalovirus infection in the spleen and its relationship to immunosuppression. *Infect. Immun.* **32**: 1067–1072.
MCFARLAND, H. F. (1974) The effect of Measles virus infection on T and B lymphocytes in the mouse. I. Suppression of helper cell activity. *J. Immun.* **113**: 1978–1983.
MCGREGOR, D. D., LOGIE, P. S. and CARMICHAEL, L. E. (1976) The mediator of cellular immunity. XII. Inhibition of activated T cells by Newcastle disease virus. *J. exp. Med.* **144**: 627–643.
MCLAREN, C., CHENG, H., SPICER, D. L. and TOMPKINS, W. A. F. (1976) Lymphocyte and macrophage responses after Vaccinia virus infection. *Inf. Immun.* **14**: 1416–1421.
MARBROOK, J. (1967) Primary immune response *in vitro* of spleen cells. *Lancet* **ii**: 1279–1281.
MASCIO, A. A. and CEGLOWSKI, W. S. (1975) Friend leukemia virus induced suppression of lymphocyte mediated cytotoxicity. *Fedn Proc.* **34**: 973.
MEDZON, E. L. and VAS, S. F. (1964) Studies on *in vitro* antibody production. II. The effect of Newcastle disease virus on antibody synthesis. *Can. J. Microbiol.* **10**: 535–541.
MELLA, B. and LANG, D. J. (1967) Leukocyte mitosis: suppression *in vitro* associated with acute infectious Hepatitis. *Science* **155**: 80–81.
MELLMAN, W. J. and WETTON, R. (1963) Depression of the tuberculin reaction by attenuated Measles virus vaccine. *J. Lab. clin. Med.* **61**: 453–458.
MERGENHAGEN, S. E., NOTKINS, A. L. and DOUGHERTY, S. F. (1967) Adjuvanticity of Lactic dehydrogenase virus: influence of virus infection on the establishment of immunologic tolerance to a protein antigen in adult mice. *J. Immun.* **99**: 576–581.
METCALF, D. and MOULDS, R. (1967) Immune responses in pre-leukemic and leukemic AKR mice. *Int. J. Cancer* **2**: 53–58.
MILLIAN, S. J. and SCHAEFFER, M. (1968) Antibody production by mice infected with selected murine oncogenic agents. *Cancer* **21**: 989–999.
MIMS, C. A. (1964) Aspects of the pathogenesis of viral diseases. *Bact. Rev.* **28**: 30–64.
MIMS, C. A. and WAINWRIGHT, S. (1968) The immunodepressive action of Lymphocytic choriomeningitis virus in mice. *J. Immun.* **101**: 717–724.
MINATO, N., REID, L., CANTOR, H., LENGYEL, P. and BLOOM, B. R. (1980) Mode of regulation of natural killer cell activity by interferon. *J. Exp. Med.* **152**: 124–137.
MOLOMUT, N., PADNOS, M. and SMITH, L. W. (1965) A lymphopenic filterable agent derived from tissue cell cultures of murine carcinoma. *J. natn. Cancer Inst.* **34**: 403–413.
MORGINI, P. K. A. and ROSENBERG, L. T. (1976) Inhibition of lymphocyte trapping by a passenger virus in murine ascitic tumors: characterization of lactic dehydrogenase virus (LDV) inhibitory component and analysis of the mechanism of inhibition. *J. exp. Med.* **143**: 100–113.
MORSE, H. C., III, CROSS, S. S. and BACKER, P. J. (1976) Neonatal infection with mouse thymic virus: effects on cells regulating the antibody response of type III pneumococcal polysaccharide. *J. Immun.* **116**: 1613–1617.
MORTENSEN, R. F., CEGLOWKSI, W. S. and FRIEDMAN, H. (1973a) Leukemia virus induced immunosuppression. IX. Depression of delayed hypersensitivity and MIF production after infection of mice with Friend leukemia virus. *J. Immun.* **111**: 1810–1819.
MORTENSEN, R. F., GEGLOWSKI, W. S. and FRIEDMAN, H. (1973b) Leukemia virus induced immunosuppression. X. Depression of T cell-mediated cytotoxicity after infection of mice with Friend leukemia virus. *J. Immun.* **112**: 2077–2086.
NOTKINS, A. L. (1965) Lactic dehydrogenase virus. *Bact. Rev.* **29**: 143–160.
NOTKINS, A. L., MERGENHAGEN, S. E., RIZZO, A. A., SCHEELE, C. and WALDMAN, T. A. (1966) Elevated γ-globulin and increased antibody production in mice infected with lactic dehydrogenase virus. *J. exp. Med.* **123**: 347–364.

NOTKINS, A. L., MERGENHAGEN, S. E. and HOWARD, R. J. (1970) Effect of virus infections on the function of the immune system. *Ann. Rev. Microbiol.* **24**: 525–538.

ODAKA, T., ISHII, H., YAMAURO, K. and YAMAMOTO, T. (1966) Inhibitory effect of Friend leukemia virus infection on the antibody formation to sheep erythrocytes in mice. *Jap. J. exp. Med.* **36**: 277–290.

OLD, L., BENACERRAF, B., CLARKE, D. A. and GOLDSMITH, M. (1960) The reticuloendothelial system and the neoplastic process. *Ann. N.Y. Acad. Sci.* **88**: 264–280.

OLDSTONE, M. B., TISHON, A. and CHILLER, J. M. (1974) Chronic virus infection and immune responsiveness. II. Lactic dehydrogenase virus infection and immune response to non-viral antigens. *J. Immun.* **112**: 370–375.

OLSON, G. B. (1973) Effect of various viruses on responsiveness of mouse lymphocytes to phytohemagglutinin stimulation. *Inf. Immun.* **7**: 438–444.

OLSON, G. B., DENT, P. B., RAWLS, W. E., SOUTH, M. A., MONTGOMERY, J. R., MELNICK, J. L. and GOOD, R. A. (1968) Abnormalities of *in vitro* lymphocyte responses during Rubella virus infections. *J. exp. Med.* **128**: 47–68.

OSBORN, J. E., BLAZKOVEC, A. A. and WALKER, D. L. (1968) Immunosuppression during acute murine cytomegalovirus infection. *J. Immun.* **100**: 835–844.

OSBORN, J. E. and MEDDARIS, D. N., JR (1967) Suppression of interferon and antibody and multiplication of Newcastle disease virus in cytomegalovirus infected mice. *Proc. Soc. exp. Biol. Med.* **124**: 347–353.

PADNOS, M., MOLOMUT, N. and HOFER, R. (1969) Antibody formation in mice with viral lymphopenia. *Fedn. Proc.* **28**: 430.

PARODI, A. S., NOTA, N. R., DEGUERRERO, L. B., FIGERIO, M. J. and WEISSENBACHER, M. (1967) Inhibition of immune response in experimental hemorrhagic fever (Junin virus). *Acta Virol.* **11**: 120–125.

PATHAK, R. N., RAMA RAO, G. V. S. V. and THOMPKINS, W. A. F. (1974) *In vitro* cellular immunity to unrelated pathogens in chickens infected with Fowlpox virus. *Inf. Immun.* **10**: 34–41.

PAYNE, L. N. (1970) Immunosuppressive effects of avian oncogenic viruses. *Proc. R. Soc. Med.* **63**: 16–19.

PELED, L. and HARAN-GHERA, N. (1971) Immunosuppression by Radiation leukemia virus and its relation to lymphatic leukemia development. *Int. J. Cancer* **8**: 97–106.

PELED, L. and HARAN-GHERA, N. (1974) The cellular basis of immunosuppression caused by the Radiation leukemia virus. *Immunology* **26**: 323–329.

PERKINS, E. H., MACKINODAN, T. and UPTON, A. C. (1969) Impairment of differentiation and proliferation of immunocompetent and spleen colony corming cells in mice of high leukemia strain. *Fedn Proc.* **28**: 499.

PERRYMAN, L. E., BANKS, K. L. and MCGUIRE, T. C. (1975) Lymphocyte abnormalities in Aleutian disease virus infection of mink: decreased T lymphocyte responses and increased B lymphocyte levels in persistent viral infection. *J. Immun.* **115**: 22–27.

PERRYMAN, L. E., HOOVER, E. A. and YOHR, D. S. (1972) Immunologic reactivity of the cat: immunosuppression in experimental Feline leukemia. *J. natn. Cancer Inst.* **49**: 1357–1365.

PETERSON, R. D. A., HENDRICKSON, R. and GOOD, R. A. (1963) Reduced antibody forming capacity during the incubation period of passage A leukemia in C_3H mice. *Proc. Soc. exp. Biol. Med.* **114**: 517–520.

PETERSON, R. D. A., PURCHASE, H. G., BURMESTER, B. R., COOPER, M. D. and GOOD, R. A. (1966) Relationships among visceral lymphomatosis bursa of Fabricius and bursa dependent lymphoid tissue of the chicken. *J. natn. Cancer Inst.* **36**: 585–598.

PINCUS, T., ROWE, W. P., STABLES, P. J. and TALAL, N. (1970) Inability to induce tolerance to bovine gamma globulin in mice infected at birth with Lymphocytic choriomeningitis virus. *Proc. Soc. exp. Biol. Med.* **133**: 986–988.

PORTER, D. D., DIXON, F. U. and LARSON, A. E. (1974) Metabolism and function of gamma globulin in Aleutian disease of mink. *J. exp. Med.* **121**: 889–900.

PORTER, D. D. and LARSEN, A. E. (1965) Aleutian disease of mink. *Prog. med. Virol.* **18**: 32–47.

PURCHASE, H. G., CHUBB, R. C. and BIGGS, P. M. (1968) Effect of Lymphoid leukosis and Marek's disease on the immunological responsiveness of the chicken. *J. natn. Cancer Inst.* **40**: 583–592.

RANSOM, J. P., GOGMAN, J. M. and TULVE, S. (1969) Formation of antibodies against Salmonella lipopolysaccharides during a latent infection by Friend murine leukemia virus. *Cancer Res.* **29**: 1407–1415.

ROSENBERG, G. L., SNYDERMAN, R. and NOTKINS, A. L. (1974) Production of chemotactic factor and lymphotoxin by human leukocytes stimulated with Herpes simplex virus. *Inf. Immun.* **10**: 111–115.

RUBIN, A. D. (1966) Lymphocyte RNA synthesis in Infectious mononucleosis: the response to phytohemagglutinin *in vitro*. *Blood* **28**: 602–605.

SALAMAN, M. H. and WEDDERBURN, N. (1966) The immunodepressive effect of Friend virus. *Immunology* **10**: 445–458.

SCHMID, F. A. and HUTCHISON, D. J. (1968) Lymphoreticular system response in AKR/J and C57Bl/J mice. *Cancer Res.* **28**: 869–873.

SCHNEIDER, M. and DORE, J. F. (1969) Effet de l'injection d'un virus leucemogene murin (Friend) sur les réactions immunitaires de souris sensibles et résistantes à ce virus. *Revue fr. Etud. clin. Biol.* **14**: 1010–1014.

SCHWAB, J. H. (1975) Suppression of the immune response by microorganisms. *Bact. Rev.* **39**: 121–143.

SCOTT, G. H. and WALKER, J. S. (1976) Immunoglobulin bearing cells in lungs of mice infected with Influenza virus. *Inf. Immun.* **13**: 1525–1527.

SEIDEL, H. J. and LAUENSTEIN, K. (1969) Immunosuppressive effects of leukemia viruses. Studies with Rauscher virus in mice resistant to leukemia. *Z. Krebsforsch.* **72**: 219–225.

SELGRADE, M. K., AHMED, A., SELL, K. W., GERSHWIN, M. E. and STEINBERG, A. D. (1976) Effect of murine cytomegalovirus on the *in vitro* responses of T and B cells to mitogens. *J. Immun.* **116**: 1459–1465.

SIEGEL, B. V. and MORTON, J. I. (1966a) Depressed antibody response in the mouse infected with Rauscher leukemia virus. *Immunology* **10**: 559–562.

SIEGEL, B. V. and MORTON, J. I. (1966b) Serum agglutinin levels to sheep red blood cells in mice infected with Rauscher virus. *Proc. Soc. exp. Biol. Med.* **123**: 467–470.

SIEGEL, B. V. and MORTON, J. I. (1967) Influence of immunologic hyperstimulation on murine viral leukemogenesis. *Blood* **29**: 585–593.

SIEGEL, B. V. and MORTON, J. I. (1976) Tumor virus effects on immunocyte precursor cells. Hemopoietic stem cell behavior and leukemogenic susceptibility. *Ann. N.Y. Acad. Sci.* **276**: 442–454.
SIEGEL, B. V., NEHER, G. H. and MORTON, J. I. (1969) Quantitation and ultrastructure of immunodepression in murine virus induced leukemia. *Lab. Invest.* **20**: 347–352.
SNODGRASS, M. J., LOWREY, D. S. and HANNA, M. G., JR (1972) Changes induced by Lactic dehydrogenase virus in thymus and thymus-dependent areas of lymphatic tissue. *J. Immun.* **108**: 877–892.
SPECTER, S., PATEL, N. and FRIEDMAN, H. (1976a) Immunosuppression induced *in vitro* by cell-free extracts of Friend leukemia virus infected splenocytes. *J. natn. Cancer Inst.* **56**: 143–147.
SPECTER, S., PATEL, N. and FRIEDMAN, H. (1976b) Peritoneal exudate cell induced restoration of antibody formation by leukemia virus suppressed spleen cell cultures. *Proc. Soc. exp. Biol. Med.* **151**: 163–167.
STARR, S. and BERKOVICH, S. (1964) Effects of Measles, gamma globulin modified Measles and vaccine Measles on the tuberculin test. *New Engl. J. Med.* **270**: 386–391.
STRAUSS, R. R., JACOBS, A. A., PAUL, B. B. and SBARRA, A. J. (1972) The role of the phagocyte in host-parasite interactions. XXXIV. The effect of phagocytizable particles and phytohemagglutinin-P on DNA synthesis by spleen cells from leukemic and non-leukemic AKR mice. *J. Ret. End. Soc.* **11**: 277–292.
STRINGFELLOW, D. A. and GLASGOW, L. A. (1974) Hyporeactivity due to infection: recognition of a transferable hyporeactivity factor in the serum of Encephalomyocarditis cirus-infected mice. *Inf. Immun.* **10**: 1337–1342.
SULLIVAN, J. L., BARRY, D. W., ALBRECHT, P. and LUCAS, S. J. (1975) Inhibition of lymphocyte stimulation by Measles virus. *J. Immun.* **114**: 1458–1461.
THEIS, G. A., MCBRIDE, R. A. and SCHURMAN, L. W. (1975) Depression of *in vitro* responsiveness to phytohemagglutinin in spleen cells cultured from chickens with Marek's disease. *J. Immun.* **115**: 848–853.
TIMONEN, T., ORTALDO, J. R. and HERBERMAN, R. B. (1981) Characteristics of human large granular lymphocytes and relationship to natural killer and K cells. *J. Exp. Med.* **153**: 569–582.
TOMPKINS, W. A. F., SCHULTZ, R. M. and RAMA RAO, G. V. S. V. (1973) Depressed cell-mediated immunity in newborn rabbits bearing fibroma virus-infected tumors. *Inf. Immun.* **7**: 613–619.
TURNER, W. and CHIRIGOS, M. A. (1969) Enhancement of murine sarcoma virus (Moloney) infection and tumorigenesis *in vivo* by coinfection with Rauscher leukemia virus. *Cancer Res.* **29**: 1956–1960.
TWOMEY, J. J. (1974) Abnormalities in the mixed leukocyte reaction during Infectious Mononucleosis. *J. Immun.* **112**: 2278–2281.
UTERMOHLEN, V. and ZABRISKIE, T. B. (1973) A suppression of cellular immunity in patients with multiple sclerosis. *J. exp. Med.* **138**: 1591–1596.
VESIKARI, T. and BUOMOVICI-KLEIN, E. (1975) Lymphocyte responses to Rubella antigen and phytohemagglutinin after administration of the RA27/3 strain of live attentuated Rubella vaccine. *Inf. Immun.* **11**: 748–753.
VON PIRQUET, C. (1908) Das Verhalten der Kutanen Tuberculin-Reaktion Wahrend der Masern. *Dt. med. Wschr.* **34**: 1297–1300.
WAGNER, H. N., MASHARIO, I. and HORNICK, R. B. (1963) Studies of the reticuloendothelial system (RES). II. Changes in the phagocytic capacity of the RES in patients with certain infections. *J. clin. Invest.* **42**: 427–434.
WEDDERBURN, N. and SALAMAN, M. H. (1968) The immunodepressive effects of Friend virus. II. Reduction of splenic hemolysin producing cells in primary and secondary responses. *Immunology* **15**: 439–454.
WEIGLE, W. O. (1971) Immunologic unresponsiveness. In: *Immunobiology*, pp. 123–134, GOOD, R. A. and FISHER, D. W. (eds). Sinauer Assoc., Stamford, Connecticut.
WEISLOW, O. S. and WHEELOCK, E. F. (1975) Depression of humoral immunity to sheep erythrocytes *in vitro* by Friend virus leukemic spleen cells: induction of resistance by Statolon. *J. Immun.* **114**: 211–215.
WHEELOCK, E. F., TOY, S. T., WEISLOW, O. S. and LEVY, M. H. (1974) Restored immune and non-immune functions in Friend virus leukemic mice treated with Statolon. *Prog. exp. Tumor Res.* **19**: 369–390.
WILLEMS, F. Th. C., MELNICK, J. L. and RAWLS, W. E. (1969) Viral inhibition of the phytohemagglutinin response of human lymphocytes and application to viral hepatitis. *Proc. Soc. exp. Biol. Med.* **130**: 652–661.
WILLIAMS, R. C., JR, KENYON, A. J. and HUNTLEY, C. C. (1968) Immunoglobulins, viruses, and speculations on their interrelationships in certain human and animal disease states. *Blood* **31**: 522–535.
WOODRUFF, J. F. and WOODRUFF, J. J. (1975a) The effect of viral infections on the function of the immune system. In: *Viral Immunology and Immunopathology*, pp. 393–418, NOTKINS, A. L. (ed). Academic Press, New York.
WOODRUFF, J. F. and WOODRUFF, J. J. (1975b) Interaction of Myxo and Paramyxoviruses with murine lymphocytes. In: *The Immune System and Infectious Diseases*, 4th Int. Convoc. Immunol., Buffalo, N.Y., pp. 118–129. Karger, Basel.
YAMANOUCHI, K., FUKUDA, A., KOBUNE, F., YOSHIKAWA, Y. and CHINO, F. (1974) Pathogenesis of Rinderpest virus infection in rabbits. II. Effect of Rinderpest virus on the immune functions of rabbits. *Inf. Immun.* **9**: 206–211.
ZATZ, M. M., GOLDSTEIN, A. L. and WHITE, A. (1973a) Lymphocyte populations of AKR/J mice. I. Effect of aging on migration patterns, response to PHA and expression of theta antigen. *J. Immun.* **111**: 1514–1518.
ZATZ, M. M., WHITE, A. and GOLDSTEIN, A. L. (1973b) Lymphocyte populations of AKR/J mice. II. Effect of leukemogenesis on migration patterns, response to PHA and expression of theta antigen. *J. Immun.* **111**: 1519–1525.

CHAPTER 6

MODULATION OF IMMUNITY AND HOST RESISTANCE BY MICRO-ORGANISMS

JOHN B. HIBBS, JR.,* JACK S. REMINGTON† and CARLETON C. STEWART‡

*Veterans Administration Hospital, Salt Lake City, Utah, and Division of Infectious Diseases, Department of Medicine, University of Utah, Salt Lake City, Utah, USA.

†Division of Allergy, Immunology and Infectious Diseases, Palo Alto Medical Research Foundation, Palto Alto, California, and Department of Medicine, Division of Infectious Diseases, Stanford University, California, USA.

‡Section of Cancer Biology, Division of Radiation Oncology, Malinckrodt Institute of Radiology, Washington University School of Medicine, Missouri, USA.

1. INTRODUCTION

Suter (1956) classified microbial pathogens into three groups based on whether their proliferation in the tissues of the infected host was extracellular or intracellular. The first group, the obligate extracellular pathogens, parasitize the extracellular environment. This group of pathogens do not have the biochemical know-how to escape lytic mechanisms present within the vacuolar system of phagocytic cells. Their proliferation rapidly ceases once they have been incorporated into secondary lysosomes of polymorphonuclear leukoytes (PMNs) or mononuclear phagocytes. Therefore, virulence of this group of pathogens depends largely on their ability to evade phagocytosis. For the host to recover from infection with this group of pathogens, certain critical events must occur; for example, specific opsonizing and complement fixing immunoglobulin must appear in the extracellular fluids and Fc and C3 receptor bearing PMNs must mobilize at the infection sites. The Fab portion of specific immunoglobulin combines with antigenic determinants present on the surface of the extracellular pathogen. This is followed by attachment of the immunoglobulin-particulate antigen complex to PMN plasma membrane Fc receptors (or C3 receptors when complement component C3 is an intermediary). Driven by metabolic energy produced by the PMN, the extracellular pathogen attached to plasma membrane Fc and C3 receptors is incorporated into a phagocytic vacuole and undergoes rapid lysis following fusion of the phagocytic vacuole with primary and secondary lysosomes. Examples of extracellular pathogens include *Streptococcus pyogenes* (group A hemolytic streptococcus), *Streptococcus pneumoniae*, and *Hemophilus influenzae.*

The second group of microbial pathogens; the facultative intracellular parasites, survive and proliferate within mononuclear phagocytes as well as in the extracellular environment. Examples include *Mycobacterium tuberculosis*, *Mycobacterium bovis* (strain BCG), *Listeria monocytogenes*, *Francisella tularensis*, brucella species, salmonella species as well as the pathogenic fungus *Histoplasma capsulatum*.

The obligate intracellular parasites are the third group. They survive and proliferate only within the intracellular environment of the infected host. Examples are chlamydiae, rickettsiae and viruses, as well as the protozoans, *Toxoplasma gondii*, *Besnoitia jellisoni* and *Trypanosoma cruzi*. The point for emphasis is that both facultative and obligate intracellular parasites survive and produce disease in the infected host by proliferating in the intracellular environment. In many situations this includes survival and proliferation within mononuclear phagocytes. Therefore the relatively straightforward defensive measure that is successful in controlling proliferation of obligate extracellular pathogens—sequester them in secondary lysosomes of a phagocytic cell—will not control the proliferation of facultative and obligate intracellular pathogens.

In many cases such as in the development of resistance to *M. tuberculosis*, the production of immunoglobulin specific for the antigens of the invading intracellular pathogen may be an epiphenomenon unrelated to the acquisition of host resistance. However, in other situations the production of immunoglobulin specific for antigenic determinants of intracellular pathogens may cooperate with and supplement other host resistance mechanisms that make the intracellular environment inhospitable for the survival and proliferation of intracellular pathogens. For example, *in vitro*, specific antibody may inhibit absorption of virus to cells that lack Fc receptors on their surface (Silverstein, 1970). Also, it has been demonstrated *in vitro* that some viruses can enter host cells by endocytosis. In certain cases, with vaccinia virus as an example, the virus is unable to penetrate the cytoplasm from its location in the endocytic vacuole if it is coated with specific immunoglobulin. Specific antibody can also induce phagocytic vacuoles containing viable virulent toxoplasma trophozoites to fuse with primary and secondary lysosomes (Jones, 1975). In addition, if the classical complement pathway is activated by certain types of immunoglobulin attached to microbial antigens, or if the alternate complement pathway is directly activated by surface characteristics of some pathogenic micro-organisms, their extracellular lysis may result (Pillemer *et al.*, 1954; Wardlaw and Pillemer, 1956; Fearon and Austen, 1977; Fearon, 1978).

To summarize, the proliferation of obligate extracellular micro-organisms can be restrained by extracellular factors that promote their rapid clearance from the extracellular spaces by phagocytic cells, particularly PMNs. In a normal host, clearance of obligate extracellular pathogens from the extracellular spaces by phagocytic cells is the equivalent of their clearance from the host. On the other hand, clearance of intracellular pathogens from the extracellular environment by mononuclear phagocytes is not necessarily equivalent to clearance from host tissues. Indeed, in the nonimmune animal with low natural host resistance, endocytosis by mononuclear phagocytes gives certain intracellular pathogens access, to an environment absolutely essential for their survival and proliferation. Resistance in the infected mammalian host is expressed only when the intracellular milieu, particularly the intracellular milieu of mononuclear phagocytes, is altered in such a way that survival and proliferation of the intracellular pathogen within the intracellular habitat is prevented.

Our knowledge of the cellular and molecular basis for the homeostatic mechanisms that make the intracellular habitat inhospitable for survival and proliferation of intracellular pathogens is still uncomfortably vague. However, one point is clear, intracellular survival and proliferation of microbial pathogens is prevented and homeostasis maintained in the mammalian host by physiologic perturbations that can produce far reaching and surprisingly nonspecific effects. In this review we will discuss our current understanding of known causes and effects of these physiologic perturbations that occur in the tissues when the host develops resistance to the survival and proliferation of an intracellular microbial pathogen. We will emphasize the central role of mononuclear phagocytes and the importance of their state of differentiation in the expression of resistance to intracellular pathogens. In addition, we will describe experimental evidence suggesting that nonspecific modulation of immunity and host resistance by intracellular pathogens also has a genesis in mononuclear phagocytes that have responded to differentiation signals generated by the host response to intracellular pathogens present in the tissues. It appears that in the course of acquiring phenotypic properties necessary for the control of survival and proliferation of intracellular micro-organisms, mononuclear phagocytes also develop a capability for nonspecific modulation of immunity and host resistance to other physiologic and pathologic stimuli.

2. THE HOST RESPONSE TO INTRACELLULAR MICRO-ORGANISMS RESULTS IN INCREASED NONSPECIFIC RESISTANCE TO TAXONOMICALLY AND ANTIGENICALLY UNRELATED INTRACELLULAR MICRO-ORGANISMS

A striking feature of acquired resistance to intracellular pathogens is nonspecificity of expression when tested under proper experimental conditions. It was noted more than 40 years ago that animals infected with the tubercle bacillus had increased resistance to the unrelated pathogen *Brucella abortus* (Pullinger, 1936). Since that time many other examples of cross resistance between infections caused by intracellular pathogens have been described. For example, mice infected with *B. abortus* have increased resistance to *M. tuberculosis* (Nyka, 1956). Howard *et al.*, (1959) described increased resistance to *Salmonella enteritidis* in mice infected with BCG. Mackaness and his colleagues noted that mice infected with brucella, salmonella, or BCG have a marked resistance to sub-lethal infection with listeria (Mackaness, 1964; Blanden *et al.*, 1966; Collins *et al.*, 1966; Blanden *et al.*, 1969). Mice with listeria infection were also highly resistant to salmonella (Blanden *et al.*, 1966). Nonspecific resistance that had waned could be stimulated again by a second injection of the homologous organism (Mackaness, 1964; Coppel and Youmans, 1969).

Nonspecific resistance to taxonomically and antigenically different micro-organisms crosses phylogenetic lines. Remington and his colleagues demonstrated increased nonspecific resistance to facultative intracellular bacteria and viruses in mice with chronic infection with toxoplasma or besnoitia, both obligate intracellular protozoans (Ruskin and Remington, 1968; Ruskin *et al.*, 1969; Remington and Merigan, 1969). Mice with chronic toxoplasma infection had increased resistance to listeria, salmonella, besnoitia and Mengo virus. Likewise, mice with chronic besnoitia infection had increased resistance to infection with listeria, salmonella, brucella, toxoplasma and Mengo virus. In addition, mice with sublethal listeria infection showed increased resistance to challenge with toxoplasma or Mengo virus. Mice with chronic toxoplasma or besnoitia infection as well as mice with sublethal infection were also found to have increased resistance to the fungus *Cryptococcus neoformans* (Gentry and Remington, 1971). Chronic infection with toxoplasma enhanced resistance of mice to infection with the helminth *Schistosoma mansoni* (Mahmoud *et al.*, 1976). Finally, infection with BCG also increases nonspecific resistance to phylogenetically unrelated micro-organisms. For example, mice with BCG infection have increased resistance to Mengo virus (Old *et al.*, 1961) or Herpesvirus hominis type 2 (Glasgow *et al.*, 1977). In addition, chronic BCG infection confers increased resistance to murine malaria (Clark and Allison, 1976) as well as babesia species, which are also hemoprotozoans (Clark and Allison, 1976; Clark *et al.*, 1977).

3. THE MACROPHAGE IS THE EFFECTOR CELL IN EXPRESSION OF INCREASED NONSPECIFIC RESISTANCE TO INTRACELLULAR MICRO-ORGANISMS—THE CONCEPT OF ACQUIRED CELLULAR IMMUNITY

The term *acquired cellular immunity* describes a mechanism of resistance evoked in a mammalian host against micro-organisms that survive and proliferate in the intracellular environment. It has been succinctly defined by Mackaness (1971) as '.... a mechanism of defense in which a specifically committed lymphocyte serves as the immunologic go between that enables mononuclear phagocytes to perform their microbicidal functions'. Acquired cellular immunity differs from the classical concept of immunity in which a specific immunoglobulin interferes with infectivity and pathogenicity by combining with a micro-organism or its products. The concept of acquired cellular immunity, at least as expressed at the effector level by macrophages, conforms closely to Metchnikoff's (1893) original concept of resistance to infectious disease, i.e. that enhanced phagocytic and digestive power of leukocytes is the critical event that results in recovery of the host.

Early *in vitro* studies implicated mononuclear phagocytes as effector cells capable of the intracellular destruction of facultative intracellular pathogens (Lurie, 1942; Suter, 1953; Mackaness, 1954, 1962, 1964; Elberg *et al.*, 1957; Elberg, 1960; Mitsuhashi *et al.*, 1961). One important observation made in these early experiments was that cross resistance between infections with facultative intracellular bacteria noted *in vivo* could at times be observed *in vitro*. Elberg and his co-workers (1957, 1960) demonstrated that peritoneal macrophages harvested from rabbits infected with BCG restricted the intracellular proliferation of both *Brucella melitensis* and *M. tuberculosis*.

In a series of experiments Mackaness (1962, 1964, 1969) and Mackaness *et al.* (1966) elucidated the immunologic basis of acquired cellular immunity. He used the term 'activated' to describe macrophages with modified functional capability that included increased microbicidal activity. In studies of resistance to intracellular bacteria in mice, he showed that macrophages can be recruited and activated by an immunologic reaction but, as participant cells in that reaction, utilize nonimmunologic mechanisms of response. He demonstrated that expression of acquired resistance to intracellular bacteria depends on three factors: (1) recognition residing in specifically immune lymophocytes, (2) the presence in the tissues of bacteria which can act as a specific antigenic stimulus for the immune lymphocytes, and (3) the mobilization and activation of macrophages with increased microbicidal activity; these macrophages are the effector cells in the expression of this resistance. For the appearance of a local and/or systemic population of activated macrophages in the host, the first two factors must coexist in the tissues. As the bacteria, which are the specific stimulus for the sensitized lymphocytes, are cleared from the tissues by activated macrophages, the sensitized lymphocytes produce less and less macrophage-activating factor(s) and macrophage function gradually reverts to normal. Mackaness also showed that, although the induction of acquired resistance to intracellular bacteria was highly specific (characterized by immunologic reactivity of the host and the presence of specific microbial antigens), its expression was nonspecific (mediated by a population of activated macrophages). For example, macrophages activated by an immune response to one intracellular bacteria (e.g. *L. monocytogenes*) had an increased nonspecific microbicidal activity for other intracellular bacteria (e.g. *Salmonella typhimurium*). Therefore immunologic factors, particularly and specifically sensitized lymphocytes, were shown to have an essential role in the induction and maintenance of acquired cellular resistance to facultative intracellular bacteria. These studies clearly demonstrate a point that deserves emphasis: specific inducing antigen must persist if nonspecific resistance is to continue to be enhanced. Adoptive transfer experiments showed that when spleen cells from BCG immunized, tuberculin-sensitive animals are transferred to normal recipients, they confer tuberculin-sensitivity but do not cause activation of recipient macrophages or increase nonspecific resistance to listeria infection. If recipients of BCG-immune lymphoid cells are injected with a small dose of BCG, macrophages in the peritoneal cavity become activated within 24–48 hr and the animal acquires a highly significant level of nonspecific resistance to listeria challenge. However, if the transferred spleen cells are obtained from non-sensitized donors, or if the eliciting dose of BCG is not given to the recipients, macrophages do not become activated and nonspecific resistance to listeria does not develop. Studies by North (1970a, b, 1973) demonstrated the critical importance of T-lymphocytes for rapid mobilization and activation of mononuclear phagocytes at infected foci for the development of acquired immunity to the facultative intracellular bacteria *L. monocytogenes*.

Using mice with chronic infection caused by the protozoans toxoplasma or besnoitia, Remington and his colleagues (Ruskin *et al.*, 1969; Remington and Merigan, 1969; Gentry and Remington, 1971; Williams *et al.*, 1976) showed a direct correlation between *in vivo* expression of increased specific and nonspecific resistance to intracellular infection and enhanced *in vitro* ability of monolayers of activated macrophages from these mice to inhibit proliferation and survival of homologous as well as a variety of unrelated intracellular pathogens. These authors (Ruskin *et al.*, 1969; Remington and Merigan, 1969) could not implicate a role for circulating antibody or interferon in the expression of specific or nonspecific resistance during chronic protozoan infection in mice. Experiments reported by Frenkel (1967) are also of interest. He showed in adoptive transfer studies that specifically sensitized lymphocytes from hamsters with chronic besnoitia infection strongly protected recipients against besnoitia challenge whereas neither lymphocytes from normal animals nor immune serum were protective. Therefore, it has been demonstrated in hamsters that acquired immunity to an intracellular protozoan infection can be passively transferred with specifically sensitized lymphocytes, and it has been demonstrated in mice that macrophages from animals with chronic protozoan infection can be activated and will restrict survival and proliferation of unrelated micro-organisms (e.g. listeria) *in vitro*. Taken together, these findings suggest that animals with chronic intracellular protozoan infection have similar mechanisms for acquiring and expressing acquired cellular resistance to the homologous infecting protozoan, as well as for acquiring and expressing nonspecific resistance to phylogenetically unrelated intracellular pathogens as was described earlier by Mackaness in the bacteria–bacteria model. In addition, Blanden (1970, 1971a, b) showed that acquired cellular immunity was the major mechanism of resistance and recovery from a generalized virus infection in mice. He provided experimental evidence that recovery from ectromelia infection was independent of circulating antibody but absolutely dependent on both T-lymphocytic activities and the mobilization of mononuclear phagocytes in infected tissues. Furthermore, Blandon and Mims (1973), using mice with generalized virus infection, demonstrated another characteristic of acquired cellular immunity, increased nonspecific resistance to taxonomically unrelated intracellular pathogens; mice with ectromelia or lymphocytic choriomenigitis virus infections had increased nonspecific resistance to listeria infection.

The studies described above clearly show that a two cell system—lymphocytes and mononuclear phagocytes—is required for the expression of acquired cellular immunity to intracellular pathogens. Mononuclear phagocytes, the effector cells that express increased resistance to intracellular pathogens, are mobilized at sites of infection and are functionally modified by secretory products of sensitized lymphocytes responding to specific antigen. *In vitro* experiments have demonstrated that sensitized lymphocytes responding to specific antigen, T-lymphocytes responding to Con A, or B lymphocytes responding to bacterial lipopolysacchride (LPS), secrete a lymphokine(s) that delivers a signal inducing activation of mononuclear phagocytes as well as physiologic modification that enables mononuclear phagocytes to nonspecifically kill or inhibit the proliferation of intracellular pathogens (Patterson and Youmans, 1970; Krahenbuhl and Remington, 1971; Godal *et al.*, 1971; Simon and Sheagren, 1972; Fowles *et al.*, 1973; Anderson and Remington, 1974; Anderson *et al.*, 1976; Williams and Remington, 1977; Nogueria and Cohn, 1978). These findings suggest that any agent capable of inducing a pleiotypic response of T-lymphocytes or B-lymphocytes that includes secretion of lymphokines with macrophage activating factor (MAF) activity can also, under appropriate physiologic or pathologic conditions, nonspecifically enhance the ability of mononuclear phagocytes to restrict survival and proliferation of intracellular pathogens.

4. THE HOST RESPONSE TO INTRACELLULAR INFECTION RESULTS IN INCREASED RESISTANCE TO NEOPLASIA

It has been known for many years that microbes or their components will enhance host resistance to neoplastic disease under appropriate experimental conditions. For example, infection with intracellular agents can stimulate increased resistance to tumor growth. Induced are infections with the facultative intracellular bacteria, BCG (Old *et al.*, 1959, 1961; Mathé *et al.*, 1969a, b; Zbar *et al.*, 1970a–c; Morton *et al.*, 1970; Larson *et al.*, 1971) and *S. enteritidis* (Hardy and Kotlarski, 1971), the lactic dehydrogenase elevating virus (Riley, 1966), and M-P virus (Molomut and Padnos, 1965), filterable hemolytic anemia virus (Sachs *et al.*, 1960), and protozoa (Hibbs *et al.*, 1971; Lunde and Gelderman, 1971).

In addition to infection with live intracellular organisms, resistance to tumor growth has been conferred by killed micro-organisms or microbial components which cause reticuloendothelial stimulation, have immunologic adjuvant action, and induce macrophage activation, i.e., macrophage differentiation toward the nonspecifically tumoricidal state. Included are the dead organisms (*Corynebacterium parvum* (Halpern *et al.*, 1966; Woodruff and Boak, 1966) *Bordetella pertussis* (Sinkovics *et al.*, 1970) and *Mycobacterium butryicum* (Regelson and Munson, 1970; Hibbs *et al.*, 1972a), or their products zymosan (Bradner *et al.*, 1958), methanol-insoluble fraction of BCG (Weiss *et al.*, 1961), and endotoxin (Shear, 1944)).

It is evident that a great number and variety of microbial agents or their products are capable, under defined experimental conditions, of stimulating nonspecific host resistance to allogeneic or syngeneic tumor growth. However, the possibility that host resistance to intracellular micro-organisms and neoplasia may share common underlying mechanisms of expression was first suggested by Zbar and his co-workers as well as by our own experiments.

Zbar *et al.*, (1970a, b, c) showed that rejection of syngeneic tumor grafts in guinea pigs required several steps. Recognition, the first step resides in sensitized lymphocytes and is specific, but tumor cell destruction, the second step, was found to be nonspecific. These workers demonstrated that close contact between sensitized cells, sensitizing antigen, and the antigenically unrelated tumor cells was required to nonspecifically suppress growth of antigenically unrelated tumor cells. These results showed a requirement for the first two factors described by Mackaness (sensitized lymphocytes and specific antigen) and in addition suggested the involvement of a third nonspecific factor.

In a series of studies, we provided strong evidence that the nonspecific component in mediating tumor resistance in mice is a population of activated macrophages (Hibbs *et al.*, 1971, 1972b) (see next section). Our results suggested that the mechanisms of host resistance to intracellular pathogens is related to those for neoplasia and that the activated macrophage is a common effector arm for expression of this resistance. *In vivo* experiments showed that mice chronically infected with intracellular protozoa had increased resistance to autochthonous and transplanted tumors (Fig. 1). In this experimen-

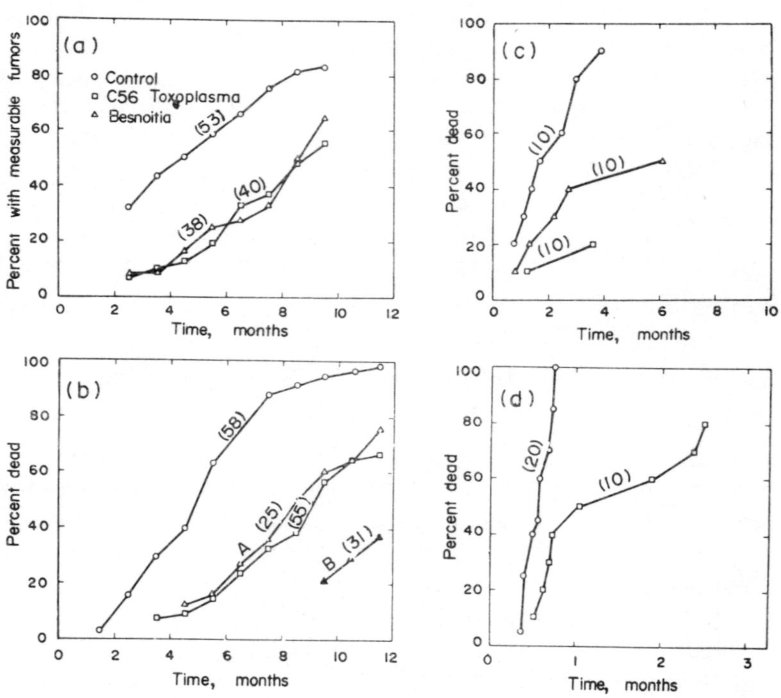

FIG. 1. Effect of chronic intracellular protozoan infection on autochthonous and transplanted tumors in mice. a—Incidence of spontaneous mammary tumor in C_3H/He mice. b—Incidence of death due to spontaneous leukemia in AKR mice. The difference between subgroup (△) and subgroup (▲) was the interval between infection and treatment with sulfadiazine, 48 hr in (△) and 96 hr in (▲). c—Incidence of death due to Friend leukemia in Swiss-Webster mice. d—Incidence of death due to sarcoma-180 in ascites form in Swiss-Webster mice. In a and b, time 0 = date of infection. In c and d, time 0 = date of tumor transplant. Figures in parentheses = number of mice. (○) = controls; (□) = chronically infected with C56 strain of *Toxoplasma gondii*; (△) = chronically infected with *Besnoitia jellisoni*. (Reprinted from Hibbs, Lambert and Remington, 1971, with permission of the publisher.)

tal model the protozoan antigens persist in the tissues for an extended period but the mice remain healthy. This provides the necessary context, coexistence of specific antigen and sensitized lymphocytes, for the expression of acquired as well as nonspecific resistance to intracellular bacteria and tumors. We observed an impressive delay in time to death due to spontaneous leukemia in AKR mice with chronic protozoan infection. In one group of mice infected with *B. jellisoni* mice did not die of leukemia until 10 months after chronic infection was established. By that time 97 per cent of control mice had died of leukemia.

Challenge with *L. monocytogenes* was used to determine whether mice infected with protozoa were resistant to a phylogenetically unrelated intracellular pathogen. Mice of the C_3H/He and AKR strains were selected randomly from groups of mice being followed for the development of spontaneous neoplasia. They were challenged with listeria 6 weeks after initiation of protozoan infection. Other experimental groups were inoculated with listeria the same day that tumor cells were grafted into other mice from the same group. Mice that had increased nonspecific resistance to neoplasia also expressed increased resistance to listeria challenge (Table 1) (Hibbs *et al.*, 1971). Therefore, in addition to stimulating nonspecific resistance to a phylogenetically unrelated intracellular pathogen, chronic infection with intracellular protozoa also stimulates nonspecific resistance to both autochthonous and transplanted neoplastic growth.

TABLE 1. *Challenge of Experimental Groups of Mice with* Listeria monocytogenes

Tumor evaluated	Strain of mice*	Experimental group†	Per cent survival	Death (days after challenge)‡ 2	3	4	5	6	7	8
Mammary carcinoma	C_3H/He	Control	0	1	7	2				
		Tg	60			1	1	1	1	
		Bj	80			1			1	
AKR leukemia	AKR	Control	0	10						
		Tg	60			2	1	1		
		Bj	80					1		1
Friend leukemia	SW	Control	10	1	5	3				
		Tg	90				1			
		Bj	70				1	1	1	
Sarcoma-180	SW	Control	10	3	2	3	1			
		Tg	90				1			

*All were females.

†Control = mice inoculated with saline or Hank's balanced salt solution; Bj = mice chronically infected with *B. Jellisoni*; Tg = mice chronically infected with *T. gondii.*

‡Numbers in columns show number of mice that died on each day.

(Reprinted from Hibbs, Lambert and Remington, 1971, with permission of the publisher.)

In other experiments we demonstrated that intraperitoneal (i.p.) inoculation of complete Freunds adjuvant (CFA) a water-in-oil emulsion which contains suspended killed *M. butryicum*, is also effective in inducing nonspecific resistance to listeria infection and to neoplasia (Hibbs *et al.*, 1972a). The mycobacterial antigens present in the CFA emulsion persist in the peritoneal cavity for a prolonged period providing an ongoing stimulus for specifically sensitized T-lymphocytes which maintain, via secretion of molecules with MAF-like activity, a population of macrophages in an ongoing state of activation. This, like the chronic protozoan infection model, provides the necessary context for expression of nonspecific resistance to intracellular micro-organisms. To evaluate nonspecific resistance to an unrelated intracellular organism, we challenged mice with the facultative intracellular bacterium, *L. monocytogenes.* Mice were pretreated with CFA, incomplete Freunds adjuvant (ICFA), or Hanks balanced salt solution (HBSS) 10 weeks before listeria challenge. All strains of mice pretreated with CFA showed significantly greater survival or prolonged time to death following i.p. inoculation with listeria (Fig. 2a). CFA stimulated marked resistance to listeria while ICFA and HBSS controls were not protected. On the same day that the SW mice (Fig. 2a) were challenged with listeria, other

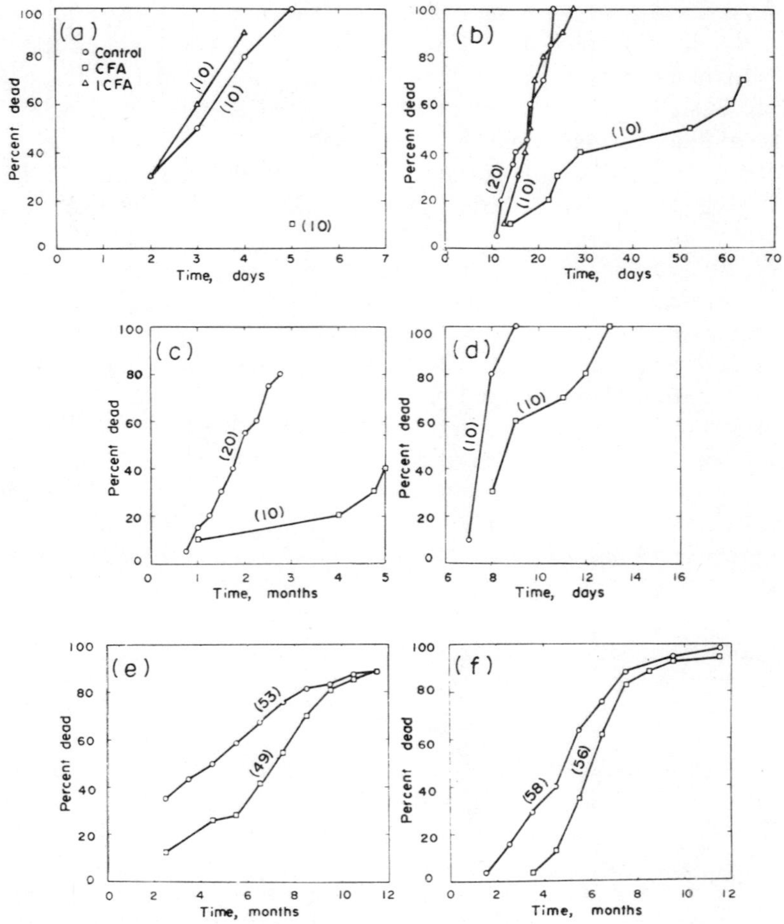

FIG. 2. Effect of CFA on resistance to listeria, transplanted tumors, and autochthonous tumors in mice. a—Incidence of death after i.p. inoculation of 1.7×10^7 listeria organisms in Swiss–Webster mice. b—Incidence of death after i.p. inoculation of 1×10^6 sarcoma-180 cells in Swiss–Webster mice. c—Incidence of death after i.p. inoculation of a 10 per cent suspension of Friend leukemia virus-infected spleen cells in Swiss–Webster mice. d—Incidence of death after i.p. inoculation of 1×10^5 leukemia L1210 cells in DBA/2 mice. e—Incidence of palpable spontaneous mammary tumors in C_3H/He mice. f—Incidence of death due to spontaneous leukemia in AKR mice. in a, time 0 = day of listeria challenge. In b, c and d, time 0 = day of tumor transplant. In e and f, time 0 = day of inoculation of CFA or HBSS. Figures in parentheses = number of mice. (Reprinted from Hibbs, Lambert and Remington, 1972a, with permission of publisher.)

mice from the same pretreatment groups were grafted with 1×10^6 sarcoma-180 cells i.p. Mice pretreated with CFA showed significantly greater survival (e.g. at 28 days $P = <0.001$), and time to death was longer than for the ICFA and HBSS controls (Fig. 2b). Greater survival and prolonged survival were noted in SW mice which 11 weeks after pretreatment with CFA, received an i.p. inoculation of 0.2 ml of a 10 per cent suspension of spleen cells infected with Friend leukemia virus (e.g. at 2.7 months $P = <0.001$) (Fig. 2c); and delayed time to death was also noted in DBA/2 mice grafted with 1×10^5 leukemia L1210 cells i.p. 9 weeks after pretreatment with CFA (e.g. at 9 days $P = <0.04$) (Fig. 2d).

CFA also stimulated increased host resistance to autochthonous tumors for mammary adenocarcinoma in C_3H/He mice (e.g. at 5.5 months $P = <0.001$) (Fig. 2e), and thymic lymphoma in AKR mice (e.g. at 4.5 months $P = <0.001$) (Fig. 2f). The protective effect against these spontaneous tumors appeared to be inversely proportional to the time interval following administration of CFA. For example, palpable mammary tumors in C_3H/He mice were initially suppressed by CFA treatment, but 11 months following CFA administration tumor incidence was identical to that of HBSS controls.

In the two *in vivo* experimental models we used to study nonspecific resistance to intracellular infection and neoplasia, mice with chronic intracellular protozoan infection or pretreated with CFA; parallel results were obtained. This suggested that the great variety of micro-organisms or their components that induce increased nonspecific host resistance to intracellular infection or neoplasia may also be able to activate a system of host cells capable of inhibiting the intracellular-replication and survival of intracellular pathogens as well as the extracellular replication and survival of neoplastic cells.

5. THE MACROPHAGE IS THE EFFECTOR CELL IN EXPRESSION OF INCREASED NONSPECIFIC RESISTANCE TO NEOPLASTIC CELLS

It is now clear that when macrophages undergo a functional modification termed activation, during acquisition of cellular immunity to intracellular micro-organisms, they also become capable of causing a nonspecific nonphagocytic extracellular stasis or lysis of neoplastic cells in addition to a nonspecific intracellular stasis or lysis of phagocytized intracellular micro-organisms.

Normal mouse peritoneal macrophages are not tumoricidal under usual or unstressed physiologic conditions as shown by their interaction with tumor cells *in vitro* (Hibbs *et al.*, 1972b, c). Indeed, modification of macrophage function is fundamental to the development of tumoricidal potential by activated macrophages. We found that chronic infection with a variety of phylogenetically unrelated micro-organisms including *T. gondii*, *B. jellisoni*, *L. monocytogenes* and BCG, induces in mice a population of activated peritoneal macrophages that are nonspecifically tumoricidal when tested *in vitro* (Hibbs *et al.*, 1972b, c; Hibbs, 1973, 1975). These results suggested that stimuli induced by the host reaction to infection were important in the acquisition of tumoricidal potential by activated macrophages.

Independently, Alexander and Evans (1971), as well as Keller and Jones (1971), provided similar experimental evidence showing that tumoricidal activated macrophages were produced in response to heterologous inducing agents—endotoxin and the nematode, *Nippostrongylus brasiliensis*, respectively. It has since been shown that other microbial agents administered to experimental animals will likewise induce the mobilization of a population of activated macrophages that are nonspecifically cytotoxic for tumor cells *in vitro*. Included are complete Freund's adjuvant (Hibbs *et al.*, 1972d), *C. parvum* (Scott, 1974; Krahenbuhl *et al.*, 1976), and *Corynebacterium granulosum* (Basic *et al.*, 1974).

Figure 3 is a macroscopic view of the cytotoxic effect of activated peritoneal macrophages from mice with chronic BCG infection; this photo demonstrates the requirement for intimate contact between activated macrophages and tumorigenic BALB/3T12 target cells. In all situations, BALB/3T12 cells have completely overgrown and formed a multilayer over the normal macrophages. On the other hand, wherever the BALB/3T12 cells come into contact with BCG-activated macrophages, there is a marked cytotoxic effect. Furthermore, it can be seen that wherever a narrow strip of adherent macrophages was removed from the culture dish with a rubber policeman prior to BALB/3T12 cell challenge, the macrophage-free substrate is overgrown with a multilayer of target cells, even though they are surrounded by viable fully cytotoxic BCG-activated macrophages. Microscopically, the BALB/3T12 cells grew to the immediate edge of the macrophage-free areas.

An additional characteristic of the activated macrophage cytotoxic reaction is that neoplastic cells are destroyed or their growth slowed under *in vitro* conditions in which non-neoplastic cells are spared and grow to confluency (Hibbs, 1974a). In our initial studies we observed that the cytolytic effect of activated macrophages was selective (Hibbs *et al.*, 1972b, c; Hibbs, 1973, 1974a). Activated peritoneal macrophages from mice with chronic toxoplasma, besnoitia, listeria, or BCG infection did not destroy contact-inhibited allogeneic fibroblast or kidney cell strains that have surfaces of high immuno-

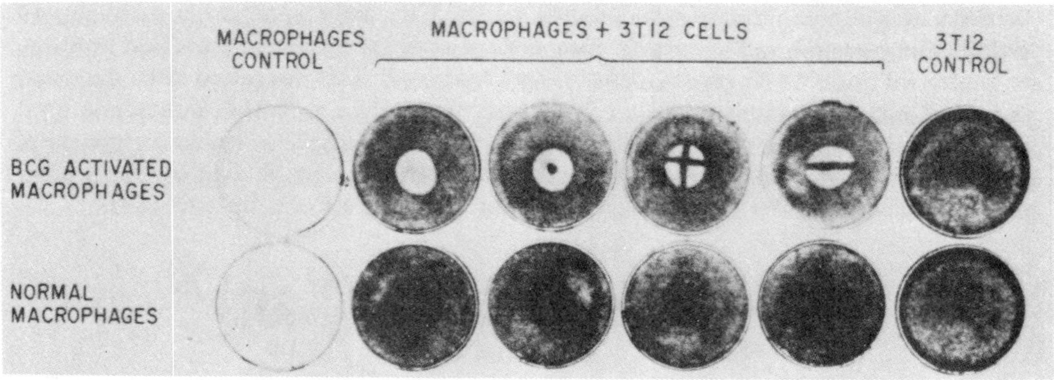

FIG. 3. Photo of Petri dishes demonstrating the importance of activated macrophage-tumor target cell contact in macrophage mediated cytotoxicity. The cytotoxicity test was performed as previously described (Hibbs, 1974b) with several minor modifications. Briefly, peritoneal cells from BCG-infected or normal BALB/c mice (6×10^5) in 0.1 ml of Dulbecco's modification of Eagle medium with 10 per cent fetal bovine serum, streptomycin (100 μg/ml), and penicillin (100 unit/ml) (complete medium) were added to the center of 35 mm Falcon plastic Petri dishes for one hour at 37°C in air with 5 per cent CO_2 to allow for adherence of macrophages. Each Petri dish was then washed with Hanks' balanced salt solution to remove nonadherent cells so that the central monolayer of adherent macrophages was restricted to the size of the 0.1 ml drop in which they were added to the Petri dish. The peripheral portion of the Petri dish remains free of macrophages. A rubber policeman was then used to remove a narrow strip of adherent macrophages from the centrally located monolayer and several varieties of mcarophage-free areas were produced on different macrophage monolayers. Target cells (tumorigenic BALB/3T12 cells, 1×10^5) were added in 2 ml of complete medium and attached evenly to the bottom of the Petri dish. The dishes were stained with Giémsa after 60 hr of culture. The multilayer of 3T12 target cells stain darkly.

genic potential, but were markedly cytolytic to both syngeneic and allogeneic tumorigenic cell lines. These experiments suggest that neoplastic cells are either more susceptible to the cytolytic effect of activated macrophages than non-neoplastic cells, or that they elicit nonimmunologic recognition and subsequent destruction by activated macrophages which are not triggered by non-neoplastic cells.

To test this hypothesis, we studied the cytotoxic activity of activated mouse macrophages against mouse embryo fibroblasts before and after spontaneous transformation of the fibroblasts *in vitro* (Hibbs *et al.*, 1972c). We found that activated C_3H/He macrophages did not destroy two allogeneic fibroblast cell strains differing from them at a strongly antigenic H-2 locus. In contrast, these macrophages were markedly cytolytic for the same allogeneic fibroblasts (and also for syngeneic fibroblasts) after the fibroblasts had spontaneously developed abnormal growth properties that included loss of contact inhibition of cell division. Because H-2 antigens are more immunogenic than tumor specific transplantation antigens or fetal antigens expressed on tumor cells, this study strongly suggests that a change associated with the acquisition of abnormal growth properties by target cells, rather than a change in antigens, is responsible for the increased susceptibility of tumor cells to destruction by activated macrophages.

Studies from several laboratories have confirmed that activated macrophages nonspecifically kill syngeneic or allogeneic neoplastic cells under *in vitro* conditions in which normal syngeneic or allogeneic target cells are spared (Holtermann *et al.*, 1973; Basic *et al.*, 1974; Cleveland *et al.*, 1974; Kaplan *et al.*, 1974; Meltzer *et al.*, 1975a,b; Piessens *et al.*, 1975; Fidler, 1978). This provides an element of selectivity to the activated macrophage tumoricidal reaction; in addition, it raises the possibility that a target cell change (or changes) occurs at the time of neoplastic transformation, is expressed as part of the neoplastic phenotype; and may be important in making neoplastic cells more susceptible to the cytotoxic effect of activated macrophages.

In the mouse at least, merely inducing a sterile inflammatory exudate in the peritoneal cavity with agents such as starch, mineral oil, thioglycollate broth, or 10 per cent peptone is not sufficient stimulus to convert macrophages into tumoricidal cells (Hibbs *et al.*,

1972b, 1977; Hibbs, 1974b; Cleveland *et al.*, 1974). This suggests that the macrophage may require a chemical signal(s) produced as a result of a specific immunologic response to antigens of the inducing micro-organism and that this signal mediates the acquisition of tumoricidal properties by macrophages. Piessens and his colleagues (1975) demonstrated that normal guinea-pig macrophages become cytolytic for syngeneic tumor cells after they have been activated *in vitro* by lymphokine-rich supernatants prepared from sensitized lymphocytes responding to specific antigen unrelated to the tumor cells. Likewise, Ruco and Meltzer (1977) used supernatants of PPD-stimulated BCG immune spleen cells to induce the *in vitro* differentiation of macrophages to the nonspecific tumoricidal level. This simulates the *in vivo* production of tumoricidal activated macrophages in BCG infected animals, when BCG and specifically sensitized lymphocytes co-exist in the tissues. Furthermore, Fidler (1975) observed that lymphokine-rich supernatants produced by sensitized lymphocytes responding to specific syngeneic tumor antigens will induce macrophages to nonspecifically kill neoplastic cells; this suggested that tumoricidal activated macrophages could be produced *in vivo* as a component of the host response to syngeneic tumor growth. Indeed, this was demonstrated by Russell and McIntosh (1977); they observed that spontaneously regressing Moloney sarcomas contained activated macrophages that were nonspecifically cytotoxic for neoplastic cells

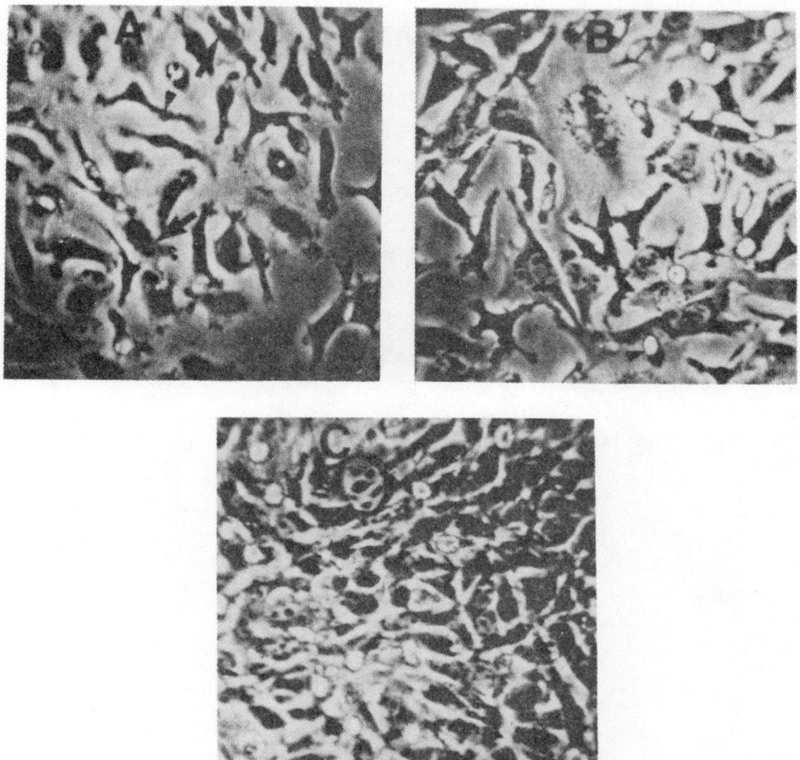

FIG. 4. Macrophage colony incubated with 3T12 tumor cells and 5 per cent normal mouse serum added to the culture medium. Photomicrographs were obtained from a time lapse movie. Tumor cells are best identified in the following sequences by their prominent nucleoli (arrow). Macrophages appear more elongated (pointer). A—Obtained 2 hr after addition of 5 per cent normal mouse serum and tumor cells, shows the edge of an intact macrophage colony. Tumor cells have attached and are distributed uniformly. Approximate edge of colony runs from bottom center to upper right corner. B—Obtained 20 hr later, colony has become completely disorganized. Tumor cells (arrow) have increased in number through proliferation, but macrophages are interacting with them. Some macrophages appear 'rounded up' and refractile on top of the tumor cells (pointer), while those still attached are spread out. C—After 45 hr of culture, a confluent monolayer of tumor cells is shown. Macrophages have been displaced from the dish and appear as small 'rounded up' and refractile cells on top of the tumor cells. (Reprinted from Stewart, Adles and Hibbs, 1978, with permission of the publisher.)

when tested *in vitro*. Therefore, there is a striking parallel between the *in vivo* and *in vitro* expression of increased nonspecific resistance to intracellular micro-organisms and neoplastic cells. Both require the presence of an immunologic event in which specific antigen interacts with sensitized lymphocytes. Soluble lymphokine-like molecules with MAF activity are secreted by the responding sensitized lymphocytes. MAF then interacts with macrophages and induces their differentiation to the activated level. Activated, but not normal macrophages are capable, under the appropriate environmental conditions, of nonspecific restriction of the intracellular survival and proliferation of intracellular micro-organisms as well as the nonphagocytic and nonspecific extracellular restriction of survival and proliferation of neoplastic cells. The experimental evidence accumulated thus far suggests that the physiologic mechanisms responsible for generation of activated macrophages capable of mediating nonspecific resistance against intracellular micro-organisms and neoplastic cells are similar if not identical. It appears likely that one or several lymphokines derived from sensitized lymphocytes responding to specific antigen induces macrophage differentiation toward the tumoricidal level and that such lymphokine exposed macrophages are capable of mediating nonspecific stasis and lysis of neoplastic cells.

In experiments using colonies of pure macrophages as effector cells, we avoided the problem of possible contamination with non-macrophage cell types that could cooperate with lymphokines as intermediaries in the macrophage activation process or act as effector cells in the mediation of stasis and lysis of neoplastic target cells (Stewart *et al.*, 1978). The results showed that all macrophage colonies exposed to MAF-rich serum from BCG infected mice were capable, through a nonphagocytic mechanism of lysing syngeneic or allogeneic tumor target cells which they contacted (Figs 4 and 5). In addition, activated clones mouse macrophages which had mediated a cytotoxic effect on EMT-6 mammary carcinoma cells were also capable of phagocytosing heat-killed *Candida albicans* at the termination of the assay (Fig. 6). Tumor cell lysis was documented by time lapse cinemicrography. It is significant that the tumor cell killing function of pure macrophage colonies was inducible, nonphagocytic and nonspecific.

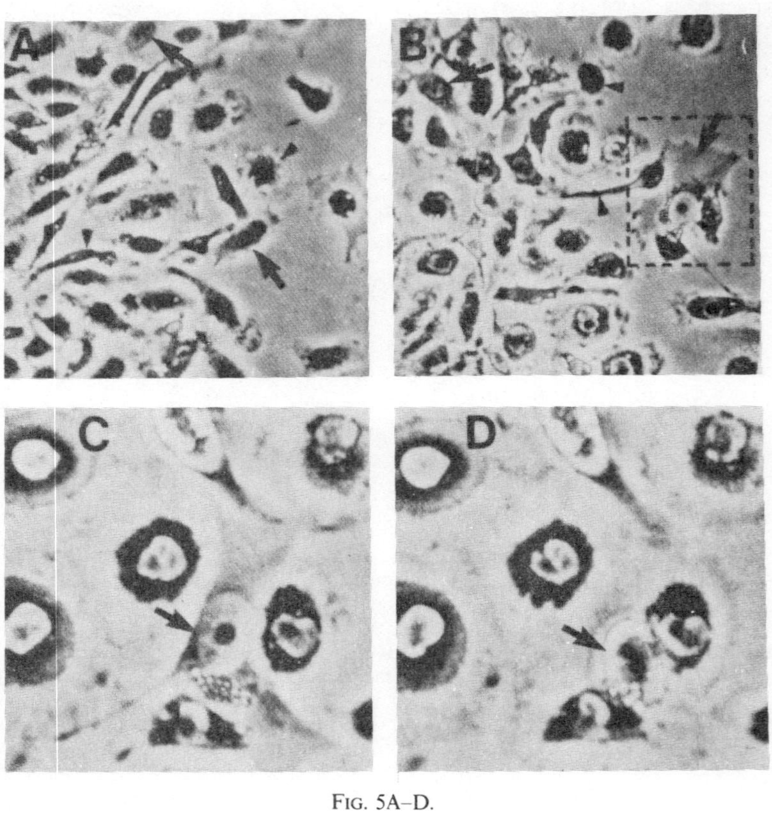

FIG. 5A–D.

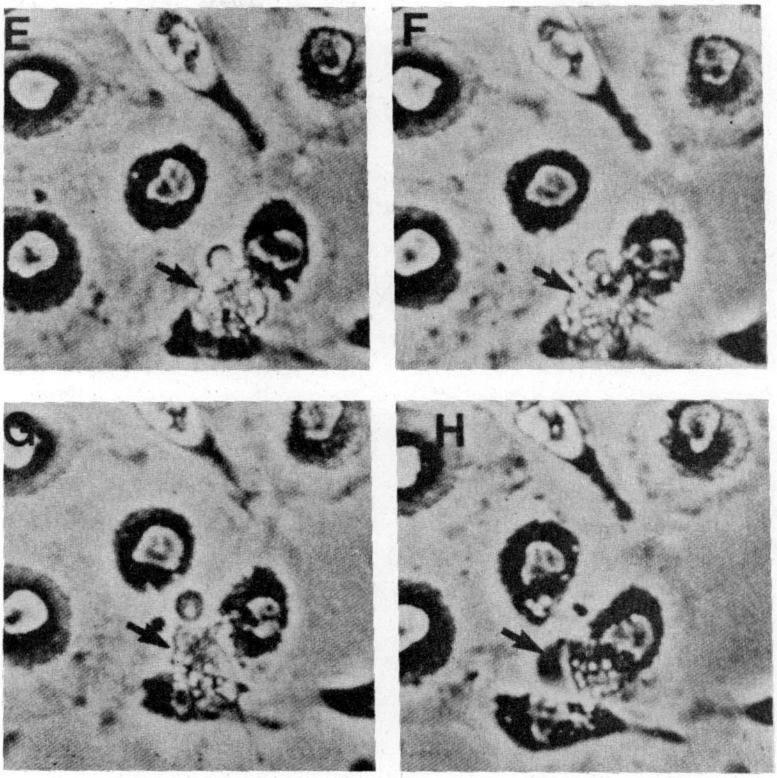

FIG. 5E–H.

FIG. 5. Macrophage colony incubated with 3T12 tumor cells and 5 per cent MAF-rich serum. A—Obtained 2 hr after addition of serum and tumor cells, shows the edge of the macrophage colony. Approximate edge runs from top to bottom and 2/3 in from the left. Tumor cells are best identified by their prominent nucleoli (arrow). Note that the morphology of the macrophages (pointer) at this time is similar to those shown in Fig. 1A. B—20 hr later, the original organization of the colony is still intact compared to Fig. 1B, but some macrophages have migrated out and interact with the tumor cells. Note the dramatic change in morphology of the macrophages (pointer) to more epithelioid like cells with organelles radially arranged around the nucleus. Dotted line shows area which has been enlarged for subsequent frames shown in Figs 2C, D, E, F and H; interval between frames is 20 min. C—44 hr after addition of tumor cells and serum (24 hr after Fig. 2B). Sequence of cytolysis (zeiosis) for this tumor cell (arrow) is shown here and in subsequent figures. Spread-out tumor cell has three macrophages attached. D—Tumor cell 'rounds up'. E, F and G—multiple blebs of cytoplasm are found all over the tumor cell. H—Dead tumor cell has become detached from the dish: a lytic bleb can be seen at arrow. (Reprinted from Stewart, Adles and Hibbs, 1978, with permission of the publisher.)

Nonspecific resistance to tumor cell growth tends to be restricted anatomically and is associated with the presence of a local population of activated macrophages. Both human studies (Klein, 1968; Morton *et al.*, 1970) and animal studies (Zbar *et al.*, 1970a, b, c) have suggested that the expression of nonspecific resistance to neoplasia may not be systemically expressed but may be limited by anatomical restrictions. Our experiments provide evidence that the anatomical restrictions often observed in nonspecific stimulation of host resistance is due to the distribution of the heterologous inducing antigen, e.g. BCG, and the population of nonspecifically tumoricidal activated macrophages mobilized in response to the heterologous inducing agent (Hibbs, 1975). We also found that local persistence of inducing antigen is required for the continued presence of a population of cytotoxic activated macrophages in an anatomical compartment, e.g. in mice, high levels of BCG tend to remain localized in the anatomical compartment(s) into which they were administered. Likewise, the presence of nonspecifically tumoricidal macrophages in the tissue (when BCG is the inducing micro-organism) tends to be a local phenomenon, also confined to the anatomical compartment(s) that contains high levels of inducing antigen (see Table 2). To further clarify this phenomenon, we related the number of viable BCG organisms present in the peritoneal cavity with the route of BCG

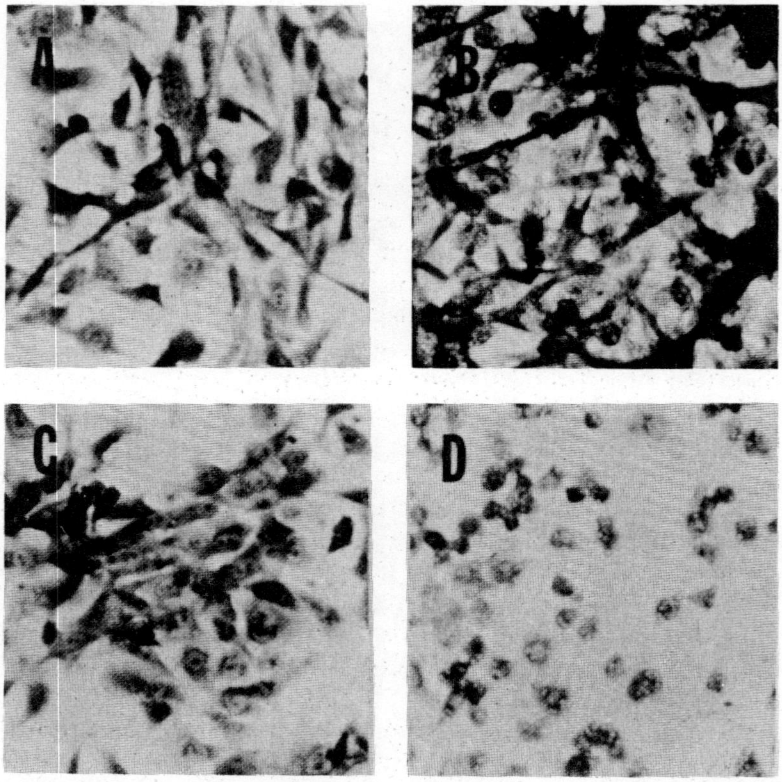

FIG. 6. Photomicrographs of EMT-6 cells cultured in either 5 per cent MAF serum or normal mouse serum with and without colony macrophages. The EMT-6 cells were cultured for 70 hr in medium containing either 5 per cent mouse serum or 5 per cent MAF-serum. Thirty mins prior to rinsing and staining the culture plates with methylene blue, 10^8 heat-killed bakers' yeast and 10 per cent reconstituted guinea-pig complement were added. A—EMT-6 cells were cultured without macrophages but in the presence of 5 per cent normal mouse serum. Note that the tumor cells have not phagocytized the yeast. B—EMT-6 cells were cultured with macrophage colonies and 5 per cent normal mouse serum. The field shown is over the top of a macrophage colony. Note that the tumor cells have overgrown the colony. The macrophages among the tumor cells have ingested yeast. C—EMT-6 cells were cultured without macrophages but with 5 per cent MAF-serum. Note that none of the cells have phagocytized the yeast and that a nearly confluent monolayer of tumor cells has been achieved, indicating this serum was not cytocidal. D—EMT-6 cells were cultured with macrophage colonies and 5 per cent MAF-serum. The field is at the edge of the clone. Note that the macrophages have all phagocytized the yeast. A few scattered viable tumor cells remain which have not phagocytized yeast. (Reprinted from Stewart, Adles and Hibbs, 1978, with permission of the publisher.)

TABLE 2. *Correlation of BCG in Peritoneal Lymph Nodes with the* in vitro *Cytotoxic Effect of Peritoneal Macrophages and Resistance to i.p. Grafts of S180*

Group	Route of administration of BCG*	Colonies of BCG cultured from peritoneal lymph nodes†	Cytotoxic effect of peritoneal macrophages for 3T12 target cells‡	Result of i.p. graft of 4×10^5 S180 cells; No. of mice dead of tumor growth/No. of mice tested
A	Control	0	0	20/20
B	BCG i.p.	3 to 4+	4+	9/20 ($P < 0.001$)
C	BCG i.v.	0 to 1+	0	20/20
D	BCG i.m.R.	0 to 1+	0	19/20

*Intraperitoneal (i.p.), intravenous (i.v.), and right gastrocnemius muscle (i.m.R.).

†Quantitation of BCG growth: 0, no growth; 1+, 1–5 colonies per Petri dish; 2+, 6–20 colonies per Petri dish; 3+, 21–50 colonies per Petri dish; 4+, 51–100 colonies per Petri dish.

‡Cytotoxic effect of macrophages for 3T12 cells; 0, multilayer of 3T12 cells among macrophages (no cytotoxic or cytoastatic effect); 1+, patchy areas of confluent 3T12 growth among macrophages (slight cytostatic effect); 2+, 10–20 3T12 cells per 430X field among macrophages (cytostatic effect); 3+, 3–9 3T12 cells per 430X field among macrophages (cytotoxic effect); 4+, 2 or fewer 3T12 cells per 430X field among macrophages (marked cytotoxic effect). The results are given as the range obtained from three separately performed experiments.

(Reprinted from Hibbs, 1975, with permission of the publisher.)

administration. Between 21 and 100 BCG colonies were cultured from peritoneal lymph nodes of mice receiving BCG intraperitoneally, while none of the mice that received BCG in the right gastrocnemius muscle or by the lateral tail vein grew more than two colonies of BCG from peritoneal lymph nodes. Furthermore, *in vitro* cytotoxicity tests showed that mice infected with BCG by the i.p. route had peritoneal macrophages that were highly tumoricidal while peritoneal macrophages from mice infected with BCG by the lateral tail vein or in the right gastrocnemius muscle were not cytotoxic. In this same study we also noted that the *in vivo* expression of nonspecific resistance to tumor growth in the peritoneal cavity correlated with the presence of inducing antigen (BCG) in high levels and with activated peritoneal macrophages with nonspecific cytotoxic effect for tumorigenic cells *in vitro* (Hibbs, 1975).

In nonspecific tumor cell destruction the cytotoxic activated macrophages induced by a heterologous antigen, (e.g. BCG), were present in the tissues before the tumor cells were grafted and could be detected after the tumor cells had been rejected (Hibbs, 1975). This continuing presence may be due to the fact that the specific antigen (BCG) which induced the production of cytotoxic activated macrophages remains in the tissues and continues to stimulate the chemical signal (lymphokine(s) with macrophage activating properties) that maintains macrophage activation even after the tumor cells have been destroyed. Krahenbuhl and Remington (1974), using listeria infection in mice, found a correlation between the presence of inducing antigen in the tissues (listeria organisms) and the presence of activated peritoneal macrophages with *in vitro* inhibiting effects for tumor cell growth.

Thus it appears that the inducing antigen must be continually present if a population of cytotoxic activated macrophages is to persist in the tissues. If a heterologous antigen, e.g. BCG, is the major stimulus for the mobilization and activation of tumoricidal macrophages *in vivo*, then nonspecific resistance will tend to be expressed where high levels of inducing antigen are present. This would explain why nonspecific resistance induced by a heterologous inducing agent such as BCG is often expressed most effectively only in tissues which contain high levels of the heterologous inducing agent.

On the other hand, specific tumor resistance is not restricted anatomically and is expressed regardless of the location of tumor growth because the inducing antigen is a structural component of the tumor target cell. We also noted that the rejection of an allogeneic lymphoma in mice induces transiently a population of activated macrophages with nonspecific tumoricidal potential (Hibbs, 1975).

It is possible to view the host response to tumor growth as a focusing and amplifying process for mobilization of tumoricidal activated macrophages. In nonspecific resistance, tumoricidal activated macrophages are recruited in response to a heterologous inducing agent as BCG, but it is obvious that there will be less chance that tumor target cells will escape destruction when the antigen inducing the mobilization is a component of the tumor cell itself. Therefore, if a heterologous inducing agent such as BCG has immunologic adjuvant action in addition to the ability to recruit tumoricidal activated macrophages directly, increased sensitization to tumor antigens may occur. In this case, lymphocytes sensitized to tumor antigens will cooperate with lymphocytes which are secreting mediators in response to the heterologous inducing agent (BCG); this cooperation will markedly improve the focusing and amplification of the mobilization of tumoricidal activated macrophages in all areas of tumor growth. However, depending on the timing and method of inoculation, an increased response to tumor specific antigens may not occur following the administration of agents such as BCG, *C. parvum*, or intracellular protozoans. Indeed, the host response to these agents may produce an environment of suppressed rather than enhanced response to specific antigenic stimulation (see following sections).

Finally, as mentioned above, the nonspecific destruction of syngeneic or allogeneic neoplastic cells by activated macrophages involves close contact between effector and target cell and appears to be mediated by molecules derived from the activated macrophage vacuolar system by a mechanism that does not involve phagocytosis (Hibbs,

1974a). The exact manner of transfer of cytotoxic molecules from the activated macrophage to the tumor target cell as well as the exact molecular mechanism(s) of the cytotoxic effect(s) is not presently understood.

6. THE HOST RESPONSE TO INTRACELLULAR INFECTION RESULTS IN A SUPPRESSED RESPONSE TO SPECIFIC IMMUNOLOGIC STIMULI

It is evident that a great variety of agents are capable, under certain experimental conditions, of stimulating nonspecific host resistance to intracellular micro-organisms or allogeneic or sygeneic tumor growth. However, most of these agents, in addition to inducing a population of activated macrophages, are able to stimulate other resistance factors of the host and their actual mechanism of action in increasing tumor resistance could be the result of stimulation of one of several host effector pathways (reviewed by Murahata and Mitchell, 1976). It has been generally believed that treatment of animals with these agents induces an augmented response to unrelated antigens subsequently administered. Indeed, enhanced development of an immune response to challenge with a non-cross reacting antigen appears to contribute to increased resistance in animals treated with many of these agents (reviewed by Yashphe, 1971). However, caution should be exercised in attributing the increased resistance to tumor growth stimulated by these agents, in all circumstances, to an enhanced immune response to tumor antigens.

In fact, we have evidence that in mice with chronic infection with the intracellular protozoans toxoplasma and besnoitia, the ability to express increased nonspecific resistance to intracellular micro-organisms and neoplasia coexists with a state of suppressed reactivity to specific antigens (Hibbs *et al.*, 1973).

TABLE 3. *Effect of Chronic Protozoan Infection on Resistance to* L. monocytogenes (*a Facultative Intracellular Bacterium*), *as well as* S. pneumoniae, *and* K. pneumoniae (*Extracellular Bacteria*)

Bacteria challenge*	Experimental group†	Per cent survival	Day of death after challenge					
			2	3	4	5	6	7
Listeria monocytogenes	Control	0		3	7			
	Chronic toxoplasma infection	90					1	
	Chronic besnoitia infection	100						
Streptococcus pneumoniae	Control	10	4	4	1			
	Chronic toxoplasma infection	0	10					
	Chronic besnoitia infection	10	7	2				
Klebsiella pneumoniae	Control	20		1	6	1		
	Chronic toxoplasma infection	0	7	3				
	Chronic besnoitia infection	0	8		2			

*Bacteria were cultured for 16 hr in trypticase soy broth at 37°C. After centrifugation at 4000 *g* for 10 min. at 4°C, they were washed three times in 0.15 M NaCl and adjusted to an appropriate concentration by measuring turbidity in a spectrophotometer at 620 mu and diluting appropriately in Hanks' balanced salt solution. The actual number of bacteria per ml was determined by plating on trypticase soy agar and counting the number of colonies at 24 hr at 37°C. The LD_{100} for each bacterium was determined and administered to the experimental groups. Swiss Webster female mice were used.

†Infection with toxoplasma or besnoitia was initiated 8 weeks prior to bacterial challenge as previously described (Hibbs *et al.*, 1971). Two weeks prior to bacterial challenge the mice were boosted with the appropriate intracellular protozoan as described (Hibbs *et al.*, 1971).

(From Hibbs, Lambert and Remington, unpublished data.)

We examined nonspecific resistance to a facultative intracellular bacteria, *L. monocytogenes* and to two obligate extracellular bacteria, *S. pneumoniae* and *Klebsiella pneumoniae*, in control mice and in mice with chronic infection with the obligate intracellular protozoans toxoplasma and besnoitia. As is apparent from the data in Table 3 the mice with chronic toxoplasma or besnoitia infection resisted challenge with an LD1000 of listeria. However, virtually all control mice as well as mice with chronic protozoan infection succumbed to *S. pneumoniae* or *K. pneumoniae.* In fact, mice with chronic protozoan infection died more rapidly when infected with obligate extracellular bacteria than did normal control animals. These results suggest that chronic intracellular infection with protozoa selectively confers increased nonspecific resistance to micro-organisms that survive and proliferate in the intracellular environment. These mice are as susceptible as normal control mice to obligate extracellular bacteria whose virulence is due to factors that impair clearance from the tissues by host phagocytic defense cells.

TABLE 4. *Effect of Chronic Toxoplasma Infection on the Response to an Intraperitoneal Graft of S180 cells**

Experimental groups†	Number dead/number grafted	Per cent survival
SWR/J Female		
Control	10/10	0
SWR/J Female		
Chronic toxoplasma infection	4/10	60
Chronic besnoitia infection	3/10	70
C_3H/He Female		
Control	10/10	0
C_3H/He Female		
Chronic toxoplasma infection	6/10	40
Chronic besnoitia infection	5/10	50

*Sarcoma 180 (S180) cells growing in the ascites form were harvested from the peritoneal cavity of an ICR mouse after 7 days of growth. A suspension of 4×10^5 S180 cells was prepared to deliver the desired number of cells in 0.1 ml of Hanks' balanced salt solution.

†Mice were infected with the C_{56} strain of toxoplasma or besnoitia as previously described (Hibbs *et al.*, 1971) 8 weeks prior to tumor grafting. Two weeks before tumor graft the toxoplasma-infected mice were boosted with 5×10^3 trophozoites i.p. of the RH strain of toxoplasma.

(From Hibbs, Lambert and Remington, unpublished data.)

Next, mice with chronic intracellular protozoan infection and normal control mice were given intraperitoneal grasts of sarcoma-180 cells. There is an impressive increased survival four months after grafting the S-180 cells in the group of mice that had chronic infection with toxoplasma or besnoitia (Table 4). In these experiments, as we noted previously, there is a strong correlation between expression of increased nonspecific resistance to an intracellular pathogen and increased nonspecific resistance to neoplastic cells.

Next we examined *in vitro* the nonspecific tumoricidal properties of peritoneal macrophages from toxoplasma or besnoitia-infected mice as well as normal control mice. Peritoneal macrophages from mice with chronic protozoan infection were activated and were markedly cytolytic for syngeneic or allogeneic tumorigenic target cells, but either had no effect or were only cytostatic for normal syngeneic or allogeneic fibroblasts (Table 5). Normal control peritoneal macrophages did not inhibit the growth of tumorigenic or normal target cells. The tumorigenic target cells grew to a multilayer and the normal fibroblasts to a monolayer after 72 hr of culture with peritoneal macrophages from normal mice. As we noted in earlier experiments, the *in vivo* expression of increased

TABLE 5. *Effect of Normal and Activated Macrophages on Normal and Tumorigenic Cells* in vitro*

Effector cells	Target cells					
Source of peritoneal macrophages	Sarcoma KHT (H-2^k)	L Cell (H-2^k)	Balb/c 3T12 (H-2^d)	C_3H/He MEF† (H-2^k)	DBA/2 MEF (H-2^d)	Balb/c MEF (H-2^d)
SWR/J Female						
Control (H-2^q)	0	0	0	0	0	0
SWR/J Female						
Chronic toxoplasma infection	4+	4+	4+	0–1+	0–1+	0–1+
Chronic besnoitia infection	4+	4+	4+	0–2+	0–1+	0–2+
C_3H/He Female						
Control (H-2^k)	0	0	0	0	0	0
C_3H/He Female						
Chronic toxoplasma infection	4+	4+	4+	0–1+	0–1+	0–1+
Chronic besnoitia infection	4+	4+	4+	1–2+	0–1+	0–1+

*Cytotoxicity test was performed as previously described (Hibbs, 1974b). The results are given as the range obtained from three experiments which were performed separately.
†MEF = normal mouse embryo fibroblasts.
Symbols used:
0 = multilayer of tumorigenic target cells or confluent monolayer of normal target cells among activated macrophages (AM).
1+ = patchy areas of confluent target cell growth among AM (slight cytostatis).
2+ = 10–20 target cells per 400X field among AM (cytostatis).
3+ = 3–9 target cells per 400X field among AM (cytotoxic effect).
4+ = 2 or less target cells per 400X field among AM (marked cytotoxic effect).
(From Hibbs, Lambert and Remington, unpublished data.)

nonspecific resistance to neoplasia correlates with the *in vitro* ability of peritoneal macrophages to nonspecifically kill as well as suppress proliferation of neoplastic cells.

Next we determined the rate of rejection of normal skin grafts when donor and recipient mice differed at the major histocompatibility locus. We found that both groups

TABLE 6. *Effect of Chronic Toxoplasma Infection on the Rejection of Allografts of Normal Skin*

Experimental groups*†	Average weight (g)	Graft	Number	Day of rejection	Mean survival time (days)
SWR/J Female Control (H-2q)	26	Primary	10	(1 × 10) (3 × 11) (6 × 12)	11.5 ± 1.5
SWR/J Female Chronic toxoplasma infection	25.8	Primary	11	(1 × 14) (1 × 15) (1 × 17) (1 × 18) (2 × 19) (1 × 20) (1 × 21) (2 × 22) (1 × 23)	19.1 ± 5.0
C_3H/He Female Control (H-2^k)	25.1	Primary	10	(2 × 10) (6 × 11) (2 × 12)	11.0 ± 1.0
C_3H/He Female Chronic toxoplasma infection	24.5	Primary	10	(1 × 13) (2 × 14) (1 × 16) (1 × 18) (1 × 19) (2 × 21) (2 × 22)	18.0 ± 5.0
SWR/J Female Control	—	Secondary	6	(2 × 7) (1 × 8) (3 × 9)	8.2 ± 1.2
SWR/J Female Chronic toxoplasma infection	—	Secondary	7	(2 × 5) (3 × 6) (1 × 12) (1 × 13)	7.6 ± 5.6

*Mice were infected with the C_{56} strain of toxoplasma as previously described (Hibbs *et al.*, 1971) 7 weeks prior to primary skin grafting. Two weeks before primary skin grafting the toxoplasma-infected mice boosted with 5×10^3 trophozoites i.p. of the RH strain of toxoplasma.
†Second-set grafts were applied approximately 3 weeks after rejection of primary grafts.
(From Hibbs, Lambert and Remington, unpublished data.)

of mice with chronic toxoplasma infection showed impaired rejection of primary grafts of normal skin ($P = <0.001$), when compared to normal control mice (Table 6). However, there was no significant difference in the second set rejection between toxoplasma infected and normal mice. These results demonstrate a dramatic difference in the response to neoplastic grafts (enhanced rejection) and normal grafts (suppressed rejection) in mice with chronic toxoplasma infection.

We then tested the response of mice with chronic toxoplasma infection and of normal control mice to tetanus toxoid, a thymus dependent antigen, using methods described previously by Ipsen (1954, 1959). The group of mice with chronic toxoplasma infection did not mount an effective primary response to tetanus toxoid, in these mice the effective dose 50 (ED_{50}) of tetanus toxoid (22LF/ml) was greater than 0.1 ml per mouse which was the highest immunizing dose used (Table 7). The ED_{50} for primary immunization of normal control mice was 0.0053 ml per mouse of tetanus toxoid (22LF/ml). However, toxoplasma infection had no effect on the secondary response to tetanus toxoid. The ED_{50} of tetanus toxoid was the same for normal mice and mice with chronic toxoplasma infection following secondary immunization.

We also tested another thymus dependent antigen, sheep red blood cells (SRBC), and obtained results identical to those achieved for grafts of normal skin and tetanus toxoid (Table 8). The primary response of mice with chronic toxoplasma and besnoitia infection

TABLE 7. *Effect of Chronic Toxoplasma Infection on Primary Immunization with Tetanus Toxoid*

Primary immunization of uninfected mice
ED_{50} = 0.0053 ml/mouse of tetanus toxoid 22Lf/ml*

Dose of toxoid/ mouse†	No. of mice	Day of death after inoculation 2	3	4	5	6	7	Survivors With tetanus	Survivors Without tetanus	Mean score
0.1000	3								3	6
0.0500	3								3	6
0.0250	3								3	6
0.0125	3								3	6
0.0064	3	1							2	4
0.0032	3	2			1					1.3
0.0016	3	3								0
No toxoid	3	3								0
Score		0	2	2	3	3	3		6	

Primary immunization of mice with chronic toxoplasma infection
ED_{50} = >0.1 ml/mouse of tetanus toxoid 22Lf/ml*

Dose of toxoid/ mouse†	No. of mice	Day of death after inoculation 2	3	4	5	6	7	Survivors With tetanus	Survivors Without tetanus	Mean score
0.1000	3	1						2		3
0.0500	3		2					1		2.0
0.0250	3	1	1					1		1.7
0.0125	3	2					1			1.3
0.0064	3	3								0
0.0032	3	3								0
0.0016	3	3								0
No toxoid	3	3								0
Score		0	2	2	3	3	3	4	6	

*The bioassay for tetanus antitoxin is a modification of the method described by Ipsen (1959). Swiss Webster female mice were infected with the C_{56} strain of toxoplasma as previously described (Hibbs *et al.*, 1971), 8 weeks prior to primary immunization with tetanus toxoid. Two weeks before primary immunization the mice were boosted with 5×10^3 trophozoites of the RH strain of toxoplasma.

†Tetanus toxoid was obtained through the courtesy of Dr. Leo Levine, Department of Public Health, Boston, Mass. The tetanus was diluted to give the appropriate dose for each group of Swiss Webster mice and was administered s.c. in the right flank. Challenge with 15 MLD of tetanus toxin (also kindly supplied by Dr. Levine) was 14 days after immunization with tetanus toxoid.

(From Hibbs, Lambert and Remington, unpublished data.)

TABLE 8. *Effect of Chronic Toxoplasma and Besnoitia on Primary and Secondary Immunization with Sheep Red Blood Cells (SRBC)*

		Hemagglutinin titers*			
		Primary response‡		Secondary response§	
Group†	Number of mice	i.p.	i.v.	i.p.	i.v.
Normal controls	12	9(9–10)	8(7–10)	12(12–13)	11(10–12)
Chronic toxoplasma infection‖	12	7(4–8)	6(4–9)	12(11–13)	11(10–12)
Chronic besnoitia infection‖	12	6(3–8)	5(4–7)	12(11–13)	12(11–13)

*All groups were immunized with 0.2 ml of a 10 per cent suspension of SRBC.

†Log_2 of reciprocal of highest serum dilution showing complete agglutination Median (range).

‡Mice bled 7 days after primary injection of SRBC.

§Mice received a second 0.2 ml injection of 10 per cent SRBC 12 days after the primary immunization and bled 3 days after.

‖Infection with toxoplasma or besnoitia was initiated 8 weeks before primary immunization with SRBC as previously described (Hibbs *et al.*, 1971). Two weeks prior to SRBC immunization the mice were boosted with the appropriate protozoan as described (Hibbs *et al.*, 1971).

(From Hibbs, Lambert and Remington, unpublished data.)

was suppressed when compared to normal control mice, but the secondary response of mice with chronic protozoan infection was normal. The purpose of these studies was to help clarify the relative role of cytotoxic activated macrophages in host resistance to neoplasia. It had previously been documented that chronic infection with intracellular protozoan parasites enhances the listericidal (Ruskin *et al.*, 1969) and tumoricidal capabilities of activated macrophages (Hibbs *et al.*, 1972b). We wanted to determine in a series of parallel experiments if other components of the host response to non-self were enhanced in mice with chronic protozoan infection. If specific immune responses were markedly enhanced, this could explain, either partially or entirely, why these mice show increased resistance to tumor development without participation of cytotoxic activated macrophages. However, our experiments show that increased nonspecific resistance to tumor development in mice with chronic protozoan infection is not associated with increased reactivity of cellular (skin allograft rejection) and humoral (antibody response to SRBC and tetanus toxoid) immune responses. In fact, the results show that chronic intracellular protozoan infection induces a state of immunosuppression. These findings lend circumstantial evidence to the idea that activated macrophages participate at the effector level in the expression of increased nonspecific resistance to tumor growth in mice with chronic protozoan infection; these same data are against the possibility that increased resistance to tumor growth in these mice is due solely to an augmented immune response to tumor-associated antigens. Therefore, chronic infection with toxoplasma or besnoitia activate host macrophages which are the effector cells in the mediation of nonspecific resistance to intracellular pathogens and neoplasia. At the same time, chronic intracellular protozoan infection suppresses specific immunologic reactions.

It is important to distinguish which effector mechanism—specific or nonspecific—is responsible for the expression of resistance in a given experimental situation. However, it is clear that nonspecific macrophage mediated effector function and specifically mediated effector functions can coexist and function effectively in the same host with chronic intracellular protozoan infection as is demonstrated by the normal secondary immune responses to rejection of normal skin grafts, secondary hemagglutinin response to SRBC, and secondary antitoxin response to tetanus toxoid. In pathological conditions in which both specific and nonspecific mechanisms are important, as in resistance to neoplastic growth or intracellular micro-organisms, it is likely that the most effective host response will occur when both mechanisms of resistance interact in a cooperative rather than antagonistic fashion.

Suppression of primary immune responses has been demonstrated in infections with other protozoans. Strickland *et al.* (1973) reported depressed levels of hemagglutinins, hemolysins, and spleen plaque-forming cells in mice with chronic toxoplasma infection challenged with sheep erythrocytes. Also, Huldt *et al.* (1973) showed that mice with chronic toxoplasma infection had reduced immunological reactivity to SRBC and polio virus vaccine. The latter group noted that the weight of the thymus gland was markedly reduced in relation to body weight in mice with chronic toxoplasma infection. In addition, they determined that decreased thymus size was not due to adrenocortical hyperactivity. Neither of these groups measured secondary immune responses in mice with chronic toxoplasma infection.

McGregor and Barr (1962) suggested that malaria infection in African children may have an immunosuppressive effect. Subsequently, a number of studies demonstrated that plasmodium infection in mice can produce immunosuppression (Salaman *et al.*, 1969; Barker, 1971; Greenwood *et al.*, 1971; Voller *et al.*, 1972; Viens *et al.*, 1974; Weidanz and Rank, 1975; McBride *et al.*, 1977; McBride and Micklem, 1977). The primary humoral antibody response to SRBC, tetanus toxoid, type III pneumococcal vaccine, bovine serum albumin, and pertussis vaccine was found to be diminished in mice with malaria. However, not all immune responses were found to be suppressed in these studies. For example, the primary humoral response to ΦX-174 bacteriophage, keyhole limpet hemocyanin, and human serum albumin were normal. Also the rejection of primary skin allografts was not prolonged in mice with malaria. Greenwood *et al.* (1972) confirmed that children with acute malaria have a diminished antibody response to tetanus toxoid.

Chronic *Trypanosoma congolense* infection in rabbits suppressed skin test reactivity to mycobacterial proteins as well as peripheral blood lymphocyte responses to purified protein derivative and phytohemagglutinin. Supernatant fluids of antigen-stimulated lymphnode cell cultures from *T. congolense*-infected rabbits also did not have migration inhibitory factor activity but did have normal levels of blastogenic factor activity (Mansfield and Wallace, 1974). It has been clearly documented that *Trypanosoma brucei* infection in mice suppresses thymus-dependent antibody responses (Goodwin *et al.*, 1972; Longstaffe *et al.*, 1973; Murry *et al.*, 1973). Finally, Purvis (1977) showed that *Babesia microti* infection in mice is accompanied by a marked depression in the ability to elicit an IgM as well as an IgG antibody response to SRBC. Correlated with the gradual disappearance of the parasites from the blood there was a slow return to normal immune responsiveness. Contact sensitivity to oxazolone and allograft survival were not affected by *B. microti* infection.

In addition to protozoans, infection with other micro-organisms has been shown to produce suppression of immune responses (reviewed by Bullock, 1976). Virus infection can have a profound effect on immunologic reactivity. (Reviewed by Notkins *et al.*, 1970.) For example, influenza infection in humans decreased skin test reactivity (Read *et al.*, 1972) and Cytomegalovirus infection in mice markedly lowered resistance to *Pseudomonas aeruginosa*, *Staphylococcus aureus* and *C. albicans* (Hamilton *et al.*, 1976, 1977). Starr and Berkovich (1964) noted that children with tuberculosis who contracted measles had suppressed skin test reactions to tuberculin proteins for as long as 42 days after the appearance of the rash. It has also been reported that measles infection reduces the response of peripheral blood lymphocytes to suboptimal concentrations of phytohemagglutinin as compared to cells from normal subjects (Finkel and Dent, 1973). Hall and Kantor (1972) showed that mumps infection in guinea-pigs produced depressed reactivity to skin test antigens. However, skin test sensitivity could be adoptively transferred to normal recipients from previously sensitized animals with active mumps infection even though the donors were anergic to the antigens at the time of transfer. These results suggest that the environment produced by active mumps infection produced suppression of immunologic reactivity. Blair *et al.* (1971) demonstrated that mice infected with the mammary tumor virus (MTV) were less vigorous in humoral antibody response and cell mediated immune response to unrelated antigens than were syngeneic MTV-free controls. Immunologic deficiency could be detected in mice neonatally infected with MTV as well as adult animals soon after introduction of the virus.

Chronic helminth infection can also have a suppressive effect on immunologic responsiveness. *Mesocestoides coiti*-infected mice developed fewer antibody secreting cells to

SRBC (a thymus-dependent antigen) and dinitrophenylated Ficoll (a thymus-independent antigen) if the antigen was inoculated into an anatomical compartment containing the cestode parasites (Mitchell and Handman, 1977). Infection with two other helminths has also been shown to cause immunosuppression in mice. *Schistosoma mansoni* infection suppressed *in vitro* responses of spleen and lymphnode cells to the T-cell mitogens phytohemagglutinin and concanavalin A (Pelley *et al.*, 1976), and *Trichinella spiralis* infection inhibited the hemagglutinin response to SRBC (Faubert and Tanner, 1971). Systemic mycotic infection in man has also been reported to produce immunosuppression. Cantanzaro *et al.* (1974) have reported depression of responsiveness to skin test antigens in patients with disseminated coccidioidomycosis.

Complete Freund's adjuvant and BCG are well established adjuvants (reviewed by Murahata and Mitchell, 1976, and pp. 275ff in this volume). However, in properly designed experiments these and other bacterial adjuvants such as *C. parvum* can depress rather than enhance immunologic responses (reviewed by Schwab, 1975). Scott (1972a) demonstrated that mice that had been inoculated with *C. parvum* 7 days earlier exhibited suppressed phytohemagglutinin, mixed lymphocyte, and graft vs host reactivity. Also, depending on the timing of administration, BCG either enhanced or suppressed skin allograft rejection in mice (Zschiesche and Heinecke, 1973). Mice infected with *Mycobacterium lepraemurium* had a depressed response to SRBC (Watson *et al.*, 1975), and peripheral blood mononuclear cells from patients with leprosy had decreased responsiveness to phytohemagglutinin, streptolysin O, and purified protein derivative (Bullock and Fasal, 1971).

It is apparent that infection with pathogens from many of the major taxonomic groups of micro-organisms can produce measurable depression of immunologic reactivity. It is interesting and significant that many of the microbes that produce immunosuppression have also been shown, under appropriate experimental conditions, to induce increased nonspecific resistance to intracellular infection and neoplastic growth.

7. THE MACROPHAGE IS AN EFFECTOR CELL CAPABLE OF SUPPRESSING IMMUNOLOGIC RESPONSES

Scott (1972b) demonstrated that a micro-organism (*C. parvum*) capable of increasing nonspecific resistance to infection and neoplasia as well as acting as an immunologic adjuvant can also suppress mitogen and antigen triggered lymphocyte responses. He noted that spleen cells and blood lymphocytes from mice pretreated with *C. parvum* were refractory or markedly unresponsive to stimulation with phytohemagglutinin *in vitro*. In addition, Scott observed that mice pretreated with *C. parvum* had impaired mixed lymphocyte and graft-versus-host (GVH) reactivity (Scott, 1972a). He demonstrated in these studies that the suppressive effect of *C. parvum* on the phytohemagglutinin responsiveness of T-lymphocytes was mediated by macrophages that were functionally modified by the presence of *C. parvum* in the tissues. Utilizing adoptive transfer experiments, Loose *et al.* (1972) showed that the profound reduction in splenic plaque forming cells in mice infected with *Plasmodium berghei* was due to functional changes in the macrophages of the infected animals. Subsequent studies have confirmed that macrophages activated by the host response to micro-organisms or their products can produce immunosuppression. Mokyr and Mitchell (1975) demonstrated suppression of lymphocyte responses by macrophages from BCG infected mice. Kirchner *et al.* (1975a), in studies that carefully characterized the suppressor cells as macrophages, showed that spleen cells from *C. parvum* treated mice strongly depressed responses to the T-lymphocyte mitogens phytohemagglutinin and Concanavalin A. The response to the B-lymphocyte mitogen, bacterial endotoxin, was also strongly inhibited in mice injected with 2.1 mg of *C. parvum.* However, after injection of one-tenth of this dose, a relative sparing of the reponse to bacterial endotoxin was noted, whereas the response to phytohemagglutinin was still suppressed. Work in other laboratories has confirmed that *C. parvum* induced immunosuppression in mice is mediated by macrophage effector cells (Lee and Berry, 1977; Wing and Remington, 1977; Bash, 1978). Klimpel and Henney (1978) reported that BCG infection in mice induced the appearance of suppressor macrophages which inhibited T-lymphocyte proliferation as well as the differentiation of T-lymphocytes to cytotoxic effector cells via a process that did not require proliferation. Bennett *et al.* (1978) showed that splenic macrophages from BCG-treated mice prevented the *in vitro* sensitization of both T and non-T cytotoxic cells. The suppressor cells were present in normal bone marrow and were attracted to the spleen by intravenous BCG. It has been noted that infection with the intracellular protozoan *T. brucei* induced a population of macrophages that suppressed both T- and B-lymphocyte responses (Eardley and Jayawardena, 1977). Wing and Remington (1977) demonstrated that activated peritoneal macrophages harvested from toxoplasma infected mice were effective suppressors of Concanavalin A induced lymphocyte transformation. These results strongly suggest that the immunosuppression documented in mice with chronic toxoplasma or besnoitia infection could be mediated by activated macrophage suppressor cells. Other studies also suggest that activated macrophages suppress DNA synthesis in lymphocytes stimulated by antigen or mitogen under *in vitro* conditions that are similar to those in which activated macrophages have been shown to kill or inhibit the proliferation of neoplastic cells (Keller, 1975; Baird and Kaplan, 1975, Baird and Kaplan, 1977a, b).

It is possible that immunosuppression mediated by activated macrophages could be responsible for enhancing tumor growth in certain circumstances. Piessens *et al.* (1970) have reported a possible example in rats infected with BCG. The experimental design may be one of the major determinants of whether resistance to neoplastic growth is increased or decreased following administration of micro-organisms or micro-organism components. For a detailed discussion of immunosuppression mediated by macrophages, see Oehler *et al.* (1978).

8. DOES MACROPHAGE ACTIVATION INDUCED BY SOLUBLE LYMPHOCYTE PRODUCTS (LYMPHOKINES) RESULT IN ACQUISITION OF AN INCREASED POTENTIAL FOR EXPRESSION OF IMMUNOSUPPRESSIVE AS WELL AS TUMORICIDAL EFFECT BY ACTIVATED MACROPHAGES?

It is well established that both T- and B-lymphocytes respond to specific antigen or nonspecific mitogens by secreting lymphokines capable of inducing macrophage activation (Reviewed by David and David, 1972; David, 1975; Cohen, 1977) and that lymphokine activated macrophages can nonspecifically kill neoplastic cells *in vitro* (Piessens *et al.*, 1975; Fidler, 1975). Supernatants of PPD-stimulated BCG immune spleen cell cultures (Ruco and Meltzer, 1977; 1978; Ruco *et al.*, 1978) or serum from mice with chronic BCG infection injected i.v. with old tuberculin (Hibbs *et al.*, 1977) contain lymphokines which induce macrophage differentiation to the nonspecifically tumoricidal state. Tadakuma *et al.* (1976) examined the biochemical and biophysical properties of soluble immune response suppressor (SIRS) present in a supernatant rich in lymphokines and able to suppress plaque-forming cell responses to SRBC by murine spleen cells *in vitro*. The SIRS was obtained from supernatant fluids of murine spleen cell cultures incubated with Concanavalin A for 48 hr; these cultures were also found to contain macrophage migration inhibition factor (MIF). These workers were unable to dissociate SIRS activity from MIF activity and suggest that SIRS and MIF may be the same factor. This possibility is supported by studies which demonstrated that intravenously administered MIF significantly suppressed the ability of animals to express delayed hypersensitivity (Yoshida and Cohen, 1974). In addition, macrophage activating factor (MAF), which induces macrophage differentiation to the nonspecifically tumoricidal state, cannot be dissociated from MIF activity, suggesting that these two factors are also similar if not identical (Churchill *et al.*, 1975). Therefore, it is possible that SIRS, MIF and MAF activities reside in the same molecule or family of molecules. If so, the same signal or signals that induce macrophage differentiation to the nonspecifically tumoricidal state could also induce macrophages to suppress not only lymphocyte proliferation, but possibly also certain differentiated functions of lymphocytes not dependent on proliferation. The ability of suppressor activated macrophages to suppress lymphocyte proliferation and possibly differentiation could be an expression of a mechanism for negative feedback regulation of macrophage mobilization and activation of foci of antigenic stimulation within the tissues; if this is so, it is a manifestation of normal homeostasis. According to this hypothesis, local suppression of lymphocyte mediated recruitment and activation of macrophages within infected or antigen containing tissue would occur when a critical number of adequately activated (differentiated in terms of microbicidal or tumoricidal capability) macrophages had arrived at the involved site. Such negative feedback control could assure economical utilization of components of the acquired cellular immune response as well as minimize or prevent host mediated damage to normal cells within the infected or antigen containing tissue.

This view has been supported in other experimental situations, besides chronic intracellular microbial infection, or the presence of certain killed microbial agents, or their products within the tissues; e.g. suppressor macrophages have been identified in mice undergoing GVH reactions and mice bearing the highly antigenic Moloney sarcoma. These three experimental situations—presence of microbial agents in the tissues, the GVH reaction, and regressing Moloney sarcomas—all have in common strong stimulation of cellular immunity and as a result all cause mobilization of large numbers of activated macrophages within tissues involved in the pathologic process.

Induction of a GVH reaction in mice produces increased resistance to the facultative intracellular bacterium *L. monocytogenes*, and peritoneal macrophages from these mice have a greatly increased capacity to destroy another facultative intracellular bacterium, *Salmonella typhimurium* (Blandon, 1969). In addition, mice undergoing a GVH reaction have a markedly depressed humoral antibody response to SRBC, keyhold limpet hemocyanin, and bovine serum albumin (Koltay *et al.*, 1965; Blanden, 1969), as well as a delay in primary and secondary allograft rejection (Lapp and Moller, 1969). It was demonstrated that spleen cells from mice undergoing GVH reactions were able to suppress the plaque forming response of normal spleen cells to SRBCs (Sjoberg, 1971) and that depletion of macrophages (phagocytic cells) but not T-lymphocytes reversed the immunosuppression (Sjoberg, 1972).

Moloney sarcomas are highly antigenic and induce a strong cellular immune response in syngeneic hosts. Spontaneously regressing Moloney sarcomas contain a high percentage of macrophages that are nonspecifically tumoricidal when tested *in vitro* (Russell and McIntosh, 1977). Progressing Moloney sarcomas also contain large numbers of macrophages, but when macrophages derived from progressing Moloney sarcomas are tested *in vitro* they do not kill tumor cells. However, macrophages derived from progressing Moloney sarcomas are activated because they can be made nonspecifically tumoricidal *in vitro* if a small amount of bacterial endotoxin (1–10 ng/ml) is added to the culture medium (Russell *et al.*, 1977). Therefore, mice bearing regressing or progressing Moloney sarcomas have a large population of activated macrophages that have been generated by the host response to tumor specific or virus specific antigens and interestingly enough, the macrophages isolated from spontaneously regressing sarcomas are more highly activated than those isolated from progressing sarcomas. Spleen cells from mice bearing regressing Moloney sarcomas have a suppressed response to phytohemagglutinin. In a series of extensive studies it has been clearly documented that adherent and phagocytic cells mediate the immunosuppression in these mice (Kirchner *et al.*, 1974, 1975a, b; Glaser *et al.*, 1976). It is significant that the peak suppressor cell activity occurred 14 days after virus inoculation and was coincident with the peak of the primary cellular immune response. Separate subpopulations of activated macrophages may be responsible for immunosuppression and tumoricidal effect. Because of the highly pleiotypic nature of the macrophage activation response, it is possible that the immunosuppressive effects of macrophages could be expressed at differentiation stages that precede acquisition of nonspecific tumoricidal stage of macrophage differentiation.

9. THERE ARE A NUMBER OF BIOCHEMICAL MECHANISMS THAT POTENTIALLY COULD HAVE A ROLE IN PRODUCING IMMUNOSUPPRESSION INDUCED BY ADMINISTRATION OF MICROBIAL AGENTS

There are probably a number of mechanisms at work in the immunosuppression noted in animals with chronic infection with intracellular micro-organisms or after administration of certain killed micro-organisms or their components. Indeed, a number of potential mechanisms have been elucidated in *in vitro* models, but the biological significance of each is difficult to assess at the present time (reviewed by Nelson, 1976; Oehler *et al.*, 1978; Allison, 1978). We will discuss molecular mechanisms identified as a possible explanation for inhibition of proliferation of normal target cells as well as inhibition of proliferation and/or lysis of neoplastic cells.

The secretion of arginase by macrophages and the subsequent depletion of the culture medium of arginine can be responsible for suppressing lymphocyte or neoplastic cell proliferation in some *in vitro* models (Kung *et al.*, 1977; Currie, 1978). Opitz *et al.* (1975a, b) noted that macrophages secrete thymidine into the culture medium. They also made the important observation that thymidine secreted by macrophages into the culture medium competes with and inhibits the incorporation of ^{3}H-thymidine into cells undergoing DNA synthesis. The amount of thymidine elaborated by macrophages is sufficient to inhibit the growth of EL-4 murine lymphoma cells which are extremely sensitive to thymidine blockade. Although sufficient 'cold' thymidine is present to inhibit ^{3}H-thymidine uptake, other dividing cells, unlike EL-4 cells, are not susceptible to thymidine blockade by concentrations of thymidine achieved in macrophage culture supernatant fluid (Stadecker *et al.*, 1977). The relevance to *in vivo* lymphocyte function of experimental results that are produced by secretion of arginase or thymidine by macrophages in 'closed' *in vitro* systems is not clear. However, in view of these findings, *in vitro* studies of activated macrophage produced stasis or lysis of target cells can be unambiguously interpreted only if the possible influence of arginase and thymidine secretion is evaluated in the experimental protocol.

Macrophages synthesize and secrete the second, third, and fourth components of complement (Brade *et al.*, 1977; Littman and Ruddy, 1977; reviewed by Colten, 1974) as well as factor B of the alternate complement pathway (Bentley *et al.*, 1977). The extent to which macrophages utilize complement components as cytotoxic effector molecules is not known. However, it has been demonstrated that the complement cleavage product C3a, produced by endotoxin activated macrophages can lyse neoplastic cells (Ferluga *et al.*, 1978) as well as lymphocytes stimulated to undergo blast transformation (Ferluga *et al.*, 1976). Therefore, the elaboration of C3a, or possibly other complement components, by activated macrophages is a potential effector mechanism capable of inhibiting the growth of or lysing of micro-organisms, neoplastic cells and stimulated lymphocytes.

Macrophages are capable of synthesis and release of prostaglandins *in vitro* (Myatt *et al.*, 1975; Gordon *et al.*, 1976; Humes *et al.*, 1977; Glatt *et al.*, 1977; Kurland and Bockman, 1978). Adherent cell populations that are presumably macrophages have been demonstrated to suppress, via prostaglandin release, mitogen induced lymphocyte proliferation as well as production of migration inhibition factor (Gordon *et al.*, 1976; Goodwin *et al.*, 1977a, b). It is of interest that E series prostaglandins are more effective in suppressing mitogen induced T-lymphocyte proliferation than in suppressing mitogen induced B-lymphocyte proliferation. The suppressor effect is eliminated by pre-treatment of macrophages (adherent cells) with the cyclo-oxygenase inhibitor indomethacin. The elaboration and release of prostaglandins by macrophages is an attractive feedback control mechanisms of possible biologic significance for regulation of lymphocyte function and, ultimately, macrophage activity.

Cultured mouse peritoneal macrophages (Glasgow and Habel, 1963) or rabbit alveolar macrophages (Acton and Myrvik, 1966) are capable of interferon synthesis and release. Bacterial endotoxin exposure induces rabbit peritoneal macrophages to release interferon

(Smith and Wagner, 1967). In addition, BCG infection in mice induces splenic macrophages to secrete type II (immune) interferon (Neumann and Sorg, 1977). These latter workers demonstrated that unfractionated spleen cells release type II interferon upon exposure to mitogens or specific antigen. When adherent spleen cells were removed, interferon production was greatly reduced and lymphocyte proliferation was markedly increased. Brodeur and Merigan (1975) showed that type I (L cell) interferon suppressed *in vivo* antibody response to SRBC and bacterial endotoxin. Both primary and secondary responses were affected. Subsequent work demonstrated that type II interferon was more immunosuppressive than type I interferon (Sonnenfeld *et al.*, 1977). Taken together these results suggest that interferon can produce immunosuppression, that macrophages are capable of interferon secretion, and that interferon production by macrophages is an inducible function dependent on the state of macrophage differentiation. It has also been reported that interferon can induce macrophages to differentiate to the nonspecifically tumoricidal state (Schultz *et al.*, 1977). Therefore, it is possible that molecules with interferon like activity are capable of inducing macrophage activation toward the tumoricidal stage as well as acting as negative feedback inhibitors in the regulation of lymphocyte function.

Lipoproteins have immuno-regulatory activity in addition to transport function. Chisari *et al.* (1976) after isolating an abnormal minor species of low density lipoprotein (LDL) from the serum of patients with acute hepatitis B as well as patients with chronic active hepatitis, found that it inhibited the formation of sheep erythrocyte rosettes with T-lymphocytes. Subsequently, Curtiss and Edgington (1976) identified a discrete subpopulation of LDL (LDL–In) in normal human serum which inhibited, at low concentrations, phytohemagglutinin, pokeweed mitogen, and allogeneic stimulation of human lymphocytes *in vitro*. These workers also showed that an appropriate concentrations unfractionated LDL or high density lipoprotein (HDL) suppressed lymphocyte proliferation responses. Others have showed that very low density lipoprotein (VLDL), intermediate density lipoprotein (IDL), LDL and HDL inhibit antigen and mitogen induced DNA synthesis by lymphocytes (Morse *et al.*, 1977; Waddell *et al.*, 1976). VLDL, IDL and LDL obtained by sequential ultracentrifugation of human plasma without further subfractionation, all have the potential to inhibit lymphocyte proliferation. Furthermore, Curtiss *et al.* (1977) demonstrated that intravenous administration of human LDL–In to mice suppressed the primary anti-SRBC hemagglutination response. The activity of the administered LDL–In was influenced by the dose of antigen, e.g. maximal inhibition of hemagglutination response was obtained with low antigen doses. Both *in vivo* and *in vitro* LDL–In is a potent inhibitor of primary lymphocyte responses to lectins and antigens while it has no demonstrable effect on secondary responses (Curtiss and Edgington, 1977; Edgington *et al.*, 1977). It is of interest that we found that chronic infection with the intracellular protozoans, toxoplasma or besnoitia, inhibited primary but not secondary immune responses (see Section 6). It is possible, although there is no experimental evidence to support this, that chronic intracellular infection can produce immunosuppression by modulating the interaction of immuno-regulatory lipoproteins with immunocompetent cells and/or by increasing the quantity of lipoproteins present in the plasma and interstitial fluids.

10. CONCLUSION

It is clear from data presented in this review that the presence of microbial agents within the tissues can activate a macrophage mediated host defense mechanism that inhibits cellular proliferation and, in certain situations, causes cellular lysis. Examples include: (1) nonspecific inhibition of proliferation and survival of intracellular microorganisms within the vacuolar apparatus of activated macrophages, (2) nonspecific inhibition of proliferation and survival of neoplastic cells in close contact with activated macrophages, and (3) nonspecific inhibition by activated macrophages of lymphocyte proliferation and possibley certain types of lymphocyte differentiation not dependent on proliferation. It will be necessary to characterize relevant biochemical effectors and their mechanism of action in the control of both normal and neoplastic cell growth mediated by macrophages as well as the environmental factors that regulate this macrophage function if continuing progress is to be made in this area of biology. It is possible that similar mechanisms may be utilized by macrophages to control the intracellular growth of intracellular micro-organisms, to inhibit the extracellular growth of neoplastic cells, and to suppress immunologic responses dependent on lymphocyte function.

Acknowledgements—Supported by grants from the Veterans Administration, Washington, D.C., and the National Institute of Health.

REFERENCES

ACTON, J. D. and MYRVIK, Q. N. (1966) Production of interferon by alveolar macrophages. *J. Bact.* **91**: 2300.

ALEXANDER, P. and EVANS R. (1971) Endotoxin and double stranded RNA render macrophages cytotoxic. *Nature New Biol.* **232**: 76.

ALLISON, A. C. (1978) Mechanisms by which activated macrophages inhibits lymphocyte responses. *Immunological Rev.* **40**: 3.

ANDERSON, S. E. JR. and REMINGTON, J. S. (1974) Effect of normal and activated human macrophages on *Toxoplasma gondii. J. Exp. Med.* **139**: 1154.

ANDERSON, S. E. JR., BAUTISTA, S. and REMINGTON, J. S. (1976) Induction of resistance to *Toxoplasma gondii* in human macrophages by soluble lymphocyte products. *J. Immunol.* **117**: 381.

BAIRD, L. G. and KAPLAN, A. M. (1975) Immunoadjuvant activity of pyran copolymer—I. Evidence for direct stimulation of T-lymphocytes and macrophages. *Cellular Immunol.* **20**: 167.

BAIRD, L. G. and KAPLAN, A. M. (1977a) Macrophage regulation of mitogen-induced blastogenesis—I. Demonstration of inhibitory cells in the spleens and peritoneal exudages of mice. *Cellular Immunol.* **28**: 22.

BAIRD, L. G. and KAPLAN, A. M. (1977b) Macrophage regulation of mitogen-induced blastogenesis—II. Mechanism of inhibition. *Cellular Immunol.* **28**: 36.

BARKER L. R. (1971) Experimental malaria: effects upon the immune response to different antigens. *J. infect. Dis.* **123**: 99.

BASH, J. A. (1978) Suppression of rat T cell proliferation by *Corynebacterium parvum*: T cell requirement for induction. *J. Reticuloendothelial Soc.* **23**: 63.

BASIC, I., MILAS, L., GRDINA, D. J. and WITHERS, H. R. (1974) Destruction of hamster ovarian cell cultures by peritoneal macrophages from mice treated with *Corynebacterium granulosum. J. natn. Cancer Inst.* **52**: 1839.

BENNETT, J. A., RAO, V. S. and MITCHELL, M. S. (1978) Systemic Bacillus Calmette-Guérin activates natural suppressor cells. *Proc. Nat. Acad. Sci.* U.S.A. **75**: 5142.

BENTLEY, C., HADDING, U., BITTER-SUERMANN, D. and BRADE, V. (1977) Effect of *in vivo* stimulation of mice on the secretion of factor B of the alternative complement pathway by peritoneal macrophages. *Eur. J. Immunol.* **7**: 183.

BLAIR, P. B., KRIPKE, M. L., LAPPE, M. A., BONHAG, R. S. and YOUNG, L. (1971) Immunologic deficiency associated with mammary tumor virus (MTV) infection in mice: hemagglutinin response and allograft survival. *J. Immunol.* **106**: 364.

BLANDEN, R. V. (1969) Increased antibacterial resistance and immunodepression during graft-versus-host reactions in mice. *Transplantation* **7**: 484.

BLANDEN, R. V. (1970) Mechanism of recovery from a generalized viral infection: mousepox—I. The effects of anti-thymocyte serum. *J. Exp. Med.* **132**: 1035.

BLANDEN, R. V. (1971a) Mechanism of recovery from a generalized viral infection: mousepox—II. Passive transfer of recovery mechanisms with immune lymphoid cells. *J. Exp. Med.* **133**: 1074.

BLANDEN, R. V. (1971b) Mechanism of recovery from a generalized viral infestion: mousepox—III. Regression of infectious foci. *J. Exp. Med.* **133**: 1090.

BLANDEN, R. V., LEFFORD, M. J. and MACKANESS, G. B. (1969) The host response to Calmette-Guérin bacillus infection in mice. *J. Exp. Med.* **129**: 1079.

BLANDEN, R. V., MACKANESS, G. B. and COLLINS, F. M. (1966) Mechanisms of acquired resistance in mouse typhoid. *J. Exp. Med.* **124**: 585.

BLANDEN, R. V. and MIMS, C. A. (1973) Macrophage activation in mice infected with ectromelia or lymphocytic choriomeningitis viruses. *Aust. J. exp. Biol. med. Sci.* **51**: 393.

BRADE, V., HALL, R. E. and COLTEN, H. R. (1977) Biosynthesis or pro-C3, a precursor of the third component of complement. *J. Exp. Med.* **146**: 759.

BRADNER, W. T., CLARKE, D. A. and STOCK, C. C. (1958) Stimulation of host defense against experimental cancer—I. Zymosan and sarcoma 180 in mice. *Cancer Res.* **18**: 347.

BRODEUR, B. R. and MERIGAN, T. C. (1975) Mechanism of the suppressive effect of interferon on antibody synthesis *in vivo. J. Immunol.* **114**: 1323.

BULLOCK, W. E. (1976) Allergy and infection. *Adv. Internal Med.* **21**: 149.

BULLOCK, W. E. JR. and FASAL, P. (1971) Studies of immune mechanisms in leprosy—III. The role of cellular and humoral factors in impairment of the *in vitro* immune response. *J. Immunol.* **106**: 888.

CATANZARO, A., SPITLER, L. and MOSER, K. M. (1974) Immunotherapy of coccidioidomycosis. *J. Clin. Invest.* **54**: 690.

CHISARI, F. V., ROUTENBERG, J. A. and EDGINGTON, T. S. (1976) Mechanisms responsible for defective human T-lymphocyte sheep erythrocyte rosette function associated with hepatitis B virus infections. *J. Clin. Invest.* **57**: 1227.

CHURCHILL, W. H. JR., PIESSENS, W. F., SULIS, C. A. and DAVID, J. R. (1975) Macrophages activated as suspension cultures with lymphocyte mediators devoid of antigen become cytotoxic for tumor cells. *J. Immunol.* **115**: 781.

CLARK, I. A. and ALLISON, A. C. (1976) Protection of mice against *Babesia* and *Plasmodium* with BCG. *Nature* **259**: 309.

CLARK, I. A., WILLIS, E. J., RICHMOND, J. E. and ALLISON, A. C. (1977) Suppression of babesiosis in BCG-infected mice and its correlation with tumor inhibition. *Infection and Immunity* **17**: 430.

CLEVELAND, R. P., MELTZER, M. S. and ZBAR, B. (1974) Tumor cytotoxicity *in vitro* by macrophages from mice infected with *Mycobacterium bovis* strain BCG. *J. natn. Cancer Inst.* **52**: 1887.

COHEN, S. (1977) The Role of cell-mediated immunity in the induction of inflammatory responses. *Am. J. Path.* **88**: 502.

COLLINS, F. M., MACKANESS, G. B. and BLANDEN, R. V. (1966) Infection-immunity in experimental salmonellosis. *J. Exp. Med.* **124**: 601.

COLTEN, H. R. (1974) Biosynthesis of serum complement. *Progr. Immunol.* **1**: 183.

COPPEL, S. and YOUMANS, G. P. (1969) Specificity of the anamnestic response produced by *Listeria monocytogenes* or *Mycobacterium tuberculosis* to challenge with *Listeria monocytogenes. J. Bacteriol.* **97**: 127.

CURRIE, G. A. (1978) Activated macrophages kill tumor cells by releasing arginase. *Nature* **273**: 758.

CURTISS, L. K. and EDGINGTON, T. S. (1976) Regulatory serum lipoproteins: Regulation of lymphocyte stimulation by a species of low density lipoprotein. *J. Immunol.* **116**: 1452.

CURTISS, L. K. and EDGINGTON, T. S. (1977) Effect of LDL–In, a normal immunoregulatory human serum low density lipoprotein, on the interaction of macrophages with lymphocytes proliferating in response to mitogen and allogeneic stimulation. *J. Immunol.* **118**: 1966.

CURTISS, L. K., DEHEER, D. H. and EDGINGTON, T. S. (1977) *In vivo* suppression of the primary immune response by a species of low density serum lipoprotein. *J. Immunol.* **118**: 648.

DAVID, J. R. (1975) Macrophage activation by lymphocyte mediators. *Fedn Proc.* **34**: 1730.

DAVID, J. R. and DAVID, R. R. (1972) Cellular hypersensitivity and immunity. *Prog. Allergy* **16**: 300.

EARDLEY, D. D. and JAYAWARDENA, A. N. (1977) Suppressor cells in mice infected with *Trypanosoma brucei. J. Immunol.* **119**: 1029.

EDGINGTON, T. S., HENNEY, C. H. and CURTISS, L. K. (1977) The bioregulatory properties of serum low density lipoprotein inhibitor (LDL–In) on the generation of killer T cells. In *Leukocyte Culture Conference* 11th, p. 736, Tucson, Arizona. *Regulatory mechanisms in lymphocyte activation*, LUCAS, D. O. (ed.). Academic, Press, N.Y.

ELBERG, S. S. (1960) Cellular immunity. *Bact. Rev.* **24**: 67.

ELBERG, S. S., SCHNEIDER, P. and FONG, J. (1957) Cross immunity between *Brucella melitensis* and *Mycobacterium tuberculosis*, intracellular behavior of *Brucella melitensis* in monocytes from vaccinated animals. *J. Exp. Med.* **106**: 545.

FAUBERT, G. and TANNER, C. E. (1971) *Trichinella spiralis*: inhibition of sheep hemagglutinins in mice. *Exp. Parasital* **30**: 120.

FEARON, D. T. (1978) Regulation by membrane sialic acid of BIH-dependent decay-dissociation of amplification C3 convertase of the alternate complement pathway. *Proc. Natn. Acad. Sci. U.S.A.* **75**: 1971.

FEARON, D. T. and AUSTEN, F. K. (1977) Activation of the alternate complement pathway with rabbit erythrocytes by circumvention of the regulatory action of endogenous control proteins. *J. Exp. Med.* **146**: 22.

FERLUGA, H., SCHORLEMMER, H. U., BAPTISTA, L. and ALLISON, A. C. (1976) Cytolytic effects of the complement cleavage products C3a. *Br. J. Cancer* **34**: 626.

FERLUGA, J., SCHORLEMMER, U., BAPTISTA, L. C. and ALLISON, A. C. (1978) Production of the complement cleavage product, C3a, by activated macrophages and its tumorolytic effects. *Clin. Exp. Immunol.* **31**: 512.

FIDLER, I. J. (1975) Activation *in vitro* of mouse macrophages by syngeneic, allogeneic, or xenogeneic lymphocyte supernatants. *J. natn. Cancer Inst.* **55**: 1159.

FIDLER, I. J. (1978) Recognition and destruction of target cells by tumoricidal macrophages. *Israel J. Med. Sci.* **14**: 177.

FINKEL, A. and DENT, P. B. (1973) Abnormalities in lymphocyte proliferation in classical and atypical measles. *Cell. Immunol.* **6**: 41.

FOWLES, R. E., FAJARDO, I. M. LEIBOWITCH, J. L. and DAVID, J. R. (1973) The enhancement of macrophage bacteriostatis by products of activated lymphocytes. *J. Exp. Med.* **138**: 952.

FRENKEL, J. K. (1967) Adoptive immunity to intracellular infection. *J. Immunol.* **98**: 1309.

GENTRY, L. O. and REMINGTON, J. S. (1971) Resistance against cryptococcus conferred by intracellular bacteria and protozoa. *J. Infect. Dis.* **123**: 22.

GLASER, M., KIRCHNER, H., HOLDEN, H. T. and HERBERMAN, R. B. (1976) Inhibition of cell-mediated cytotoxicity against tumor-associated antigens by suppressor cells from tumor-bearing mice. *J. natn. Cancer Inst.* **56**: 865.

GLASGOW, L. A. and HABEL, K. (1963) Interferon production by mouse leukocytes *in vitro* and *in vivo. J. Exp. Med.* **117**: 149.

GLASGOW, L. A., FISCHBACH, J., BRYANT, S. M. and KERN, E. R. (1977) Immunomodulation of host resistance to experimental viral infections in mice: effects of *Corynebacterium acnes*, *Corynebacterium parvum*, and *Bacillus Calmette-Guérin. J. Infect. Dis.* **135**: 763.

GLATT, M., KALIN, H., WAGNER, K. and BRUNE, K. (1977) Prostaglandin release from macrophages: an assay system for anti-inflammatory drugs *in vitro. Agents and Actions* **7**: 321.

GODAL, T., REES, R. J. W. and LAMVIK, J. O. (1971) Lymphocyte-mediated modification of blood-derived macrophage function *in vitro*; inhibition of growth of intracellular mycobacteria with lymphokines. *Clin. Exp. Immunol.* **8**: 625.

GOODWIN, J. S., BANKHURST, A. D. and MESSNER, R. P. (1977a) Suppression of human T-cell mitogenesis by prostaglandin. *J. Exp. Med.* **146**: 1719.

GOODWIN, J. S., MESSNER, R. P., BANKHURST, A. D., PEAKE, G. T., SAIKI, J. H. and WILLIAMS, R. C. JR. (1977b) Prostaglandin-producing suppressor cells in Hodgkin's disease. *New Engl. J. Med.* **297**: 963.

GOODWIN, L. G., GREEN, D. G., GUY, M. W. and VOLLER, A. (1972) Immunosuppression during trypanosomiasis. *Br. J. Exp. Path.* **53**: 40.

GORDON, D., BRAY, M. A. and MORLEY, J. (1976) Control of lymphokine secretion by prostaglandins. *Nature* **262**: 401.

GREENWOOD, B. M., PLAYFAIR, J. H. L. and TORRIGIANI, G. (1971) Immunosuppression in murine malaria. I. General characteristics. *Clin. Exp. Immunol.* **8**: 467.

GREENWOOD, B. M., BRADLEY-MOORE, A. M., PALIT, A. and BRYCESSON, A. D. M. (1972) Immunosuppression in children with malaria.-*Lancet*, **i**: 169.

HALL, C. B. and KANTOR, F. S. (1972) Depression of established delay hypersensitivity by mumps virus. *J. Immunol.* **108**: 81.

HALPERN, B. N., BIOZZI, G., STIFFEL, C., MOUTON, D., MORAND, J., BOUTHILLIER, Y. and DECREUSFOND, C. (1966) Inhibition of tumour growth by administration of killed *Corynebacterium parvum. Nature* (Lond.) **212**: 853.

HAMILTON, J. R., OVERALL, J. C. JR. and GLASGOW, L. A. (1976) Synergistic effect on mortality in mice with murine cytomegalovirus and *Psudomonas aeruginosa, Staphylococcus*, or *Candida albicans* infections. *Infection and Immunity* **14**: 982.

HAMILTON, J. R., OVERALL, J. C. JR. and GLASGOW, L. A. (1977) Synergistic infection with murine cytomegalovirus and *Candida albicans* in mice. *J. Infect. Dis.* **135**: 918.

HARDY, D., KOTLARSKI, I. (1971) Resistance of mice to Ehrlich ascites tumour after immunization with live *Salmonella enteritidis* 11RS. *Aust. J. exp. Biol. med. Sci.* **49**: 271.

HIBBS, J. B. JR. (1973) Activated macrophage nonimmunologic recognition: target cell factors to contact inhibition. *Science* **180**: 868.

HIBBS, J. B., JR. (1974a) Discrimination between neoplastic and nonneoplastic cells *in vitro* by activated macrophages. *J. Natn. Cancer Inst.* **53**: 1487.

HIBBS, J. B., JR. (1974b) Heterocytolysis by macrophages activated by Bacillus Calmette-Guérin: lysosome exocytosis into tumor cells. *Science* **184**: 468.

HIBBS, J. B., (1975) Activated macrophages as tumoricidal effector cells—II. Requirement for local persistence of inducing antigen. *Transplantation* **19**: 81.

HIBBS, J. B., JR., LAMBERT, L. H., JR. and REMINGTON, J. S. (1971) Resistance to murine tumors conferred by chronic infection with intracellular protozoa, *Toxoplasma gondii*, and *Besnoitia jellisoni. J. Infect. Dis.* **124**: 587.

HIBBS, J. B., JR., LAMBERT, L. H., JR. and REMINGTON, J. S. (1972a) Adjuvant induced resistance to tumor development in mice. *Proc. Soc. exp. Biol. Med.* **139**: 1053.

HIBBS, J. B., LAMBERT, L. H., JR. and REMINGTON, J. S. (1972b) Possible role of macrophage mediated nonspecific cytotoxicity in tumor resistance. *Nature New Biol.* **235**: 48.

HIBBS, J. B., JR. LAMBERT, L. H., JR. and REMINGTON, J. S. (1972c) Control of carcinogenesis: A possible role for the activated macrophage. *Science* **177**: 998.

HIBBS, J. B., JR., LAMBERT, L. H., JR. and REMINGTON, J. S. (1972d) *In vitro* nonimmunologic destruction of cells with abnormal growth characteristics by adjuvant activated macrophages. *Proc. Soc. exp. Biol. Med.* **139**: 1049.

HIBBS, J. B., JR., LAMBERT, L. H., JR. and REMINGTON, J. S. (1973) Activated macrophage nonspecific tumor resistance associated with immunosuppression. *J. Reticuloendothel. Soc.* **13**: 368.

HIBBS, J. B., JR., TAINTOR, R. R., CHAPMAN, H. A., JR. and WEINBERG, J. B. (1977) Macrophage tumor killing: influence of the local environment. *Science* **197**: 279.

HOLTERMANN, O. A., KLEIN, E. and CASALE, G. P. (1973) Selective cytotoxicity of peritoneal leucocytes for neoplastic cells. *Cellular Immunol.* **9**: 339.

HOWARD, J. G., BIOZZI, G., HALPERN, B. N., STIFFEL, C. and MOUTON, D. (1959) The effect of mycobacterium tuberculosis (BCG) infection on the resistance of mice to bacterial endotoxin and *Salmonella enteritidis* infection. *Br. J. exp. Path.* **40**: 281.

HULDT, G., GARD, S. and OLOVSON, S. G. (1973) Effect of *Toxoplasma gondii* on the thymus. *Nature* (Lond.) **244**: 301.

HUMES, J. L., BONNEY, R. J., RELUS, L., DAHLGREN, M. E., SADOWSKI, S. J., KUEHL, F. A., JR. and DAVIS, P. (1977) Macrophages synthesize and release prostaglandins in response to inflammatory stimuli. *Nature (Lond.)* **269**: 149.

IPSEN, J. (1954) Inherent immunizability to tetanus toxoid, based on studies in pure inbred mice. *J. Immunol.* **72**: 243.

IPSEN, J. (1959) Differences in primary and secondary immunization of inbred mouse strains. *J. Immunol.* **83**: 448.

JONES, T. C. (1975) Phagosome-lysosome interaction with toxoplasma. In *Mononuclear Phagocytes in Immunity, Infection, and Pathology*, p. 595, VAN FURTH, R. (ed.). Blackwell Scientific Publications, Oxford.

KAPLAN, A. M., MORAHAN, P. S. and REGELSON, W. (1974) Induction of macrophage-mediated tumor-cell cytotoxity by pyran copolymer. *J. Natn. Cancer Inst.* **52**: 1919.

KELLER, R. (1975) Major changes in lymphocyte proliferation evoked by activated macrophages. *Cellular Immunol.* **17**: 542.

KELLER, R. and JONES, V. E. (1971) Role of activated macrophages and antibody inhibition and enhancement of tumour growth in rats. *Lancet* **ii**: 847.

KIRCHNER, H., HOLDEN, H. T. and HERBERMAN, R. B. (1975a) Splenic suppressor macrophages induced in mice by injection of *Cornebacterium parvum. J. Immunol.* **115**: 1212.

KIRCHNER, H., MUCHMORE, A. V., CHUSED, T. M., HOLDEN, H. T. and HERBERMAN, R. B. (1975b) Inhibition of proliferation of lymphoma cells and lymphocytes by suppressor cells from spleens of tumor-bearing mice. *J. Immunol.* **114**: 206.

KLEIN, E. (1968) Tumors of the skin—X. Immunotherapy of cutaneous and nucosal neoplasms. *N.Y. J. Med.* **68**: 900.

KLIMPEL, G. R. and HENNEY, C. S. (1978) BCG-induced suppressor cells—I. Demonstration of a macrophage-like suppressor cell that inhibits cytotoxic T-cell generation *in vitro*. *J. Immunol.* **120**: 563.

KOLTAY, M., KINSKY, R. G., ARNASON, B. G. and SCHAFFNER, J. B. (1965) Immunoglobulins and antibody formation in mice during the graft versus host reaction. *Immunology* **9**: 581.

KRAHENBUHL, J. L. and REMINGTON, J. S. (1971) *In vitro* induction of nonspecific resistance in macrophages by specifically sensitized lymphocytes. *Infection and Immunity* **4**: 337.

KRAHENBUHL, J. L. and REMINGTON, J. S. (1974) The role of activated macrophages in specific and nonspecific cytostasis of tumor cells. *J. Immunol.* **113**: 507.

KRAHENBUHL, J. L., LAMBERT, L. H. and REMINGTON, J. S. (1976) Effects of *Corynebacterium parvum* treatment and *Toxoplasma gondii* infection on macrophage-mediated cytostasis of tumour target cells. *Immunology* **31**: 837.

KUNG, J. Y., BROOKS, D. N., JAKWAY, J. B., LEONARD, L. L. and TALMAGE, D. W. (1977) Suppression of *in vitro* cytotoxic response by macrophages due to induced arginase. *J. Exp. Med.* **146**: 665.

KURLAND, J. I. and BOCKMAN, R. (1978) Prostaglandin E production by human blood monocytes and mouse peritoneal macrophages. *J. Exp. med.* **147**: 952.

LAPP, W. S. and MOLLER, G. (1969) Prolonged survival of H-2 incompatible skin allografts on F_1, animals treated with parental lymphoid cells. *Immunology* **17**: 339.

LARSON, C. L., USHIJIMA, R. N., FLOREY, J. J., BAKER, R. E. and BAKER, M. B. (1971) Effect of BCG on Friend disease virus in mice. *Nature New Biol.* **229**: 243.

LEE, K. C. and BERRY, D. (1977) Functional heterogeneity in macrophages activated by *Corynebacterium parvum*: characterization of subpopulations with different activities in promoting immune responses and suppressing tumor cell growth. *J. Immunol.* **118**: 1530.

LITTMAN, B. H. and RUDDY, S. (1977) Production of the second component of complement by human monocytes: Stimulation by antigen-activated lymphocytes or lymphokines. *J. Exp. Med.* **145**: 1344.

LONGSTAFFE, J. A., FREEMAN, J. and HUDSON, K. M. (1973) Immunosuppression in trypanosomiasis: Some thymus dependent and thymus independent responses. *Trans. R. Soc. Trop. Med. Hyg.* **67**: 264.

LOOSE, L. D., COOK, J. A. and LUZIO, N. R. D. (1972) Malarial immunosuppression—A macrophage mediated defect. *Proc. helminth. Soc. Wash.* **39**: 484.

LUNDE, M. N. and GELDERMAN, A. H. (1971) Resistance of AKR mice to lymphoid leukemia associated with a chronic protozoan infection, *Besnoitia jellisoni*. *J. Natn. Cancer Inst.* **47**: 485.

LURIE, M. B. (1942) Studies on the mechanism of immunity in tuberculosis: The fate of tubercle bacilli ingested by mononuclear phagocytes derived from normal and immunized animals. *J. Exp. med.* **75**: 247.

MACKANESS, G. B. (1954) The growth of tubercle bacillus in monocytes from normal and vaccinated rabbits. *Am. Rev. Tuberc.* **69**: 495.

MACKANESS, G. B. (1962) Cellular resistance to infection. *J. Exp. Med.* **116**: 381.

MACKANESS, G. B. (1964) The immunologic basis of acquired cellular resistance. *J. Exp. Med.* **120**: 105.

MACKANESS, G. B. (1969) The influence of immunologically committed lymphoid cells on macrophage activity *in vivo*. *J. Exp. Med.* **129**: 973.

MACKANESS, G. B. (1971) Resistance to intracellular infection. *J. Infect. Dis.* **123**: 439.

MACKANESS, G. B., BLANDEN, R. V. and COLLINS, F. M. (1966) Host-parasite relations in mouse typhoid. *J. Exp. Med.* **124**: 573.

MAHMOUD, A. A. F., WARREN, K. S. and STRICKLAND, G. T. (1976) Acquired resistance to infection with *Schistosoma mansoni* induced by *Toxoplasma gondii*. *Nature* **263**: 56.

MANSFIELD, J. M. and WALLACE, J. H. (1974) Suppression of cell-mediated immunity in experimental African typanosomiasis. *Infection and Immunity* **10**: 335.

MATHE, G., AMIEL, J. L., SCHWARZENBERG, L., SCHNEIDER, M., CATTAN, A., SCHLUMBERGER, J. R., HAYAT, M. and DE VASSAL, F. (1969a) Active immunotherapy for acute lymphoblastic leukemia. *Lancet* **i**: 697.

MATHE, G., POUILLART, P. and LAPEYRAQUE, F. (1969b) Active immunotherapy to L1210 leukemia applied after the graft of tumour cells. *Br. J. Cancer* **23**: 814.

MCBRIDE, J. S., MICKLAM, H. S. and URE, J. M. (1977a) Immunosuppression in murine malaria—I. Response to type III pneumococcal polysaccharide. *Immunology* **32**: 635.

MCBRIDE, J. S. and MICKLEM, H. S. (1977b) Immunosuppression in murine malaria—II. The primary response to bovine serum albumin. *Immunology* **33**: 253.

MCGREGOR, I. A. and BARR, M. (1962) Antibody response to tetanus toxoid innoculation in malarious and non-malarious children. *Trans. R. Soc. Trop. Med. Hyg.* **56**: 364.

MELTZER, M. S., TUCKER, R. W., SANFORD, K. K. and LEONARD, E. J. (1975a) Interaction of BCG-activated macrophages with neoplastic and non-neoplastic cell lines *in vitro*: Quantitation of the cytotoxic reaction by release of tritiated thymidine from prelabeled target cells. *J. Natn. Cancer Inst.* **54**: 1177.

MELTZER, M. S., TUCKER, R. W. and BREUER, A. C. (1975b) Interaction of BCG-activated macrophages with neoplastic and nonneoplastic cell lines *in vitro*. Cinemicrographic analysis. *Cellular Immunol.* **17**: 30.

METCHIKOFF, E. (1893) *Lecures in the comparative pathology of inflamation.* Kegan, Paul, Trench and Co., London.

MITCHELL, G. F. and HANDMAN, E. (1977) Studies on immune responses to larval cestodes in mice: A simple mechanism of non-specific immunosuppression in Mesocestoides corti-infected mice. *Ajebak* **55**: 615.

MITSUHASHI, S., SATO, I. and TANAKA, T. (1961) Experimental salmonellosis Intracellular growth of *Salmonella enteridis* ingested in mononuclear phagocytes of mice,, and cellular basis of immunity. *J. Bacteriol.* **81**: 863.

MOKYR, M. B. and MITCHELL, M. S. (1975) Activation of lymphoid cells by BCG *in vitro*. *Cell. Immunol.* **15**: 264.

MOLOMUT, N. and PADNOS, M. (1965) Inhibition of transplantable and spontaneous murine tumours by the M-P virus. *Nature* **208**: 948.

MORSE, J. H., WITTE, L. D. and GOODMAN, D. S. (1977) Inhibition of lymphocyte proliferation stimulated by lectins and allogeneic cells by normal plasma lipoproteins. *J. Exp. Med.* **146**: 1791.

MORTON, D. L., EILBER, F. R., MALMGREN, R. A. and WOOD, W. C. (1970) Immunological factors which influence response to immunotherapy in malignant melanoma. *Surgery* **68**: 158.

MURAHATA, R. I. and MITCHELL, M. S. (1976) Modulation of the immune response by BCG: A review. *Yale J. Biol. Med.* **49**: 283.

MURRY, P. K., URGUHART, G. M. and JENNINGS, F. W. (1973) The response of mice infected with *T. brucei* to the administration of sheep erythrocytes. *Trans. R. Soc. Trop. Med. Hyg.* **67**: 267.

MYATT, L., BRAY, M. A. and GORDON, D. (1975) Macrophages in intrauterine contraceptive devices produce prostaglandins. *Nature (Lond.)* **257**: 227.

NELSON, D. S. (1976) Nonspecific immunoregulation by macrophages and their products. In *Immunobiology of the Macrophage*, p. 235, NELSON, D. S. (ed.). Academic Press, N.Y.

NEUMANN, C. and SORG, C. (1977) Immune interferon—I. Production by lymphokine-activated murine macrophages. *Eur. J. Immunol.* **3**: 719.

NOGUERIA, N. and COHN, Z. A. (1978) *Tryponosoma cruzi*: *in vitro* induction of macrophage microbicidal activity. *J. Exp. Med.* **148**: 288.

NORTH, R. J. (1970a) The relative importance of blood monocytes and fixed macrophages to the expression of cell-mediated immunity to infection. *J. Exp. Med.* **132**: 521.

NORTH, R. J. (1970b) Suppression of cell-mediated immunity to infection by an antimitotic drug. Further evidence that migrant macrophages express immunity. *J. Exp. Med.* **132**: 535.

NORTH, R. J. (1973) The importance of thymus derived lymphocytes in cell mediated immunity to infection. *Cellular Immunol.* **7**: 166.

NOTKINS, A. L., MERGENHAGEN, S. E. and HOWARD, R. J. (1970) Effect of virus infections on the function of the immune system. *A. Rev. Microbiol.* pp. 525–538.

NYKA, W. (1956) Enhancement of resistance to tuberculosis in mice experimentally infected with *Brucella abortus*. *Am. Rev. of Tuber.* **73**: 251.

OEHLER, J. R., HERBERMAN, R. B. and HOLDEN, H. T. (1978) Modulation of immunity by macrophages. *Pharmac. Ther. A.* **2**: 551.

OLD, L. J., BENACERRAF, B., CLARK, D., CARSWELL, E. A. and STOCKERT, E. (1961) The role of the reticuloendothelial system in the host reaction to neoplasia. *Cancer Res.* **21**: 1281.

OLD, L. J., CLARKE, D. A. and BENACERRAF, B. (1959) Effect of Bacillus Calmette-Guérin infection on transplanted tumours in the mouse. *Nature* **184**: 291.

OPITZ, H. G., NIETHAMMER, D., LEMKE, H., FLAD, H. D. and HUGET, R. (1975a) Inhibition of ^{3}H-thymidine incorporation by lymphocytes by a soluble factor from macrophages. *Cellular Immunol.* **16**: 379.

OPITZ, H. G., NEITHAMMER, D. and JACKSON, R. C. (1975b) Biochemical characterization of a factor released by macrophages. *Cellular Immunol.* **18**: 70.

PATTERSON, R. J. and YOUMANS, G. P. (1970) Demonstration in tissue culture of lymphocyte-mediated immunity to tuberculosis. *Infection and Immunity* **1**: 600.

PELLEY, R. P., RUFFIER, J. J. and WARREN, K. S. (1976) Suppressive effect of a chronic Helminth infection, *Schistosomiasis mansoni*, on the *in vitro* responses of spleen and lymph node cells to the T-cell mitogens phytohemagglutinin and concanavalin A. *Infection and Immunity* **13**: 1176.

PIESSENS, W. F., CHURCHILL, W. H. JR and DAVID, J. R. (1975) Macrophages activated *in vitro* with lymphocyte mediators kill neoplastic but not normal cells. *J. Immunol.* **114**: 293.

PIESSENS, W. F., LACHAPELLE, F. L., LEGROS, N. and HEUSON, J. C. (1970) Facilitation of rat mammary tumour growth by BCG. *Nature* **228**: 1210.

PILLEMER, L., BLUM, L., LEPOW, I. H., ROSS, D. A., TODD, E. W. and WARDLAW, A. C. (1954) The properdin system and immunity—I. Demonstration and isolation of a new serum protein, properdin, and its role in immune phenomena. *Science* **120**: 279.

PULLINGER, E. J. (1936) The influence of tuberculosis on the development of *Brucella abortus* infection. *J. Hyg. Comb.* **36**: 456.

PURVIS, A. C. (1977) Immunodepression in *Babesia microti* infections. *Parasitology* **75**: 197.

REED, W. P., OLDS, J. W. and KISCH, A. L. (1972) Decreased skin-test reactivity associated with influenza. *J. infect. Dis.* **125**: 398.

REGELSON, W. and MUNSON, A. E. (1970) The reticuloendothelial effects of interferon inducers: Polyanionic and non-polyanionic prophylaxis against micro-organisms. *Ann. N.Y. Acad. Sci.* **173**: 831.

REMINGTON, J. S. and MERIGAN, T. C. (1969) Resistance to virus challenge in mice infected with protozoa or bacteria. *Proc. Soc. exp. Biol. Med.* **131**: 1184.

RILEY, V. (1966) Spontaneous mammary tumors: Decrease in incidence in mice infected with the LDH virus. *Science* **153**: 1657.

RUCO, L. P. and MELTZER, M. S. (1977) Macrophage activation for tumor cytotoxicity: Induction of tumoricidal macrophages by supernatants of PPD-stimulated Bacillus Calmette-Gúerin-immune spleen cell cultures. *J. Immunol.* **119**: 889.

RUCO, L. P. and MELTZER, M. S. (1978) Macrophage activation for tumor cytotoxicity: Increased lymphokine responsiveness of peritoneal macrophages during acute inflammation. *J. Immunol.* **120**: 1054.

RUCO, L. P., MELTZER, M. S. and ROSENSTREICH, D. L. (1978) Macrophage activation for tumor cytotoxicity: Control of macrophage tumoricidal capacity by the LPS gene. *J. Immunol.* **121**: 543.

RUSKIN, J. and REMINGTON, J. S. (1968) Immunity and intracellular infection: Resistance to bacteria in mice infected with a protozoan. *Science* **160**: 72.

RUSKIN, J., MCINTOSH, J. and REMINGTON, J. S. (1969) Studies on the mechanism of resistance of phylogenetically diverse intracellular organisms. *J. Immunol.* **103**: 252.

RUSSELL, S. W., DOE, W. F. and MCINTOSH, A. T. (1977) Functional characterization of a stable, noncytolytic stage of macrophage activation in tumors. *J. Exp. Med.* **146**: 1151.

RUSSELL, S. W. and MCINTOSH, A. T. (1977) Macrophages isolated from regressing Moloney sarcomas are more cytotoxic than those recovered from progressing sarcomas. *Nature* **268**: 69.

SACHS, J. H., CLARK, R. F. and EGDAHL, R. H. (1960) The induction of immunity with a new filterable agent. *Surgery* **48**: 244.

SALAMAN, N. H., WEDDERBURN, N. and BRUCE-CHWATT, L. J. (1969) The immuno-depressive effect of a murine plasmodium and its interaction with murine oncogenic virus. *J. Gen. Microbiol.* **59**: 391.

SCHULTZ, R. M., PAPAMATHEAKIS, J. D. and CHIRIGOS, M. A. (1977) Interferon: An inducer of macrophage activation by polyanions. *Science* **197**: 674.

SCHWAB, J. H. (1975) Suppression of the immune response by micro-organisms. *Bacteriological Rev.* **39**: 121.

SCOTT, M. T. (1972a) Biological effects of the adjuvant *Corynebacterium parvum*—I. Inhibition of PHA, mixed lymphocyte and GVH reactivity. *Cellular Immunol.* **5**: 459.

SCOTT, M. T. (1972b) Biological effects of the adjuvant *Corynebacterium parvum*—II. Evidence for macrophage-T-cell interaction. *Cellular Immunol.* **5**: 469.

SCOTT, M. T. (1974) *Corynebacterium parvum* as a therapeutic anti-tumor agent in mice II local injection. *J. Natn. Cancer Inst.* **53**: 861.

SHEAR, M. J. (1944) Chemical treatment of tumors—IX. Reactions of mice with primary subcutaneous tumors to injection of a hermorrhage-producing bacterial polysaccharide. *J. Natn. Cancer Inst.* **4**: 461.

SILVERSTEIN, S. (1970) Macrophages and viral immunity. *Seminars in Hematology* **7**: 185.

SIMON, H. B. and SHEAGREN, J. N. 1972) Enhancement of macrophage bactericidal capacity by antigenically stimulated immune lymphocytes. *Cellular Immunol.* **4**: 163.

SINKOVICS, J. G., AHEARNS, J. J., SHIRATO, E. and SCHULLENBERGER, C. C. (1970) Viral leukemogenesis in immunologically and hematologically altered mice. *J. reticuloendoth. Soc.* **8**: 474.

SJOBERG, O. (1971) Antigenic competition *in vitro* of spleen cells subjected to a graft-versus-host reaction. *Immunology* **21**: 351.

SJOBERG, O. (1972) Effect of allogeneic cell interaction on the primary immune response *in vitro. Clin. exp. Immunol.* **12**: 365.

SMITH, T. J. and WAGNER, R. (1967) Rabbit macrophage interferons—I. Conditions for biosynthesis by virus-infected and uninfected cells. *J. Exp. Med.* **125**: 559.

SONNENFELD, G., MANDEL, A. D. and MERIGAN, T. C. (1977) The immunosuppressive effect of type II mouse interferon preparations on antibody production. *Cellular Immunol.* **34**: 193.

STADECKER, M. J., CALDERON, J., KARNOVSKY, M. and UNANUE, E. (1977) Synthesis and release of thymidine by macrophages. *J. Immunol.* **119**: 1738.

STARR, S. and BERKOVICH, S. (1964) Effects of measles, gammaglobulin-modified measles and vaccine measles on the tuberculin test. *New Engl. J. Med.* **270**: 386.

STEWART, C. C., ADLES, C. and HIBBS, J. B. JR. (1978) Cloned macrophages can be induced to kill tumor cells. *J. reticuloendoth. Soc.* **24**: 107.

STRICKLAND, G. T., PETTITT, L. E. and VOLLER, A. (1973) Immunodepression in mice infected with *Toxoplasma gondii. Am. J. Trop. Med. Hyg.* **22**: 452.

SUTER, E. (1953) Multiplication of tubercle bacilli within mononuclear phagocytes in tissue cultures derived from normal animals vaccinated with BCG. *J. Exp. Med.* **97**: 235.

SUTER, E. (1956) Interaction between phagocytes and pathogenic micro-organisms. *Bacteriol. Rev.* **20**: 94.

TADAKUMA, T., KUHNER, A. L., RICH, R. R., DAVID, J. R. and PIERCE, C. W. (1976) Biological expressions of lymphocyte activation—V. Characterization of a soluble immune response suppressor (SIRS) produced by concanavalin A-activated spleen cells. *J. Immunol.* **117**: 323.

VIENS, P., TARZAALI, A. and QUEVILLON, M. (1974) Inhibition of the immune response to pertussis vaccine during *Plasmodium berghei yoelii* infection in mice. *Amer. J. Trop. Med. Hyg.* **23**: 846.

VOLLER, A., GALL, D. and MANAWADU, B. R. (1972) Depression of the antibody response to tetanus toxoid in mice infected with malaria parasites. *Z. Tropenmed. Parasit.* **23**: 152.

WADDELL, C. C., TAUNTON, O. D. and TWOMEY, J. J. (1976) Inhibition of lymphoproliferation by hyperlipoproteinemic plasma. *J. of clin. Invest.* **58**: 950.

WARDLAW, A. C. and PILLEMER, L. (1956) The properdin system and immunity—V. The bactericidal activity of the properdin system. *J. Exp. Med.* **103**: 553.

WATSON, S. R., SLJIVIC, V. S. and BROWN, I. N. (1975) Defect of macrophage function in the antibody response to sheep erythrocytes in systemic *Mycobacterium lepraemurium* infection. *Nature* **256**: 206.

WEIDANZ, W. P. and RANK, R. G. (1975) Regional immunosuppression induced by *Plasmodium berghei yoelii* infection in mice. *Infection and Immunity* **11**: 211.

WEISS, D. W., BONHAG, R. S. and DE OME, K. B. (1961) Protective activity of fractions of tubercle bacilli against isologous tumours in mice. *Nature* **190**: 889.

WILLIAMS, D. M. and REMINGTON, J. S. (1977) Effect of human monocytes and macrophages on *Trypanosoma cruzi. Immunology* **32**: 19.

WILLIAMS, D. M., SAWYER, S. and REMINGTON, J. S. (1976) Role of activated macrophages in resistance of mice to infection with *Trypanosoma cruzi. J. infect. Dis.* **134**: 610.

WING, E. J. and REMINGTON, J. S. (1977) Studies on the regulation of lymphocyte reactivity by normal and activated macrophages. *Cellular Immunol.* **30**: 108.

WOODRUFF, M. F. A. and BOAK, J. L. (1966) Inhibitory effect of injection of *Corynebacterium parvum* on the growth of tumor transplants in isogenic hosts. *Br. J. Cancer* **20**: 345.

YASHPHE, D. J. (1971) Immunological factors in nonspecific stimulation of host resistance to syngeneic tumors. *Israel J. Med. Sci.* **7**: 90.

YOSHIDA, T. and COHEN, S. (1974) Lymphokine activity *in vivo* in relation to circulating monocyte levels and delayed skin reactivity. *J. Immunol.* **112**: 1540.

ZBAR, B., BERNSTEIN, I., TANAKA, T. and RAPP, H. J. (1970a) Tumor immunity produced by the intradermal inoculation of living tumor cells and living *Mycobacterium bovis* (Strain BCG). *Science* **170**: 1217.

ZBAR, B., WEPSIC, H. T. and RAPP, H. V. (1970b) Tumor-graft rejection in syngeneic guinea pigs: Evidence for a two-step mechanism. *J. Natn. Cancer Inst.* **44**: 473.
ZBAR, B., WEPSIC, H. T., RAPP, H. J., STEWART, L. C. and BORSOS, T. (1970c) Two-step mechanism of tumor graft rejection in syngeneic guinea pigs—II. Initiation of reaction by a cell fraction containing lymphocytes and neutrophils. *J. Natn. Cancer Inst.* **44**: 701.
ZSCHIESCHE, W. and HEINECKE, H. (1973) Effects of variable Bacillus Calmette-Guérin regimens on skin graft rejection. *Transplantation* **15**: 172.

CHAPTER 7

MODULATION OF IMMUNITY BY BACILLUS CALMETTE–GUÉRIN (BCG)*

MALCOLM S. MITCHELL* AND RICHARD I. MURAHATA**
** University of Southern California, Los Angeles, USA*
*** Armour-Dial Research Laboratory, Arizona, USA*

1. INTRODUCTION

Bacillus Calmette–Guérin (BCG), an attenuated strain of *Mycobacterium bovis*, was developed as a vaccine against human tuberculosis by Calmette and Guérin at the Pasteur Institute in 1908. Particularly within the past 20 years, BCG has received considerable attention in completely different roles, as an immunological modulator and an 'antitumor' agent. Investigations with this agent in the immunotherapy of cancer have met with some success in different animal systems and with limited success in several trials in man. The majority of this work has been done empirically, with the regression of the tumor or survival of the animal as the endpoint, with relatively less attention to measurement of antitumor immunity. Since the effects of BCG on the immune response are multifaceted, a clearer understanding of what is known of its mechanisms of action may lead to a more rational basis for its use, not only in cancer immunotherapy but also in other immunological applications.

In this review we will first describe some of the effects of BCG on broad phenomena, such as the rejection of tumors and the synthesis of antibody and cell-mediated immunity, and then try to indicate what is known of the specific cellular mechanisms by which it may act.

ANTITUMOR EFFECTS

It is an interesting irony that, while the antitumor effects of BCG have rekindled scientific interest in the whole field of immunological modulation, it is precisely those effects that are the least well understood immunologically. The complexity of the immune response to tumors and the wide variation in modes of administration of BCG account for much of the difficulty. While our subsequent discussion of the effects of BCG on defined populations of lymphoid cells may shed some light on this issue, a general categorization of the antitumor applications may be useful because of their practical importance.

Several broad distinctions might be made. It is important to distinguish between the use of BCG directly into a site of tumor growth (intralesional or intratumoral BCG) and BCG given by vaccination into uninvolved skin or by injection (systemic BCG). In addition, the administration of BCG as a *prophylaxis*, during the period of induction of a tumor or before an inoculum of cells has become a palpable tumor, is distinct from *therapy* of an established tumor. Finally, the use of BCG alone as a nonspecific stimulator of the reticuloendothelial system or of 'immunity' should be distinguished from its use as an *adjuvant*, in conjunction with antigen (tumor cells). The importance of recognizing such categories as these is considerable when attempt-

* *Abbreviations used:* B cells: 'Bursa'-dependent lymphocytes; BCG: Bacillus Calmette-Guérin, strain of *Mycobacterium bovis;* CMI: cell-mediated immunity; Con A: concanavalin A; DMC: delipidated (lipid-free) mycobacterial cells, derived from BCG by exhaustive chloroform-methanol extraction; LPS: lipopolysaccharide (endotoxin); MER: methanol-extraction residue of BCG; MOPC: mineral oil-induced plasmacytoma; NK cells: natural killer cells; PFC: plaque-forming cells; PHA: phytohemagglutinin; PPD: purified protein derivative of *Mycobacterium tuberculosis;* RES: reticuloendothelial system; SRBC: sheep red blood cells; T cells: thymus-dependent lymphocytes.

ing to decide whether on balance BCG is a significant antitumor agent, since it is not a cytotoxic chemical but simply a modifier of the host's intrinsic antitumor response, the effects of which are highly dependent upon scheduling.

Nearly 20 yr ago, Old *et al.* (1959) and Biozzi and co-workers (Biozzi *et al.*, 1959; Halpern *et al.*, 1959) independently showed that BCG increased the resistance of rats and mice to several transplantable tumors, especially lymphomas. BCG was given before or concomitantly with the tumor and thus was an effective immunoprophylactic agent. Mathé (1969) later began treatment of mouse leukemia L1210 with BCG immediately after inoculation of the cells and found that 20 per cent of the mice could be cured if 10^4 tumor cells or fewer were used. Leukemia–lymphomas in mice are the most responsive of tumors to prophylaxis with BCG; Mathé *et al.* (1974) have prolonged survival by systemic pretreatment with BCG before L1210, and have found the established lymphomas frequently responsive to BCG and many other adjuvants (Mathé *et al.*, 1973). The growth of mouse lymphomas has either been inhibited by BCG or unaffected, but never enhanced, whereas solid tumors have been enhanced occasionally.

BCG given systemically inhibited the induction of tumors by methylcholanthrene (Lavrin *et al.*, 1973; Tokunaga *et al.*, 1974) if mice were treated 2 weeks before or after the application of the carcinogen. When the tumors became palpable, treatment was usually ineffective. The growth of methylcholanthrene-induced tumors was not prevented completely but was at least considerably delayed, even in experiments where the final incidence of tumors was the same as in controls (Lavrin *et al.*, 1973). A transient suppression of carcinogen- and virus-induced tumors was also reported earlier by Old *et al.* (1961). The incidence of 'spontaneous' AKR leukemia was prevented by repeated injection of BCG (Ungaro *et al.*, 1973), and MER prevented radiation virus-induced leukemia (Haran-Ghera and Weiss, 1973). All of these data on systemic prophylaxis suggest that many of the effects of BCG on tumors cannot be explained by local granuloma formation and nonspecific destruction of 'innocent' bystander tumor cells, factors which may account, in part, for its intralesional effects. In fact, Old *et al.* (1961) attributed the prophylactic effects to systemic stimulation of the RES, which in broad outline may be correct, with cellular details that we will consider shortly.

Much of the work on immunotherapy of established tumors by BCG has dealt with direct intralesional injection, especially with the transplantable line 10 hepatocarcinoma in the guinea pig (Zbar *et al.*, 1970, 1971, 1972). This tumor, when injected intradermally into the animal, grows progressively, spreads first to regional lymph nodes and is very weakly antigenic for the syngeneic host, thus mimicking many of the attributes of human tumors. The growth of established tumor grafts could be suppressed by intralesional injection of living BCG organisms (Zbar and Tanaka, 1971; Zbar *et al.*, 1970, 1971, 1972, 1973). Bekierkunst (1976) has recently achieved similar results with killed BCG coated with 'cord factor' (trehalose-6,6′-dimycolate) emulsified in mineral oil. Even at a time when the tumor had spread microscopically to regional lymph nodes, intralesional BCG not only caused regression of the treated nodule but also cured approximately 50–60 per cent of the animals. Systemic immunity appeared in these cured guinea pigs after regression of the injected nodules had occurred (Zbar *et al.*, 1973). Interestingly, systemic resistance to the tumor was not induced by such common methods as the injection of killed tumor cells alone or excision of a primary nodule. To further measure the systemic consequences of intralesionally administered BCG, Zbar and co-workers (1970, 1973; Bartlett and Zbar, 1972) injected a mixture of hepatoma cells and living BCG intradermally and measured the ability of guinea pigs to reject various doses of tumor cells elsewhere. They were able to achieve immunity that was tumor-specific and systemic (against small numbers of tumor cells) by mixing BCG with the tumor, but not by injecting each separately. The systemic effect of intralesional BCG is found only after immunity to the tumor has developed, since uninjected contralateral nodules usually do not regress at the same time as the injected tumor.

In mice the efficacy of intralesional BCG or BCG–tumor cell mixtures in producing regression of tumors is far more variable than in the guinea pig. In one study, BCG therapy did not influence the growth of a sarcoma or a carcinoma but cured 2/3 of the mice whose melanomas were injected intralesionally (Faraci and Schour, 1974). Prolonged survival but no cures was produced by intralesional injection into primary methylcholanthrene-induced tumors in these mice. Hawrylko and Mackaness (1973) and Hawrylko (1975) reported that optimal immunization against a mastocytoma occurred when killed tumor cells were injected into a site 'prepared' by injection with BCG 10 days before, i.e. prophylaxis, whereas immunotherapy was ineffective. Even in other experiments where tumor growth was inhibited by immunological adjuvants, the development of systemic immunity in the mouse was inconsistent (Bartlett *et al.*, 1972; Meltzer and Leonard, 1973; Ruskin and Remington, 1971). Bartlett *et al.* (1976) have noted that the ratio of BCG to tumor cells, specifically to LSTRA lymphoma in an experimental inoculum (or by extension, in an injected lesion), was a key determinant of whether systemic immunity developed in the mouse. High ratios favored local rejection but gave suboptimal systemic immunization, whereas low ratios favored systemic immunity at the expense of local rejection.

In patients with melanoma, intralesional therapy with BCG is effective in treating approximately one-half the patients (Morton *et al.*, 1970; Pinsky, 1973), but only 15 per cent of uninjected lesions regress, and only those in the immediate vicinity of the injected nodules. Furthermore, metastatic melanoma frequently develops in individuals whose injected nodules regressed completely. In hamsters, BCG therapy of established tumors or prophylaxis with BCG–tumor cell mixtures was generally ineffective (Fortner *et al.*, 1974).

Thus, while intralesional therapy is often effective and has provided interesting therapeutic models, even when it is useful it is not necessarily conducive to systemic immunity and certainly is not dependent upon it. The site of inhibition of a tumor is characterized histologically by an intense chronic type of inflammatory exudate, consisting predominantly of lymphocytes and macrophages (Hanna *et al.*, 1972a, b; Nathanson, 1972; Lieberman *et al.*, 1974). Granuloma formation is common at these sites. Although the inflammatory response to BCG may be necessary for the expression of tumor resistance, it may not be sufficient, since other inflammatory agents do not have similar effectiveness and may even accelerate tumor growth (Hanna *et al.*, 1972b). Anitgenicity of the adjuvant may be essential for its activity. The most effective BCG preparations are those that are most antigenic (Mackaness *et al.*, 1973). BCG apparently elicits a profound reaction to itself as an antigen, which leads to inflammation and necrosis that encompasses the foreign (tumor) cells in the vicinity and may lead to a systemic state of resistance. All of these activities probably involve the macrophages and lymphocytes in the reactive lesion, with immunity resulting from the sensitization of sufficient memory T-cells.

BCG–tumor cell vaccines deserve further attention because of their potential importance in man, in whom most immunotherapy has thus far been with BCG alone. These combined vaccines offer the possibility of systemic immunization and a true adjuvant effect of the BCG on immunity to an immunogen, but it is apparent from animal studies that the predictability of their success is uncertain. Baldwin and Pimm (1973) found that experimental pulmonary metastases from rat hepatoma could be restricted by BCG or mixtures of BCG and tumor cells, but that metastases were increased with some tumors, those of weak antigenicity. Bekierkunst (1975) has prepared an effective vaccine for the prevention of guinea pig hepatoma, consisting of live hepatoma cells, killed BCG organisms, cord factor and mineral oil, which obviates the need for living BCG. In rats and rabbits, BCG–polyoma cell vaccines have been used to produce 'unblocking' factor in the serum, which then purportedly counteract the deleterious effects of the 'blocking' factor on CMI in those animals (Bansal and Sjögren, 1972). Whether mixtures of BCG and tumor cells in slow release emulsions will prove to be the only effective preventatives, or whether schemes in which pretreatment with BCG is a prominent feature, such as that of Hawrylko and Mackaness (1973), will be effective, remains to be seen.

BCG has not conclusively prevented the development of cancer in man, despite evidence of such an effect in animals. Although two epidemiological studies have suggested that the incidence of leukemia was decreased in children who had received BCG vaccination for tuberculosis (Davignon *et al.*, 1970; Rosenthal *et al.*, 1972), controlled trials where the entrants into the study were randomly assigned have failed to confirm a significantly lower incidence (Comstock *et al.*, 1971, 1975). In fact, in the study of Comstock *et al.* (1975), an excess of lymphosarcoma and Hodgkin's disease was found, together with a slight decrease in the incidence of leukemia.

Deleterious effects have been observed in the tumor-bearing host, particularly when BCG has been given after the tumor was well established. Enhancement of tumor growth in animals has been described by several investigators (Piessens *et al.*, 1971; Bansal and Sjögren, 1973; Lavrin *et al.*, 1973; Mathé *et al.*, 1973) and has been reported anecdotally in man (Levy *et al.*, 1972). BGC cell walls also have enhanced tumor growth when BCG was given to rats prior to a Morris hepatoma (Wepsic *et al.*, 1976). Pretreatment with complete Freund's adjuvant has had similar adverse consequences with virus-induced and carcinogen-induced transplantable tumors (Alford *et al.*, 1969; Meltzer and Leonard, 1973). The explanation for enhancement is uncertain but may involve the stimulation of serum 'blocking factors', antibody–antigen complexes that antagonize CMI to the tumor *in vitro* and presumably *in vivo* as well. Blocking factors were in fact demonstrated with BCG-enhanced polyoma tumors and in a patient with metastatic melanoma after intratumor BCG (Levy *et al.*, 1972; Bansal and Sjögren, 1973). However, the appearance of blocking activity in the serum coincident with metastasis in BCG-treated subjects may be more the consequence of tumor growth than its cause, since soluble tumor antigen shed into the circulation could then elevate blocking activity (Mitchell *et al.*, 1977). Another possible explanation for enhancement by BCG is the induction of suppressor cells, either directly or through immune complexes (Gershon *et al.*, 1974). Finally, the related phenomenon of antigenic competition, which involves suppressor T cells, might be of importance in the enhancement of some tumors. Several groups have reported that BCG has antigenic similarity to some tumors (Borsos and Rapp, 1973; Minden *et al.*, 1976). Whether this helps to explain some of BCG's protective and therapeutic properties and its tumor-enhancing effects under certain conditions is a matter for conjecture. Since some solid tumors have been enhanced by BCG, it is important to recognize that treatment with systemic BCG, particularly if gross tumor is present, not only may be futile but also potentially dangerous.

EFFECTS ON ANTIBODY SYNTHESIS

One of the earliest known effects of tuberculous infection on immunity was the augmentation of antibody synthesis noted by Lewis and Loomis (1924) with SRBC in the guinea pig. Three years later, Dienes and Schoenheit (1927) found increased immunity when ovalbumin or timothy pollen was injected into the granulomatous lesion. Since then, many others have demonstrated the adjuvancy of BCG or its derivatives on antibody synthesis (Miller *et al.*, 1973; Paranjpe and Boone, 1974; Sparks and Breeding, 1974; Steinkuller *et al.*, 1969). Miller *et al.* (1973), in a particularly careful study, found that if the injection of BCG preceded immunization of mice with SRBC by 14 days, maximal augmentation of immunity was achieved. DNA synthesis and cell proliferation were increased in lymphoid tissue after the administration of BCG and appeared to be correlated with its adjuvant effects. Expansion of the pool of antibody-forming cells, B cells, is one possible explanation of BCG's adjuvancy; similar findings by Yashphe and colleagues with MER (1969, 1972) support this. Yet it is uncertain whether the effects on B cells are direct or are mediated through helper T cells. PPD, lipid-free BCG [also termed delipidated mycobacterial cells (DMC)] (Mitchell *et al.*, 1975) and other mycobacterial fractions, principally peptidoglycans, (Damais *et al.*, 1975) are B cell mitogens *in vitro* and may have similar activity *in vivo*. Nevertheless, the necessity for the presence of T cells for many substances to act as adjuvants (Allison and Davies, 1971; Taub and Gershon, 1972) and the important modulatory role of the T cell in antibody production suggest that indirect effects of BCG on antibody formation through the T cell must be considered. Among the many soluble factors released by T cells is one that stimulates antibody synthesis by B cells. This material was elicited by re-exposure to T cells, previously sensitized to BCG *in vivo*, to the same adjuvant (more precisely PPD) *in vitro* (Maillard and Bloom, 1972). The specific immune response of memory T cells reacting to BCG as an antigen led to nonspecific immunostimulation of antibodies to SRBC, via the action of the mediator. Expansion of the pool of helper T cells, in addition to the pool of B cells, is another likely effect, supported by the findings of Kitamura *et al.* (1976). These workers found that living BCG greatly enhanced the response to hamster RBC in SL mice, whose degree of immunity depends sensitively upon helper T cell function. Moreover, BCG stimulation obviated the need for carrier-priming in the response of these mice to the hapten TNP, again suggesting the recruitment of helper T cells. Jacobs *et al.* (1975), studying unimmunized mice, found that MER-treated mice had more theta antigen-positive cells binding SRBC than did controls, direct evidence that helper T cells reactive with antigen were increased by this BCG derivative. The mitogenic effects of BCG on T cells *in vitro* (Mokyr and Mitchell, 1974), with a probable counterpart *in vivo* (Mitchell *et al.*, 1973), may well underlie the expansion and recruitment of these helper T cells. However, since some investigators have failed to observe mitogenic effects of BCG or MER on T cells (Bekierkunst, 1976; Ben-Efraim, 1977), further confirmation must be sought before this explanation can be considered plausible.

BCG also has had immunosuppressive effects on antibody synthesis at certain dosage schedules. Those schedules of BCG that favor delayed hypersensitivity tend to depress antibody synthesis (Mackaness *et al.*, 1974). Repeated scarification of guinea pigs with BCG augmented delayed sensitivity to SRBC but decreased antibody formation (Peters *et al.*, 1974). Our own unpublished observations on hemagglutinin titers in mice to SRBC confirm these data, since mice given 1×10^7 viable BCG i.p. 14 and 4 days before, if SRBC had titers of 1:2, compared with 1:16 for controls without BCG. BCG failed to augment cytotoxic antibody titers against H-2d alloantigens when given 10 days before irradiated H-2d (L1210) tumor cells, a schedule that augmented CMI to the same antigens (Murahata and Mitchell, 1982a, b). Whether suppressor cells of the T cell or macrophage series were stimulated by BCG, accounting for its failure to augment immunity, was not demonstrated in these experiments. Such a mechanism is possible, since suppressor cells, particularly macrophages, can be induced by BCG (see discussion below) (Mitchell *et al.*, 1973; Florentin *et al.*, 1976; Bennett and Mitchell, 1978).

Effects on Cell-Mediated Immunity

As previously mentioned, the adjuvant effect of an active tuberculous infection on cell-mediated immunity was first noted by Dienes and Schoenheit (1927), who found that increased delayed hypersensitivity reactions to ovalbumin and timothy pollen were induced by injecting these soluble antigens into a tuberculous lesion. Freund's complete adjuvant augments delayed hypersensitivity to soluble antigens because of its content of killed mycobacteria (Nelson and Boyden, 1964). BCG or its derivatives potentiate cell-mediated immunity (CMI) to protein antigens (Meyer *et al.*, 1975), to haptens conjugated with normally non-immunogenic carrier molecules (Kuperman *et al.*, 1972), and to poorly immunogenic tumor lines (Hawrylko, 1975). The wax D fractions from several human types of mycobacterium tuberculosis could mimic the adjuvant effect of the whole killed mycobacteria, including the production of corneal hypersensitivity, when injected together with a protein antigen in a water-in-oil emulsion. However, wax D from BCG apparently lacks a critical peptide component, which causes it to be inactive (White *et al.*, 1964).

The survival of skin grafts is profoundly affected by the administration of BCG (Balner *et al.*, 1962; Vitale and Allegretti, 1963; Peters *et al.*, 1974; Zschiesche and

Heinecke, 1973). Accelerated rejection of these skin grafts usually has been produced by pretreatment with BCG, particularly with allografts. However, Zschiesche and Heinecke (1973) found that syngeneic male to female skin grafts were rejected in an accelerated fashion if BCG were administered 21 or 28 days before grafting, but prolongation of graft survival was produced by BCG given twice, 36 and 7 days before grafting. This prolongation was not found with allogeneic skin grafts, while the accelerated rejection was also demonstrable with allografts. Significantly, mice that received BCG twice had a more pronounced stimulation of the phagocytic activity of their RES than those who received BCG once, and yet had prolonged graft survival. A likely explanation for this paradox is that suppressor macrophages were induced concomitantly with killer and phagocytic macrophages.

The survival of solid spleen allografts and isografts was decreased markedly by BCG, whereas dispersed syngeneic or allogeneic spleen cells survived normally *in vivo* despite pretreatment of recipients with BCG (Biozzi *et al.*, 1964). The initial engraftment was unaffected, suggesting that BCG increased the proliferation of immunocompetent lymphocytes following recognition of antigen. Nonspecific RES stimulation does not seem to be of primary importance in the accelerated rejection of allografts and isografts produced by BCG and its derivatives (Steinkuller and Burton, 1966), since the maximal resistance to isografts induced by MER occurs after RES activity has returned to normal. In addition, RES stimulation has been associated with decreased rapidity of rejection (Zschiesche and Heinecke, 1973), not necessarily accelerated rejection. Splenectomy alone between BCG administration and skin grafting abolishes the accelerated rejection (Balner *et al.*, 1962) but this does not provide conclusive evidence for or against the importance of the RES.

ANTAGONISM OF IMMUNOSUPPRESSION BY BCG

Among the most interesting and potentially exploitable effects of BCG and its derivatives, particularly MER, is their ability to reverse or protect against the immunosuppressive effects of various agents. MER caused nearly complete reversal of the immunosuppressive effects of antithymocyte serum on the circulating antibody response to SRBC, whether given before or after the antithymocyte serum (Weiss, 1972). In addition, MER protected against the suppressive effects of cortisone acetate on the appearance of rosette-forming cells, after immunization with SRBC. The immunosuppression caused by antilymphocyte serum on the response to allogeneic cells, as measured by spleen cell-mediated cytotoxicity against ^{51}Cr-labeled targets, was similarly affected (Kuperman *et al.*, 1973).

BCG pretreatment increased the number of plaque-forming cells directed against sheep RBC and could partially protect against or reverse the immunosuppressive effect of methylcholanthrene (Stjernsward, 1966). The combination of BCG and methylcholanthrene resulted in approximately the same number of antibody-producing cells as in immunized controls given neither agent. BCG also conferred long-lasting protection against the immunosuppressive effects of the cytotoxic antimetabolite cytosine arabinoside (cytarabine, ara-C). Spleen cell-mediated immunity to allogeneic leukemia L1210, measured by a 48-hr growth inhibition assay, was significantly decreased by cytarabine, 20 mg/kg/day for 5 days, but was the same as in immunized controls in the group pretreated 10 days before the antigen with intravenous BCG (Murahata and Mitchell, 1976a, b; 1982a, b). Treatment with BCG after chemotherapy caused a transient but significant reversal of immunosuppression. Investigation into the type of lymphoid cell affected by cytarabine and BCG thus far suggests that the same cell diminished by the former is increased by the latter, and that it is a member of the monocytic series (Murahata and Mitchell, 1982b) (see further discussion under Effects on Macrophages).

Pretreatment with BCG was apparently able to protect against the immunosuppressive effects of the alkylating agent cyclophosphamide, since mice could be made resistant to the induction of a tumor by Moloney sarcoma virus, or could be immunized against challenge by a Moloney sarcoma virus-induced tumor even in the face of cyclophosphamide chemotherapy (Houchens *et al.*, 1973, 1974). It is possible, however, since specific *in vitro* measurement of immunity was not made in these studies, that these effects may have been due in part to the induction of interferon. Yet further support for an immunostimulatory antagonism of immunosuppression comes from studies of Mathé and colleagues on immunity to leukemia L1210. The therapeutic benefit from high, toxic doses of cyclophosphamide against syngeneic L1210 leukemia in mice could be increased by subsequent treatment with BCG (Mathé *et al.*, 1974). The increased efficacy of combined therapy was attributed by the authors to a myeloprotective effect of BCG but could just as well have resulted from reversal of immunosuppression. In contrast to studies with Moloney sarcoma virus and allogeneic L1210, pretreatment with BCG appeared to *increase* the number of drug-related deaths attributable to cyclophosphamide. Whether this effect was ascribable to the induction of DNA synthesis in myeloid or lymphoid cells, thereby increasing their susceptibility to the cytotoxic effects of cyclophosphamide, was not established.

Reversal of immunosuppression was also found in antigen–antibody-induced suppression of macrophage receptors for cytophilic antibody (Mitchell, 1976). In this system, peritoneal macrophages from mice treated 10 days previously with specific immune complexes were unable to attach cytophilic antibody to leukemia L1210 *in vitro*. This suppression can be prevented or reversed by the injection of viable BCG 5 days before or after suppressive treatment (Rao and Mitchell, 1981). Since 'suppressor' T cells are intimately involved in this phenomenon (Gershon *et al.*, 1974; Rao *et al.*, 1977), it is not clear whether the protection and reversal effected by BCG are mediated through T cells or are direct effects on the macrophage membrane. Direct effects of BCG on the membrane may play a role in the resistance of spleen cells to immunosuppression by antilymphocyte serum, since isolated cells treated with MER *in vivo* were more resistant to cytolysis *in vitro* by antilymphocyte serum and complement (Kuperman *et al.*, 1973).

It should be noted for balance that in our studies, pretreatment with BCG failed to antagonize the immunosuppression of cytotoxic antibody production by cytarabine. Furthermore, T cell-mediated cytolysis was *diminished* by pretreatment with BCG, which potentiated the suppressive effects of cytarabine in this system (Murahata and Mitchell, 1982a). The induction of suppressor macrophages by BCG is a mechanism we strongly suspect was responsible here, as it is *in vitro*, for the decreased generation of cytolytic T cells (Bennett *et al.*, 1978).

2. EFFECTS ON SPECIFIC TYPES OF LYMPHOID CELL

Stimulation of Effector Macrophages

In its activity as a protective vaccination against *M. tuberculosis*, BCG presumably acts to increase specific cell-mediated immunity to that organism, with which it shares antigenic cross-reactivity (Mackaness, 1964). However, in addition, alveolar macrophages from rabbits injected with BCG show an increased ability to inhibit nonspecifically the growth of intracellular organisms other than mycobacteria, with an accompanying increase in the content of lysosomal hydrolases (Leake and Myrvik, 1968). Nonspecific cytotoxicity to unrelated bacteria can also be induced in macrophages from animals immunized with *M. tuberculosis*, *Listeria monocytogenes*, *Brucella abortus* or *Toxoplasma gondii* (Ruskin and Remington, 1971). With BCG, the rate and onset and the strength of cytotoxicity depend upon the vaccinating dose and require the development of a delayed sensitivity reaction to BCG itself. Heat-killed BCG are ineffective in the induction of nonspecific antimicrobial cytotoxicity; chronic infection with living bacteria is required. Alternatively, the persistance of mycobacteria can be accomplished by the injection of killed organisms in complete Freund's adjuvant (Ruskin and Remington, 1971). Protection against *M. tuberculosis* can be achieved by nonviable BCG, with BCG cell walls attached to oil droplets, or a combination of peptidoglycolipid cell wall skeleton attached to a lipid component (Ribi *et al.*, 1975).

BCG increases the random migration, chemotaxis and pinocytosis of macrophages in the guinea pig (Poplack *et al.*, 1976) and increases chemotaxis in the macrophages of the mouse (Meltzer *et al.*, 1975). There was an increase in chemotaxis effected by several strains of BCG, beginning 4 days after the mycobacteria and lasting through day 21. Pinocytic capacity was increased only briefly during the third and fourth weeks after inoculation (Poplack *et al.*, 1976).

Mice inoculated with BCG have an accelerated rate of clearance of *Escherichia coli* endotoxin and of carbon particles by macrophages of the RES (Howard *et al.*, 1959). BCG-infected animals also clear *Salmonella enteritidis* more rapidly than control animals and catabolize denatured albumin more rapidly. BCG protects against staphylococcus and *Candida* even in immunosuppressed mice, suggesting that BCG-stimulated macrophages are involved (Shea *et al.*, 1975).

Although there is a wide-ranging protective effect against microbes, ranging from bacteria to viruses, BCG does not cause macrophage-mediated protection against all organisms. BCG-activated macrophages capable of destroying *Listeria* cannot kill *Yersinia tularensis* (Myrvik, 1972). Furthermore, even where BCG is protective, the mechanism may not involve the macrophage. Pretreatment with BCG completely prevented the infection usually caused in CBA mice by *Babesia* and *Plasmodium* (Clark *et al.*, 1976). Yet these protozoa were killed intraerythrocytically after their appearance in the peritoneum, and immunity was long-lived, suggesting that mediators released from immunized T cells were involved. Salvin *et al.* (1973) have in fact found substances in the serum of BCG-infected mice with interferon and migration-inhibitory activity, after restimulation with BCG, tuberculin, or certain unrelated antigens. BCG protects against the local growth and 'metastasis' of *Echinococcus* hydatid cysts (Rau and Tanner, 1975), in much the same manner as against metastatic tumor cells (Baldwin and Pimm, 1973), but has no effect against *Treponema pallidum* infection (Graves *et al.*, 1975). Thus, even though stimulation of CMI may be involved in the effects of BCG, that does not necessarily mean that macrophage-mediated killing is involved in all instances, nor that the stimulation of CMI will lead to nonspecific protection against all organisms.

Hibbs *et al.* (1972a, b; 1973), Cleveland *et al.* (1974) and Holtermann *et al.* (1973) have shown that BCG-activated macrophages are capable of recognizing and destroying a variety of neoplastic cells. With few exceptions (McLaughlin *et al.*, 1972), these activated macrophages can discriminate between neoplastic and non-neoplastic (usually nontransformed fibroblast) cells. In general, early passages of embryo cells, which show little contact inhibition, are susceptible to killing by BCG-activated macrophages, while later passages are minimally affected (Cleveland *et al.*, 1974; Holtermann *et al.*, 1973). Peritoneal macrophages induced by substances such as starch, mineral oil or thioglycollate were not nonspecifically tumoricidal, even though these frequently appeared morphologically 'activated'. This is an *in vitro* correlation of the earlier observations that activation of macrophages is necessary but not sufficient for the expression of the tumoricidal effects of BCG. The manner in which BCG-activated macrophages discriminate between tumor cells and normal cells is uncertain; whether discrimination involves recognition of the antigenic structure or another characteristic, such as the proliferative rate of the neoplastic cells, has not been conclusively established. Evans and Alexander (1972) have shown that specific recognition of tumor antigens on a syngeneic tumor by macrophages in tumor-immunized mice can be promorted through an 'arming factor' from T cells, but that BCG-nonspecifically-activated macrophages, lacking the specific arming factor, kill a variety of tumor cells. It should be noted, too, that cytophilic antibody derived from B cells constitutes another such arming factor (Granger and Weiser, 1966). Thus, a relative discrimination is possible in BCG-activated macrophages and to a much greater degree in 'armed, activated' macrophages.

BCG injected intravenously into mice also stimulates splenic mononuclear cells, which may be monocytes (macrophages), to become cytotoxic to tumor cells even if they have not previously been exposed to the tumor (Mitchell *et al.*, 1973). In our original experiments, BCG augmented CMI to P815Y mastocytoma cells, as measured by a 48 hr microcytotoxicity assay, when given with suboptimal doses of tumor cells to allogeneic mice (Mitchell *et al.*, 1973). Controls given BCG alone, however, had the same degree of CMI as those given BCG and alloantigen. The 'pseudoimmune' mononuclear cells involved in CMI were at first assumed to be T cells, since they were not significantly reduced by adherence to glass or plastic surfaces and since T cells were known to be effector cells in a 6-hr ^{51}Cr-release assay with the same alloantigenic system (Brunner *et al.*, 1970). However, further work has shown that these mononuclear cells are not sensitive to anti-Thy-1 serum, are developed even in thymus-deprived mice and have a range of killing (several types of tumor cell but not normal fibroblasts) that suggest they are in the monocytic series (Kinder and Mitchell, unpublished data). They are detectable only by a 48-hr growth inhibition assay, not by a 6-hr ^{51}Cr-release assay. We have found that very similar cells are elicited by BCG given to mice 10 days before alloantigen. The major difference is the specificity of the cytotoxicity these cells display toward the immunogen, when alloantigenic (L1210) cells are given in conjunction with BCG (Murahata and Mitchell, 1976a, b, 1978). The mononuclear cells produced by BCG and alloantigen are insensitive to anti-Thy-1 serum, undetectable by 6-hr ^{51}Cr-release, unaffected by glass and plastic adherence and resistant to 500 r and 1000 r *in vitro* radiation. Evidence for surface immunoglobulin was equivocal. Nylon wool columns trap some of the cells, but many others pass through, and even the adherent cells are readily elutable. Perhaps the most direct evidence that the cells are not T cells, but depend upon T cells for their specificity, comes from experiments in which the cells were partially depleted by treatment with carbonyl iron and a magnet. Repletion of the cells removed by this procedure could be accomplished with purified macrophages from the peritoneum of *normal* mice. Treatment of the spleen cells with anti-Thy-1 serum prevented repletion by normal peritoneal cells, whereas anti-Thy-1 treatment of the peritoneal cells had no effect. Since the splenic effector cells were not killed by silica but were depleted by carbonyl iron magnet treatment, they were most probably not phagocytic but rather adherent to the outside of the carbonyl iron particle. The weight of evidence thus far suggests that the cell induced by BCG and alloantigen is of the monocytic series, armed specifically by a T cell factor.

Kiessling *et al.* (1976) and Herberman *et al.* (1975) have described nonadherent 'natural killer' cells in the peritoneal exudate of mice, which cause a low background level of cytotoxicity against foreign cells in unimmunized mice. The 'natural killer' (NK) cell lacks the markers characteristic of classical T or B cells and is also not a mature macrophage, since it is nonadherent and nonphagocytic. Trypsinization markedly decreases its function, which is also labile at 37°C. BCG, but not proteose peptone or thioglycollate broth, can increase the activity of peritoneal cells with similar characteristics (Wolfe *et al.*, 1976), although cells stimulated by BCG cannot be called 'natural', strictly speaking, since the term applies to an ostensibly uninduced population. These peritoneal cells were cytotoxic in a 4-hr ^{51}Cr-release assay and thus are different from the nonadherent, nonphagocytic inhibitory spleen cells evoked by BCG and alloantigen described above. Yet the nonadherent, nonphagocytic peritoneal NK cell may well be related to the nonadherent, nonphagocytic splenic mononuclear cell, with both representing varieties of immature macrophage lacking many of the features of the fully developed cell. Peritoneal adherent cells capable of killing allografted tumor cells in a 16-hr ^{51}Cr-release assay were increased by treatment with intraperitoneal BCG, as well as other adjuvant substances (Schultz *et al.*, 1976). The specificity of these cells was not tested after the administration of antigen and adjuvant, making it difficult to relate them further to our splenic mononuclear effector cells. Cytotoxic peritoneal exudate macrophages and NK cells were induced by the i.p. injection of BCG into nude rats, indicating that the induction was independent of the thymus (Gray and Brooks, 1980). The increase in NK cell activity following i.p. BCG was dependent upon the presence of macrophages. Cell-free supernatant fluids derived from 24-hr cultures of BCG-induced peritoneal exudate cells were also effective in increasing NK activity (Tracey, 1979). Nathan *et al.* (1976, 1977) have described a related peritoneal nonphagocytic adherent cell that was cytotoxic to tumor cells, induced by BCG alone. They believe that this subpopulation of peritoneal cells is not a variety of macrophage but rather a peculiar B cell, but none of their data completely rules out the former possibility. The same group had previously reported that several tumor lines were enhanced in their growth by normal peritoneal cells *in vitro* but less enhanced by cells from BCG-treated mice (Nathan and Terry, 1975).

The low level of 'nonspecific' background inhibitory activity against tumor cells found in the peritoneum or spleen of the mouse may simply reflect the few killer cells present, which may be 'natural' or induced by the normal microflora impinging upon the animals. Expansion by BCG or other adjuvants of this subpopulation of inhibitory cells thus may lead to a population that is grossly cytotoxic to tumor cells rather than stimulatory.

STIMULATION OF AFFERENT MACROPHAGES

BCG also influences macrophages that are involved in the afferent arm of immunity. Lymphocyte-activating factor (LAF, or Interleukin-1), a substance that causes proliferation of T cells in mice (Gery and Waksman, 1972; Gery *et al.*, 1972), is produced by such macrophages in the peripheral blood, peritoneum or spleen of several species of animals. The spleen of a BCG-treated mouse produces 2- to 3-fold more LAF than a comparable normal spleen (Mitchell *et al.*, 1973), in proportion to the increased percentage of macrophages. Purified adherent cells from the BCG-treated spleen produce increased amounts of LAF, again in proportion to their increased number. BCG treatment of splenic cells *in vitro* leads to a 20-fold increase in the amount of LAF produced (Mokyr and Mitchell, 1975), while various derivatives of BCG, such as MER and lipid-free mycobacteria, stimulate splenic macrophages 3- to 6-fold above baseline *in vitro* (Mitchell *et al.*, 1975). LAF may be responsible for the mitogenic effect of BCG on T cells, acting as an intermediary stimulator and expander of the number of reactive T cells. It has been postulated that the profound amplification of cellular immunity produced by BCG may depend on such proliferation-inducing mediators, produced not only by macrophages but by T cells as well (Gery and Waksman, 1972; Mokyr and Mitchell, 1975). Yashphe, Weiss and co-workers have also obtained some evidence that MER acts to improve the processing or presentation of antigen (SRBC) by macrophages (Weiss, 1972). By analogy with other adjuvants, such as *B. pertussis* and *E. coli* LPS, which clearly augment antibody production in part through stimulation of antigen laden macrophages (Unanue *et al.*, 1969; Spitznagel and Allison, 1970), BCG and its derivatives may improve the presentation of antigen in more immunogenic form or may alter the macrophage membrane to permit more avid association with antibody-producing (B) cells.

INDUCTION OF SUPPRESSOR ADHERENT CELLS

In addition to its stimulation of afferent and effector macrophages, BCG can also elicit suppressor adherent cells that are most likely macrophages. These suppressor adherent cells induced in BCG-treated mice inhibit the response to the mitogens Con A and PHA by splenic T cells (Mitchell *et al.*, 1973; Florentin *et al.*, 1976). Their partial depletion by adherence to glass led to improvement in the response to both mitogens, both in normal mice and especially in BCG-treated mice where their suppressive activity was greatly increased. The effect on the response of spleen cells to B-cell mitogens, such as LPS, was impossible to measure accurately because sticky B cells were removed by glass adherence, too. BCG is itself a mitogen for splenic T cells (Mokyr and Mitchell, 1975; Bekierkunst, 1975). The response to BCG of normal spleen cells was improved by removal of adherent cells by serial adsorptions to plastic, reducing their percentage from 10 to 1 per cent (Mokyr and Mitchell, 1975). Together with evidence that a very small percentage of macrophages is required for BCG to stimulate T cells (Mokyr and Mitchell, 1975) and Waksman's complementary evidence on the optimal percentage of macrophages needed to permit a response to

PHA (1–5 per cent) (Folch *et al.*, 1972), these data indicate that a concentration of 5–10 per cent of macrophages (the normal range) may in fact be supraoptimal and thereby suppressive. By increasing both the number and activation of macrophages, BCG may act to inhibit mitogenic responses.

Direct evidence for adherent suppressor cells activated in the spleen by BCG has come from independent coincidental investigations of Bennett, Mitchell and colleagues (Bennett *et al.*, 1978; Bennett and Mitchell, 1979, 1980; Bennett *et al.*, 1981a, b) and of Klimpel and Henney (1978). These laboratories found that the *in vitro* immunization of C57BL/6 mouse spleen cells by allogeneic P815Y tumor cells was abrogated by a large dose of BCG administered approximately 1 to 6 weeks earlier. Two $\times 10^7$ viable units of intravenous BCG, or more, attracted 'natural suppressor cells', i.e. suppressor cells shown to be present in normal bone marrow, from the bone marrow to the spleen. There they were activated by the BCG and proliferated during the second week after BCG. Only nylon-adherent, anti-Thy 1-resistant spleen cells from BCG treated spleens were effective suppressors. Admixture of these cells with normal spleen cells, at a ratio as low as 1:10, significantly inhibited the ability of the latter to be immunized by the alloantigenic tumor cells. These adherent suppressor cells, which seem to be a variety of macrophage block the development of cytotoxic T-cells and non T killer cells, very likely by inhibiting proliferation. The same mechanism would explain their antagonism of the response to mitogens. The nonadherent cells from BCG-treated spleen had the capacity to be immunized once removed from the presence of the adherent cells. Furthermore, once cytotoxic cells were already generated, the adherent cells had no effect on their activity. Specifically, either the addition of adherent suppressor cells to sensitized T-cells or the removal of adherent cells once immunization was achieved each failed to influence the cytotoxicity against the target cells. These natural suppressor cells release prostaglandins and can be inhibited by prostaglandin antagonists, such as indomethacin.

There was a strong correlation between suppressor cell activity against T cell immunization *in vitro,* and the presence of granulocyte-macrophage colony forming units (CFU-C). In fact these may represent two different functions of the same cell (Bennett and Marsh, 1980). It is uncertain whether a soluble principle is produced by the suppressor cells which might explain their actions. BCG-induced suppressor macrophages can suppress both cytotoxic lymphocyte formation and the generation of PFC *in vitro.* However, the supernatant fluids derived from the suppressor cells were effective only against the generation of PFC. These results seem to indicate a different mechanism or different macrophage subpopulations involved into suppressor activities (Klimpel *et al.*, 1979). It is suggested in both systems, however, that the principal mode of action of the suppressor cell is the inhibition of production of a helper factor produced by Lyt 1+ helper T cells (Klimpel, 1979).

An attempt to reconcile these findings with the experiments of Braun *et al.* (1978) showing an *augmentation* of anamnestic immunization *in vitro* by BCG, has led to the discovery of two strains of BCG that differ remarkably in their ability to induce suppressor cells. Braun *et al.* (1978) found that with the mineral oil induced plasmcytoma (MOPC)-315, BALB/c mice given Phipps BCG intraperitioneally while bearing the primary tumor had spleen cells that were enhanced in their ability to respond to a rechallenge with MOPC-315 cells *in vitro.* A collaborative study of several batches of this strain of BCG in comparison with the Tice BCG used by Bennett and colleagues showed that Phipps strains 734 and 724 had purely augmentative effects when given *in vivo,* while Phipps strain A-8 and Tice BCG induced suppressor cells. These effects were demonstrable in both the syngeneic (MOPC-BALB/c) and allogeneic (P815Y-C57BL/6) systems (Mokyr *et al.*, 1980).

The adjuvanticity usually seen *in vivo* after administration of BCG is probably always the vector sum of several opposing forces, of which the negative vector is the induction of suppressor adherent cells. The strength of immunogenicity of the antigen, and more importantly the timing, dose and strain of BCG are certainly other factors influencing the outcome of immodulation. The concomitant presence of macrophage-like killer cells in the same spleen that contains suppressor cells indicates that several types of macrophage activity are elicited. There may well be distinct subpopulations of macrophages akin to those found with lymphocytes: afferent (helper), effector (cytotoxic) and suppressor, perhaps with identifying phenotypic markers analogous with the Ly antigens. The alternative, that different types of assay measure different properties of the same population of macrophages, has not been ruled out, however. This issue of subgroups of macrophages is considered in more detail in another review in this volume (p. 35ff).

ALTERATION OF LYMPHOCYTE TRAPPING

The concentration ('trapping') of peripheral blood lymphocytes in the spleen and lymph node can be altered by BCG. Zatz (1976) found that splenic trapping of ^{51}Cr-labeled lymphocytes in the mouse was increased briefly in the spleen 1–2 days after BCG, then again 3 weeks later, whereas in lymph nodes there was persistent trapping. Either intravenously or subcutaneously administered BCG increased trapping in lymph nodes, but intravenous BCG *decreased* splenic trapping. The macrophage has been implicated in this process of concentrating lymphocytes by BCG (Frost and Lance, 1974), although Zatz (1976) believes that T cells also are involved. Whether suppressor macrophages or suppressor T cells might be involved in the 'negative trapping' in the spleen is a matter for further study. Whole, viable BCG cells are not required to augment trapping. With techniques similar to those of Zatz, Ogura *et al.* (1975) showed in the tumor-bearing rat that BCG cell walls attached to oil droplets increased the influx of lymphocytes into the regional lymph node to a greater extent than that induced by the AH-130 hepatoma alone. The immunosuppression caused by BCG in the treatment of adjuvant arthritis in rats may be due to altered lymphocyte traffic, as Sutherland *et al.* (1979) have postulated.

EFFECTS ON T CELLS

BCG is mitogenic for T cells (Mokyr and Mitchell, 1975), stimulating not only splenic nonadherent cells enriched for T cells but also thymus cells in the Swiss CD-1 and inbred C3H mouse. A critical concentration of macrophages of approximately 0.25–0.5 per cent is required for this effect, since removal of macrophages (below 0.25 per cent) abolishes the mitogenic effect of BCG and reconstitution to 0.5 per cent restores it (Mokyr and Mitchell, 1975). Thus, the effect on T cells may be indirect through the macrophage, which is similar to findings on the mitogenicity of PHA (Levis and Robbins, 1970). Bekierkunst (1976a) was, for reasons not immediately apparent, unable to stimulate thymic T cells with BCG unless they were admixed with spleen cells. MER stimulated T cells *in vitro*, but DMC failed to do so (Mitchell *et al.*, 1976), perhaps indicating a requirement for lipid. The dose–response curves described for spleen and thymus cells with BCG resemble those for other T cell mitogens, such as Con A, with inhibitory effects at the highest concentration (250×10^5 viable units per ml) and a rather sharp optimum at approximately 1×10^6 viable units per ml.

The relationship of the mitogenicity or antigenicity of adjuvants and their activity as adjuvants is not entirely clear, but it appears that many adjuvant substances are either mitogens or antigens (Mokyr and Mitchell, 1975; Skidmore *et al.*, 1975). Specific desensitization to BCG abolished its intratumoral effect (Zbar *et al.*, 1971). Moreover, the strains of BCG that were most antigenic were also the strongest adjuvants *in vivo* (Mackaness *et al.*, 1973). Many, but not all, peptidoglycans isolated from mycobacteria that have adjuvancy have been mitogenic, particularly B cell mitogens acting on spleen cells from the nude mouse (Damais *et al.*, 1975). Some strong mitogens, such as Con A and PHA, have predominantly immunosuppressive effects *in vivo* (Elves, 1967) or *in vitro* (Peavy and Pierce, 1974), which have been due to the production of suppressor T cells in at least one circumstance (Peavy and Pierce, 1974). Mitogenicity for lymphocytes not always correlated with the production of specific lymphocyte-made mediators or the development of cytotoxic effector cells (Williams and Granger, 1969; Klein, 1971; Kirkpatrick, 1971; Asherson *et al.*, 1973), but the incorporation of ^{3}H-thymidine into the DNA of lymphocytes may constitute a simple means by which rapid screening of substances for possible adjuvancy can be achieved.

Although our early experiments with BCG *in vivo* were interpreted as showing improved spleen T cell-mediated cytotoxicity against allogeneic tumor cells, it is now evident that the effector cell does not kill within 4–6 hr and is not sensitive to anti-theta serum, making it unlikely that it is a T cell. Cell-mediated cytotoxicity measured by ^{51}Cr-release within 6 hr was unchanged in mice given 1×10^7 BCG 10 days before alloantigen, when tested 14 days after antigen (Murahata and Mitchell, 1978). Pretreatment with complete Freund's adjuvant virtually abolished the cytotoxic T cell response to alloantigens in mice, although the memory function of T cells was unaltered (Reinisch *et al.*, 1976). It is probable that scheduling is once again of considerable importance in determining whether and how BCG affects the function of T cells. Braun *et al.* (1978) have augmented the anamnestic *in vitro* response of mouse splenic T cells to syngeneic MOPC tumor cells by pretreatment with BCG *in vivo*, 11 days before the start of incubation. It is also likely that many of the effects of BCG on allografts and tumors *in vivo* depend upon the augmented proliferation of sensitized T cells, judging from extensive histological observations (Zbar *et al.*, 1971; Hanna *et al.*, 1972a; Mackaness *et al.*, 1973) even though the direct demonstration of increased number and activity of T cells by *in vitro* assays has not always been possible.

Priming of Mice for Production of 'Tumor Necrosis Factor' (TNF)

Tumor necrosis factor (TNF) is a glycoprotein of 150,000 da that is released into the serum of mice pretreated with intravenous BCG 2 weeks before intravenous stimulation with *E.coli* LPS (Carswell *et al.*, 1975; Green *et al.*, 1976). As its name states, this material causes hemorrhagic necrosis of several transplantable mouse tumors *in vivo* or in culture, but normal embryo fibroblasts are unaffected. BCG pretreatment is essential for endotoxin challenge to be effective in eliciting TNF. However, other agents causing reticuloendothelial proliferation, such as *C. parvum* or zymosan, can substitute for BCG. While the origin of TNF is undetermined, it may come from the activated macrophages present in abundance in the spleen of BCG-primed animals. Since the spectrum of activity of TNF resembles that of BCG-activated macrophages, sparing nontransformed cells, it is possible that TNF is one of the soluble mediators released during the destruction of tumor cells, which under ordinary circumstances are not found in the serum but only in the immediate vicinity of the rejection reaction. The physiological significance of TNF release is open to question, particularly since the mice producing the substance are frequently moribund of endotoxin shock, but its potential efficacy as passive immunotherapy of tumor-bearing mice is a matter of considerable interest.

Effects on Interferon, Colony-stimulating Factor and Pyrogens

While interferon and colony-stimulating factor are not really immunological mediators, their stimulation represents 'paraimmunological' effects of immunological modulators that may also be exploitable therapeutically. These substances appear to be members of a family of macrophage-made materials, of which LAF is another example. BCG can induce interferon activity (Salvin *et al.*, 1973), which is made by both lymphocytes and macrophages, a property shared by many other immunological modulators (Grossberg, 1972). In fact, agents first identified as inducers of interferon, such as poly I:C and poly A:U, and the fluorenone derivatives have many properties of adjuvance, suggesting that each class of agent be investigated routinely for the other property. Whether any additional therapeutic gain will be realized from antitumor therapy with BCG against tumors caused by oncogenic viruses remains to be seen.

Colony stimulating factor, which stimulates the growth of myeloid colonies from the bone marrow in agar culture, has been increased by BCG in the dog (Kelly, Marsh and Mitchell, unpublished data), and by the adjuvants LPS and *C. parvum* in the mouse (Sheridan and Metcalf, 1972; Wolmark and Fisher, 1974). It is likely that other such trophic and regulatory substances are produced by macrophages, and that stimulators of macrophages such as BCG and its fractions will prove useful as augmentors of their production. Antagonism of the myelosuppressive effects of chemotherapy is one such use. An increase in suppressor substances from macrophages would also be predicted by this reasoning, and from the known effects on BCG in eliciting suppressor macrophages.

Pyrogenic substances produced by lymphocytes represent another paraimmunological response, which often accompanies immunity and can be induced by immune complexes among other stimuli (Atkins *et al.*, 1972). It is of interest not only that BCG is itself pyrogenic, like many similar organisms, but that there appears to be a general correlation between the adjuvanticity of components of bacterial cell walls and their pyrogenic effects (Kotani *et al.*, 1976). However, if the two properties prove inextricably linked, this would obviously be a hinderance to the isolation of nontoxic components with immunomodulatory capacity.

3. FRACTIONS OF BCG

A number of derivatives of BCG have been produced in an attempt to find fractions that share the beneficial attributes of BCG but lack its toxicity. We will exclude MER from this discussion, since it has been reviewed in detail elsewhere (Ben-Efraim, 1977 and this volume, p. 303ff). Lipid-free derivatives prepared from BCG or related mycobacteria have been capable of protecting against several ascites leukemias and Ehrlich ascites carcinoma in mice (Hiu, 1972; Chedid *et al.*, 1973; Mathé *et al.*, 1973). Although lipid-free mycobacterial cell walls and lipid-depleted cell walls (also known as cell wall skeletons) are effective against dispersed tumors, the effectiveness of fractions against solid tumors, particularly by the intratumoral route, appears to depend upon the additional presence of lipid. Ribi and co-workers physically reattached cell walls and cell wall skeletons to oil droplets and found their activity restored to that of whole BCG against solid tumors (Ribi *et al.*, 1973; Zbar *et al.*, 1972). Not only are BCG cell walls in saline ineffective, but pretreatment with them creates an unresponsive state to cell walls in oil, which abrogates the latter's specific antituberculous protection, minimizes granuloma formation and causes a loss of footpad swelling on challenge with PPD (Meyer *et al.*, 1974). Lipid-free cell wall skeletons have afforded some protection against tumors when mixed with autologous mammary tumor cells and reinjected, but systemic immunity was not produced since new mammary tumors arose despite rejection of the primary (Tokuzen *et al.*, 1975).

The contribution of lipid to the therapeutic effects of BCG may be its ability to elicit granulomas, both 'nonallergic' and immunologically determined. Highly refined fractions of BCG are apparently incapable of evoking a strong inflammatory response. While that may lessen their toxicity, it is also a therapeutic drawback. BCG cell walls attached to mineral oil increase the trapping of lymphocytes into the draining lymph node, to a greater extent than that caused by the tumor alone (Ogura *et al.*, 1975). Tumor growth and metastasis to the lymph node were both suppressed in those experiments. The granuloma formation caused or abetted by lipid may depend upon stimulation of T cells, with their subsequent elaboration of soluble mediators. Some evidence for the necessity of lipid in the stimulation of T cells comes from experiments on the mitogenicity of BCG and its lipid-free fraction, DMC. DMC was incapable of stimulating T cells in contrast to BCG, which was a strong T cell mitogen (Mitchell *et al.*, 1975). Ineffectiveness against solid tumors of lipid-poor fractions might be an *in vivo* reflection of their inability to stimulate T cells. The rejection of dispersed tumors and leukemias in mice seems to depend more critically upon antibody and non-T cells (Alexander *et al.*, 1966; Deegan and Mitchell, unpublished data). Therefore, cell walls, as water-soluble, lipid-free supernatants fractions of sonicated BCG, and lipid-depleted organisms, which are all stimulants of splenic B cells (Mitchell *et al.*, 1975; Baker *et al.*, 1975), would be expected to have activity against them. Yamamura *et al.* (1976) were able to increase significantly specific T cell-mediated cytotoxicity to a suboptimal dose of P815-X2 mastocytoma cells by the administration of lipid-free cell wall skeletons together with mineral oil. Background cytotoxicity with P815-X2 alone, by ^{51}Cr-release, was 15 per cent, whereas skeleton-oil-treated mice had 66–100 per cent lysis. The contribution of oil droplets in inducing T cell-mediated lysis was considerable, since oil alone (with P815-X2 cells) improved lysis to a level of 48–84 per cent. While there was clearly an augmentative effect on T cells from admixing cell wall skeletons with the oil, the authors unfortunately did not test what effect cell wall skeletons by themselves had on immunity. Thus, the lipid intrinsic to BCG has effects that can be mimicked and thus elucidated by admixture with oil.

Ribi *et al.* (1973) have diagrammed the structure of the cell wall skeleton, which exists as an insoluble polymer, a peptidoglycolipid, as follows:

	ester linkage		(1) phosphodiester? (2) glycosidic?	
[MYCOLIC ACID]$_x$	⟶	[ARABINOGALACTAN]$_y$	⟶	[MUCOPEPTIDE]$_z$
C_{76}–C_{84} *a*-C_{24} branch *b*-OH		D-Arabinose D-Galactose		*N*-acetyl-glucosamine *N*-glycolyl-muramic acid Alanine Glutamic acid Diaminopimelic acid

It appears that one component lost in the removal of 'free lipids' from BCG or its cell wall is the trehalose–mycolic acid ester trehalose-6, 6′-dimycolate, known as 'cord factor' (Lederer, 1976) or as 'P_3' (Ribi *et al.*, 1973). This mycolate component appears to be capable of inducing granulomata by itself, although these are more transient than with the whole organism, and are ineffective at causing complete regression. When added back to cell wall skeletons in oil, P_3 caused tumors that were unresponsive to the skeletons alone to be successfully refected (Ribi *et al.*, 1973; Meyer *et al.*, 1974). Even when BCG is simply killed and lyophilized, cord factor may be lost, since the addition of cord factor to such BCG in oil or aqueous medium restored its capacity as an antitumor agent in intratumoral therapy and as a vaccine (Bekierkunst, 1975, 1976).

A variety of combinations of P_3 with other bacterial materials has been examined for antitumor properties, upon intralesional injection. With the guinea pig line 10 hepatoma, Ribi and co-workers have found that a combination of P_3 and a glycolipid from Salmonella a *Re*-mutant, particularly when given as an emulsion, were particularly effective in causing regression of the tumor. *Re* glycolipid with cell wall skeletons of BCG were also effective, causing nearly 100% regressions if either of them was given in an oil-water emulsion (Ribi, personal communication). In these studies large amounts of material (150 to 350 μg) have been injected, and exclusively intratumorally, so that it is difficult to be certain that there would be persistent, long-lived systemic immunity generated the tumor would be killed and that there would be a persistent, long-lived systemic immunity generated if the materials were given systemically instead. The amounts injected, represent more than the amounts 150 to 350 μg starting dose of the components contained in the whole BCG usually injected. Also, most of the tumors tested have been relatively immunogenic. In these studies, the administration of materials has been exclusively by the intratumoral route. Whether any of these components cell wall, cell wall skeleton or P_3, can boost the specific immunity to the tumor-associated antigens has not been conclusively tested, although it is likely that the peptidoglycan-containing portions are true adjuvants. Endotoxin contamination, and the endotoxin properties of some of the fractions, as well as the *Re* glycolipid, may also prove to be problems in translating these results to the clinic.

The component responsible for the adjuvanticity of BCG may be a small peptide present in the peptidoglycan (mucopeptide) portion of the cell wall. Although mycobacteria were not specifically the subject of their investigation, Fleck *et al.* (1974) found with several Gram-positive and negative bacteria that the smallest bacterial structures containing adjuvant activity were peptides of the general form,

L-Ala–D-Glu ——— R_3–D-Ala,

where R_3 was either a meso-diaminopimelic acid or an *N*-substituted L-lysine residue. Muramyl dipeptides closely resemble the active portion of mycobacterial peptidoglycan which is largely responsible for its modulatory capacity. These materials are water-soluble and active orally (Chedid *et al.*, 1976, 1977). Synthetic muramyl dipeptides, analogous with material from bacterial cell walls, including mycobacteria, have had adjuvant effects on antibody synthesis and delayed sensitivity (Kotani *et al.*, 1976) and have protected nonspecifically against Klebsiella infection, possibly through macrophages (Chedid *et al.*, 1976, 1977). These muramyl dipeptides are closely related to the peptides studied by Fleck *et al.* (1974). One strongly adjuvant member of the series, which is the limit peptide of BCG, has the form:

N-acetylmuramyl–L-Ala–D-Glu–NH_2.

This is commonly the material referred to as MDP. It is of interest that synthetic muramyl dipeptides with D-alanine instead of the natural L-isomer depress the immune response rather than augment it (Chedid *et al.*, 1976). Both the cell wall skeleton, with its peptidoglycan, and P_3 appear to be necessary for the effective intratumoral therapy of guinea pig hepatoma and long-lived subsequent systemic protection (Ribi *et al.*, 1973).

The series of MDP's developed by Chedid and his collaborators have greatly expanded our understanding of the chemical basis for the adjuvanticity of BCG. Unlike many derivatives of BCG, MDPs can substitute for whole BCG in minuscule amounts, increasing both nonspecific immunity (through macrophages) and specific immunity when given with antigen. MDPs can stimulate macrophages to release prostaglandins, endogenous pyrogen, and lymphocyte activating factor, and can activate macrophages to kill tumor cells *in vitro*. Longer derivatives in the series are more easily phagocytized and hence are the most effective in stimulating macrophages.

MDP inhibited the migration of macrophages from guinea pigs or rats *in vitro*, an effect that was shown not to be due to migration inhibitory factor from lymphocytes. The stereochemistry required for adjuvanticity was also required for the inhibition of migration and the investigators suggest that the same change of the membrane has caused inhibition of migration might be related to the adjuvant effect of the material (Nagao *et al.*, 1979). However another group (Galelli *et al.*, 1980) found no correlation between the structures required for adjuvanticity and the activation of macrophages as measured by an inhibition of tumor growth *in vitro*. Direct effects on the macrophage membrane are nevertheless of undoubted importance in the activities of BCG and its various fractions. In fact changes in the externally disposed membrane proteins of macrophages have been demonstrated with BCG and other adjuvant materials (Kan-Mitchell *et al.*, 1980). Cytolytic T-cells specific for an antigenic target are increased after antigen given with MDP. When conjugated to the synthetic carrier, T, G A–L, MDP obviates the need for Freund's adjuvant in several test systems of antibody production. The most exciting aspect of the MDPs from a theoretical stand-point is that they offer the opportunity to manipulate the critical structure responsible for adjuvancy of mycobacteria, and thus to modulate biological activity towards various types of lymphoid cells. One can thereby learn the critical determinants that affect such activity. Thus many that will prove useful clinically will undoubtedly not be the naturally occurring dipeptides of microorganisms, but rationally designed derivatives. They appear to have very low toxicity in early clinical trials, and can be used systemically by a variety of routes.

Thus, since BCG is a complex biological material, it is not unlikely that attempts to isolate portions possessing specific properties, such as granuloma formation, adjuvancy, and perhaps even cross-antigenicity with certain tumor cells, will be a fruitful way to continue in the development of BCG as a therapeutic agent.

4. CLINICAL IMMUNOTHERAPY WITH BCG

Several concise reviews have dealt specifically with clinical immunotherapy and should be consulted for more extensive information (Bast *et al.*, 1974; Mastrangelo *et al.*, 1976). Our aim here is to point out a few representative studies that have suggested the clinical efficacy of BCG in the treatment of human tumors and those that have measured the immunological consequences of BCG in man.

Therapeutic Trials

The three neoplastic diseases that have received the most attention from immunotherapists have been acute myelogenous leukemia, malignant melanoma, and most recently, lung cancer. After induction of a remission by intensive chemotherapy, Crowther and colleagues (1973) administered BCG alone or with allogeneic tumor cells as maintenance therapy. These groups compared favorably with one given only chemotherapy, although none of the regimens significantly prolonged survival. In subsequent trials by the same group (Hamilton-Fairley, 1977), an advantage was demonstrated for a regimen of chemoimmunotherapy, combining cytotoxic agents and BCG by vaccination plus irradiated allogeneic leukemic cells, over a regimen involving chemotherapy alone. Both the duration of remission and survival were prolonged by the addition of immunotherapy to chemotherapy, in part because subsequent remission was more easily induced in patients given regimens including immunotherapy than in those maintained on chemotherapy alone (Freeman *et al.*, 1973). BCG has been used alone successfully as maintenance therapy (Gutterman *et al.*, 1974), although the lack of concurrent controls in that study hinders definite conclusions about its efficacy. Vogler and Chan (1974) intensively pretreated patients with BCG for 4 weeks before maintenance chemotherapy with methotrexate and found a significantly longer duration of remission in that group, compared with one given chemotherapy. Of the many studies with immunotherapy, involving BCG with or without irradiated leukemic cells, very few have relied exclusively upon immunotherapy for maintenance. Freeman *et al.* (1973) found no difference in the duration of the first remission but increased survival in the eight patients given immunotherapy with BCG and leukemic cells, mainly because of a high rate of reinduction of remission.

Recently the Manchester group reported a successful use of BCG and allogeneic leukemic cells given as the only therapy during remission. Patients receiving immunotherapy without concomitant chemotherapy had a significant longer remission and survival from remission than the randomized control group. While the differences in the duration of the first remission and the survival from remission were modest, on the order of 16 weeks and 45 weeks respectively, the clear demonstration that immunotherapy alone may be successful in this setting is worthy of note (Harris *et al.*, 1982).

The same benefit of immunotherapy has not been reproducibly demonstrated in acute lymphocytic leukemia of children (Leukaemia Committee, 1971; Heyn *et al.*, 1973; Leventhal *et al.*, 1973), despite Mathé's original encouraging report (Mathé *et al.*, 1969). Perhaps because chemotherapy alone is so effective in this disease, the additional benefit bestowed by BCG has been difficult to prove.

Melanoma has been treated by intralesional injection of BCG, which is effective in ameliorating tumor nodules in approximately 60 per cent of the patients treated (see Table 1 in Bast *et al.*, 1974). Whether this is truly an augmentation of tumor-specific immunity is debatable, since the intense local inflammatory response accompanying rejection of the tumor is usually limited to the injected nodule or closely situated neighboring lesions. Distant visceral metastases, if present situated have rarely been affected, and if absent, have developed despite regression of injected nodules. Thus, systemic immunity may be irrelevant in the response to injected nodules, just as in the guinea pig hepatoma model, with direct local activation of macrophages and perhaps T cells causing rejection. Nonspecific augmentation of systemic immunity to melanoma by vaccination with BCG, after surgical removal of a primary melanoma and tumor-containing regional lymph nodes, has been attempted by several groups. Gutterman *et al.* (1973) found that using BCG with scarification was effective in prolonging the disease-free period in those who had a primary tumor of the trunk or extremities, but not the head and neck. Historical controls rather than a concomitant, randomly assigned control group were used for comparison. The ostensible superiority of the BCG regimen in prolonging remission may have been due to its intralymphatic spread and consequent local antitumor effects, rather than systemic augmentation of immunity, since no BCG was applied in the head and neck region. Although the period of follow-up was only 2 yr, and strict randomization was not performed, the study of Eilber *et al.* (1976) is nonetheless encouraging. While 42 control patients had a median duration of remission of 8 months, 84 subjects given BCG by multiprong vaccination for as long as 2 yr had a significantly longer disease free interval, with a projected median exceeding 42 months. Prospective randomized trials with BCG alone or combined with irradiated allogeneic cells are in progress, and should help to define the true efficacy of BCG. Thus far, it is apparent that the cure of microscopic metastases in melanoma by vaccination with BCG has been an elusive goal, but that significant advances have been made.

One of the most encouraging recent reports on immunotherapy with BCG has been that of McKneally *et al.* (1982), who randomized 66 patients with bronchogenic carcinoma of the lung, stages I–III from 1973–1977. Those patients with stage I (localized) cancer who received a single postoperative intrapleural injection of Tice BCG, 10^7 viable units, had a significantly lower rate of metastasis than those not receiving BCG. Eleven of the 30 had a recurrence of disease vs 20 of 36 controls, all of whom have died. Unfortunately, patients with stage II or III cancer were not benefited by intrapleural BCG. All BCG-treated patients also received isoniazid to control spread of the mycobacteria. Such studies as these deserve, and are in fact receiving, wider randomized trials for confirmation. Attempts to inject BCG directly into lung tumors prior to surgery have been performed at Yale and UCLA (Matthay *et al.*, 1982; Holmes *et al.*, 1982). The treatment was generally well tolerated and the desired infiltrates of lymphoid cells were induced in both studies. However, the one randomized study found no difference in mortality and disease-free intervals (Matthay *et al.*, 1982), while the other, non-randomized, study noted what appeared to be a difference in disease-free survival at a median follow-up of 15 months (55% vs. 37% for the surgery alone group). (Holmes *et al.*, 1982). These three investigations represent a significant use of regionally administered BCG for its antitumor effects, primarily against tumor in regional lymph nodes and perhaps also against microscopic visceral metastases.

The local use of BCG in the treatment of superficial bladder cancers (Morales and Ersil, 1982; Pinsky *et al.*, 1982) represents another clinical application of this material. Among the few randomized trials that have been performed with systemically administered BCG, it appears that ovarian cancer is benefited by the addition of BCG to combination chemotherapy (Alberts *et al.*, 1982). Furthermore, complete responses were more uniformly achieved when BCG was added to combination chemotherapy for diffuse histiocytic lymphoma but not for other cell types, in a large-scale study by the Southwest Oncology Group (Jones, 1982). Nevertheless, the survival of patients was improved for both diseases, diffuse histiocytic and nodular lymphoma, when BCG was given with chemotherapy at the outset of treatment.

IMMUNOLOGICAL EFFECTS OF BCG IN MAN

While the clinical efficacy of BCG has been suggested in several studies, it is noteworthy that the immunological correlates of a beneficial response generally have been lacking. Most studies that have measured immunity in patients treated with BCG have assessed nonspecific immunocompetence with microbial antigens to which the patients were presumed to be sensitized, such as candida, mumps, trichophyton and

PPD. Fewer studies have used the ability of a patient to be sensitized to a new skin test antigen, such as dinitrochlorobenzene (DNCB), as a measurement of increased immunocompetence. While Chess *et al.* (1973) found an increase in the magnitude of established delayed hypersensitivity reactions after patients had been treated with BCG, Mavligit *et al.* (1976) found no such effect. Furthermore, the latter group, studying 103 melanoma patients without gross evidence of disease, found no change in the number of patients who were able to be sensitized to DNCB, nor in the intensity of reaction to the chemical. Lui *et al.* (1975) found no correlation between the effectiveness of BCG as immunotherapy and its effects on general immunocompetence, which was generally unaltered.

Lieberman *et al.* (1974) studied six patients with cutaneous melanoma treated with intralesional BCG, of whom four had a good regression of injected nodules. Three of the four responders had an increase in their *in vitro* blastogenic response to melanoma antigens and all four had an increased response to the T cell mitogen phytohemagglutinin. The two nonresponders showed no such increases. Leukocyte migration inhibition in the presence of melanoma antigens was absent before therapy but was present in two of the four responders afterwards. Rosette-forming cells were also increased in the responders, but only in one of the two nonresponders. These results suggest that intralesional BCG *per se* did not routinely cause an increase in specific and nonspecific parameters of CMI but that it did so primarily in responders to therapy, perhaps indicating that the improved disease status was contributory to the improved immunological response.

'Tumor-specific' immunity has been measured in several studies, especially in patients receiving intralesional BCG. In general, those patients with a favorable response to BCG have had lymphocyte-mediated cytotoxicity to melanoma cells, but elevation of that response was not always achieved by BCG treatment even in responding patients (Seigler *et al.*, 1972, 1973; Nathanson and Clark, 1973; Bornstein *et al.*, 1973). With melanoma patients, Shibata *et al.* (1976) found that oral BCG increased CMI to allogeneic targets in four of seven patients but increased antibodies in only one of fourteen. We have studied the effect of BCG on the reactivity of a patient to autochthonous or allogeneic melanoma cells, i.e. 'tumor-specific' cell-mediated immunity. Mononuclear cells from the peripheral blood were tested in seven patients given intradermal or intralesional Tice strain BCG 1×10^6–2×10^7 viable units (Mitchell *et al.*, 1977). CMI was not increased in the patients receiving intralesional BCG, despite the disappearance of the injected lesions in two of the four patients, and was increased by a mean of 20 per cent above baseline in the intradermally inoculated group, with a return to baseline despite continued therapy. In a larger study recently completed (Mitchell, Merrill and Mokyr, unpublished data), 25 melanoma patients given Tice BCG by multiprong inoculation for 18 months showed a poor correlation between their clinical response, i.e. prolongation of the disease-free interval, and the augmentation of CMI, which was inconsistent. Only six of twenty-five had a sustained elevation of CMI greater than 20 per cent above baseline, thirteen had no significant change, three had a transient decrease in CMI with subsequent recovery, and the remaining three had a sustained decrease below their pretreatment level. Despite these *in vitro* findings, the same group has had improved median survival (33 months) compared with historical controls that were cited above, and the majority of the group are still disease-free 2–3 yr after the study. It is entirely possible that measurement of the reactivity of regional lymph nodes is a more accurate reflection of the effectiveness of BCG given into the skin, but obviously these nodes are inaccessible for serial studies of immunity. Notwithstanding the important and unresolved question of whether the cell-mediated cytotoxicity assay is a valid measurement of tumor-specific immunity, our results with the technique thus far have failed to provide evidence that BCG given into the skin of melanoma patients is capable of improving their CMI to homologous tumor cells.

While it has been claimed that improved survival has been produced by BCG in hematopoietic neoplasms, it remains uncertain whether improvement in the clinical response is immunologically mediated. Tumor-specific responses in leukemia are difficult to measure; one of the few studies attempting to do so, in chronic myelocytic leukemia (Ramachandar *et al.*, 1975), claimed that seven of eight patients who developed circulating antibodies to leukemic cells after BCG *plus* allogeneic irradiated myeloblasts had stability of their disease. In this setting, with antigen, BCG was designed to be used as a true adjuvant, rather than as a non specific stimulator of the RES. However, there was no proof that BCG *augmented* immunity, since no controls were given myeloblasts alone for comparison.

HAZARDS AND TOXICITY

Local reactivity to BCG depends upon the number of injections and the route of administration. Intradermal inoculations produce ulcerations locally, occasionally with regional lymphadenopathy, which may take several months to heal completely. With malaise lasting 24 hr, sometimes with a low-grade fever, is the most usual accompaniment of multiprong (Heaf-gun) vaccination and is somewhat more severe with intradermal administration (Sparks, 1973). No more than approximately 2×10^7 BCG viable organisms are tolerable intradermally, because of the severity of the local inflammation and ulceration, in contrast to 5×10^8 viable organisms applied to the skin by multiprong vaccination. However, the number of organisms actually entering the skin after the multiprong technique may be less than 2×10^7. Intralesional inoculation of BCG probably is tantamount to injection into the circulation, since tumor nodules are highly vascular. Thus, the number and severity of the complications by this route are greater. Fever in the range of 40°, chills, severe malaise, and anaphylactic reactions have been seen after intratumoral injection (Sparks, 1976). Granulomatous hepatitis has been documented by biopsy in approximately 12 per cent of patients receiving intralesional BCG (Hunt *et al.*, 1973), a process which appears to be allergic in nature, since viable organisms have not been recovered from the lesions. At least two patients have died from massive Shwartzman-like reactions after repeated intralesional injections (McKhann *et al.*, 1975). BCG sensitizes mice to the effects of bacterial endotoxin (Suter *et al.*, 1958) and presumably does so in man. It is these reactions, more severe in the tuberculin positive or repeatedly BCG-vaccinated individual, that have stimulated the search for less toxic fractions that retain the beneficial effects of the whole organism. Enhancement of tumor growth by intradermally administered BCG has been suggested but not proved in man (Levy *et al.*, 1972).

5. CONCLUSIONS AND PROJECTIONS

BCG has been a useful immunological modulator, whose specific properties are only now being elucidated well after its value has been established empirically. Regardless of its future rule as an adjunct in the treatment of cancer or other diseases, BCG can serve as an important prototype of a microbial modulator. Its activities in lymphoid and myeloid cells may be important indicators of which properties should be sought when screening similar agents for adjuvancy or suppressive effects. From the clinical point of view, the further development of fractions of BCG that mimic its effects but lack its toxicity would be most desirable.

Modulation of immunity by BCG is the vectorial sum of its many effects on influx, trapping and activation of lymphocytes and macrophages. Most of its overall effects have augmented immunity, but when suppressive activities are specifically measured, it is clear that they often co-exist with adjuvant effects. It is likely, although perhaps a little disheartening, that carefully controlled 'scientific empiricism' will be required to determine the appropriate dosage schedules to achieve the desired effects, since there appears to be no single schedule that invariably causes adjuvancy. For this reason, measurement of the immune response to the specific antigen in question (e.g. tumor cells) is mandatory in clinical immunotherapy trials, to provide a firmer base on which to judge the success or failure of the regimen.

Finally, the use of BCG as an adjuvant to specific antigen at appropriate schedules will almost surely be examined in man, when purified tumor antigens are available. This exploitation of the potential of BCG for increasing a specific immune response rather than simply its capacity as a chronic inflammatory stimulus locally or a 'nonspecific' stimulant of systemic immunity may prove to be a most important means of enabling the host to attack his tumor systemically and thus more completely.

Acknowledgements—Supported in part by Grants CA-13105 USPHS and IM-50, American Cancer Society and a Research Career Development Award CA-70,982 (Dr. Mitchell).

REFERENCES

ALEXANDER, P., CONNELL, D. I. and MIKULSKA, Z. B. (1966) Treatment of murine leukemia with spleen cells or sera from allogeneic mice immunized against tumor. *Cancer Res.* **26**: 1508–1515.

ALFORD, T. C., HOLLINSHEAD, A. and HUEBNER, R. (1969) Paradoxical effect of Freund's complete adjuvant upon transplantation efficiency of adenovirus-induced tumour cells. *J. gen. Virol.* **5**: 541–543.

ALLISON, A. C. and DAVIES, A. J. S. (1971) Requirement of thymus-dependent lymphocytes for potentiation by adjuvants of antibody formation. *Nature, Lond.* **233**: 330–332.

ASHERSON, G. L., FERLUGA, J. and JANOSSY, G. (1973) Nonspecific cytotoxicity by T cells activated with plant mitogens *in vitro* and the requirement for plant agents during the killing reaction. *Clin. exp. Immunol.* **15**: 573–589.

ATKINS, E., FELDMAN, J. D., FRANCIS, L. and HURSH, E. (1972) Studies on the mechanism of fever accompanying delayed hypersensitivity. The role of the sensitized lymphocyte. *J. exp. Med.* **135**: 1113–1132.

BAKER, L. A., SHARPTON, T., MINDEN, P. and CAMPBELL, P. A. (1976) Adjuvant and mitogenic properties of a supernatant fraction of sonically-treated *Mycobacterium bovis* (BCG). *Infect. Immunol.* **14**: 83–87.

BALDWIN, R. W. and PIMM, M. V. (1973) BCG immunotherapy of pulmonary growths from intravenously transferred rat tumour cells. *Br. J. Cancer* **27**: 48–54.

BALNER, H., OLD, L. J. and CLARKE, D. A. (1962) Accelerated rejection of male skin isografts by female C57BL mice infected with Bacillus Calmette–Guérin (BCG). *Proc. Soc. exp. Biol. Med.* **109**: 58–62.

BANSAL, S. C. and SJÖGREN, H. O. (1972) Counteraction of the blocking of cell-mediated tumor immunity by inoculation of unblocking sera and splenectomy: immunotherapeutic effects on primary polyoma tumors in rats. *Int. J. Cancer* **9**: 490–509.

BANSAL, S. C. and SJÖGREN, H. O. (1973) Effects of BCG on various facets of the immune response against polyoma tumors in rats. *Int. J. Cancer* **11**: 162–171.

BARTLETT, G. L., PURNELL, D. M. and KREIDER, J. W. (1976) BCG inhibition of murine leukemia: local suppression and systemic tumor immunity require different doses. *Science, Wash.* **191**: 299–301.

BARTLETT, G. L. and ZBAR, B. (1972) Tumor-specific vaccine containing *Mycobacterium bovis* and tumor cells: safety and efficacy. *J. Natn. Cancer Inst.* **48**: 1709–1926.

BARTLETT, G. L., ZBAR, B. and RAPP, H. J. (1972) Suppression of murine tumor growth by immune reaction to the *Bacillus Calmette–Guérin* strain of *Mycobacterium bovis. J. natn. Cancer Inst.* **48**: 245–257.

BAST, R. C., JR., ZBAR, B., BORSOS, T. and RAPP, H. J. (1974) BCG and Cancer. *New Engl. J. Med.* **290**: 1413–1420, 1458–1469.

BEKIERKUNST, A. (1975) Immunotherapy and vaccination against cancer with non-living BCG and cord factor (trehalose-6,6′-dimycolate). *Int. J. Cancer* **16**: 442–447.

BEKIERKUNST, A. (1976a) Immunotherapy of cancer with non-living mycobacteria and cord factor (trehalose-6,6′-dimycolate) in aqueous medium. *J. natn. Cancer Inst.* **57**: 963–964.

BEKIERKUNST, A. (1976b) Stimulation of lymphocyte proliferation by killed mycobacteria and other bacterial species. *Infect. Immunol.* **14**: 28–32.

BEN-EFRAIM, S. (1977) Methanol extraction residue: effects and mechanisms of action. *Pharmac. Ther.* **1**: 383–410.

BENNETT, J. A., MARSH, J. C. and MITCHELL, M. S. (1981) Suppressor macrophages: Their induction, characterization and regulation. In: *Modulation of Cellular Immunity in Cancer by Immune Modifiers,* M. A. Chirigos, M. S. Mitchell, M. J. Mastrangelo and M. Krim (eds.), pp. 9–26. New York, Raven.

BENNETT, J. A. and MITCHELL, M. S. (1979) Induction of suppressor cells by intravenous administration of Bacillus Calmette-Guerin (BCG) and its modulation by cyclophosphamide. *Bio-chem. Pharmacol.* (Arnold Welch Festschrift). **28**: 1947–1952.

BENNETT, J. A. and MITCHELL, M. S. (1980) Systemic administration of BCG activates natural suppressor cells in the bone marrow and stimulates their migration into the spleen. In: *Neoplasm Immunity: Experimental and Clinical,* R. G. Crispen (ed.), pp. 61–83. New York–Amsterdam–Oxford: Elsevier-North Holland.

BENNETT, J. A., RAO, V. S., KEMP, J. D. and MITCHELL, M. S. (1981) Selectivity in the effects of indomethacin on BCG-activated suppressor cell populations. *J. Immunopharm.* **3**: 221–239.

BERD, D. and MITCHELL, M. S. (1976) Immunological enhancement of leukemia L1210 by *Corynebacterium parvum. Cancer Res.* **36**: 4119–4124.

BIOZZI, G., STIFFEL, C., HALPERN, B. N. and MOUTON, D. (1959) Effet de l'inoculation du bacille de Calmette–Guérin sur le developpement de la tumeur ascitique d'Ehrlich chez la souris. *C.R. Séanc. Soc. Biol.* **153**: 987–989.

BIOZZI, G., STIFFEL, C., MOUTON, D., BOUTHILLIER, Y. and DECREUSEFOND, C. (1964) Survival of spleen cells transplanted into syngeneic and allogeneic mice during stimulation of the reticuloendothelial system induced by *Myco tuberculosis* (BCG) infection. *Br. J. exp. Pathol.* **45**: 357–363.

BORNSTEIN, R. S., MASTRANGELO, M. J. and SULIT, H. (1973) Immunotherapy of melanoma with intralesional BCG. *Natn. Cancer Inst. Monogr.* **39**: 213–220.

BORSOS, T. and RAPP, H. J. (1973) Brief communication: antigenic relationship between *Mycobacterium bovis* (BCG) and a guinea pig hepatoma. *J. natn. Cancer Inst.* **51**: 1085–1086.

BRAUN, D. P., MOKYR, and DRAY, S. (1978) Generation of anti-MOPC 315 cytotoxicity in uneducated or *in vitro* educated spleen cells from normal or MOPC-315 tumor-bearing mice pretreated *in vivo* with BCG. *Cancer Res.* (In press).

BRUNNER, K. T., MAUEL, J., RUDOLF, H. and CHAPUIS, B. (1970) Studies of allograft immunity in mice. I. Induction, development and *in vitro* assay of cellular immunity. *Immunology* **18**: 501–515.

BRUNNER, K. T., MAUEL, J. and SCHINDLER, R. (1966) *In vitro* studies of cell-bound immunity: cloning assay of the cytotoxic action of sensitized lymphoid cells on allogeneic target cells. *Immunology* **11**: 499–506.

CARSWELL, E. A., OLD, L. J., KASSEL, R. L., GREEN, S., FIORE, N. and WILLIAMSON, B. (1975) An endotoxin-induced serum factor that causes necrosis of tumors. *Proc. natn. Acad. Sci.* **72**: 3666–3670.

CHEDID, L., AUDIBERT, F., LEFRANCIER, P., CHOAY, J. and LEDERER, E. (1976) Modulation of the immune response by a synthetic adjuvant and analogs. *Proc. natn. Acad. Sci.* **73**: 2474–2475.

CHEDID, L., LAMENSANS, A. and PARANT, F. (1973) Protective effects of delipidated mycobacterial cells and purified cell walls against Ehrlich carcinoma and a syngeneic lymphoid leukemia in mice. *Cancer Res.* **33**: 2187–2195.

CHEDID, L., PARANT, M., PARANT, F., LEFRANCIER, P., CHOAY, J. and LEDERER, E. (1977) Enhancement of nonspecific immunity to *Klebsiella pneumoniae* infection by a synthetic immunoadjuvant (*N*-acetyl muramyl-L-alanyl-D-isoglutamine) and several analogs. *Proc. natn. Acad. Sci.* **74**: 2089–2093.

CHESS, L., BOCK, G. N., UNGARO, P. C. *et al.* (1973) Immunologic effects of BCG in patients with malignant melanoma: specific evidence for stimulation of the 'secondary' immune response. *J. natn. Cancer Inst.* **51**: 57–65.

CLARK, I. A., ALLISON, A. C. and COX, F. E. (1976) Protection of mice against Babesia and Plasmodium with BCG. *Nature, Lond.* **259**: 309–311.

CLEVELAND, R. P., MELTZER, M. S. and ZBAR, B. (1974) Tumor cytotoxicity *in vitro* by macrophages from mice infected with *Mycobacterium bovis* strain BCG. *J. natn. Cancer Inst.* **52**: 1887–1895.

COMSTOCK, G. W., LIVESAY, V. T. and WEBSTER, R. G. (1971) Leukaemia and BCG. *Lancet* **2**: 1062–1063.

COMSTOCK, G. W., MARTINEZ, I. and LIVESAY, V. T. (1975) Efficacy of BCG vaccination in prevention of cancer. *J. natn. Cancer Inst.* **54**: 835–839.

CROWTHER, D., POWLES, R. L., BATEMAN, C. J. *et al.* (1973) Management of adult acute myelogenous leukaemia. *Br. Med. J.* **1**: 131–137.

DAMAIS, C., BONA, C., CHEDID, L. *et al.* (1975) Mitogenic effect of bacterial peptidoglycans possessing adjuvant activity. *J. Immunol.* **115**: 268–271.

DAVIGNON, L., LEMONDE, P. and ROBILLARD, P. (1970) BCG vaccination and leukaemia mortality. *Lancet* **2**: 638.

DIENES, L. and SCHOENHEIT, E. W. (1927) Local hypersensitiveness. I. Sensitization of tuberculous guinea pigs with egg white and timothy pollen. *J. Immunol.* **14**: 9–42.

EILBER, F. R., MORTON, D. L., HOLMES, E. C., SPARKS, F. C. and RAMMING, K. P. (1976) Adjuvant immunotherapy with BCG in treatment of regional lymph node metastases from malignant melanoma. *New Engl. J. Med.* **294**: 237–240.

ELVES, M. W. (1967) Suppression of antibody production by phytohaemagglutinin. *Nature, Lond.* **213**: 495–496.

EVANS, R. and ALEXANDER, P. (1972) Mechanism of immunologically specific killing of tumor cells by macrophages. *Nature, Lond.* **236**: 168–170.

FAIRLEY, G. H. (1976) Immunotherapy in the management of myelogenous leukemia. *Archs intern. Med.* **136**: 1406–1412.

FARACI, R. P. and SCHOUR, L. (1974) Malignant melanoma: specific immunity induced by Bacillus Calmette–Guérin in BALB/c mice. *Science, Wash.* **185**: 68–70.

FLECK, J., MOCK, M., TYTGAT, F., NAUCIEL, C. and MINCK, R. (1974) Adjuvant activity in delayed hypersensitivity of the peptidic part of bacterial peptidoglycans. *Nature, Lond.* **250**: 517–518.

FLORENTIN, I., HUCHET, R., BRULEY-ROSSET, M., HALLE-PANNENKO and MATHÉ, G. (1976) Studies on the mechanisms of action of BCG. *Cancer Immunol. Immunother.* **1**: 31–40.

FOLCH, H., YOSHINAGA, M. and WAKSMAN, B. H. (1972) Regulation of lymphocyte responses *in vitro*. III. Inhibition by adherent cells of the T-lymphocyte response to phytohemagglutinin. *J. Immunol.* **110**: 835–839.

FORTNER, G. W., HANNA, M. G., JR. and COGGIN, J. H., JR. (1974) Differential effects of two strains of BCG on transplantation immunity to SW40-induced tumors in hamsters. *Proc. Soc. exp. Biol. Med.* **147**: 62–67.

FREEMAN, C. B., HARRIS, R., GEARY, C. G. *et al.* (1973) Active immunotherapy used alone for maintenance of patients with acute myeloid leukaemia. *Br. med. J.* **4**: 571–573.

FROST, P. and LANCE, E. M. (1974) The relation of lymphocyte trapping to the mode of action of adjuvants. In: *Immunopotentiation*, WOLSTENHOLME, G. E. W. and KNIGHT, J. (eds.) pp. 29–45. Elsevier–North Holland, Amsterdam.

GALELLI, A., LEGARREC, Y., CHEDID, L., LEFRACIER, P., DERRIEN, M. and LEVEL, M. (1980). Macrophage stimulation *in vitro* by an inactive muramyl dipeptide derivative after conjugation to a multi-poly (DL-alanyl)-poly (L-lysine) carrier. *Infect. Immun.* **28**: 1–5.

GERSHON, R. K., MOKYR, M. B. and MITCHELL, M. S. (1974) Activation of suppressor T cells by tumour cells and specific antibody. *Nature, New Biol.* **250**: 594–596.

GERY, I., BAER, A., STUPP, Y. and WEISS, D. W. (1974) Further studies on the effects of the methanol extraction residue fraction of the tubercle bacilli on lymphoid cells and macrophages. *Israel J. med. Sci.* **10**: 984–991.

GERY, I. and EIDINGER, D. (1977) Selective and opposing effects of cytochalasin B and other drugs on lymphocyte responses to different doses of mitogens. *Cell. Immunol.* **30**: 147–155.

GERY, I., GERSHON, R. K. and WAKSMAN, B. H. (1972) Potentiation of the T-cell response to mitogens. I. The responding cell. *J. exp. Med.* **136**: 128–142.

GERY, I. and WAKSMAN, B. H. (1972) Potentiation of the T-cell response to mitogens. II. The cellular source of potentiating mediator(s). *J. exp. Med.* **136**; 143–155.

GRANGER, G. A. and WEISER, R. S. (1966) Homograft target cells: contact destruction *in vitro* by immune macrophages. *Science, N.Y.* **151**: 97–99.

GRAVES, S. R. and JOHNSON, R. C. (1975) Effect of pretreatment with *M. bovis* (strain BCG) and immune syphilicic serum on rabbit resistance to *Treponema pallidum. Infect. Immunol.* **12**: 1029–1036.

GRAY, J. D. and BROOKS, C. G. (1980) The induction of cytotoxic macrophages and natural killer cells in congenitally athymic nu/rnu rats. *Cell. Immunol.* **53**: 405–412.

GREEN, S., DOBRJANSKY, A., CARSWELL, E. A., KASSEL, R. L., OLD, L. J., FIORE, N. and SCHWARTZ, M. K. (1976) Partial purification of a serum factor that causes necrosis of tumors. *Proc. natn. Acad. Sci.* **73**: 381–385.

GROSSBERG, S. E. (1972) The interferons and their inducers: molecular and therapeutic considerations. *New Engl. J. Med.* **287**: 127–128.

GUTTERMAN, J. U., HERSH, E. M., RODRIGUEZ, V. *et al.* (1974) Chemoimmunotherapy of adult acute leukaemia. Prolongation of remission in myeloblastic leukaemia with BCG. *Lancet* **2**: 1405–1409.

GUTTERMAN, J. U., MAVLIGIT, G. M., BLUMENSHEIN, G., BURGESS, M. A., MCBRIDE, C. M. and HERSH, E. M. (1976) Immunotherapy of human solid tumors with Bacillus Calmette–Guérin: Prolongation of disease-free interval and survival in malignant melanoma, breast, and colorectal cancer. *Ann. N.Y. Acad. Sci.* **277**: 135–158.

GUTTERMAN, J. U., MAVLIGIT, G. M. and MCBRIDE, C. (1973) Active immunotherapy with BCG for recurrent malignant melanoma. *Lancet* **1**: 1208–1212.

GUTTERMAN, J. U., MAVLIGIT, G. M., REED, R. *et al.* (1975) Immunology and immunotherapy of human malignant melanoma: historic review and perspectives for the future. *Semin. Oncol.* **2**: 155–174.

HALPERN, B. N., BIOZZI, G., STIFFEL, C. and MOUTON, D. (1959) Effet de la stimulation du système réticuloendothélial par l'inoculation du bacille de Calmette–Guérin sur le dévelopement de l'épithelioma atypique T-8 de Guérin chez le rat. *C.r. Séanc. Soc. Biol.* **153**: 919–923.

HANNA, M. G., JR., ZBAR, B. and RAPP, H. J. (1972a) Histopathology of tumor regression after intralesional injection of *Mycobacterium bovis*. I. Tumor growth and metastasis. *J. natn. Cancer Inst.* **48**: 1441–1455.

Idem (1972b) II. Comparative effects of vaccinia virus, oxazolone, and turpentine. *J. natn. Cancer Inst.* **48**: 1697–1707.

HARAN-GHERA, N. and WEISS, D. W. (1973) Effect of treatment of C57BL mice with the methanol extraction residue fraction of BCG on leukomogenesis induced by the radiation leukemia virus. *J. natn. Cancer Inst.* **50**: 229–234.

HARRIS, R., ZUHIE, S. R., FREEMAN, C. B., READ, A. P., MACIVER, J. E., GEARY, C. G., DELAMORE, W., and TOOTH, J. A. (1982) A successful randomized trial of immunotherapy alone vs no-maintenance treatment in acute myelogenous leukemia. *In: Immunotherapy of Human Cancer.* Terry, W. D. and Rosenberg, S. A. (eds.), pp. 11–16. Excerpta Medica, New York.

HAWRYLKO, E. (1975) Immunopotentiation with BCG: dimensions of a specific anti-tumor response. *J. natn. Cancer Inst.* **59**: 1189–1197.

HAWRYLKO, E. and MACKANESS, G. B. (1973) Immunopotentiation with BCG. IV. Factors affecting the magnitude of an antitumor response. *J. natn. Cancer Inst.* **51**: 1683–1688.

HERBERMAN, R. B., NUNN, M. E., HOLDEN, H. T. and LAVRIN, D. H. (1975) Natural cytotoxic reactivity of mouse lymphoid cells against syngeneic and allogeneic tumors. II. Characterization of effector cells. *Int. J. Cancer* **16**: 230–239.

HEYN, R., BORGES, W., JOO, P. *et al.* (1973) BCG in the treatment of acute lymphocytic leukemia (ALL). *Proc. Am. Ass. Cancer Res.* **14**: 45.

HIBBS, J. B., JR. (1973) Macrophage non-immunologic recognition: Target cell factors related to contact inhibition. *Science, N.Y.* **180**: 868–870.

HIBBS, J. B., JR., LAMBERT, L. H., JR. and REMINGTON, J. S. (1972) Possible role of macrophage mediated nonspecific cytotoxicity in tumour resistance. *Nature, New Biol.* **235**: 48–50.

HIU, I. J. (1972) Water-soluble and lipid-free fraction from BCG with adjuvant and antitumour activity. *Nature, New Biol.* **238**: 241–242.

HOLMES, E. C., RAMMING, K. P., GOLUB, S. H., EDELSTEIN, R., NIITSUMA, M., BEIN, M. and COULSON, W. (1982) Intralesional BCG in pulmonary tumors. *In: Immunotherapy of Human Cancer* Terry, W. D. and Rosenberg, S. A. (eds.), pp. 81–86. Excerpta Medica, New York.

HOLTERMANN, O. A., KLEIN, E. and CASALE, G. P. (1973) Selective cytotoxicity of peritoneal leucocytes for neoplastic cells. *Cell Immunol.* **9**: 339–352.

HOUCHENS, D. P., GASTON, M. R., KINNEY, Y. and GOLDIN, A. (1974) Prevention of cyclophosphamide immunosuppression by Bacillus Calmette–Guérin. *Cancer Chemo. Rep.* **58**: 931–933.

HOUCHENS, D. P., GOLDBERG, A. I., GASTON, M. R. KONDE, M. and GOLDIN, A. (1973) Studies of the effects of Bacillus Calmette–Guérin on Moloney sarcoma virus-induced tumors in normal and immunosuppressed mice. *Cancer Res.* **33**: 685–691.

HUNT, J. S., SILVERSTEIN, M. C. and SPARKS, F. C. (1973) Granulomatous hepatitis: a complication of BCG immunotherapy. *Lancet* **2**: 820–821.

JACOBS, D. M., PASS, E., ABRAHAM, C. and WEISS, D. W. (1978) Studies on the influence of the methanol extraction residue tubercle bacillus fraction on immunological responsiveness of mice. Effects on antibody formation to a soluble protein and a T-independent antigen, delayed hypersensitivity to sheep erythrocytes and numbers of antigen-reactive lymphoid cells. *Israel J. med. Sci.* **14**: 60–74.

JULIUS, M. H., SIMPSON, E. and HERZENBERG, L. A. (1973) A rapid method for the isolation of functional thymus-derived murine lymphocytes. *Eur. J. Immunol.* **3**: 645–649.

KIESSLING, R., PETRAYNI, G., KARRE, K., JONDAL, M., TRACEY, D. and WIGZELL, H. (1976) Killer cells: a functional comparison between natural, immune T-cell and antibody-dependent *in vitro* systems. *J. exp. Med.* **143**: 772–780.

KIRKPATRICK, C. H. (1971) Chronic mucocutaneous candidiasis model-building in cellular immunity. *Ann. Intern. Med.* **79**: 955–978.

KITAMURA, Y., NOMOTO, K., TORISU, M. and TAKEYA, K. (1976) Effects of BCG (Bacillus Calmette–Guérin) vaccines on immune responses in mice. *Japan. J. Microbiol.* **20**: 303–308.

KLEIN, W. J., JR. (1971) Lymphocyte-mediated cytotoxicity *in vitro*. Effect of enhancing antisera. *J. exp. Med.* **134**: 1238–1252.

KLIMPEL, G. R. (1979) Soluble factors from BCG-induced suppressor cells inhibit *in vitro* PFC responses but not cytotoxic responses. *Cell. Immunol.* **53**: 405–412.

KLIMPEL, G. R., OKADA, M. and HENNEY, C. S. (1979) Inhibition of *in vitro* cytotoxicity responses by BCG-induced macrophage-like suppressor cells. II. Suppression occurs at the level of a 'helper' T cell. *J. Immunol.* **123**: 350–357.

KOTANI, S., WATANABE, Y., SHIMONO, T. *et al.* (1976) Correlation between the immunoadjuvant activities and pyrogenicities of synthetic *N*-acetylmuramyl-peptides or -amino acids. *Biken J.* **19**: 9–13.

KUPERMAN, O., FEGIS, M. and WEISS, D. W. (1973) Reversal by the MER tubercle bacillus fraction of the suppressive effects of heterologous antilymphocyte serum (ALS) on the allograft reactivity of mice. *Cell. Immunol.* **8**: 484–489.

LAVRIN, D. H., ROSENBERG, S. A., CONNOR, R. J. and TERRY, W. T. (1973) Immunoprophylaxis of methylcholanthrene induced tumors in mice with Bacillus Calmette–Guérin and methanol-extracted residue. *Cancer Res.* **33**: 472–477.

LEAKE, E. S. and MYRVIK, Q. M. (1968) Changes in morphology and in lysozyme content of free alveolar cells after intravenous injection of killed BCG in oil. *J. Reticuloendothel. Soc.* **5**: 33–53.

LEDERER, E. (1976) Cord factor and related trehalose esters. *Chem. Phys. Lipids* **16**: 91–106.

Leukaemia Committee (1971) Treatment of acute lymphoblastic leukaemia: comparison of immunotherapy (BCG), intermittent methotrexate, and no therapy after a five-month intensive cytotoxic regimen (Concord trial): preliminary report to the Medical Research Council by the Leukaemia Committee and the Working Party on Leukaemia in Childhood. *Br. med. J.* **4**: 189–194.

LEVENTHAL, B. G., LEPOURHEIT, A., HALTERMAN, R. H. *et al.* (1973) Immunotherapy in previously treated acute lymphatic leukemia. *Natn. Cancer Inst. Monogr.* **39**: 177–187.

LEVIS, W. R. and ROBBINS, J. H. (1970) Effect of glass-adherent cells on the blastogenic response of 'purified' lymphocytes to phytohemagglutinin. *Exp. Cell Res.* **61**: 153–158.

LEVY, N. L., MAHALEY, M. S. and DAY, E. D. (1972) Serum-mediated blocking of cell-mediated antitumor immunity in a melanoma patient; association with BCG immunotherapy and clinical deterioration. *Int. J. Cancer* **10**: 244–248.

LEWIS, P. A. and LOOMIS, D. (1924) Allergic irritability: the formation of anti-sheet hemolytic amboceptor in the normal and tuberculous guinea pig. *J. exp. Med.* **40**: 503–515.

LIEBERMAN, R., EPSTEIN, W. and FUDENBERG, H. H. (1974) Immunopathologic changes in patients with cutaneous malignant melanoma following intratumoral inoculation of BCG: correlation with cell-mediated immunity. *Int. J. Cancer* **14**: 401–416.

LUI, V. K., KARPUCHAS, J., DENT, P. B. *et al.* (1975) Cellular immunocompetence in melanoma: effect of extent of disease and immunotherapy. *Br. J. Cancer* **32**: 323–330.

MACKANESS, G. B. (1964) The immunological basis of acquired cellular resistance. *J. exp. Med.* **120**: 105–120.

MACKANESS, G. B., AUCLAIR, D. J. and LAGRANGE, P. H. (1973) Immunopotentiation with BCG. I. Immune response to different strains and preparation. *J. natn. Cancer Inst.* **51**: 1655–1667.

MACKANESS, G. B., LAGRANGE, P. H. and ISHIBASHI, T. (1974) The modifying effect of BCG on the immunological induction of T cells. *J. exp. Med.* **139**: 1540–1552.

MAILLARD, J. and BLOOM, B. R. (1972) Immunological adjuvants and the mechanism of cell cooperation. *J. exp. Med.* **136**: 185–190.

MASTRANGELO, M. J., BERD, D. and BELLET, R. E. (1976) Critical review of previously reported clinical trials of cancer immunotherapy with non-specific immunostimulants. *Ann. N.Y. Acad. Sci.* **277**: 94–122.

MATHÉ, G., AMIEL, J. L., SCHWARZENBERG, L. *et al.* (1969) Active immunotherapy for acute lymphoblastic leukaemia. *Lancet* **1**: 697–699.

MATHÉ, G., HALLE-PANNENKO, O. and BOURUT, C. (1974) Immune manipulation by BCG administered before or after cyclophosphamide for chemoimmunotherapy of L1210 leukaemia. *Eur. J. Cancer* **10**: 661–666.

MATHÉ, G., KAMEL, M., DEZFULIAN, M., HALLE-PANNENKO, O. and BOURUT, C. (1973) An experimental screening system for 'systemic adjuvants of immunity' applicable in cancer immunotherapy. *Cancer Res.* **33**: 1987–1997.

MATHÉ, G. POUILLART, P. and LAPEYRAQUE, F. (1969) Active immunotherapy of L1210 leukaemia applied after the graft of tumour cells. *Br. J. Cancer* **23**: 814–824.

MATTHAY, R. A., MAHLER, D. A., MITCHELL, M. S., CARTER, D. H., LOKE, J., BECK, G. J., REYNOLDS, H. Y. and BAUE, A. E. (1982) Intratumoral BCG immunotherapy prior to surgery for carcinoma of the lung: preliminary results. *In: Immunotherapy of Human Cancer,* Terry, W. D. and Rosenberg, S. A. (eds.), pp. 69–79. Excerpta Medica, New York.

MAVLIGIT, G. M., GUTTERMAN, J. U. and HERSH, E. M. (1976) Effect of BCG (Tice strain) on primary sensitization to 2,4-dinitrochlorobenzene and on established delayed hypersensitivity in human malignant melanoma. *J. natn. Cancer Inst.* **57**: 749–751.

McKhann, C. F., Hendrickson, C. G., Spitler, L. E. *et al.* (1975) Immunotherapy of melanoma with BCG: two fatalities following intralesional injection. *Cancer* **35**: 514–520.

McKneally, M. F., McIlduff, J. B., Older, T. M., Foster, E. O., Alley, R. D. and Linenger, L. (1982) Four-year follow-up on the Albany experience with intrapleural BCG in lung cancer. *In: Immunotherapy of Human Cancer,* Terry, W. D. and Rosenberg, S. A. (eds.), pp. 87–92. Excerpta Medica, New York.

Meltzer, M. S., Jones, E. E. and Boetcher, D. A. (1975) Increased chemothactic responses of macrophages from BCG-infected mice. *Cell. Immunol.* **17**: 268–276.

Meyer, T. J., Anacker, R. L. and Ribi, E. (1974) Effects of pretreatment of mice with BCG cell walls in saline on subsequent vaccination with BCG oil droplet vaccination. *Cell. Immunol.* **14**: 52–65.

Meyer, T. J., Ribi, E. and Azuma, I. (1974) Biologically active components from mycobacterial cell walls. II. Suppression and regression of strain-2 guinea pig hepatoma. *J. natn. Cancer Inst.* **52**: 103–111.

Miller, T. E., Mackaness, G. B. and Lagrange, P. H. (1973) Immunopotentiation with BCG. II. Modulation of the response to sheep red blood cells. *J. natn. Cancer Inst.* **51**: 1669–1676.

Minden, P., Sharpton, T. R. and McClatchy, J. K. (1976) Shared antigens between human malignant melanoma cells and *Mycobacterium bovis* (BCG). *J. Immunol.* **116**: 1407–1414.

Mitchell, M. S. (1976) Role of 'suppressor' T-lymphocytes in antibody-induced inhibition of cytophilic antibody receptors. *Ann. N.Y. Acad. Sci.* **276**: 229–241.

Mitchell, M. S., Kirkpatrick, D., Mokyr, M. B. and Gery, I. (1973) On the mode of action of BCG. *Nature, New Biol.* **243**: 216–218.

Mitchell, M. S., Mokyr, M. B. and Davis, J. M. (1977) Effect of chemotherapy and immunotherapy on tumor-specific immunity in melanoma. *J. clin. Invest.* **57**: 517–526.

Mitchell, M. S., Mokyr, M. B. and Kahane, I. (1975) Effect of fractions of BCG on lymphoid cells *in vitro. J. natn. Cancer Inst.* **55**: 1337–1343.

Mokyr, M. B. and Mitchell, M. S. (1975) Activation of lymphoid cells by BCG *in vitro. Cell. Immunol.* **15**: 264–273.

Mokyr, M. B., Bennett, J. A., Braun, D. P., Hengst, J. C. D., Mitchell, M. S. and Dray, S. (1980). Opposite effects of different strains or batches of the same strain of BCG on the *in vitro* generation of syngeneic and allogeneic anti-tumor cytotoxicity. *J. Natl. Cancer Inst.* **64:** 339–344.

Morton, D. L., Eilber, F. R., Malmgren, R. A. and Wood, W. C. (1970) Immunological factors which influence response to immunotherapy in malignant melanoma. *Surgery* **68**: 158–164.

Murahata, R. I. and Mitchell, M. S. (1976a) Antagonism of the immunosuppressive effects of cytarabine (ara-C) by Bacillus Calmette–Guérin (BCG). *Proc. Am. Ass. Cancer. Res.* **17**: 83.

Murahata, R. I. and Mitchell, M. S. (1976b) Antagonism of immunosuppression by BCG. In: *The Macrophage in Neoplasia,* Fink, M. A. (ed.) pp. 263–265. Academic Press, New York.

Murahata, R. I. and Mitchell, M. S. (1982) Modulation of cell-mediated immunity by BCG. I. Antagonism and potentiation of immunosuppression caused by cytarabine. *J. Natl. Cancer Inst.* **69:** 607–612.

Murahata, R. I. and Mitchell, M. S. (1982b) Modulation of cell-mediated immunity by BCG. II. Induction of specific, nonadherent non-T killer cells by BCG and alloantigen. *J. Natl. Cancer Inst.* **69:** 613–618.

Myrvik, Q. M. (1972) Function of the alveolar macrophage in immunity. *J. Reticuloendothel. Soc.* **11**: 459–468.

Nagao, S., Tanaka, A., Yamamoto, Y., Koga, T., Onoue, K., Shiba, T., Kusumoto, K. and Kotani, S. (1979) Inhibition of macrophage migration by muramyl peptides. *Infect. Immun.* **24:** 308–312.

Nathan, C. F., Asofsky, R. and Terry, W. D. (1977) Characterization of the nonphagocytic adherent cell from the peritoneal cavity of normal and BCG-treated mice. *J. Immunol.* **118**: 1612–1621.

Nathan, C. F., Hill, V. M. and Terry, W. D. (1976) Isolation of a subpopulation of adherent peritoneal cells with anti-tumour activity. *Nature, Lond.* **260**: 146–148.

Nathan, C. F. and Terry, W. D. (1975) Differential stimulation of murine lymphoma growth *in vitro* by normal and BCG-activated macrophages. *J. exp. Med.* **142**: 887–902.

Nathanson, L. (1972) Regression of intradermal malignant melanoma after intralesional injection of *Mycobacterium bovis* strain BCG. *Cancer Chemother. Rep.* **56**: 659–665.

Nathanson, L. and Clark, A. (1973) *In vitro* assay of cell mediated immunity in BCG therapy of malignant melanoma: a preliminary report. *Natn. Cancer Inst. Monogr.* **39**: 221–224.

Nelson, D. S. and Boyden, S. V. (1964) The cutaneous reactivity of guinea pigs to pure protein antigens. I. A critical evaluation of methods for the induction of delayed-type hypersensitivity to pure proteins. *Int. Archs. Allergy appl. Immun.* **25**: 279–303.

Oehler, J. R., Herberman, R. B. and Holden, H. T. (1978) Modulation of immunity by macrophages. *Pharmacol. Therap.* **2**: 551–593.

Ogura, T., Azuma, I., Nishikawa, H. *et al.* (1975) Effect of oil-attached BCG cell wall on the kinetics of lymphocytes in the tumor-draining node. *Gann* **66**: 349–354.

Old, L. J., Benacerraf, B., Clarke, D. A., Carswell, E. A. and Stockert, E. (1961) The role of the reticuloendothelial system in the host reaction to neoplasia. *Cancer Res.* **21**: 1281–1300.

Old, L. J., Clarke, D. A. and Benacerraf, B. (1959) Effect of Bacillus Calmette–Guérin infection on transplanted tumours in the mouse. *Nature, Lond.* **184**: 291–292.

Paranjpe, M. S. and Boone, C. W. (1974) Stimulated growth of syngeneic tumors at the site of an ongoing delayed hypersensitivity reaction to tuberculin in BALB/c mice. *J. natn. Cancer Inst.* **52**: 1297–1299.

Peavy, D. L. and Pierce, C. W. (1974) Cell-mediated immune responses *in vitro.* I. Suppression of the generation of cytotoxic lymphocytes by concanavalin A and concanavalin B-activated spleen cells. *J. exp. Med.* **140**: 356–369.

Peters, L. C., Hanna, M. G., Jr., Gutterman, J. U., Mavligit, G. M. and Hersh, E. M. (1974) Modulation of the immune response of guinea pigs by repeated BCG scarification. *Proc. Soc. exp. Biol. Med.* **147**: 344–349.

Piessens, W. F. Heimann, R., Legros, N. and Henson, J. C. (1971) Effect of bacillus Calmette-Guérin on mammary tumor formation and cellular immunity in dimethylbenz (a) anthracene-treated rats. *Cancer Res.* **31**: 1061–1065.

PINSKY, C., HIRSHAUT, Y. and OETTGEN, H. (1973) Treatment of malignant melanoma by intratumoral injection of BCG. *Natn. Cancer Inst. Monogr.* **39**: 225–228.

POPLACK, D. G., SHER, N. A., CHAPARAS, S. D. and BLAESE, R. M. (1976) The effect of *Mycobacterium bovis* (Bacillus Calmette–Guérin) on macrophage randome migration, chemotaxis and pinocytosis. *Cancer Res.* **36**: 1233–1237.

RAMACHANDAR, K., BAKER, M. A. and TAUB, R. N. (1975) Antibody responses to leukemia-associated antigens during immunotherapy of chronic myelocytic leukemia. *Blood* **46**: 845–854.

RAO, V. S. and MITCHELL, M. S. (1981) BCG prevents suppression of macrophage-mediated immunity induced by immune complexes. *Proc. Amer. Assoc. Cancer Res.* **22**: 274.

RAO, V. S., MOKYR, M. B., GERSHON, R. B. and MITCHELL, M. S. (1977) Specific T cell-dependent, antigen-antibody induced suppression of macrophages: abrogation by nonspecifically stimulated T cells. *J. Immunol.* **118**: 2117–2124.

RAU, M. E. and TANNER, C. E. (1975) BCG suppresses growth and matastasis of hydatid infections. *Nature, Lond.* **256**: 318–319.

REINISCH, C. L., GLEINER, N. A. and SCHLOSSMAN, S. F. (1976) Adjuvant regulation of T cell function. *J. Immunol.* **116**: 710–715.

RIBI, E. E., MEYER, T. J., AZUMA, I. *et al.* (1973) Mycobacterial cell wall components in tumor suppression and regression. *Natn. Cancer Inst. Monogr.* **39**: 115–119.

RIBI, E., MEYER, T. J., AZUMA, I., PARKER, R. and BREHMER, W. (1975) Biologically active components from mycobacterial cell walls. IV. Protection of mice against aerosol infection with virulent Mycobacterium tuberculosis. *Cell. Immunol.* **16**: 1–10.

ROSENTHAL, S. R., CRISPEN, R. G. and THORNE, M. G. (1976) BCG vaccination and leukemia mortality. *J. Am. med. Ass.* **222**: 1543–1544.

RUSKIN, J. and REMINGTON, J. S. (1971) Resistance to intracellular infection in mice immunized with toxoplasma vaccine and adjuvant. *J. Reticuloendothel. Soc.* **9**: 465–479.

SALVIN, S. B., YOUNGNER, J. S. and LEDERER, W. H. (1973) Migration inhibitory factor and interferon in the circulation of mice with delayed hypersensitivity. *Infect. Immunol.* **7**: 68–75.

SCHULTZ, R. M., PAPMATHEAKIS, J. D., STYLOS, W. A. and CHIRIGOS, M. A. (1976) Augmentation of specific macrophage-mediated cytotoxicity: correlations with agents which enhance antitumor resistance. *Cell. Immunol.* **25**: 309–316.

SEIGLER, H. F., SHINGLETON, W. W., METZGAR, R. S. *et al.* (1972) Nonspecific and specific immunotherapy in patients with melanoma. *Surgery* **72**: 162–174.

SEIGLER, H. F., SHINGLETON, W. W. and METZGAR, R. S. (1973) Immunotherapy in patients with melanoma. *Ann. Surg.* **178**: 352–359.

SHER, N. A., CHAPARAS, S. D., GREENBERG, L. D. and BERNARD, S. (1975) Effects of BCG, Corynebacterium parvum and methanol-extraction residue in the reduction of mortality from Staphylococcus aureus and Candida albicans infections in immunosuppressed mice. *Infect. Immunol.* **12**: 1325–1330.

SHERIDAN, J. W. and METCALF, D. (1972) Studies of the bone marrow colony stimulating factor (CSF): relationship of tissue CSF to serum CSF. *J. cell. Physiol.* **80**: 129.

SHIBATA, H. R., JERRY, L. M. and LEWIS, M. G. (1976) Immunotherapy of human malignant melanoma with irradiated tumor cells, oral Bacillus Calmette–Guérin, and levamisole. *Ann. N.Y. Acad. Sci.* **277**: 355–366.

SKIDMORE, B. J., CHILLER, J. M., MORRISON, D. C. and WEIGLE, W. O. (1975) Immunologic properties of bacterial lipopolysaccharides (LPS): correlation between the mitogenic, adjuvant, and immugenic activities. *J. Immunol.* **114**: 770–775.

SPARKS, F. C. (1976) Hazards and complications of BCG immunotherapy. *Med. Clins N. Am.* **60**: 499–509.

SPARKS, F. C. and BREEDING, J. H. (1974) Tumor regression and enhancement resulting from immunotherapy with Bacillus Calmette–Guérin and neuraminidase. *Cancer Res.* **34**: 3262–3269.

SPARKS, F. C., SILVERSTEIN, M. J., HUNT, J. S. *et al.* (1973) Complications of BCG immunotherapy in patients with cancer. *New Engl. J. Med.* **289**: 827–830.

SPITZNAGEL, J. and ALLISON, A. C. (1970) Mode of action of adjuvants: retinol and other lysosome-labilizing agents and adjuvants. *J. Immunol.* **104**: 119–127.

STEINKULLER, C. B. and BURTON, D. (1966) Immunology of spontaneous mammary tumors in mice. Mode of action of a tumor protective fraction of tubercle bacilli (MER). *Proc. Am. Ass. Cancer Res.* **7**: 68.

STEINKULLER, C. B., KRIGBAUM, L. G. and WEISS, D. W. (1969) Studies on the mode of action of the heterologous immunogenicity of a methanol-insoluble fraction of attenuated tubercle bacilli (BCG). *Immunology* **16**: 255–275.

STJERNSWARD, J. (1966) Effect of Bacillus Calmette–Guérin infection and/or methylcholanthrene on the antibody forming cells measured at the cellular level by a hemolytic plaque test. *Cancer Res.* **26**: 1591–1594.

SUTER, E., ULLMAN, G. E. and HOFFMAN, R. G. (1958) Sensitivity of mice to endotoxin after vaccination with BCG (Bacillus Calmette–Guérin). *Proc. Soc. exp. Biol. Med.* **99**: 167–169.

SUTHERLAND, R. I. L., SPADARO-ANTONELLI, M. S., LAWRENCE, V. J. W. and QUAGLIATA, F. (1979) Immunosuppressive activity of BCG: Effect of adjuvant disease, lymphocyte subpopulations, and homing of thoracic duct cells in rats. *Infec. Immun.* **25**: 310–319.

TOKUNAGA, T., YAMAMOTO, S., NAKAMURA, R. M. and KATAOKA, T. (1974) Immunotherapeutic and immunoprophylactic effect of BCG on 3-methylcholanthrene-induced autochthonous tumors in Swiss mice. *J. natn. Cancer Inst.* **53**: 459–463.

TOKUZEN, R., OKABE, M. and NAKAHARA, W. (1975) Effect of Nocardia and Mycobacterium cell wall skeletons on autochthonous tumor grafts. *Gann* **66**: 433–435.

TRACEY, D. E. (1979) The requirement for macrophage in the augmentation of natural killer cell activity by BCG. *J. Immunol.* **123**: 840–845.

UNANUE, E. R., ASKONAS, B. A. and ALLISON, A. C. (1969) A role of macrophages in the stimulation of immune responses by adjuvants. *J. Immunol.* **103**: 71–78.

UNGARO, P. C., DRAKE, W. P. and MARDINEY, M. R. (1973) Repetitive administration of BCG in prevention and treatment of spontaneous leukemia of AKR mice. *J. natn. Cancer Inst.* **50**: 125–128.
VITALE, B. and ALLEGRETTI, N. (1963) Influence of Bacillus Calmette–Guérin infection on the intensity of the homograft rejection in rats. *Nature, Lond.* **199**: 507–509.
VOGLER, W. R. and CHAN, Y. K. (1974) Prolonging remission in myeloblastic leukaemia by Tice strain Bacillus Calmette–Guérin. *Lancet* **2**: 128–131.
WEISS, D. W. (1972) Nonspecific stimulation and modulation of the immune response and of states of resistance by the methanol-extraction residue fraction of tubercle bacilli. *Natn. Cancer Inst. Monogr.* **35**: 157–171.
WEPSIC, H. T., HARRIS, S. SANDER, J., ALAIMO, J. and MORRIS, H. (1976) Enhancement of tumor growth following immunization with Bacillus Calmette–Guérin cell walls. *Cancer Res.* **16**: 1950–1953.
WHITE, R. G., JOLLÈS, P., SAMOUR, D. and LEDERER, E. (1964) Correlation of adjuvant activity and chemical structure of wax D fractions of mycobacteria. *Immunology* **5**: 158–171.
WILLIAMS, T. W. and GRANGER, G. A. (1969) Lymphocyte *in vitro* cytotoxicity: correlation of derepression with release of lymphotoxin from human lymphocytes. *J. Immunol.* **103**: 170–177.
WOLFE, S. A., TRACEY, D. E. and HENNEY, C. S. (1976) Induction of 'natural killer' cells by BCG. *Nature, Lond.* **262**: 584–586.
WOLMARK, N. and FISHER, B. (1974) The effect of a single and repeated administration of *Corynebacterium parvum* on bone marrow macrophage colony production in syngeneic tumor-bearing mice. *Cancer Res.* **34**: 2869–2872.
YAMAMURA, Y., AZUMA, I., TANIYAMA, T. *et al.* (1976) Immunotherapy of cancer with cell wall skeleton of *Mycobacterium bovis*—Bacillus Calmette–Guérin. Experimental and clinical results. *Ann. N.Y. Acad. Sci.* **277**: 209–226.
YASHPHE, D. J. (1972) Modulation of the immune response by a methanol-insoluble fraction of attenuated tubercle bacilli (BCG). II. Relationship of antigen dose to heightened primary and secondary immune response to sheep red blood cells. *Clin. exp. Immunol.* **12**: 497–506.
YASHPHE, D. J., STEINKULLER, C. B. and WEISS, D. W. (1969) Modulation of immunological responsiveness by pretreatment with a methanol-insoluble fraction of killed tubercle bacilli. *Israel J. med. Sci.* **5**: 259–266.
ZATZ, M. D. (1976) Effects of BCG on lymphocyte trapping. *J. Immunol.* **116**: 1587–1592.
ZBAR, B., BERNSTEIN, I. D., BARTLETT, G. L., HANNA, M. D., JR. and RAPP, H. J. (1972) Immunotherapy of cancer: regression of intradermal tumors and prevention of growth of lymph node metastases after intralesional injection of living *Mycobacterium bovis. J. natn. Cancer Inst.* **49**: 119–130.
ZBAR, B., BERNSTEIN, I. D. and RAPP, H. J. (1971) Suppression of tumor growth at the site of infection with living Bacillus Calmette–Guérin. *J. natn. Cancer Inst.* **46**: 831–839.
ZBAR, B., BERNSTEIN, I., TANAKA, T. and RAPP, H. J. (1970) Tumor immunity produced by the intradermal inoculation of living tumor cells and living *Mycobacterium bovis* (strain BCG). *Science* **170**: 1217–1218.
ZBAR, B. and RAPP, H. J. (1973) An experimental model for immunotherapy of cancer. *Natn. Cancer Inst. Monogr.* **39**: 3–6.
ZSCHIESCHE, W. and HEINECKE, H. (1973) Effects of variable Bacillus Calmette–Guérin regimen on skin graft rejection. *Transplantation* **15**: 172–173.

CHAPTER 8

METHANOL EXTRACTION RESIDUE: EFFECTS AND MECHANISMS OF ACTION

SHLOMO BEN-EFRAIM*

Department of Human Microbiology, Sackler School of Medicine, Tel-Aviv University, Ramat-Aviv, Tel-Aviv 69978, Israel

1. INTRODUCTION

The immune response is the outcome of interaction between various types of immunocompetent cells, particularly macrophages and lymphocytes (Sjöberg *et al.*, 1972). Macrophage activity is thought to be nonspecific (Alexander and Evans, 1971), although specific excitation by a 'macrophage arming factor' released from sensitized splenocytes has also been implicated (Evans *et al.*, 1973). The contribution of lymphocytes is represented by the presence of clones which react specifically with the stimulating antigen (Ada, 1970). Macrophage and especially lymphocyte populations of cells are heterogeneous and comprise functionally different cells (Roitt *et al.*, 1969). The big classes of 'T' and 'B' cells are divided into certain subclasses (Raff, 1971; Cantor and Asofsky, 1972; Basten *et al.*, 1971). The T cells are usually considered responsible for development of cell-mediated immunity (CMI) and for the 'helper effect' required for the elicitation of the antibody response to T-dependent antigens (Raff, 1970; Greaves *et al.*, 1974). The B cell population includes the antibody-forming cells and is thus involved in the humoral antibody response (Greaves *et al.*, 1974). These conclusions are based on experiments on the effect of selective cell depletion on the immune response and on cases of immune deficiencies.

The dualism of lymphocytes is also reflected in their potential responses: they can be either stimulated and develop an immune response, or they can be specifically paralysed. Moreover, in addition to 'active' lymphocytes (developing an immune response), evidence has accumulated in recent years of a 'suppressor' cell population which interferes with the function of active lymphocytes (Gershon *et al.*, 1972; Dutton, 1975). Suppressor cells have been found particularly among the T-cell population (Gershon *et al.*, 1972; Dutton, 1975). It seems, therefore, that the outcome of stimulation by immunogens is determined to a large extent not only by the degree of cooperation within the chain macrophage-T and B cells, but also by the interplay between active and suppressor populations of lymphocytes (Jerne, 1973). This interplay will determine in part whether an immunological response or immunological paralysis will emerge following antigenic stimulation.

The immunologic capacity of the organism can be affected by substances classified as 'adjuvants'. This effect, defined as 'immunomodulation', is usually expressed by immunopotentiation, but under certain conditions may lead to immunosuppression (Allwood and Asherson, 1971). The immunopotentiation effect can be selective, that is, it can divert the response to a certain type (CMI or humoral antibody response), or to a certain class of antibodies IgM, IgG, etc.). Immunosuppression may be expressed by deviation in the type of immune response elicited (Allwood and Asherson, 1971) and may be related to stimulation of suppressor T cells

---

* Professor of Immunology, Tel-Aviv University, Israel. The experimental and clinical studies with MER related to my own work and to the research of Professor D. W. Weiss and co-workers (since 1969) were supported by U.S. Public Health Service Contract NO1-CB-2208 and NO1-12127; Concern Foundation, Inc.; Lautenberg Endowment; Cancer Research Institute, New York; Leukemia Research Foundation, Inc.; The National Council for Research and Development, Israel and the GSF München, Germany; Hematology Research Foundation; Tisch Circle of Friends; Dr. 'I' Fund, The Ahmanson Foundation, Los Angeles; Chief Scientist's Office, Ministry of Health, Jerusalem; Katzenelbogen Award, Tel-Aviv.

(Gefford and Orbach-Arbouys; Uciyama and Jacobs, 1978) or suppressor B cells (Gill and Liew, 1979). The effect of immunomodulators on the immune response is dependent on a series of factors concerned with the adjuvant (chemical structure, quantity and route of immunization). The property of certain immunomodulators to selectively affect the immunological response is of course important in those cases in which a preferential potentiation in the type of immune response (i.e. CMI *vs* antibody response) is desired.

Thus, three main partners in the development of the immunological response are the immunogen itself, the immunocompetent system and the modulator. Several possibilities can be considered for explaining the immunomodulating effect. The modulator may act directly or via influence on other cell types of the different populations of immunocompetent cells and, thus, affect the development or expression of the immunological response. In this way administration of immunomodulators may impinge on the reticuloendothelial system (RES) and macrophage function (clearance, processing, release of lymphocyte-activating factors), lymphocyte functions (proliferation and stimulation of T or B cells), as well as the degree of cooperation between the various types of cells. During recent years it has also been reported that immunomodulating agents may either augment (Pioch *et al.*, 1979; Tracey, 1979) or depress (Lotzova and Gutlerman, 1979) natural killer (NK) cell activity. These effects are of importance in view of the assumption that NK cells could present an important part of immunosurveillance and tumor defense mechanisms. Another possibility which has to be considered is the presence of shared antigens between the adjuvant and the antigen complex used for immunization (Elberg *et al.*, 1957; Minden *et al.*, 1972; Borsos and Rapp, 1973; Bucans and Hanna, 1974; Minden *et al.*, 1974a). In this case the response to the immunogenic complex will be augmented by the mere addition of certain antigens to the immunizing mixture. Finally, the immunomodulator may act directly on the cell antigen entity by altering the cell membrane. Such a change can result in increase of immunogenicity of the cell or render the cell more susceptible to killing by already existing humoral or cellular immune mechanisms. Thus, it was shown that metabolic inhibitors, proteolytic enzymes and X-ray increased the sensitivity of tumor cells to killing by antibody plus complement, whereas L-epinephrine, insulin, hydrocortisone and prednisolone increased their sensitivity (Ohanian, 1977). Changes in physical properties of the cell membrane may also affect the susceptibility of cells to immune attack (Ohanian, 1977). A possible effect of immunomodulators on target cells may be important with regard to their use as immunotherapeutic agents in cases of cancer.

Mycobacteria have been the most extensively studied group of organisms for their immunomodulating ability. One of the first observations in this respect, reported some 50 years ago, was that injection of antigens directly into the tuberculous lesions of guinea pigs produced a modified immunologic response (Dienes and Schoenheit, 1927). Later on, Freund (1951) described an adjuvant-containing mineral oil-detergent mixture which killed mycobacteria; Freund's complete adjuvant (FCA) has proved useful until today as an immunopotentiator, although certain immunosuppressive effects have also been reported. Mycobacterial strains alone, and especially the attenuated bovine-type Bacillus Calmette-Guerin (BCG), were shown to act as immunostimulators (Bast *et al.*, 1974a, b). Extensive work has been done on the chemical isolation and characterization of the active adjuvant principle of mycobacteria from the cell wall. A chloroform-soluble peptidoglycolipid fraction called Wax D was claimed to be the active component by some authors (Raffel, 1950) while its activity was denied by others (Freund and Stone, 1959). Subfractionation of Wax D after acetylation yielded seven subfractions, three of which were reported to be active as adjuvant in guinea pigs (Tanaka *et al.*, 1968). Contradictory findings were reported in another work in which acetylated Wax D and its subfractions were all completely inactive as adjuvants (White, 1967). An adjuvant-active glycolipid-lacking peptide moiety was recently separated from Wax D preparation of *M. tuberculosis* strain *Aogama B* (Kumazawa *et al.*, 1976). A similar preparation obtained from Wax D of *M. bovis* BCG was not adjuvant active (Kumazawa *et al.*, 1976). In both cases the adjuvant activity was tested in guinea pigs using hen egg-white lysozyme as antigen and incorporating the fraction in oil-detergent mixture (Freund's incomplete adjuvant).

Another fraction isolated from BCG which was water soluble and lipid free was reported to possess adjuvant and antitumor activity (Hui, 1972). Other purified mycobacterial cell wall components showing immunostimulating and tumor therapeutic activity were described recently. These include a peptido-glycolipid cell wall skeleton CWS-I′ (Meyer *et al.*, 1974), a toxic free lipid 'P3' cord factor (Azuma *et al.*, 1974), and a sulpholipid fraction (Goren, 1974). Efforts have been made during recent years to delineate the portion of mycobacterial cell wall that is essential for its adjuvant activity. A synthetic N-acetylmuramyl-dipeptide was shown to be the minimal structure required for eliciting the adjuvant effects ascribed to mycobacterial cell walls in FCA (for Review see Parant, 1979).

The classical purified protein derivative (PPD) of mycobacteria was also shown to stimulate the immunological response *in vivo* (Diamantstein *et al.*, 1976) or *in vitro* (Kreisler and Möller, 1974) to sheep red blood cells (SRBC) and to act as a B cell mitogen (Sultzer and Nilsson, 1972). Under certain conditions, PPD and other B cell mitogens suppressed the immune response *in vivo* to SRBC, thus showing the importance of defining strict schedules for immunostimulation by various substances (Diamantstein *et al.*, 1976).

The topic of the present review is MER (methanol extraction residue), one of the mycobacterial fractions studied extensively over the last 20 years. The preparation, properties and various activities of MER have been described in a series of monographs (Yashpe, 1971; Weiss and Yashpe, 1973; Weiss, 1976). The purpose of the review is to determine to what extent the mode of action of MER is understood at the present time. The first part will cover the MER effects in experimental systems (*in vivo* and *in vitro*) and in human cancer patients. The second part is a critical appraisal of the mode of action of MER in light of the present knowledge on its immunomodulatory effects and its activity on various types of immunocompetent cells.

2. EFFECTS OF MER ON STATES OF RESISTANCE AND IMMUNOLOGICAL REACTIVITY

2.1 Experimental Studies

2.1.1. *Antimicrobial Activity*

MER fraction was first developed in an effort to produce a nonliving vaccine against tuberculous infection. This problem received much attention in the 1950s, especially at the Rockefeller Institute in New York and the Sir William Dunn School of Pathology, University of Oxford, England.

Vaccination with a suspension of avirulent tubercle bacilli killed by exposure to 2 per cent phenol markedly increased the resistance of mice to tuberculous infection (Weiss and Dubos, 1955). Similarly, a vaccine prepared from phenol-killed human tubercle bacilli was found to be effective in prolonging the survival time of guinea pigs infected by inhalation of a cloud of virulent tubercle bacilli (Weiss and Wells, 1960a). A crude methanol extract of the phenol-killed, acetone washed tubercle bacilli was found capable of eliciting in mice (Weiss and Dubos, 1956) and in guinea pigs (Weiss and Wells, 1960b) a low degree of enhanced resistance against subsequent infection with living tubercle bacilli. The immunogenic power of residues of MER was found to be much higher than that of the methanol extract (Weiss and Wells, 1960b). The degree of protection provided by MER preparation against subsequent infection with tubercle bacilli in guinea pigs was approximately of the same order as that of the living BCG vaccine. The possibility that the protective activity of the methanol extract was due to contamination by MER could not be ruled out. This could occur either by addition of a certain antigenic fraction to the extract, or (in a retrospective view) by addition of a nonspecific immunomodulator to the immunizing mixture. In this respect it is noteworthy that combinations of methanol extract preparations with small quantities of their residues (MER-like fraction) appeared to be synergistic in their protective effects in guinea pigs (Weiss and Wells, 1960b).

The possible use of MER as a tool for increasing nonspecific antimicrobial activity emerged from fortuitous observations in guinea pigs in the mid 1950s. It turned out that guinea pigs treated with MER were almost wholly immune to an epidemic of *Pasteurella pseudotuberculosis,* which was highly virulent for untreated animals (Weiss and Yashpe, 1973). This observation led to a long series of experiments on the protective activity of MER against certain bacterial infections, and raised the question as to whether the effect of MER is due to shared antigens with different bacterial species, or to a nonspecific stimulation of the immunocompetent system.

One of the first experimental models used was mice infected with the low virulent strain EV76 of *Pasteurella pestis* (Weiss, 1960). This model was chosen in view of previous reports (Girard and Grumbach, 1958) of an increase in resistance of mice infected with tubercle bacilli to experimental inoculation with *P. pestis*. Methanol extract as well as MER of killed tubercle bacilli increased the resistance of mice to infection with the strain EV76 *P. pestis* (Weiss, 1960). Additional experiments showed that the protective effect of MER is exerted towards a large variety of virulent bacterial strains. Thus, MER treatment heightened the resistance in mice against subsequent challenge with several strains of *Klebsiella, Streptococcus pyogenes, Diplococcus pneumoniae, Staphylococcus aureus, Proteus mirabilis, Pseudomonas aeruginosa* and *Salmonella typhimurium* (Weiss *et al.*, 1964). Protection against experimental *Klebsiella* infection is now used as a standard bio-assay for MER activity (Weiss and Yashpe, 1973). Recently a new experimental system was devised to assess the protective effect of BCG, *C. parvum* and MER towards infections (Sher *et al.*, 1975). An immuno-suppressive state was created in CDF mice by treatment with cyclophosphamide (CY). CY-treated mice were more susceptible to infection with *S. aureus* and *Candida albicans* (Sher *et al.*, 1975). The effect of MER was tested against *S. aureus* septicemia in CY-treated mice. A significant protective, dose-dependent effect was observed when MER was given 25 days prior to challenge (Sher *et al.*, 1975).

Enhanced resistance to certain bacterial infections following MER treatment might be related to the presence of shared antigens between MER and various bacterial species. A broad range of shared antigens and cross-reactivity between *Mycobacterium tuberculosis* and other bacterial species was reported. This includes cross-immunity between *Brucella melitensis* and *Mycobacterium tuberculosis* (Elberg *et al.*, 1957) and shared antigens between BCG and *Listeria monocytogenes, B. abortus, S. typhimurium*, or *E. coli* (Minden *et al.*, 1960, 1972). MER is derived from BCG organisms and it is possible therefore that some of the shared antigens with other bacterial species are present in this fraction. As far as we know there has been no systematic study on the antigenic make-up of MER, including the occurrence of shared antigens with various bacterial species. Thus, it is difficult at this stage to evaluate the role of such hypothetical shared antigens in the protective effect of MER towards bacterial infections.

2.1.2. *Effects of MER on Immunologic Responsiveness to Particulate and Soluble Antigens*

The observations on the antimicrobial activity of MER raised several questions:

(a) Is the effect of MER due to nonspecific immunomodulation of the response towards various *unrelated* antigens?
(b) What is the role played by 'shared antigens' in the immunomodulatory effect of MER?
(c) What are target cells (macrophages, various types of lymphocytes) of MER activity?
(d) Is the effect of MER on the development of various types of immune responses a selective one? If so, it should be possible to devise conditions for preferential potentiation of certain immune responses: CMI or antibody response (including the immunoglobulin-type of antibodies elicited).
(e) What is the role played by immunological memory to MER in the immunomodulatory effect of the agent? This possibility should be considered in view of the fact that MER is an immunogenic fraction derived from BCG *Mycobacterium* strain.

It was hoped that some of these questions could be answered by testing the effect of MER on the immunological response towards a battery of particulate and soluble antigens, including compounds containing chemically well-defined haptenic determinants.

Antigenic entities included in this study were sheep or mouse red blood cells and bacteriophage T_2 as particulate antigens, bovine gamma globulin (BGG), conjugates of proteins with dinitrophenyl (DNP), the pneumococcal polysaccharide type III (S III), conjugate of trinitrophenyl with *E. coli* lipopolysaccharide (TNPLPS), monovalent hapten dinitrophenyl-glycine (DNP-Gly) as soluble antigens, and contact sensitizers like dinitrofluorobenzene

(DNFB) and dinitrochlorobenzene (DNCB). The effect of MER treatment on the antibody response (antibody-forming cells, titers and types of antibodies formed) and on CMI (delayed type hypersensitivity (DH) and contact sensitization) was evaluated.

The effect of MER on CMI and on humoral antibody response was evaluated in both *in vivo* and *in vitro* systems.

In vivo studies

2.1.2.1. *Effect on antibody-forming cells.* The effect of MER treatment on the number of spleen cells producing 19S and 7S antibodies, following antigenic stimulation, was evaluated by using SRBC as antigen. The MER activity was determined according to a number of variables: (a) number of injections and timing of MER treatment (before, simultaneous with or after immunization); (b) strain and age of mice; (c) phase of the immune response (primary or secondary); (d) antigen dose; and (e) time elapsed after immunization.

The results indicate that treatment by two injections of MER on days 14 and 3 before immunization was optimal for stimulation of the early primary response (Steinkuller *et al.*, 1969). The number of both 19S and 7S antibody-producing cells was raised (Yashpe *et al.*, 1969). The rise in the number of PFC was found to be specific on the basis of its inhibition by anti SRBC passive antibody (Yashpe and Weiss, 1970). The stimulatory effect of MER was more evident when a low dose (4×10^7 SRBC) of antigen was used (Yashpe *et al.*, 1969) as compared with a higher dose: 2×10^9 SRBC (Steinkuller *et al.*, 1969). The increase in number of SRBC-PFC in MER-treated mice was observed already at 18 hr after immunization, and was still detectable up to 21 days afterwards (Yashpe *et al.*, 1969). In certain cases, an early increase in the number of SRBC-PFC was observed in spleens of nonimmunized mice treated with MER. This increase may be due to polyclonal proliferation (including antigen-reactive cells), induced by MER.

Treatment with MER before the first immunization resulted in a lowered spleen content of both 19S and 7S antibody-producing cells following a second immunizing injection (Yashpe *et al.*, 1969). A similar immunodepressing effect was observed when MER was given after the first immunization, on days 14 and 3 before the second immunization (Yashpe *et al.*, 1969).

Older mice (10 weeks old) seemed to be more susceptible to the immunopotentiating effect of MER than younger ones (8 weeks old). The age influence was more marked in Swiss albino mice than in Balb/c strain. In the young Swiss mice the splenic content of PFC was even depressed in MER-treated mice (Steinkuller *et al.*, 1969). However, in another test system (Pass *et al.*, 1975), treatment with MER potentiated immunological responsiveness in young mice to an otherwise tolerogenic administration of nonaggregated BGG. Thus, the effect of MER in young mice may depend on the strain used, the nature of the test antigen, and the parameters of treatment with the agent. An increase in multiplication of specific PFC by MER treatment in animals immunized with SRBC was also described in rats. (Esher *et al.*, 1973).

MER-treated mice showed also an appreciably enhanced PFC response to TNP hapten when coupled to SRBC (Jacobs *et al.*, 1978). On the other hand, MER had only little influence on the specific TNP-PFC response elicited by the T-independent antigen TNP-LPS (Jacobs *et al.*, 1978). It seems unlikely that MER effect towards immunological response against a simple hapten like TNP is due to sharing of antigenic components between MER and the immunogen. It is also of interest that MER had little effect on the response to the same hapten when presented as a T-independent antigen entity.

2.1.2.2. *Effect on circulating antibodies.* The experiments on the effect of MER on appearance, levels and types of circulating antibodies against SRBC paralleled those onPFC, and were also extended to other species (guinea pigs in addition to mice and rats).

Data on MER activity towards the production of antibodies to SRBC were in good agreement with its effect on specific PFC levels. Thus, prior treatment with MER potentiated the primary antibody response to SRBC in mice (Yashpe and Weiss, 1970; Yashpe and Haran-

Ghera, 1970) and rats (Esher *et al.*, 1973). The increase in the immune response in MER-treated mice was antigen dose-dependent (Yashpe and Haran-Ghera, 1970). Administration of MER between primary and secondary immunization with SRBC delayed and depressed significantly the secondary hemagglutination response (Yashpe and Weiss, 1970). The primary response to SRBC was not affected by one or two doses of MER given after immunization (Yashpe and Weiss, 1970).

MER also potentiated the immune response to other particulate and soluble antigens. Thus, the circulating hemagglutinin response to allogeneic red blood cells was markedly increased in MER-treated mice (Steinkuller *et al.*, 1969). The effect of MER was long lasting and was evident even when an interval of 59 days elapsed between the treatment and immunization (Steinkuller *et al.*, 1969).

Several points were raised in connection with the immunomodulatory effect of MER on the antibody response to various antigens. Prior treatment with MER augmented the antibody response to phage T_2, similar to its effect on SRBC (Yashpe and Weiss, 1970). However, the effect of MER treatment on the secondary immune response to phage T_2 differed from that observed with SRBC: instead of depression of the secondary response, administration of MER either prior to first immunization with T_2 phage or in the interval between two such immunizations, heightened the secondary antiphage reaction. This finding indicates that, in addition to the MER effect on the immunocompetent cells, the nature of the antigen involved should also be considered a factor in the outcome of the immunomodulation process.

The experiments on the effect of MER activity on the immune response to soluble antigens were important for several reasons: (a) to create conditions in which the possibility of presence of antigens common to MER and the test immunogen is unlikely; (b) to find out if MER can stimulate the immune response to poor or nonimmunogenic substrates; and (c) to determine the selective effect of MER on either cell-mediated immunity or antibody response.

Balb/c mice pretreated with MER gave a primary response to soluble BGG, while BGG itself in saline solution was nonimmunogenic (Jacobs *et al.*, 1978; Pass and Yashpe, 1971). The secondary response to BGG in MER-treated mice was markedly higher than in untreated mice, after boosting with alum-precipitated BGG.

Experiments were performed in guinea pigs on the effect of MER on the primary immune response to DNP protein conjugates (Kuperman *et al.*, 1972; Ben-Efraim *et al.*, 1973, 1974). The results can be summarized as follows:

Prior treatment with MER saline suspension potentiated the antibody response to the DNP hapten when the specific immunogenic stimulus was strong: 10 μg DNP-HSA (Ben-Efraim *et al.*, 1973) or 100 μg DNP-GPA (Ben-Efraim *et al.*, 1974). Pretreatment with MER incorporated in Freund's Incomplete Adjuvant was not effective, thus suggesting that a good systemic distribution of MER is required for its effect. Moreover, pretreatment with FCA 14 days before immunization did not affect the immunological reactivity, and administration of FCA 7 days before the antigen had only a slight potentiating effect on the immune response (Ben-Efraim *et al.*, 1973). When administered either in saline together with the antigen or after immunization, MER was ineffective. These results indicate the importance of variables like timing of MER treatment and antigen dose in the immunomodulation process. They also supply a strong argument in favor of the assumption that the activity of MER is not due to the presence of shared antigens with the immunogen, because in this system the immunomodulatory effect of MER was exerted against a simple haptenic determinant.

Recent studies have added a new feature to the spectrum of activity of MER towards soluble antigens. Pretreatment with MER prevented the establishment of immune paralysis by threshold doses of the T independent antigen, the pneumococcal polysaccharide type III and by a paralyzing dose of 100 μg TNP-LPS (Ben-Efraim *et al.*, 1979). It is of interest to mention that bacterial adjuvants like FCA and *C. parvum* and B-cell mitogens (PPD, LPS, DS) were not effective (Ben-Efraim *et al.*, 1979).

2.1.2.3. *Effect on T-cell function and CMI.* The effect of MER on the carrier function (helper T cells) and on delayed type hypersensitivity (DH) reaction was determined in guinea pigs (Kuperman *et al.*, 1972; Ben-Efraim *et al.*, 1973, 1974). The main conclusion was that under certain conditions the effect of MER on CMI can be dissociated from its effect on the antibody response. Thus, pretreatment with MER potentiated the DH response towards low doses of allogeneic DNP-globulin (10 μg DNP-GPG) and xenogeneic DNP-protein (1 μg DNP-HSA). On the other hand, as reported above, pretreatment with MER potentiated the antibody response to strong immunogenic stimuli of the same antigens. Treatment with MER simultaneous with or after immunization was not effective (Ben-Efraim *et al.*, 1973).

The development of the DH response was partially inhibited in MER-treated guinea pigs when DNP-HSA in FCA was used for sensitization. MER was administered (2 mg/ml i.p.) on days −1, 0, +1, 2, 3 and 4 relative to the day of immunization with 1 μg or 5 μg of DNP-HSA in FCA (Ben-Efraim *et al.*, 1974).

The carrier function of BGG (given 21 days before immunization with DNP-BGG) in the immune response of guinea pigs towards the DNP hapten linked to BGG by MER was not promoted by MER treatment (Ben-Efraim *et al.*, 1974). Immunopotentiation of the antibody response to BGG by MER has already been described (Pass *et al.*, 1975; Jacobs *et al.*, 1978; Pass and Yashpe, 1971). In 'carrier' experiments, a relatively high dose (50 μg) of BGG was used. Therefore, it is possible that MER selectively promoted the antibody response to BGG instead of its carrier function.

The main conclusion from the experiments on the effect of MER on defined particulate and soluble antigens is that the immunological responses to a variety of antigens can be qualitatively and quantitatively modulated by the use of the agent MER. The immunomodulatory effect is dependent on the time of MER treatment, nature and dose of antigen used.

Recently (Jacobs *et al.*, 1978) the effect of MER on CMI in C57B1 mice was evaluated. DH footpad reactions were elicited by immunization with low doses ($5 \times 10^5 - 1 \times 10^7$) of SRBC. MER (0.4 mg/mouse) was usually given on the same day and by the same route (i.p. or s.c.) as the antigen. The bleedings and tests for footpad swelling were performed 4 days later. The results obtained were similar to those described in guinea pigs (Kuperman *et al.*, 1972; Ben-Efraim *et al.*, 1973). Mice treated with MER gave greater footpad reactions than untreated mice after immunization with limiting doses of SRBC, whereas the antibody response was not affected (Jacobs *et al.*, 1978).

Another system of CMI in which MER was assayed is contact hypersensitivity (CH) to DNFB. Two preparations (A and B), both orginated from the same master lot, were tested. One preparation failed consistently to potentiate CH reactivity in Balb/c mice, whereas the other proved significantly efficacious (Zimber *et al.*, 1981a). Pretreatment with each of the two preparations (A and B) restored significantly the ability of animals immunosuppressed by drug treatment to respond to DNFB sensitization (Zimber *et al.*, 1977, 1981b). This applies to CY induced immunosuppression in guinea pigs (Zimber *et al.*, 1977) and mice (Zimber *et al.*, 1977, 1981b) and to CY, methotrexate (MTX) or 5-fluorouracil (5-FU) suppressed mice (Zimber *et al.*, 1981b). Hapten-induced tolerance and potentiation of DNFB sensitization by CY in guinea pigs and mice were not influenced by MER treatment (Zimber *et al.*, 1977, 1981b).

In vitro systems

The study on the effect of MER on the immunological response is of importance because it can throw light on the direct interaction between the immunomodulator and immunocompetent cells and on the impact of the agent on selected subpopulations of cells.

The effect of MER on either antibody response or cell mediated immune response *in vitro* was evaluated.

2.1.2.4. *Effect on antibody response in vitro.* MER potentiated the primary antibody response *in vitro* by mouse spleen cells to SRBC and to TNP hapten when conjugated with SRBC (Ben-Efraim and Diamantstein, 1975; Ben-Efraim *et al.*, 1980). Numbers of specific PFC to either SRBC or TNP hapten (Ben-Efraim and Diamantstein, 1975; Ben-Efraim *et al.*, 1980) were increased and antibody (hemolysin) titers to SRBC were markedly raised in cultures containing MER. The potentiating effect of MER on the specific PFC response to

SRBC *in vitro* was also observed in macrophage depleted spleen cell cultures (Ben-Efraim *et al.*, 1980) and in intact spleen cell suspensions originated from nude mice (Ben-Efraim and Diamantstein, 1975). Immunopotentiating activity of MER for SRBC was found to be dependent on the quantity of MER added to the cultures (Ben-Efraim *et al.*, 1980) and to the time of MER addition: maximal effect when added simultaneously with antigen presentation (Ben-Efraim *et al.*, 1980). MER also facilitated induction of specific PFC to the monovalent hapten DNP-glycine and had no effect on the response to the T-independent entity TNP-LPS (Ben-Efraim *et al.*, 1980). Attempts were made recently to characterize the immunocyte population affected by MER in the *in vitro* induction of PFC response to SRBC. Reconstruction experiments were performed, adding enriched peritoneal macrophages (M) or T-spleen lymphocytes (T) from normal or MER-treated Balb/c to selectively depleted syngeneic splenocyte cultures sensitized with SRBC. M and T cells from MER treated donors were superior to populations from untreated animals in restoring responsiveness to SRBC in depleted cultures (Halperin *et al.*, 1980).

In another series of experiments, no difference was found in the number of SRBC-PFC between cultures containing B cells from MER treated or untreated mice (Dar, Halperin, Ben-Efraim and Weiss, unpublished) and supplied with normal M and T cells. Incubation of normal peritoneal macrophage cultures with MER induced release of soluble factors(s) that facilitated the primary antibody response *in vitro* to SRBC in macrophage depleted cultures. Addition of SRBC to the macrophage cultures did not result in release of active factors(s) and did not influence the MER effect. The active supernatants also had a synergistic effect on PHA stimulation of mouse thymocytes.

2.1.2.5. *Effect on CMI in vitro.* The effect of MER on CMI *in vitro* was studied in a system of unidirectional mixed lymphocyte-tumor cell cultures. Addition of small amounts of MER potentiated appreciably the elicitation of cytotoxic reactivity of splenocytes or lymph node cells from normal donor C57B1/6, Balb/c and strain A mice against mitomycin C-inactivated leukemia cells of both syngeneic and allogeneic origin (Kedar *et al.*, 1978). On the other hand, higher quantities of MER had a strong suppressive effect. The effects of MER were observed only when the agent was present during the initial 24–48 hours of the 6-day culture. MER affected generation of cytotoxic lymphocytes *in vitro* primarily by the nylon nonadherent cell population.

The conclusion from *in vitro* experiments is that MER can affect both antibody response and CMI. This can be shown either by adding MER to the cultures or by using for cultures immunocompetent cells from MER-treated donors.

2.1.3. *Antitumor Activity in Experimental Systems*

Certain basic principles should be considered for experimentation and evaluation of MER effect on appearance, development and regression of tumors. The first basic assumption is that tumor cells contain new antigenic fractions not present in the surrounding normal cells (Prehn and Main, 1957). These fractions should be able to elicit an immunological response either in the tumor-bearing host or in other allogeneic and syngeneic individuals. The existence of tumor-associated antigens has been demonstrated in several experiments performed under carefully controlled conditions of isogenicity of tumor donor and test animals (Klein *et al.*, 1963) or by transfer of tumor on the same animals: autologous transfer (Klein *et al.*, 1960).

The proof of immunogenicity of certain tumors raised a second question about the existence of a system of immunological surveillance intended to eliminate modified cells, including the tumor ones (Burnet, 1971). If this is the case, the development of a tumor would be related to some escape from the immunosurveillance mechanism (Klein, 1973). Consequently, decrease in the immunocompetence would facilitate the spontaneous appearance and growth of tumors, while restoration of the immunocompetence ability would increase the chance of tumor regression.

A new aspect was added by data showing that the immunological response against tumor cells not only may lead to tumor rejection (cytotoxic effect), but, under certain conditions, may increase the chance of tumor take and development (enhancement effect) (Hellström and

Hellström, 1969). While not a general rule, it is usually assumed that the cell-mediated immune response and IgM type response are expressed by cytotoxic activity, while certain IgG types of antitumor antibodies exhibit enhancing activity. On the other hand, other experiments (Linna *et al.*, 1974) question the role of antibodies in the enhancement effect. This is based on findings showing that bursectomized birds which are totally agammaglobulinemic and incapable of making antibodies, nonetheless develop potent blocking factors to tumor antigens. It seems that the interfering factors are, in this case, soluble tumor antigens. Soluble tumor antigens are today widely considered a possibility in tumor enhancement (Treves *et al.*, 1976a). In view of this, it is possible that treatment with MER leads to an increased liberation of soluble tumor antigens by potentiating cytotoxic damage to target cells. Therefore, the effectiveness of immunomodulators should be judged not only by overall increase in the immune response to tumor cells, but also by their ability to potentiate selectively the antitumor cytotoxic activity of the immunocompetent system.

The effect of immunomodulators on the host-tumor relationship can be evaluated in three situations: (a) protective effect on subsequent tumor challenge; (b) reduction in the incidence of spontaneous developing tumors; and (c) therapeutic value in tumor-bearing animals.

The first situation is similar to that encountered in experiments on the modulation of the immune response towards bacteria and more defined antigen entities. The second situation can be compared with the MER effect on naturally occurring infections, and the last one (therapeutic value) is more relevant to the use of immunomodulators in cancer patients.

The results of experiments on the effect of MER treatment in all three situations are compiled accordingly.

2.1.3.1. *Effect on tumor challenge.* The first experiments on the protective activity of MER against isologous tumors were performed in Balb/c Crgl and C3H Crgl strains of mice (Weiss *et al.*, 1961). The tumors tested were uterine sarcoma in Balb/c mice and mammary carcinoma or osteogenic sarcoma in C3H mice. The experimental procedure was i.p. injection of various MER quantities (0.25–1.0 mg), followed a month later by subcutaneous transplantation of isologous tumors. MER exerted a marked protective effect expressed by reduction in the number of deaths, failure of the malignant isografts to develop, and slower rate of growth of tumors. The dose of MER was critical, and its efficiency was at least that of living BCG or more. These studies were later extended to additional strains of mice and various isografts of neoplastic tissue. Protection of Balb/c mice by MER-pretreatment against challenge with an isograft of uterine sarcoma was confirmed (Weiss *et al.*, 1966a). The dose of MER used was critical: a quantity of 0.5 mg was highly protective, but larger quantities were ineffective in preventing growth of tumors. Administration of MER after implantation of the tumor was either ineffective or only slightly retarded the tumor development. Pretreatment with MER also had a protective effect against growth of isografts of other neoplastic tissues. Thus, prior administration of MER protected C3H mice against challenge with hepatoma or osteogenic sarcoma, and considerably delayed the development of mammary carcinoma isografts in R III mice (Weiss *et al.*, 1966a). Some retardation in the development of osteogenic sarcoma in C3H mice was also observed in animals receiving MER after the implantation of the tumor (Weiss *et al.*, 1966a). An interesting observation was that pretreatment with MER enhanced the rate of development of isografts of fibrosarcoma in Balb/c or DBA/2 mice (Weiss *et al.*, 1966a). The enhancement may result from selective increase in the production of enhancing antibodies in MER-treated animals. It is also possible that the optimal conditions for MER administration (time, dosage) are different for this type of tumor than for the previously mentioned tumors.

Pretreatment with MER was usually more effective than with living BCG in raising the resistance of mice against isografts of neoplastic tissue. An exception to these findings is the case of myeloid leukemia isograft in C57B1 mice: living BCG treatment induced protection, while MER was ineffective (Weiss *et al.*, 1966a).

The role played by the route of administration and the type of the tumor in the outcome of the immunomodulatory effect of MER was emphasized in an additional work (Mathe *et al.*, 1973). Pretreatment with MER at 2.5 days before implantation delayed the L1210 leukemia mortality in DBA × C57B1/6F_1 mice when given s.c. and was ineffective when injected i.v., i.p. or i.d. Lewis's solid tumor mortality is delayed by i.v. pretreatment with MER, but unaffected by i.p. i.d. or s.c. injection. Intradermal injection of MER enhanced the mortality following implantation of ICIG CI_1 (Mathe *et al.*, 1973).This tumor was originally induced with dimethyl benzene anthracene (DMBA) and was found to be sensitive to immunological enhancement.

The occasional enhancement effect of MER pretreatment on the development of transplanted syngeneic tumors was also stressed by other authors (Jacobs and Kripke, 1974). The effect was observed in Balb/cfC3H (MTV+) and Balb/c (MTV−) hosts challenged with (MTV+) mammary tumor. MER treatment simultaneously with specific tumor immunization had no effect on the development of protective immune response. MER administered prophylactically prolonged the survival of Balb/c mice challenged with transplants of syngeneic MPC-11 plasmacytomas (producing and nonproducing myeloma proteins) to a moderate but significant extent (Stupp *et al.*, 1978). Prophylactic administration of MER combined with CY treatment after tumor implantation was more effective than CY alone in the case of MPC-11 nonproducing strain (Stupp *et al.*, 1978). Injection of MER at the time of tumor challenge was without effect on CY therapy (Stupp *et al.*, 1978).

The effect of MER on the growth of tumors has also been examined in other species. Thus, pretreatment with MER prevented the development of line-10 hepatocarcinoma in syngeneic strain 2 of guinea pigs (Minden *et al.*, 1974; Wainberg *et al.*, 1976a, b). Simultaneous administration of MER with isogeneic sarcoma or hepatoma restricted their subcutaneous growth in inbred Wistar rats (Hopper *et al.*, 1975). Treatment of three-month-old chickens with MER prior to challenge infection with Rous sarcoma virus had an interesting effect on the development of tumors: initial appearance of the tumors was not affected but a substantial proportion (38 to 58%) of the chickens pretreated with MER showed complete and long-lasting regression of the neoplasms (Markson *et al.*, 1978). The efficacy of MER treatment was dependent on site of injection (near the site of viral challenge), quantity and time of administration (Markson *et al.*, 1978).

The general conclusion which can be drawn from experiments on the effect of MER on subsequent tumor challenge are in certain aspects similar to those encountered with soluble and particulate antigens. Timing and dose of MER, as well as the nature of the antigen, are important in the delineation of the MER effect. It is difficult to draw a parallel between the selective effect of MER on CMI *vs* antibody response towards soluble antigens on one side, and protection *vs* enhancement effect towards tumors on the other. It is possible that the enhancement effect of MER is due to selective increase of antitumor antibody response, but the complexity of tumor antigenic material does not permit a final conclusion on this point.

Stimulation of cellular immunological responsiveness against tumor cells by MER was also shown to occur by *in vitro* tests (Kuperman *et al.*, 1972). Inbred C3Hf and C57B1 male mice were given MER several days before administration of an allogeneic Balb/c plasma cell tumor. Lymphoid cells were harvested from MER-treated mice and from injected mice as controls. The tumor damage induced *in vitro*, as expressed by per cent ^{51}Cr released by contact with lymph node cells from mice pretreated with MER, was higher than that by lymphoid cells taken from saline controls.

2.1.3.2. *Effect on spontaneous tumor development*. Hopes about the preventive effect of immunomodulators (including MER) on spontaneous tumor development are based on the assumption that appearance of tumors is due to some deficiency in the immunosurveillance mechanism. This deficiency reflects a certain decrease in the immunocompetence which might be restored to normal levels by the immunomodulator.

Data on the protection afforded by MER against naturally-occurring bacterial lethal infections have already been reported (Weiss and Yashpe, 1973). A similar process of nonspecific increase in the potential of immunological responsiveness could also be beneficial in delaying development of spontaneous tumors.

Administration of MER prevented or retarded the development of spontaneous tumors in several systems. Monthly i.p. injections of MER (2.5–5 mg), during the first several months of life, reduced the incidence of palpable spontaneous mammary carcinomas in C3H mice (Cohen *et al.*, 1975; Weiss *et al.*, 1964). Larger doses might enhance the tumor development

(Weiss, 1967). Another study was performed to determine whether MER treatment can effect the development of the preneoplastic alveolar nodules of murine mammary carcinoma (Weiss *et al.*, 1966b). Three-week-old C3H female mice received isologous pituitary implants into a mammary fat pad in order to stimulate lobular alveolar development of the mammary gland, followed by injections of MER. After 3 months the mammary fat pads carrying the implanted pituitaries were removed, and 1 month later the mammary glands were harvested and counted for nodules. Treatment with MER results in marked inhibition of spontaneous nodulogenesis, thus showing activation of the immunological response.

Isogeneic skin grafting to promote the rapid development of papillomas in 3-methylcholantrene-initiated mouse skin was used as another system for testing MER activity (Lappe, 1968). Treatment with MER 4 or 15 days before grafting delayed the appearance of papillomas and decreased their incidence. The results were interpreted as proof that increase in the immunologic competence by MER results in better immunologic surveillance against papillomas.

An attempt to determine the effect of MER on host-virus relationship leading to progressive neoplasia was made in the case of leukemogenesis, induced by the radiation leukemia virus in C57Bl/6 mice (Haran-Ghera and Weiss, 1973). The effect of MER was tested by treatment either before or after infection with RLV leukemia virus. MER treatment before virus inoculation resulted in enhancement of leukemia development (higher per cent leukemia incidence and shortening of the mean latent period to onset of palpable leukemias). Marked protection on C57Bl/6 mice against the leukemogenic action of the RLV was obtained by giving MER after infection with RLV, provided that at least two injections were given later than 30 days after infection. The system employed included two components as possible targets for the MER activity: the virus itself and the neoplastic cells. It is difficult to conclude against which of these components (or both) the MER exerted its effect. The enhancing effect of MER treatment before infection with RLV suggests that the degree of virus replication is not impaired by MER, and that MER activity is expressed only in the presence of a certain number of neoplastic cells. The preventive effect of MER, when given after infection with RLV, could be due to increased immunological response, either against certain tumor-associated antigen(s) at a stage when tumor cells are already present (at least 30 days after infection with RLV), or against the virus itself leading to its eradication.

An approach intended to draw a better parallel between experimental conditions and clinical situations was recently described (Treves *et al.*, 1976b). The effect of MER on the development of spontaneous pulmonary metastases was tested before or after surgical removal of syngeneic implants of lung carcinoma 3LL in C57Bl mice. Injection of MER either 2 days before or 1 day after the tumor removal prevented spreading of metastases in most of the treated mice. The MER treatment was not effective when administered on day −6 or day +3 in relation to tumor removal (day 0). Injection of 0.1 mg MER directly in the primary tumor implants or two to three injections of 0.5 mg each administration between days −3 and +13 was also not effective. The conclusion of these experiments is that MER prevents the development of metastases and stresses again the importance of dose and timing for achieving an optimal effect.

2.1.3.3. *Immunotherapeutic studies.* The ultimate aim of experimental models is to mimic as much as possible spontaneously occurring neoplasia in man, and to test under these conditions the therapeutic value of certain treatments. This implies use of therapeutic agents after the tumor has reached a detectable size and use of combined treatments: immunotherapy, chemotherapy and irradiation. Therefore, immunotherapeutic studies with MER were performed in tumor-bearing animals and the effect of combined treatments (MER + irradiation, MER + chemotherapeutic agent; and MER + irradiation + chemotherapy) was evaluated. The experimental conditions included either established isografts or simulated local recurrence of tumors in mice, established isografts in guinea pigs, and Rous sarcomas in chickens.

A study was carried out on the effect of MER alone, or as a component in combined treatment, on development of neoplastic isografts and newly-initiated simulated local recurrence tumors in Balb/c and C3HeB mice (Yron *et al.*, 1973). The tumors used were of isogenic origin and included: (a) benzo (α)pyrene-induced fibrosarcoma in C3HeB males; (b) 3-methyl-cholantrene-induced fibrosarcoma in Balb/c females; (c) a mammary adenocarcinoma originated in an outgrowth of a hyperplastic alveolar nodule appearing in hormonally hyperstimulated Balb/c female (D7T4S tumor, MTV-); (d) a mammary adenocarcinoma which developed spontaneously in a multiparous Balb/cfC3H (MTV +). The therapeutic irradiation was by means of X-rays: 2000 or 3000 R in 4–6 min at the tumor site. The chemotherapeutic agents employed were CY, 5-FU, vinblastine sulfate, MTX and thioTEPA. MER given alone had a protective effect (retarded tumor development and prolonged host survival) in only a few cases. In contrast, MER combined with irradiation or chemotherapy (CY, MTX, 5-FU) significantly inhibited tumor growth rate and extended the life of the hosts, without negative effects.

The therapeutic effect of MER alone and in combination with X-ray treatment was retested over a broad spectrum of experimental circumstances (Yron *et al.,* 1975). Two mammary carcinomas, one infected with MTV and one free of this agent, were used as established isografts or simulated local recurrence implants in Balb/c mice. Combined therapy with MER and irradiation again proved to be more successful than MER alone. Smaller quantities of MER given in one treatment were more effective than larger doses. It is of interest that the therapeutic action of MER was at least as satisfactory and usually even more effective when given distal to the tumor site, as compared with direct introduction of MER into the tumor. This point was also stressed in another work with the same tumor model (Cohen *et al.,* 1975).

The question of efficiency of combined chemoimmunotherapy with MER as compared with MER alone was reinvestigated in another work (Cohen *et al.,* 1976). The experimental model used consisted of simulated local recurrence challenge with either a MTV + mammary carcinoma or MTV − mammary carcinoma (tumor D7T4S), in Balb/c mice. The results again demonstrated the superiority of a combined chemoimmunotherapeutic regimen over MER alone in animals challenged with the MTV + carcinoma. Two additional points are noteworthy from this work: (a) combined intervention of MER + 5-FU was synergistic, while combination with CY or MTX was no more effective than CY or MTX alone; and (b) none of the chemoimmunotherapeutic regimens were more effective in mice challenged with D7T4S tumor, than the chemotherapeutic treatment alone. These findings indicate that the synergistic effect of chemoimmunotherapy with MER is dependent on the drug nature and type of tumor used.

The effect of MER + CY therapy as compared with CY only, was also evaluated in Balb/c mice bearing plasma cell tumors. When MER was introduced at the time of tumor challenge or thereafter to animals also treated with CY, the therapeutic response was not appreciably different from that of mice under therapy with CY only (Stupp *et al.,* 1978).

The assumption on which the authors of the above-mentioned works base their studies is that MER stimulates the immunologic apparatus nonspecifically and thus promotes beneficial anti-tumor immunity. It is possible that this effect is better manifested when reduction in the tumor mass is achieved by additional treatments (irradiation, chemotherapy). It is also possible that MER protects against toxic side-effects of other therapy on hematopoietic tissue. Factors such as MER dose, time, site and number of injections also seem to play a role in the expression of the protective effect.

Immunotherapy studies with MER were recently carried out in guinea pigs (Wainberg *et al.,* 1976b, c, 1977). The model system studied was the inbred strain 2 guinea pigs and a diethylnitrosamine-induced, transplantable line 10 hepatocarcinoma. MER was given (0.5–1.0 mg) 7 days after injection of tumor cells, either directly into the growing tumor nodules, or into the opposite flank.

Several points must be mentioned from the experiments performed in guinea pigs. In contrast to the results obtained in mice (Cohen *et al.,* 1975; Weiss *et al.,* 1964), MER had a protective effect only when injected directly into growing tumor nodules and had no effect on tumor development when administered distally. Repeated skin tests with tumor extracts led to abolishment of effective antitumor immunity and permitted tumor recurrence. The mechanism of this effect is still obscure. It is possible that repeated skin testing may either lead to the formation of antibodies enhancing to tumor growth, or that free soluble tumor antigen may interfere with effective antitumor immunity by reacting with the antibodies or the lymphocytes. From the practical point of view, these results raise the question of the safety of repeated skin testing with human tumor antigens in patients. Immunotherapy with MER was more effective in mediating tumor regression in strain 2 guinea pigs obtained from the Weizmann Institute of Science in Israel and the National Jewish Hospital, Denver, Colorado, than in animals obtained from the National Institutes of Health, Bethesda (Wainberg *et al.*, 1976b, 1977). Certain differences in the antigenic make-up were detected between the colonies of strain 2 as reflected in skin graft tests. It was suggested that the difference in MER effectiveness may be due to some genetic drift reflected either by increase in antigenicity of line 10 tumor cells in animals of Israeli and Denver origin, or by changes in NIH guinea pigs relative to histocompatibility antigenic expression of line 10 tumor cells. Another explanation put forth by the authors was that MER, like BCG (Borsos and Rapp, 1973), shares antigens with line 10 tumor cells and may, under certain circumstances, stimulate the formation of antibodies enhancing tumor growth.

The findings on vertical transmission of tumor resistance in guinea pigs (Wainberg *et al.*, 1976c) are relevant here. Resistance to the transplantable guinea pig line 10 hepatocarcinoma from MER-treated tumor resistant mothers has been demonstrated in the second and third generation offsprings. The mechanism for this resistance transmission is poorly understood. It is not due to passage of antitumor protective antibodies by nursing, and probably not by a mere presence of MER. One possibility suggested by the authors is transportation across the placental barrier of antitumor antibodies and/or specifically sensitized small lymphocytes.

The effect of therapeutic treatment with MER on Rous sarcoma of chickens induced by the Rous sarcoma virus was investigated recently (Markson and Weiss, 1980). Multiple concurrent injections of MER at the site of palpable Rous sarcomas developing in chickens following infection with the Rous sarcoma virus resulted in permanent regression of the neoplasms in 25 of 76 subjects (Markson and Weiss, 1980). Administration of MER in a single injection in the tumor area was effective in only 2 of 54 birds (Markson and Weiss, 1980).

A new parameter concerning the effect of MER treatment on tumor induction and development was studied recently (Kollmorgen *et al.*, 1979). The combined effects of diet and MER on DMBA-induced mammary carcinoma in Sprague-Dawley female rats was evaluated. MER protected rats from DMBA-induced mammary carcinoma when given either before the carcinogen or within two weeks after exposure to DMBA (Kollmorgen *et al.*, 1979). Combination of low fat diet and MER therapy provided maximum protection (Kollmorgen *et al.*, 1979).

Some general conclusions can be drawn from immunotherapeutic studies performed with MER in experimental animals (mice, guinea pigs, chickens and rats):

(a) Combined treatment (MER + irradiation; MER + chemotherapy; MER + irradiation + chemotherapy) was usually more effective than treatment with MER alone. The protective effect was dependent on the drug and type of tumor used.

(b) MER treatment was more efficient in mice when given at a distal site, while in guinea pigs it was necessary to inject directly into the tumor in order to achieve protection. Moreover, substrains of guinea pigs of the same inbred line differed in regard to the antitumor protection provided by MER treatment. In another system (Markson and Weiss, 1980) it seemed important also to inject at the site of the tumor multiple concurrent injections instead of a single injection of MER, in order to obtain significant regression of the neoplasms.

(c) The degree of efficiency of MER treatment can be influenced by the kind of diet used. A low fat diet seems more beneficial in this respect than a high fat diet (Kollmorgen *et al.*, 1979).

(d) Offspring from tumor-bearing MER-treated animals were more resistant to tumor challenge than control animals. This finding suggests that the protective effect of MER is due to increase in antitumor immunity transferred to the offspring, and not to a direct interaction between MER and the tumor.

2.2. Immunotherapy in Man

2.2.1. *General Comments*

Clinical trials on the effectiveness of MER treatment are subject to certain obvious ethical considerations and conditions peculiar to human beings. Some of the relevant limitations can be summarized as follows:

2.2.1.1. *Safety of use.* The main dangers are the possible occurrence of severe undesirable reactions to MER itself and induction of tumor enhancement instead of tumor regression in the MER-treated cancer patients. The first aspect is related to intrinsic properties of MER, i.e. to the fact that a high proportion of human beings are sensitive to various mycobacterial components (including MER) and to the physical state of MER (particulate agent in suspension). Therefore the occurrence of nonspecific reactions and of specific immunological reactions (especially DH) should be considered.

Occurrence of side effects following MER administration by various routes has been examined. I.d. injection of MER was usually well tolerated. Febrile reaction attributable to MER i.d. therapy were mild and infrequent (Moertel *et al.*, 1975a; Izak *et al.*, 1977; Jackson *et al.*, 1979). Local skin reactions varying in severity from small reddened papules, through white or yellow pustules to draining ulcerations were quite frequent (Grimm, 1979; Denefrio, 1979; Robinson *et al.*, 1979; Sterchi *et al.*, 1980; Cooper *et al.*, 1980). With repeated MER treatment the severity of reactions tended to increase, probably because DH was induced (Moertel *et al.*, 1975). Usually the cutaneous reactions were tolerable and acceptable to patients (Moertel *et al.*, 1975a; Grimm, 1979; Robinson *et al.*, 1979) especially if the treatment dose of MER was determined for each patient according to its skin reactivity (Robinson *et al.*, 1979). An interesting observation reported was that i.d. injection of MER in melanoma or breast carcinoma patients can cause systemic granuloma which on X-ray can mimic recurrent malignancy or an infectious process (Denefrio, 1979). Use of ethyl chloride spray for lessening of the pain induced by i.d. MER was recommended (Stein *et al.*, 1978). Intralesional injection of MER in cutaneous malignant melanoma was followed by erythema, pustule formation and ulceration at injection sites and very seldom by transient nausea, vomiting, hypotension, lethargy, cyanosis and hepatic dysfunction (Krown *et al.*, 1977).

MER has proven to be well tolerated when administered systemically (Vogl *et al.*, 1977). Administration i.v. of MER did not cause acute changes in blood pressure or pulse, did not alter serum levels of alkaline phosphate, transaminase or creatinine, and did not affect blood counts (Vogl *et al.*, 1978). Hematological effects of i.v. injection of MER were determined in cytopenic patients (Quesada and Hersh, 1980). I.v. MER therapy was associated with correction of neutropenia and leukopenia, increase in absolute neutrophilic count, increase or decrease in platelet counts in various patients (Quesada and Hersh, 1980). Fever, chills and malaise occurred in all patients (Quesada and Hersh, 1980).

Effects of oral administration of MER was recently investigated (Bartal *et al.*, 1980). Patients with non oat cell lung cancer were given oral MER for 30 days. No changes attributed to MER therapy were found in the routine blood test, X-ray and scanning (Bartal *et al.*, 1980).

The second possibility (tumor enhancement) has not yet been encountered in any instance of therapeutic employment of MER in the several forms of human malignancy examined. This may not be surprising in view of the available experimental information. Experiments performed with mammary tumors in mice showed that MER induced tumor enhancement only when given before challenge with the tumor (Weiss *et al.*, 1966a). Moreover, MER used therapeutically in conjunction with chemotherapy or irradiation never led to enhancement in animal models.

2.2.1.2. *Heterogeneity of the test groups.* The human population involved in clinical trials is very heterogeneous in regard to genetic background, medical care, social conditions, previous contact with *Mycobacterium* species, etc. It is also difficult to choose appropriate controls for the MER-treated groups. All these restrictions interfere with the interpretation of MER immunotherapeutic effectiveness.

2.2.1.3. *Use of combined treatments.* For obvious ethical reasons, the only criterion for use or discontinuation of a certain treatment lies in the evaluation of its safety and therapeutic efficiency. Therefore, the MER treatment is usually given with other types of treatment, including radiation, immunosuppressive drugs, etc. Encouraging data were obtained from experiments carried out in mice and guinea pigs. Addition of MER to irradiation or chemotherapeutic treatment in mice was in certain cases more effective than treatment without MER. It was also found (Stupp *et al.*, 1976) that MER administration restored the ability of CY-treated mice to respond immunologically to SRBC. Pretreatment with MER prevented induction of immunosuppression of CH to DNFB by CY in guinea pigs (Zimber *et al.*, 1977) and CY, MTX or 5-FU in mice (Zimber *et al.*, 1977, 1981b). These findings indicate that the immunosuppressive effects of widely used cytotoxic drugs can be counterbalanced by treatment with MER.

2.2.1.4. *MER-tumor relationship.* In many instances, tumors in patients are already far advanced when treatment is initiated. At this stage, the tumor(s) mass is great and it is possible that impairment of immunocompetence either by the tumor itself or by other treatments was inflicted. The optimal experimental conditions for MER effect, especially on CMI, are treatment before the antigen challenge and small antigen dose. Therefore, the clinical conditions under which MER is required to 'act' are very different from those found optimal for experimental animals. Whenever possible, it may be desirable to withhold MER treatment until tumor mass is reduced maximally by conventional means.

2.2.1.5. *'Unexpected' discontinuation of MER treatment.* The schedule of MER treatment is largely dependent on the willingness of the patient to cooperate, the physician-patient relationship, the necessity for other drastic treatment which might interrupt the scheduled MER injection, etc.

While these factors do hinder somewhat the use of MER in cancer patients, controlled clinical trials with MER are widely in progress both in Israel and the United States with a large variety of cases, including acute myelocytic leukemia (AML) and various kinds of solid tumors.

2.2.2. *Effect in AML*

The survival time in adult patients with AML treated with MER plus chemotherapy and chemotherapy alone was determined in studies performed in Israel (Weiss, 1976; Izak *et al.*, 1977; Weiss *et al.*, 1975) and elsewhere (Cuttner *et al.*, 1975; Bekesi *et al.*, 1976, 1977). The patients were treated with MER once monthly for 2 years, in addition to standard maintenance and reinduction chemotherapy. In some patients who showed a marked decline in the immunologic function, MER treatment was continued beyond the 2-year period. In a study of twenty-two patients on MER + chemotherapy and eighteen on chemotherapy alone (Weiss *et al.*, 1975) the remission and survival times of MER-treated patients were significantly prolonged. The immunological capacity improved as reflected in an increased ability to respond to hemocyanin antigenic stimulus and an increase in PHA lymphocyte stimulation *in vitro*.

Clinical trials were also performed in the United States on the effect of chemoimmunotherapy with MER in AML (Cuttner *et al.*, 1975, Bekesi *et al.*, 1976, 1977). In one trial (Cuttner *et al.*, 1975) six patients were treated with chemotherapy alone and five received an additional monthly i.d. injection of MER on multiple sites, for several months. The remission in MER-treated patients was between 92 to 193 days as opposed to 63 to 162 days in the chemotherapy group, and their abilities to respond to five recall antigens increased from 1 to 3 in the pre-MER period to 3–5 after MER treatment. In another trial (Bekesi *et al.*, 1976), with fifty-three patients, the effect of three types of treatments was evaluated: chemotherapy alone (control group), chemotherapy + immunization with neuraminidase (N'ase)-treated allogeneic myeloblasts with or without MER (immunized groups). The median remission duration of the control group was 20 weeks, whereas in the immunized group it was more than 78 weeks. Patients from the immunized groups had a longer survival time: five of thirty-two patients died by 90 weeks compared with seventeen of twenty-one in the control group. An additional trial along the same lines was conducted in AML patients (Bekesi *et al.*, 1977). All patients received cyclical maintenance chemotherapy (cytosine arabinoside and daunorubicin). One group was kept on chemotherapy alone, another group received also N'ase treated myeloblasts and a third was given cells + MER. Patients receiving cells as immunogen showed significant improvement. Cells + MER did not improve remission over that from cells alone (Bekesi *et al.*, 1977). The data presented (Bekesi *et al.*, 1977, 1978) do not provide clear evidence on the difference between the MER-treated immunized group and immunized group not treated with MER.

In continuation of a previous trial (Weiss *et al.*, 1975) a total of 35 AML cases were examined to determine the possible relationship between the degree of immune reactivity and clinical state in AML. A highly significant correlation was observed between the T-cell functions (PHA stimulation, mixed lymphocyte reaction) and the clinical state. Higher T-cell reactivity was associated with longer duration of remission and survival, while levels of B-cell functions (Ig production, antibody response to hemocyanin) were not correlated to the course of the disease. Addition of MER to the chemotherapy resulted in a significant increase in T-cell functions as well as in longer duration of remission and survival. The MER administration had apparently no effect on the humoral immune response and Ig levels of AML patients. Although the remission lymphocytes from MER-treated patients were better stimulated by this compound or PPD than cells isolated during relapse, their response was still far below that observed for cells from normal donors. The main conclusion of the authors is that clinical improvement in AML patients by MER administration may be due to restoration of T-cell function (Izak *et al.*, 1977).

2.2.3. *Effect in Solid Tumors*

Clinical trials with MER were also performed with patients suffering from melanoma, lung carcinoma, bladder carcinoma, colon carcinoma, larynx carcinoma and several other carcinomata (Weiss, 1976; Robinson *et al.*, 1975). The effects of MER therapy were evaluated with regard to increase in overall reactivity of the immunocompetent system and to clinical improvement of treated patients. The clinical trials included groups of various types of solid tumors.

Clinical trials on effectiveness of MER treatment in metastatic melanoma were conducted in Israel (Robinson *et al.*, 1975) and in the United States (Grimm, 1979; Denefrio, 1979; Sterchi *et al.*, 1980; Krown *et al.*, 1976, 1977; Kostinas *et al.*, 1978). The trial done in Israel (Robinson *et al.*, 1975) included 6 melanoma patients as a part of a group of 27 cancer patients with various types of tumors. MER was apparently well tolerated and improved skin test response to recall antigens: PPD, streptokinase and *Candida* (Robinson *et al.*, 1975). In view of the small number of patients it is difficult to evaluate the effect of MER on the progression of the disease. Preliminary results were reported from a clinical trial in the United States with MER in metastatic melanoma (Krown *et al.*, 1976). Eight patients received daily injections of MER into the lesions. The side effects to MER were graded as mild in four cases, moderate in three and severe in one patient. The therapeutic effect was evaluated as complete regression in one case, partial regression in six other cases, and progression of lesions in one of the cases. The authors concluded that apparently 'MER is tolerated reasonably well and may be useful in the treatment of cutaneous melanoma metastases'. In another study (Krown *et al.*, 1977) MER was injected intralesionally in 18 patients with cutaneous malignant melanoma. The author concluded that 'MER is capable of destroying metastatic lesions of malignant melanoma after direct injection' (Krown *et al.*, 1977). The effect of MER addition to chemotherapy in stage III and IV melanoma was evaluated in a clinical trial involving 116 patients (Kostinas *et al.*, 1978). No significant difference was found between the group receiving chemotherapeutic drugs only (procarbazine, vinblastine and dactinomycin) and the group also receiving MER (Krown *et al.*, 1977). Similar results were reported in a trial including 43 patients with locally resected stage II and III malignant melanoma: addition of immunotherapy with MER to dacarbazine (DTIC) did not affect the median time to relapse (Denefrio, 1979). In a recent trial (Sterchi *et al.*, 1980), the effects of DTIC with and without MER on recurrence of malignant melanoma was reinvestigated. Fifty-seven patients with locally resected stage II (37 patients) and stage III (20 patients) were distributed at random in two groups: DTIC alone or DTIC + MER. The study revealed no significant difference between MER treated vs untreated group (Sterchi *et al.*, 1980).

A first trial on the effect of MER on advanced gastrointestinal cancer was performed in a group of 40 patients, all previous chemotherapy failures (Moertel *et al.*, 1975a, b), MER raised immunocompetence levels as expressed by increased reactivity to recall antigens and to DNCB challenge, increase in lymphocyte blastogenesis to mitogens, elevation of immunoglobulin levels and of T and B cells (Moertel *et al.*, 1975a, b). It was concluded that MER is a potent stimulus of cellular and humoral immunity and that this stimulation may result in antineoplastic effect (Moertel *et al.*, 1975a, b). Comparison between radio-chemotherapy and radio-chemotherapy + MER in colo-rectal cancer was done in a group of 53 patients (Robinson *et al.*, 1979). Addition of MER led to increase in immunological reactivity (skin tests to recall antigens, lymphocyte stimulation by mitogens and antigens) and to significant longer disease-free interval, lower recurrence rate and better survival (Robinson *et al.*, 1979). Adjuvant therapy with or without MER was also evaluated in 394 patients with surgically curable colon cancer (Lokich, 1979). The groups compared were 5-FU plus MeCCNV, MER, 5-FU plus MeCCNV plus MER and an untreated control group. No significant differences between the treated groups with regard to period of time until recurrence or survival were found during a median follow up period of 13 months (Lokich, 1979).

Several trials were conducted on the effect of combined chemotherapy and MER in breast cancer. The first study was carried out with twenty-four patients, of which eleven were classified in stage II, three in stage III and ten in stage IV (Perloff *et al.*, 1978). All patients with stage III and stage IV regressed, and only one of eleven stage II patients had relapses. *In vivo* assays of reactivity to five recall antigens and *in vitro* examination of B and T cells and of lymphocyte blastogenesis showed improvement in the immunologic function. Local ulcerations were observed in twenty-two patients injected with 200 μg MER, and in eight cases reduction in MER dose was felt necessary. The treated patients developed skin reactivity to minute doses of MER. Therefore, addition of MER to the therapeutic regimen seemed to improve the clinical condition and the immunologic function.

The second study determined the effects of MER and BCG addition to chemotherapy in fifty-two breast cancer patients (Tashima *et al.*, 1976). The main conclusion was that both additions (MER or BCG) had a beneficial effect, without significant differences between the two immunotherapeutic agents. In a later trial (Perloff *et al.*, 1978) the effect of i.d. immunotherapy with MER was studied in 49 cancer patients, 45 of whom were women with breast carcinoma in stages II, III and IV. First injections of MER induced DH to the agent as shown in a second titration (Perloff *et al.*, 1978). It is suggested that skin reactions to MER may be useful for titration of immunotherapy doses (Perloff *et al.*, 1978). Chemotherapy alone (cytoxan, 5-FU and prednisone) was compared with chemotherapy + MER treatment in 71 post-menopausal women with measurable metastatic breast cancer (Britell *et al.*, 1979). It seems that the use of MER did not affect the response rate, time to progression or survival of breast cancer patients receiving chemotherapy (Britell *et al.*, 1979). Another parameter investigated was impact of prior radiotherapy to frequency and duration of response to chemotherapy with or without MER for metastatic breast cancer (Aisner *et al.*, 1979). Radiotherapy appears to impart a less favorable prognosis on response to chemotherapy with or without MER (Aisner *et al.*, 1979).

A report on a study performed in children aged 1–11 years (Necheles *et al.*, 1976) dealt with the effect of MER on the treatment of disseminated neuroblastoma. Ten children received a combined chemoimmunotherapeutic treatment including MER, while eleven comparable cases were treated with chemotherapy alone. The response rates were not significantly different between the two groups (9/10 vs 7/11). However, a substantial increase in the duration of response was observed in MER-treated children: relapse only in two children at the end of 15 months as compared with a median duration of response of 36 weeks in the chemotherapy group. Local reactions to MER were observed in all the children and in three of them there were transient systemic symptoms such as fever. It appeared that MER immunotherapy may have had a significant role in prolonging clinical response in children with widespread neuroblastoma.

Chemotherapy vs chemoimmunotherapy (including MER) for small cell carcinoma of the lung (SCC) was assayed (Aisner *et al.*, 1977). No difference in response or survival was found between the group on chemotherapy alone (CY, adriamycin and VP 16-213) and the group receiving MER (Aisner *et al.*, 1977). In another trial SCC patients treated with MER in addition to radiotherapy and chemotherapy showed a tendency for improved survival by comparison with the group nontreated with MER (Jackson *et al.*, 1979). Chemotherapy alone and chemotherapy + MER were also evaluated in previously irradiated stage III SCC of the lung (Jagathambal *et al.*, 1979). The conclusion was that MER with or without chemotherapy (vincristine-adriamycin-CY) as well as chemotherapy alone did not prolong survival of previously irradiated patients (Jagathambal *et al.*, 1979). The effect of oral administration of MER was tested in 17 patients with non oat cell lung cancer (Bartal *et al.*, 1980). It seems that some increase in general immunocompetence was observed although no regression in tumor size was seen (Bartal *et al.*, 1980).

Increase in immunocompetence in patients with advanced lung cancer following MER treatment was also mentioned in another report (Mekori *et al.*, 1980). In this case the immunological status of 29 patients receiving MER in addition to the conventional radiotherapy and/or chemotherapy was compared with immunological reactivity in 22 patients kept on radiotherapy and chemotherapy only (Mekovi *et al.*, 1980).

During the last years two clinical trials were performed in order to evaluate the benefit of MER addition to chemotherapy in advanced Hodgkin's disease. The first study included 136 patients in the beginning (Vinciguerra *et al.*, 1978) and was later extended to a total number of 180 patients (Coleman *et al.*, 1979). MER treatment was added to chemotherapy with CVPP (CCNV, Vinblastine, Procarbazine, Prednisone), BAVS (Bleomycin, Adriamycin, Vincristine, Streptozotocin) or both (CVPP + BAVS). No benefit has been seen from the addition of MER with respect to response frequency or duration of remission. In a second study (Vinciguerra *et al.*, 1978; Coleman *et al.*, 1979). (Cooper *et al.*, 1980) the effectiveness of MER in preventing relapse in patients with Hodgkin's disease who had a low tumor burden, was evaluated. Patients in complete remission following 2 years of maintenance chemotherapy were randomized to receive MER (59 patients) or no immunotherapy (70 patients). No difference in frequency of relapses was observed between the MER treated and untreated groups during a follow-up period of almost 3 years (Cooper *et al.*, 1980).

The effect of MER therapy was also evaluated in some other cases (Robinson *et al.*, 1975) of malignant neoplasia (bladder, larynx, ovary, retroperitoneal tumor, tongue) and in a group of patients with nonspecified advanced cancer and resistant to classical therapy (Vogl *et al.*, 1977).

A summary of clinical trials performed with MER is given in Table 1.

TABLE 1. *Summary of clinical trials performed with MER*

Clinical diagnosis	References
Acute myelocytic leukemia	Izak *et al.*, 1977; Weiss *et al.*, 1975; Cuttner *et al.*, 1975; Bekesi *et al.*, 1976; Bekesi *et al.*, 1977
Melanoma	Grimm, 1979; Denefrio, 1979; Sterchi *et al.*, 1980; Krown *et al.*, 1977; Robinson *et al.*, 1975; Krown *et al.*, 1976; Kostinas *et al.*, 1978
Gastrointestinal cancer	Moertel *et al.*, 1975a; Robinson *et al.*, 1979; Robinson *et al.*, 1975; Moertel *et al.*, 1975b; Lokich, 1979
Breast cancer	Denefrio, 1979; Robinson *et al.*, 1975; Perloff *et al.*, 1976; Tashima *et al.*, 1976; Perloff *et al.*, 1978; Britell *et al.*, 1979; Aisner *et al.*, 1979; Necheles *et al.*, 1976
Lung carcinoma	Jackson *et al.*, 1979; Bartal *et al.*, 1980; Robinson *et al.*, 1975; Aisner *et al.*, 1977; Jagathambal *et al.*, 1979; Mekori *et al.*, 1980
Hodgkin's	Cooper *et al.*, 1980; Vinciguerra *et al.*, 1978; Coleman *et al.*, 1979
Others or nonspecified neoplasia	Vogl *et al.*, 1978; Robinson 1975

The data reported up until now indicate that MER was usually well tolerated and increased the overall activity of the immunocompetent system, especially cellmediated immunological response. MER had an apparently beneficial effect in certain cases of cancer, but it is still difficult to draw final conclusions. This in view of scarcity of data and because in certain trials 'hopeless' cases which failed to respond to other kinds of therapy, were included. More strictly controlled trials are required in order to evaluate the effectiveness of MER treatment in various clinical types of neoplasia.

3. MODE OF ACTION STUDIES

3.1 General Comments on the Action of Immunomodulators

Several explanations have been put forth for the activity of immunomodulators. It is worthwhile to mention briefly the prevailing concepts in this field before discussing the various interpretations for MER activity.

Reports on the immunopotentiating effect of certain substances have appeared since 1926. Adbsorption of antigen to insoluble particles of aluminium phosphate was shown markedly to increase the immune response (Ramon, 1926; Glenny *et al.*, 1926). In 1953, Freund described potentiation of the immune response by incorporating an aqueous solution of the antigen in an oil emulsion containing mycobacterial organisms (Freund, 1953). These findings indicated the presence of immunomodulators in the mycobacterial cell complex. Freund (1953) also first suggested the possible mode of action of immunopotentiators. He proposed several means of immunopotentiation: (a) protracted antigenic stimulus resulting from the slow release of antigen from the site injected with the antigen-adjuvant mixture (depot effect); (b) stimulation of RES; and (c) direct action on the lymphocytes involved in the immune response.

The first possibility is more relevant to adjuvants given simultaneously with the antigen in the same mixture, which change the physical nature of the antigen (from soluble to particles). The 'depot effect' is less likely to play a role if the adjuvant is injected separately or after the antigen injection. The other two possibilities (RES stimulation and effect on lymphocytes) were extensively studied and are more relevant to the MER mechanism of activity.

3.1.1. *Stimulation of the RES*

Involvement of the phagocytic activity of the RES in the response to antigenic challenge seems well established. Experimental data showed that the intravascular clearance of a particulate antigen proceeds according to the same laws which govern the phagocytosis of inert colloidal material (Halpern *et al.*, 1957). Different rates of clearance may be manifested towards different particulate substances (Filkins and Di Luzio, 1966) indicating that RES function measured by carbon clearance is not necessarily equivalent to its activity in relation to specific antigens. However, stimulations of the phagocytic activity of the RES is usually associated with marked elevations in antibody response (Cutler, 1960; Halpern, 1959; Wooles and Di Luzio, 1963) and augmentation of resistance to infections (Weiss *et al.*, 1964; Old *et al.*, 1960). It seems plausible that immunomodulators may stimulate the RES function and promote in this way the immune response. It was shown (Rupp *et al.*, 1960) that i.v. injection of FCA stimulates the RES of the rabbit as expressed by marked proliferation of the reticuloendothelial cells, vascular endothelium and the interstitial connective tissues, in a variety of organs. It is of interest that, in this case, FCA was injected systemically and the tissue reaction was found in various organs. BCG itself (Biozzi *et al.*, 1954) and *C. parvum* (Halpern *et al.*, 1964) have been shown to exert a powerful stimulating effect on the RES, expressed by hyperplasia and increased phagocytic activity.

Stimulation of RES by immunomodulators may also result in more effective processing, leading to more extensive stimulation, and to overall increase in macrophage function (cytotoxic effects, enzyme activity). The results reported, although clearly indicating activation of macrophages by immunomodulators, do not provide direct evidence for more effective processing of the antigen. *B. pertussis* and berryllium sulfate were shown to exert their promoting effect on antibody producing cells and antibody titers only after their uptake by macrophages (Unanue *et al.*, 1969). However, the adjuvant action was not conditioned by the presence of antigen and adjuvant in the same macrophage. The overall catabolism and antigen retention was also not significantly altered in the presence of adjuvants (Unanue *et al.*, 1969). The authors suggested three interpretations for their findings: (a) change in the fate of antigen in macrophages (less likely); (b) macrophages act as effective carriers of adjuvants to a critical anatomical site; and (c) adjuvants may exert a cytotoxic effect on macrophages leading to the appearance of 'altered' macrophages able to stimulate the proliferating activity of the surrounding antigen sensitive lymphoid cells. The last possibility might be in line with more recent reports showing induced release of lymphocyte active factors from macrophages by mitogens (Gery and Waksman, 1972a, b). Other authors reported increase in production of lysosomal enzymes, chemotactic activity towards macrophages, and in killing capacity of these cells in the presence of immunomodulators. Production of lysosomal enzymes by guinea pig peritoneal macrophages was increased by factors from strains of Corynebacterium (Wilkinson *et al.*, 1973). This effect was associated with chemotactic activity for macrophages (Wilkinson *et al.*, 1973). BCG-infested mice showed a greater chemotactic response *in vitro* of peritoneal macrophages than the response of macrophages from uninfected mice (Meltzer *et al.*, 1975a). Increase in the cytotoxic activity to tumor cells of peritoneal macrophages originated from mice treated with *C. parvum* or BCG was also reported (Halpern *et al.*, 1973; Meltzer *et al.*, 1975b).

An adverse effect on macrophage function has been suggested recently (Murahata and Zighelboim, 1979a; Murahara and Zighelboim, 1979b). I.v. administration of *C. parvum* to mice resulted in marked inhibition of memory cell-mediated cytotoxic response to alloantigens. This impairment seems due to generation of suppressor macrophages by *C. parvum* (Murahata and Zighelboim, 1979a). The inhibitory effect was restricted to cell mediated type immune response and was expressed only by spleen cell populations (Murahata and Zighelboim, 1979b).

Stimulation of the RES function by immunomodulators seems to be well established. It is likely that this effect plays a role in the promotion of the immune response. However, recent findings reported in this field suggest that under certain conditions, the effect of immunomodulators on macrophage function may be expressed by inhibition (instead of promotion) of immune response. It is also possible that direct effects on lymphocyte populations are involved as alternative or additional ways for immunomodulation.

3.1.2. *Effect on Lymphocyte Populations*

Modulation of typical T cell functions, including cytotoxic effect, graft rejection, delayed hypersensitivity and helper effect, has been reported by numerous workers. However, evidence is still scarce on whether this effect is related to mitogenic stimulation of T cells by immunomodulators. CBA mouse T lymphocytes stimulated by Con A showed an increased cytotoxicity in the presence of PHA against DBA-1 mastocytoma (Asherson *et al.*, 1973). On the other hand, Con A and PHA do not act usually as immunopotentiators, and under certain circumstances they exhibit an immunosuppressive effect (Egan *et al.*, 1974; Chan, 1969). It was reported (Chen and Leon, 1976) that Con A enhances the *in vitro* immune response to the T independent antigen dextran by facilitating the release of active soluble T-cell products. The adjuvant poly(A)-poly(U) increased the incorporation of thymidine into lymphocytes from sensitized subjects exposed *in vitro* to tuberculin (Friedman *et al.*, 1969) and also in mixed leukocyte responses (Allison, 1973), but removal of adherent cells (mostly macrophages) decreased the stimulating effect (Allison, 1973). The polysaccharide lentinan potentiated selectively the T-cell function in the immune response to SRBC (Dresser, 1972) and had a marked antitumor activity (Maeda *et al.*, 1973). Other typical CMI responses, such as skin graft rejection and skin DH, were not affected by lentinan (Maeda *et al.*, 1973). According to the authors (Maeda *et al.*, 1973) the target for immunopotentiation by lentinan remains unclarified.

Adjuvant regulation of T-cell function may involve selective effect on various functionally distinct subpopulations of T cells. Thus FCA was found to suppress the generation of cytolytic T cells, whereas helper T cell function was augmented (Reinisch *et al.*, 1976). Immunomodulators like BCG (Geffard and Orbach-Arbouys, 1976) and LPS (Uchiyama and Jacobs, 1978) were shown to induce stimulation of suppressor T cells.

More convincing evidence is available on the relationship between direct mitogenic effect on B cells and immunomodulatory activity. B-cell mitogens such as LPS (Andersson *et al.*, 1972a) polyanions, PPD were shown to potentiate the immune response *in vivo* (Diamantstein *et al.*, 1976) and *in vitro* (Kreisler and Möller, 1974). The immunopotentiating effect was in direct relation to the mitogenic effect (Vogt *et al.*, 1973). It was also evident in nude mice lacking functionally active T cells (Bullock and Andersson, 1973) and towards isolated haptens *in vitro* (Watson *et al.*, 1973). On the basis of these data it was assumed that B-cell mitogens bypass the T-cell function in T-B cell coordination by giving to the B antigen reactive cells a second stimulation signal usually provided by T cells or their soluble factors (Watson *et al.*, 1973). It was also reported (Diamantstein *et al.*, 1976) that B-cell mitogens can suppress the immune response when administered several days before the injection of the antigen. Some immunomodulatory effects of B-cell mitogens may be due to selective stimulation of B-cell subpopulations. Thus, LPS appears to induce a population of specific suppressor B cells which are capable of regulating T-cell function (Gill and Liew, 1979). Polyanions and LPS seem to act on subpopulations of B-cells of different stages of maturity (Diamantstein *et al.*, 1974). The capsular polysaccharide of *Klebsiella pneumoniae* had different effects on the functions of various subpopulations of B cells involved in the immune response to T dependent antigen (Nakashima *et al.*, 1979).

The effect of immunomodulators on other lymphocyte subpopulations (non T or B cells) has also been reported. BCG was shown to stimulate NK cell activity (Pioch *et al.*, 1979; Tracey, 1979) whereas glucan depressed the activity of NK cells (Lotzova and Gutterman, 1979). Finally, it was claimed that BCG stimulates the proliferation of granulocyte-macrophage colony-forming cells (Bennett and Marsh, 1980).

Recently (Emeson, 1980) adjuvant-induced selective recruitment of specifically reactive lymphocytes to the injected sites was reported and this was suggested as a probable mechanism of adjuvant action.

In conclusion, evidence is accumulating on the direct or indirect effect of various immunomodulators on different populations of lymphoid cells. It seems probable that most immunomodulators act on more than one type of cell (macrophages, T and B cells) and affect the interaction between various populations and subpopulations of immunocompetent cells.

3.2. Mechanisms of MER Activity

It is worthwhile to emphasize certain properties of MER fraction which may be relevant to its activity.

3.2.1. *Properties of MER*

(a) MER is a particulate, heterogenous preparation, probably containing several components. It may possibly contain more than one active principle, and its activity may therefore be an expression of additive or synergistic effects.

(b) MER is a fraction with intrinsic immunogenicity derived from tubercle bacilli which are widely spread in nature. Previous contact of the organism with tubercle bacilli is highly probable, and may provide an immunogenic stimulus towards one of the antigenic components of MER. This is probably the case in a high proportion of human beings as reflected by the tuberculin test. Therefore, the possibility of antigenic stimulation by MER in an already sensitized host should be taken into consideration.

(c) In a large variety of experimental systems, MER activity is better expressed when administered a few days before immunization. This finding indicates the need of a latent period for the establishment of MER effect and a systemic mode of action. The possibility of a 'depot effect' by MER is almost ruled out, in view of the fact that it seems unnecessary to inject MER simultaneously with the antigen.

(d) Experiments performed in animals as well as immunotherapeutic studies in man have shown that MER modulates both CMI and antibody responses. Therefore, the effect of MER (direct or indirect) is exerted at the functional level of T cells and B cells as well.

In view of these considerations, the effect of MER on the various types of immunocompetent cells and its relation to the immunomodulatory activity will be discussed.

3.2.2. *Effect of MER on Morphology and Function of Lympoid-RES*

Morphological changes in lymphoid organs and stimulation of RES function were observed in MER-treated mice. Frequent increase in the size, weight and number of nucleated cells of spleens followed treatment with MER when two injections were given (Steinkuller *et al.*, 1969). These findings were correlated with the effect of MER pretreatment on the specific immune response to SRBC (PFC). In certain cases, a single injection of MER three days prior to immunization increased the numbers of PFC without changing substantially the total numbers of nucleated cells in the spleens (Steinkuller *et al.*, 1969). Two prior injections of MER increased both the total cell content of the spleen as well as the specific immune response. However, the increase in the numbers of PFC occurred earlier and was relatively greater than the increase in the total numbers of nucleated spleen cells (Steinkuller *et al.*, 1969). Apparently, the kinetics of the MER immunomodulatory activity differed from that of the morphological changes induced in the lymphoid organ.

The relation between stimulation of RES clearing function and immunopotentiation by MER seems to be a more complex one. MER considerably enhanced total and functional carbon clearing activity as early as two hours after treatment (Steinkuller *et al.*, 1969). The mean K (phagocytic clearance value) returned to normal within the next eight hours, and rose again, remaining above normal until 70 hours afterwards. It seems therefore that at an optimal time for antigen injection (three days after MER administration), the RES clearing activity is normal. It is possible that pretreatment with MER has the effect of preconditioning the RES for an increased anamnestic response induced by the antigen. This assumption is strengthened by the finding that a second injection of MER led to an immediate steep peaking of K (Steinkuller *et al.*, 1969).

It has been argued that different rates of clearance may be manifested towards different substances (Filkins and Di Luzio, 1966). It was therefore of interest to determine the rate of clearance of the antigen affected by the MER administration. Experiments were performed with the soluble antigen BCG protein in mice (Jacobs *et al.*, 1978). Pretreatment with MER stimulated the antibody synthesis to this antigen. The radio-labeled antigen ^{125}I-BGG was taken up more by the mesenteric lymph node, lungs and gut of MER-treated mice two hours after antigen injection, but was subsequently eliminated more quickly from these organs and blood. Certain interpretations of these changes in terms of immunopotentiating effect were given. It is possible that more effective early uptake of the antigen will permit a ready access to immunocompetent cells, while the subsequent rapid elimination will prevent establishment of tolerance by an antigen excess (Weiss and Yashpe, 1973).

3.2.3. *Effect on Macrophages*

The findings on facilitation of RES function by MER indicate that one of the target cells of MER activity might be the macrophage. Therefore, investigations were carried out on the effect of MER on macrophage physiology. Cell populations composed mostly of macrophages were used. The effect of MER administration on the production of lymphocyte-activating factor (LAF) by macrophages and on their enzymatic, phagocytic and killing activities were determined.

In vivo *administration*

3.2.3.1. *Effect on LAF production.* Glass-adherent peritoneal cells (mostly macrophages), originated from MER-treated and control mice, were examined for their ability to produce

LAF (Gery *et al.*, 1975). LAF is known to stimulate T cells and to potentiate their response to mitogens (Gery and Waksman, 1972a, b). Peritoneal cells from MER-treated mice produced significantly more LAF than untreated controls. These data strongly suggest a direct effect of MER on macrophages. The further increase of thymocyte response to PHA when either Con A or LPS were added to the LAF-producing cultures may be interpreted in various ways: (a) increase in LAF production in the presence of Con A or LPS (such an effect was reported for LPS (Gery and Waksman, 1972a, b); (b) synergistic effect in combinations LAF-Con A-PHA (all three factors react on various subpopulations of T cells); and (c) synergistic effect of LPS on either LAF or PHA activity. B-cell mitogens like dextran sulfate were reported to act synergistically in increasing the T cell response to PHA (Blitstein-Willinger *et al.*, 1976). However, in this case, LPS did not affect the response to PHA (Blitstein-Willinger *et al.*, 1976).

3.2.3.2. *Effect on lysosomal enzyme activities.* Macrophage lysosomal enzyme activity has been associated with phagocytic and effector cell capacities of macrophages towards pathogenic microorganisms and neoplastic target cells (Axline and Cohn, 1970; Gershon *et al.*, 1967; Hard, 1970). Therefore, it seems likely that potentiation of macrophage function by MER should be related to increase in their lysosomal enzyme levels. Experimental evidence was recently brought on this point (Yagel *et al.*, 1975). The activities of all the four enzymes tested (acid phosphatase, glucoronidase, cathepsin D and lysozyme) were markedly elevated in the cell lysates of peritoneal macrophages derived from MER-treated mice (Yagel *et al.*, 1975).

3.2.3.3. *Effect on phagocytic, bacteriostatic and bactericidal activity.* The effect of MER on these activities was tested by using peritoneal macrophages from MER-treated mice and *Staphylococcus* or *Listeria* as test organisms (Gallily *et al.*, 1976, 1977). Treatment with MER resulted in appreciable increase in the capacity of peritoneal macrophages to phagocytize living radioactively labeled staphylococci *in vitro,* to inhibit their intracellular multiplication, and to kill the engulfed bacteria.

The effect of MER on macrophage potency was selective (Gallily *et al.*, 1977). Thus, phagocytosis of living *S. albus* and *S. aureus* organisms, but not of *Listeria monocytogens* was enhanced (Gallily *et al.*, 1977). Macrophage from MER-treated mice displayed a significant facility to reduce the viability of intracellular *S. albus* and *L. monocytogenes* but not of *S. aureus* (Gallily *et al.*, 1977).

3.2.3.4. *Effect on antibody response.* Peritoneal cells or macrophage enriched fractions (glass-wool adherent) from MER-treated mice were markedly more effective than similar populations from normal donors in reconstituting the capacity of primary antibody response *in vitro* to SRBC in macrophage depleted cultures (Halperin *et al.*, 1980).

3.2.3.5. *Effect on tumor cells.* Early experiments showing nonspecific increase in the ability of cells from lymphoid organs of MER-treated animals to damage tumor cells were reported with C57B1 mice and plasmacytoma (Kuperman *et al.*, 1972). In these experiments no attempts were made to separate the cell population into lymphocytes and macrophage components. Therefore, no direct indication was obtained on the macrophage role in the increased cytotoxic effect. More recent experiments (Weiss *et al.*, 1976) were more conclusive concerning the increase in cytotoxic activity of macrophages derived from MER-treated animals. In this study, special care was taken to avoid the possibility that cancer cells may be injured as bystanders of specific interactions between mycobacterial antigens and immune elements. For this purpose, the effect of MER on immunocompetent cells was evaluated in irradiated recipients which received cells from MER-treated donors. The recipients afterwards received a challenge injection of allogeneic plasma tumor cells. The spleen cells from MER treated mice induced in the recipient hosts of the same strain subsequently exposed to the allogeneic PCT a heightened degree of cytotoxic reactivity against the tumor cells. In additional experiments, an attempt was made to determine the nature of cells responsible for the heightened degree of cytotoxic activity. Splenocyte suspensions originating either from MER treated mice or saline injected mice, were separated into adherent (presumably macrophage) and non-adherent (presumably lymphocyte) cell populations. The separated populations were then injected into irradiated recipients of the same strain in four combinations: both macrophages and lymphocytes from MER treated mice; both cell populations from saline injected animals; macrophages from MER treated mice and lymphocytes from saline injected animals; and, macrophages from saline mice and lymphocytes from MER treated animals. Afterwards, the recipients received living PCT cells. Eight days later, the animals were killed and the splenocyte suspensions were tested for anti-PCT reactivity *in vitro*. The results obtained show that both macrophages and lymphoid cells from mice subjected to MER treatment can evoke in recipients sensitized to the PCT a potentiated splenocyte toxicity for the tumor cells, the macrophage population displaying a more consistent and larger transfer effect. These findings indicate a direct effect of MER on macrophages and a possible (direct or indirect) influence of MER on a cytotoxic lymphocyte population.

3.2.3.6. *In vitro studies*. The above described effects point out that the macrophage is one of the target cells for MER activity. The experiments reported were based on treatment with MER *in vivo* followed by determinations of macrophage activities *in vitro*. It would be of interest to examine the effect of MER added directly to the macrophage population *in vitro*. First attempts were made by testing potentiation of the *in vitro* generation of cytotoxic effector cells against EL4 mouse leukemia (Weiss *et al.*, 1976). Splenocytes incubated in the presence of MER showed increased cytotoxicity, thus suggesting a direct effect on MER on effector cells. The effect of MER was dose and time dependent.

In another series of experiments (Kedar *et al.*, 1978), the effect of MER on the cytotoxic response *in vitro* against EL4 leukemia cells was evaluated. The addition of small amounts of MER to the cultures potentiated appreciably the elicitation of cytotoxic activity, whereas higher quantities had a strong suppressive effect. MER also induced some cytotoxic capacity in normal murine and human lymphoid cells not exposed to specific tumor cell stimulation. The population of cells affected by MER was the nylon nonadherent fraction. The mechanisms envisaged (Kedar *et al.*, 1978) for explaining MER stimulating activity were: (a) direct effect on development of cytotoxic precursor cells by amplification of helper T-cell function or abrogation of suppressor cell activity; (b) activation of residual macrophages still present in the nylon nonadherent fraction; (c) activation of NK cells; (d) sensitization of lymphoid cells to the MER itself; (e) mitogenicity of MER on certain lymphoid cell populations. The suppressive action exerted by large amounts of MER may be due (Kedar *et al.*, 1978) to antigenic competition between target cell antigens and antigenic determinants of MER, induction of suppressor cells, or toxicity of MER for macrophages.

Addition of MER *in vitro* to macrophage monolayer increased hydrolytic enzyme activity (acid phosphatase, β-glucoronidase, cathepsin D and lysozyme) (Gallily and Weiss, 1977). However, exposure of mouse peritoneal macrophages *in vitro* to MER failed to heighten their phagocytic and bacteriostatic activities toward *Staphylococcus albus* (Gallily *et al.*, 1981).

Incubation of normal peritoneal macrophage cultures with MER induced release of soluble factor(s) that facilitated the primary antibody response *in vitro* to SRBC in macrophage depleted cultures and had a synergistic effect on PHA stimulation of mouse thymocytes (Dar, Halperin, Ben-Efraim and Weiss, unpublished).

On the basis of data accumulated in *in vitro* experiments, it seems likely that the macrophage can be directly affected by contact with MER. However, increase in some macrophage activities was found only in macrophages taken from MER treated animals and were not induced by *in vitro* contact of MER with the cells.

3.2.4. *Effect on T Cells*

Stimulation of activities attributed to T cells by MER treatment is well documented. This applies to studies on DH and CH reactions in guinea pigs (Kuperman *et al.*, 1972; Ben-Efraim *et al.*, 1973; Zimber *et al.*, 1977) and mice (Jacobs *et al.*, 1978; Zimber *et al.*, 1977, 1981a, b), increase in resistance of guinea pigs (Minden *et al.*, 1974b; Wainberg *et al.*, 1976a, b, c) and mice (Weiss *et al.*, 1961, 1966) to transplanted syngeneic tumors, immunotherapeutic effect in man (Izak *et al.*, 1977) and animals, and stimulation of cytotoxic activity towards target tumor cells (Kuperman *et al.*, 1972; Kedar *et al.*, 1978). However, it is not yet clear whether MER has a direct effect on T cells or whether its activity on these cells is mediated via other cells, probably macrophages.

Experiments were performed on the mitogenic effect of MER *in vitro* on thymocytes, MER did not stimulate ^{3}HThy incorporation, either in Balb/c thymocytes (Ben-Efraim and Diamantstein, 1975) or in guinea pig thymocytes (Ben-Efraim *et al.*, 1976). On the other hand, it was claimed (Mitchell *et al.*, 1975) that MER increased the thymidine incorporation *in vitro* in thymus cells originated from the C3H/He and Swiss CD-1 mouse strains. The mouse strains used in this work were different from those used in the previously mentioned research (Ben-Efraim and Diamantstein, 1975). It is possible that immunocompetent cells originated from various strains of mice differ in their ability to become stimulated by certain mitogens. Moreover, the experimental set-up was different from that used in the work with the Balb/c strain (Minden *et al.*, 1974b): time of incubation with ^{3}HThy was 24 hr instead of 4 hr (Mitchell *et al.*, 1975). The optimal concentration found for the MER mitogenic effect on thymus cells was relatively high: 250 μg MER/5 $\times 10^{6}$ cells per culture (Mitchell *et al.*, 1975). The effect of MER on ^{3}HThy incorporation was also tested in human peripheral blood lymphocytes (Ben-Efraim and Diamantstein, unpublished). The data showed significant increase in ^{3}HThy incorporation, both by MER (stimulation index (SI) up to twenty-two times depending on MER dose; 0.5–15 μg per culture) and PPD (SI = 55 for 10 μg per culture), in cells originated from tuberculin positive individuals. MER and PPD had no stimulating effect on cells derived from tuberculin-negative persons. These results show that at least in two species (guinea pig, mouse), MER seems not to act as a direct T-cell mitogen. The effect of both MER and PPD on peripheral blood lymphocytes (up to 70 per cent T cells) in tuberculin positive individuals is probably due to antigenic stimulation resulting from previous contact with antigenic components of tubercle bacilli.

Various experimental data may be interpreted as indirect evidence on the effect of MER on T cells. In an early report (Yashpe and Haran-Ghera, 1970) it was claimed that s.c. injection of MER caused enlargement of the draining lymph nodes, due to hyperplasia of the paracortical area of the nodes. Paracortical hyperplasia is due largely to T cells, and in view of this fact it was assumed that MER may affect the T cell population (Weiss and Yashpe, 1973). On the other hand, later data (Stupp *et al.*, 1975) showed preferential increase in lymphocytes with 'B' properties in lymph nodes draining sites of MER injection.

An indirect mode of action of MER on T cells has been suggested by findings of increased LAF production by macrophages from MER-treated animals (Gery *et al.*, 1975) or macrophages treated *in vitro* with MER (Dar, Halperin, Ben-Efraim, Weiss, unpublished). It has been assumed (Gery and Waksman, 1972a) that LAF plays a role in immunopotentiation by mediating T cell mitogenesis (Allison and Davies, 1971). An indirect effect of MER on T cells (via macrophages), may also be suggested by data showing that macrophages from MER-treated animals were able to transfer passively the property of elevated cytotoxic capacity towards allogeneic plasma tumor cells (Weiss *et al.*, 1976). Additional reported findings on the interaction between MER and either ALS treatment or CY administration, indicate an effect of MER on 'active' T cell population. In mice pretreated with MER, anti-thymocyte serum (ATS) given one day prior to SRBC had little immunosuppressive activity, although ATS suppressed the antibody response in mice injected with plain saline (Yashpe and Haran-Ghera, 1970). Treatment of mice with MER markedly prevented the immunosuppressive effect elicited by heterologous ALS against allograft reactivity (Kuperman *et al.*, 1973). This effect may be due to some MER-induced change in the membrane properties or maturation stage of the cells affected by ALS, because spleen cells from MER-treated animals were more refractory to the direct cytotoxic action of ALS and complement *in vitro* (Kuperman *et al.*, 1973). It was shown (Zimber *et al.*, 1977, 1981b) that MER can prevent the immunosuppressive effect of CY on the establishment of CH to DNFB in guinea pigs and mice. CY was assumed to suppress proliferating cells, like, for example, active T cells stimulated by DNFB skin application. It is possible that the MER effect is due to correction of CY suppressive activity by mediating increase in stimulation of the active T cell population. Other data reported recently (Jacobs *et al.*, 1978) also suggest a MER effect on T cells specifically involved in the immune response: the levels of θ^+ rosette-forming cells (presumably T cells) capable of binding the antigenic entity, SRBC, were increased in mice treated with MER. It is noteworthy that the 'background' levels (in the absence of antigen) of θ^+ rosette-forming cells were not increased in MER-treated animals (Jacobs *et al.*, 1978). This finding is in line with the data on lack of mitogenic effect of MER on T cells (Ben-Efraim and Diamantstein, 1975; Ben-Efraim *et al.*, 1976). A mitogenic effect would be reflected (as is the case for B cells) by increase in background of θ^+ RFC as an expression of polyclonal proliferation characteristic for stimulation by mitogens.

New data on the effect of MER on T cells and their function have been added during recent years. Splenic lymphocytes rigorously purified after removal of macrophage cells, release, after incubation with MER, supernatants possessing phagocyte activating capability (Gallily *et al.*, 1981). This observation agrees with the concept that the principal effect of BCG and related mycobacteria is initial stimulation of T-lymphocytes resulting in the elaboration of soluble mediators that act on macrophages (Hadden *et al.*, 1977). T-enriched (nylon non-adherent, 98% of cells sensitive to anti-$Thy_{1,2}$ serum) spleen cell subpopulations originated from MER treated donors were more effective than similar subpopulations from MER untreated donors in restoring the capacity of primary antibody response *in vitro* to SRBC in cultures depleted of T cells (Halperin *et al.*, 1980). It has also been suggested that one of the mechanisms by which MER acts to elevate cytotoxic capacity *in vitro* is by amplification of helper T cell function (Kedar *et al.*, 1978).

In conclusion, the new data, in addition to earlier findings, support the assumption that some of the MER activity is exerted at the level of T cells. More data are required on the possibility of direct interaction between MER and isolated purified T-cell populations.

3.2.5. *Effect on B Cells*

Certain findings seem to favour the assumption of a direct effect of MER on B-cell population. MER activated DNA synthesis *in vitro* in spleen cells of Balb/c mice and nude mice lacking functionally active T cells (Ben-Efraim and Diamantstein, 1975) and in spleen cells of guinea pigs (Ben-Efraim *et al.*, 1976). The increase in ^{3}HThy incorporation effected by MER in spleen cells of mice was not macrophage dependent, thus suggesting that the mitogenic effect is not mediated by macrophages (Ben-Efraim and Diamantstein, 1975). Removal of B cells from the guinea pig spleen cell population was accompanied by loss of MER mitogenic activity, indicating that the B cell was the target for MER effect (Ben-Efraim *et al.*, 1976). A considerable increase in the uptake of ^{3}HThy was also found in cultures of spleen cells from MER-treated C57B1 mice, over that in the control cultures from untreated animals (Gery *et al.*, 1975).

MER increased the background of PFC *in vitro* (without addition of SRBC to the culture), and of 'B' RFC to SRBC in spleen cell population from MER-treated mice (Jacobs *et al.*, 1978). Increase in background of antigen-reactive cells is taken as an index for polyclonal proliferation of B cells characteristic for B cell mitogens (Kreisler and Möller, 1974). Moreover, MER potentiated also the specific immune response *in vitro* to SRBC in Balb/c and nude mice (Ben-Efraim and Diamantstein, 1975) and to the haptenic determinant TNP in Balb/c mice (Ben-Efraim and Diamantstein, 1975). The effect of MER in increasing the primary immune response to SRBC in nude spleen cell cultures indicate that, similar to other B cell mitogens (Andersson *et al.*, 1972b; Diamantstein *et al.*, 1971), MER may act directly on B cells by replacing some function of T-helper cells. It was also reported that MER can facilitate the antibody response *in vitro* to the monovalent hapten DNP-glycine (Ben-Efraim *et al.*, 1980). This effect is characteristic for B-cell mitogens like LPS (Watson *et al.*, 1973).

A synergistic effect between the stimulation of spleen cells by MER and LPS (another B-cell mitogen) has been reported (Gery *et al.*, 1975). The effect is similar to that described for the B-cell mitogens dextran sulfate and LPS (Watson *et al.*, 1973), and suggests accordingly that MER and LPS act on different B cell subpopulations.

The effect of MER on B-cell function is also evidenced by its ability to prevent the immunosuppressive effect of CY on the antibody response to SRBC (Stupp *et al.*, 1976). Treatment with MER restored the ability of primary response to the antigen when given 2 days after immunization (at the same time with CY). The most restorative action on secondary antibody response (2nd injection of SRBC on day 44, CY on day 46) was achieved by injecting MER at the time of primary immunization. This effect is due probably to the increase in the number of memory cells to SRBC in MER-treated animals. However, the prevention of CY suppressive effect by MER is not yet a proof of direct action of MER on B cells. The effect of amplification of the B-cell response might also be exerted via other types of immunocompetent cells.

A direct effect of MER on B-cell compartment has been suggested recently (Gallily *et al.*, 1981): separated B splenic lymphocytes, rigorously purified after removal of macrophage cells, release, after incubation with MER, supernatants possessing phagocyte activating capability. It is also of interest to mention that B splenic cells taken from MER treated donors were no more effective than B splenic cells of normal donors in developing a primary antibody response *in vitro* to SRBC. This last finding suggests that the effect of MER on B cells *in vitro* may not be paralleled by a similar effect *in vivo*. It should be pointed out that MER potentiated the primary antibody response *in vitro* (including possible effect on B cells) only when introduced to the cultures simultaneously with the antigen (Ben-Efraim *et al.*, 1980). On the other hand, MER was active *in vivo* only when administered a few days before immunization (Stein Kuller *et al.*, 1969; Ben-Efraim *et al.*, 1973).

The data available on the effect of MER on B-cell function *in vitro* seem to indicate that MER may act directly on B cells. It is still premature to conclude on whether direct interaction between MER and B cells plays a role in the immunomodulatory effect *in vivo* by this agent.

3.2.6. *Role of Shared Antigens*

The presence of antigens shared by BCG with other bacterial strains (Elberg *et al.*, 1957; Minden *et al.*, 1960, 1972) or tumor cell lines (Borsos and Rapp, 1973; Bucans and Hanna, 1974; Minden *et al.*, 1974a) has been reported. No such reports are available on a direct antigenic analysis of MER in comparison with target antigen entities. It is still possible that in certain particular cases, the immunomodulatory effect of MER is due to shared antigens between the agent and tumor cell. However, it is highly unlikely that as a general rule the MER activity is due to 'shared antigens' for the following reasons:

(a) The effect of MER is exerted towards a broad spectrum of antigens including simple haptenic determinants.

(b) There is proof of a direct effect of MER on at least two types of immunocompetent cells (macrophages and B cells).

(c) Passive transfer of cells with increased cytotoxic activity from MER-treated animals. It is most unlikely that appreciable amounts of MER could have passed to the recipient animals and still be present in the *in vitro* reaction mixture.

4. CONCLUDING REMARKS*

The first advantage claimed for MER over living BCG was that MER is a nonliving entity. Therefore, preparations of MER can be better standardized than BCG, are less prone to nonspecific contamination, and are not subjected to dangers arising from variability in host permissiveness to the multiplication and spread of living organisms, and from injection of excessive quantities of the active immunomodulator.

MER is a particulate, immunogenic, heterogeneous, chemically nondefined fraction of BCG tubercle organisms. It seems also that a large proportion of humans exhibit immunological memory toward MER in view of previous contact with mycobacterial organisms. MER fraction may also share some antigenic determinants with unrelated bacterial species and cells (including tumor cells). These properties have to be considered when dealing with various immunomodulatory effects of MER.

* The reader is also referred to recent Discussions and Reviews in this field (Weiss, 1977, 1978, 1979, 1980).

MER stimulated RES function, activated macrophages, acted as a B-cell mitogen and possibly induced release of factor(s) possessing phagocytic activating capability from B and T cells. Interaction between various populations of immunocompetent cells is probably affected by MER either by release of LAF component(s) from macrophages or release of macrophage activating factor(s) from lymphocytes. Therefore, MER has a wide spectrum of activities due either to one or more components present in the MER complex. It should also be mentioned that it is difficult to extrapolate on the real part played by MER activities shown *in vitro* on its modulatory effect *in vivo*. To this it is necessary to add that the immunomodulatory effects of MER are dependent on the dose and time of MER administration, the nature and quantity of the target antigen, and the host species. Therefore, optimal conditions for MER utilization have to be defined for each one of the systems.

Proper use of immunotherapy for beneficial effect in cancer is still highly controversial. This field is hampered by a long series of difficulties which seem almost insurmountable. Some of these difficulties are: wide variation between patient's clinical stage, need for immunopotentiation *after* and in the presence of antigenic stimulation, doubts on whether spontaneously arising neoplasms of man are immunogenic, immunosuppression (specific and nonspecific) by tumor cell components, huge mass of widespread tumor material, heterogeneity in tumor cell population, and so on.

To all this, it should be added that immunotherapy is usually performed in combination with immunosuppressive treatments, like radiotherapy and chemotherapy. In view of these limiting conditions it looks extremely difficult to obtain beneficial effects by immunotherapy with immunomodulators including MER.

Several mechanisms of activity can be envisaged for explaining immunomodulation by MER, including its immunotherapeutic effect. MER can act on various populations of immunocompetent cells, especially on macrophages. This activity may be affected by intrinsic, already existent immunological response to MER antigenic components. It might be that in those cases where MER is more effective when injected intralesionally, such treatment induces migration of immunocompetent cells: macrophages and lymphocytes (committed or noncommitted toward MER antigenic components) at the tumor site. Another possibility is that MER acts directly on tumor cells and renders them more sensitive to already existing immune killing mechanisms. MER may also exert a beneficial effect by bestowing marked, nonspecific protection against microbial pathogens and thus reducing the hazard of infection in cancer patients debilitated by the disease and by immunosuppressive treatment. The possibility of shared antigens between MER and tumor cells seems less likely as a general process of MER intervention, although it may still play a role in certain cases.

The interrelation between MER and chemotherapy is not yet fully understood. As was mentioned in this review, MER may counterbalance the immunosuppressive effect of certain drugs on antibody response or cell-mediated immune response in experimental animals. Concerning cancer patients, it has been reported that immunological intervention by MER in AML was beneficial when combined with a certain schedule of chemotherapy, but had no effect when another chemotherapeutic schedule was used. This finding suggests some selective effect of MER on the activity of various drugs.

Immunoprophylaxis of cancer is still in an embryonic stage, in view of lack of clear determination of 'high risk' populations. It is known that certain immunomodulators including MER can heighten natural resistance to bacterial infections, prevent or delay appearance of spontaneous tumors, and increase the chance of specific immunization against tumors in experimental animals. Therefore, if ways of predicting development of tumors will improve, it might be that immunomodulators will help in prevention or delay in appearance of clinically declared cancer in highly exposed human populations.

A new, exciting possibility was suggested for the employment of MER. It was found that MER can potentiate the sensitization *in vitro* of cytotoxic effector cells against murine leukemia cells. This opens the way for use of enriched populations of cytotoxic effector cells in passive/adoptive immunotherapy if adequate methods of mass preparation and preservation can be formulated.

Much effort has been made during recent years in preparing and testing activity of synthetic adjuvants in a series of experimental *in vivo* and *in vitro* systems. These compounds are highly purified and well defined chemically. Unfortunately, very little is known on whether synthetic adjuvants can be used and are effective in humans. It might be that the 'defects' inherent in classical immunomodulators, including MER, are translated to advantages when it comes to their use in humans. This applies to physical form, heterogeneity in number of active principles and ways of activity, intrinsic immunogenicity and occurrence of immunological memory toward immunomodulating agents.

Acknowledgements—I am deeply indebted to Professor David W. Weiss for his continuous interest and advice during the preparation of this manuscript.

REFERENCES

ADA G. L. (1970) Antigen cells in tolerance and immunity. *Transpl. Rev.* **5:** 105–129.

AISNER, J., ESTERHAY, R. J. JR. and WIERNIK, P. H. (1977) Chemotherapy vs. chemoimmunotherapy for small cell carcinoma of the lung. *Proc. Am. Soc. Clin. Oncol.* **18:** 310.

AISNER, J., WEINBERG, V., WIERNIK, P. H., LESNICK, G., PERLOFF, M., WEISS, R. B., ELLISON, R. R., YATES, J. and GINSBERG, S. J. (1979) Frequency and duration of response to combination chemotherapy for metastatic breast cancer: impact of prior radiotherapy (RT). *Proc. Am. Soc. Clin. Oncol.* **20:** 421.

ALEXANDER, P. and EVANS, R. (1971) Endotoxin and double-stranded RNA render macrophages cytotoxic. *Nature New Biol.* **232:** 76–78.

ALLISON, A. C. and DAVIES, A. J. S. (1971) Requirement of thymus-dependent lymphocytes for potentiation by adjuvants of antibody formation. *Nature Lond.* **223:** 330–332.

ALLISON, A. C. (1973) Effect of adjuvants on different cell types and their interactions in immune responses. In: *Immunopotentiation,* A Ciba Foundation Symposium, pp. 73–94, WOLSTENHOLME, G. E. W. AND KNIGHT, J. (Eds). Elsevier, Associated Scientific Publishers, Amsterdam.

ALLWOOD, G. G. and ASHERSON, G. L. (1971) Depression of delayed hypersensitivity by pretreatment with Freund-type adjuvants. I. Description of the phenomenon. *Clin. exp. Immunol.* **9:** 249–258.

ANDERSSON, J., SJÖBERG, O. and MÖLLER, G. (1972a) Induction of immunoglobulin and antibody synthesis *in vitro* by lipopolysaccharides. *Eur. J. Immunol.* **2:** 349–353.

ANDERSSON, J., SJÖBERG, O. and MÖLLER, G. (1972b) Mitogens as probes for immunocyte activation and cellular cooperation. *Transpl. Rev.* **11:** 131–177.

ASHERSON, G. L., FERLUGA, J. and JANOSSY, G. (1973) Nonspecific cytotoxicity by T cells activated with plant mitogens *in vitro* and the requirement for plant agents during the killing reaction. *Clin. exp. Immunol.* **15:** 573–589.

AXLINE, S. G. and COHN, Z. A. (1970) *In vitro* induction of lysozomal enzymes by phagocytosis. *J. exp. Med.* **131:** 1239–1260.

AZUMA. I., RIBI, E. E. and MEYER, TH. J. (1974) Biologically active components from mycobacterial cell walls. I. Isolation and composition of cell wall skeleton and component P_3. *J. Nat. Cancer Inst.* **52:** 95–101.

BARTAL, A., MORDOHOVICH, D., LICHTIG, C., MEKORI, T. and ROBINSON, E. (1980) Oral administration of MER-BCG preclinical and clinical studies. *Proc. Am. Soc. Clin. Oncol.* **21:** 458.

BAST, R. C. JR., ZBAR, B., BORSOS, R. and RAPP, H. J. (1974a) BCG and Cancer. *New Engl. J. Med.* **290:** 1413–1420.

BAST, R. C. JR., ZBAR, B., BORSOS, R. AND RAPP, H. J. (1974b) BCG and Cancer. *New Engl. J. Med.* **290:** 1458–1469.

BASTEN, A., MILLER, J. F. A. P., WARNER, N. L. and PYE, J. (1971) Specific inactivation of thymus-derived (T) and non-thymus (B) lymphocytes by ^{125}I-labeled antigens. *Nature New Biol.* **231:** 104–106.

BEKESI, J. G., HOLLAND, J. F., CUTTNER, J., SILVER, R., COLEMAN, M., JAROWSKI, C. and VINCEGUERRA, V. (1976) Immunotherapy in acute myelocytic leukemia (AML) with Neuraminidase treated allogeneic myeloblasts with or without MER. *Proc. Am. Soc. Clin. Oncol.* **17:** 184.

BEKESI, J. G., HOLLAND, J. F., CUTTNER, J., GLIDEWELL, O., KRULL, R., JAROWSKI, C., COLEMAN, M. and SILVER, R. (1977) Chemoimmunotherapy in acute myelocytic leukemia. *Proc. Am. Soc. Clin. Oncol.* **18:** 198.

BEN-EFRAIM, S., CONSTANTINI-SOUROJON, M. and WEISS, D. W. (1973) Potentiation and modulation of the immune response of guinea pigs to poorly immunogenic protein-hapten conjugates by pretreatment with the MER fraction of attenuated tubercle bacilli. *Cell. Immuol.* **7:** 370-379.

BEN-EFRAIM, S. and DIAMANTSTEIN, T. (1975) Mitogenic and adjuvant activity of a methanol extraction residue (MER) of tubercle bacilli on mouse lymphoid cells *in vitro*. *Immunol. Comm.* **4:** 565-577.

BEN-EFRAIM, S., TEITELBAUM, R., OPHIR, R., KLEINMAN, R. and WEISS, D. W. (1974) Nonspecific modulation of immunological responsiveness in guinea pigs and mice by the MER mycobacterial fraction: Influence of conditions of MER treatment and specific immunization, and effect of MER on early stages in the immune response. In: *Immunological Parameters of Host-Tumor Relationships,* Vol. III, pp. 158–169, WEISS, D. W. (Ed). Academic Press, New York (and *Isr. J. Med. Sci.* **10:** 972–983).

BEN-EFRAIM, S., ULMER, A., SCHMIDT, M. and DIAMANTSTEIN, T. (1976) Differences between lymphoid cell populations of guinea pigs and mice as determined by the response to mitogens *in vitro*. *Intl. Arch. Allerg. Imm.* **51:** 117–130.

BEN-EFRAIM, S., OPHIR, R., TEITELBAUM, R., ZIMBER, CH, BARBASH, G. and WEISS, D. W. (1979) Effect of the MER tubercle bacillus fraction on the responsiveness of mice to T-independent antigens. *Int. Arch. Allergy appl. Immunology* **58:** 110–118.

BEN-EFRAIM, S., SARIR, C., DAR, O., BARBASH, G., GROVER, N. and WEISS, D. W. (1980) Effects of the MER tubercle bacillus fraction on the production of antibodies *in vitro*. *Cell. Immunol.* **50:** 314–326.

BENNETT, J. A. and MARSH, J. C. (1980) Relationship of Bacillus Calmette-Guerin induced suppressor cells to hematopoietic precursor cells. *Cancer Res.* **40:** 80–85.

BLITSTEIN-WILLINGER, E., SCHULTZ, G. and DIAMANTSTEIN, T. (1976) Changes in thymocyte reactivity to lectins by B-cell mitogens of the type of sulphated polyanions. *Immunology* **30:** 529–535.

BIOZZI, G., BENACERRAF, B., GRUMBACH, F., HALPERN, B. N., LEVADITI, J. and RIST, N. (1954) Etude de l'activite granulopexique du S.R.E. au cours de l'infection tuberculeuse chez la souris. *Ann. Inst. Pasteur* **87:** 291–301.

BORSOS, T. and RAPP, H. J. (1973) Antigenic relationship between *Mycobacterium bovis* (BCG) and a guinea pig hepatoma. *J. Nat. Cancer Inst.* **51:** 1085–1086.

BRITELL, J. C., BISEL, H., AHMAN, D. L. and FRYTAK, S. (1979) Cytoxan, 5-fluorouracil and prednisone (CFP) and immunotherapy in advanced breast cancer. *Proc. Am. Soc. Clin. Oncol.* **20:** 396.

BUCANS, C. and HANNA, M. G. JR. (1974) Immunoelectromicroscopic analysis of surface antigens common to *Mycobacterium bovis* (BCG) and tumor cells. *J. Nat. Cancer Inst.* **53:** 1313–1323.

BULLOCK, W. W. and ANDERSSON, J. (1973) Mitogens as probes for immunocyte regulation: specific and non-specific suppression of B cell mitogenesis. In: *Immunopotentiation,* A Ciba Foundation Symposium, pp. 173–183, WOLSTENHOME, G. E. W. and KNIGHT, J. (Eds). Elsevier, Associated Scientific Publishers, Amsterdam.

BURNET, F. M. (1971) Immunological surveillance in neoplasia. *Transpl. Rev.* **7:** 3–25.

CANTOR, H. and ASOFSKY, R. (1972) Synergy among lymphoid cells mediating the graft-vs-host response. III. Evidence for interaction between two classes of thymus-derived cells. *J. exp. Med.* **135:** 764–779.

CHAN, P. C. Y. (1969) Immunosuppressive action of phytohemagglutinin. Effect on peritoneal macrophages. *Int. Arch. Allergy* **36:** 486–496.

CHEN, J. C. and LEON, M. A. (1976) The immune response to dextran in Balb/c mice. I. Modification of 'Thymus-Independent' response by the T cell mitogen Concanavalin A. *J. Immunol.* **116:** 416–422.

COLEMAN, M., VINCIGUERRA, V. P., RAFLA, S. and STUTZMAN, M. (1979) Combination chemoimmunotherapy in advanced recurrent Hodgkin's disease: a randomized study of the cancer and leukemia group B (CALG B). *Proc. Am. Soc. Clin. Oncol.* **20:** 428.

COHEN, D., YRON, I., HABER, M., ROBINSON, E. and WEISS, D. W. (1975) Effects of treatment with the MER tubercle bacilli fraction on the survival of mice carrying mammary tumor isografts: Injection of MER at the tumor site or at distal location. *Brit. J. Cancer* **32:** 483–490.

COHEN, D., YRON, I., HABER, M., GROVER, N. and WEISS, D. W. (1976) Chemoimmunotherapy of syngeneic mouse mammary carcinomas employing MER. *Ann. N.Y. Acad. Sci.* **277:** 185–208.

COOPER, M. R., PAJAK, T. F., GOTTLIER, A. and HOLLAND, J. F. (1980) Effect of methanol extraction residue of Bacillus Calmette-Guerin (MER–BCG) in advanced Hodgkin's disease. *Proc. Am. Soc. Clin. Oncol.* **21:** 467.

CUTLER, J. L. (1960) The enhancement of hemolysin production in the rat by zymosan. *J. Immunol.* **84:** 416–419.

CUTTNER, J., HOLLAND, J. F. and BEKESI, J. G. (1975) Chemoimmunotherapy of acute myelocytic leukemia. *Proc. Am. Soc. Clin. Oncol.* **16:** 264.

DENEFRIO, J. (1979) Systemic epitheloid granulomata following immunotherapy with methanol extraction residue of Bacillus Calmette-Guerin (MER). *Proc. Am. Soc. Clin. Oncol.* **20:** 386.

DIAMANTSTEIN, T., WAGNER, B., L'AGE-STEHR, J., VEYSE, I., ODENWALD, M. V. and SCHULTZ, G. (1971) Stimulation of humoral antibody formation by polyanions. III. Restoration of the immune response to sheep red blood cells by polyanions in thymectomized and lethally irradiated mice protected with bone marrow cells. *Eur. J. Immunol.* **1:** 302–304.

DIAMANTSTEIN, T., BLITSTEIN-WILLINGER, E. and SCHULTZ, G. (1974) Polyanions and lipopolysaccharide act on different subpopulations of B-cells. *Nature New Biol.* **250:** 596–597.

DIAMANTSTEIN, T., KEPPLER, W., BLITSTEIN-WILLINGER, E. and BEN-EFRAIM, S. (1976) Suppression of the primary immune response *in vivo* to sheep red blood cells by B-cell mitogens. *Immunology* **30:** 401–407.

DIENES, L. and SCHOENHEIT, E. W. (1927) Local hypersensitiveness. I. Sensitization of tuberculous guinea pigs with egg-white and timothy pollen. *J. Immunol.* **14:** 9–42.

DRESSER, D. W. (1972) The role of T cells and adjuvant in the immune response of mice to foreign erythrocytes. *Eur. J. Immunol.* **2:** 50–57.

DUTTON, R. W. (1975) Suppressor T cells. *Transpl. Rev.* **26:** 39–55.

EGAN, H. S., REEDER, W. J. and EKSTEDT, R. D. (1974) Effect of Concanavalin A *in vivo* in suppressing the antibody response in mice. *J. Immunol.* **112:** 63–69.

ELBERG, S. S., SCHNEIDER, P. and FONG, J. (1957) Cross-immunity between *Brucella melitensis* and *Mycobacterium tuberculosis*. Intracellular behavior of *Brucella melitensis* in monocytes from vaccinated animals. *J. exp. Med.* **106:** 545–554.

EMESON, E. E. (1980) Adjuvant-induced selective recruitment of specifically reactive lymphocytes: a probable mechanism of adjuvant action. *J. Immunol.* **124:** 2222–2230.

ESHER, H. J., VALENTINE, E. A., TAYLOR, D. J. and BOGDEN, A. E. (1973) Immunoadjuvant activity of bacterial fractions on antibody-forming cells during the primary immune response period. *Immunol. Comm.* **2:** 585–595.

EVANS, R., COX, H. and ALEXANDER, P. (1973) Immunologically specific activation of macrophages armed with the specific macrophage arming factor. *Proc. Soc. Exp. Biol. N.Y.* **143:** 256–259.

FILKINS, J. P. and DI LUZIO, N. R. (1966) Mechanism of gelatin inhibition of reticuloendothelial function. *Proc. Soc. Exp. Biol. Med. N.Y.* **122:** 177–180.

FRIEDMAN, H. M., JOHNSON, A. G. and PAN, P. (1969) Stimulating effect of polynucleotides on short term leukocyte cultures. *Proc. Soc. Exp. Biol. Med.* **132:** 916–918.

FREUND, J. (1951) The effect of paraffin oil and mycobacteria on antibody formation and sensitization. *Am. J. Clin. Pathol.* **21:** 645–656.

FREUND, J. (1953) The response of immunized animals to specific and nonspecific stimuli. In: *Nature and Significance of the Antibody Response,* pp. 46–48, PAPPENHEIMER, A. J. JR. (Ed). Columbia University Press, New York.

FREUND, J. and STONE, S. H. (1959) The effectiveness of tuberculoglycolipid as an adjuvant in eliciting allergic encephalomyelitis and aspermatogenesis. *J. Immunol.* **82:** 560–567.

GALLILY, R., YAGEL, S. and WEISS, D. W. (1976) Potentiated lysosomal enzyme, bacteriostatic and bactericidal activities of peritoneal macrophages of mice treated with the MER fraction of tubercle bacilli. In: *The Reticuloendothelial system in health and disease,* pp. 351–361, REICHERT, G. M., ESCOBAR, M. R. and FRIEDMAN, H. (Eds). Plenum Press, New York.

GALLILY, R. and WEISS, D. W. (1977) Effects of the MER immunomodulator on macrophages. Studies *in vitro* and *in vivo*. *Isr. J. Med. Sci.* **13:** 1047.

GALLILY, R., DOUCHAN, Z. and WEISS, D. W. (1977) Potentiation of mouse peritoneal antibacterial functions by treatment of the donor animals with the methanol extraction residue fraction of tubercle bacilli. *Infect. Immun.* **18:** 405–411.

GALLILY, R., STAIN, I. and WEISS, D. W. (1981) Mouse macrophage functions under influence of factors released by spleen cells preincubated with the MER tubercle bacillus fraction. *Immunopharmacol.* **3:** 221–231.

GEFFARD, M. and ORBACH-ARBOUYS, S. (1976) Enhancement of T suppressor activity in mice by high doses of BCG. *Cancer Immunol. Immunother.* **1:** 41–43.

GERSHON, R. K., CARTER, R. L. and LANE, N. J. (1967) Studies on homotransplantable lymphoma in hamsters. IV. Observations on macrophages in the expression of tumor immunity. *Am. J. Pathol.* **51:** 1111–1133.

GERSHON, R. K., COHEN, P., HENCIN, R. and LIEBHABER, S. A. (1972) Suppressor T cells. *J. Immunol.* **108:** 586–590.

GERY, I. and WAKSMAN, B. H. (1972a) Potentiation of the T-lymphocyte response to mitogens. I. The responding cell. *J. exp. Med.* **136:** 128–142.

GERY, I. and WAKSMAN, B. H. (1972b) Potentiation of the T-lymphocyte response to mitogens. II. The cellular source of potentiating mediators. *J. exp. Med.* **136:** 143–155.

GERY, I., BAER, A., STUPP, Y. AND WEISS, D. W. (1975) Further studies on the effects of the Methanol Extraction Residue fraction of tubercle bacilli on lymphoid cells and macrophages. In: *Immunological Parameters of Host-Tumor Relationships*, pp. 170–177, *Vol.* III, WEISS, D. W. (Ed). Academic Press, New York.

GILL, H. K. and LIEW, F. Y. (1979) Regulation of delayed-type hypersensitivity. IV. Antigen-specific suppressor cells for delayed-type hypersensitivity induced by lipopolysaccharide and sheep erythrocytes in mice. *Eur. J. Immunol.* **9:** 101–106.

GIRARD, G. and GRUMBACH, F. (1958) L'infection tuberculeuse de la souris entraine sa resistance a l'infection pesteuse experimentale. *Compt. Rend. Soc. Biol.* **152:** 280–284.

GLENNY, A. T., POPE, C. G., WADDINGTON, H. and WALLACE, U. (1926) Immunological notes. XVII–XXIV. *J. Pathol.* **29:** 31.

GOREN, M. B. (1974) Sulfatide III of *M. tuberculosis:* Structure and biological activity. In: *International Symposium on Immunostimulants*, Proceedings, Paris.

GREAVES, M. F., OWEN, J. J. T. and RAFF, M. C. (1974) General effector functions of T and B lymphocytes *in vivo*. In: *T and B Lymphocytes: Origins, Properties and Roles in Immune Responses*, pp. 81–84, Exerpta Medica, Amsterdam.

GRIMM, R. A. (1979) Dacarbazine and immunotherapy with the methanol extraction residue of BCG in stage II and II melanoma. *Proc. Am. Soc. Clin. Oncol.* **20:** 374.

HADDEN, J. W., DELMONTE, L. and OETTGEN, H. F. (1977) Mechanisms of immunopotentiation. In: *Immunopharmacology*, pp. 279–317, HADDEN, J. W., COFFEY, R. G. and SPREAFICO, F. (Eds). Plenum Medical Book Company, New York.

HALPERIN, D., DAR, O., BEN-EFRAIM, S. and WEISS, D. W. (1980) MER effects on immunocyte function in antibody production *in vitro*. *Isr. J. Med. Sci.* **16:** 808.

HALPERN, B. N. (1959) The role and function of the reticuloendothelial system in immunological processes. *J. Pharm. Pharmac.* **11:** 321–338.

HALPERN, B. N., BIOZZI, G., BENACERRAF, B. and STIFFEL, C. (1957) Phagocytosis of foreign red blood cells by the reticulo-endothelial system. *Am. J. Physiol.* **189:** 520–526.

HALPERN, B. N., PREVOT, A. R., BIOZZI, G., STIFFEL, C., MOUTON, D., MORARD, J. C., ROUTHILLIER, Y. and DECREUSEFOND, C. (1964) Stimulation de l'activite phagocitaire du systeme reticuloendothelial provoquee par *Corynebacterium parvum*. *J. Reticuloendothel. Soc.* **1:** 77–96.

HALPERN, B., FRAY, A., CREPIN, Y., PLATICA, O., LORINET, A. M., RABOURDIN, A., SPARKOS, L. AND ISAC, R. (1973) *Corynebacterium parvum*, a potent immunostimulant in experimental infections and in malignancies. In: *Immunopotentiation*, A Ciba Foundation Symposium, pp. 217–234, WOLSTENHOLME, G. E. W. and KNIGHT, J. (Eds). Elsevier, Associated Scientific Publishers, Amsterdam.

HARAN-GHERA, N. and WEISS, D. W. (1973) Effect of treatment of C57Bl/6 mice with the MER fraction of BCG on leukemogenesis by the Radiation Leukemia Virus (RLV). *J. Natl. Cancer Inst.* **50:** 229–234.

HARD, G. C. (1970) Some biochemical aspects of the immune macrophage. *Br. J. Exp. Pathol.* **51:** 97–105.

HELLSTRÖM, I. and HELLSTRÖM, K. E. (1969) Studies on cellular immunity and its serum-mediated inhibition on Moloney-virus-induced monkey sarcoma. *Int. J. Cancer* **4:** 587–600.

HUI, I. J. (1972) Water-soluble and lipid-free fraction from BCG with adjuvant and antitumor activity. *Nature New Biol.* **238:** 241–242.

HOPPER, D. G., PIMM, M. V. and BALDWIN, R. W. (1975) Methanol extraction residue of BCG in the treatment of transplanted rat tumors. *Brit. J. Cancer* **31:** 176–181.

HOWARD, J. G., BIOZZI, G., HALPERN, B. N., STIFFEL, C. and MOUTON, D. (1959) The effect of Mycobacterium tuberculosis (B.C.G.) infection on the resistance of mice to bacterial endotoxin and Salmonella enteriditis injection. *Br. J. Expt. Pathol.* **40:** 281–290.

IZAK, G., STUPP, Y., MANNY, N., ZAJCEK, G. and WEISS, D. W. (1977) The immune response in acute myelocytic leukemia. The effect of MER on T- and B-cell functions and their relation to the course of the disease. *Proc. Int. Symp. on Malignant Proliferative Disease*, IZAK, G. (Ed). Academic Press, New York (and *Isr. J. Med. Sci.* **13:** 677–693.

JACKSON, D. V., RICHARDS, F. II, MUSS, H. B., COOPER, M. R., WHITE, D. R. and SPURR, C. L. (1979) Immunotherapy of small cell carcinoma of the lung (SCC): a randomized study. *Proc. Am. Soc. Clin. Oncol.* **20:** 367.

JACOBS, D., PASS, E., ABRAHAM, C. and WEISS, D. W. (1978) Studies on the influence of the MER tubercle bacillus fraction on immunological responsiveness of mice. Effects on antibody formation to a soluble protein and a T-independent antigen, delayed hypersensitivity to sheep erythrocytes, and numbers of antigen-reactive lymphoid cells. In: *Immunological Parameters of Host-Tumor Relationships*, pp. 60–74, Vol. V, WEISS, D. W. (Ed). Academic Press, New York (and *Isr. J. Med. Sci.* **14:** 60–75).

JACOBS, D. M. and KRIPKE, M. L. (1974) Accelerated development of transplanted mammary tumors in mice pretreated with the methanol extraction residue of BCG and prevention of acceleration by concomitant specific immunization. *J. Nat. Cancer Inst.* **52:** 219–224.

Jagathambal, K., Cortes, E. P., Mundia, A., Khan, F., Steinberg, H., Garvey, J., Akbiyik, N., Aral, I., Wesseley, Z., Rai, K. and Sawitsky, A. (1979) Immunochemotherapy in previously irradiated stage III squamous cell carcinoma (SCC) of the lung: a randomized study. *Proc. Am. Soc. Clin. Oncol.* **20:** 412.

Jerne, N. K. (1973) The immune system. *Sci. Am.* **229:** 52–60.

Jerne, N. K., Nordin, A. A. and Henry, C. (1963) The agar plaque technique for recognizing antibody-producing cells. In: *Cell bound Antibodies,* pp. 109, Amos, B. and Koprowski, H. (Eds). Wistar Institute Press, Philadelphia.

Kedar, E., Nahas, F., Unger, E. and Weiss, D. W. (1978) *In vitro* induction of cell-mediated immunity to murine leukemia cells. III. Effect of methanol extraction residue fraction of BCG on the generation of cytotoxic lymphocytes against leukemia. *J. Nat. Cancer Inst.* **60:** 1097–1106.

Klein, G. (1973) Tumor immunology. *Transpl. Proc.* **5:** 31–41.

Klein, G., Sjögren, H. O., Klein, E. and Hellström, K. E. (1960) Demonstration of resistance against methylcholanthrene-induced sarcomas in the primary autochtonous host. *Cancer Res.* **20:** 1561–1572.

Klein, G., Sjögren, H. O. and Klein, E. (1963) Demonstration of host resistance against sarcomas induced by implantation of cellophane films in isologous (syngeneic) recipients. *Cancer Res.* **23:** 84–92.

Kollmorgen, G. M., Sansing, W. A., Lehman, A. A., Longley, R., Fischer, G. and McCay, P. B. (1979) Effect of diet and MER on DMBA-induced mammary carcinoma. *Proc. Am. Soc. Clin. Oncol.* **20:** 41.

Kostinas, J. E., Leone, L. A. and Rege, V. B. (1978) Procarbazine, Vinblastine and Dactinomycin in stage III and IV melanoma with or without MER. *Proc. Am. Soc. Clin. Oncol.* **19:** 355.

Kreisler, J. M. and Möller, G. (1974) Effect of PPD on the specific immune response to heterologous red cells *in vitro.* J. Immunol. **112:** 151–161.

Krown, E. S., Pinsky, M. C., Hirshaut, Y. and Oettgen, H. F. (1976) Intralesional injection of MER in metastic melanoma. *Proc. Am. Fed. Clin. Res.* **24:** 377A.

Krown, S. E., Pinsky, C. M., Hirshaut, Y., Wantebo, H. J. and Oettgen, H. F. (1977) Intralesional injection of MER in cutaneous malignant melanoma. *Proc. Am. Soc. Clin. Oncol.* **18:** 431.

Kumazawa, Y., Shibusawa, A., Suzuki, T. and Mizunoe, K. (1976) Separation of an adjuvant-active glycolipid lacking peptide moiety from Wax D preparation of Mycobacterium tuberculosis strain Aoyama B. *Immunochemistry* **13:** 173–177.

Kuperman, O., Yashpe, D. J., Ben-Efraim, S., Sharf, S. and Weiss, D. W. (1972) Nonspecific stimulation of cellular immunological responsiveness by a mycobacterial fraction. *Cell. Immunol.* **3:** 277–282.

Kuperman, O., Feigis, M. and Weiss, D. W. (1973) Reversal by the MER tubercle bacillus fraction of the suppressive effects of heterologous antilymphocytic serum (ALS) on the allograft reactivity of mice. *Cell Immunol.* **8:** 484–489.

Lappe, M. A. (1968) Evidence for the antigenicity of papillomas induced by 3-Methylcholanthrene. *J. Nat. Cancer Inst.* **40:** 823–846.

Linna, T. J., Hu, C. and Thompson, K. D. (1974) Development of systemic and local tumors induced by avian reticuloendotheliosis virus after thymectomy or bursectomy. *J. Nat. Cancer Inst.* **53:** 847–854.

Lokich, J. J. (1979) Adjuvant therapy for surgically curable colon cancer: a controlled study of chemo and immune therapy. *Proc. Am. Soc. Clin. Oncol.* **20:** 423.

Lotzova, E. and Gutterman, J. U. (1979) Effect of glucan on natural killer (NK) cells: further comparison between NK cell and bone marrow effector cell activities *J. Immunol.* **123:** 607–611.

Maeda, Y. Y., Hamuro, J., Yamada, Y., Ishimura, K. and Chihara, G. (1973) The nature of immunopotentiation by the antitumour polysaccharide lentinan and the significance of biogenic amines in its action. In: *Immunopotentiation,* A Ciba Foundation Symposium, pp. 259–281, Wolstenholme, G. E. W. and Knight, J. (Eds). Elsevier, Associated Scientific Publishers, Amsterdam.

Markson, Y. and Weiss, D. W. (1980) Effect of therapeutic treatment with the MER tubercle bacillus fraction on Rous sarcomas of chickens induced by the Rous sarcoma virus. *Cancer Immunol. Immunother.* **9:** 159–162.

Markson, Y., Dolsansky, F. and Weiss, D. W. (1978) Effects of prophylactic treatment with the methanol extraction residue fraction of tubercle bacilli (MER) on the development of Rous sarcomas of chickens following challenge with the Rous sarcoma virus. *Isr. J. Med. Sci.* **14:** 51–59.

Mathe, G., Moamena, K. and Dezfulian, M. (1973) An experimental screening for 'systemic adjuvants of immunity' applicable in cancer immunotherapy. *Cancer Res.* **33:** 1987–1997.

Meltzer, M. S., Jones, E. E. and Boetcher, D. A. (1975a) Increased chemotactic response of macrophages from BCG-infected mice. *Cell. Immunol.* **17:** 268–276.

Meltzer, M. S., Tucker, R. W., Sanford, K. K. and Leonard, E. J. (1975b) Interaction of BCG activated macrophages with neoplastic and nonneoplastic cell lines *in vitro:* quantitation of the cytotoxic reaction by release of tritiated thymidine from prelabeled target cells. *J. Nat. Cancer Inst.* **54:** 1177–1184.

Mekori, T. Segal, R., Bartal, A., Cohen, Y. and Robinson, E. (1980 Immune investigations and therapy in patients with advanced lung cancer. *Cancer Immunol. Immunother.* **7:** 251–255.

Meyer, Th. J., Ribi, E. E. and Azuma, I. (1974) Biologically active components from Mycobacterial cell walls. II. Suppression and Regression of Strain-2 guinea pig hepatoma. *J. Nat. Cancer Inst.* **52:** 103–111.

Minden, P., McClatchy, J. K., Cooper, R., Bardana, E. J. and Farr, R. S. (1960) Shared antigens between *Mycobacterium bovis* (BCG) and other bacterial species. *Science* **176:** 1060–1061.

Minden, P., McClatchy, J. K. and Farr, R. S. (1972) Shared antigens between heterologous bacterial species. *Infect. Immun.* **6:** 574–582.

Minden, P., McClatchy, J. K. and Wainberg, M. (1974a) Shared antigens between *Mycobacterium bovis* (BCG) and neoplastic cells. *J. Nat. Cancer Inst.* **53:** 1325–1331.

Minden, P., Wainberg, M. and Weiss, D. W. (1974b) Protection against guinea pig hepatomas by pretreatment with subcellular fractions of *Mycobacterium bovis* (BCG). *J. Nat. Cancer Inst.* **52:** 1643–1645.

Mitchell, M. S., Birnbaum-Mokyr, M. and Kahane, I. (1975) Stimulation of lymphoid cells by components of BCG. *J. Nat. Cancer Inst.* **55:** 1337–1343.

Moertel, C. G., Ritts, R. E. Jr., Schutt, A. J. and Hahn, R. G. (1975a) Clinical studies of methanol extraction residue fraction of Bacillus Calmette-Guerin as an immunostimulant in patients with advanced cancer. *Cancer Res.* **35:** 3075–3083.

MOERTEL, C. G., RITTS, R. E., SCHUTT, A. J. and HAHN, R. G. (1975b) A phase I study of methanol extraction residue of BCG (MER-BCG). *Proc. Am. Ass. Cancer Res.* **16:** 143.

MURAHATA, R. I. and ZIGHELBOIM, J. (1979a) Inhibition of memory cell-mediated cytotoxic response by systemic administration of *Corynebacterium parvum. Cell. Immunol.* **42:** 289–297.

MURAHATA, R. I. and ZIGHELBOIM, J. (1979b) Inhibition of cell-mediated cytotoxicity to tumor alloantigens by systemic administration of *Corynebacterium parvum. Cancer Immunol. Immunother.* **6:** 101–106.

NAKASHIMA, I., YOKOCHI, T., NAGASE, F. and KATO, N. (1979) Different effects of the capsular polysaccharide of *Klebsiella pneumoniae* on the functions of various subpopulations of B cells in the immune response of mice to T-dependent antigen. *Microbiol. Immunol.* **23:** 273–286.

NECHELES, T. F., RAUSEN, A., KING, F. and POCHEDLY, C. (1976) MER/BCG in the treatment of disseminated neuroblastoma. *Proc. Am. Soc. Clin. Oncol.* **17:** 258.

OHANIAN, S. H., SCHLAGER, S. I. and BORSOS, T. (1977) Molecular interaction of cells with antibody and complement: Influence of metabolic and physical properties of the target on the outcome of humoral immune attack. In: *Contemporary Topics in Molecule Immunology*, pp. 153–180, REISFELD, R. A. and INMAN, F. P. (eds.). Plenum Press, New York.

OLD, L. J., CLARKE, D. A. and BENACERRAF, B. (1960) Mengo virus infection in B.C.G. or zymosan treated mice. *Fedn Proc.* **19:** 208–211.

PARANT, M. (1979) Biologic properties of a new synthetic adjuvant, muramyl dipeptide (MDP). In: *Springer Semin. Immunopathol.*, pp. 101–118, Springer-Verlag, Berlin.

PASS, E. and YASHPE, D. J. (1971) Stimulation of antibody synthesis to soluble bovine gamma globulin (BCG) by a methanol-extraction residue (MER) of BCG. *Isr. J. Med. Sci.* **7:** 609–610.

PASS, E., JACOBS, D. M. and WEISS, D. W. (1975) Modulation of the immune response by a methanol-insoluble fraction of attenuated tubercle bacilli (BCG). (Personal communication.)

PERLOFF, M., HOLLAND, J. F. and BEKESI, J. G. (1976) Chemoimmunotherapy of breast cancer. *Proc. Am. Soc. Clin. Oncol.* **17:** 308.

PERLOFF, M., BUSHKIN, E., HOLLAND, J. F. and DORPH, D. (1978) Dose response curves during intradermal immunotherapy. *Proc. Am. Soc. Clin. Oncol.* **19:** 350.

PIOCH, Y., GERBER, M. and SERROU, B. (1979) Natural killer-like activity induced in spleen by IP injection of BCG. *Cancer Immunol. Immunother.* **7:** 181–184.

PREHN, R. T. and MAIN, J. M. (1957) Immunity to methylcholanthrene-induced sarcomas. *J. Nat. Cancer Inst.* **18:** 769–778.

QUESADA, J. and HERSH, E. (1980) Hematological effects of intravenous methanol extraction residue of BCG (IV MER) in cytopenic patients. *Proc. Am. Soc. Clin. Oncol.* **21:** 204.

RAFF, M. C. (1970) Role of thymus-derived lymphocytes in the secondary humoral immune response in mice. *Nature Lond.* **226:** 1257–1258.

RAFF, M. C. (1971) Evidence for subpopulation of mature lymphocytes within mouse thymus. *Nature New Biol.* **229:** 182–184.

RAFFEL, S. (1950) Chemical factors involved in the induction of infectious allergy. *Experimentia* **6:** 410–419.

RAMON, G. (1926) L'anatoxine diphterique et les anatoxines en general. Etude experimentale (Revue). *J. Med. Franc.* **15:** 381.

REINISCH, C. L., GLEINER, N. A. and SCHLOSSMAN, S. F. (1976) Adjuvant regulation of T cell function. *J. Immunol.* **116:** 710–715.

ROBINSON, E., BARTAL, A., COHEN, Y. and HAAS, R. (1975) Preliminary report on the effect of methanol extraction residue of BCG (MER) on cancer patients. *Brit. J. Cancer* **32:** 1–4.

ROBINSON, R., BARTAL, A., COHEN, Y. and MEKORI, T. (1979) Adjuvant therapy in colo-rectal cancer (a randomized trial comparing radio-chemotherapy and radio-chemotherapy combined with the methanol extraction residue of BCG (MER). *Proc. Am. Soc. Clin. Oncol.* **20:** 408.

ROITT, I. M., GREAVES, M. F., TORRIGIANI, G., VROSTOFF, J. and PLAYFAIR, J. H. L. (1969) The cellular basis of immunological responses. *Lancet* **II:** 367–376.

RUPP, J. C., MOORE, R. D. and SCHOENBERG, M.D. (1960) Stimulation of the reticuloendothelial system in the rabbit by Freund's adjuvant. *Arch. Pathol.* **70:** 43–49.

SHER, N. A., CHAPARAS, S. D., GREENBERG, L. E. and BERNARD, S. (1975) Effects of BCG, *Corynebacterium parvum*, and Methanol Extraction Residue in the reduction of mortality from *Staphylococcus aureus* and *Candida albicans* infections in immunosuppressed mice. *Infect. Immun.* **12:** 1325–1330.

SJÖBERG, O., ANDERSSON, J. and MOLLER, G. (1972) Requirement for adherent cells in the primary and secondary immune responses *in vitro*. *Eur. J. Immunol.* **2:** 123–126.

STEIN, J., MARCHIONY, A., MUNDIA, A. and CORTES, E. P. (1978) Ethyl chloride spray (ECS) and the reduction of pain by intradermal immunotherapy. *Proc. Am. Soc. Clin. Oncol.* **19:** 357.

STEINKULLER, C. G., KRIGBAUM, L. G. and WEISS, D. W. (1969) Studies on the mode of action of the heterologous immunogenicity of a methanol-insoluble fraction of attenuated tubercle bacilli (BCG). *Immunology* **16:** 255–275.

STERCHI, J. M., COLE, W., RICHARDS, F. II, MUSS, H. B., WHITE, D. R., COOPER, M. R. AND SPURR, C. L. (1980) Dacarbazine (DTIC) and immunotherapy with the methanol extraction residue of BCG (MER) in stage II and stage II melanoma. *Proc. Am. Soc. Clin. Oncol.* **21:** 363.

STUPP, Y., NAVOK, T. and GERY, I. (1975) Preferential increase in lymphocytes with 'B' properties in lymph nodes draining sites of adjuvant injection. *Isr. J. Med. Sci.* **11:** 1383.

STUPP, Y., SALTOUN, R. and WEISS, D. W. (1976) Prevention by the MER tubercle bacillus fraction of immunosuppression induced by cancer chemotherapeutic agents. I. Antibody response of mice treated with cyclophosphamide. *Cancer Immunol. Immunotherap.* **1:** 219–226.

STUPP, Y., MANNY, N., SHLOMAI, Z., GROVER, N., WEISS, D. W. and IZAK, G. (1978) Effect of treatment with the MER tubercle bacillus fraction on syngeneic plasma cell tumors of BALB/c mice. *Cancer Immunol. Immunother.* **3:** 189–193.

SULTZER, B. M. and NILSSON, B. S. (1972) PPD tuberculin—a B-cell mitogen. *Nature New Biol.* **240:** 198–200.

TAKASUGI, M. and HILDEMANN, W. H. (1969a) Regulation of immunity toward allogeneic tumors in mice. I. Effect of antiserum fractions on tumor growth. *J. Nat. Cancer Inst.* **41:** 843–856.

TAKASUGI, M. and HILDEMANN, W. H. (1969b) Regulation of immunity toward allogeneic tumors in mice. II. Effect of antiserum and antiserum fractions on cellular and humoral response. *J. Nat. Cancer Inst.* **43:** 857–867.

TANAKA, K., TANAKA, A. and SUGIYAMA, K. (1968) Immunological adjuvants. I. Adjuvant activity and immunogenicity of acetylated Wax D and its subfractions. *Int. Arch. Allergy* **34:** 495–506.

TASHIMA, C. K., BLUMENSCHEIN, G. R. and GUTTERMAN, J. U. (1976) Comparison of adriamycin combination drug program with BCG immunotherapy vs MER immunotherapy for metastatic breast cancer. *Proc. Am. Soc. Clin. Oncol.* **17:** 288.

TRACEY, D. E. (1979) The requirement for macrophages in the augmentation of natural killer cell activity by BCG. *J. Immunol.* **123:** 840–845.

TREVES, A. J., COHEN, I. R. and FELDMAN, M. (1976a) A syngeneic metastatic tumor model in mice: the natural immune response and its manipulation. *Isr. J. Med. Sci.* **12:** 369–383.

TREVES, A., COHEN, I., FELDMAN, M. and WEISS, D. W. (1976b) Effect of treatment with MER on the development of spontaneous pulmonary metastases from syngeneic implants of tumor 3LL in C57B1 in mice. *Isr. J. Med. Sci.* **12:** 384–387.

UCHIYAMA, T. and JACOBS, D. M. (1978) Modulation of immune response by bacterial lipopolysaccharide (LPS): cellular basis of stimulatory and inhibitory effects of LPS on the *in vitro* IgM antibody response to a T-dependent antigen. *J. Immunol.* **121:** 2347–2351.

UNANUE, E. R., ASKONAS, B. A. and ALLISON A. C. (1969) A role of macrophages in the stimulation of immune responses by adjuvants. *J. Immunol.* **103:** 71–78.

VINCIGUERRA, V. P., COLEMAN, M. and RAFLA, S. (1978) A randomized trial of chemoimmunotherapy in advanced, recurrent Hodgkin's disease. *Proc. Am. Soc. Clin. Oncol.* **19:** 321.

VOGT, W., RÜHL, H., WAGNER, B. and DIAMANTSTEIN, T. (1973) Stimulation of DNA synthesis in mouse lymphoid cells by polyanions *in vitro*. II. Relationship between adjuvant activity and stimulation of DNA synthesis by polyanions. *Eur. J. Immunol.* **3:** 493–496.

VOGL, S. E., LUMB, G., BEKESI, J. G. and HOLLAND, J. F. (1977) Preclinical study of IV administration of methanol extraction residue of Bacillus Calmette-Guerin. *Cancer Treat. Rpts.* **61:** 901–903.

VOGL, S. E., PERLOFF, M., HOLLAND, J. F. and BEKESI, J. G. (1978) Phase I trial of intravenous (iv) administration of the methanol extraction residue of Bacillus Calmette-Guerin (MER). *Proc. Am. Soc. Clin. Oncol.* **19:** 382.

WAINBERG, M. A., DEUTSCH, V. and WEISS, D. W. (1976a) Stimulation of antitumor immunity in guinea-pigs by methanol extraction residue of BCG. *Brit. J. Cancer* **34:** 500–508.

WAINBERG, M. A., MARGOLESE, R. G. and WEISS, D. W. (1976b) Tumor immunoprophylaxis and immunotherapy in guinea pigs treated with the methanol extraction residue (MER) of BCG. In: *BCG in Cancer Immunotherapy*, pp. 39–50, LA MOUREUX, G., TURCOTTE, R. and PORTELANCE, V. (eds.) Grune and Stratton, New York.

WAINBERG, M., MINDEN, P. and WEISS, D. W. (1976c) Vertical transmission of tumor resistance in guinea pigs. *Nature* **259:** 213–215.

WAINBERG, M. A., MARGOLESE, R. G. and WEISS, D. W. (1977) Differential responsiveness of various substrains of inbred strain 2 guinea pigs to immunotherapy with the methanol extraction residue (MER) of BCG. *Cancer Immunol. Immunother.* **2:** 101–108.

WATSON, J., TRENKNER, E. and COHN, M. (1973) The use of bacterial lipopolysaccharides to show that two signals are required for the induction of antibody synthesis. *J. exp. Med.* **138:** 699–714.

WEISS, D. W. (1960) Enhanced resistance of mice to infection with *Pasteurella pestis* following vaccination with fractions of phenol-killed tubercle bacilli. *Nature* **186:** 1060–1061.

WEISS, D. W. (1967) Immunology of spontaneous tumors. In: *Proceedings of the Fifty Berkeley Symposium on Mathematical Statistics and Probability*, pp. 657–706, LECAM, L. and NEWMAN, J. (eds.). University of California Press, Berkeley.

WEISS, D. W. (1976) MER and other mycobacterial fractions in the immunotherapy of cancer. In: *Symposium on Immunotherapy in Malignant Disease*, pp. 473–497, Vol. 60. Medical Clinics of North America.

WEISS, D. W. (1977) Aspects of immunotherapy of cancer with BCG and mycobacterial fractions. (Invited Commentary) *World J. Surgery* **1:** 579–583.

WEISS, D. W. (1978) Host mechanisms for control of tumor growth that can be modulated by nonspecific immunotherapy. In: *Immunotherapy of Human Cancer*, pp. 41–61, HERSH, E. M. and SINKOVICS, J. G. (eds.). Raven Press, New York.

WEISS, D. W. (1979) Approaches to 'nonspecific' immunotherapy of cancer with microbial immunomodulators. In: *The role of nonspecific immunity in the prevention of cancer*, pp. 177–209, SELA, M. (ed.). Pontificia Academia, Scientiarum, Vatican City.

WEISS, D. W. (1980) Tumor antigenicity and approaches to tumor immunotherapy—an outline. *Curr. Topics in Microbiol. and Immunol.* Springer-Verlag, Berlin **89:** 1–83.

WEISS, D. W., FAULKIN, L. J. JR. and DEONE, K. B. (1964) Acquisition of heightened resistance and susceptibility to spontaneous mouse mammary carcinomas in the original host. *Cancer Res.* **24:** 732–741.

WEISS, D. W., BONHAG, R. S. and LESLIE, P. (1966a) Studies on the heterologous immunogenicity of a methanol-insoluble fraction of attenuated tubercle bacilli (BCG). II. Protection against tumor isografts. *J. exp. Med.* **124:** 1039–1065.

WEISS, D. W., LAVRIN, D. H., DEZFULIAN, M., VAAGE, J. and BLAIR, P. G. (1966b) Studies on the immunology of spontaneous mammary carcinomas of mice. In: *Viruses Inducing Cancer*, pp. 138–168, BURDETTE, W. J. (ed.). University of Utah Press, Salt Lake City.

WEISS, D. W., STUPP, Y., MANNY, N. and IZAK, G. (1975) Treatment of acute myelocytic leukemia (AML) patients with the MER tubercle bacillus fraction. A preliminary report. *Transl. Proc.*, pp. 545–552, Vol. III, No. 1, Supp. 1, SCHLESINGER, M. and BILLINGHAM, R. E. (eds.). Grune and Stratton, New York.

WEISS, D. W., KUPERMAN, O., FATHALLAH, N. and KEDAR, E. (1976) Mode of action of mycobacterial fractions in anti-tumor immunity: Preliminary evidence for a direct nonspecific stimulatory effect of MER on immunologically reactive cells. *Ann. N.Y. Acad. Sci.* **276:** 536–549.

WHITE, R. G. (1967) Characterization of mycobacterial components of adjuvant mixture. In: *Adjuvants of Immunity*, pp. 49. Karger, Basel, New York.

WEISS, D. W. and DUBOS, R. J. (1955) Antituberculous immunity induced in mice by vaccination with killed tubercle bacilla or with a soluble bacillary extract. *J. exp. Med.* **101:** 313–330.

WEISS, D. W. and DUBOS, R. J. (1956) Antituberculous immunity induced by methanol extracts of tubercle bacilli—its enhancement by adjuvants. *J. exp. Med.* **103:** 73–85.

WEISS, D. W. and WELLS, A. Q. (1960a) Vaccination against tuberculosis with nonliving vaccines. II. Vaccination of guinea pigs with phenol-killed tubercle bacilli. *Am. Rev. Resp. Dis.* **81:** 518–538.

WEISS, D. W. and WELLS, A. O. (1960b) Vaccination against tuberculosis with nonliving vaccines. III. Vaccination of guinea pigs with fractions of phenol-killed tubercle bacilli. *Am. Rev. Resp. Dis.* **82:** 339–357.

WEISS, D. W. and YASHPE, D. J. (1973) Nonspecific stimulation of antimicrobial and antitumor resistance and of immunologic responsiveness by the MER fraction of tubercle bacilli. In: *Dynamic Aspects of Host Parasite Relationship,* pp. 163–223, Vol. 1, ZUCKERMAN, A. and WEISS, D. W. (eds.). Academic Press, New York.

WEISS, D. W., BONHAG, R. S. and DEOME, K. B. (1961) Protective activity of fractions of tubercle bacilli against isologous tumors in mice. *Nature* **190:** 889–891.

WEISS, D. W., BONHAG, R. S. and PARKS, J. A. (1964) Studies on the heterologous immunogenicity of a methanol-insoluble fraction of attenuated tubercle bacilli (BCG). I. Antimicrobial protection. *J. exp. Med.* **119:** 53–70.

WILKINSON, P. C., O'NEILL, G. J., MCINROY, R. J., CATER, J. C. and ROBERTS, J. A. (1973) Chemotaxis of macrophages: the role of a macrophage-specific cytotoxin from anaerobic corynebacteria and its relation to immunopotentiation *in vivo*. In: *Immunopotentiation,* A Ciba Foundation Symposium, pp. 121–135, WOLSTENHOLME, G. E. W. and KNIGHT, J. (eds.). Elsevier, Associated Scientific Publishers, Amsterdam.

WOOLES, W. R. and DI LUZIO, N. R. (1963) Reticuloendothelial function and the immune response. *Science* **142:** 1078–1080.

YAGEL, S., GALLILY, R. and WEISS, D. W. (1975) Effect of treatment with the MER fraction of tubercle bacilli on hydrolytic lysomal enzyme activity of mouse peritoneal macrophages. *Cell. Immunol.* **19:** 381–386.

YASHPE, D. J. (1971) Immunological factors in non-specific stimulation of host resistance to syngeneic tumors. *Isr. J. Med. Sci.* **7:** 90–107.

YASHPE, D. J. and HARAN-GHERA, N. (1970) Modulation of the immune response by a methanol extraction residue of BCG. Studies on the mode of action. *Isr. J. Med. Sci.* **6:** 446.

YASHPE, D. J. and WEISS, D. W. (1970) Modulation of the immune response by a methanol-insoluble fraction of attenuated tubercle bacilli (BCG). I. Primary and secondary responses to sheep red blood cells and T_2 phage. *Clin. exp. Immunol.* **7:** 269–281.

YASHPE, D. J., STEINKULLER, C. and WEISS, D. W. (1969) Modulation of immunological responsiveness by pretreatment with a methanol-insoluble fraction of killed tubercle bacilli. *Isr. J. Med. Sci.* **5:** 259–266.

YRON, I., WEISS, D. W., ROBINSON, E., COHEN, D., ADELBERG, M. G., MIKORI, T. and HABER, M. (1973) Immunotherapeutic experiments in mice with the MER fraction of BCG: Studies with solid tumors. *Nat. Cancer Inst. Monog.* **39:** 33–54.

YRON, I., COHEN, D., ROBINSON, E., HABER, M. and WEISS, D. W. (1975) Effects of MER and therapeutic irradiation against established isografts and simulated local recurrence of mammary carcinomas. *Cancer Res.* **35:** 1779–1790.

ZIMBER, CH., BEN-EFRAIM, S. and WEISS, D. W. (1977) Prevention by MER tubercle bacillus fraction of immunosuppression induced by cancer chemotherapeutic agents. II. Contact hypersensitivity in guinea pigs and mice treated with cyclophosphamide. *Cancer Immunol. Immunother.* **3:** 35–42.

ZIMBER, CH., BEN-EFRAIM, S. and WEISS, D. W. (1981a) Variable nonspecific immunopotentiating efficacy of two preparations of MER: effect on contact hypersensitivity of mice to dinitrofluorobenzene. *Cancer Immunol. Immunother.* **10:** 211–215.

ZIMBER, CH., BEN-EFRAIM, S. and WEISS, D. W. (1981b) Prevention by the MER tubercle bacillus fraction of immunosuppression induced by cancer chemotherapeutic agents. III. Contact hypersensitivity to dinitrofluorobenzene in mice treated with methotrexate, 5-fluorouracil or cyclophosphamide, or exposed to dinitrobenzene-sulfonate. *Cancer Immunol. Immunother.* **10:** 147–155.

NOTE ADDED IN PROOF

We have investigated recently (Ben-Efraim, S., Halperin, D., Reuben, C., Dat, O., and Weiss, D. W., *Cell. Immunol.*, 1984, **86:** 33–45) the effect of MER on the generation of primary antibody responsiveness *in vitro* to sheep red blood cells in cell reconstitution experiments employing enriched populations of mouse macrophages and of T and B lymphocytes. Enriched populations were incubated *in vitro* with MER for 48 hours or were collected from MER-treated donors. Macrophages and T cells that had been exposed to MER *in vivo* or *in vitro* and their supernatants demonstrated a markedly greater effect than nonexposed cells in the generation of direct plaque-forming cells upon antigenic stimulation of the cultures with SRBC. In contrast, PFC production was not stimulated in B-lymphocyte populations that had been in contact with the agent.

CHAPTER 9

IMMUNOBIOLOGY OF *CORYNEBACTERIUM PARVUM*

JACOB ZIGHELBOIM* and DAVID BERD**

**University of California, Los Angeles, USA*
***Thomas Jefferson University, Pennsylvania, USA*

1. INTRODUCTION

The injection of laboratory animals with anaerobic coryneform bacteria results in interesting biologic effects, the most important being the modulation of immune function. A series of reports published over the last 10 years document the ability of these organisms to modify several cell types (M. T and B lymphocytes and NK cells) and to stimulate and/or inhibit diverse components of the immune response.

This review summarizes the effects of anaerobic coryneform bacteria on the immune response and explores the cellular mechanism whereby these effects are mediated. Technical variables, in particular dose, route, and schedule of administration, are not presented in detail. Most studies have used doses of 10–70 mg/kg (0.2–1.4 mg for a 20 g mouse) of killed bacteria given either intravenously (I.V.) or intraperitoneally (I.P.) in a single injection. Only where variability of dose, route and schedule are specially relevant will specific details be presented.

TAXONOMY OF ANAEROBIC CORYNEFORM BACTERIA

Prevot (1975) was the first to observe that the organs of animals and humans naturally infected or injected with killed suspensions of anaerobic coryneforms displayed 'histioreticulosis with large multinuclear macrophages showing intense hyperergia'. He characterized this phenomenon as 'lethal stimulation of the RES (reticuloendothelial system)'. Although many strains of anaerobic coryneforms produce this effect, he chose for more detailed studies strain 936B, which he identified as *Corynebacterium parvum*. Significant activity was also associated with a separate strain identified as *C. granulosum*.

The physiologic effects of these organisms have been tested using killed (heat and/or formalin) preparations of bacteria from several sources, including The American Type Culture collection, The National Type Culture collection (Great Britain), and The Merieux Institute (Lyon, France). These preparations are usually referred to as *'C. parvum'*. There is considerable doubt, however, about the existence of *C. parvum* as a taxonomic entity. Johnson and Cummins (1972) examined the biochemical characteristics, cell wall composition, and DNA homology of a large number of strains of anaerobic coryneforms. Most met the criteria for classification under the genus *Propionibacterium* (not *Corynebacterium*). Five distinct groups were identified: (1) acnes-type I; (2) acnes—type II; (3) avidum) (4) granulosum; and (5) 'classical' propionibacteria. Strains labelled *'C. parvum'* belong to one of the first four groups and in themselves do not constitute a distinct taxonomic entity. All but the last group include organisms active as reticuloendothelial stimulants, immunologic adjuvants, and against malignant tumors (O'Neill *et al.*, 1973; McBride *et al.*, 1975a).

The designation *'C. parvum'* identifies, therefore, bacterial preparations (usually killed) that contain one of a number of anaerobic coryneforms. Their biologic properties may vary depending on the species contained in the preparation. For example, Berek *et al.* (1983) showed that on a per weight basis *P. acnes* I has more potent antitumor effects than *P. acnes* II in a murine teratocarcinoma model. Fortunately, most of the work to be discussed here involves suspensions of killed organisms supplied by either the Burroughs-Wellcome Co. (*P.*

acnes I) or the Merieux Institute (*P. avidum*) which have equivalent antitumor activity and biologic properties (Fisher *et al.*, 1975). For the sake of simplicity the term *'C. parvum'* will be used throughout this review.

2. MORPHOLOGIC ALTERATIONS FOLLOWING *C. PARVUM*

One of the most striking consequences of *C. parvum* inoculation is the development of hyperplasia of central and peripheral lymphoid organs. In mice, a single injection given I.V. or I.P. (in doses ranging from 0.1 to 2.8 mg) produces a three- to seven-fold increase in the weight of the spleen within two weeks (Castro, 1974a; Milas *et al.*, 1975; Greenberg and Dimitrov, 1976; Halpern *et al.*, 1973; Toujas *et al.*, 1975). Liver weights also increase about two-fold, while lung weights increase only slightly (Castro, 1974a; Scott and Warner, 1976; Brozovic *et al.*, 1975). Chronic low-dose administration is almost as effective as a single high dose (Scott and Warner, 1976). Subcutaneous administration generally causes less splenomegaly (at most two-fold) (Scott and Warner, 1976; Bomford and Olivotto 1974) and oral administration is without effect (Sadler and Castro, 1976). Subcutaneous injection of *C. parvum* causes regional lymphadenopathy while non-regional nodes are less affected (Castro, 1974a; Milas *et al.*, 1975). All hyperplastic organs remain enlarged for several weeks and return to normal by 4–6 weeks (Milas *et al.*, 1975).

Localization and degree of lymphoid hyperplasia following *C. parvum* inoculation may be reflective of the tissue distribution of the bacterium. Intravenous or I.P. administration of radiolabelled *C. parvum* is followed by rapid accumulation within the reticuloendothelial cells of liver and spleen where it remains for a long time (Dimitrov *et al.*, 1977). Subcutaneous or footpad inoculation is associated with localization at the injection site, with small amounts reaching regional lymph nodes or the systemic circulation. As expected, this route of administration causes little or no hepatosplenomegaly.

The number of nucleated cells extractable from enlarged spleens is about twice the number extracted from normal spleens (Warr and James, 1975; Mantovani *et al.*, 1976; Biozzi *et al.*, 1968), or higher (Milas *et al.*, 1975). The number of nucleated cells per mg of spleen, however, is lower than normal, suggesting that a significant proportion of the weight increment is due to fluid, erythrocytes, or cells not readily extractable by the usual methods.

Most of the information on *C. parvum* induced lymphoid hyperplasia has been derived from studies in mice where strain differences are rare. Rats respond similarly (Brozovic *et al.*, 1975), while rabbits failed to demonstrate organ enlargement (Pinckard *et al.*, 1968). There is no report of hepatosplenomegaly occurring in humans, although the latter have always received proportionately lower doses of *C. parvum* than mice.

The histology of the hyperplastic organs is noteworthy of comment. An example of a spleen from a *C. parvum*-treated mouse is shown in Fig. 1. Moderate hyperplasia of the follicles and marked congestion of the pulp is readily noted. Lymph nodes draining *C. parvum* injection sites have enlarged germinal centres, expansion of their paracortical areas, and large numbers of macrophages in the sinuses (O'Neill *et al.*, 1973). The histologic changes in liver are presented in Fig. 2. As shown, lymphocytic infiltration and granuloma formation are prominent.

Single cell suspensions from spleens of *C. parvum*-treated mice consist predominantly of small lympocytes (80–90%) (Greenberg and Dimitrov, 1976) and macrophages (15–20%) (Mantovani *et al.*, 1976). Macrophages do not appear activated, i.e. they are generally small and contain small amounts of vacuolated cytoplasm. Neutrophils and uncharacterized blastic cells (probably hematopoietic) are more conspicuous than in normal spleens.

The lymphocyte populations detected in spleen and lymph nodes from *C. parvum*-treated mice differ from normal. Theta-bearing T-cells are decreased by about 50% after a single I.V. or I.P. bolus (Mantovani *et al.*, 1976; Castro, 1974a), but not following chronic administration (even though the total administered dose is the same) (Likhite, 1975). Percent of Fc-R cells (determined by formation of erythrocyte-antibody rosettes) is usually unchanged (Mantovani *et al.*, 1976). Considering the increase in total lymphocytes, the absolute number of T cells in the spleen remains the same as normal while the absolute number of B cells is twice

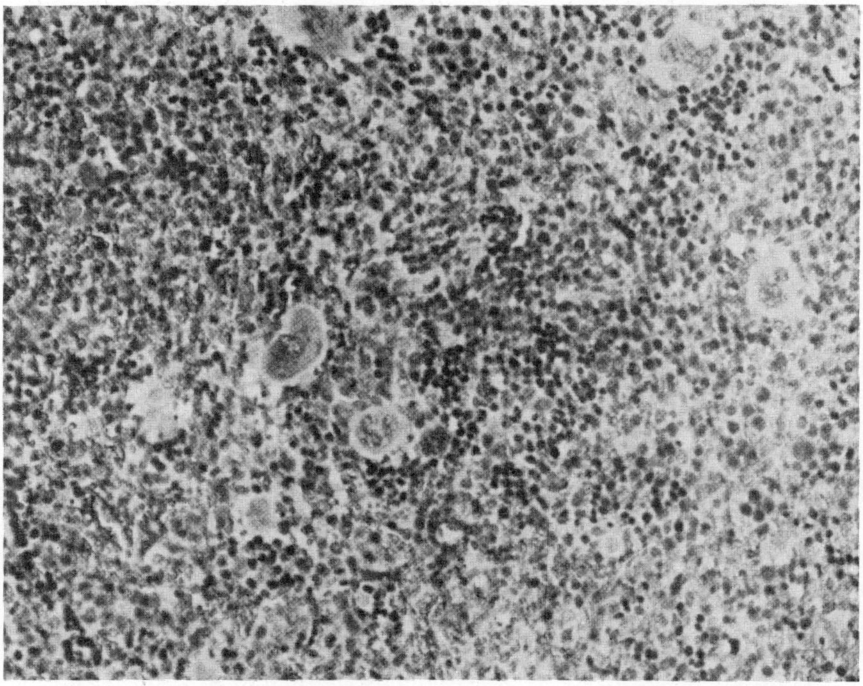

FIG. 1. Spleen of mouse given *C. parvum* 0.5 mg i.v. 7 days before, showing intense hematopoietic activity. The dark cells are erythroblasts, and the large multinucleated cells are megakaryocytes.

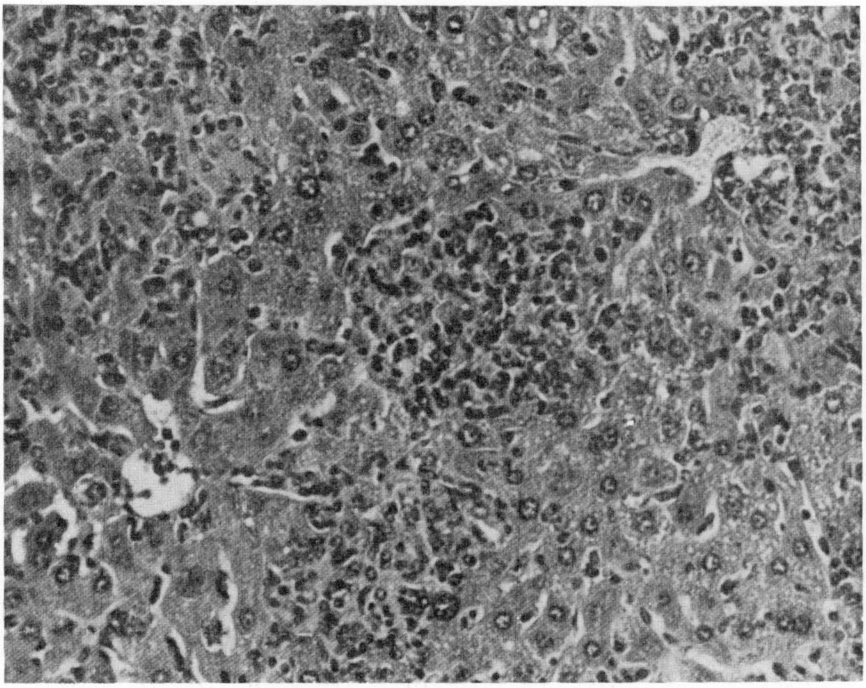

FIG. 2. Liver of mouse given *C. parvum* 0.5 mg i.v. 7 days before, showing mononuclear cell infiltration with formation of granulomas.

normal. In lymph nodes the relative proportion of T cells decreases slightly (Castro, 1974a; Likhite, 1975) while their absolute number is increased.

Intraperitoneal *C. parvum* causes a brisk exudation of cells into the peritoneal cavity which usually peaks 6–12 hours following inoculation. The number of nucleated cells increases 3–6-fold (Kirchner *et al.*, 1975a; McBride *et al.*, 1975a; Lichtenstein *et al.*, 1983c). During the first 24 hours the predominant cells are neutrophils. This component declines subsequently and is substituted by a mononuclear population composed of 50–70% macrophages. Many macrophages have phagocytosed neutrophils and some are large, vacuolated cells. A subset of macrophages recruited into the P.C. acquire tumoricidal properties, as demonstrated by their ability to lyse tumor targets *in vitro.* T lymphocytes and NK effector cells are also recruited into the peritoneal cavity. The mononuclear exudate usually peaks between 72 and 96 h following *C. parvum* inoculation and persists for 1 to 3 weeks. Peritoneal exudate does not develop after intravenous injection (Olivotto and Bomford, 1974).

The component(s) of the bacterium responsible for the hyperplastic changes described before have not been well defined. Pringle and Cummins (1981) showed that modification of ionizable groups on the surface of the bacteria decreases its RES stimulation ability. In fact a correlation seems to exist between amino or carboxyl group modification and loss of activity. It appears that only the amino groups associated with cell wall carbohydrates (and not those associated with surface proteins) are involved in RES stimulation. Two types of treatments markedly decrease the bacteria's ability to produce splenomegaly. One involves cleaving bonds between carbon atoms containing oxidizable functions and the second consists of extraction of cell wall polysaccharides.

Periodate oxidation, an example of the first type of treatment, and exposure to hydrochloric acid (extracts polysaccharides) caused profound losses of RES stimulatory activity. Based on these results it is tempting to assume that cell wall polysaccharides play an important role in the induction of splenomegaly. Extracted polysaccharides by themselves, however, do not induce splenomegaly. These results suggest that RES stimulation does not depend upon a particular chemical grouping on the cell wall but rather on the integrity of complex molecules such as peptidoglycan-polysaccharide complexes.

3. MODULATION OF RETICULOENDOTHELIAL FUNCTION

C. parvum increases the speed with which colloidal carbon particles are cleared from the circulation (Halpern *et al.,* 1964). This alteration is primarily mediated by enhanced phagocytosis of carbon particles by RES macrophages, especially in liver and spleen (Stiffel *et al.,* 1970). A number of reports have confirmed this observation and further demonstrated that carbon clearance was 4 to 5 times above normal 1 week following *C. parvum* inoculation (Halpern *et al.,* 1973; McBride *et al.,* 1975a; O'Neill *et al.,* 1973). This effect does not simply reflect liver and spleen enlargement. Carbon clearance returns to normal 2 weeks after *C. parvum* inoculation, at a time when splenomegaly was maximal (Halpern *et al.,* 1973). Moreover, some strains of anaerobic coryneforms can cause hepatosplenomegaly without increasing carbon clearance. The reverse situation, i.e. increased clearance without organ enlargement, however, it quite unusual (O'Neill *et al.,* 1973; McBride *et al.,* 1975a). *C. parvum* probably augments particle clearance by increasing the number of tissue macrophages as well as enhancing their phagocytic capacity.

Antigens like sheep red blood cells may also be cleared more rapidly in *C. parvum*-treated, non-immune mice (Warr and Sljivic, 1974). Howard *et al.,* (1973a) reported, however, that other antigens like pneumococcal polysaccharides were not cleared more rapidly than normal. Furthermore, 6–10 days following administration the antigen reappeared in blood, possibly due to enhanced exocytosis by *C. parvum*-stimulated tissue macrophages.

4. RESISTANCE TO INFECTIOUS AGENTS

C. parvum inoculation can render animals less susceptible to a variety of lethal infections. For example, mice given *C. parvum* 14–28 days before injection with *Brucella abortus* have bacterial counts in the spleen that approximate 0, while controls have counts in the order of 10^3-10^4 (Halpern *et al.,* 1973). Pretreatment with *C. parvum* can also prevent mortality from *Salmonella enteriditis* (Collins and Scott, 1974). Other infectious agents resisted more effectively in *C. parvum*-treated animals include *Bordetella pertussis, Staphylococcus aureus* (Sher *et al.,* 1975), *Candida albicans* (Sher *et al.,* 1975) and *Listeria monocytogenes* (Swartzberg *et al.,* 1975; Ruitenberg and van Norle Jansen, 1975; Tuttle and North, 1975). *C. parvum* can also increase resistance to intracellular parasites like *Toxoplasma gondii* (Swartzberg *et al.,* 1975), *Plasmodium berghei* (Nussenzweig, 1967), and *Mengo virus* in mice (Halpern *et al.,* 1973).

Intravenous and intraperitoneal administration of *C. parvum* protects mice against infection with herpes virus I (Kirshner *et al.,* 1977). Intraperitoneal injection 3 days before inoculation with HSV I resulted in decreased mortality from encephalitis (90% in control compared to 30% in immunoprophylaxed mice) (Szmigielski *et al.,* 1982). Protection was also reported against murine hepatitis virus infection in strains susceptible to the virus. Subcutaneous injection of *C. parvum* together with live or attenuated virus vaccines causes a significant enhancement of the immune response manifested by higher titers of antiviral antibodies.

The protective effects seen with *C. parvum* may reflect macrophage and/or NK activation as well as interferon production.

On occasions *C. parvum* can decrease host resistance to infections. Purnell (1976) reported that mice given *C. parvum* 3 days before or simultaneously with *Aspergillus nidulans* had shortened survival compared to controls. Histopathologically the *C. parvum*-injected mice had enhanced invasion of brain, kidneys, and heart by the fungus. Rats given *C. parvum* show delayed expulsion of *Trichinella spiralis* worms from their gastrointestinal tract, an effect that seems to be T cell dependent (Ruitenberg and Steerenberg, 1973). Administration of *C. parvum* 1 day after (as opposed to pretreatment as noted above) challenge with *S. enteriditis* decreased mice survival (Collins and Scott, 1974). Similarly *C. parvum*-treated mice failed to develop immunity against *T. cruzi.*

Resistance to infectious agents involves macrophages (phagocytosis and cytocidal effects), T cells (helper activity for antibody and/or direct cytotoxicity) and non-specific cytotoxic effectors (NK and ADCC). *C. parvum,* depending on the *in vivo* conditions, may enhance and/or suppress these components of host defense leading to either enhanced or decreased resistance.

5. ANTITUMOR ACTIVITY

Interest in *C. parvum* stems primarily from its ability to inhibit the growth of malignant tumors. The discussion that follows summarizes the antitumor effects of *C. parvum* in a variety of murine and human tumors. Woodruff and Boak (1966) were the first to use *C. parvum* for the control of a transplantable syngeneic murine tumor. They reported that I.V. administration 2 days before or 8–12 days after subcutaneous inoculation of tumor cells significantly delayed the appearance of the neoplasm and prolonged survival. Similarly, Halpern *et al.* (1966) reported 90% cures in mice injected simultaneously with Ehrlich ascites tumor cells and *C. parvum.* These findings have been amply confirmed and extended by many investigators (Table 1).

C. parvum has been most effective when given before, simultaneously, or shortly after tumor inoculation. Prolonged survival and cures have been reported, however, in mice bearing small (5–10 mm) subcutaneous tumors when directly inoculated with *C. parvum* (Scott, 1976; Woodruff and Dunbar, 1975; Likhite and Halpern, 1974) or given the bacteria together with cytotoxic drugs, i.e. cyclophosphamide (Fisher *et al.,* 1975, 1976a).

C. parvum can also control the growth of intraperitoneal tumors. Knapp and Berkowitz (1976), Bast *et al.,* (1979) and Berek *et al.,* (1983) showed that formalin killed *C. parvum* can cure over 60% of C3H/FeJ mice injected with a poorly immunogenic ovarian teratocarcinoma (MOT). The bacterium was most effective when injected 24 to 48 h after tumor inoculum.

Strongly immunogenic tumors seem to respond better to systemic *C. parvum* than weakly immunogenic tumors. Smith and Scott (1972) showed prolonged survival in mice challenged with an immunogenic radiation induced leukemia but not in those inoculated with a less immunogenic variant of the same neoplasm.

TABLE 1. *Inhibition of Tumor Growth by* C. parvum[1]

	C. parvum administration		Tumor transplantation			
Dose[2] (mg)	Route[3]	Day[4]	Type	Route	Results	References
0.5	i.v., i.p., s.c.	−2 or 3 to 8	Sarcoma—chemically induced	s.c.	Prolonged survival	Woodruff and Dunbar, 1975; Woodruff and Boak, 1966
0.25	i.v.	3 to 13	Sarcoma—chemically induced	s.c.	50% complete regression	Milas *et al.*, 1974a
0.25	i.v., s.c.	−7	Sarcoma—chemically induced	i.v.	Suppression of lung metastases	Milas *et al.*, 1974b
1.4	i.p.	−1	Sarcoma—chemically induced	i.p.	Prevention of mortality	Castro, 1974b
0.7	i.l.	3	Sarcoma—chemically induced	s.c.	No growth	Woodruff and Dunbar, 1975
0.5	i.v.	−2 or 8	Mammary carcinoma	s.c.	Prolonged survival	Woodruff and Boak, 1966
0.4	i.p.	0 or 14	Mammary carcinoma	s.c.	Slower growth	Likhite, 1975; Likhite and Halpern, 1974
0.4	i.l.	14	Mammary carcinoma	s.c.	Complete regression	Likhite and Halpern, 1974
0.4	Mixed	0	Mammary carcinoma	s.c.	Complete regression	Likhite, 1975
0.7	Mixed	0	Mammary carcinoma	s.c.	No growth	Purnell *et al.*, 1976
0.4	i.v., i.p.	−7	Lewis lung	s.c.	Prolonged survival	Mathé *et al.*, 1973
0.7	i.v., i.p.	0	Lewis lung	s.c.	Slower growth	Sadler and Castro, 1976
0.25	i.p.	0	Ehrlich ascites	i.p.	Decreased mortality	Halpern *et al.*, 1966
0.7	i.p., i.v.	−5	Mastocytoma P815Y	i.p.	Prolonged survival	Scott, 1975a
0.07	i.l.	2	Mastocytoma P815Y	s.c.	44% complete regression	Scott, 1976
0.14	i.p.	1	Melanoma B16	i.p.	Prolonged survival	Houchens *et al.*, 1976
1.4	i.v., i.p.	−7	Leukemia-radiation induced	i.p.	Prolonged survival	Smith and Scott, 1972
0.14	i.p.	−7 or 1	Leukemia-P388	i.p.	Prolonged survival	Houchens *et al.*, 1976

[1]All data pertain to syngeneic tumors in mice.

[2]If multiple dosages tested, lowest effective dose is listed; all results are from single doses of Cp.

[3]Abbreviations: i.v.—intravenous, i.p.—intraperitoneal, s.c.—subcutaneous, i.l.—intralesional, mixed—mixed and injected with tumor cells.

[4]Tumor given day 0.

Regression of tumors following intralesional injection of *C. parvum* is usually associated with the development of specific immunity (Likhite and Halpern, 1974; Scott, 1974c). Lymphocytes (but not serum) from these mice can prevent tumor growth in naive, non-immune recipients.

C. parvum can also act as an adjuvant in tumor vaccines. Mice injected with a mixture of *C. parvum* and viable or irradiated tumor cells can develop specific resistance to tumor rechallenge (Scott, 1975b; Likhite, 1975). Mice cured of subcutaneous tumor by surgery and given systemic *C. parvum* develop resistance to tumor rechallenge (Purnell *et al.*, 1976) and to the development of lung metastases (Proctor *et al.*, 1973), while mice treated with surgery alone do not. This occurrence, however, was not seen in all tumor systems examined. Purnell *et al.*, (1976) and Woodruff *et al.*, (1976) reported, in fact, opposite effects, i.e. less resistance to rechallenge.

The effect of *C. parvum* on the growth of allogeneic tumors is equally complex. *C. parvum* pretreatment of allogeneic (H-2 compatible) Balb/C mice 7 days before inoculation of L1210 leukemic cells resulted in 100% cures (compared to 0% in controls) (Houchens *et al.*, 1976). Mantovani *et al.*, (1976) reported, however, that *C. parvum* could either decrease or increase mortality of H-2 incompatible C3H mice inoculated with L1210 cells. Berd and Mitchell (1976) reported that H2 incompatible C57BL/6 mice given *C. parvum* 7 days before L1210 exhibited enhanced tumor growth. Eventually all mice rejected the tumor inoculum, although the *C. parvum*-treated mice took longer. These findings are not peculiar to L1210 leukemia. Murahata and Zighelboim, (1980) reported delayed rejection of a P815 mastocytoma tumor cell rechallenge in allogeneic mice inoculated with *C. parvum* 9 days after a subcutaneous inoculum of P815 cells. The delayed rejection coincided with decreased memory cytotoxicity in spleen and the development of suppressor macrophages.

6. ANTITUMOR EFFECTS IN MAN

C. parvum has been tested in a large number of human tumors. Almost invariably the agent was administered to patients with advanced disease by either the intravenous or subcutaneous route. These clinical studies gave disappointing results.

Preclinical studies in murine systems revealed, however, that *C. parvum* given intraperitoneally caused powerful inflammatory responses (Lichtenstein *et al.*, 1983c) and the recruitment and activation of macrophages and NK cells (Lichtenstein *et al.*, 1983c). These results suggested that intraperitoneal administration of *C. parvum* could effectively control intraperitoneal cancer, i.e. ovarian carcinoma and other tumors that metastasize to the peritoneal cavity.

Intraperitoneal *C. parvum* in humans has been effective in two clinical conditions: (a) in advanced ovarian cancer resistant to chemotherapy and (b) in patients with minimal residual disease after cytoreductive surgery and 8–12 cycles of systemic chemotherapy. Mantovani *et al.*, (1981) reported that 3/8 patients with advanced ovarian cancer resistant to chemotherapy had complete disappearance of ascites following I.P. *C. parvum*. An additional 2 patients showed marked reduction, while 3 patients had no response. These results encouraged Bast *et al.*, (1983) to conduct a phase I–II intraperitoneal *C. parvum* in patients with advanced ovarian cancer who had residual cancer following cytoreductive surgery and systemic combination chemotherapy. Fifty percent of the treated patients demonstrated >50% reduction of intraperitoneal tumor. Two had complete responses and one had disappearance of macroscopic disease.

The clinical impact and significance of these antitumor effects is being examined in a phase II trial.

Mignot *et al.*, (1981) reported lower relapse rates in patients injected with *C. parvum* in the neighbourhood of operable carcinomas of the uterine cervix. This study accrued 43 patients whose cancers were confined to the cervix, upper part of the vagina and parametrial region. The patients were randomly allocated to receive either immunotherapy (as a single injection of 2 mg *C. parvum* in the neighbourhood of the tumor) 10 days before surgery or surgery alone.

The relapse rate in patients pretreated with *C. parvum* was 5% compared to 29% in the controls. These results are better then achieved with any other form of therapy. Administration of *C. parvum* in the neighbourhood of a cervix carcinoma slowed down the growth of the tumor and might have increased its curability.

7. MODULATION OF THE IMMUNE RESPONSE

EFFECTS OF C. PARVUM ON ANTIBODY RESPONSES TO T CELL DEPENDENT ANTIGEN

C. parvum can markedly augment antibody responses to T dependent antigens (Playfair and Purves, 1971). Howard *et al.*, (1973b) reported that *C. parvum* given I.P. 4 days before a large (10^5 or 10^6 cells) inoculum of sheep red blood cells increased the number of plaque-forming cells (PFCs) per spleen 2–10 times above control levels. If *C. parvum* was given 7 days after antigen the number of indirect and direct PFCs remained elevated (while the latter were decreasing in controls). Other investigators report similar results (Greenberg and Dimitrov, 1976; James *et al.*, 1974; Castro, 1974a; Mathe *et al.*, 1973). When PFCs are expressed per 10^6 spleen cells rather than per spleen, the increase is less striking and at times the values are less than in controls (James *et al.*, 1974; Warr and James, 1975). The timing of *C. parvum* and antigen administration critical. The adjuvant effect diminishes if *C. parvum* is given simultaneously or 1–3 days after sheep red blood cells (James *et al.*, 1974; Mathe *et al.*, 1973; Warr and Sljivic, 1974; Warr and James, 1975).

A parallel effect was noted when measuring titer of agglutinating antibody to sheep erythrocytes. In *C. parvum*-pretreated mice, the antibody titers were four- to eight-fold higher, and both mercaptoethanol-sensitive and resistant antibody levels were increased (Biozzi *et al.*, 1968; McBride *et al.*, 1975a; Warr and Sljivic, 1974; Howard *et al.*, 1973b).

Secondary responses are less influenced by pretreatments with *C. parvum* either before priming (Warr and Sljivic, 1974) or after the second dose of antigen (Biozzi *et al.*, 1968).

Warr and Sljivio (1974) reported depressed antibody response to sheep red cells following *C. parvum*. They found that *C. parvum* given before a low dose (10^6 cells) of antigen caused a marked decrease in the number of direct PFCs per spleen; this was not noted when a high dose (10^8 cells) was used. The significance of this observation is not clear. Variations in technique could account for the discrepancies.

C. parvum also increases the antigen binding capacity (ABC) of antibodies generated against BSA in mice. Relative binding affinity, a measure of quality of antibody, was not changed (James *et al.*, 1974). In rabbits, titers of hemagglutinating antibody increased four-fold by pretreatment with *C. parvum* while the secondary response increased to a lesser extent (Halpern *et al.*, 1973).

Centrifuged BSA is less immunogenic in rabbits than whole BSA. Pretreatment with *C. parvum* results in a four-fold increase in ABC with centrifuged BSA but has no effect on the ABC to whole BSA (Pinckard *et al.*, 1967a); the antibody produced has increased binding affinity as well. Administration of *C. parvum* simultaneously with antigen did not affect antibody titer (Pinckard *et al.*, 1967b).

The effect of *C. parvum* on induction of tolerance was investigated using the BSA system. Injection of centrifuged BSA renders adult rabbits tolerant to highly immunogenic alum-precipitated BSA. Pretreatment with *C. parvum* prevented the development of tolerance (Pinckard *et al.*, 1968). These effects were inconsistent and dependent on the system tested. For example, *C. parvum* did not interfere with the development of high dose tolerance to pneumopolysaccharide or reversed tolerance in neonatal animals (Pinckard *et al.*, 1967c).

C. parvum acts as an adjuvant to other T dependent antigens, i.e. rat red blood cells (Howard *et al.*, 1973b), keyhole limpet hemocyanin (KLH) (Weiner and Bandieri, 1975), ovalbumin (O'Neill *et al.*, 1973) and picrylated albumin (Neveu *et al.*, 1964). With the latter two antigens, it is most effective when admixed with incomplete Freund's adjuvant and given together with antigen.

Antibody responses to tumor cell antigens are probably T dependent. C57BL/6 mice challenged with allogeneic L1210 leukemia develop complement dependent cytotoxic antibody against histocompatibility antigens on the tumor cells. Mice given *C. parvum* I.V. (1.0 to 0.1 mg) 7 days before tumor cells show profound suppression of the antibody response (Berd and Mitchell, 1976) and enhanced tumor growth. Mantovani *et al.*, (1976), using the same tumor model in C3H mice (also allogeneic), reported no change in cytotoxic antibody titer. The titer of antibodies capable of participating in antibody dependent cellular cytotoxicity was similarly unaffected.

Occasionally *C. parvum* can also cause inhibition of antibody responses to T dependent antigens, i.e. tetanus toxoid. *C. parvum*-pretreated mice require greater doses of tetanus toxoid for protection against the toxin (Knight and Lucken, 1975).

Effects of C. parvum on Antibody Responses to T Independent Antigens

C. parvum can have either adjuvant or suppressive effects on antibody responses to T independent antigens. Warr and Sljivic, (1974) and Howard *et al.*, (1973a) demonstrated that *C. parvum* given 4 days before type III pneumococcal polysaccharide causes an increase in the number of direct PFCs per spleen. This effect was noted over a broad range of SIII doses (2 to 10 μg). Large doses (i.e. 500 μg), however, were tolerogenic in either control or *C. parvum*-pretreated mice, while lower doses (<2 μg) had no adjuvant effect (Howard *et al.*, 1973a, b; James *et al.*, 1974). Antibody responses to dinitrophenol (DNP) coupled with leven were also enhanced by prior treatment with *C. parvum* (Del Guercio and Leuchars, 1972).

Under special circumstances, antibody responses can be suppressed. Simultaneous administration with SIII caused marked suppression of direct PFCs (Howard *et al.*, 1973a, b). Mice given *C. parvum* and challenged with live *Salmonella enteriditis* show delayed and diminished antibody response to the pathogen (Collins and Scott, 1974).

In summary, *C. parvum* augments antibody responses to T-dependent and independent antigens. Primary responses are more affected than secondary responses. Under certain conditions, however, responses to either type of antigen and to tumor-associated antigens can be significantly suppressed.

8. DELAYED HYPERSENSITIVITY

Addition of *C. parvum* to a mixture of incomplete Freund's adjuvant (IFA) and antigen amplifies the delayed hypersensitivity (DH) response induced by antigen and IFA alone (Degrand and Raynaud, 1973; Neveu *et al.*, 1964). Similarly, administration of *C. parvum* after sensitization also enhanced DH responses to tumor cells even in immunocompromised (thymectomy and antithymocyte serum) mice (Likhite, 1975).

By contrast, animals given *C. parvum* 4–10 days before the sensitizing antigen showed suppressed DH. Guinea pigs sensitized with bovine gamma globulin (BGG) mixed with *C. parvum* in IFA develop DH to BGG. When sensitization is preceded by injection of *C. parvum* the response is decreased by 50% (Asherson and Allwood, 1971). DH responses to *Salmonella enteriditis* are also abrogated by pretreatment with *C. parvum* (Collins and Scott, 1974). Scott, (1974a) reported suppression of DH to sheep red blood cells in mice. Suppression was schedule-dependent, i.e. induced by a single high dose of *C. parvum* but not seen with chronic low dose administration (Scott and Warner, 1976).

Modulation of DH responses by *C. parvum* depends on when and how the agent is given. Systemic administration before sensitization regularly suppressed DH. Lymphoid cells from suppressed animals were less efficient than normal cells in reconstituting DH response in suppressed animals (Allwood and Asherson, 1971). These results imply inhibition at the central or effector level of the immune response, probably due to depression of T cell activity.

9. MECHANISM OF ACTION

The preceding sections have focused on the effects of *C. parvum* on cellular and humoral immunity and have highlighted some of its most striking biologic effects. This section attempts to provide the cellular and biochemical basis for the effects described. The leading hypothesis is that *C. parvum* effects are mediated via stimulation and activation of macrophages which then directly or via soluble mediators influence T and B lymphocytes, and NK cells.

10. EFFECTS ON MACROPHAGES

C. parvum directly stimulates macrophage function. As a result these cells undergo morphological changes, increase their acid phosphatase activity, produce interferon and acquire tumoricidal capacity (Buck and Kelley, 1980). The morphologic changes frequently noted include increased spreading and increments in the proportion of vacuoles and granules. These changes correlate best with acquisition of tumoricidal properties. The components on the microbial cell wall responsible for inducing these changes are heat stable and refractory to extraction by methanol-chloroform, dilute acid, and butanol.

Mechanical disruption of the cells results in complete loss of macrophage activating capacity suggesting that neither the cell wall nor the cytoplasmic fractions are capable of activating macrophages by themselves.

Clearly, the components of the bacterium cell responsible for macrophage activation must be encountered in an arrangement present only in intact cells.

C. parvum also stimulates macrophage production. Forty-eight hours after *C. parvum* administration there is a four-fold increase in the number of macrophage colony forming cells in bone marrow (Dimitrov *et al.*, 1975). This probably reflects direct stimulation of macrophage precursors as well as increased production of colony stimulating factor.

Macrophages are responsible for lymphocyte trapping seen after *C. parvum* inoculation. Frost and Lance (1973) observed that a variety of immune adjuvants, when injected subcutaneously cause trapping of intraveneously injected normal syngeneic lymphocytes in regional lymph nodes. *C. parvum* was the most effective of the agents tested, causing four times more trapping than complete Freund's adjuvant. The ability to cause trapping was transferred by peritoneal cells or by adherent cells from spleen suspensions suggesting it was macrophage mediated. Lymphocyte trapping was also increased in liver, lung (Warr and Sljivic, 1974) and spleen (Scott, 1974a).

Development of adjuvanticity corresponds temporarily with the height of reticuloendothelial stimulation (Howard *et al.*, 1973a). *C. parvum* strains most effective as adjuvants are also most effective in increasing liver and spleen weights. Strains that induce the greatest degree of splenomegaly also have the most potent antitumor effects (McBride *et al.*, 1975a). There are exceptions, however, i.e. Pinchard *et al.*, (1968) and Pinckard and Halonen (1971) found a strain of *C. parvum* able to cause an adjuvant effect without increasing liver and spleen weights in rabbits and mice.

There is direct evidence that the adjuvant effect of *C. parvum* on T dependent antigens is mediated via macrophage stimulation. Weiner (1975) studied plaque-forming cells to sheep red blood cells *in vitro*. Spleen cells from mice treated with *C. parvum* produced two to three times more plaques per culture than normal spleen cells. Response of normal spleen cells depleted of macrophages could be restored by adding peritoneal macrophages from *C. parvum*-treated mice but not by macrophages from normal or thioglycollate-treated mice. These macrophages retained their restorative capacity for up to 40 days after a single injection of *C. parvum*. In the same system other investigators have documented that immune augmentation is mediated by adherent, radioresistant cell fractions (Watson and Sljivic, 1976).

Weiner and Bandieri (1975) demonstrated that macrophages from mice treated with *C. parvum* take up KLH at the same rate as normal cells but degrade it more slowly. As a result, they retain three times as much antigen on their surface as normal macrophages. This increase in surface antigen may provide more effective immunologic triggering of lymphocytes and on all likelihood is responsible for the adjuvant effect.

The role of macrophages in the adjuvant effects of *C. parvum* to T independent antigens is less clear. Howard *et al.*, (1973a) treated mice with *C. parvum* and lethal irradiation followed by reconstitution with normal spleen cells and one day later mice were challenged with SIII. It was expected that splenocytes of *C. parvum*-treated mice would contain normal lymphocytes and a population of stimulated radioresistant macrophages that would augment the antibody response. These mice showed almost complete suppression of plaque-forming cells to SIII compared to untreated irradiated and reconstituted animals. These results are consistent with the *in vitro* observation of Diener *et al.*, (1970) that macrophages adherent to plastic dishes are unnecessary for the antibody response to T independent antigens and when in excessive numbers can suppress the response. More recently Gorczynski (1976) identified a subpopulation of macrophages sensitive to antimacrophage serum, but not adherent to plastic dishes that can augment the antibody response to a T independent antigen *in vitro*. *C. parvum* may exert adjuvanticity by stimulating this subpopulation. The possibility that *C. parvum* directly stimulates antibody-producing (B) cells is discussed in the next section.

Macrophages are important mediators of the antitumor effects mediated by *C. parvum*. Four to ten days after the I.P. administration of *C. parvum* peritoneal cells are cytotoxic to tumor cells *in vitro* (Table 2). Intravenous injection produces similar results (Olivotto and Bomford, 1974) while subcutaneous administration is ineffective (Scott and Warner, 1976). In some of the systems summarized in Table 2 the effector cell has not been identified. In others, however (Ghaffer *et al.*, 1974, 1975; Jones *et al.*, 1975; Kirchner *et al.*, 1975a; Olivotto and Bomford, 1974; Schultz *et al.*, 1976), the effector cells have been shown to be adherent, phagocytic radioresistant cells (Basic *et al.*, 1975), insensitive of anti-theta serum, and sensitive to carageenan (Kirchner *et al.*, 1975a).

As indicated in Table 2, peritoneal macrophages from *C. parvum*-treated mice are cytotoxic to many cultured tumor cell lines. Basic *et al.*, (1975) showed that non-neoplastic murine cells, i.e. fibroblasts, kidney cells, and erythrocytes, are not lysed by these macrophages. Jones *et al.*, (1975) described cytolysis of syngeneic and allogeneic embryo cells. The degree of cytolysis was low, and the target cells used were in the second to sixth tissue culture generation which might have changed their antigenicity.

The mechanism by which *C. parvum* stimulates macrophages to become cytotoxic is unknown. This simplest hypothesis is that direct activation of normal, mature macrophages takes place. This idea is supported by observations that activation is not decreased in mice depleted of T cells. Lymphocytes or serum from *C. parvum*-treated mice do not confer cytotoxicity to normal macrophages *in vitro* (Ghaffer *et al.*, 1975).

Chapes and Haskill (1982) observed strong correlations between macrophage cytotoxicity and the intracellular localization of *C. parvum* following intraperitoneal inoculation. Separation of these peritoneal macrophages by velocity sedimentation revealed that the most rapidly sedimenting (largest) macrophages (which contain the highest number of bacteria) had the highest cytotoxic activity. Experiments using FACS analysis of macrophages exposed to fluorescinated *C. parvum (in vivo)* revealed that the cells containing fluorescent labeled *C. parvum* were highly cytotoxic, while those free of *C. parvum* were less. These results suggest that direct processing of the bacterium by macrophages is important in the development of the cytolytic state. Interestingly, mixing *C. parvum in vitro* with normal macrophages does not elicit their cytotoxic program. Macrophages induced by I.P. injections of mineral oil and mixed with *C. parvum in vitro* do become cytotoxic. This suggests that development of cytotoxicity requires two types of activating stimuli; one taking place *in vivo*.

The requirement for *in vivo* stimulation is consistent with the observations of Fisher and Wolmark (1976) that *C. parvum* may act on macrophage precursors rather than on their mature counterparts. When bone marrow cells from tumor-bearing mice are cultured *in vitro*, the macrophages isolated from the colonies are cytotoxic to tumor cells. The administration of *C. parvum* to these mice results in an increased number of cytotoxic macrophages grown from colony-forming cells *in vitro*. The proportion of macrophages that are cytotoxic is not increased, however. This indicates that *C. parvum* stimulates precursors of all macrophages, including those whose progeny become cytotoxic.

TABLE 2. *Cytotoxicity of Peritoneal Macrophages Induced by* C. parvum

C. parvum[1] administered	Purification of effector cells	Target cell	Detection of cytotoxicity	Degree of cytotoxicity	References
i.p.	A	Sarcoma—CI	C	100%	Basic *et al.*, 1975
i.p.	A	Sarcoma—CI	PL—IUDR	90%	Ghaffar *et al.*, 1975
i.p.	A	Sarcoma—CI	PL—IUDR	90–95%	Ghaffar *et al.*, 1974
i.p.	None	Sarcoma—CI	PL—IUDR	95%	McBride *et al.*, 1975a
i.v.	A	Sarcoma—S	C, PL—H	95%	Olivotto and Bomford, 1974
i.p.	None	Mastocytoma—P815Y	PL—H	100%	Scott, 1975a
i.v.	?	Leukemia—RI	PL—H	90%	Scott and Warner, 1976
i.p.	A, anti-theta	Lymphoma—MV	PL—H	80%	Kirchner *et al.*, 1975a
i.p.	A	Leukemia—MV	Cr	36%	Fray *et al.*, 1975
i.p.	A	Leukemia—MV—allo	Cr	15%	Schultz *et al.*, 1976
i.p.	A	Embryo cells	Cr	[2]	Jones *et al.*, 1975
i.p.	A, I	Fibroblasts, kidney cells, erythrocytes	C	0	Basic *et al.*, 1975

[1]Abbreviations: i.p.—intraperitoneally; i.v.—intravenously; A—adherence; I—irradiation; CI—chemically induced; S—spontaneous; MV—Moloney virus induced; allo—allogeneic; RI—radiation induced; C—counting; PL—post-labeling; H—^{3}H-thymidine; Cr—^{51}Cr; IUDR—^{125}IUDR.

[2]Not indicated by percentage—see text.

C. parvum-stimulated macrophages may also exhibit cytotoxicity *in vivo*. ^{51}Cr-labeled tumor cells injected into mice treated with *C. parvum* are lysed within 24 h as measured by appearance of ^{51}Cr in the urine (Bomford and Olivotto, 1974). This is too short a time for the generation of immune lymphocytes, so that non-specifically activated cells seem the most likely effector population. Of course, other cells such as neutrophils could account for the findings. Haskill *et al.*, (1980) showed that in the C3H mammary carcinoma system intratumor injection of *C. parvum* caused tumor regression via generation of macrophages active in ADCC.

Additionally it has been shown that total body irradiation with 800 R one day before administration of *C. parvum* eliminates its antitumor effect. Irradiation the same day or one day after has no effect (Bomford and Olivotto, 1974). This suggests participation of rapidly proliferating but inherently radioresistant cells (i.e. macrophages). Furthermore, treatment of mice with gold salts (McBride *et al.*, 1975c) or rifampin (Fisher *et al.*, 1976b) partially abrogates the antitumor activity of *C. parvum*. Both agents allegedly act specifically on macrophages. Rifampin in fact decreases the number of cytotoxic macrophages grown from colony-forming cells.

The tumoricidal effects mediated by activated macrophages require live cells (Ghaffar *et al.*, 1974) and macrophage: tumor cell ratios higher than 10:1 (Ghaffar *et al.*, 1975; Kirchner *et al.*, 1975a). Supernatant fluids from macrophage cultures are inactive (Ghaffar *et al.*,1975; Jones *et al.*, 1975; Olivotto and Bomford, 1974). Macrophage-induced lysis of tumor cells is slow, with minimal ^{51}Cr being detected at 6–8 h (Jones *et al.*, 1975; Schultz *et al.*, 1976). The antitumor effects are primarily cytostatic and best assessed by examining the effects of *C. parvum*-treated macrophages on tumor DNA synthesis (measured by uptake of ^{3}H thymidine or ^{125}IUdR).

There is no direct evidence that macrophages are operative in the resistance to infectious agents, although it seems probable they are important.

Macrophages stimulated by *C. parvum* may participate in the resistance to infectious agents via production and release of interferon. Stimulation of C57B1/6 mouse spleen cells with *C. parvum* results in the production of two classes of interferon, i.e. interferon alpha/beta and interferon gamma. Kinetic studies showed that interferon alpha/beta activity peaked at 12–24 hours, while interferon gamma peaked at 48–72 hours. Non-adherent cells are the major producers of interferon alpha/beta and thymocytes are of interferon gamma. Treatment with monoclonal anti-Thy 1.2 antibody and complement reduced the production of interferon gamma but had little effect on the production of interferon alpha/beta. These results suggest that T cells produce interferon gamma and non-adherent non-T cells produce interferon alpha/beta (Evans and Johnson, 1981).

It has been shown that *C. parvum*-induced production of interferon by human peripheral leukocytes (Berek *et al.*, 1983; Biozzi *et al.*, 1968; Bomford and Olivotto, 1974), and mouse spleen cells (Bomford and Christie, 1971; Brozovic, Sljivic and Warr, 1975). The role of interferon in the biologic effects attributed to *C. parvum* is worth examining.

Systemic administration of *C. parvum* also causes the appearance in spleen of adherent phagocytic macrophage-like cells capable of suppressing several T cell functions *in vitro* (Kirchner *et al.*, 1975a; Scott, 1972b; Lichtenstein *et al.*, 1981a, b). The *in vivo* role of these type of suppressor cells remains poorly defined. Their role in suppressing primary and/or memory cytotoxicity *(in vivo)* seems limited. Murahata *et al.*, (1980) demonstrated that hot phenol extracted components of *C. parvum* suppress primary and memory cytotoxicity without causing generation of suppressor macrophages. Evidently, suppression of primary and memory CTLs and induction of regulatory macrophages are not linked or interdependent.

11. LYMPHOCYTES—B CELLS

The antibody response to two T independent antigens—type 3 pneumococcal polysaccharide (SIII) and DNP-levan—is increased by pretreatment with *C. parvum*. Howard *et al.*, (1973a) reasoned that if *C. parvum* stimulates B cells directly, then the adoptive transfer of spleen cells from *C. parvum* mice would increase the number of PFCs induced by SIII in the recipients. This was not the case, and in fact recipients of *C. parvum* spleen cells produced fewer plaques than recipients of normal spleen cells. Furthermore, if pretreatment with *C. parvum* were to increase the number of B splenocytes stimulated to make antibody to SIII, then PFCs would appear more rapidly in pretreated mice. Instead, the kinetics of PFCs development was identical in *C. parvum*-treated and control animals. These results reduce the likelihood that direct stimulation of B cells is the mechanisms responsible for the enhanced response to SIII.

C. parvum has variable effects on B cells responsiveness to mitogens. Splenocytes of treated mice show impaired blastogenesis to pokeweed mitogen (Milas *et al.*, 1975; Scott, 1972a), while lymph node cells respond more vigorously (Milas *et al.*, 1975). Responsiveness of spleen cells to lipopolysaccharide (LPS) is suppressed by high doses (2.1 mg) of *C. parvum* (Howard *et al.*, 1973a; Kirchner *et al.*, 1975a).

12. LYMPHOCYTES—T CELLS

C. parvum has multiple effects on T lymphocyte function. *C. parvum* causes marked decreases in thymus weight and a relative decrease in the number of T cells in spleen and lymph nodes. In thymectomized mice treated with antilymphocyte serum, *C. parvum* produces increases in the relative number of T cells in these organs; this is presumed to be due to direct stimulation of residual T cell populations (Likhite, 1975).

C. parvum influences many immune functions mediated by T cells, i.e. delayed hypersensitivity rections; mitogenic responses to policlonal mitogens (PHA and concanavalin A); mixed lymphocyte responses (MLR); graft versus host reactions (GVH); skin graft rejection; and lymphocyte mediated cytolysis. Scott (1972a) observed that seven days after administration spleen cells failed to respond to PHA. Marked depression of this response was also noted in lymphocytes from peripheral blood. This effect is somehow restricted as immunologically inert bacterium, i.e. *C. diphtheriae* are not suppressive.

Other investigators (Kirchner *et al.*, 1975a; Milas *et al.*, 1975) have made similar observations using Con A. Kirchner *et al.*, (1975a) reported that high dose *C. parvum* (2.0 mg) suppressed responses to PHA, Con A, and the B cell mitogen LPS, while low dose (0.2 mg) only suppressed responses to Con A and PHA. Very low doses (0.035 and 0.0025 mg) are either ineffective or may increase mitogen responses (Milas *et al.*, 1975; Scott and Warner, 1976).

Pretreatment of recipients (F1 hybrids) with *C. parvum* dramatically decreased the severity of GVH disease, as measured by decreased mortality and prolongation of survival (Howard *et al.*, 1967). This protection could not be adoptively transferred. Subsequently, Scott (1972a) and Mathe *et al.*, (1973) showed that the severity of GVH was also decreased when *C. parvum* was administered to donor mice. The best explanation for these observations is that *C. parvum* suppresses donor T cells responsible for GVH.

C. parvum can also inhibit the ability of mice to reject skin grafts (Castro, 1974a; Colapinto, 1975; Iossifides *et al.*, 1964; Milas *et al.*, 1975). Survival time for allogeneic grafts, (both H2 incompatible) is prolonged by 25–100%. Survival time of syngeneic male to female grafts may be slightly prolonged or shortened, depending on when *C. parvum* is administered (Colapinto, 1975).

Kirchner *et al.*, (1975b) showed that killer T cells cytotoxic (by ^{51}Cr release) to a virus-induced tumor could be generated by culturing spleen cells *in vitro* with the tumor cells. The degree of cytotoxicity generated by spleen cells from *C. parvum*-treated mice was strikingly lower than in normal spleen cells. Berd and Mitchell (1976) made similar observations *in vivo*. Mice injected with allogeneic leukemia cells develop splenic T cells cytotoxic *in vitro*. Pretreatment with *C. parvum* significantly diminished cytotoxicity. Suppression of cytotoxicity in both systems could be partially explained by dilution of T cells in *C. parvum* spleens, but the results obtained when varying the spleen cell/target cell ratio and the inhibition of normal spleen cells when adding *C. parvum* spleen cells suggest alternative mechanism(s). Suppression of the generation or the activity of cytotoxic T cells seems more probable. To that effect Murahata and Zighelboim (1979) demonstrated that systemic administration of *C. parvum* following subcutaneous immunization of C57B1/6 mice with allogenic P815 (H-2d) tumor cells impaired expression of primary cell mediated cytotoxicity in spleen. Additionally, these splenocytes have reduced ability to generate memory cytotoxicity when restimulated *in vitro* or *in vivo* with the appropriate alloantigens (Murahata and Zighelboim, 1979; Murahata and Zighelboim, 1980). Decreased memory cytotoxicity following rechallenge with intraperitoneal P815 mastocytoma was detected in spleen and mesenteric lymph nodes. Peritoneal cavity lymphocytes only expressed a slight decrease in cytotoxicity. By contrast, serum levels of cytotoxic antibodies to the same alloantigens (H-2d) were unaffected, suggesting that the bacterium had selective effects on the cellular immune response.

The effect of *C. parvum* on primary and memory cytotoxic immune responses were dependent on the dose and route of administration of the bacterium (Lichtenstein *et al.*, 1980). Only systemic administration (I.V. or I.P.) caused suppression of the primary and memory cytotoxic responses. Injection of *C. parvum* either subcutaneously or admixed with tumor cells had lesser or no effects.

The effects of *C. parvum* on primary and memory cytotoxicity seemed to be mediated by different components of the bacterium cell wall. These were dissociatable chemically and pharmacologically. Hot phenol-water extraction of killed *C. parvum* cells generated a residue fraction which upon treatment with metaperiodate lost its ability to suppress memory but not primary cytotoxic responses. This fractionation procedure also generated a fraction that had the opposite effects, i.e. selectively inhibited primary but not memory cytotoxicity. These results indicate that generation of primary and memory cytotoxicity are not linked (Murahata and Zighelboim, 1980).

Systemic *C. parvum* also suppresses cytotoxic immune responses to syngeneic virus-induced tumors or minor histocompatibility antigens (Lichtenstein *et al.*, 1983a). A single I.V. injection of *C. parvum* to B10.BR ($H\text{-}2^k$) mice primed with allo-identical CBA/J ($H\text{-}2^k$) spleen cells inhibits a subsequent secondary *in vitro* generation of CTLs. The inhibitory effect was possibly induced by (specific and/or non-specific) regulatory cells present in the spleen of these mice.

Other evidence, although a bit circumstantial, for direct effect of *C. parvum* on T lymphocytes is provided by the work of Halpern and Fray (1969) on NZB mice. These animals spontaneously develop hemolytic anemia which generally begins at about five months of age. In contrast, NZB mice given *C. parvum* develop this condition at 6–8 weeks, an age when the disease is never seen in untreated mice. The authors attributed this observation to a stimulation of anti-erythrocyte antibody by *C. parvum*. More recent experiments (Krakauer *et al.*, 1976) suggest, however, that auto-immunity in these mice is due to a loss of T suppressors of anti-self immune responses.

As described above, *C. parvum* suppresses many T cell functions under experimental conditions. This suppression seems to be mediated by regulatory cells. Splenocytes may play an important role. Scott (1974a) observed that suppression of DH to sheep erythrocytes was prevented by splenectomy. Splenectomy, however, did not neutralize the inhibitory effects of *C. parvum* on allogeneic skin graft rejection (Milas *et al.*, 1975). Other effects of *C. parvum* on T cell functions may be indirect, i.e. via activated macrophages. Spleen cell response to mitogens can be restored by depletion of an adherent, phagocytic and radioresistant cell population insensitive to anti-theta serum (Kirchner *et al.*, 1975a; Scott, 1972b). Moreover, adherent cells from *C. parvum* spleen when mixed with normal spleen cells markedly suppressed their mitogen responsiveness. *C. parvum*-stimulated adherent-phagocytic cells can also suppress generation of cytotoxic T cells *in vitro* (Kirchner *et al.*, 1975b). But in the *in vivo* system of Berd and Mitchell (1976) depletion of adherent cells did not restore cytotoxicity nor did mixing *C. parvum* adherent cells with cytotoxic cells.

This evidence overwhelmingly supports the idea of a population of macrophages stimulated by *C. parvum* that actively suppress responsiveness of B cells to mitogens and inhibit the maturation of T lymphocytes to cytotoxic cells. T cells that have already differentiated into killer cells, however, are not interfered. Whether this mechanism applied to the other immunosuppressive effects of *C. parvum* and whether it is operative *in vivo* are unanswered questions.

13. NK CELLS

C. parvum has been reported to cause marked augmentation (Gallagher, M. T. *et al.*, 1979; Djeu *et al.*, 1979) as well as marked suppression (Ojo *et al.*, 1978; Savary and Lotzova, 1978) of NK cell activity. These discordant results may reflect the use of strains of *C. parvum* with different immunologic properties. This theory was confirmed by Nasrallah *et al.*, (1980) on NK cell activity in mice inoculated with different strains of *C. parvum*.

Recently, Lichtenstein *et al.*, (1983b) showed that intraperitoneal injection of *C. parvum* cells into naive rats caused marked augmentation of NK activity among PEC. Comparable effects were obtained following injection of HCL modified cells or cell wall components obtained following extractive treatment of whole cells with pyridine. The boosting effect was first noticed on day three following inoculation and usually lasted for 3–4 weeks. How *C. parvum* causes augmentation of NK activity is still unknown. Stimulation of interferon production is one of the most likely possibilities.

14. CONCLUDING REMARKS

It is simplistic to characterize *C. parvum* as an immunostimulant. Clearly, *C. parvum* influences humoral and cellular immune responses to a variety of antigens. These responses are either amplified or suppressed depending on the experimental conditions. Commenting on this point, Mathe *et al.*, (1973) proposed that *C. parvum* (and similar materials) be referred to as an immunomodulator. Even this term is imprecise, since some of its most striking biologic effects, i.e. antitumor and anti-microbial activities could have nothing to do with modulation of immune function. After all, antitumor activity persists in the face of severe immunosuppression, e.g. T cell deprived mice. Similarly, *C. parvum* increase resistance to infectious agents while simultaneously decreasing the host immune responses to the specific pathogen.

Perhaps Prevot's original appellation of 'reticulostimulant' is most accurate. *C. parvum* stimulates the bone marrow to generate macrophages and directly activates these calls morphologically and functionally (chemotaxis, lymphocyte trapping, particle clearance). The activated macrophages mediate non-specific anti-microbial and anti-tumor activity which is non-immunologic in nature and influences the immune system by modulating (enhancing or suppressing) lymphocyte functions. The physiologic outcome may be resistance to infection or susceptibility to infection, tumor inhibition or tumor enhancement, adjuvanticity or immunosuppression, depending on the experimental conditions.

The information derived from experimental systems should guide us in exploring the clinical applications of *C. parvum*. The most obvious of these is the treatment of malignant tumors. It is probable that it will be effective only in patients with very small tumor burdens or when given with tumoricidal agents. Moreover, *C. parvum* may impair the induction of tumor-specific immunity by vaccines. Enhancement of human tumors is also possible, although this could be detected only by carefully controlled studies.

C. parvum may have other clinical applications, particularly in organ transplantation, i.e. delay the rejection of visceral allografts in humans. Transplantation of allogeneic bone marrow to patients treated with *C. parvum* is an interesting possibility, since the severity of the graft versus host reaction might be decreased.

Finally, it is apparent that the biologically active material we refer to as *C. parvum* may be derived from several species of anaerobic coryneform bacteria. These organisms reside as saprophytes in the bodies of animals and humans (Rogosa *et al.*, 1974). One cannot help but wonder if they are constantly affecting subtle but significant changes in our immune function, and, more specifically, whether they modulate our response to malignant tumors.

REFERENCES

ALLWOOD, G. G. and ASHERSON, G. L. (1971) Depression of delayed hypersensitivity by pretreatment with Freund-type adjuvants. II. Mechanism of the phenomenon. *Clin. Exp. Immunol.* **9:** 259–266.

ASHERSON, G. L. and ALLWOOD, G. G. (1971) Depression of delayed hypersensitivity by pretreatment with Freund-type adjuvants. I. Description of the phenomenon. *Clin. Exp. Immunol.* **9:** 249–258.

BASIC, I., MILAS, L., GRDINA, D. J. and WITHERS, H. R. (1975) *In vitro* destruction of tumor cells by macrophages from mice treated with *C. granulosum. J Natl. Cancer Inst.* **55:** 589–596.

BAST, R. C., BEREK, J. S., OBRIST, R., GRIFFITH, C. T., BERKOWITZ, R. S., HACKER, N. F., PARKER, L., LAGASSE, L. D. and KNAPP, R. C. (1983) Intraperitoneal immunology of human ovarian carcinoma with *Corynebacterium parvum. Cancer Res.* **43:** 1395–1401.

BAST, R. C., KNAPP, R. C., MITCHELL, A. K., THURSTON, J. G., TUCKEE, R. W. and SCHOLSSMAN, S. F. (1979) Immunology of a murine ovarian carcinoma with *Corynebacterium parvum* and specific hetero antiserum. I. Activation of peritoneal cells to mediate antibody mediated cellular cytotoxicity. *J. Immunol.* **132:** 1945–1951.

BERD, D. A. and MITCHELL, M. S. (1976) Immunological enhancement of leukemia L1210 by *Corynebacterium parvum* in allogeneic mice. *Cancer Res.* **36:** 4119–4124.

BEREK, J. S., LICHTENSTEIN, A. K., LAGASSE, L., NEIBERG, R. and ZIGHELBOIM, J. (1983) Immunotherapy with biochemically dissociated *C. parvum* fractions. Submitted for publication.

BIOZZI, G., STIFFEL, C., MOUTON, D., BOUTHILLIER, Y. and DECREUSEFOND, C. (1968) A kinetic study of antibody producing cells in the spleen of mice immunized intravenously with sheep erythrocytes. *Immunology* **14:** 7–20.

BOMFORD, R. and OLIVOTTO, M. (1974) The mechanism of inhibition by *Corynebacterium parvum* of the growth of lung nodules from intravenously injected tumor cells. *Int. J. Cancer* **14:** 226–235.

BROZOVIC, B., SLJIVIC, V. S. and WARR, G. W. (1975) Haematological changes and iron metabolism in rats. *Br. J. Exp. Pathol.* **56** (2): 183–192.

BUCK, G. E. and KELLEY, M. T. (1980) Investigation of the component of propionibacterium acnes *(Corynebacterium parvum)* responsible for macrophage activation. *Infection and Immun.* **27:** 620–627.

CASTRO, J. E. (1974a) The effect of *Corynebacterium parvum* on the structure and function of the lymphoid system in mice. *Eur. J. Cancer* **10:** 115–120.

CASTRO, J. E. (1974b) Antitumor effects of *Corynebacterium parvum* in mice. *Eur. J. Cancer* **10:** 121–127.

CHAPES, S. K. and HASKILL, S. (1982) Role of *Corynebacterium parvum* in the activation of peritoneal macrophages. *Cell Immunol.* **70:** 65–75.

COLAPINTO, N. D. (1975) Skin grafting across the H–Y barrier and the effect of biological adjuvants. *Proc. R. Soc. Lond. Ser. B,* **189:** 107–119.

COLLINS F. M. and SCOTT M. T. (1974) Effect of *Corynebacterium parvum* treatment on the growth of *Salmonella enteriditis* in mice. *Infec. Immunity* **9:** 863–869.

DEGRAND, F. and RAYNAUD, M. (1973) Quantitative effect of *Mycobacteria* and of anaerobic *Corynebacteria* upon immunogenic activity of azobenzearsonate-N-acetyl-L-tyrosine in guinea pigs. *Eur. J. Immunol.* **3:** 660–661.

DEL GUERCIO, P. and LEUCHARS, E. (1972) The immune response in mice to the haptenic determinant DNP coupled to a thymus-independent carrier (Levan). *J. Immunol.* **109:** 951–956.

DIENER, E., SHORTMAN, K. and RUSSELL, P. (1970) Induction of immunity and tolerance *in vitro* in the absence of phagocytic cells. *Nature* **225:** 731–732.

DIMITROV, N. V., ANDRE, S., ELIOPOULOS, G. and HALPERN, B. (1975) Comparative studies on the effect of *Corynebacterium parvum* on bone-marrow cell colony formation *in vitro*. In: *Corynebacterium parvum. Applications in Experimental and Clinical Oncology,* pp. 173–180. HALPERN, B. (ed.). Plenum Press, New York.

DIMITROV, N. V., GREENBERG, CH.S. and DENNY, T. (1977) Organ distribution of *Corynebacterium parvum* labelled with iodine-125. *J. Natl. Cancer Inst.* **58:** 287–294.

DJEU, J. Y., HEMBAUGH, J. A., HOLDEN, H. T. and HERBERMAN, R. B. (1979) Augmentation of mouse natural killer cell activity by interferon and interferon inducers. *J. Immunology* **122:** 175–181.

EVANS, S. R. and JOHNSON, H. M. (1981) The induction of at least two distinct types of interferon in mouse spleen cell cultures by *Corynebacterium parvum. Cell Immunol.* **64:** 64–72.

FISHER, B. and WOLMARK, N. (1976) Correlation of antitumor chemoimmunotherapy with bone marrow macrophage precursor cell stimulation and macrophage cytotoxicity. *Cancer Res.* **36:** 2241–2247.

FISHER, B., WOLMARK, N., RUBIN, H. and SAFFER, E. (1975) Further observations on the inhibition of tumor growth by *Corynebacterium parvum* and cyclophosphamide. I. Variation in administration of both agents. *J. Natl. Cancer Inst.* **55:** 1147–1153.

FISHER, B., RUBIN, H., SAFFER, E. and WOLMARK, N. (1976a) Further observations of the inhibition of tumor growth by *Corynebacterium parvum* with cyclophosphamide. II. Effect of cortisone acetate. *J. Natl. Cancer Inst.* **56:** 571–574.

FISHER, B., RUBIN, H. and WOLMARK, N. (1976b) Further observations on the inhibition of tumor growth by *Corynebacterium parvum* with cyclophosphamide. IV. Effect of rifampin on tumor growth inhibition, bone marrow macrophage precursor stimulation, and macrophage cytotoxicity. *J. Natl. Cancer Inst.* **57:** 317–322.

FRAY, A., SPARROS, LORINET, A. M. and HALPERN, B. (1975) Nonspecific cytotoxic activity of peritoneal exudate cells against isogenic tumoral cells in animal treated with *Corynebacterium parvum*. In: *Corynebacterium parvum. Applications in Experimental and Clinical Oncology,* pp. 181–186. HALPERN, B. (ed.). Plenum Press, New York.

FROST, P. and LANCE, E. M. (1973) The relation of lymphocyte trapping to the mode of action of adjuvants. In: *Immunopotentiation.* Ciba Foundation Symposium 18, pp. 29–38. Associated Scientific Publisher, Amsterdam.

GALLAGHER, M. T., NASRALLAH, A. G., DATTA, S. K., PRIEST, E. L., WEAVER, J. E. and TRENTIN, J. T. (1979) Stimulation of natural killer cell activity in infant, aged and low responder strain mice by *Corynebacterium parvum. Fed. Proc.* **38:** 1278.

GHAFFAR, A., CULLEN, R. T., DUNBAR, N. and WOODRUFF, M. F. A. (1974) Anti-tumor effect *in vitro* of lymphocytes and macrophages from mice treated with *Corynebacterium parvum. Br. J. Cancer* **29:** 199–205.

GHAFFAR, A., CULLEN, R. T. and WOODRUFF, M. F. A. (1975) Further analysis of the anti-tumor effect *in vitro* of peritoneal exudate cells from mice treated with *Corynebacterium parvum. Br. J. Cancer* **31:** 15–24.

GORCZYNSKI, R. M. (1976) Control of the immune response: Role of macrophages in regulation of antibody- and cell-mediated immune responses. *Scand. J. Immunol.* **5:** 1031–1047.

GREENBERG, C. S. and DIMITROV, N. V. (1976) The effect of hydrocortisone on the immune response of mice treated with *Corynebacterium parvum. Clin. Immunol. Immunopath.* **5:** 264–271.

HALPERN, B. and FRAY, A. (1969) Declenchement de l'anemie hemolytique autoimmune chez de jeunes souriceaux NZB par l'administration de *Corynebacterium parvum*. *Ann. Inst. Pasteur* **117:** 778–789.

HALPERN, B., PREVOT, A. R., BIOZZI, G., STIFFEL, C., MOUTON, D., MORARD, J. C., BOUTHILLIER, Y., and DECREUSEFOND, C. (1964) Stimulation de l'activite du systeme reticuloendothelial provoquee par *Corynebacterium parvum*. *J. Reticuloendothel. Soc.* **1:** 77–96.

HALPERN, B. N., BIOZZI, G., STIFFEL, C. and MOUTON, D. (1966) Inhibition of tumor growth by administration of killed *Corynebacterium parvum*. *Nature* **212:** 853–854.

HALPERN, B., FRAY, A., CREPIN, Y., PLATICA, O., LORINET, A. M., RABOURDIN, A., SPARROS, L. and ISAC, R. (1973) *Corynebacterium parvum*, a potent immunostimulant in experimental infections and in malignancies. In: *Immunopotentiation,* Ciba Foundation Symposium 18, pp. 217–236. Associated Scientific Publishers, Amsterdam.

HASKILL, S., RITTER, F. and BECKER, S. (1980) Effect of *C. parvum* on intratumor immunity to the T1699 mammary adenocarcinoma. *J. Immunol.* **125:** 454–458.

HOUCHENS, D. P., JOHNSON, R. K., OVEJERA, A., GASTO, M. R. and GOLDIN, A. (1976) Effects of *Corynebacterium parvum* alone and in combination with adriamycin in experimental tumor systems. *Cancer Treat. Rep.* **60:** 823–828.

HOWARD, J. G., BIOZZI, G., STIFFEL, C., MOUTON, D. and LIACOPOULOS, P. (1967) an analysis of the inhibitory effect of *Corynebacterium parvum* on graft-versus-host disease. *Transplantation* **5:** 1510–1524.

HOWARD, J. G., CHRISTIE, G. H. and SCOTT, M. T. (1973a) Biologic effects of *Corynebacterium parvum*. IV. Adjuvant and inhibitory activities on B lymphocyts. *Cell. Immunol.* **7:** 290–310.

HOWARD, J. G., SCOTT, M. T. and CHRISTIE, G. H. (1973b) Cellular mechanisms underlying the adjuvant activity of *Corynebacterium parvum*: Interaction of activated macrophages with T and B lymphocytes. In: *Immunopotentiation.* Ciba Foundation Symposium 18, pp. 101–116. Associated Scientific Publisher, Amsterdam.

IOSSIFIDES, I. A., GUTZAIT, L., BRAND, M. and TOCANTINS, L. M. (1964) Enhanced survival of skin homografts in mice with a bacterial infection. *Ann. N.Y. Acad. Sci.* **114:** 487–495.

JAMES, K., GHAFFAR, A. and MILNE, I. (1974) The effect of transplanted methycholanthrene induced fibrosarcoma and *Corynebacterium parvum* on the immune response of CBA and A/HeJ mice to thymus dependent and independent antigens. *Br. J. Cancer* **29:** 11–20.

JOHNSON, J. L. and CUMMINS, C. S. (1972) Cell wall composition and deoxyribonucleic acid similarities among the anaerobic coryneforms, classical propionibacteria, and strains of *Arachnia propionica*. *J. Bacteriol.* **109:** 1047–1065.

JONES, J. T., MCBRIDE, W. H. and WEIR, D. M. (1975) The *in vitro* killing of syngeneic cells by peritoneal cells from adjuvant-stimulated mice. *Cell. Immunol.* **18:** 375–383.47.

KIRCHNER, H., HOLDEN, H. T. and HERBERMAN, R. B. (1975a) Splenic suppressor macrophages induced in mice by injection of *Corynebacterium parvum*. *J. Immunol.* **115:** 1212–1216.

KIRCHNER, H., GLASER, M. and HERBERMAN, R. B. (1975b) Suppression of cell-mediated tumor immunity by *Corynebacterium parvum*. *Nature* **257:** 396–397.

KIRSHNER, H., HIRT, M. M., BECKER, H. and MUNK, K. (1977) Production of an antiviral factor by murine spleen cells after treatment with *Corynebacterium parvum*. *Cellular Immunol.* **31:** 172–176.

KNAPP, R. C. and BERKOWITZ, R. S. (1976) *Corynebacterium parvum* as an immunotherapeutic agent in an ovarian cancer model. *Am. J. Obstet. Gynecol.* **128:** 782–786.

KNIGHT, P. A. and LUCKEN, R. N. (1975) The effects of *Corynebacterium parvum* suspension on the response to tetanus toxoid. In: *Corynebacterium parvum. Applications in Experimental and Clinical Oncology,* pp. 91–99. HALPERN, B. (ed.). Plenum Press, New York.

KRAKAUER, R. S., WALDMANN, T. A. and STROBER, W. (1976) Loss of supressor T cells in adult NZB/NZW mice. *J. Exp. Med.* **144:** 662–673.

LICHTENSTEIN, A. K., ALI, M., MACK, P. and ZIGHELBOIM, J. (1983a) Regulation of cytotoxic reactivity to minor histocompatibility antigens by administration of *Corynebacterium parvum*. *Transplantation,* in press.

LICHTENSTEIN, A. K., BEREK, J. S. and ZIGHELBOIM, J. (1983c). Role of neutrophils in antitmor effects of intraperitoneal *C. parvum*. Submitted for publication.

LICHTENSTEIN, A., BICK, A., CANTRELL, J. and ZIGHELBOIM, J. (1983b) Augmentation of NK activity by *Corynebacterium parvum* fractions *in vivo* and *in vitor*. *Int. J. Immunopharm.* In press.

LICHTENSTEIN, A., MURAHATA, R., SUGASAWARA, R. and ZIGHELBOIM, J. (1981a) Suppressor T cells and suppressor macrophages induced by *Corynebacterium parvum*. *Cell. Immunol.* **58:** 257–268.

LICHTENSTEIN, A., MURAHATA, R., TERPENNING, M., CANTRELL, J. and ZIGHELBOIM, J. (1981b) Activation and mechanism of action of suppressor macrophages. *Cell. Immunol.*

LICHTENSTEIN, A., MURAHATA, R. and ZIGHELBOIM, J. (1980) Inhibition of cell-mediated cytotoxicity by *Corynebacterium parvum*. *Cancer Immunol. Immunother.* **8:** 39–44.

LIKHITE, V. V. (1975) Rejection of mammary adenocarcinoma cell tumors in DBA/2 mice immunocompromised by thymectomy and treatment with antithymocyte serum. *J. Immunol.* **114:** 1736–1741.

LIKHITE, V. V. and HALPERN, B. N. (1974) Lasting rejection of mammary adenocarcinomacell tumors in DBA/2 mice with intratumor injection of killed *Corynebacterium parvum*. *Cancer Br.* **34:** 341–344.

MANTOVANI, A., SESA, C., PERI, G., ALLAVENA, P., INTRONA, M., POLENTARUTTI, N. and MANGIONI, C. (1981) Intraperitoneal administration of *Corynebacterium parvum* in patients with ascitic ovarian tumors resistant to chemotherapy: effects on cytotoxicity of tumor-associated macrophages and NK cells. *Int. J. Cancer* **27:** 437–446.

MANTOVANI, A., TAGLIABUE, A., VECCHI, A. and SPREAFICO, F. (1976) Effect of *Corynebacterium parvum* on cellular and humoral antitumoral immune effector mechanisms. *Eur. J. Cancer* **12:** 113–123.

MATHE, G., KAMEL, M., DEZFULIAN, M., HALLE-PANNENKO, O. and BOURUT, C. (1973) An experimental screening for systemic adjuvants of immunity applicable in cancer immunotherapy. *Cancer Res.* **33:** 1987–1997.

MCBRIDE, W. H., DAWES, J., DUNBAR, N., GHAFFAR, A. and WOODRUFF, M. M. A. (1975A) A comparative study of anaerobic coryneforms. Attempts to correlate their anti-tumor activity with their serological properties and ability to stimulate the lymphoreticular system. *Immunology* **28:** 49–58.

McBride, W. H., Tuach, S. and Marmion, B. P. (1975b) The effects of gold salts on tumor immunity and its stimulation by *Corynebacterium parvum*. *Br. J. Cancer* **32:** 550–567.

McBride, W. H., Tuach, S. and Marmion, B. P. (1975c) The effect of gold salts on tumor immunity and its stimulation by *Corynebacterium parvum*. *Br. J. Cancer* **32:** 558–567.

Mignot, M. H., Lens, J. W., Drexhage, H. A., von Blomberg, B. M. E., Flier, V. D., Cort, J. and Stolk, G. (1981). Lower relapse rates after neighborhood injection of *Corynebacterium parvum* in operable cervix carcinoma.

Milas, L., Hunter, N., Basic, I. and Withers, H. R. (1974a) Complete regressions of an established murine fibrosarcoma induced by systemic application of *C. granulosum*. *Cancer Res.* **34:** 2470–2475.

Milas, L., Gutterman, J. U., Bais, I., Hunter, N., Mavligit, G., Hersh, E. M. and Withers, R. R. (1974b) Immunoprophylaxis and immunotherapy for a murine fibrosarcoma with *C. granulosum* and *C. parvum*. *Int. J. Cancer* **14:** 493–503.

Milas, L., Basic, I., Kogelnik, H. D. and Withers, H. R. (1975) Effects of *Corynebacterium granulosum* on weight and histology of lymphoid organs, response to mitogens, skin allografts and a syngeneic fibrosarcoma in mice. *Cancer Res.* **35:** 2365–2374.

Murahata, R. I. and Zighelboim, J. (1979) Inhibition of memory cell-mediated cytotoxic response by systemic administration of *Corynebacterium parvum*. *Cell. Immunol.* **42:** 289–279.

Murahata, R. I., Cantrell, J., Lichtenstein, A. and Zighelboim, J. (1980) Dissociation of biological activites of *Corynebacterium parvum* by chemical fractionation. *Int. J. Immunopharmac.* **2:** 47–53.

Murahata, R. I. and Zighelboim, J. (1980) Systemic administration of *Corynebacterium parvum* during sensitization to tumor alloantigen modified response to rechallenge. *Cancer Immunol. Immunother.* **8:** 257–261.

Nasrallah, A. G., Gallagher, M. T., Priest, E. L. and Trentin, J. J. (1980) Comparative effects of different strains of *Corynebacterium parvum* on natural cell mediated cytotoxicity. *Cancer Res.* **40:** 4159–4164.

Neveu, T., Branellec, A. and Biozzi, G. (1964) Proprietes adjuvantes de *Corynebacterium parvum* sur la production d'anticorps et su l'induction de l'hypersensibilite retardee envers les proteines conjuguees. *Ann. Inst. Pasteur* **106:** 771–777.

Nussenzweig, R. S. (1967) Increased nonspecific resistance to malaria produced by administration of killed *Corynebacterium parvum*. *Exp. Parasitol.* **21:** 224–231.

Ojo, E., Haller, O., Kimura, A. and Wigzell, H. (1978). An analysis of conditions allowing *Corynebacterium parvum* to cause either augmentation of inhibition of natural killer cell activity against tumor cells in mice. *Int. J. Cancer* **21:** 444–452.

Olivotto, M. and Bomford, R. (1974) *In vitro* inhibition of tumor cell growth and DNA synthesis by peritoneal and lung macrophages from mice injected with *Corynebacterium parvum*. *Int. J. Cancer* **15:** 478–488.

O'Neill, G. J., Henderson, D. C. and White, R. G. (1973) The role of anaerobic coryneforms on specific and non-specific immunological reactions. I. Effect on particle clearance and humoral and cell-mediated immunological responses. *Immunology* **24:** 977–995.

Pinckard, R. N. and Halonen, M. (1971) The enhancement of rabbit anti-BSA IgE, homocytotropic antibody production by *Corynebacterium parvum* strain 10387. *J. Immunol.* **106:** 1602–1608.

Pinckard, R. N., Weir, D. M. and McBride, W. H. (1967a) Factors influencing the immune response. I. Effects of the physical state of the antigen and of lymphoreticular cell proliferation on the response to intravenous injection of bovine serum albumin in rabbits. *Clin. Exp. Immunol.* **2:** 331–341.

Pinckard, R. N., Weir, D. M. and McBride, W. H. (1967b) Factors influencing the immune response. II. Effects of the physical state of the antigen and of lymphoreticular cell proliferation on the response to intraperitoneal injection of bovine serum albumin in rabbits. *Clin. Exp. Immunol.* **2:** 343–350.

Pinckard, R. N., Weir, D. M. and McBride, W. H. (1967c) Effects of *Corynebacterium parvum* on immunological unresponsiveness to bovine serum albumin in the rabbit. *Nature* **215:** 870–871.

Pinckard, R. N., Weir, D. M. and McBride, W. H. (1968) Factors influencing the immune response. III. The blocking effect of *Corynebacterium parvum* upon the induction of acquired immunological unresponsiveness to bovine serum albumin in the adult rabbit. *Clin. Exp. Immunol.* **3:** 413–421.

Playfair, J. H. L. and Purves, E. C. (1971) Antibody formation by bone marrow cells in irradiated mice. I. Thymus dependent and thymus independent responses to sheep erythrocytes. *Immunology* **21:** 113–121.

Prevot, A. R. (1975) Bacteriological aspects of anaerobic corynebacteria in relation to RES stimulation. In: *Corynebacterium parvum. Applications in Experimental and Clinical Oncology*, pp. 3–10. Halpern, B. (ed.). Plenum Press, New York.

Pringle, A. T. and Cummins, C. S. (1981) The cell surface of propionibacterium acnes: effect of specific chemical modification of the ability of vaccines to produce splenomegaly in mice. *Can. J. Microbiol.* **28:** 375–382.

Proctor, J., Reudenstam, C. M. and Alexander, P. (1973) Increased incidence of lung metastases following treatment of rats bearing hepatomas with irradiated tumor cells and the beneficial effect of *Corynebacterium parvum* in this system. *Biomedicine* **19:** 248–252.

Purnell, D. M. (1976) Enhancement of tissue invasion in murine aspergillosis by systemic administration of suspensions of killed *Corynebacterium parvum*. *Am. J. Pathol.* **83:** 547–555.

Purnell, D. M., Otterstrom, J. R., Bartlett, G. L. and Kreider, J. W. (1976) Antitumor activity of killed *Corynebacterium parvum* suspensions in a murine mammary adenocarcinoma (CaD2) system. *J. Natl. Cancer Inst.* **56:** 1171–1175.

Rogosa, M., Cummins, C. S., Lelliot, R. A. and Keddie, R. M. (1974) Coryneform group of bacteria. In: *Bergey's Manual of Determinative Bacteriology*, p. 640. Buchanan, R. E. and Gibbons, N. E. (eds.). William and Wilkins, Baltimore.

Ruitenberg, E. J. and Steerenberg, P. A. (1973) Possible immunosuppressive effect of *Corynebacterium parvum* on infection with *Trichinella spiralis*. *Nature New Biol.* **242:** 149–150.

Ruitenberg, E. J. and van Noorle Jansen, L. M. (1975) Effect of *Corynebacterium parvum* on the course of a *Listeria monocytogenes* injection in normal and congenitally athymic (nude) mice. *Zbl. Bact. Hyg. I. Abt. Orig.* **A 231:** 197–205.

Sadler, T. E. and Castro, J. E. (1976) Lack of immunological and antitumor effects of orally administered *Corynebacterium parvum* in mice. *Br. J. Cancer* **31:** 359–363.

SAVANY, C. A. and LOTZOVA, E. (1978) Suppression of natural killer cell cytotoxicity by splenocytes from *Corynebacterium parvum* injected bone marrow-tolerant and infant mice. *J. Immunol.* **120:** 239–243.

SCHULTZ, R. M., PAPAMATHEAKIS, J. D., STYLOS, W. A. and CHIRIGOS, M. A. (1976) Augmentation of specific macrophage-mediated cytotoxicity: correlation with agents which enhance antitumor resistance. *Cell. Immunol.* **25:** 309–316.

SCOTT, M. T. (1972a) Biological effects of the adjuvant *Corynebacterium parvum*. I. Inhibition of PHA, mixed lymphocyte and GVH reactivity. *Cell. Immunol.* **5:** 459–468.

SCOTT, M. T. (1972b) Biological effects of the adjuvant *Corynebacterium parvum*. II. Evidence for macrophage-T-cell interaction. *Cell. Immunol.* **5:** 469–479.

SCOTT, M. T. (1974a) Depression of delayed-type hypersensitivity by *Corynebacterium parvum*: Mandatory role of the spleen. *Cell. Immunol.* **13:** 251–263.

SCOTT, M. T. (1974b) *Corynebacterium parvum* as a therapeutic antitumor agent in mice. I. Systemic effects from intravenous injection. *J. Natl. Cancer Inst.* **53:** 855–860.

SCOTT, M. T. (1974c) *Corynebacterium parvum* as a therapeutic antitumor agent in mice. II. Local injection. *J. Natl. Cancer Inst.* **53:** 861–865.

SCOTT, M. T. (1975a) *In vivo* cortisone sensitivity of nonspecific antitumor activity of *Corynebacterium parvum* activated mouse peritoneal macrophages. *J. Natl. Cancer Inst.* **54:** 789–792.

SCOTT, M. T. (1975b) Potentiation of the tumor-specific immune response by *Corynebacterium parvum*. *J. Natl. Cancer Inst.* **55:** 65–72.

SCOTT, M. T. (1976) Failure of *Corynebacterium parvum* presensitization to modify the antitumor effects of systemic and local therapeutic injections of *Corynebacterium parvum* in mice. *J. Natl. Cancer Inst.* **56:** 675–677.

SCOTT, M. T. and WARNER, S. L. (1976) The accumulated effects of repeated systemic or local injections of low doses of *Corynebacterium parvum* in mice. *Cancer Res.* **36:** 1335–1338.

SHER, N. A., CHAPARAS, S. D., GREENBERG, L. E. and BERNARD, S. (1975) Effects of BCG, *Corynebacterium parvum*, and Methanol-Extraction Residue in the reduction of mortality from *Staphlococcus aureus* and *Candida albicans* infection immunosuppressed mice. *Infec. Immunity* **12:** 1325–1330.

SMITH, S. E. and SCOTT, M. T. (1972) Biological effects of *Corynebacterium parvum*: III. Amplification of resistance and impairment of active immunity to murine tumors. *Br. J. Cancer* **26:** 361–367.

SIFFEL, C., MOUTON, D. and BIOZZI, G. (1970) Kinetics of the phagocytic function of reticuloendothelial macrophages *in viv*. In: *Mononuclear Phagocytes*, pp. 335–381. VAN FURTH, R. (ed.). Blackwell Scientific Publications, Oxford and Edinburgh.

SWARTZBERG, J. E., KRAHENBUHL, J. L. and REMINGTON, J. S. (1975) Dichotomy between macrophage activation and degree of protection against *Listeria monocytogenes* and *Toxoplasma gondii* in mice stimulated with *Corynebacterium parvum*. *Infec. Immunity* **12:** 1037–1043.

SZMIGIELSKI, S., ROSZKOWSKI, W., ROSZKOWSKI, K., KO, H. L., JELJASZEWICZ, J. and PULVENER, B. (1982) Experimental immunostimulation by prepionibacteria. In: *Bacteria and Cancer*, pp. 129–147. JELJASZEWICZ, J., PULVENER, B. and ROSZKOWSKI, W. (eds.). Academic Press, London.

TOUJAS, L., DAZORD, L. and GUEFFI, J. (1975) Kinetics of proliferation of bone marrow cell lines after injection of immunostimulant bacteria. In: *Corynebacterium parvum. Applications in Experimental and Clinical Oncology*, pp. 117–125. HALPERN, B. (ed.). Plenum Press, New York.

TUTTLE, R. L. and NORTH, R. J. (1975) Mechanisms of antitumor action of *Corynebacterium parvum*: nonspecific tumor cell destruction at site of an immunologically mediated sensitivity reaction to *Corynebacterium parvum*. *J. Natl. Cancer Inst.* **55:** 1403–1411.

WARR, G. W. and SLJIVIC, V. S. (1974) Enhancement and depression of the antibody response in mice caused by *Corynebacterium parvum*. *Clin. Exp. Immunology* **17:** 519–532.

WARR, G. W. and JAMES K. (1975) Effect of *Corynebacterium parvum* on the class and subclass of antibody produced in the response of different strains of mice to sheep erythrocytes. *Immunology* **28:** 431–441.

WATSON, S. R. and SLJIVIC, V. S. (1976) The role of macrophages in the adjuvant effect on antibody production of *Corynebacterium parvum*. *Clin. Exp. Immunology* **17:** 141–149.

WEINER, E. (1975) The role of macrophages in the amplified *in vitro* response to sheep red blood cells by spleen cells from *Corynebacterium parvum* treated mice. *Cell. Immunology* **19:** 1–7.

WEINER, E. and BARDIERI, A. (1975) Modifications in the handling *in vitro* of ^{125}I-labeled keyhole limpet haemocyarin by peritoneal macrophages from mice pretreated with the adjuvant *Corynebacterium parvum*. *Immunology* **29:** 265–274.

WOODRUFF, M. F. A. and BOAK, J. L. (1966) Inhibitory effect of injection of *Corynebacterium parvum* on the growth of tumor transplants in isogeric hosts. *Br. J. Cancer* **20:** 345–355.

WOODRUFF, M. F. A. and DUNBAR, N. (1975) Effect of local injection of *Corynebacterium parvum* on the growth of a murine fibrosarcoma. *Br. J. Cancer* **32:** 34–41.

WOODRUFF, M. F. A., GHAFFAR, A., DUNBAR, N. and WHITEHEAD, V. L. (1976) Effect of *Corynebacterium parvum* on immunization with irradiated tumor cells. *Br. J. Cancer* **33:** 491–495.

CHAPTER 10

MODULATION OF THE IMMUNE RESPONSE BY CHEMOTHERAPY

Donald P. Braun and Jules E. Harris

Section of Medical Oncology, Department of Medicine, Department of Immunology, Rush-Presbyterian-St. Luke's Medical Center, 1753 West Congress Parkway, Chicago, Illinois 60612 U.S.A.

1. INTRODUCTION

Several decades of investigation have amply demonstrated that the immune response may be modified by various forms of drug treatment. Such modification may impair or augment immune function. Relevant factors in considering drug induced immunosuppression include: (1) the pharmacological action of the drug; (2) the pharmacokinetics of the drug; (3) the dosage and schedule of drug administration; (4) the nature of the immune response investigated; and (5) the influence of antigen administration schedule. Suppression of the immune response by drugs has been extensively reviewed (Schwartz, 1968; Hersch, 1974; Bach, 1975).

The past decade has seen important advances in our appreciation of the complex interactions between various subsets of T-cells, B-cells and macrophages during the immune response. Immunological responses were once considered simply as products of B-cells or T-cells. Those same responses are now considered as products of multiple positive and negative interactions between components of immunological circuits. Thus, the elicitation of a single recognized immune effector function such as IgG antibody synthesis is today known to be influenced by at least two kinds of T-cells (helper and suppressor), an array of antigen-specific B-cells, one or more kinds of macrophages and a growing multitude of serum substances (Waldman and Howard, 1979). The emphasis and intent of this review will be to describe how the multiple interacting components of the antigen-specific immune response may be altered by drugs.

2. DRUGS EFFECTS ON AFFERENT IMMUNE RESPONSES

The afferent limb of the immune response is triggered by exposure to antigenic material through injection, inhalation, ingestion or absorption. Inflammatory processes mediated by granulocytic, monocytic and lymphocytic components in conjunction with serum constituents culminate in antigen degradation and transport of antigenic materials to peripheral lymphatic organs (i.e. nodes or spleen) via lymphatic drainage (nodes) or blood circulation (spleen). In those organs, antigen is trapped at the surface of phagocytic cells for presentation to immunocompetent antigen-specific lymphocytes which are continuously in flux between lymph and blood. Interaction between membrane-bound antigen and specific but uncommitted lymphocyte is mediated by lymphocyte membrane receptors for determinants on antigenic molecules and on the surface of macrophages. Modulation of the afferent portion of the immune response by drugs would be affected by agents which influence monocyte/macrophage number and function, B-cell number and function or T-cell number and function in the context of antigen uptake, processing and presentation.

2.1. MONOCYTE/MACROPHAGE COMPONENTS

Alkylating agents in appropriate dose and schedule decrease both macrophage number and function in the absence of intentional antigenic stimulation. The most widely studied agent in this class is cyclophosphamide, an agent with activity in most phases of the immune response. In mice, cyclophosphamide decreases the number of peritoneal macrophages following injection of proteose peptone (Gadeberg *et al*., 1975) and decreases bacterial and viral uptake by the peritoneal cells (Gadeberg *et al*., 1975; Rhodes *et al*., 1975; Kabiri and Hadalgh, 1977). Inhibition of digestion by peritoneal macrophages following cyclophosphamide treatment has also been reported (Pereverseva, 1978). Cyclophosphamide treatment of mice prior to antigen injection has led to inhibition of antigen clearance from serum and markedly reduced antigen retention in the spleen. Drug treatment after antigen prevented antigen clearance from serum but did not effect antigen retention in the spleen (Nettesheim and Hammons, 1970). Antigen localization by dendritic reticulum cells may be resistant to cyclophosphamide (Miller *et al*., 1979). Cyclophosphamide treatment has led to decreased macrophage number and function in guinea pig peripheral blood (Hunninghake and Fauci, 1976) and human peripheral blood (Deinard *et al*., 1974; Smith *et al*., 1979). This results from decreased bone marrow stem cell production and maturation. The effect is at least partly responsible for the therapeutic efficacy of cyclophosphamide in the control of a variety of experimentally produced inflammatory disease states (Chang, 1977b). Bronchial alveolar macrophage numbers may be relatively resistant to cyclophosphamide. Administration of varying doses of cyclophosphamide sufficient to produce peripheral blood leukopenia did not decrease alveolar macrophage number in rats (Sharbaugh and Grogan, 1969), guinea pigs (Hunninghake and Fauci, 1977a; Pennington, 1978) or dogs (Lockhard *et al*., 1971; Reynolds *et al*., 1976). Impairment of antigen ingestion and degradation were noted with certain of those treatment regimens (Sharbaugh and Grogan, 1969; Lockhard *et al*., 1971; Hunninghake and Fauci, 1977a). Reduction of macrophage number and function by other alkylating agents such as nitrogen mustard (Netzel *et al*., 1977), and chlorambucil (Hersh and Freireich, 1968) has also been been reported.

Agents which inhibit DNA synthesis may also reduce macrophage number and function by impairment of macrophage production. Early studies demonstrated that agents such as 6-mercaptopurine, azathioprine, methotrexate and hydroxyurea prevent monocyte exudation during inflammatory responses (Page *et al*., 1962; Hersh *et al*., 1966; Hurd and Ziff, 1968). Utilizing a skin window technique, Hersh and coworkers (Hersh *et al*., 1966) showed a marked reduction of monocyte infiltration at 8 and 24 hr following surgical trauma in rabbits treated with either 6-MP or methotrexate. This was not necessarily associated with granulocytopenia or lymphopenia. Drug effects ceased within 5 days following treatment. Subsequent studies by Hurd and Ziff (Hurd and Ziff, 1968) attributed these effects to a suppression of bone marrow monocyte production. Van Furth and coworkers (Van Furth *et al*., 1975) demonstrated that azathioprine arrests the cell cycle of promonocytes thereby delaying mitosis. Treatment of mice with even low doses of azathioprine was found to increase cell cycle time of promonocytes by over 5 hr and led to a reduction of monocyte production by 70 per cent. Consistent with this observation is the finding that methotrexate or azathioprine decreases the accumulation of macrophages into the mouse peritoneal cavity following injection of irritants without altering the functional capacities of those cells (Gadeberg *et al*., 1975). Their therapeutic efficacy in the treatment of inflammatory diseases is also in keeping with that observation (Chang, 1977a). Alveolar macrophages are sensitive to treatment with DNA synthesis inhibitors. For example, rabbits given twice weekly doses of methotrexate exhibited progressive declines in alveolar macrophage number/gram tissue as early as one month after initiation of treatment without concomitant declines in peripheral blood monocyte, lymphocyte or granulocyte numbers (Sieger, 1977). Bacterial clearance by macrophages was not reduced until 6 months of treatment and was then attributed to decreased phagocytosis.

The steroid hormones were among the first agents to demonstrate immunomodulatory activity against macrophages (Vernon, 1969). Both reductions in macrophage number (Gadeberg *et al.*, 1975) and alteration of macrophage function (Fauci and Dale, 1974a,b) have been described with these agents. The effects seen are clearly dose related. Doses of cortisone in excess of 10 mg/kg markedly decreased antigen absorption and digestion in guinea pigs, rats and mice while doses below 5 mg/kg enhanced phagocytosis (Vernon, 1969). Nicol and coworkers (Nicol *et al.*, 1967) demonstrated that cortisol and prednisolone have greater anti-phagocytic activity than does cortisone. Multiple effects of these agents on most phases of the inflammatory process have been well documented (Hersh and Bodey, 1970). Steroid hormones also alter antigen localization in lymphoid tissues, increasing localization in the liver while decreasing localization in the spleen (Warr and Sljivic, 1973; Sljivic and Warr, 1973). Cortisone acetate given prior to antigen enhances antigen clearance from serum and reduces antigen retention in spleen (Nettesheim and Hammons, 1970). Drug treatment following antigen inhibits splenic antigen retention. A modification of membrane structure by the steroids is one means by which these agents distort macrophage function. In this regard, cortisone reportedly inhibits the binding of IgG-coated human erythrocytes to the macrophage Fc receptor and inhibits the binding of IgM-C3b-coated erythrocytes to the macrophage C3b receptor (Sljivic and Warr, 1973). In guinea pigs, cortisone acetate inhibited the clearence by splenic macrophages of guinea pig erythrocytes sensitized with low amounts of rabbit antibodies and the clearance by liver and splenic macrophages of erythrocytes sensitized with greater amounts of antibodies (Atkinson and Frank, 1974). Bronchial alveolar macrophage number and function were variably affected by cortisone in some studies, while cortisone in combination with cyclophosphamide drastically altered both the number and function of these cells (Pennington, 1977; Pennington, 1978). Absolute numbers of alveolar macrophages appear less sensitive to steroids than do lymphocytes (Reynolds *et al.*, 1976).

Actinomycin D and puromycin, antibiotics that inhibit RNA and protein synthesis respectively also suppress macrophages. Actinomycin D given prior to antigen reduces splenic retention without altering serum antigen clearance (Nettesheim and Hammons, 1970). Drug treatment following antigen inhibits serum antigen clearance without altering splenic antigen retention. Administration of these drugs to rabbits completely depressed monocyte inflammatory exudation; 5-fluorouracil was ineffective in similar experiments (Page *et al.*, 1964). Carminomycin, bleomycin and Actinomycin D-treated mice experienced impairment of phagocytosis by peritoneal macrophages without significant changes in the digestive activity of those cells (Nikulina, 1978). Cytochalasin B interacts with membrane structures and will inhibit the binding of peripheral blood monocytes to IgG sensitized erythrocytes (Atkinson and Parker, 1977), depress macrophage phagocytic function (Malawista *et al.*, 1971) and retard macrophage motility (Snyderman, 1971). Cytochalasins A and E irreversibly block the binding of sensitized erythrocytes to rabbit alveolar macrophages while cytochalasins D and B do so reversibly (Atkinson and Parker, 1977). Vinblastine and colchicine may also inhibit the membrane function of macrophages and like the cytochalasins, interefere with macrophage–erythrocyte binding. The target of that interference, however, appears to be the C3b receptor (Atkinson and Parker, 1977).

2.2. Lymphocyte Components

Lymphocytes that participate in the afferent portion of the immune response are immunocompetent but uncommitted. Their development is independent of antigen at this stage and their intermitotic interval is long. The majority of these cells circulate between blood and lymph until antigen triggering occurs. They then home to relevant peripheral lymphoid organs. Lymphocyte homing patterns following antigen injection have been reported to be altered by steroids (Zatz, 1975). This aspect of lymphoid sensitivity to drugs has not, however, been extensively investigated. Drug modulation of lymphocytes during the afferent portion of the immune response would be reflected by alteration of lymphocyte numbers, distribution and/or subset proportions in the absence of antigenic stimulation. Selectivity of drug action against lymphocyte subsets has been reported in many studies and may be attributed to either or both intrinsic differential sensitivity or differential recovery kinetics on the part of B and T cells.

The effects of cyclophosphamide on lymphocytes in the absence of intentional antigenic stimulation have been determined for most lymphoid tissue including lymph nodes, spleen, peripheral blood, bone marrow and thymus in a wide variety of animal species. Early studies by Turk and Poulter demonstrated that cyclophosphamide in a dose of 300 mg/kg given 3 times on alternating days exhaustively depleted lymphocytes from B-dependent areas in lymph nodes and spleen without substantially affecting lymphocytes in the T-dependent areas of those tissues (Turk and Poulter, 1972). Such treatments also depleted lymphocytes from the cortical region of thymus, the site of immature thymocyte development, without a drastic effect on the medullary areas of the thymus, the site of more mature thymocytes in that organ. These findings were confirmed by Stockman and coworkers (Stockman *et al.*, 1973) who also demonstrated that T-cell recovery in these organs was rapid (within 3 days following cessation of drug) while B-cell recovery was prolonged (14 days after drug). Those early studies demonstrating a greater relative sensitivity of B cells than T cells to cyclophosphamide have been repeatedly confirmed. However, some qualifcations are now in order. Dumont (1974) studied the repopulation by B and T cells of mouse spleen following a single injection (300 mg/kg) of cyclophosphamide. Total spleen nucleated cell numbers were reduced to 5 per cent of normal within 2 days following drug treatment and were found to recover and rebound to twice normal levels within 12 days. Normal cell numbers were reestablished within 30 days. B cell numbers declined to less than 3 per cent of normal within one day following drug treatment with recovery beginning on day 15 and normal levels reestablished by day 30. Two populations of T cells, characterized by different electrophoretic mobilities were also studied (Dumont and Barrois, 1975). The slower of these T cell populations was diminished on day 1, but recovered rapidly beginning on day 8. The faster of these T cell populations did not decline until day 8 and began to recover only on day 16. Normal numbers and proportions of these 2 different T cells populations was not restored until day 30. An alteration of thymic functions by cyclophosphamide may also contribute to the drug-induced reduction of lymphocytes. This was shown in studies by Kolb (1977) who demonstrated that cyclophosphamide depletes B cells completely from spleens of normal mice within 2 days but absolute numbers of T cells are also substantially diminished. When analyzed by electrophoretic mobility, both slow-moving B cells and faster-moving T cells declined uniformly. Following splenic atrophy, a period of hypertrophy was seen characterized by intense regeneration of Ig−+ cells and a relative paucity of Thy 1.2−+ cells. At this time, only one population of cells with an intermediate electrophoretic mobility between that of mature B and T cells was detectable. In T cell deficient ('B') mice treated with cyclophosphamide, the period of regeneration was characterized by the development of increased numbers of Ig−+ cells and null cells demonstrating a single peak of electrophoretic mobility similar to that seen during this period in normal drug-treated mice. Normal levels of T and B cells in both types of mice were restored by 16 days after drug treatment. Cyclophosphamide may reduce lymphocyte number in some lymphoid tissues more than in others. Thus, total lymphocytes following cyclophosphamide treatment reached nadir levels of 5 per cent of normal by day 3 in thymus, bone marrow, spleen and lymph nodes but repopulation kinetics differed markedly in each of those tissues (Willers and Sluis, 1975). Thymus lymphocytes exhibited rebound-overshoot recovery of lymphocyte numbers reaching normal levels on day 14 and twice normal levels by day 21. Bone marrow lymphocytes rapidly recovered to normal levels by day 7 with no accompanying rebound overshoot past normal pretreatment levels. Spleen cells recovered to normal levels by day 11, overshot to almost twice normal levels by day 14, and declined to subnormal levels by day 21. Lymph node lymphocyte number remained at subnormal levels reaching only 30 per cent of normal by day 21. In the lymph nodes and spleen, B cells were reduced to a greater extent than T cells. The injection of antigen during nadir periods hastened lymphocyte repopulation in those organs. Cyclophosphamide was also found to reduce total lymphocytes in mouse peripheral blood with nadirs of 5 per cent of normal being reached within 4 days of drug treatment. Relative increases in T cells were noted in these studies. Antigen injection accelerated recovery of lymphocyte numbers to normal levels (Mackiewicz *et al.*, 1978).

A greater relative sensitivity of B cells as compared to T cells following cyclophosphamide has been reported in the peripheral blood, lymph nodes, bone marrow and spleen for most other species studied (Johansen *et al.*, 1974; Revell, 1974; Scheper *et al.*, 1975; Burroughs and Cidlowski, 1978; Revell, 1978). Again, immature thymocytes appear more sensitive than do mature thymocytes. Low doses of cyclophosphamide (50–100 mg/kg) decrease B cell numbers without altering T cell numbers in guinea pig blood, lymph nodes and thymus (Revell, 1978). Restoration of T cell occurs faster than restoration of B cells (Winkelstein, 1977). In man, cyclophosphamide may differentially diminish B cells greater than T cells at therapeutically-employed doses and differential recovery kinetics are often seen Dewys *et al.*, 1970; Clements *et al.*, 1973; Harris *et al.*, 1973; Hurd, 1973; Harris *et al.*, 1976). Some preferential reduction in B cell percentages was seen in one study *in vitro* with human peripheral blood lymphocytes (Johansen *et al.*, 1974) at doses which killed 60 per cent of the cells while in a different study (Ohnuma *et al.*, 1978) no preferential effects were seen at similar toxic doses. Null cells in man may be relatively resistant to cyclophosphamide (Ritter, 1976). Although less well studied, other alkylating agents such as BCNU, methyl-CCNU and nitrogen mustard (Abb *et al.*, 1977; Ghaffar *et al.*, 1978; Stylos *et al.*, a, b) decrease lymphocyte, T cell and B cell numbers in most lymphoid tissues of normal hosts following drug injection. Some differential sensitivity for subsets of T cells as defined by mitogen responsiveness has been seen (Stylos *et al.*, 1978a, b).

Lymphocytes participating in the afferent portion of the immune response are not actively mitotic. Still, agents that inhibit DNA synthesis can, with appropriate dose, deplete lymphocytes, in the absense of antigenic stimulation. This may in fact be due to actions against dividing cells since the normal host is continuously producing lymphocytes. Different populations of lymphocytes in unstimulated host have been described which may be distinguished in terms of their mitotic characteristics. For example, studies by Bach and Dardenne (1973) demonstrated a differential sensitivity of mouse T cells to azathioprine. Spleen and thymus cells were found to be long-lived, dependent on thymic hormone stimulation, rarely recirculating and highly sensitive to the effects of azathioprine. In contrast, lymph node and peripheral blood T cells were long-lived, recirculated continuously, were independent of thymic hormone and minimally sensitive to azathioprine. In guinea pigs, azathioprine treatment depleted splenic leukocytes by only 30 per cent without altering the relative proportion of T and B cells (Johansen *et al.*, 1974). Relatively high doses of 6-MP (100 mg/kg) or methotrexate (75 mg/kg) did not significantly alter lymphocyte numbers or T and B cell proportions in the peripheral blood or lymph nodes of treated guinea pigs. Significant leukopenia in rats has been observed, however, with comparable doses of methotrexate (Leme *et al.*, 1977). Cytosine arabinoside (Ara-C) did not reduce the percentage or absolute number of B cells in the spleens of normal mice (Albert-Hoadach *et al.*, 1978), whereas 5-fluorouracil substantially depleted thymus cells in rats (Ogiso *et al.*, 1978). In another study, adriamycin gave a transient decline in peripheral blood B cells without affecting T cells, 5-fluorouracil had no effect (Ezdinli *et al.*, 1978). Studies in children with acute lymphocytic leukemia in stable remission demonstrated no alteration of lymphocytes, T cells, B cells or null cells when methotrexate, 6-MP or Ara-C were used as maintenance therapy (Ritter, 1976). Cyclophosphamide was found to produce a substantial decrease in both percentage and absolute number of T and B cells in those children leading to a relative increase in null cells. Similar studies have documented relative resistance of T cells to long term maintenance therapy possible due to their sequestration in bone marrow (Borella *et al.*, 1972; Green and Borella, 1973; Borella and Green, 1978). *In vitro* studies with normal human lymphocytes demonstrated selective sensitivity of T cells to Ara-C and B cells to 5-fluorouracil (Ohnuma *et al.*, 1978).

Steroid hormones influence lymphocyte numbers in various lymphatic tissues. This in some cases, may be attributable to redistribution of cells rather than to their direct destruction. Reports of possible selectivity of steroids against T cells as compared to B cells are contradictory. Thus, hydrocortisone acetate reduced lymphocyte numbers in guinea pig lymph nodes within 2 days and in peripheral blood within 5 days following drug treatment without altering the relative T and B cell proportions in those tissues (Winkelstein, 1977). Similar findings were reported for guinea pig spleen cells (Johansen *et al.*, 1974) and for porcine lymph node and peripheral blood cells (Brownlie *et al.*, 1978). No selective decrease of T or B cells were seen with human peripheral blood cells *in vitro* (Ohnuma *et al.*, 1978). On the other hand, Fauci and coworkers (Fauci and Dale, 1974a, b; Fauci and Dale, 1975; Fauci, 1975; Yu *et al.*, 1974) demonstrated selective depletion of T cells from the peripheral blood of both guinea pigs and man. Kinetic studies with Cr^{51}labelled lymphocytes in both species indicated that hydrocortisone-induced lymphopenia was not due to cell destruction, but rather to alteration in lymphocyte circulation leading to sequestration of cells from the peripheral blood in other lymphoid tissues, particularly the bone marrow. Haynes and Fauci extended these findings in man with a study of the differential sensitivity of human T cell subsets to corticosteroid treatment (Haynes and Fauci, 1978). T cells with membrane receptors for the Fc portion of IgM (T_M cells) or T cells lacking Fc receptor were depleted from the blood of normal subjects receiving hydrocortisone while T cells with membrane receptor for the Fc portion of IgG (T_G cells) were not affected. Similarly, Dumont and coworkers demonstrated in the mouse a differential sensitivity to hydrocortisone of 2 electrophoretically distinct populations of thymus cells (Dumont and Sabolovic, 1973; Dumont and Barrois, 1975). Thymus cells with rapid electrophoretic mobility were characterized as having high H-2 density, low theta density and minimal TL antigens and could function in the graft vs host response, T-dependent antibody synthesis and PHA-induced lymphoproliferation. These cells which were considered mature thymocytes were resistant to elimination by hydrocortisone. Immature thymocytes with slower electrophoretic mobility were characterized as having moderate H-2 density, high TL antigens and were depleted by treatment with hydrocortisone. Greater sensitivity of immature thymocytes than mature thymocytes to depletion by hydrocortisone was also reported by Lee (Lee, 1977). He suggested, however, that relatively more B cells than T cells were eliminated from the spleens of treated mice.

Anti-tumor antibiotics. mitotic inhibitors and certain enzymes such as asparaginase are known to alter lymphocyte numbers in the absence of antigenic stimulation. Carminomycin, an agent with proliferation inhibitory capacity, depleted lymphocytes from the thymus and spleens of mice reversibly (Goldberg *et al.*, 1977) as did rubidomycin (Liashenko *et al.*, 1979) and bleomycin (Mori *et al.*, 1977). Streptozotocin depletes lymphocytes from the peripheral blood and thymus tissues of mice and reduces their spontaneous DNA synthesis (Nevalainen and Hoftiezer, 1977). *In vitro* studies with human peripheral blood lymphocytes did not demonstrate a differential sensitivity of T and B cells to bleomycin and daunorubicin while asparaginase appeared highly selective for T cells (Ohnuma *et al.*, 1978). Cyclosporin A and niridazole may also exhibit preferential effects against T cells (Mottironi *et al.*, 1978; White *et al.*, 1979a, b). In one study vinblastine reduced by 50 per cent the number of lymphocytes in guinea pig spleen and thymus without differentially affecting T or B cells. On the other hand, *in vitro* studies with vinblastine at 60 per cent lethal doses appeared to preferentially destroy human T cells (Johansen *et al.*, 1974). Those results were in contrast to studies by Ohnuma and coworkers in which neither vinblastine nor vincristine appeared to be selective against B or T cells (Ohnuma *et al.*, 1978).

2.3. Immunocompetence

Apart from altering lymphocyte numbers in the absence of antigenic stimulation, drugs can also alter lymphocyte immunocompetence for afferant processes. Those processes are technically difficult to dissect away from early steps conventionally included in the central portion of the immune response since immunocompetence for antigen is tested in antigen-stimulated systems. Generally, studies entail transfer of lymphoid cells from drug-treated donors to anergic recipients followed by challenge with antigen. For example, spleen cells from mice treated with cyclophosphamide 5, 7, 11, 14 or 21 days prior to transfer were found to be unable to restore immune responsiveness for antibody synthesis to anergic mice (Willers and Sluis, 1975). Partial restoration was achieved with drug-treated donor spleen cells in combination with normal bone marrow cells indicating again, a relative sensitivity of B cells to cyclophosphamide. Lymph node cell immunocompetence apparently recovered faster than that of spleen cells since lymph node cells from donors treated 14 or 21 days prior to transfer were able to restore immunocompetence to the anergic recipient. Yet, even in that situation full restoration of responsiveness required bone marrow cells from normal donors. Similar approaches have been used to demonstrate (1) inhibition of B cell immunocompetence by 6-MP or 6-TG early after antigen injection; (2) inhibition of splenic lymphocyte immunocompetence by vinblastine; (3) inhibition of B cells by actinomycin D; (4) inhibition of T cell and B cell immunocompetence by Methotrexate; and (5) inhibition of resting B cells by procarbazine (Santos and Owens, 1966; Sycklocha *et al.*, 1966; Sterzl, 1970; Kaufman, 1971; Liske, 1973; Zaitsevskaia *et al.*, 1977).

The molecular processes required for lymphocyte immunocompetence are not known. One processes which is beginning to receive attention is that of antigen-macrophage binding by lymphocytes. Agents which interfere with membrane functions and structures including the cytochalasins, vinblastine and colchicine, or the steroid hormones have been found to interfere with lymphocyte binding to antigen-pulsed macrophages. For example. cytochalasin B treatment of lymph node or peritoneal lymphocytes obtained from guinea pigs prevented subsequent DNA synthesis when treated cells were added to PPD-pulsed syngeneic macrophages (Rosenthal *et al.*, 1975). Cytochalasin B did not interfere with macrophage binding to antigen and did not prevent stimulation of drug treated lymphocytes by mitogen-pulsed macrophages. Vinblastine and colchicine were found to exert similar effects in separate studies but appeared to interfere with afferent processes that were independent of antigen (Lipsky and Rosenthal, 1975).

3. DRUG EFFECTS ON CENTRAL IMMUNE RESPONSES

The central portion of the immune response is its productive phase. Antigen-specific but uncommitted lymphocytes arrested from recirculation by specific binding to antigenic and macrophage determinants during the afferent response enter a DNA synthesis phase. This is followed by differentiation and proliferation of cells committed along regulatory or effector pathways. Modulation by chemotherapy of the central portion of the immune response would be affected by agents which modify either or both (1) cellular DNA synthesis and (2) differentiation of suppressor cells, helper cells and effector B and T cells. Since these events are dependent upon antigen, antigen timing in relation to drug administration is a primary determinant of drug action. Clearly, any agent that can interfere with cell division as is the case with the majority of drugs used for cancer chemotherapy can influence the immune response by terminating or distorting the proliferation of antigen-triggered cells.

3.1. Modulation of Cellular DNA Synthesis

Selectivity of drug action on B cell or T cell DNA synthetic responses has been described for many agents. This may, in fact, reflect differences in recovery kinetics or differential stimulation of B cells and T cells by antigens or mitogens relative to effective drug concentration rather than differences in intrinsic sensitivity of the cells to drug. Thus, experiments employing levels or types of antigen which stimulate T cells greater and faster than B cells might well result in apparent selective effects by drug against T cells. Under other circumstances, the same drug might exhibit greater activity against B cells. In a study (Ohnuma *et al.*, 1978) of the selectivity of action against human spontaneous B cell and T cell DNA synthesis *in vitro*, a selective inhibition of B cells greater than that for T cells with 5-fluorouracil was found; selective inhibition of T cells greater than B cells was seen with Ara-C and asparaginase. No selectivity of action was seen with cortisone, azathioprine, bleomycin, cyclophosphamide, cis-platinum, daunorubicin, vinblastine or vincristine. Clearly, reports of selectivity by drugs *in vivo* must must be analyzed in relation to all aspects of the test system before intrinsic differential sensitivity can be accepted.

Alkylating agents such as cyclophosphamide or BCNU depress both T cell and B cell DNA synthesis following stimulation with antigen or mitogen. Some differences may be seen which depend on the lymphoid tissue studied. For example, BCNU treatment of mice resulted in a decline of splenic T cell DNA synthesis following PHA or Con A stimulation. This was found in association with diminished LPS induced B cell DNA synthesis. PHA and LPS responses recovered within 10 days but the Con A response was still substantially depressed at that time. PHA responsiveness was completely and permanently abolished by cyclophosphamide in thymus cells while the effect on Con A responsiveness was temporary (Ritter, 1976). Selective suppression of B cell DNA synthesis greater than T cell DNA synthesis has been reported with the alkylating agents (Stockman *et al.*, 1973). Still, enhancement of LPS-induced DNA synthesis at a time of depressed PHA and Con A responsiveness has also been observed (Snippe *et al.*, 1976). Cyclophosphamide treatment of mice appeared to decrease PHA-induced DNA synthetic responses in lymph node lymphocytes greater than in splenic lymphocytes (Scheiffarth *et al.*, 1973). Differences may also be observed which depend on whether antigen-induced or mitogen-induced DNA synthesis is studied. Thus, cyclophosphamide treatment of guinea pigs sensitized with tuberculin led to a suppression of PPD-induced DNA synthesis in spleen, lymph node and peripheral blood cells while the responsiveness of lymphocytes from those tissues to PHA and Con A remained normal (Balow *et al.*, 1975). Relative differences between *in vivo* and *in vitro* activities have already been suggested. In this regard, cyclophosphamide decreased DNA synthesis in PHA-stimulated peripheral blood lymphocytes to a greater extent relative to controls *in vivo* than *in vitro* (Astaldi *et al.*, 1969). Depression of mitogenic factor production by cyclophosphamide has been reported (Ashworth, 1977). Both cyclophosphamide and BCNU have been observed to enhance lymphocyte DNA synthesis under appropriate conditions of drug dose and antigen administration schedule (Ghaffar *et al.*, 1978; Karp *et al.*, 1977; Mansour and Nelson, 1977).

Agents which directly inhibit DNA synthesis alter proliferation of T cells and B cells following antigen or mitogen stimulation. Administration of these agents following antigen stimulation supresses most T and B cell DNA synthetic responses if adequate dosage of drug is achieved. Administration prior to antigen has little effect or may lead to enhancement of immune response. Reports of the differential sensitivity of T and B cell DNA synthesis with these agents are subject to all of the constraints on interpretation previously mentioned. One study using normal human lymphocytes *in vitro* estimated that Ara-C was 50 times more inhibitory to spontaneous T cell proliferation *in vitro* than to B cell proliferation (Ohnuma *et al.*, 1978). On the other hand, a relatively greater effect on T cells over B cells following treatment with 5-fluorouracil has been reported in studies of cancer patients (Nordman *et al.*, 1978). Methotrexate treatment of rats resulted in an initial enhancement of PHA-induced proliferative responses within 24 hr of drug injection followed by a decline of responsiveness associated with lymphopenia. The kinetics of this effect differed when peripheral blood lymphocytes were compared to splenic lymphocytes, depression of responsiveness being seen at 72 and 96 hr respectively (Mansour *et al.*, 1978). Methotrexate treatment of mice has also been reported to augment the

PHA responsiveness of spleen cells within 5 days following drug treatment (Orbach-Arbouys and Castes, 1979). The proliferation of B cells following antigen injection is most affected when methotrexate is administered 48 hr after antigen (Santos and Owens 1964). Possible membrane modification by methotrexate may also contribute to a loss of proliferative responsiveness in lymphocytes secondary to direct effect on DNA synthesis (Hoffmann *et al.*, 1977). In guinea pigs, 6-MP modified antigen-induced peripheral blood lymphoproliferation in association with depressed development of delayed type hypersensitivity and antigen-stimulated MIF production; (Scherbaum and Ambrosius, 1978) in a similar study, antigen-stimulated lymphoproliferation but not DTH or MIF production was resistant to that drug (Zweiman and Phillips, 1970). PHA-induced proliferation of mouse lymph node cells may be more sensitive to 6-MP than spleen cells (Scheiffarth *et al.*, 1973). Cis-platinum inhibits Con A-induced T cell proliferation greater than LPS-induced B cell proliferation in mouse spleen lymphocytes; the difference in sensitivity here was attributed to a faster recovery of B cells as compared to T cells for all drug doses tested (Wierda and Pazdernik, 1979). In drug comparison studies, 5-fluorouracil was found to depress the *in vitro* proliferative response of PHA stimulated peripheral blood cells from normal humans to a greater extent than did cyclophosphamide, colchicine, vinblastine, prednisolone or daunorubicin (Astaldi *et al.*, 1969). A similar effect was seen with peripheral blood lymphocytes taken from cancer patients treated with these drugs. Cyclophosphamide was more effective than 6-MP in depressing the PHA-induced lymphoproliferation of mouse lymph node and spleen cells (Scheiffarth *et al.*, 1973). As with many of these agents, 5-fluorouracil in low doses was found to enhance PHA and Con A stimulation of lymphocytes in mice and humans (Berenbaum, 1979). Five-bromodeoxyuracil in amounts sufficient to prevent IgM synthesis following LPS or sheep erythrocyte stimulation of mouse spleen cells did not reduce DNA synthesis in those cells (Bachvaroff and Rapaport, 1977).

As expected, mitotic inhibitors such as vinblastine, vincristine or colchicine exert significant modulatory effects on lymphoproliferation during the central portion of the immune response. Differential sensitivity of T cells has been reported in some studies (Johansen *et al.*, 1974) while differential sensitivity of B cells has been seen in others (Crum *et al.*, 1977). A lack of differential effects was seen when spontaneous T and B cell proliferation was considered in studies of human cells *in vitro* (Ohnuma *et al.*, 1978). Both mitogen and antigen-induced DNA synthesis may be inhibited or enhanced depending on drug dose and timing (Astaldi *et al.*, 1969; Leford and McGregor, 1977).

Other agents important in inhibiting cellular DNA synthesis during the central portion of the immune response include anti-tumor antibiotics, most notably actinomycin D (Kaufman, 1971) which may have greater effects against B cells than T cells. Streptozotocin, however, may effect T cells preferentially (Nevalainen and Hoftiezer, 1977) while carminomycin and rubomycin exerted equivalent suppressive effects on both T cells and B cells (Shapovalova *et al.*, 1979). Cyclosporin A has demonstrated marked selectivity for T cell DNA synthesis in most studies (White *et al.*, 1979a, b; Brent, 1979).

Inhibition of lymphoproliferation by steroid hormones may preferentially effect T cells as already discussed in the consideration of drug effects on events in earlier phases of the immune response. Thus, methylprednisolone can inhibit DNA synthetic responses to alloantigens (Rosenberg and Lysz, 1977; Gerber *et al.*, 1978). Con A and PHA (Gerber *et al.*, 1978), contact skin sensitizing antigens (Venetianer *et al.*, 1978) and tumor antigens (Schechter and Feldman, 1977). Kinetic studies of the inhibitory effects of hydrocortisone administered 2 days prior, simultaneously with or 1–2 days following antigen administration demonstrated marked impairment of DNA synthesis at those times while enhancement was seen with longer pretreatment or post-treatment intervals (Dumont and Barrois, 1975; Gerber *et al.*, 1978).

3.1.1. *Differentiation of Suppressor Cells*

Cyclophosphamide has become the standard agent for demonstrating drug sensitivity of suppressor cell development. Effective doses in most species encompass a broad range from 5 mg/kg to 200 mg/kg and antigen dose and timing are critical considerations in most studies (Schwartz *et al.*, 1978; Rollinghoff *et al.*, 1977; Glaser, 1979; Sy *et al.*, 1977; Mitsuoka *et al.*, 1976; Germain and Benacerraf, 1978; Hengst *et al.*, 1980). Generally, for effects on suppressor cells to be seen cyclophosphamide is administered 1–2 days prior to antigen injection. While most studies have demonstrated effects against suppressor T cells, suppression by macrophages (Hengst *et al.*, 1980) and B cells (Katz *et al.*, 1974) may also be modified with cylcophosphamide.

Virtually any immune response that is subject to regulation by suppressor T cells may be augmented by eliminating those cells with cyclophsophamide. Antibody responses can be augmented following cyclophosphamide administration. Some of the more interesting examples showing this effect include: (1) primary PFC responses to hapten-modified syngeneic cells (Cheung *et al.*, 1978); (2) antibody responses of highly restricted heterogeneity (here, cyclophosphamide treatment increased the magnitude of heterogeneity, (Kipps *et al.*, 1978); (3) hapten-specific restricted IgE responses (here cyclophosphamide converted nonresponder or low responder mouse strains to responders (Chiorazzi *et al.*, 1977); (4) IgM responses to T independent antigens (Duclos *et al.*, 1977); and (5) secondary IgG responses to Ir gene-restricted antigens (here, cyclophosphamide eliminated suppressor cells which prevented cooperation between primed cells and antigen-pulsed nonresponder macrophages (Germain and Benacerraf, 1978). Similarly, delayed type hypersensitivity and contact sensitivity reactions can be agumented by pretreatment of the host with cyclophosphamide. Some examples here include augmentation of responses to methylated human serum albumin (Mitsuoka *et al.*, 1976), DNP-BSA (Attallah *et al.*, 1979), sheep erythrocytes (Gill and Liew, 1978), Dinitrofluorobenzene (Sy *et al.*, 1977), oxazolone (Asherson *et al.*, 1979), and picyril chloride (Nakano and Nakano, 1978). Tolerance induction with low doses of antigen (Asherson *et al.*, 1979) or high doses of antigen (Schwartz *et al.*, 1978; Sy *et al.*, 1977) may be modulated by cyclophosphamide elimination of suppressor cells while established tolerance may be broken by cyclophosphamide (Polak and Turk, 1974). Cyclophosphamide eliminates suppressor cells which maintain specific unresponsiveness to grafts (Wood and Monaco, 1977) and can modulate the graft vs host reaction (Bonavida and Hutchinson, 1978). Cyclophosphamide appears to eliminate suppressor cells which control the induction of autoreactive T cells (L'age-Stehr and Diamanstein, 1978). Both T dependent and B dependent mitogen responses can be increased following elimination of suppressor cells with cyclophosphamide (Bash *et al.*, 1976; Rook and King, 1978). Of potential importance for the design of combined chemotherapy-immunotherapy regimens for the treatment of cancer is the observation that cyclophosphamide can also decrease *adherent* suppressor cells induced by BCG (Bennett and Mitchell, 1979).

Elimination of suppressor T cells by cyclophosphamide has been associated with the augmentation of cytotoxic T cell induction. Thus, Rollinghoff and coworkers demonstrated augmentation of the *in vivo* generation of cytotoxicity against TNP-conjugated syngeneic spleen cells or against allogeneic P815 and E14 tumors following cyclophosphamide treatment of CBA mice (Rollinghoff *et al.*, 1977). Augmentation depended upon the dose of cyclophosphamide administered (100 mg/kg being optimal) and the timing of treatment (cyclophosphamide treatment 2 days prior to immunization being optimal). The effects of cyclophosphamide treatment were abolished by normal T cells but not by normal B cells. Glaser reported similar findings in a syngeneic SV-40-induced murine tumor system (Glaser, 1979). Evidence has been obtained suggesting that the precursors of suppressor cells controlling cytotoxic cell induction are more sensitive to cyclophosphamide than are the precursors of the cytotoxic cells themselves (Ferguson and Simmons, 1978).

Several studies have indicated that the expression of suppressor cell activity may depend on cells which amplify this process. Effects on these cells by cyclophosphamide were studied by Sy and coworkers (Sy *et al.*, 1979). Lymph node cells from mice sensitized with supraoptimal doses of dinitrofluorobenzene inhibited the elicitation of contact sensitivity in normal recipients simultaneously receiving immune lymph node cells. However, pretreatment of the donors of the immune cells with cyclophosphamide prevented suppression of their transfer activity by suppressor cells obtained from the supraoptimally sensitized donors. Suppression was restored by addition of immune lymph node cells from non-drug treated donors but not by normal lymph node cells. The accessory cell for suppressor cell activity was found to be a T cell which was induced by antigen and was eliminated by cyclophosphamide treatment or thymectomy. Interestingly, Cone and coworkers presented evidence suggesting that cyclophosphamide may also augment cells that amplify suppressor cell activity (Cone *et al.*, 1977). These cells were antigen-specific, adherent to nylon and their production was inhibited by doses of sheep erythrocytes which were optimal for stimulation of B cells. Cyclophosphamide pretreatment prevented high dose inhibition of their production. A synthesis of these concepts was advanced by Schwartz and coworkers (Schwartz *et al.*, 1978) resulting from studies of the regulation of delayed-type hypersensitivity to sheep erythrocytes in mice. These authors suggested that since cyclophosphamide tended to agument the responsiveness of hosts sensitized with supraoptimal doses of antigen while often diminishing responsiveness of optimally sensitized hosts, the action of this drug may not necessarily be directed only against suppressor cells but rather, against either positive or negative regulatory cells depending upon the conditions of the system.

It would be erroneous, however, to suggest that all suppressor cells are susceptible to cyclophosphamide. Gill and Liew (Gill and Liew, 1978) suggested that cyclophosphamide inhibited precursors of suppressor cells but had little effect on suppressor cells which had already encountered antigen. They showed that cyclophosphamide eliminated suppressor cells in mice if given 2 days prior or simultaneously with sheep erythrocytes but had little effect in abolishing the passive transfer of suppression mediated by cells from antigen-stimulated donors. Direct evidence for elimination of suppressor cells by early cyclophosphamide treatment was obtained by demonstrating absence of those cells in the spleens of drug-treated mice when the cellular composition of the spleens of those animals was analyzed by Ficoll density gradient techniques. In studies by Bonavida and coworkers (Bonavida, 1977; Bonavida *et al.*, 1979) cyclophosphamide treatment following antigen injection failed to eliminate suppressor cells that suppressed nonspecifically, the *in vitro* generation of cytotoxic cells. In an *in vivo* test system, cyclophosphamide treatment 2 or 4 days following antigen failed to eliminate cells which suppressed the production of IgM and IgG anti-tumour antibodies and delayed by several days the appearence of cytotoxic lymphocytes. Further experiments in that system indicated that cyclophosphamide treatment following antigen injection can, rather than eliminating suppression, actually induce suppressor cell activity. Injection of cyclophosphamide 2–6 days following a secondary alloimmunization suppressed the generation of cell-mediated cytotoxicity but not secondary cytotoxic antibody production. Furthermore, those cells elicited by cyclophosphamide treatment following secondary antigen injection could suppress the activity of normal cells in the mixed lymphocyte reaction. In a different study, pretreatment of normal mice with cyclophosphamide elicited spleen cells which suppressed normal cellular responses to mitogens *in vitro* (Rook and King, 1978). Those cells were not sensitive to mitomycin C, adherent to nylon, and when added to normal cells in low numbers, enhanced rather than suppressed reactivity.

Although cyclophosphamide modulation of suppressor cells has received the broadest experimental attention, there is evidence as well for modulation of suppressor cells by other agents. The ability of corticosteroids to modulate suppressor cell activity has been demonstrated in studies of the graft vs host reaction and tolerance induction. Cohen and associates (Cohen *et al.*, 1970) showed that pretreatment of donor mice with hydrocortisone prior to transfer of thymus, spleen or bone marrow cells enhanced the subsequent graft vs host reaction in recipients. T cell-deprived 'B' mice that were reconstituted with thymus cells from hydrocortisone treated donors were resistant to the induction of tolerance (Zan-Bar *et al.*, 1975a, b; Nachtigal *et al.*, 1975). Similarly, hydrocortisone administration to the recipients of spleen extracts prevented the subsequent tolerance of skin grafts (Rieger *et al*., 1978). Resistence and possible enhancement of mature suppressor cell activity following hydrocortisone treatment of tolerant hosts was observed during attempts to adoptively transfer tolerance (Nachtigal *et al*., 1975). Hydrocortisone treatment of mice was found to substantially augment lymphoproliferative response to T cell mitogens and alloantigens (Dumont and Barrois, 1975; Gerber *et al*., 1978; Stavy *et al*., 1974). Facilitation of tumor allografts in hosts treated with methylprednisolone has also been observed (Gerber *et al*., 1978).

The augmentation of cytotoxic T cell responses *in vivo* and *in vitro* following hydrocortisone treatment has been attributed to the elimination of suppressor cell precursors. Schechter and Feldman (Schechter and Feldman, 1977) reported that hydrocortisone could prolong the survival of C57B1 mice inoculated with syngeneic Lewis Lung Carcinoma cells. Treatment with drug 3–5 days following tumor cell inoculation proved to be more effective than treatment given prior to or simultaneously with tumor cell inoculation. Hydrocortisone-resistant spleen cells which recovered 2–3 days after drug treatment of tumor-bearing mice proved to be actively suppressive when transfered with tumor cells to normal recipients. This indicated a relative resistance of mature suppressor cells to this drug. A subsequent study of these investigators (Schecter and Feldman, 1978) demonstrated *in vitro* recovery of cytotoxicity in the spleens of hydrocortisone-treated tumor-bearing mice. Suppressor cells normally arising during the *in vitro* generation of cytotoxic cells in the mixed lymphocyte culture reaction were not found when spleen cells from steroid-treated mice were used in the reaction (Al-Adra and Pilarski, 1978). The observation of Haynes and Fauci (Haynes and Fauci, 1978) that T_G cells persist in the blood of normal humans receiving hydrocortisone is of interest since that T cell subset is known to function as a suppressor cell of antibody synthesis (Moretta *et al*., 1976; Moretta *et al*., 1977).

Agents which inhibit DNA synthesis have also demonstrated suppressor cell modulatory effects. In one study, administration of methotrexate to rats during the induction of adjuvant-induced arthritis was found to delay the onset of the disease and to augment the normally diminished PHA and Con A responsiveness of spleen cells from adjuvant-injected hosts (Kourounakis and Kapusta, 1977). Augmentation was also obtained by *in vitro* incubation of methotrexate with spleen cells from experimental animals during mitogen-induced lymphoproliferation assays. B cell mitogen responsiveness was not, however, augmented. Two types of suppressor cells were characterized in the system, one being adherent to glass but not plastic and sensitive to methotrexate *in vitro* and the other being adherent to both glass and plastic and insensitive to methotrexate *in vitro. In vivo* treatment of arthritic rats with methotrexate led to the elimination of both kinds of suppressor cells in host spleens. In other studies (Orbach-Arbouys and Castes, 1979), a single injection of methotrexate intraperitoneally led to enhancement of subsequent PHA-induced lymphoproliferation, graft vs host reactivity and primary PFC responses to sheep erythrocytes. Optimum augmentation was achieved with a 5 day interval between methotrexate injection and subsequent *in vitro* assessment. When suppressor cells were induced by high doses of BCG 14 days prior to testing, methotrexate treatment of mice 8 days following BCG injection abrogated suppression. Similar results were obtained by adult thymectomy. Methotrexate was also seen to eliminate cells regulating induced contact sensitivity to oxazolone (Griswold and Walz, 1978). Azathioprine and 6-MP have both shown modulatory activity against suppressor cells (Demetriu and Fauci, 1979; Hollowell *et al*., 1979). In man, azathioprine inhibits the *in vitro* generation of suppressor cells by Con A and the action of naturally occuring suppressor cells in the peripheral blood of persons who are poor pokeweed mitogen responders (Demetriu and Fauci, 1979).

The antibody responses in mice to antigens such as diptheria toxoid, human gamma globulin and TNP haptens can be augmented by treatment of responders with mitotic poisons such as colchicine or vinblastine (Shek and Coons, 1978; Parks *et al*., 1979). In studies by Shek and Coons (Shek and Coons, 1978) administration of colchicine at the same time as antigen elevated titers of specific antibody 3–7 fold in the primary response and more than 15 fold in the secondary response. The number of PFCs seen in the spleens of drug-treated mice was double that seen in untreated mice for primary responses and 5 fold that seen in untreated mice for secondary responses. Studies by Parks and coworkers (Parks *et al.*, 1979) demonstrated enhancement of PFC formation in response to aggregated human gamma globulin in mice treated with colchicine from one day prior to one day following the injection of 100 μg of antigen. Augmentation of responsiveness in mice receiving 400 μg of aggregated human gamma globulin was not achieved with any colchicine treatment schedule. Tolerance induction by disaggregated human gamma globulin was not prevented in spleens of mice receiving colchine 3 hr after tolerogen injection. These data suggested that colchicine probably destroyed antibody synthesizing cells and suppressor cells in the donor since anergic mice receiving mixtures of spleen cells from drug-treated tolerized mice and normal mice gave enhanced PFC responses to antigenic challenge while mice receiving normal spleen cells and spleen cells from mice rendered tolerant but not treated with drug were completely suppressed. Colchicine treatment of mice receiving tolerized spleen cells together with normal spleen cells and an immunizing dose of antigen followed 10 days later by a secondary challenge with antigen eliminated the activity of mature suppressor cells. This led to a vigorous secondary PFC response.

Tolerance induction to human gamma globulin in the mouse may also be blocked by puromycin aminonucleoside. Thymus cells from mice obtained 24 hr following drug and tolerogen injection were unable to transfer tolerance to anergic recipients simultaneously receiving normal bone marrow cells (Maserang and Hyde, 1977). Thymus cells from donor mice rendered tolerant 48–72 hr prior to puromycin injection were able to transfer tolerance. Amphotericin B treatment together with injection of dinitrofluorobenzene or TNP-human serum albumin led to increased primary and secondary PFC responses and to augmented delayed hypersensitivity through elimination of suppressor cells (Blanke *et al.*, 1977). Tilorone HCl treatment of mice 2 or 4 days prior to spleen cell transfer to F_1 hybrid recipients increased subsequent graft vs host reactivity (Zschiesche *et al.*, 1977). On the other hand, Procarbazine together with donor tissue extracts and ALS may create long-lasting responsiveness to allografts by the enhancement of suppressor cells (Brent and Opara, 1979a, b).

Several studies have now demonstrated that suppressor macrophages may also be modified by chemotherapy. Hengst and associates (Hengst *et al.*, 1980) reported that low dose cyclophosphamide treatment of plasmacytomatous mice early during tumor growth was less effective than was the same treatment given later during tumor growth. The results seen were atributed to several actions of the drug including (1) reduction in glass adherent cells from spleens of drug treated tumor bearing mice and (2) reduction of tumor cells from spleens of drug treated tumor bearing mice. It was suggested that the time interval between tumor innoculation and drug treatment rather than initial tumor size was critical for successful therapy.

In cancer patients the effects of combination chemotherapy have only begun to be studied for their effects on host suppressor cell mechanisms. Short intensive courses of cancer chemotherapy have been shown to suppress immune function transiently—this is followed by rebound overshoot recovery of responsiveness in those patients who mount an objective tumor reduction response (Harris *et al.*, 1973). Braun and coworkers (Braun *et al.*, 1980a, b) demonstrated that the occurrence of rebound overshoot was attributed to drug induced reduction in monocyte suppressor function in solid tumor cancer patients. The reduction seen was attributed to either or both a reduction in relative numbers of macrophages following drug treatment or a reduction in suppressor function without concommittant reduction in macrophage numbers following drug treatment. Recovery of indomethacin-sensitive monocyte suppressor function was responsible for the eventual decline in immune function seen following drug induced rebound overshoot. Both single agent therapy with methotrexate and a variety of combination chemotherapy regimens were found to reduce monocyte suppressor cells and lead to the rebound overshoot phenomenon.

3.1.2. *Differentiation of Helper Cells*

Cyclophosphamide under appropriate conditions of dose and schedule can also eliminate helper T cells. In one study, helper cells were induced in mice by pretreatment with PHA or sheep erythrocytes. Five days later (when maximal splenic DNA synthesis was elicited) cyclophosphamide was given. The antibody production, as measured by indirect PFC techniques, was depressed for 18 days. Antibody production could be completely restored by sheep erythrocyte-activated T cells but not with activated B cells (Schwarze, 1977). The timing of cyclophosphamide administration for reduction of helper cell activity was found to be critical in studies by Van den Broek and Kenning (Van den Broek and Keuning, 1977). Those workers found that helper cells for anti-sheep erythrocyte antibody synthesis were eliminated only when cyclophosphamide was administered 1–3 days following antigen injection. Studies by Bonavida and associates (Bonavida *et al.*, 1979) demonstrated that cyclophosphamide administration 2 days following secondary immunization of mice with allogeneic tumor cells did not eliminate helper cells for cytotoxic antibody production even though cell-mediated cytotoxicity was significantly diminished. Possible induction of cells which enhance the mitogen responses of normal cells *in vitro* by pretreatment of mice with cyclophosphamide has been reported (Rook and King, 1978).

Methotrexate treatment of donor mice followed by transfer of lymphocytes to anergic syngeneic recipients subsequently challenged with sheep erythrocytes led to substantially reduced PFC responses (Zaitsevskaia *et al.*, 1977). Responsiveness was restored by normal thymocytes but not by B cells, indicating a reduction of helper cells in the drug-treated donors. The reduction of helper cells by 6-MP has been observed and even greater reductions by the DNP-derivative of 6-MP have been found (Malberg *et al.*, 1978). On the other hand the treatment of human peripheral blood cells with azathioprine followed by pokeweed mitogen stimulation demonstrated relative resistance of helper cells to this drug (Demetriu and Fauci, 1979). Helper T cells do not appear sensitive to mitomycin C (Waldman, 1978).

Hydrocortisone treatment of mice was found to concentrate helper cell and cytotoxic cell precursors in their spleens but an accessory cell needed for elicitation of cytotoxicity was eliminated (Lee, 1977). This accessory cell appeared to be a macrophage and its action was restored by either normal peritoneal macrophages or 2 mercaptoethanol. Haynes and Fauci, however, have reported the selective elimination of the T_M cell from the peripheral blood of hydrocortisone-treated normal humans (Haynes and Fauci, 1978). This cell is known to serve as a helper cell for pokeweed mitogen-induced antibody synthesis (Moretta *et al.*, 1976; Moretta *et al.*, 1977).

None of the mitotic inhibitors have demonstrated any definitive selective modulatory activity against helper cells. For example, spleen cells from mice treated with sheep erythrocytes showed enhanced secondary PFC responses *in vitro* when challenged with antigen in the presence of increasing concentrations of vinblastine (Minato and Katsura, 1978). Attempts to induce net helper effects by elimination of suppressor cells in tolerant rendered mice by colchicine have failed (Parks *et al.*, 1979) but simultaneous elimination of helper cells by drug was not proven. That helper T cells need not proliferate to exert biological activity has been suggested and may explain the lack of effects of these agents in those studies (Minato and Katsura, 1978).

The antitumor antibiotics, adriamycin and daunorubicin were found to eliminate T cells which had helper function for cytotoxic antibody synthesis in mice (Orsini and Mihich, 1975). Their action in that study proved to be superior to that of methotrexate or Ara-C. Cyclosporin A was found to block helper T cell function for antibody responses to DNP-KLH in rats without altering lymphoproliferative responses to B cell mitogens (Burckhardt and Guggenheim, 1979). Elimination of antigen-specific helper cells for mixed lymphocyte responses by cyclosporin A has been suggested. This is based on the observation that following drug treatment, responses to the original stimulator were diminished while responses to third party cells were unaffected and suppressor cell activity was maintained (White *et al.*, 1979a). Reduction of helper cell activity by combination chemotherapy has been observed in human cancer patients (Athanassiades *et al.*, 1978).

3.1.3. *Differentiation of Effector Cells*

The notion of hierarchy of drug sensitivty for different kinds of immune responses has been suggested by many studies (Mitchell *et al.*, 1969). The rank order for decreasing sensitivity to drug-induced suppression is development of newly acquired cellular hypersensitivity, primary antibody synthesis, secondary or memory antibody synthesis and established cellular immunity. For this relationship to be maintained, precursors of effector cells must be more sensitive to drugs than are mature effector cells. Discussion of the sensitivity to drugs of precursor cell differentiation to mature effector cells has formed the basis for most reviews of immunosuppressive agents. This review, however, is concerned primarily with the modulation of immunity by drugs and not simply its suppression. The differentiation of effector cells during the central portion of the immune response will be considered in light of the observations made concerning the drug sensitivity of the regulatory cells that control that process.

Greater sensitivity to drug modification on the part of suppressor cell development as compared to effector cell development would be expected in situations where impairment of suppressor cells leads to augmented effector reactions. This could result from either or both a selective differential sensitivity of suppressor cell precursors to a particular drug or to accelerated recovery of helper and effector cell precursors as compared to suppressor cell precursors following drug treatment. Drug dosage and schedule in relation to antigen administration are primary considerations in the analysis of drug effects on effector cell development.

2.1.3.1. *Effector B cells.* Most comparative studies have shown that primary antibody responses are more sensitive to drug-induced suppression than are secondary antibody responses. This may be related in part to different mitotic requirements for expression of effector function on the part of uncommitted B cells and memory B cells. Miller and Cole (1967) demonstrated the resistance of memory B cells in rat lymph nodes to doses of cyclophosphamide, prednisone, 6-MP and Actinomycin D which abolished primary antibody synthesis. By serially studying the longevity of radiolabelled B cells obtained from drug-treated rats after secondary immunological stimulation, they confirmed that the number of labelled lymphocytes seen was stable for several months during the period encompassing nodal lymphocyte depletion and subsequent repopulation. During this period, serum agglutinin titres for specific antigen did not deviate from those of control animals. Other relevant factors which need to be considered in investigations of drug modulation of B cell differentiation include (1) the T cell dependence of the B cell response under investigation; (2) the participation of regulatory cells in the response; and (3) the nature of the response studied including the class of antibodies produced and characteristics of their biological activities.

Berenbaum has recently recorded the results of an extensive study of drug action on T dependent and T independent antibody synthesis (Berenbaum, 1979b). He has classified drugs into two categories, designated Class I and Class II, depending upon when, in relation to antigen injection, drug treatment leads to immunosuppression. Class I agents inhibit antibody synthesis when given prior to or following antigen injection. Class II agents are effective only when drug is given following antigen.

The alkylating agents have been classified as Class I agents for T dependent and T independent antibody synthesis (Berenbaum, 1979b). These agents which include cyclophosphamide, melphalan, susulfan, mitoclomine and nitrogen mustard inhibited T dependent (sheep erythrocyte) and T independent (LPS) primary PFC development in mouse spleen cells when given from a period of 6 days prior to 2 days following antigen injection. Cyclophosphamide, melphalan, nitrogen mustard and busulfan depressed T dependent and T independent responses equally while mitoclomine suppressed the T independent response greater than the T dependent response. Increasing the dose of these agents prolonged the effective interval prior to antigen injection during which suppression could be obtained. Since augmentation of response was not seen in that study, conclusions about helper and suppressor cell modulation were not possible.

Factors such as the timing and dose of drug and antigen administration may together affect helper and supressor T cells more than having any direct effect against B cells. For example, pretreatment of animals with cyclophosphamide in doses that do not eliminate B cells will generally spare helper T cells while often eliminating suppressor T cells. In Kerckhaert *et al.* (1977) the dosage requirements were determined for suppression or augmentation of T dependent antibody synthesis to sheep erythrocytes in mice. Suppression was achieved by cyclophosphamide in doses of 300 mg/kg and 200 mg/kg when administered 8 hr before antigen injection, while a dose of 100 mg/kg led to enhancement. Studies by Schwarze (1977) indicated that the precursors of B cells for T dependent antibody synthesis may be less sensitive to cyclophosphamide than are helper T cells. The administration of drug to mice 5 days after antigen injection suppressed PFC formation. This was restored completely by antigen-activated T cells. Antigen-activated B cells had no effect on restoration indicating a sparing of B effector cells in the drug-treated mice.

Since suppressor cells may exert their effects on B cell responses either by inhibiting the induction of helper T cells or by inhibiting helper T cell–B cell interaction, augmentation of B cell differentiation by drugs might reflect modulation of either or both of these functions. Chiorozzi and his associates (1977) suggested that elimination of suppressor cells by cyclophosphamide leads to enhancement primarily through permitting helper T cell differentiation to proceed (Chiorozzi *et al.*, 1977). The interference of T cell–B cell cooperation by suppressor cell is less sensitive to drug effects.

T independent antibody responses may also be modulated by cyclophosphamide actions directed against T cells. In Duclos *et al.* (1977) it was demonstrated that low dose cyclophosphamide pretreatment of mice (20 mg/kg) daily for 4 days prior to injection of a T independent antigen resulted in enhanced IgM synthesis in normal mice but suppressed IgM synthesis in nude mice. These data suggested T cell regulation of B cell differentiation following drug treatment as a major factor determining the kinetics of recovery of B cells. In Snippe *et al.* (1978) it was demonstrated, however, that restoration of the direct PFC response to a T independent antigen occured more rapidly in nude mice than in their heterozygous littermates. Restoration of the indirect PFC response was more rapid in the Nu/+ mice. Cyclophosphamide suppression of anti-sheep erythrocyte antibody synthesis in situations where drug is given after antigen has been found to depress and prolong IgM synthesis while completely blocking IgG antibody synthesis (Liske, 1973).

Although primary antibody synthesis is more sensitive to suppression than secondary antibody synthesis under most conditions, Herrlinger reported that cyclophosphamide can eliminate secondary responses more effectively than primary responses to T dependent antigens in rats (Herrlinger and Muller-Ruchholtz, 1978) with appropriate manipulation of drug and antigen timing. When cyclophosphamide was used to completely abolish IgM and IgG synthesis in sensitized mice, IgM responses were found to recover faster than IgG responses (Herrlinger and Muller-Ruchholtz, 1978). Suppression of memory cells for IgG antibody synthesis by cyclophosphamide is optimal when drug is given between 10 and 14 days after antigen (Speirs *et al.*, 1978).

Cyclophosphamide may effect the development of certain B cells differently than other B cells. Cyclophosphamide administration to guinea pigs has been found to suppress Arthus-mediating skin sensitizing antibodies to ovalbumin without altering the development of antibodies to DNP-Bovine gamma globulin (Maguire *et al.*, 1979). In that study, effects of suppressor B cells were suggested. Similarly, hemagglutinating antibody synthesis appears less sensitive to suppress by cyclophosphamide than does synthesis of skin sensitizing antibodies (Noble *et al.*, 1977). The possibility that cyclophosphamide may alter membrane immunoglobulin turnover has also been suggested (Shand and Howard, 1978).

Agents which interfere with cellular proliferation either by inhibition of DNA synthesis or inhibition of mitosis have been classified as Class II agents for T dependent and T independent antibody synthesis (Berenbaum *et al.*, 1979b). Such agents which include 6-MP, 6-TG, 5-FU, methotrexate, vincristine and vinblastine were found to interfere with both kinds of antibody synthesis only when administered one or two days following antigen injection. Increasing the dose of these agents increased the magnitude of suppression but was ineffective in prolonging the effective post-antigen injection drug treatment interval. A moderate degree of selectivity against T dependent antibody synthesis was seen in that study with the Class II agents.

Many studies with this class of agents confirm the hierarchic scheme of drug sensitivity already mentioned—that is, they inhibit the differentiation of B cells for primary antibody responses better than for secondary antibody responses. Again, constraints to this order are imposed when drug dose and antigen timing are manipulated. Some selectivity for primary IgM and IgG synthesis has been demonstrated with these agents and may reflect modulation activity against helper T cells coincident with direct effects against B cells (Malberg *et al.*, 1978). In this context, Zaitsevskaia and coworkers (Zaitsevskaia *et al.*, 1977) demonstrated that methotrexate can suppress splenic B cell differentiation by effects against against both helper T cells and B cells. In that study, spleen cells from drug-treated donors elicited minimal antibody forming PFCs when transferred to anergic donors. Partial restoration of the response was seen by transfer of bone marrow cells alone while complete restoration required transfer of both thymocytes and bone marrow cells. In Griswold *et al.* (1972) it was demonstrated that suppression of both 19s and 7s PFC production occurred in mice treated with Ara-C early (day 1 or 2) or late (day 6 through 10) following injection of sheep erythrocytes. IgG PFCs were inhibited to a greater extent by early drug treatment than by late drug treatment. IgM PFCs were inhibited equally by either treatment schedule. This suggests that inhibition of DNA synthesis is not the sole explanation for the depression of antibody production seen with these drugs. Evidence bearing on this consideration was presented by Bachvaroff and coworkers (Bachvaroff and Rapaport, 1977) who demonstrated that bromodeoxyuracil can prevent IgM production in LPS-stimulated or sheep erythrocyte stimulated B cells without affecting DNA or RNA synthesis. Interference with secretion of IgM appeared to be responsible.

Comparative studies of the effects of various agents on B cell differentiation and antibody production indicate that class II agents are more effective in suppressing IgE synthesis than cyclophosphamide or rapamycin (Martel *et al.*, 1977). Comparisons within this class of agents have also been performed. They show prolonged depressive effects of actinomycin D when that drug is given for up to 7 days following antigen injection (Youmans and Youmans, 1978). 5-Fluorodeoxyuracil was effective only when administered simultaneously or no later than 18 hr following antigen. Methotrexate depresses antibody production best when administered 48 hr after antigen in mice, guinea pigs and rats (Berenbaum, 1962; Friedman *et al.*, 1961; Santos and Owens, 1966). Pharmacokinetic considerations are therefore, of primary importance in determining the effects of these agents on effector B cell differentiation.

Several kinds of antibodies may also be differentially affected by Class II drugs. Ossler and associates (Ossler *et al.*, 1977) demonstrated that 6-MP affects the production of individual populations of IgG_2 complement-binding antibodies in different manners. Treatment of guinea pigs with 6-MP daily for 7 days after antigen injection resulted in complete suppression of IgG_2 antibovine gamma globulin antibody production, with no effect on IgG_2 anti-DNP antibody production and enhancement of IgG_2 anti-human serum albumin antibody production.

Mitotic inhibitors also modulate effector B cell differentiation both at the level of regulatory cells and by direct effects on B cells. Helper cells and precursor B cells do not appear sensitive to these agents under conditions which eliminate suppressor cells even when drug administration is delayed until the time of antigen injection (Shek and Coons, 1978). Studies of dose dependency of modulation indicate that precursor B cell differentiation may be less sensitive to these agents than helper T cells (Leonteva *et al.*, 1977). Synchronization of helper T cells and B cells by vincristine following antigen stimulation has been described and renders those cells susceptible to destruction by other drugs (Schwarze, 1978). This method appears to be suitable for the induction of specific B cell tolerance. Kinetic studies of the effects of methotrexate and vinblastine on B cell differentiation in mice treated with drug 2 or 3 days after antigen injection revealed that recruitment of precursor B cells and helper T cells into spleen tissues was not sensitive to drug. However, alternating patterns of enhanced and depressed PFC production were seen in the spleens of drug-treated mice suggesting that one effect of drug treatment is disruption of helper T cell-B cell interaction (Romanycheva *et al.*, 1978).

Steroid hormones have been classified as Class I agents for T dependent and T independent antibody synthesis since steroids given prior to or following antigen injection leads to a suppression of B cell differentiation (Berenbaum, 1979b). Hydrocortisone is more inhibitory to T dependent responses than T independent responses. Maximum activity against sheep erythocyte responses were seen when drug was administered 1 or 2 days prior to antigen while maximum effectiveness against LPS responses were seen when drug was given 1 day following antigen. Dual and opposing effects of methylprednisolone on B cell differentiation were demonstrated by Saxon *et al.* (Saxon *et al.*, 1978) in humans. *In vivo* drug treatment of normal humans reduced the ability of B cells to respond *in vitro* to helper T cells during pokeweed mitogen-induced antibody synthesis but also eliminated suppressor T cells for this reaction. Lipsky and coworkers (Lipsky *et al.*, 1978) demonstrated augmentation of mitogen-induced antibody synthesis in human peripheral blood cells through elimination of suppressor cells by hydrocortisone. Again, greater sensitivity of suppressor cells to drug treatment as compared to helper T cell and B cell precursors was suggested.

Inhibitors of RNA or protein synthesis including streptozotocin, chloramphenicol and cycloheximide appear to suppress B cell differentiation best when administered from 4–7 days following antigen (Youmans and Youmans, 1978). In contrast, cis-platinum can suppress B cell differentiation when administered from 2 days prior to 2 days following antigen injection (Wierda and Pazdernik, 1979).

Asparaginase was found to suppress IgG antibody production without effecting IgM production (Schaffner and Hadge, 1977). This may reflect an action against helper T cells since this agent was found to be highly selective against T cells (Ohnuma *et al.*, 1978). Continued use of asparaginase *in vivo* may be limited by the appearence of inactivating antibodies for this enzyme (Mehta *et al.*, 1977). Augmentation of B cell responses has been reported with amphotericin B by a mechanism attributed to direct modification of B cell membrane sterols (Blanke *et al.*, 1977).

2.1.3.2. *Effector T Cell Development*. Mature effector T cells which differentiate during the central phase of the immune response mediate one form of cell-mediated cytotoxicity, delayed type hypersensitivity, graft vs host and graft rejection reactions and production of lymphokines upon stimulation with antigen. Differentiation of these cells is under the regulatory control of suppressor and helper cells. Other studies indicate a role for B cells in regulating effector T cell differentiation although this role may be more important in the control of efferent T cell processes. The influence of drugs on effector T cell differentiation in relation to modulation by suppressor and helper cells indicates a greater drug resistance by precursors of effector T cells and helper cells as compared to precursors of suppressor cells. Still, it is important to reemphasize that drug dose and antigen timing are primary determinants of drug modulation of effector T cell development. The induction of tolerance to specific antigens may be accomplished under appropriate conditions of drug and antigen scheduling which selectively elicit suppressor cell differentiation presumably without stimulating helper and effector cell differentiation (Brent and Opara, 1979a, b).

There is experimental evidence to show that effector T cell differentiation may be suppressed by cyclophosphamide treatment prior to or following antigen injection when adequate drug doses are used (Riccardi *et al.*, 1978). With lower drug doses, however, enhancement of T cell differentiation by drug treatment prior to antigen and suppression of T cell differentiation by drug treatment following antigen is often seen. In Zimber *et al.* (1977) it was demonstrated that enhancement of contact sensitivity to dinitrofluorobenzene occurred by treatment of guinea pigs with cyclophosphamide prior to antigen and suppression of that reactivity occurred by drug post-treatment. The route of antigen injection and the use of adjuvants are important factors in this type of experiment. Immunization of mice by intracutaneous injection of sheep erythrocytes emulsified in Freund's Complete Adjuvant resulted in enhanced delayed type hypersensitivity when cyclophosphamide was administered from 7 days prior to 15 days following antigen injection (Kerckhaert *et al.*, 1977). Direct evidence for the differential sensitivity of suppressor and cytotoxic T cell precursors was described by Ferguson and Simmons (Ferguson and Simmons, 1978). Treatment of mice with 100 mg/kg of cyclophosphamide one day prior to initiating *in vitro* sensitization of cytotoxic cells led to enhanced levels of cytotoxicity in antigen-stimulated cultures of spleen cells taken from treated animals and prevented the generation of suppressor cells normally seen in unstimulated cultures. Moreover, the non-antigen stimulated cultures from drug-treated mice could act as responder cells in secondary antigen-stimulated cultures. Cells from normal mice or mice treated with only 20 mg/kg of drug could not. Cyclophosphamide pretreatment of mice has also been reported to suppress the induction of suppressor cells by thymic factors (Bach, 1979).

Differential drug effects on T cell differentiation have also been seen when comparing *in vivo* and *in vitro* systems. For example, cyclophosphamide was shown to depress cell mediated cytotoxicity against allogeneic tumor cells *in vitro* without effecting the *in vivo* rejection of those grafts (Gerber *et al.*, 1978). Similarly, depression of *in vitro* cell mediated cytotoxicity 2 weeks following cyclophosphamide treatment was associated with normal skin graft rejection (Milton *et al.*, 1976). Similar discrepencies in assays for effector T cell development have also been noted. Cyclophosphamide treatment of guinea pigs simultaneously with injection of Complete Freund's Adjuvant had no effect on the development of effector T cells for PPD-stimulated MIF production but completely abolished effector cell responses for PPD-stimulated blastogenesis (Winkelstein *et al.*, 1973). Differential cyclophosphamide sensitivity of cytotoxic T cell development for allogeneic cells and hapten-modified syngeneic cells has been reported (Hurme, 1979). This perhaps indicates distinct drug sensitivities of regulatory cells for allogeneic and H-2 restricted responses. Greater cyclophosphamide sensitivity of effector T cell development in lymph node cells as compared to spleen cells (Scheiffarth *et al.*, 1973) or peripheral blood cells (Ashworth, 1977) has also been suggested.

The widely held belief that cyclophosphamide preferentially inhibits B cells has led to the suggestion that some of the modulatory effects on T cell differentiation seen following treatment with cyclophosphamide are due to actions directed against B cells. In La Grange *et al.* (1974) it was argued that cyclophsophamide pretreatment of mice augments delayed type hypersensitivity to sheep erythrocytes by suppressing the production of blocking antibody. Parker and Turk (Parker and Turk, 1978) demonstrated augmentation of delayed type hypersensitivity to ovalbumin in guinea pigs following a drug treatment which eliminated Arthus-mediating antibodies to that antigen. In contrast, cyclophosphamide intensified the generation of contact sensitivity in B cell deficient mice (Macguire *et al.*, 1979). Pacha and associates (Pacha *et al.*, 1979) demonstrated complete suppression of the development of MIF reactivity to microbial antigens in infected rabbits following cyclophosphamide treatment but with no effect on specific antibodies. It was reported in Bonavida *et al.* (1979), that cyclophosphamide treatment 2–6 days following secondary immunization of mice with allogeneic tumor cells depressed cell-mediated cytotoxicity but not secondary antibody production. Askenase and associates (1975) demonstrated agumentation of delayed type hypersensitivity following cyclophosphamide treatment of mice without altering specific antibody production.

As is the case for effector B cell differentiation, effector T cell differentiation is most effected by drugs which inhibit DNA synthesis when drug is given following antigen administration. The hierarchic relationships for drug sensitivity of T effector cell function are generally maintained for agents that suppress cellular proliferation. Mitchell and De Conti (1970) demonstrated depression of the development of contact sensitivity to DNCB in cancer patients treated with 5-fluorouracil but maintenance or enhancement of delayed hypersensitivity to recall antigens. This basic relationship suggests that interference with dividing T cells is primarily responsible for drug modulation with this class of agents. Thus, cells mediating delayed hypersensitivity in rats are inhibited by Vinblastine (Leford and McGregor, 1978) or actinomycin D (Youmans and Youmans, 1978) when drug is given following antigen. Skin graft rejection is inhibited by carminomycin injected within one week following graft application (Shapovalova *et al.*, 1979). On the other hand, 6-MP treatment of guinea pigs following tuberculin immunization has been reported to depress the development of skin test reactivity to PPD without affecting the development of PPD-induced lymphoproliferation (Zweiman and Phillips, 1970). In other studies, 6-MP treatment led to concomittant depression of the development of skin test, MIF and lymphoproliferative reactivity to antigen (Scherbaum and Ambrosius, 1978). Relative resistance of memory cells for cytotoxic T cell development as compared to precursor cells was seen in studies by Jacobs and associates (Jacobs *et al.*, 1977). In that study, azathioprine depressed tumor rejection in unsensitized rats when given after a primary challenge but did not alter tumor rejection following a secondary challenge. The induction of cytotoxic T cell development by polyclonal activators is abolished *in vitro* by Ara-C or hydroxyurea (Igarashi, 1977).

The early injection of agents which interfere with lymphoid cell DNA synthesis following exposure to antigen may lead to enhancement due to elimination of suppressor cells. This suggests that precursor cells for these distinct T cell functions are differentially affected by this class of agents. Additional evidence for this has been seen in cases where drugs in combination with immunostimulants lead to greater enhancement of response than treatment with immunostimulants alone. Methotrexate treatment of guinea pigs one day following oxazolone sensitization depressed resultant contact sensitivity but enhancement of responsiveness was seen following treatment with levamisole. This enhancement was greater than that seen with levamisole treatment alone suggesting either drug-induced elimination of suppressor cells or recovery of effector cells more rapid than recovery of suppressor cells following immunostimulation (Griswold and Walz, 1978). Synergism between drugs such as Methotrexate, AraC, and 5-FU and Immunostimulation has been seen in a number of systems with appropriate timing of drug and immunostimulant administration (Sparks *et al.*, 1977). Elimination of B cell functions which interfere with T cell development has not been extensively attempted with this class of agents. That this approach might be possible is suggested by observations that agents such as Ara-C do not interfere with the development of graft rejection in doses which completely depress IgM and IgG synthesis (Griswold *et al.*, 1972). The apparent selectivity of 5-fluorouracil for B cell function has been discussed above. It may be a suitable drug to use in attempting to develop methods to enhance T cell responses. On the other hand, azathioprine may inhibit the *in vitro* generation of cytotoxic T cells in doses that do not effect the development of cytotoxic antibodies (Rollingoff *et al.*, 1973).

Augmentation of T effector cell differentiation by the elimination of suppressor cells with steroid hormones has already been considered as have the effects of these agents on helper cells. Greater sensitivity to these drugs on the part of suppressor cell precursors as compared to effector cell precursors is thus assumed. It has been directly demonstrated for cytotoxic T cell development (Hirano and Nordin, 1976) and for the graft vs host reaction (Cohen *et al.*, 1970). Mature suppressor cells, however, do not appear sensitive to hydrocortisone (Schechter and Feldman, 1977; Nachtigal *et al.*, 1975). Suppression of the *in vitro* generation of cytotoxic T cells in mixed lymphocyte cultures with human peripheral blood cells was achieved with methylprednisolone but evidence was obtained suggesting elimination of proliferating effector cells was not responsible (Rosenberg and Lysz, 1977). This is not, though, the case in the mouse where hydrocortisone appears to directly suppress T cell development (Claman *et al.*, 1971). Augmentation of cellular proliferation during *in vitro* development of cytotoxic T cells has also been described (Stavy *et al.*, 1974). Mature effector T cells exhibit some sensitivity to hydrocortisone *in vivo* but are much less sensitive than are precursor effector T cells. Thus, in Venetianer *et al.* (1978) it was demonstrated that hydrocortisone treatment of guinea pigs 3 days after oxazolone sensitization reduced the development of delayed sensitivity and antigen-induced proliferative responses in regional lymph nodes, while drug treatment prior to antigen completely abolished the development of this reactivity. Discordance between the effects of methylprednisolone on cytotoxic T cell development and graft rejection have been observed (Gerber *et al.*, 1978). The ability of these agents to alter lymphocyte populations in various tissues without direct destruction of cells probably also contributes to the modulation effects on T cell development that have been reported. In some cases, concentration of precursor effector and helper cells in certain lymphoid tissues may result from drug treatment (Lee, 1977).

The selective depression of effector T cell development by agents which may preferentially effect T cells has been studied. Cyclosporin A substantially inhibits the development of tuberculin skin test sensitivity, the graft vs host reaction and graft rejection without altering effector B cell differentiation (White *et al.*, 1979a). The development of antigen induced proliferation appears to be more sensitive to cyclosporin A than does the development of antigen induced MIF reactions (White *et al.*, 1979a). Asparaginase is also reported in a number of studies to exhibit selectivity for effector T cell development (Holland and Ohnuma, 1979) although one study demonstrated depression of B cell function without alteration of graft vs host reactivity (Mehta *et al.*, 1977). The development of delayed type hypersensitivity may be more sensitive to chloramphenicol than to streptozotocin or cycloheximide. Actinomycin D appears more effective than any of those agents on the delayed type hypersensitivity reaction (Youmans and Youmans, 1978). Vigorous and persistent depression of graft rejection, *in vitro* generation of cytotoxic T cells, delayed type hypersensitivity and graft vs host reactivity have all been seen with DTIC (Giampietri *et al.*, 1978).

4. DRUG EFFECTS ON EFFERENT IMMUNE RESPONSE

The efferent portion of the immune response expresses the immune effector functions developed during the central portion of the response. Drug action during this phase of the response is often difficult to study since effects on mechanisms which regulate effector cell development and direct effects against specific effector cell function are not easily discriminated. Suppression of mature effector function is certainly possible, particularly in the case of functions whose continual expression is dependent upon ongoing clonal expansion. Most effector B cell processes are resistant to suppression by drugs. However, terminally differentiated B cells or plasma cells are short-lived with half life estimates on the order of two days (Douglas, 1976). Thus, antibody synthesis can be suppressed in sensitized hosts by drugs which inhibit immune cell clonal expansion. This is seen in cases where long term immunosuppressive therapy leads to decreased levels of serum immunoglobulin (Fauci *et al.*, 1971; Borella and Webster, 1971). This may also be seen in certain forms of resistance to infection. For example, resistance of rats to *Trichinella spiralis* is mediated by mature B cells and T cells but effector B cells are delivered to the sites of infection while still in active cycle. Hence, those B cells are susceptible to vinblastine while the mature effector T cells are not (Crum *et al.*, 1977). Drugs that interfere with metabolic processes needed for effector function such as protein synthesis can also suppress mature responses (Moody *et al.*, 1977).

Memory antibody synthesis and established cellular immunity are relatively resistant to drug suppression. Many of the studies concerned with drug modulation for this phase of the immune response have been performed *in vitro*. Some caution is needed, however, in interpreting the results of experiments where drugs are added to *in vitro* assay systems since the drug may alter target cell susceptibility apart from direct actions against effector cells. An example of this is the increased susceptibility of target cells to lysis by lymphotoxin caused by a number of drugs (Sawada *et al.*, 1977).

4.1. MATURE EFFECTOR T CELLS

Effector T cells mediate at least one form of cellular cytoxicity and elaborate lymphokines when exposed to sensitizing antigen. Their combined participation with macrophages and accessory cells in the delayed type hypersensitivity reaction, tumor and graft rejection reactions, graft vs host disease and resistance to many infectious organisms can be considered in the context of T cell cytotoxicity and lymphokine production. The effector reactions of T cells are also known to be modulated by B cells or B cell derived blocking antibody. In an attempt to determine the direct effects of cyclophosphamide on established cellular immunity, Balow and associates (1977b) tested the effect *in vivo* activated cyclophosphamide on the *in vitro* responses of guinea pig lymphocytes obtained from PPD-immune animals (Balow *et al.* (1977b). *In vitro* drug treatment was found to inhibit mitogen-induced T cell proliferation and certain forms of non-T cell cytotoxicity immediately whereas depression of PPD-stimulated MIF production was not seen until after 48 hr of continuous cyclophosphamide treatment. PPD-induced blastogenesis and cytotoxic T cell activity was not tested. An earlier study by this group, testing the *in vivo* sensitivity of established delayed hypersensitivity to tuberculin in guinea pigs yielded somewhat different results (Balow *et al.*, 1975). In that study, cyclophosphamide treatment of PPD-immune guinea pigs daily for 4 days in doses of 5, 10, or 20 mg/kg/day led to a dose dependent decline in antigen-stimulated MIF production and antigen-stimulated proliferation in immune peripheral blood, lymph node and spleen cells. On the other hand, mitogen-induced T cell proliferation by PHA and Con A was not affected. Reduced T cell specific reactivity could not be atributed to drug effects on macrophages since assays were performed with mixtures of immune cells and normal PEC. Niridazole blocks the production of MIF from sensitized T cells but not the release of preformed MIF by antigen pre-pulsed immune T cells (Bernard *et al.*, 1977). Puromycin exerts comparable activity (Jones, 1976). The possibility of interference with macrophage function is an important consideration in analyzing drug modulation of T effector functions since most *in vivo* and many *in vitro* T cell assays require macrophages. Studies of delayed type hypersensitivity reactions are affected by this consideration. Treatment of guinea pigs with established cellular immunity to tuberculin by 6-MP was found to depress antigen-specific reactions without altering antigen-stimulated blastogenesis or MIF production *in vitro* (Zweiman and Phillips, 1970). In a similar study, methotrexate, cyclophosphamide and colchicine were found to strongly suppress delayed hypersensitivity to PPD in immune guinea pigs (Wojnar *et al.*, 1979). The sensitivity of macrophages to these drugs has already been discussed. Augmented monocyte recruitment into tuberculin skin tests sites has been seen following recovery from cyclophosphamide treatment in mice that had received immune lymphocytes and PPD (Milon and Marchal, 1978). Effector T cell function may be affected by B cell activity. Some aspects of this relationship have been mentioned. In addition to those studies, it was demonstrated in Katz *et al.* (1974) that the removal of B cells from guinea pig spleens by adherence to anti-IgG columns prevented suppression of delayed type hypersensitivity in recipients receiving immune T cells and antigen. Cyclophosphamide treatment of donors also effectively eliminated those supressor B cells. The increased monocyte recruitment seen during recovery from cyclophosphamide treatment (Milon and Marchal, 1978) was attributed to the suppression of a B cell dependent splenic retention of those effector cells (Marchal *et al.*, 1978). The reversal of this by drug led to augmented delayed hypersensitivity. Suppression of graft rejection by immune T cells with azathioprine was attributed in part to an azathioprine-induced alteration of the antigen/antibody ratio in the blocking factors necessary for prolonged graft survival (Diderich *et al.*, 1979). Reversal by cyclophosphamide of the action of mature suppressor cells in inhibiting the activity of effector T cells mediating delayed hypersensitivity was attributed to elimination of a drug-sensitive auxiliary cell needed for suppression (Sy *et al.*, 1979). Drug effects on cytotoxic T cells have also been described. Mature cytotoxic T cells are more resistant to immunosuppressive drugs than are their precursor cells (Cherniakhovskaia *et al.*, 1978). Cyclophosphamide was found to eliminate precursor T cells for transplantation rejection reactions without interfering with the cytotoxic responses of antigen-presensitized cells (Cherniakhovskaia *et al.*, 1978). Azathioprine treatment of mice was unable to suppress cytotoxic antibody formation or T cell activity against allogeneic cells. Hydrocortisone and methylprednisone depressed the *in vitro* generation of cytotoxic T cells by reducing the number of those cells recovered from culture but did not alter the cytotoxic capacity of those cells (Balow *et al.*, 1977a). On the other hand, cytochalasin B markedly inhibits the effector function of cytotoxic T cells apparently by inhibiting the adsorption by immune cells to target cell antigens (Golstein *et al.*, 1978). All cytochalasins block the recognition stage of T cell mediated lysis without affecting the disintegration stage; all but cytochalasin A blocked calcium-dependent steps. Cytochalasin B also blocked the lethal hit stage. Colchicine and vinblastine interfere with cytotoxic T cell lytic function but at a step distal to target cell binding (Golstein *et al.*, 1978). Reports of depression or augmentation of effector cell function in man by drugs should be interpreted in the light of all of these observations (Vetto *et al.*, 1978; Noonan *et al.*, 1977; Robinson *et al.*, 1977).

4.2. Mature Non T Cell–Non B Cell Effector Functions

Immunosuppressive drugs have been investigated for their modulation activity against the effector functions of macrophages, K cells and NK cells. Concerted efforts have been made to define the mechanisms responsible for macrophage killing, antibody-dependent cellular cytotoxicity, and spontaneous lymphocyte-mediated cytotoxicity, and to characterize the role of these functions in disease states. Membrane-bound antibody is responsible for antigen recognition and initiation of killing in some forms of these reactions, most notably in macrophage killing and ADCC.

A large study by Ehrke and coworkers (Ehrke *et al.*, 1978) tested the *in vitro* effects of 24 different drugs on 5 separate cytotoxic effector functions in mice. Effector functions studied included (1) complement-dependent cellular cytotoxicity (CDCC) against sheep erythrocytes which measures lysis by antibody secreted by effector B cells; (2) complement-independent cellular cytotoxicity (CICC), which measures lysis by non T/non B cells after interaction with target cells coated with antibody secreted by effector B cells; (3) ADCC, which measures non T/non B cell lysis of target cells passively coated with exogenous antibody; (4) complement-independent phagocytosis, which measures destruction of target cells coated with endogenous antibody; and (5) antibody-dependent phagocytosis, which measures destruction of target cells coated with exogenously added antibody. In general, inhibitors of DNA synthesis were not suppressive in any test. Phagocytic and lytic functions associated with complement-independent cytotoxicity were sensitive to protein synthesis inhibitors, anthracycline antibiotics, bleomycin, and actinomycin D among other agents tested. With the exception of complement-dependent cytotoxicity, all functions were inhibited by agents such as vinblastine that inhibited cell motility. Effects on C′-dependent cytotoxicity were attributed to increased target cell lysis by drugs. This kind of approach although limited to *in vitro* testing, will probably yield important information concerning further drug modulatory activities for cellular cytotoxicity.

Macrophages may be activated by lymphocyte-derived factors or immunostimulants such as BCG and *C. parvum*. Interestingly, cyclophosphamide treatment of mice has also been found to induce macrophage activation and killing. In one such study Schultz *et al.*, 1978; Schultz and Chirigos, 1978) it was reported that in mice the induction of macrophage cytotoxicity against MBL-3 lymphoblastoid leukemia cells could be enhanced by cyclophosphamide. This peaked 2 days after subcutaneous injection of the drug. In another study, the same group demonstrated that cyclophosphamide treatment ranging from 150–500 mg/kg abolished macrophage activation and killing induced by BCG. The induced macrophages could still be stimulated by lymphokines *in vitro* (Schultz *et al.*, 1978; Schultz and Chirigos, 1978). Adriamycin treatment of mice led to impairment of peritoneal macrophage and spleen cell macrophage activation by *C. parvum* (Mantovani *et al.*, 1977; Mantovani, 1977). Daunomycin *in vivo* or *in vitro* proved to be more inhibitory to *C. parvum*-induced macrophage activation than did adriamycin. Adriamycin and cyclophosphamide injected intraperitoneally had no effect on macrophage numbers in the peritoneal cavity but did induce macrophage killer cells (Stoychkov, 1979). This reaction was increased with higher doses of adriamycin (10 mg/kg better than 2.5 mg/kg) or lower doses of cyclophosphamide (50 mg/kg better than 300 mg/kg). Destruction of immune lymphocytes followed by release of macrophage activating factors was suggested as an explanation for this finding. Mitogen-induced cytotoxicity is also depressed by cyclophosphamide (Cherniakhovskaia *et al.*, 1978). Although adriamycin but not daunomycin appeared to spare macrophage killing in peritoneal cells, the reverse was true in splenic macrophages following peritoneal drug injection (Mantovani *et al.*, 1976). The subcutaneous injection of hydrocortisone succinate or cortisone acetate with varying schedules of administration increased the numbers of alveolar macrophages in guinea pig lung tissues coincident with peripheral blood lymphocytopenia and monocytopenia (Hunninghake and Fauci, 1977b). Hydrocortisone *in vivo* or *in vitro* did not interfere with macrophage cytotoxicity as assessed by PHA-induced or antibody-dependent macrophage cytotoxicty tests. Continued treatment with cortisone acetate caused a sharp decline in both functions. Cyclophosphamide in 2 separate schedules did not reduce guinea pig alveolar macrophage number. *In vitro* and *in vivo* exposure to 100 mg/kg cyclophosphamide did not effect PHA-induced or antibody-dependent macrophage cytotoxicity. However, *in vivo* administration of drug for 5 days at 20 mg/kg (a dose which does not decrease macrophage numbers) did substantially reduce macrophage killing (Hunninghake and Fauci, 1977a). Cortisone acetate also appears to interfere with alveolar macrophage activity by lymphocyte-derived macrophage activation factors (Hunninghake and Fauci, 1977b; Sharma and Piessens, 1978). Similarly, puromycin, pactamycin and actinomycin D prevented macrophage activating factor-induced macrophage killing of guinea pig hepatoma cells if the macrophage effectors were pretreated. They could not abolish an ongoing lytic reaction (Sharma and Piessens, 1978). This suggested that protein synthesis is needed for macrophage tumor cell binding. Mitomycin C proved ineffective in that test system but could block macrophage activation by lymphocytes if those cells were pretreated (Rilsgaard *et al.*, 1978). Cytochalasin A and B reversibly inhibited macrophage activation by macrophage activation factor and subsequent killing of guinea pig hepatoma cells through inhibition of macrophage tumor cell binding (Sharma and Piessens, 1978). Colchicine and vinblastine inhibited both binding and killing in that study. Hydrocortisone can inhibit the tumoricidal effects of interferon-activated macrophages (Hibbs, 1976), and can inhibit antibody-dependent macrophage cytotoxicity (Hunninghake and Fauci, 1977b).

Antibody-dependent cellular cytotoxicity (ADCC) is mediated by lymphoid cells that are non T/non B cells but that have Fc receptors on their surface. Colchicine, hydrocortisone and cytochalasin B have each been found to completely suppress ADCC in human peripheral blood in a dose dependent manner (Urbaniak, 1979). Actinomycin D and puromycin caused 30–50 per cent inhibition of function; mytomycin C had no effect. Cortisone acetate treatment of mice and rats was found to have no effect on ADCC function against AKR lymphoma cells in spleen and peripheral blood cells even though lymphopenia occurred with treatment. Cortisone acetate did depress ADCC function in whole spleen and macrophage-depleted spleen cells when those were tested against chicken erythrocytes (Purves and Brown, 1978). A redistribution of effector cells to bone marrow was suggested since ADCC in that tissue was found to increase by 70 per cent at the time when spleen ADCC depression occurred. One report indicates that steroid treatment of normal humans does not interfere with ADCC against erythrocytes sensitized with chicken antibodies (Scheinberg and Cathcart, 1976) while another report suggests that treatment of transplant patients with prednisolone depressed peripheral blood

ADCC to chicken erythrocytes sensitized with rabbit antibodies (Dupont *et al.*, 1977). Both hydrocortisone and methylprednisolone were found to decrease ADCC activity of human peripheral blood cells to Chang Liver cells sensitized with low amounts of antibody (Purves and Brown, 1978).

Long term azathioprine treatment of ulcerative colitis patients reportedly decreases blood ADCC levels by 25 fold within one year and also decreases PHA-induced macrophage cytotoxicity (Campbell *et al.*, 1976). Depletion of effector cells from the circulation without destruction was postulated. Four day azathioprine treatment of mice (80 mg/kg) markedly decreased ADCC to chicken erythrocytes while a single injection (80 mg/kg) had no effect. Azathioprine in that study did not effect antibody synthesis or the development of cytotoxic T cells to allogeneic tumors and did not lead to depletion of macrophages. ADCC recovered rapidly after cessation of drug (Mantovani *et al.*, 1978). Cytochalasin A and B, cycloheximide, actinomycin D and puromycin were found to decrease cytotoxic T cell and ADCC activity in parallel in a separate study (Strom *et al.*, 1975). Cycloheximide, puromycin and actinomycin D can also enhance ADCC (Moody *et al.*, 1977; Hellstrom *et al.*, 1975). The development of complement-independent cellular cytotoxicity in mice was found to increase following treatment with adriamycin or daunorubicin and this was attributed to drug-induced concentration of effector cells in the spleen. Cyclophosphamide *in vitro* was found to decrease ADCC immediately in guinea pig peripheral blood cells while melphalan treatment of tumor-bearing mice was found to depress antibody synthesis but augment ADCC (Haskill and Parthenais, 1978).

Spontaneous lymphocyte mediated cyctotoxicity is mediated by natural killer cells which are non T/non B cells but which may bear Fc receptors. The reaction does not require antibody. In one study (Mantovani *et al.*, 1978) it was reported that azathioprine or cyclophosphamide treatment of mice by various schedules substantially decreased NK activity against YAC-1 cells in mice. Recovery of normal activity occured within 7 days. Daunomycin was less effective while DTIC had no effect in that study. In Petranyi *et al.* (1978) it was reported that puromycin *in vitro* (10 μg/ml) in concentrations which decreased cytotoxic T cell activity enhanced NK activity to YAC-1 cells in mice. Less striking effects were seen when testing puromycin *in vitro* on human NK activity against K562 myeloid leukemia target cells. *In vivo* administration of cyclophosphamide to mice was found to diminish NK activity to YAC target cells by 30 per cent within one day following a high drug dose (500 mg/kg). Azathioprine (420 mg/kg) decreased this activity by 40 per cent while hydrocortisone (600 mg/kg) decreased activity by 60 per cent. Cycloheximide and colchicine were found to completely inhibit NK, ADCC and cytotoxic T cell activity in a dose dependent manner in that study. Suppression of NK activity by cytochalasins and colchicine was demonstrated in Henney *et al.* (1978). A possible augmenting role of phagocytes for NK activity was suggested by Oehler and Herberman (Oehler and Herberman, 1978) who reported that high dose cyclophosphamide or hydrocortisone depressed NK activity in rats. Poly-I-C treatment was found to restore NK activity of drug-treated hosts to a level similar to that of Poly-I-C, non-drug treated hosts. Treatment with silica in amounts which did not decrease Con A stimulation were found to decrease NK activity. This supports the view that the macrophage plays an accessory role in the development of mature NK cells from NK cell precursors. High dose treatment of hamsters with cyclophosphamide (500 mg/kg) was also found to diminish NK activity within one day following drug administration (Datta *et al.*, 1979).

5. CONCLUSIONS

The apparent selectivity of action reported for many chemotherapeutic agents against distinct immunological functions may be largely due to their modification of the complex interactions that control the development of immunity. As discussed in this review, many drugs exert modulatory activity during the afferent, central and efferent portions of the immune response. Thus, the effects of drug treatment on a dynamic and regulated physiological process such as the immune response would depend not only upon drug dose, schedule and pharmacological characteristics, but also upon the functional status of the immune system at the time of drug administration. Indeed, the functional status of the immunoregulatory cell network at the time of drug treatment may be a primary determinant of drug action. Future studies into drug modification of immunity should be directed toward developing methods to manipulate immunoregulatory cells. Questions of drug dose and schedule should be explored in the context of what is known about the immunological mechanisms operative during each phase of the immune response. That information would greatly facilitate the design of single or combination chemotherapy treatment programs for many human disease states. It would also help in cancer medicine in arranging the timing of therapies seeking to combine chemotherapy and immunotherapy. Ideally, external immunological manipulation with immunotherapy might prove most efficacious when administered at a time following drug treatment when suppressor cell mechanisms were selectively impaired. In a like manner, priming of the immune system with immunotherapy might be followed by appropriate chemotherapy to manipulate specifically only those cells responding to the external immunological stimulus. As knowledge of the cellular and biochemical events of the immune response increases, greater ability to manipulate that response through drug therapies should be realized.

REFERENCES

ABB, J., NETZEL B., RODT, H., GROSS-WILDE, H., WEGER, N. and THIERFELDER, S. (1977) Hematologic and immunologic studies in dogs given nitrogen mustard (HN3). *Blut.* **35:** 51–6.

AL-ADRA, A. R. and PILARSKI, L. M. (1978) Antigen-specific suppression of cytotoxic T cell responses in mice. I. Suppressor T cells are not cytotoxic cells. *Eur. J. Immunol.* **8:** 504–11.

ALBERT-HOADACH, A., BORELLA, L. and PINKEL D. (1978) The synergistic effect of cyclophosphamide and cytosine arabinoside on lymphocytes bearing membrane immunoglobulin. *Proc. Amer. Assoc. Cancer Res.* **19:** 130.

ASHERSON, G. L., PERERA, M. A. and THOMAS, W. R. (1979) Contact sensitivity and the DNA response in mice to high and low doses of oxazolone: Low dose unresponsiveness following painting and feeding and its prevention by pretreatment with cyclophosphamide. *Immunol.* **36:** 449–59.

ASHWORTH, L. A. (1977) Relationship between mitogenic factor and *in vitro* lymphocyte stimulation during guinea pig immune response to KLH. *Int. Arch. Allergy Appl. Imm.* **54:** 347–55.

ASKENASE, P. W., HAYDEN, B. J. and GERSHON, R. K. (1975) Augmentation of delayed type hypersensitivity by doses of cyclophosphamide which do not affect antibody responses. *J. Exp. Med.* **141:** 697–702.

ASTALDI, G., ERIDANI, S., PONTI, G. M., VALENTINE, R. and GIANGRANDE, A. (1969) Influence of antiblastic agents applied either *in vivo* or *in vitro* on human lymphocyte transormation in cell culture. *Blut.* **19:** 8–16.

ATHANASSIADES, P. H., PLATTS-MILLS, T. A. E., ASHERSON, G. L. and OLIVER, R. T. D. (1978) Effect of antileukaemic chemotherapy on helper and suppressor activity of T-cells on immunoglobulin production by B-cells. *Eur. J. Cancer* **14:** 971–6.

ATKINSON, J. P. and FRANK, M. M. (1974) Complement-independent clearance of IgG-sensitized erythrocytes: inhibition by cortisone. *Blood* **44:** 629–37.

ATKINSON, J. P. and PARKER, C. W. (1977) Modulation of macrophage Fc receptor function by cytochalasin-sensitive structures. *Cell Immunol.* **33:** 353–9.

ATTALLAH, A. M., AHMED, A. and SELL, K. W. (1979) *In vivo* induction of carrier-specific cyclophosphamide-sensitive suppressor cells for cell-mediated immunity in mice. *Int. Arch. Allergy Appl. Immunol.* **60:** 178–5.

BACH, J. F. and DARDENNE, M. (1973) Antigen recognition by T lymphocytes III. Evidence of two populations of thymus-dependent rosette-forming cells in spleen and lymph nodes. *Cell Immunol.* **6:** 394–406.

BACH, J. F. (1975) The mode of action of immunosuppressive agents. Amsterdam, North Holland.

BACH, J. F. (1979) New trends in non-antigen specific immune suppression. *Transpl. Proc.* **11:** 851–4.

BACHVAROFF, R. J. and RAPAPORT, F. T. (1977) Studies of antibody formation. III. Effects of 5-bromodeoxyuridine upon normal and neoplastic B-lymphocyte function. *Cell Immunol.* **31**(1): 98–119.

BALOW, J. E., HURLEY, D. L. and FAUCI, A. S. (1975) Cyclophosphamide suppression of established cell-mediated immunity. Quantitative vs qualitative changes in lymphocyte population. *J. Clin. Invest.* **56:** 65–70.

BALOW, J. E., HUNNINGHAKE, G. W. and FAUCI, A. S. (1977a) Corticosteroids in human lymphocyte-mediated cytotoxic reactions. *Transplant.* **23:** 322–8.

BALOW, J. E., PARILLO, J. E. and FAUCI, A. S. (1977b) Characterization of the direct effects of cyclophosphamide on cell-mediated immunologic responses. *Immunology* **32:** 899–904.

BASH, J. A., SINGERE, A. M. and WAKSMAN, B. H. (1976) The suppressive effect of immunization on the proliferative response of rat cells *in vitro*. II. Abrogation of antigen-induced suppression by selective cytotoxic agents. *J. Immunol.* **116:** 1350–3.

BENNETT, J. A. and MITCHELL, M. S. (1979) Induction of suppressor cells by intravenous administration of Bacillus Calmette-Guerin and its modulation by cyclophosphamide. *Biochem. Pharmacol.* **28:** 1947–1952.

BERENBAUM, M. C. (1962) A screen for agents inhibiting the immune response and the growth of tumors. *Nature* (London) **196:** 384–5.

BERENBAUM, M. C. (1979a) The immunosuppressive effects of 5-flurocytosine and 5-fluorouracil. *Chemotherapy* **25:** 54–9.

BERENBAUM, M. C. (1979b) Time-dependence and selectivity of immunosuppressive agents. *Immunol.* **36:** 355–65.

BERNARD, C. C., LEYDON, J. and MACKAY, I. R. (1977) Anti-T cell activity of niridazole in experimental autoimmune encephalomyelitis. *Int. Arch. Allergy, appl. Immunol.* **53:** 555–9.

BLANKE, T. J., LITTLE, J. R., SHIRLEY, S. F. and LYNCH, R. G. (1977) Augmentation of murine immune responses by amphotericin B. *Cell Immunol.* **33:** 180–90.

BONAVIDA, B. (1977) Antigen-induced cyclophosphamide-resistant suppressor T-cells inhibit the *in vitro* generation of cytotoxic cells from one-way mixed leukocyte reactions. *J. Immunol.* **119:** 1530–33.

BONAVIDA, B. and HUTCHINSON, I. V. (1978) Modulation of T-dependent cell-mediated immune responses by antigen-reactive cell opsonization and active suppression. *Transplant Proc.* **10:** 31–35.

BONAVIDA, B., HUTCHINSON, I. V. and THOMAS, A. (1979) Cyclophosphamide-sensitive and cyclophosphamide-resistant suppressor cells in the immune response to alloantigens. *Transplant Proc.* **11:** 872–7.

BORELLA, L. and WEBSTER, R. G. (1971) The immunosuppressive effects of long-term combination chemotherapy in children with acute leukemia in remission. *Cancer Res.* **31:** 420–6.

BORELLA, L., GREEN, A. A. and WEBSTER, R. G. (1972) Immunologic rebound after cessation of long term chemotherapy in acute leukemia. *Blood* **40:** 42–51.

BORELLA, L. and GREEN, A. A. (1978) Sequestration of PHA-responsive cells (T-lymphocytes) in the bone marrow of leukemic children undergoing long-term immunosuppressive therapy. *J. Immunol.* **109:** 927–32.

BRAUN, D. P., COBLEIGH, M. A. and HARRIS, J. E. (1980a) Selective effect of cytotoxic chemotherapy on immunoregulatory suppressor cells in solid tumor cancer patients: *In Chicago Symposium on Tumor Progression. Developments in Cancer Research.* (R. G. Crispen, Ed.) Elsevier/North-Holland, vol **2**; 91.

BRAUN, D. P., COBLEIGH, M. A. and HARRIS, J. E. (1980b) The 'rebound-overshoot' phenomenon: A consequence of selective cytotoxic drug effect on immunoregulatory suppressor mechanisms. *Proceedings Amer. Soc. Clin. Oncology*, **21:** 373.

BRENT, L. (1979) Immunologic manipulation: Specific mechanisms. *Transplant Proc.* **11:** 839–44.

BRENT, L. and OPARA, S. C. (1979a) Specific unresponsiveness to skin allografts in mice. V. Synergy between donor tissue extract, procarbazine hydrochloride, and antilymphocyte serum in creating a long-lasting unresponsiveness mediated by suppressor T cells. *Transplantation* **27:** 120–6.

BRENT, L. and OPARA, S. C. (1979b) Synergy between antigen, antilymphocyte serum, and procarbazine hydrochloride in murine skin allotransplantation. *Transplant Proc.* **11:** 1019–22.

BROWNLIE, S. E., CAMPBELL, J. G., HEAD, K. W., IMLAH, P., MCTAGGART, H. S. and MOVIE, J. G. (1978) The effects on prednisolone on normal pigs. *Eur. J. Cancer* **14:** 567.

BURCKHARDT, J. J. and GUGGENHEIM, B. (1979) Cyclosporin A: *In vivo* and *in vitro* suppression of rat T-lymphocyte function. *Immunology* **36:** 753–9.

BURROUGHS, S. F. and CIDLOWSKI, J. A. (1978) Glucocorticoid and mitogen sensitivity of rat splenic and thymic lymphocytes *in vitro* after *in vivo* cyclophosphamide treatment. *Cancer Res.* **38:** 4562–8.

CAMPBELL, A. C., SKINNER, J. M., MADENNAN, I. C. M. *et al.* (1976) Immunosuppression in the treatment of inflammatory bowel disease. II. The effects of azathioprine on lymphoid cell populations in a double blind trial in ulcerative colitis. *Clin. Exp. Imm.* **24:** 249–58.

CHANG, Y. H. (1977a) Mechanisms underlying the suppression of adjuvant-induced arthritis by 6-mercaptopurine. *Arth. Rheum.* **20:** 1135.

CHANG, Y. H. (1977b) Adjuvant polyarthritis I: Incorporation of quantitative measurements of humoral and cellular immune response. *J. Pharmacol. Exp. Ther.* **201:** 1–7.

CHERNIAKHOVSKAIA, I. I., FONTALIN, L. N. and RUBAKOVA, E. I. (1978) Effect of preliminary administration of allogenic cells on transplantation immunity in mice receiving cyclophosphamide. *Bull. Eksp. Biol. Med.* **85:** 192–4.

CHEUNG, N. K., SCHERR, D. H., HEGHINIAN, K. M., BENACERRAF, B. and DORF, M. E. (1978) Immune suppression *in vivo* with antigen-modified syngeneic cells. I. T-cell-mediated suppression to the terpolymer poly-(Glu, Lys, Phe). *J. Exp. Med.* **148:** 1539–49.

CHIORAZZI, N., FOX, D. A. and KATZ, D. H. (1977) Hapten-specific IgE antibody responses in mice. VII. Conversion of IgE 'nonresponder' strains to IgE 'responders' by elimination of suppressor T cell activity. *J. Imm.* **118:** 48–54.

CLAMAN, H. N., MOORHEAD, J. W. and BRENNER, W. H. (1971) Corticosteroids and lymphoid cells *in vitro* I. Hydrocortisone lysis of human guinea pig and mouse thymus cells. *J. Lab. Clin. Med.* **78:** 499–507.

CLEMENTS, P., LEVY, J. and BARNETT, E. V. (1973) Immunosuppressive effects on B-lymphocytes in rheumatoid arthritis. *Arthritis Rheum.* **16:** 537–8.

COHEN, J. J., FISCHBACH, M. and CLAMAN, H. N. (1970) Hydrocortisone resistance of graft vs host activity in mouse thymus, spleen and bone marrow. *J. Immunol.* **105:** 1146–50.

CONE, R. E., GERSHON, R. K. and ASKENASE, P. W. (1977) Nylon adherent antigen-specific rosette-forming T cells. *J. Exp. Med.* **146:** 1390–1404.

CRUM, E. D., DESPOMMIER, D. D., MCGREGOR, D. D. (1977) Immunity to Trichinella spiralis. I. Transfer of resistance by two classes of lymphocytes. *Immunol* 33: 787–95.

DATTA, S. K., GALLAGHER, M. T. and TRENTIN, J. J. (1979) Natural cell-mediated cytotoxicity in hamsters. *Int. J. Cancer* **23:** 728–34.

DEINARD, A. S., FORTUNY, I. E., THEOLOGIDES, A., ANDERSON, G. L., GOEN, J., KENNEDY, B. J. (1974) Studies on the neutropenia of cancer chemotherapy. *Cancer.* **33:** 1210–8.

DEMETRIU, A. and FAUCI, A. S. (1979) Differential sensitivity of human lymphocyte subpopulations to Azathioprine. *ransplant. Proc.* **11:** 878–81.

DEWYS, W. D., GOLDIN. A. and MANTEL, N. (1970) Hematopoetic recovery after large doses of cyclophosphamide: Correlation of proliferative state with sensitivity. *Cancer. Res.* **30:** 1692–7.

DIDERICH, P. P., BONTHIUS, F., HESSE, C. J., VAESSEN, L. M., BAMEIJER, L. D. (1979) The effect of azathioprine on the generation of passive enhancing sera. *Transplant Proc* **11**: 1418–9.

DOUGLAS, S. D. (1976) Cells involved in Immune Response. In: *Basic and Clinical Immunology*. FUDENBERG, H. H., STITES, D. P., CALDWELL, J. L. and WELLS, J. V. (Eds.), pp. 70. Lang, Los Allos, Ca.

DUCLOS, H., GALANAUD, P., DEVINSKY, O., MAILLOT, M. D., DORMONT, J. (1977) Enhancing effect of low dose cyclophosphamide treatment on the *in vitro* antibody response. *Eur. J. Imm.* **7**: 679–4.

DUMONT, F. and SABOLOVIC D. (1973) Heterogeneity of the hydrocortisone-resistant cell subpopulation in the mouse thymus. *Biomed.* **19**: 257–60.

DUMONT, A. F. (1974) Destruction and regeneration of lymphocyte populations in the mouse spleen after cyclophosphamide treatment. *Int. Arch. Allergy* **47**: 110–23.

DUMONT, A. F. and BARROIS, R. (1975) Effect of treatment with cyclophosphamide on the electrophoretic mobility and mitogen responsiveness of mouse thymus cells. *Bio. Med.* **23**: 391–5.

DUPONT, E., OPELY, G., GUSTAFSSON, L. A., MIKULSKI, S. M., TERASAKI, P. I. (1977) Depressed effector cell function in antibody-dependent cell-mediated cytotoxicity in kidney allograft recipients. *Transplant* **23**: 165–8.

EHRKE, M. J., COHEN, S. A. and MIHICH, E. (1978) Selectivity of inhibition by anticancer agents of mouse spleen immune effector functions involved in responses to sheep erythrocytes. *Cancer Res.* **38**: 521–30.

EZDINLI, E. Z., SIMONSON, K. L. and RANDALL, S. A. (1978) Comparison of the effects of single vs multiple agent chemotherapy on lymphocytes assayed by the rosette technique. *Cancer* **42**: 2234–43.

FAUCI, A. S., WOLFF, S. and JOHNSON, J. S. (1971) Effects of cyclophosphamide upon immune response in Wegener's granulomatosis. *N. Eng. J. Med.* **285**: 1493–4.

FAUCI, A. S. and DALE, D. C. (1974a) Effect of alternate-day prednisone therapy on human lymphocyte subpopulations. *Clin. Res.* **22**: 417.

FAUCI, A. S. and DALE, D. C. (1974b) The effect of *in vivo* hydrocortisone on subpopulations of human lymphocytes. *J. Clin. Inv.* **53**: 240–6.

FAUCI, A. S. (1975) Mechanisms of corticosteroid action on lymphocyte subpopulations I. Redistribution of circulating T and B lymphocytes to the bone marrow. *Immunol* **28**: 669–80.

FAUCI, A. S. and DALE, D. C. (1975) Alternate-day prednisone therapy and human lymphocyte subpopulations. *J. Clin. Inv.* **55**: 22–32.

FERGUSON, R. M. and SIMMONS, R. L. (1978) Differential cyclophosphamide sensitivity of suppressor and cytotoxic cell precursors. *Transplant* **25**: 36–38.

FRIEDMAN, R. M., BUCKLER, C. E. and BARON, S. (1961) The effect of aminomethylpteroylglutamic acid on the development of skin hypersensitivity and on antibody formation in guinea pigs. *J. Exp. Med.* **114**: 173–83.

GADEBERG, O. V., RHODES, J. M. and LARSEN, S. O. (1975) The effect of various immunosuppressive agents on mouse peritoneal macrophages and on the *in vitro* phagocytosis of Escherichia coli 04: H5 and degredation of 125 1-labelled HSA-antibody. *Immunology* **28**: 59–70.

GAUMER, H. R., SALVAGGIO, J. E., WESTON, W. L. and CLAMON, H. N. (1974) Cortisol inhibition of immunologic activity in guinea pig alveolar cells. *Int. Arch. Allergy* **47**: 797–809.

GERBER, M., ANDRESS, D., PIOCH, Y., RADAL, M. and SERROU, B. (1978) Effect of cyclophosphamide and methylprednisolone on *in vitro* cellular immune response to allogeneic tumor cells. Correlation with *in vivo* rejection. *Transplant* **26**: 142–9.

GERMAIN, R. N. and BENACERRAF, B. (1978) The involvement of suppressor T cells in Ir gene regulation of secondary antibody responses of primed (responder X nonresponder) F1 mice to macrophage-bound L-glutamic acid 600L-alanine 30-L-tyrosine. *J. Exp. Med.* **148**: 1324–37.

GHAFFAR, A., LICHTER, W., WILLHAM, L. L., SIGEL, M. M. (1978) Effect of anticancer chemotherapeutic agents on immune reactions of mice. I. Comparison of two nitrosoureas; 1,3,-Bis(2-chloroethyl)-1-nitrosourea and 1-(2-Chloroethyl)-3-(4-methylcyclohexyl)-1-nitrosourea. *J. Natl. Cancer, Inst.* **60**: 1483–7.

GIAMPIETRI, A., CIRCOLO, A., FRATI, L., BONMASSAR, E. and GOLDIN, A. (1978) Long-term inhibition of immune responses by 5-(3,3-0 Dimethyl-1-triazeno) Imidazole-4-carboxamide (DTIC). *Proc. Am. Assoc. Cancer Res.* **10**: 176.

GILL, H. K., LIEW, F. Y. (1978) Regulation of delayed-type hypersensitivity. III. Effect of cyclophosphamide on the suppressor cells for delayed-type hypersensitivity to sheep erythrocytes in mice. *Eur. J. Imm.* **8**: 172–6.

GLASER, M. (1979) Regulation of specific cell-mediated cytotoxic response against SV40-induced tumor associated antigens by depletion of suppressor T cells with cyclophosphamide in mice. *J. Exp. Med.* **149**: 774–9.

GOLDBERG, E. D., MIKHAILOVA, T. N., ZINGER, G. B., SHUBINA, T. S. and KOZLOVA, I. G. (1977) Effect of carminomycin on the immunological reactivity of the body. *Antibiotiki* **22**: 734–9.

GOLSTEIN, P., FOA, C., MACCLENNAN, I. C. (1978) Mechanism of T-cell mediated cytolysis: the differential impact of cytochalasins at the recognition and lethal hit stages. *Eur. J. Immunol.* **8**: 302–9.

GREEN, A. A. and BORELLA, L. (1973) Immunologic rebound after cessation of long-term chemotherapy in acute leukemia II. *In vitro* response to phytohemmaglutinin and antigens by peripheral blood and bone marrow lymphocytes. *Blood* **42**: 99–110.

GRISWOLD, D. E., HEPPNER, G. H. and CALABRESI, P. (1972) Selective suppression of humoral and cellular immunity with cytosine arabinoside. *Cancer. Res.* **32**: 298–301.

GRISWOLD, D. E., WATLZ, D. T. (1978) Restoration of methotrexate-suppressed oxazolone-induced contact sensitivity with levamisole. *Inflammation* **3**: 111–6.

HARRIS, J. E., BAGAI, R. C. and STEWART, T. H. M. (1973) Serial monitoring of immune reactivity in cancer patients receiving chemotherapy as a means of predicting antitumor response in *Proceedings of the Seventh Leukocyte Culture Conference*. F. DAGUILLARD (Ed) New York Academic Press, 443.

HARRIS, J. E., SENGAR, D., STEWART, T. and HYSLOP, D. (1976) The effect of immunosuppressive chemotherapy on immune function in patients with malignant disease. *Cancer* **37**: 1058–69.

HASKILL, S., PARTHENAIS, E. (1978) Immunologic factors influencing the intra-tumor localization of ADCC effector cells. *J. Immunol.* **120:** 1813–7.

HAYNES, B. B. F. and FAUCI, A. S. (1978) Immunologic factors influencing the intra-tumor localization of ADCC effector cells. *J. Clin. Inv.* **61:** 703–7.

HELLSTROM, I., HELLSTROM, K. E. and NEPOM, J. T. (1975) Increased lymphocyte-mediated destruction of tumor cells in microcytotoxicity assays seen after addition of inhibitors of protein synthesis. *Int. J. Cancer.* **16:** 830–9.

HENGST, J. C. D., MOKYR, M. B. and DRAY, S. (1980) Importance of timing in cyclophosphamide therapy of MOPC-315 tumor bearing mice. *Cancer Res.* **40:** 2135–41.

HENNEY, C. S., TRACEY, D., DURDIK, J. M., KLIMPEL, G. (1978) Natural killer cells. *In vitro* and *In vivo. Am. J. Pathol.* **93:** 459–67.

HERRLINGER, J. D., MULLER-RUCHHOLTZ, W. (1978) Different suppressive effects of combined cyclophosphamide-antigen treatment compared with exclusive cyclophosphamide treatment on primary and secondary humoral immune reactivty. *Int. Arch. Allergy Applied Imm.* **57:** 82–9.

HERSH, E. M., WONG, V. G. and FREIREICH, E. J. (1966) Inhibition of the local inflammatory response in man by antimetabolites. *Blood* **27:** 38–47.

HERSH, E. M. and FREIREICH, E. J. (1968) Host defense mechanisms and their modification by cancer chemotherapy. BUSCH H. (Ed.) *Methods in Cancer Res.* Vol. VI, page 355, Acad. Press, NY.

HERSH, E. M. and BODEY, E. P. B. (1970) Leukocytic mechanism of inflammation. *Ann. Rev. Med.* **21:** 105–32.

HERSH, E. M. (1974) Immunosuppressive agents. In: *Antineoplastic and Immunosuppressive Agents* I. SARTORELLI, A. C. and JOHNS, D. G. (Eds) Springer-Verlag, Berlin, pp. 577 (1974).

HIBBS, J. B. (1976) The macrophage as a tumoricidal effector cell: A review of *in vivo* and *in vitro* studies on the mechanism of the activated macrophage nonspecific cytotoxic reaction. In: *The Macrophage in Neoplasia.* FINK, M. (Ed.) Acad Press, New York, pp. 83.

HIRANO, T. and NORDIN, A. A. (1976) Cell-mediated immune response *in vitro* I. The development of suppressor cells and cytotoxic lymphocytes in mixed lymphocyte cultures. *J. Immunol.* **116:** 1115–22.

HOFFMANN, C. C., MOORE, K. C., SHIH, C. Y. and BLAKLEY, R. L. (1977) Scanning electron microscopy of human lymphocytes during transformation and subsequent treatment with methotrexate. *J. Cell Sci.* **28:** 151–65.

HOLLAND, J. F., OHNUMA, T. (1979) Lessons from the study of induced alterations in amino acids in patients with cancer. *Cancer Treat. Rep.* **3:** 1013–8.

HOLLOWELL, R. R., MEDZIHRADSKY, J. L. and ELION, G. M. (1979) Differential effects of 6-mercaptopurine and azathioprine on suppressor cells. *Fed Proc* **38:** 598.

HUNNINGHAKE, G. W. and FAUCI, A. S. (1976) Divergent effects of cyclophosphamide administration on mononuclear killer cells: Quantitative depletion of cell members vs qualitative suppression of functional capabilities. *J. Immunol.* **117:** 337–42.

HUNNINGHAKE, W. and FAUCI, A. S. (1977a) Immunological reactivity of the lung. IV. Effect of cyclophosphamide on alveolar macrophage cytotoxic effector function. *Clin. Exp. Imm.* **27:** 555–9.

HUNNINGHAKE, G. W. FAUCI, A. S. (1977b) Immunologic reactivity of the lung III. HUNNINGHAKE, G. W., FAUCI, A. S. (1977b) Immunologic reactivity of the lung III. Effects of corticosteroids on alveolar macrophage cytotoxic effector cell function. *J. Immunol.* **118:** 146–50.

HURD, E. R. and ZIFF, M. (1968) Studies on the anti-inflammatory action of 6-mercaptopurine. *J. Exp. Med.* **128:** 785–800.

HURD, E. R. (1973) The effect of cyclophosphamide treatment on B and T lymphocytes in patients with connective tissue diseases. *Arthritis Rheum.* **16;** 554.

HURME, M. (1979) Differential cyclophosphamide sensitivity of precursor cells in allogeneic and H-2 restricted cytotoxic responses. *J. Exp. Med.* **149;** 290–4.

IGARASHI, T., OKADA, M., KISHIMOTO, T. and YAMAMURA Y. (1977) *In vitro* induction of polyclonal killer T cells with 2-mercaptoethanol and the essential role of macrophages in this process. *J. Immunol.* **118:** 1697–1703.

JACOBS, S. C., MCLAUGHLIN, A. P. and GITTES, R. F. (1977) Effects of immunosuppression on the rejection of methylcholanthrene tumor isografts. *J. Surg. Oncol.* **9:** 353–7.

JOHANSEN, K. S., JOHANSEN, T. S. and TALMAGE, D. W. (1974) T-cell rosette formation in primates, pigs and guinea pigs. *J. Allergy and Clin. Imm.* **54:** 86–93.

JONES, B. M. (1976) Mechanisms of leukocyte migration inhibition by breast tumor cell fractions. *Br. J. Cancer* **34:** 14–9.

KABIRI, M. and HADALGH, M. D. (1977) Interaction of coxsackievirus B-3 and peritoneal exudate cells of adult mice treated with cyclophosphamide. *J. Med. Virol.* **1(3):** 183–91.

KARP, J. E., BURKE, P. J. and HUMPHREY, R. L. (1977) Induction of serum and plasma cell proliferation during chemotherapy of multiple myeloma. *Blood* **49:** 925–34.

KAUFMAN, S. J. (1971) Selective inhibition of cells in the immune response by actinomycin D. *J. Imm.* **106:** 781–85.

KATZ, S. L., PARKER, D. and TURK, J. L. (1974) B-cell suppression of delayed hypersensitivity reactions. *Nature* **251:** 550–1.

KERCKHAERT, J., HOFHUIS, F. M., WILLERS, J. M. (1977) Effects of variation in time and dose of cyclophosphamide injection on delayed hypersensitivity and antibody formation. *Cell Immunol.* **20:** 232–37.

KIPPS, T. J., BENACERRAF, B., DORF, M. E. (1978) Regulation of antibody heterogeneity by suppressor T-cells; Diminishing suppressor T-cell activity increases the number of dinitrophenyl clones in mice immunized with dinitrophenyl-poly (Glu, Lys, Phe) or dinitrophenyl-poly (Glu, Lys, Ala). *Proc. Nat. Acad. Sci. U.S.A.* **75:** 2914–7.

KOLB, J. P., POUPON, M., LESPINATS, G. M., SABOLOVIC, D. and LOISILLIER, F. (1977) Splenic modifications induced by cyclophosphamide in C3H/He, nude, and 'B'-mice. *J. Imm.* **118:** 1595–9.

KOUROUNAKIS, L. and KAPUSTA, M. A. (1977) Restoration of diminished T-cell function in adjuvant induced disease by methotrexate. Evidence for two populations of splenic T-cell suppressors. *J. Rheumatol.* **3:** 346–54.

L'AGE-STEHR, J. and DIAMANSTEIN, T. (1978) Induction of autoreactive T lymphocytes and their suppressor cells by cyclophosphamide. *Nature* **271:** 663–5.

LA GRANGE, P. H., MACKANESS, G. M. and MILLER, T. E. (1974) Potentiation of T-cell-mediated immunity by selective suppression of antibody formation with cyclophosphamide. *J. Exp. Med.* **139:** 1529–39.

LEE, K. (1977) Cortisone as a probe for cell interactions in the generation of cytotoxic T cells. Effect on helper cells, cytotoxic T cell precursors and accessory cells. *J. Immunol.* **119:** 1836–44.

LEFORD, M. J., MCGREGOR, D. D. (1978) The lymphocyte mediators of delayed hypersensitivity: The early phase cells. *Immunol.* **34:** 581–90.

LEME, J. G., BECHARA, G. H., SUDD, L. S. (1977) The proinflammatory function of lymphocytes in non-immune inflammation: Effect of steroidal and non-steroidal anti-inflammatory agents. *Br. J. Exp. Pathol.* **58:** 703–11.

LEONTEVA, T. I., MAKSIMOVA, G. F., BABICHEV, V. A., UTESHEV, B. X. (1977) Immunosuppressive properties of vinblastine and colchicine. *Tsitologia.* **19:** 186–91.

LIASHENKO, V. A., SHAPOVALOVA, S. P., ALEKSANDER, S. K. MALKOVA, I. V. (1979) Comparison of the action of carminomycin and rubomycin on the dynamics of the primary and secondary immune responses. *Antibiotiki* **24:** 449–454.

LIPSKY, P. E. and ROSENTHAL, A. S. (1975) Macrophage-lymphocyte interaction: Antigen independent binding of guinea pig, lymph node lymphocytes by macrophages. *J. Immunol.* **115:** 440–5.

LIPSKY, P. E., GINSBURG, T. W. W., FINKELMAN, F. D. and MORRISS, Z. (1978) Control of human B lymphocyte responsiveness enhanced suppressor T cell activity after *in vitro* incubation. *J. Imm.* **120:** 902–10.

LISKE, R. A. (1973) Comparative study of the action of cyclophosphamide and procarbazine on the antibody production in mice. *Clin. Exp. Immunol.* **15:** 271–80.

LOCKHARD, V. G., SHARBAUGH, R. J., ARHELGER, R. B. and GROGAN, J. B. (1971) Ultrastructural alterations in phagocytic functions of alveolar macrophages after cyclophosphamide administration. *J. Ret. Soc.* **9:** 97–104.

MACKIEWICZ, U., BRELINSKA-PECZALSKA, R., KONYS, J. (1978) The influence of cyclophosphamide on lymphnode and peripheral blood lymphocytes in mice. *Arch. Immunol. Ther. Exp.* (Warsz) **26:** 375–80.

MACGUIRE, H. C., FARRIS, L., WEIDANZ, W. (1979) Cyclophosphamide intensifies the acquisition of allergic contact dermatitis in mice rendered B-cell deficient by heterologous anti-IgM antisera. *Immunology* **37:** 367–72.

MALAWISTA, S. E., GEE, J. B. L., BENSCH, K. G. (1971) Cytochalasin B reversibly inhibits phagocytosis: Functional metabolic and ultrastructural effects in human blood leukocytes and rabbit alveolar macrophages. *Yale J. Biol. Med.* **44:** 286–300.

MALBERG, K., NUHN, P., AMBROSIUS, H. (1978) 6-(2,4-dinitrophenyl)-mercaptopurine, a stronger immunosuppressive drug than 6-mercaptopurine to primary humoral T-cell dependent immune response in mice. *Acta. Biol. Med. Ger.* **37:** 645–54.

MANSOUR, A., NELSON, D. S. (1977) Effect of cyclophosphamide treatment on the response of rat peripheral blood lymphocytes to phytohemmagglutinin. *Cell Immunol.* **30:** 272–81.

MANSOUR, A., HENDERSON, J. A., NELSON, D. S. (1978) Effect of methotrexate on the response of rat lymphocytes to phytohaemmagglutinin. *Clin. Exp. Immunol.* **34:** 393–401.

MONTOVANI, A. (1977) *In vitro* and *in vivo* cytotoxicity of adriamycin and daunomycin for murine macrophages. *Cancer Res.* **37:** 815–20.

MANTOVANI, A., TALIABUE, A. and SPREAFICO, F. (1977) The effect of adriamycin on the induction and expression of macrophage cytotoxicity. *Proc. Amer. Assoc. Cancer Res.* **18:** 34.

MANTOVANI, A., VECCHI, A., TAGLIABUE, A. and SPREAFICO, F. (1976) The effects of adriamycin and daunomycin on antitumoral immune effector mechanisms in an allogeneic system. *Eur. J. Cancer.* **12:** 371 (1976–79).

MANTOVANI, A., LUINI, W., PERI, G., VECCHI, A., SPREAFICO, F. (1978) Effect of chemotherapeutic agents on natural cell-mediated cytotoxicity in mice. *J. Natl. Cancer. Inst.* **61:** 1255–61.

MARCHAL, G., MILON, G., HURTREL, B. and LA GRANGE, P. H. (1978) Titration and circulation of cells mediating delayed type hypersensitivity in normal and cyclophosphamide treated mice during response to sheep red blood cells. *Immunol* **35:** 981–7.

MARTEL, R. R., KLICIUS, J., GALET, S. (1977) Inhibition of the immune response by rapamycin a new antifungal antibiotic. *Canadian J. Physiol. Pharmacol.* **55:** 48–51.

MASERANG, D. L., HYDE, R. M. (1977) Blockade of immune tolerance induction by puromycin aminonucleoside. *Cell Immunol.* **31:** 255–65.

MEHTA, J., KNOTTS, L. L., HAHN, B. H. (1977) Effect of altered lymphocyte function on immunologic disorders in NZN/NZW mice. *Arth. Rheum.* **20:** 65–72.

MILLER, G. A., PHIPPO, R. P., TEW, J. G. (1979) Induction of antibody synthesis by antigen retained in cyclophosphamide treated mice upon infusion of memory cells. *Fed. Proc.* **38:** 1220.

MILLER, J. J. and COLE, L. J. (1967) Resistance of long-lived lymphocytes and plasma cells in rat lymphnodes to treatment with prednisone, cyclophosphamide, 6-mercaptopurine and actinomycin-D. *J. Exp. Med.* **126:** 109–115.

MILON, G. and MARCHAL, G. (1978) Increased infiltration by monocytes in delayed type hypersensitivity site following cyclophosphamide treatment. *Immunol.* **35:** 989–95.

MILTON, J. D., CARPENTER, C. B. and ADDISON, I. E. (1976) Depressed T-cell reactivity and suppressor activity of lymphoid cells from cyclophosphamide treated mice. *Cell Immunol* **24:** 308–17.

MINATO, N., KATSURA, Y. (1978) Virus-replicating T cells in the immune response of mice. II. Characterization of T cells capable of replicating vesicular stomatitis virus. *J. Exp. Med.* **148:** 837–49.

MITCHELL, M. S., WADE, M. E., DE CONTI, R. C., BERTINO, J. R. and CALABRESI, P. (1969) Immunosuppressive effects of cytosine arabinoside and methotrexate in man. *Ann. Int. Med.* **70:** 535–47.

MITCHELL, M. S. and DE CONTI, R. C. (1970) Immunosuppression by 5-Fluorouracil. *Cancer* **26:** 884–9.

MITSUOKA, A., BABA, M. and MORIKAWA, W. (1976) Enhancement of delayed hypersensitivity by depletion of suppressor T cells with cyclophosphamide in mice. *Nature* **262**: 77–78.

MOODY, C. E., TUNTICHAROEN, M., LAUS, D. C. (1977) Increased cell-mediated lysis of chicken erythrocytes following the addition of metabolic inhibitors. *Immunology* **33**: 285–3.

MORETTA, L., FERRARINI, M., MINGARI, J. C., MORETTA, A., WEBB, S. R. (1976) Subpopulations of human T cells identified by receptors for immunoglobulins and mitogen responsiveness. *J. Immunol.* **117**: 2171–4.

MORETTA, L., WEBB, S. R., GROSSI, C. E., LYDYARD, P. M., COOPER, M. D. (1977) Functional analysis of two human T cells bearing receptors for IgM or IgG. *J. Exp. Med.* **146**: 184–200.

MORI, H., NAGAI, H., KODA, A. (1977) Effect of FT-207 on antibody formation. *Cancer and Chemotherapy* **4**: 797–4.

MOTTIRONI, V. D., RUDOFSKY, U. H., SWIFT, R. V., ESPOSITO, L. L. (1978) Niridazole inhibition of local graft vs host reaction in rat muscle. *Clin. Immunol. Immunopathol.* **10**: 158–67.

NACHTIGAL, D., ZAN-BAR, I., FELDMAN, M. (1975) The role of specific suppressor T cells in human tolerance. *Transplant Rev.* **26**: 87.

NAKANO, K., NAKANO, Y. (1978) Suppressor cells in antigenic competition in contact allergy in mice. *Immunol.* **34**: 981–7.

NETTESHEIM, P., HAMMONS, A. S. (1970) Effect of immunosuppressive agents on retention of antigen in the mouse spleen. *Pro. Soc. Ex. Biol. Med.* **133**: 696–701.

NETZEL, B., RODT, G., GROSS-WEILDE, H., WEGER, N., THIERFELDER, S. (1977) Hematologic and immunologic studies in dogs given nitrogen mustard (HN3). *Bluat*, **35**: 51–6.

NEVALAINEN, D. E., HOFTIEZER, V. (1977) The response of C3H mice to streptozotocin. I. Thymic depression and leukocyte toxicity. *Am. J. Med. Tech.* **43**: 417–418.

NICOL, T., QUANTOCK, D. C. and VERNON-ROBERTS, B. (1967) The effect of steroid hormones on local and general reticuloendothelial activity: Relation of steroid structure to function. In *The Reticuloendothelial System and Atherosclerosis.* N. R. DILUZIO and P. AOLETTI, (Ed.) pp. 221, Plenum Press, NY.

NIKULINA, L. B. (1978) Effect of actinomycin D. Carcinomycin and Bleomycin and their joint use with serotonin and zymosan on the functional state of the peritoneal macrophages. *Antibiotiki* **23**: 543–8.

NOBLE, B., PARKER, D., SCHEPER, R. J., TURK, J. L. (1977) The relation between B-cell stimulation and delayed hypersensitivity. The effect of cyclophosphamide pretreatment on antibody production. *Immunol.* **32**: 885–91.

NOONAN, F. P., HALLIDAN, W. J., WALL, D. R. and CLUNIE, G. J. A. (1977) Cell-mediated immunity and serum blocking factors in cancer patients during chemotherapy and immunotherapy. *Cancer Res.* **37**: 2473–80.

NORDMAN, E., SAARIMAA, H., TOIVANEN, A., (1978) The influence of 5-fluorouracil on cellular and humoral immunity in cancer patients. *Cancer* **41**: 64–9.

OEHLER, J. J., HERBERMAN, R. B. (1978) Natural cell-mediated cytotoxicity in rats. III. Effects of immunopharmacologic treatments on natural reactivity and on reactivity augmented by polyinosinic-polycytidylic acid. *Int. J. Cancer* **21**: 2219.

OGISO, T., NODA, N., MASUDA, H., KATO, Y. (1978) Antitumor agents. II. Effect of 5-fluorouracil and cyclophosphamide on immunological parameters and liver microsomes of tumor-bearing rats. *Jpn. J. Pharmacol.* **28**: 175–83.

Ohnuma, T., Arkin, H., Minowada, J., Holland, J. F. (1978) Differential chemotherapeutic susceptibility of human T-lymphocytes and B-lymphocytes in culture. *J. Natl. Cancer. Inst.* **60**: 749–52.

ORBACH-ARBOUYS, S. and CASTES, M. (1979) Augmentation of immune responses after methotrexate administration. *Immunol* **36**: 265–69.

ORSINI, F. and MIHICH, E. (1975) Immunosuppression by adriamycin (AM) and daunonubicin (DM). *Proc. Am. Assoc. Cancer. Res.* **16**: 130.

ORSINI, F., PAVELIC, Z., MIHICH, E., (1977) Increased primary cell-mediated immunity in culture subsequent to adriamycin or daunorubicin treatment of spleen donor mice. *Cancer Res.* **37**: 1719–26.

OSSLER, K., KROPPE, P., AMBROSIUS, H. (1977) The influence of 6-mercaptopurine on the humoral immune response in guinea pig. 2. The influence on formation of complement binding antibodies. *Aller. Immunol* (Leipz) **23**: 12–16.

PACHA, J., METZGER, M., SMOGOR, W., MICHALASKA, E., PODWINSKA, J., RUCZKOWSKA, J., (1979) Effect of immunosuppressive agents on the course of experimental syphillis in rabbits. *Arch. Immunol. Ther Exp.* (Warsz) **27**: 45–51.

PAGE, A. R., CONDI, R. M., GOOD, R. A. (1962) Effect of 6-mercaptopurine on inflammation. *Am. J. Path.* **40**, 519–30.

PAGE, A. R., CONDI, R. M., GOOD, R. A. (1964) Inhibition of the lymphocyte response to inflammation with antimetabolites. *Amer. J. Path.* **45**: 1029–44.

PARKER, D., TURK, J. C. (1978) The effect of cyclophosphamide pretreatment on B-cell stimulation: Dissociation of action on homocytotropic antibody and other B-cell functions. *Immunology* **34**: 115–21.

PARKS, D. E., SHALLER, D. A., WEIGLE, W. O. (1979) Induction and mode of action of suppressor cells generated against human gamma globulin II. Effects of colchicine. *J. Exp. Med.* **149**: 1168–79.

PENNINGTON, J. E. (1977) Bronchoalveolar cell response to bacterial challenge in the immunosuppressed lung. *Amm. Rev. Respir. Dis.* **116**(4): 885–93.

PENNINGTON, J. E. (1978) Differential effects of cyclophosphamide and cortisone acetate on bronchoalveolar phagocytic cell populations. *Ann. Rev. Respir. Dis.* **118**: 319–24.

PEREVERZEVA, E. R. (1978) The influence of cyclophosphane and phenthyrine and their combination with zymosan and serotonin on the functional features distinguishing peritoneal macrophages in mice. *Farmakol. Toksikol.* **41**(4): 422–7.

PETRANYI, G. G., GYORFFY, G., BENCZUR, M., VARGA, M., GYODI, E., ONODY, K., FUST, G., LANG, I. (1978) Features, genetics and *in vivo* importance of lymphocyte mediated natural cytotoxicity. *Panminerva Med.* **20**: 71–80.

POLAK, L. and TURK, J. L. (1974) Reversal of immunological tolerance by cyclophosphamide through inhibition of suppressor cell activity. *Nature* **249:** 654–6.

PURVES, E. C., BROWN, K. (1978) Effect of cortisone acetate on effector cells for antibody-mediated cytotoxicity in mouse and rat. *Transplantation* **25:** 7–11.

REVELL, P. A. (1974) Studies on the effect of cyclophosphamide on T and B lymphocytes in the blood, lymph nodes and thymus of normal guinea pigs. *Int. Arch. Allergy and Applied Imm.* **47;** 864–74.

REVELL, P. A. (1978) Effect of long-term cyclophosphamide treatment on T and B lymphocytes in normal guinea pigs. *Int. Arch. Allergy App. Imm.* **56:** 443–8.

REYNOLDS, H. Y., KAZMIEROWSKI, J. A., DALE, D. C. (1976) Changes in the comparison of canine respiratory cells obtained by bronchial lavage following irradiation or drug immunosuppression. *Proc. Soc. Exp. Biol. Med.* (*N.Y.*) **151:** 756–61.

RHODES, J. M., BIRCH-ANDERSON, A., RAV, H. (1975) The effect of cyclophosphamide, methotrexate and X-irradiation on the ultrastructure and endocytic capacity of murine peritoneal macrophages. *Acta. Path. Microbiol. Scan.* **A83:** 443–53.

RICCARDI, C., FIORETTI, M. C., GIAMPIETRI, A., PUCCETTI, P., GOLDIN, A. (1978) Growth and rejection patterns of murine lymphoma cells antigenically altered following drug treatment *in vivo*. *Transplant* **25:** 63–8.

RIEGER, M., GUNTER, J., KRISTOVA, A. H., HILGERT, I. (1978) Evidence of suppressor cell-mechanism of allograft tolerance induced by spleen extract and hydrocortisone. *Folia. Biol.* (PRAHA) **24:** 145–61.

RILSGAARD, S., RHODES, J. M., BENNEDSEN, J. (1978) Macrophage activation by lymphokines and after direct contact with sensitized lymphocytes: Histocompatibility requirements and the effect of inhibitors. *Scand. J. Immunol.* **7:** 209–13.

RITTER, J. (1976) Null cells in leukaemia during therapy (letter to editor). *Lancet* **2**(7996): 1204.

ROBINSON, E., BARTAL, A., COHEN, Y., HAASZ, R., MEKORI, T. (1977) Treatment of lung cancer by radiotherapy, chemotherapy and methanol extraction residue of BCG (MER). *Cancer* **4D:** 1052–9.

ROLLINGHOFF, M., SCHRADER, J., WAGNER, H. (1973) Effect of azathioprine and cytosine arabinoside on humoral and cellular immunity *in vitro*. *Clin. Exp. Immunol.* **15:** 261–9.

ROLLINGHOFF, M., STARZINSKI-POWITZ, A., PFIZENMAIER, K., WAGNER, H. (1977) Cyclophosphamide-sensitive T lymphocytes suppress the *in vivo* generation of antigen specific cytotoxic T lymphocytes. *J. Exp. Med.* **145:** 455–9.

ROMANYCHEVA, V., BABICHEV, V. A., UTESHEV, B. S., KALINKOVITCH, A. G. (1978) The kinetics of inhibition with methotrexate and vinblastine of the primary immune response to sheep red blood cells in mice (plaque-forming cells). *Folia. Biol.* (Praha) **24:** 343–54.

ROOK, G. A., KING, J. (1978) Is the adherent, non-specific 'suppressor' cell from rodent spleens an *in vitro* artefact? *Clin. Exp. Immunol.* **32:** 466–70.

ROSENBERG, J. and LYSZ K. (1977) Methylprednisolone suppression of proliferating and cytotoxic lymphocytes. *Trans. Proc.* **9,** 1055–7.

ROSENTHAL, A. S., BLAKE, J. T., LIPSKY, P. E. (1975) Inhibition of macrophage-lymphocyte interaction by cytochalasin-B during antigen recognition by T lymphocytes. *J. Immunol* **115:** 1135–9.

SANTOS, G. W., OWENS, A. H. (1964) A comparison of the effects of selected cytotoxic agents on the primary agglutinin response in rats injected with sheep erythrocytes. *Bull. John Hopkins Hosp.* **114:** 384–401.

SANTOS, G. W., OWENS, A. H. (1966) Adoptive transfer of immunologically competent cells. I. Quantitative studies of antibody formation in cyclophosphamide pretreated mice. *Bull John Hopkins Hosp.* **118:** 109–126.

SANTOS, G. W., OWENS, A. H. (1966) 19S and 7S antibody production in the cyclophosphamide or methotrexate treated rat. *Nature* (*London*), **209:** 622–4.

SAWADA, J., KISHIE, T., OSAWA, T. (1977) Effect of various reagents on the susceptibility of target cells to the cytotoxicity of guinea pig lymphotoxin (GLT). *Microbiol Immunol* **21:** 167–74.

SAXON, A., STEVENS, R. H., RAMIR, S. I., CLEMENTS, P. J., YU, D. T. Y. (1978) Glucocorticoids administered *in vivo* inhibit human suppressor T lymphocyte function and *in vitro* immunoglobulin synthesis. *J. Clin Invest* **61:** 922–30.

SCHAFFNER, H., HADGE, D. (1977) Effect of L-asparaginase on humoral immune response against protein antigens in mice. *Allerg Immunol* (Leipz) **23:** 24–33.

SCHECHTER, B., FELDMAN, M. (1977) Hydrocortisone affects tumor growth by eliminating precursors of suppressor cells. *J. Immunol.* **119:** 1563–8.

SCHECHTER, B., FELDMAN, M. (1978) *In vitro* retrieval of the cytotoxic potential of spleen cells of tumor-bearing mice. *Isr J. Med. Sci.* **14:** 131–45.

SCHEIFFARTH, F., LEYKAMS, D., WARNATZ, H., BAENKLER, H. W. (1973) Effect of cytostatic drugs on blast cell transformation of lymph node and spleen cells. *Res Exp Med* **160:** 196–205.

SCHEINBERG, M. A., CATHCART, E. S. (1976) Antibody-dependent direct cytotoxicity of human lymphocytes I. Studies on peripheral blood lymphocytes and sera of patients with systemic lupus erythematosus. *Clin. Exp. Immunol.* **24:** 317–22.

SCHEPER, R. J., BAAK, J. P. A., HIISWARA, S., VELDHUIZEN, W. (1975) RRBC and EAC rosette formation after DNCB contact sensitization and cyclophosphamide treatment of guinea pigs. *Immunol* **29:** 909–19.

SCHERBAUM, I., AMBROSIUS, H. (1978) Comparative investigations of quantitative determination of cell-mediated immunity by skin test, macrophage migration inhibition test, and lymphocyte transformation test in guinea pigs. *Aller. Imm.* (Leipz) **24:** 278–86.

SCHRIEBER, A. D., PARSONS, J., MCDERMOTT, P., COOPER, R. A. (1975) Effect of corticosteroids on the human monocyte, IgG and complement receptors. *J. Clin. Invest.* **56:** 1189–97.

SCHULTZ, R. M., PAVLIDIS, N. A., CHIRIGOS, M. A., WEISS, J. F. (1978) Effects of whole body X-irradiation and cyclophosphamide treatment on induction of macrophage tumoricidal function in mice. *Cell. Immunol.* **38:** 302–9.

SCHULTZ, R. M., CHIRIGOS, M. A. (1978) Effects of irradiation and cyclophosphamide (CY) treatments on expression of macrophage tumoricidal function in mice. *Proc. Amer. Assoc. Cancer Res.* **19:** 15.

SCHWARTZ, A., ASKENASE, P. W., GERSHON, R. K. (1978) Regulation of delayed-type hypersensitivity reactions by cyclophosphamide-sensitive T cells. *J. Immunol.* **121**: 1573–7.

SCHWARTZ, R. S. (1968) Immunosuppressive drug therapy in Human Transplantation. RAPAPORT F. T. and DAUSSET, J. (Eds.) pp. 440, Grune and Stratton, New York.

SCHWARZE, G. (1977) Drug-induced immunological unresponsiveness: Selective inhibition of T-cell, 'helper function' by cyclophosphamide in mice pretreated with phytohaemagglutinin. *Clin Exp Immunol.* **27**: 178–82.

SCHWARZE, G. (1978) Immunosuppression by means of cytostatic chemotherapy. Inhibition of antibody formation and induction of tolerance in animal experiments. *Fortschr Med* **96**: 2107–11.

SHAND, F. L., HOWARD, J. G. (1978) Cyclophosphamide inhibited B cell receptor regeneration as a basis for drug-induced tolerance. *Nature* (London) **271**: 255–7.

SHAPOVALOVA, S. P., ALEKSANDER, S. K., LIASHENKO, V., MALKOVA, Y., POVAROU, L. S. (1979) Immunodepressive action of carcinomycin and rubomycin derivatives. *Antibiotiki* **24**: 521–5.

SHARBAUGH, R. J., GROGAN, J. B. (1969) Alterations in the bactericidal capacity of the rat lung after immunosuppression. *Antimicrob Agents Chemother* **9**: 468–52.

SHARMA, S. D., PIESSENS, W. P. (1978) Tumor cell killing by macrophages activated *in vitro* with lymphocyte mediators. II. Inhibition by inhibitors of protein synthesis. *Cell Immunol* **38**: 264–75.

SHARMA, S. D., PIESSENS, W. F. (1978) Tumor cell killing by macrophages activated *in vitro* with lymphocyte mediators. III. Inhibition by cytochalasins, colchicine, and vinblastine. *Cell Immunol* **38**: 276–85.

SHEK, P. N., COONS, A. H. (1978) Effect of colchicine on the antibody response. I. Enhancement of antibody formation in mice. *J Exp Med* **147**: 1213–27.

SIEGER, L. (1977) Effects of chronic methotrexate therapy on numbers and function of rabbit alveolar macrophages. *Proc. Soc Exp Biol Med.* **156**: 406–10.

SLJIVIC, V. S., WARR, G. W. (1973) Activity of the reticuloendothelial system and the antibody response. I. The effect of stilboestriol on the immune response to sheep erythrocytes in the mouse. *Brit J Exp Path.* **54**: 69–78.

SMITH, B., STJERNSWARD, J., DOWDLE, E. *et al.* (1979) The lymphocyte: monocyte ratio: B and T cell ratio after radiotherapy, chemotherapy and surgery. *Int J Radiation Oncol Biol Phys* **5**: 1841–9.

SNIPPE, H., DAVIDSE, R. P. A., BELDER, M., WILLERS, J. M. N. (1976) Effects of cyclophosphamide treatment on the *in vitro* activity of mouse lymphoid cells after nonspecific and specific stimulation. *Int Arch Allergy Appl Imm* **50**: 536–47.

SNIPPE, H., MERCHANT, B., JOHANNESSEN, L., INMAN, J. K. (1978) Effects of cyclophosphamide on the *in vivo* response of outbred athymic (nude) mice to a thymusindependent antigen (DNP-AGG-Ficoll). *Immunol* **35**: 1009–15.

SNYDERMAN, R., GEURZ, H., MERGENHAGEN, S. E. (1971) Effect of C4 depletion on the utilization of the terminal components of guinea pig complement by endotoxin. *Nature New Biol.* **231**: 153–5.

SPARKS, F. C., ALBERT, N. E., ANDREONE, P. A., BREEDING, J. H. (1977) Effect of Bacillus calmette-guerin on immunosuppression from cyclophosphamide, methotrexate and 5-fluorouracil. *Cancer Res* **37**: 2560–4.

SPEIERS, R. S., BENSON, R. W., KNOWLES, B. J., ROBERTS, D. (1978) Models for assessing the effect of toxicants on immunocompetence in mice. II. Effect of cyclophosphamide on the antibody responses to type III pneumococcal polysaccharide and tetanus toxoid in BALB/c female mice. *J Environ Pathol Toxicol.* **1**: 791–812.

STAVY, L., COHEN, I. R., FELDMAN, M. (1974) Stimulation of rat lymphocyte proliferation by hydrocortisone during the induction of cell-mediated immunity *in vitro*. *Transplantation* **17**: 173–9.

STERZL, J. (1970) The effect of immunosuppressive drugs at various stages of differentiation of immunologically competent cells. In *Immunity, Cancer, and Chemotherapy*, E. MIHICH, (Ed.) Acad Press, NY, pp. 73.

STOCKMAN, G. D., HEIM, L. R., SOUTH, M., TRENTIN, J. J. (1973) Differential effects of cyclophosphamide on the B and T cell compartments of adult mice. *J Immunol* **110**: 277–82.

STOYCHKOV, J. N., SCHULTZ, R. M., CHIRIGOS, M. A., PAVLIDIS, N. A., GOLDIN, A. (1979) Effects of adriamycin and cyclophosphamide treatment on induction of macrophage cytotoxic function in mice. *Cancer Res* **39**: 3014–7.

STROM, T. B., GAROVOY, M. R., BEAR, R. A. *et al.* (1975) A comparison of the effects of metabolic inhibitors upon direct and antibody-dependent lymphocyte mediated cytotoxicity. *Cell Immunol* **20**: 247–56.

STYLOS, W. A., CHIRIGOS, M. A., LENGEL, C. R., LYNG, P. J. (1978a) T and B lymphocyte populations of tumor-bearing mice treated with 1,3-Bis(chloroethyl)-1-nitrosourea(BCNU) or pyran. *Cancer Immunol Immunother* **5**: 165–72.

STYLOS, W. A., CHIRIGOS, M. A., LYNG, P. G., LENGEL, C. R. (1978b) T and B lymphocyte populations of the spleen and thymus in normal and immunosuppressed BALB/c mice. *Cell Imm* **40**: 79–90.

SY, M. S., MILLER, S. D., CLAMAN, H. N. (1977) Immune suppression with supraoptimal doses of antigen in contact sensitivity. I. Demonstration of suppressor cells and their sensitivity to cyclophosphamide. *J Immunol* **119**: 240–4.

SY, M., MILLER, S. D., MOOREHEAD, J. W., CLAMAN, H. N. (1979) Active suppression of 1-Fluoro-2,4-Dinitrobenzene-immune T cells requirement of an auxiliary T cell induced by antigen. *J Exp Med* **149**: 1197–1207.

SYCKLOCHA, D., SIMINOVICH, L., TILL, J. E., MCCULLOCH, E. A. (1966) The proliferative state of antigen-sensitive precursors of hemolysin-forming cells, determined by the use of the inhibitor, vinblastine. *J Immunol* **96**: 472–77.

TURK, J. L., POULTER, L. W. (1972) Selective depletion of lymphoid tissue by cyclophosphamide. *Clin Exp Imm* **10**: 285–96.

URBANIAK, S. J. (1979) ADCC (k-cell) lysis of human erythrocytes sensitized with rhesus alloantibodies. II. Investigation into the mechanism of lysis. *Br J Haematol* **42**: 315–25.

VAN DEN BROEK, A. A., KEUNING, F. J. (1977) Effects of drugs on immune responsiveness in rabbits. *Dev. Biol. Stand* **38**: 167–72.

VAN FURTH, R., GASSMAN, A. E., DIESSELHOFF-DEN DULK, M. M. C. (1975) The effect of azothioprine (imuran) on the cell cycle of promonocytes and the production of monocytes in the bone marrow. *J Exp Med* **141:** 531–46.

VENETIANER, H., ARANYI, P., BOSZE, Z. S., FACHET, J. (1978) Sensitivity of glucocorticoids of lymphnode cells stimulated *in vivo* by oxasolone. *Scand J Immunol* **8:** 355–62.

VERNON, R. B. (1969) The effects of steroid hormones on macrophage activity. *Int Rev Cytology* **25:** 131–65.

VETTO, R. M., BURGER, D., VANDENBARK, A., FINKE, P. E. (1978) Changes in tumor immunity during therapy determined by leukocyte adherence inhibition and dermal testing. *Cancer* **41:** 1034–39.

WALDMANN, H. (1978) The influence of the major histocompatibility complex on the function of T-helper cells in antibody formation. *Immunol Rev* **42:** 202–23.

WALDMANN, H., HOWARD, J. (1979) Cellular basis of the immune response in defense and recognition IIA-cellular aspects (International Review Biochemistry, Vol 22-Lennox, ES ed.) University Park Press, Baltimore, pp. 29.

WARR, G. W., SLJIVIC, V. S. (1973) Activity of the reticuloendothelial system and the antibody response. I. Effect of stilboestriol on the immune response to sheep erythrocytes in the mouse. *Brit J Exp Path* **54:** 56–68.

WHITE, D. J., CALNE, R. Y., PLUMB, A. (1979a) Mode of action of cyclosporin A: A new immunosuppressive agent. *Transplant Proc* **11:** 855.

WHITE, J. G., PLUMB, A. M., PAWELEC, G., BRONS, G. (1979b) Cyclosporin A: An immunosuppressive agent preferentially active against proliferating T cells. *Transplant* **27:** 55.

WIERDA, D., PAZDERNIK, T. L. (1979) Suppression of spleen lymphocyte mitogenesis in mice injected with platinum compounds. *Eur. J Cancer* **16:** 1013–23.

WILLERS, J. M. N., SLUIS, E. (1975) The influence of cyclophosphamide on antibody formation in the mouse. *Ann Immunol* (Inst Pasteur) **126C:** 267–79.

WINKELSTEIN, A., JOKIPII, A. M. M., JOKIPII, L. (1973) (Short communications) Suppression of cell-mediated immunity by cyclophosphamide: It's independence of concomitant B cell response. *Cell Immunol* **9:** 477–81.

WINKELSTEIN, A. (1977) Effect of immunosuppressive drugs on T and B lymphocytes in guinea pigs. *Blood* **50:** 81–91.

WOJNAR, R. J., BRITTAIN, R. J., DZELZKALNS, E. (1979) Effect of nonsteroidal antiinflammatory and other pharmacological agents on tuberculin reaction. *J Pharm Sci* **68:** 12–15.

WOOD, M. L., MONACO, A. P. (1977) The effect of cyclophosphamide on the specific unresponsiveness to skin allografts induced in ALS-treated mice infused with donor bone marrow. *J Immunol* **118:** 1456–9.

YOUMANS, A. S., YOUMANS, G. P. (1978) Effect of metabolic inhibitors on the formation of antibody to sheep erythrocytes, on development of delayed hypersensitivity, and on the immune response to infection with mycobacterium tuberculosis in mice. *Infect Immun* **19:** 212–16.

YU, D. T. Y., CLEMENTS, D. J., PAULUS, H. E., PETER, J. B., LEVY, J. BARNETT, E. B. (1974) Human lymphocyte subpopulations effect corticosteroids. *J Clin Inv* **53:** 565–71.

ZAITSEVSKAIA, E. V., BABICHEV, V. A., MAKSIMOVA, G. F. (1977) Effect of methotrexate on the level of T- and B-lymphocytes. *Farmakol Toksikol* **40:** 322–26.

ZAN-BAR, I., NACHTIGAL, D., FELDMAN, M. (1975a) Mechanisms in immune tolerance. II. Specific immunosuppression by T lymphocytes of B memory cells in mice made tolerant to HSA. *Cell Immunol* **17:** 202–214.

ZAN-BAR, I., NACHTIGAL, D., FELDMAN, M. (1975b) Mechanism in immune tolerance III. Specific immunosuppression and the induction of tolerance: synergism and antagonism. *Cell Immunol* **17:** 215–27.

ZATZ, M. M. (1975) Effects of cortisone on lymphocyte homing. *Isr J Med Sci* **11:** 1368.

ZIMBER, C., BEN-EFRAIM, S., WEISS, D. M. (1977) Prevention by the MER tubercle bacillus fraction of immunosuppression induced by cancer chemotherapeutic agents. II. Contact hypersensitivity in guinea pigs and mice treated with cyclophosphamide. *Cancer Immunol Immunother.* **3:** 35–42.

ZSCHIESCHE, W., SLAVINA, E., LEIPONSKAYA, I. (1977) Effect of tilorone hydrochloride on graft vs host (GHV) reaction in mice. *Acta Biol Med Ger* **36:** 107–12.

ZWEIMAN, B., PHILLIPS, M. S. (1970) *In vivo* lymphocyte reactivity during depression of tuberculin hypersensitivity by 6-mercaptopurine. *Science* **169:** 284–5.

CHAPTER 11

MODULATION OF IMMUNITY BY LEVAMISOLE AND DTC

GERARD RENOUX*

Laboratoire d'Immunologie, Faculté de Médecine, 37032 Tours Cedex, France

1. INTRODUCTION

We found levamisole an almost non-toxic immunopotentiating agent whose activities are very different from those of other biological adjuvants. It represents a new step in the development of a rational, scientifically-based immunopharmacology designed to modify immune response in patients, through the development of chemically-defined substances. The oral administration of levamisole is also a practical advantage over many other immunotherapies, as many patients would prefer to receive pills instead of injections that might be painful.

As a prototype of a new class of agents, levamisole was accepted with enthusiasm or, at the other extreme, with considerable scepticism. Since the story was new, it was found both puzzling and disturbing. There was no linear dose-response effect with levamisole and the host played a major role in the responses. We entered a new field revealing many interrelationships between the immune system and other functions of the host. A route was opened by the discoveries of peptide hormones and of neurotransmitter receptors on cell membrane of lymphocytes and monocytes, and by the discovery of the general role of cyclic nucleotides in translating surface signals, particularly in lymphocytes. Levamisole, and even more DTC, could be potent tools to help in understanding these relationships.

As with all 'parents', we sometimes feared the problems our 'offspring' might cause, but toxic effects proved to be few. It is important to state here that one should try to be unprejudiced as possible in evaluating a novel approach to immunotherapy, whether one is its discoverer or a supposedly disinterested scientific investigator in the field. We discovered the activities of levamisole on immune responsiveness with a 'prepared mind' and a 7 per cent solution of an antihelminthic drug. Long ago we had found evidence for a possible role for sulfur derivatives in immunity. Indeed, a better immunization of man against rickettsial typhus was attained with a dead vaccine containing sodium ethylxanthate as an antiseptic (Durand *et al.*, 1942), and dithioglycerol favored the recovery of *Brucella*-infected animals (Renoux, 1951).

Years later, an unsuspectedly high infection rate was noted in heifers vaccinated against brucellosis and challenged by virulent *B. abortus* (Plommet *et al.*, 1970). An interference of *Coxiella burneti* infection on immunological processes was demonstrated (Renoux, 1969). On the other hand, all animals had been deparasitized with 'Nemecide'. So it was with interest that we learned in 1969 from the manufacturer (Specia) that this racemic isomer of 2,3,5, 6-tetrahydro-6-phenylimidazo(2,1-b) thiazole hydrochloride was able to interfere with the energy metabolism and possessed some cholinergic-like activities.

Prepared by a wonderful training at Rutgers University with our devoted friend Dr. Werner Braun, we appreciated the role of cyclic nucleotides and the part played by pharmacological mediators in modulating immune responses. Thus, experiments to show an effect of this sulfur-containing agent on immune responses were planned with Nemecide. The first essay consisted of an appraisal of Nemecide activity on *Brucella* immunization. Mice vaccinated with *Brucella* vaccines (H38 or B19) evidenced a better protection to virulent *B. abortus* challenge when a treatment with Nemecide (later known as tetramisole, Janssen) was given 2 days

*Associate Scientist, Memorial Sloan-Kettering Cancer Center, New York.

after vaccination. However, my wife and I decided that these findings should be checked by further experiments. We were aware of the fact that it was a new approach to immunostimulation as well as for studies in immunopharmacology. For the first time, a chemically-defined simple molecule demonstrated an activity on cells of the immune system.

The study on *Brucella* immunization was repeated and extended, and experiments with xenogenic erythrocytes as antigen were also performed. Since all data correlated, the first result on the effects of the drug on vaccination against brucellosis was then published (Renoux and Renoux, 1971).

It marked the start of an extensive interdisciplinary research effort to investigate the effects of tetramisole and its optical isomers on various host-defense mechanisms. However, conflicting data revealed an ambivalent influence of levamisole on T cell responses. We, therefore, attempted to develop a synthetic sulfur compound devoid of the inhibitory, and potentially sensitizing, effects of levamisole.

This review is intended to indicate some trends in the pharmacology and molecular biology of immunological events evoked by studies on levamisole and sodium diethyldithiocarbamate, DTC, as most publications have already been reviewed (Renoux, 1978, 1980a, b).

2. CHEMISTRY, PHARMACOLOGY AND METABOLISM OF LEVAMISOLE.

Tetramisole is a synthetic antihelmintic, first described by Thienpont *et al.*, (1966). The drug is active against most nematodes of animals and man and has been extensively and safely used in veterinary and human medicine.

Levamisole is the levo-isomer of 2,3,5, 6-tetrahydro-6-phenylimidazo(2,1-b) thiazole hydrochloride, MW 240.75. It is a stable white crystalline powder readily soluble in water. It hydrolyzes in aqueous solution, especially at high pH. The aqueous solution is acid.

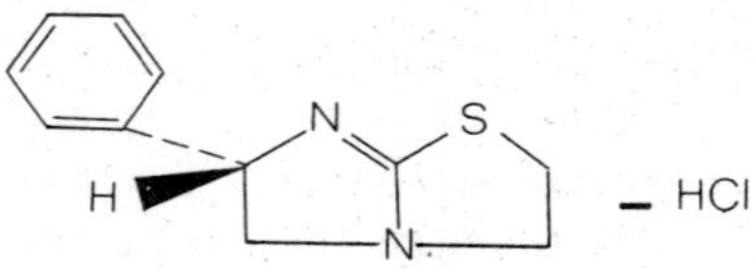

Levamisole is rapidly absorbed from the gastrointestinal tract or from the injection site. Peak blood levels of about 0.5 μg/ml are reached within 2 hours after an oral dose of 150 mg in adult men. Levamisole has in plasma a half-life of about 4 hours in man, is extensively metabolized in the liver, and completely eliminated from the body in less than 2 days (Graziani and De Martin, 1977).

Pharmacologically, both isomers stimulate parasympathetic and sympathetic ganglia, the latter effect being accompanied by an inhibition of the norepinephrine reuptake (Van Nueten, 1972). Levamisole resembles certain anti-depressant drugs (Colpaert *et al.*, 1975) and possesses some mood-elevating effect on man.

Levamisole was found to be a potent stereospecific inhibitor of furmarate reductase in several nematodes (Van den Bossche, 1972).

Levamisole is a potent inhibitor of mammalian alkaline phosphatases, except for intestinal and human placental isoenzymes. This inhibitory activity is highly specific (Van Belle, 1972, 1976).

The drug has no direct effect on bacteria, viruses and fungi (Thienpont *et al.*, 1966; Fischer *et al.*, 1975) and is not cytotoxic to normal and tumor cells in concentrations up to 100 μg/ml (Lichtenfeld *et al.*, 1974; Pabst and Crawford, 1974; Sampson and Lui, 1976). It does not appear to induce interferon production.

LD_{50} of acute toxicity for levamisole depends on the route of administration, as summarized in Table 1. In rats, daily oral administration of 100 mg/kg of levamisole for 3 months did not demonstrate any adverse effect. Prolonged treatments with doses above 20 mg/kg were convulsant in dogs and sheep (Forbes, 1972).

No carcinogenic effect, or haematological modifications were observed in 12–18-month studies in rats and dogs. Similarly, administration of levamisole 25 mg/kg for 1 month to mice

TABLE 1. *Acute Toxicity of Levamisole*

	LD_{50} (mg/kg) route of administration		
	i.v.	s.c.	oral
mice	28	121	285
rats	28	89	345

did not alter haematological parameters (Renoux *et al.*, 1977a). However, chronic treatment with a high dose of levamisole (25 mg/kg) increases the rate and intensity of spontaneous lymphomas in New Zealand Black mice, although this treatment was effective in delaying the onset of auto-immune disease (Renoux, manuscript in preparation). At daily doses between 5 and 150 mg/kg, levamisole was devoid of dysmorphogenic or toxic effects on rabbit or rat fetuses. Its prolonged administration through three generations did not modify male or female fertility in rats and rabbits.

3. EXPERIMENTAL IMMUNOMODULATION STUDIES WITH LEVAMISOLE.

In animals with a mature immune system levamisole has demonstrated a dose-dependent ability to augment the immune response to xenogenic erythrocyte or bacterial antigens, and to restore or increase host defences impaired by ageing or by immaturity of immune mechanisms (Table 2).

TABLE 2. *Effect of Levamisole on Host Defence to Infections and Responses to Xenogenic Erythrocytes*

Test	Response	Reference
Plaque-forming cells (PFC) to sheep red cells	2–7-fold increase; dose dependent IgM-PFC inhibition and IgG-PFC increase	Renoux and Renoux (1972a, 1974b, 1977a, c)
Antigenic competition and nonspecific immunity	Restoration of antibacterial immunity suppressed by a *C. burneti* infection	Renoux and Renoux (1972e)
Brucella challenge	Dose- and time-dependent stimulation of vaccinations	Renoux and Renoux (1971, 1973b)
Plasmodium berghei challenge	Enhanced defence	Desowitz (1975)
C. pseudotuberculosis challenge	Enhanced defence	Irwin and Knight (1975)
Staphylococcus or herpes infection of suckling mice	Enhanced defence	Fischer *et al.*, (1975)
Plaque-forming cells in aged mice	Restoration of immune responsiveness	Renoux and Renoux (1972b), Bruley-Rosset *et al.*, (1978)

3.1. POTENTIATION OF T-CELL ACTIVITY BY LEVAMISOLE ON NORMAL HEALTHY ANIMALS

Levamisole has little or no effect on total antibody production in healthy animals (Table 3). However, treatment of female mice and concurrent immunization with sheep erythrocytes triggers early synthesis of IgG antibodies (Renoux and Renoux, 1977d).

The effect of timing of drug administration, and of various doses, on the response of mouse spleen cells to sheep red cells was investigated by the haemolytic plaque-forming cell (PFC) assay in agar. This is a well-known macrophage and helper T-cell-induced response expressed through B-cells, thus allowing the evaluation of the competence of a range of immunocompetent cells. Levamisole had different activities according to the interval between immunization and administration. Moreover, there was a narrow range of doses which modulated the magnitude of IgM-PFC numbers. However, a dose of 25 mg/kg of levamisole, which was inhibitory for IgM-PFC, increased IgG-PFC numbers in outbred female mice (Renoux and Renoux, 1975; Renoux *et al.*, 1977a, b) and pretreatment with levamisole inhibited PFC

TABLE 3. *Influence of Levamisole on Antibody Response to Various Antigens*

Test antigen	Antibody response	Reference
Sheep red cells in mice	No modification of total levels; dose-dependent suppression or increased IgM and IgG-antibodies	Renoux and Renoux (1974b, 1975, 1977) Renoux (1974b, 1977a, b, 1979a)
Brucella in mice	Dose-dependent modification	Renoux and Renoux (1973b)
Newcastle virus in chicks	No change	Kulkani *et al.*, (1973)
Viruses and bacteria in cattle	No significant changes	Provost *et al.*, (1974)
Foot and mouth in cattle	No significant changes	Schmied and Rosenbusch (1973), De Diego *et al.*, (1974)
C. pseudotuberculosis in mice	Reduction in mean levels	Irwin and Knight (1975)

responses (Renoux and Renoux, 1974). Moreover, chronic administration of the agent induced a strong inhibition of the responses to mitogens and antigens (Renoux and Renoux, 1979a).

Also, immunomodulation was antigen-specific since the 'background' response to horse red cells was not increased, but rather suppressed. These features clearly distinguish the mode of action of sulphur derivatives from the effects of 'biological adjuvants' (Renoux and Renoux, 1974b).

A dose of 5 mg/kg of levamisole on some occasions failed to increase the immunity of outbred mice, but on others caused a significant increase in the number of spleen plaque-forming cells, when compared to untreated controls (Renoux and Renoux, 1974b). These findings prompted us to search for a possible role of host factors in modulating the effects of levamisole.

The *in vivo* effectiveness of levamisole in enhancing immune responses of normal healthy animals to bacterial or erythrocyte antigens and the rapid switch of specific antibody synthesis from IgM to IgG (Renoux and Renoux, 1977d), which is a known effect of activated T lymphocytes (Vitetta and Uhr, 1975), suggest that the amplification of the immune response is based upon T-cell activation by levamisole.

In vivo T-cell activation was also evidenced by the effect of levamisole on the graft-versus-host (GVH) reaction in F1 hybrid mice. Levamisole suppressed the GVH reaction when administered to recipient new-born F1 mice and increased the GVH response if given to the parental donor (Renoux and Renoux, 1972d). Levamisole stimulated an accelerated rejection of skin isografts in mice (Chirigos *et al.*, 1973; Renoux *et al.*, 1976c). The graft rejection system, C57BL/6 male tail skin on isogenic females, was selected with the viewpoint that the weak histocompatibility difference provided by the male H-Y antigen resembles that between autologous malignancy and the host. Accelerated graft rejection occurred with a single dose of 25 mg/kg given on the day of grafting or 7 days later, whereas a dose of 2.5 mg/kg was found inactive. Treatment with levamisole also increases delayed type hypersensitivity (DTH) to sheep red cells, another cell-mediated immune response. However, mice treated with 2.5 mg/kg of levamisole, simultaneous with erythrocyte immunization, elicited higher and longer sustained levels of DTH responses than after a treatment with 25 mg/kg of the drug (Renoux and Renoux, 1975; Renoux *et al.*, 1976c).

The capacity of levamisole to increase the number of potentially reactive T-cells is shown by significant stimulation of DNA synthesis by murine splenocytes in the presence of the drug. Antigen or mitogen does not need to be present at the time of levamisole treatment to induce an increase in cell proliferation (Renoux, 1978). These data confirm *in vitro* experiments showing enhancement of blastogenesis or increased phytohaemagglutinin (PHA) responsiveness of murine spleen cells on addition of levamisole to cell cultures (Hadden *et al.*, 1975; Merluzzi *et al.*, 1975; Sunshine *et al.*, 1977). However, B-cell-enriched spleen cells were not stimulated by levamisole (Merluzzi *et al.*, 1976).

3.2. POTENTIATION OF MACROPHAGE ACTIVITIES BY LEVAMISOLE

The ability of levamisole to augment macrophage activities is critically dose-dependent (Table 4). At adequate dosage, levamisole increases the binding of IgG and C3, and increases

TABLE 4. *Effects of Levamisole on Macrophage Function*

Test	Response	Reference
Phosphodiesterase activity and phagocytosis	Dose-related increase	Lima *et al.*, (1974)
Staphylococcus albus phagocytosis	No *in vitro* effect	Versijp *et al.*, (1975)
IgG receptor activity	*In vitro* enhancement	Schreiber *et al.*, (1975)
Chemotaxis, mobility, phagocytosis, Fc and C3 receptor activity	*In vitro* enhancement	Al-Ibrahim *et al.*, (1975), Douglas *et al.*, (1976), Schmidt *et al.*, (1976)
Listeria endocytosis	No observable effect	Renoux *et al.*, (1976a)
Listericidal capacity	Dose-related efficacy in treated mice	Renoux *et al.*, (1976a)
Leucocyte adherence	Increase after *in vivo* administration	Strecher *et al.*, (1976)

the phagocytosis and digestion of virulent *Listeria* organisms. However, Teller (personal communication) was unable to find levamisole-induced modifications of carbon clearance in outbred or inbred mice, a feature described by Hoebeke and Franchi (1973). These apparently conflicting data might indicate that the rate of uptake of inert particles could be less essential than the processing of antigen in triggering immune events.

3.3. Potentiation of the Functions of Polymorphonuclears by Levamisole

In laboratory animals levamisole can restore or increase neutrophil mobility (Anderson *et al.*, 1976), phosphodiesterase activity (Lima *et al.*, 1974), and adherence and chemotaxis (Strecher *et al.*, 1976). It has been shown that levamisole can restore the glucose metabolism (latex nitroblue tetrazolium test; latex-NBT) of the neutrophils in melanoma and lung cancer patients, and that increase in the latex-NBT responses correlates with clinical improvement (Stos, 1978).

3.4. Levamisole and Animal Tumors

The effectiveness of levamisole in potentiating cell-mediated immune responses prompted the use of levamisole in animal cancer therapy, alone or as an adjunct of chemotherapy.

Available data (review in Renoux, 1978) evidence that levamisole efficacy against tumor growth and on survival rate is dose- and time-dependent. Improvement of the clinical response was associated with a recovery of the immune capacity impaired by the cytoreductive therapy (Perk *et al.*, 1975; Woods *et al.*, 1975).

In brief, the effects of levamisole on cancerous animals are very similar to those observed in uninfected normal animals: animal strain, sex and age, antigen and dose or schedule of administration of the drug are obvious factors which determine the effectiveness of levamisole (section 3.5).

3.5. Mechanisms of Action of Levamisole

3.5.1. *Genetic and Epigenetic Control of Levamisole-induced Immunomodulation*

All experimental and clinical findings suggest that the effects of levamisole are critically dose-dependent, which has resulted in apparently conflicting data. We evaluated the antibody responses to sheep red blood cells in mice of various inbred strains treated with levamisole. These responses appear to be under polygenic control, not associated with the H-2 complex, and modified by a Y-linked component and epigenetic factors revealed by ageing. Strain, sex, age and the dose of levamisole all influenced the activity of levamisole in an interrelated manner. Effects varied from inhibited to unchanged or increased antibody responses, without a direct relationship between the genetic regulation of levamisole's effectiveness and a genotypic capacity to respond to the antigenic signal (Renoux *et al.*, 1979a).

3.5.2. *Protective Influence of Levamisole Metabolites*

A metabolite of levamisole, dl-2-oxo-3-(2-mercaptoethyl)-5-phenyl-imidazolidine (OMPI), is formed from the opening of the sulphur-containing ring. OMPI is nearly 100 times more active *in vitro* than levamisole in enhancing the polymerisation rate of tubulin (De Brabander *et al.*, 1978) and protecting gluthathione-depleted cells from auto-oxidative necrosis. It has thus been proposed that levamisole may act through OMPI in enhancing leucocyte functions by scavenging deleterious oxidative radicals and by enhancing microtubule integrity and functions.

However, the above data do not demonstrate whether or not these effects were associated with the activities of imidazole, still structurally present in OMPI. They do not clarify the role of OMPI on *in vitro* and *in vivo* assayed immune responses, as it seems unlikely than an intact microtubular system is a strict requirement for signal transmission in lymphocyte activation (Betel and Martijnse, 1976).

3.5.3. *Effect of Levamisole on Cyclic Nucleotides*

The cyclic nucleotides, adenosine monophosphate (c AMP) and guanosine monophosphate (c GMP), mediate the actions of hormones and hormone-like substances acting at the cell surface. In the immune system, cell proliferation is associated with a high intracellular level of c GMP, and increased levels of c AMP serve as an inductive signal in the differentiation of lymphocytes (Hadden, 1977; Strom *et al.*, 1977). Increased levels of c GMP appear to be the signal to neoplastic cells for continuous division in the absence of the 'stop' signal of c AMP (Pastan *et al.*, 1975; Sheppard, 1972). The intracellular ratio of c AMP/c GMP determines the pathway a precursor antibody-forming cell follows (Watson, 1975).

Levamisole contains an imidazole moiety, a cholinergic agent which causes an elevation of c GMP levels. For this reason, similar *in vitro* activities associated with cholinergic-like effects on lymphocyte functions are shared by levamisole and imidazole. Increases in phytohaemagglutinin-induced proliferation and in c GMP levels, and decreases in c AMP levels occur (Hadden *et al.*, 1975). However, imidazole does not increase delayed hypersensitivity to sheep red blood cells, does not induce T-cell differentiation *in vivo*, does not induce the serum factor which appears after treatment with levamisole (or sodium diethyldithiocarbamate), and clearly divides treated animals into responders and non responders (Renoux and Renoux, 1977b).

In addition, levamisole has time- and dose-dependent regulatory characteristics which enhance or inhibit immune responses against a variety of antigens. Immunoenhancement of immunodepression might, therefore, be predicted from the effects of the agent on cyclic nucleotides. Differentiation of lymphocytes is a prerequisite to trigger, regulate and express an immune response, even though expression is associated with a specific clonal proliferation. Thus, cholinergic agents (or adjuvants) increasing c GMP levels might enhance immune responses or mitogen-induced proliferation by favouring the clonal proliferation triggered by the simultaneous presence of a stimulus. During repeated administration these agents will cause immunodepression, or even suppression, by preventing differentiation of new precursor cells, probably by maintaining low intracellular levels of c AMP (or low c AMP/c GMP ratio). Striking in these regards is the finding that imidazole blocks the induction of prothymocytes and pro-B-cells to differentiation (Scheid *et al.*, 1978), an unexplained contrast with the increased c GMP level associated with the activity of thymopoietin, a synthetic thymic hormone (Sunshine *et al.*, 1978).

3.5.4. *Mediation through Serum Factors Induced by the Sulphur Moiety*

Levamisole immunopotentiation can be transferred by a serum factor obtained from animals after treatment with the drug. In transfer experiments this factor increased the immune response to sheep erythrocytes in recipient mice and induced regression of the tumor in leukaemic AKR mice, even when leukaemic mice failed to respond directly to treatment with levamisole (Renoux *et al.*, 1975, 1977b).

Enhancement of immune response to erythrocytes and destruction of tumours by responder serum was not due simply to transfer of residual levamisole, since serum from comparably treated nonresponder animals had no effect. It is not due to serum complement, since AKR mice are C5-deficient and heating at 56°C does not reduce the activity. This factor is active across species, since the serum of levamisole-treated rabbits stimulated immune responses in mice.

In addition, levamisole (and sodium diethyldithiocarbamate) induces *in vivo* thymocyte differentiation from precursor spleen cells of congenitally thymusless *nu/nu* mice. In such experiments these sulphur drugs stimulated the production of a serum factor that enhanced immunity *in vivo* and evoked thymocyte differentiation *in vitro* (Renoux and Renoux, 1977b).

In summary, the effects of levamisole on the immune system occur as the result of interactions between the T-cell recruiting activities induced by its sulphur moiety and the cholinergic effect of its imidazole ring. A complex relationship between host, antigen and levamisole is responsible for modifying the activities of many cellular systems in the host. The result of levamisole administration depends upon the dose of the agent, the time of administration with respect to the antigen, and the genetic control of the host.

4. CLINICAL USE OF LEVAMISOLE

Short of aspirin, no compound has seen experimental application in as many diseases as levamisole.

A number of studies report efficacy of levamisole in such diverse disorders as chronic and recurrent bacterial infections including leprosy and brucellosis, chronic and recurrent viral infections, particularly herpes (Hadden *et al.*, 1976b; Werner, 1979), and lupus erythematosus (Gordon and Yanagihara, 1977). All these diseases are known to be associated with immunologic disturbance. Rheumatoid arthritis seems to be the disease where the most encouraging results are obtained supporting favourable comparison with penicillamine, both in patient improvement and side effects.

The majority of trials with levamisole in cancer patients have been performed without reference to the immune status of the patient before treatment, without periodic monitoring to evaluate the effectiveness of the drug and without testing the potential beneficial effect of doses other than the standard 150 mg, thus forgetting that individual factors may modulate the activity of levamisole. In brief, indiscriminate testing with levamisole has led to anarchy, and conflicting data, that have unjustifiably dampened the confidence in levamisole, as well as in the value of immunotherapy. The need for cooperative trials and careful appraisal of treatment strategies can be examplified from the experience with levamisole treatment of acute non-lymphocytic leukemia. In two studies (Chang *et al.*, 1978; Thorling *et al.*, 1978) levamisole administered within intermittent high dose chemotherapy, did not benefit the patients. In two other studies (Lethinen *et al.*, 1978; Pavlovsky *et al.*, 1978), the patients received continuous chemotherapy and levamisole, and in these trials levamisole prolonged significantly the duration of complete remission. In all four studies, there is no report of agranulocytosis due to levamisole, in contrast to the reports about other malignancies and rheumatoid arthritis.

The general feeling is that the still unsufficient cognizance of the mode of action of levamisole on the immune system and other regulatory systems and inaccurately prepared clinical trials, have lead to results open to personal interpretation. Nevertheless, the available evidence suggests that levamisole has increased the survival of most cancer patients. To appreciate the benefit, one should keep in mind that conventional therapies are still unable to modify the survival rate of patients not receiving an immunostimulant drug.

In general, the use of levamisole is safe with mild side-effects such as nervousness, insomnia, gastrointestinal upset, and alteration in taste and smell; however, some of these effects were also described in placebo-treated patients. More important are skin rash, febrile illness, polyarthralgia, myalgia and malaise which may be due to sensitization by levamisole (Turck and Parker, 1979). The treatment of patients with rheumatoid polyarthritis has often resulted in neutropenia and sometimes agranulocytosis, if the levamisole therapy was unduly continued. Having the HLA-B27 phenotype seems to increase such a risk and corticosteroid treatment may aggravate the condition. Since these symptoms disappear after drug administration is stopped, they can be prevented by hematologic monitoring of patients.

The immunopharmacology of levamisole has revealed the complexities of the biological pathways underlying the clinical effectiveness of agents proposed as immunopotentiators, immunostimulants or immunomodulators. It has shown the role of host factors in modulating the influence of immunostimulants (Renoux *et al.,* 1979a), and the further need for specific immuno-assays to evaluate and monitor the clinical efficacy of an agent. Levamisole has open the way for the development of chemically-definded compounds as biological response modifiers.

5. CHEMISTRY, METABOLISM AND PHARMACOLOGY OF SODIUM DIETHYLDITHIOCARBAMATE, DTC

The development of DTC resulted from the search for a synthetic, chemically-defined compound, devoid of the ambivalent effect of levamisole on T cells, which effect was thought to drive from the imidazole nucleus and from the sensitizing effect of thiazole or benzole rings.

DTC, M.W. 171 (Fig. 1), is obtained by reacting diethylamine with carbon disulphide in the presence of sodium hydroxide. It is readily soluble in water, buffers, or culture media.

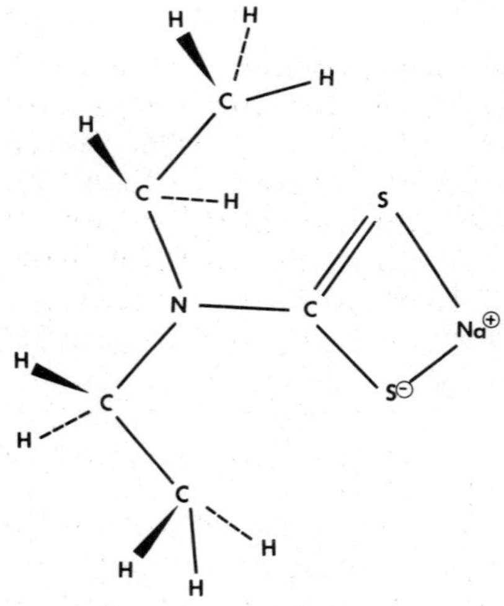

171,27

$C_5H_{10}NS_2Na$

FIG. 1. Formula of sodium diethyldithiocarbamate (DTC).

The pharmacology and toxicology of DTC have been extensively studied, as DTC is a chelating agent used in the treatment of nickel poisoning and a tool to study metalloenzymes (Albert, 1973; 'Nickel', 1975; Sunderman, 1979). DTC is absorbed from the gastrointestinal tract or from the injection site in about 5 minutes. DTC is rapidly metabolized and its plasma half-life is less than 20 minutes. Consequently, DTC will not interfere with other drugs, such as barbitrates, if administered after a 3-hour interval.

Purified and lyophilized DTC (Institut Mérieux) is essentially devoid of toxicity and side-effects for use as an immunopotentiator at doses of 0.5 to 25 mg/kg (Table 5).

The pharmacology of DTC has extensively been studied, and recently reviewed (Renoux, 1982). Administration to animals of large doses (above 200 mg/kg) evidences a number of

TABLE 5. *Toxicities of DTC (LD_{50} mg/kg)*

		i.v.	oral
Acute	mice	>1000	1870
	rats	>1000	2830
	dogs	>1000	>500
Chronic	rabbits	>100/day	>100/day
(4 months)	dogs	>100/day	>100/day

activities: inhibition of the dopamine-beta-hydroxylase, and concomitant depression in brain norepinephrine levels; potentiation of barbital sleep; retrograde amnesia of trained passive avoidance; a dose of 680 mg/kg produces cerebral seizure activity. All these effects are transient and recovery to normal occurs within 24 to 48 hours after administration of the agent.

The effects of DTC on catecholamine levels, and liver microsomal enzymes are interesting data, as it is almost a rule in pharmacological studies that the effect of low doses contrasts with the activity of high doses.

5.1. Absence of Carcinogenicity. Anti-cancer Effects. Radio-protective Properties

A recent Report (National Cancer Institute, 1979) relaters a bioassay of DTC conducted by administering the chemical in feed for 104–109 weeks to rats and mice. Survivals of the rats and mice were not affected, and no clinical signs could be related to administration of the drug. The high dose (about 140 mg per day) prolonged the survival of female mice. No tumors occurred at incidences that were significantly higher in the dosed groups than in the control groups. In addition, the incidence of some spontaneous tumors was lower in the dosed groups than in the corresponding control groups.

DTC exerts a protective effect against a variety of chemically-induced malignant tumors, such as tumors resulting from exposure to polycyclic hydrocarbons (Wattenberg, 1974), diemethylhydrazine-induced colonic cancer (Fiala *et al.*, 1977a; Wattenberg, 1975; Wattenberg and Fiala, 1978) or liver hepatoma due to azodyes (Fiala *et al.*, 1977b). DTC was found to be a free radical scavenger (Lutz *et al.*, 1973), protecting rats against the carcinogenic effects of dimethylnitrosamine, likely by preventing DNA strand breaks, or through the effects of DTC on liver enzymes to modify the metabolic pathways of carcinogens (Abanoni *et al.*, 1977; Sarma *et al.*, 1974). In addition, administration of DTC to rats inhibits the nephrotoxicity and the gastro-intestinal toxicity of *cis*-platinum without altering its anti-tumor efficacy (Borch and Pleasant, 1979; Borch *et al.*, 1980).

The doses employed in these studies (200–540 mg/kg) were higher than the doses (0.5 to 25 mg/kg) tested for activity on the immune system.

The beneficial influences of DTC against the lethal effects of ionizing radiations have been reviewed by Strömme and Eldjarn (1966). DTC was found a protective agent better than cysteamine, dimethyldithiocarbamate or tetraethylthiuram disulfide.

In addition, DTC has *in vivo* and *in vitro* antibiotic effects against a variety of bacteria, fungi and parasites (review in Renoux, 1982).

5.2. Anabolic Effect of DTC

At the doses tested for augmenting activities, 0.5 to 25 mg/kg, DTC does not modify the weight of treated animals in comparison with saline-treated controls. In contrast, a treatment with DTC suppresses the wasting disease induced in mice by injecting 2 mg of PMF, a phenol-fraction from *Brucella melitensis* (Renoux and Renoux, 1979b). A single administration of 2.5 mg/kg DTC is sufficient to prevent emaciation. Furthermore, DTC-treated mice at the time of PMF injection, exhibited 25 days later a weight increase of 4–5 g per animal above that of saline-treated controls. The unique anabolic effect of DTC on animals stressed by a toxic bacterial fraction, might be of interest for the potential use of the agent in infected patients.

5.3. Anti-toxic Effects of DTC

A number of studies (review in Renoux, 1982) show that DTC, through its action on monooxygenases, prevents and even cures the development of chemically-induced diabetes and protects liver cells against drug (chloroform, carbon tetrachloride, vinyl chloride, paracetamol, bromobenzene, benzo(a) pyrene) induced damages.

5.4. Influences of DTC on Mouse Spleen Weight or Lymphocyte Numbers

In contrast with immunoadjuvants of bacterial origin, DTC does not modify the spleen weight in treated mice. If any effect, DTC, administered at the time of immunization, would induce a mere splenocontraction, in comparison with control animals immunized with sheep red blood cells, SRBC. The treatments with DTC leave unchanged the total number of nucleated spleen cells. However, such treatments result in an increased percent of live cells, in comparison with controls (Renoux and Renoux, 1979b). The cell-protective effect of DTC might have a relationship with its radio-protective efficacy.

The data evidence that the immunostimulation afforded by DTC is not associated with a random proliferation of cells involved in the immune system.

5.5. Toxico-pharmacology of Purified DTC in Man

All of these data, including the immunological findings, were found sufficiently promising to suggest Phase I trials of the purified and lyophilized DTC (Institut Mérieux). Informed consent was obtained from 29 volunteers: 16 male patients, 38–73 years of age, affected with chronic bronchitis and 13 cancer patients of either sex, 48–83 years old.

The data can be simply summarized as follows. The slow intravenous administration of 0.5–5 mg/kg body weight of DTC was devoid of toxicity, and untoward effects, or changes in clinical, hematological, and biochemical parameters. Similar results were obtained on 12 additional chronic bronchitis patients, and are observed in a current double-blind study on the effects of weekly-repeated treatment with 5 mg/kg DTC where, at present, no clinical differences are observed among patients (Renoux and Renoux, 1981; Renoux *et al.*, 1980d).

Immunostimulant doses of purified DTC are devoid of toxicity, adverse effects on brain activity, and synergic activity with sedatives and anesthetics. DTC should be slowly administered, in more than 20 minutes, if administered by the intravenous route. Current studies (Dr. Lemarié) indicate that oral, aerosol or intrathecal administration of DTC can be as safe and as active as intravenous injection.

6. EXPERIMENTAL IMMUNOMODULATION STUDIES WITH DTC

As a biological response modifier, DTC demonstrates a unique influence on the T-cell lineage.

6.1. Potentiation of T-cell Activities by DTC on Normal Healthy Animals

DTC induces the production of only IgG α-SRBC circulating antibodies as early as 6 days after immunization (Renoux and Renoux, 1979b). A single administration in a range of doses between 0.5 and 25 mg/kg at different time intervals in relation to the antigenic stimulus (10^8 SRBC) in various mouse strains, elicits a marked increase in the number of IgM- and of IgG-plaque forming spleen cells, whereas the non-specific IgM antibody response to horse red cells is abolished (Renoux and Renoux, 1977a, b; Renoux *et al.*, 1977c). The data were extended by showing that in C3H/He or in BALB/c mice, increased IgG-α SRBC responses, a T-cell triggered event, are evident as early as day 2 in treated mice of both strains, and sustained for the 7 days of observation, in comparison with untreated controls (Renoux and Renoux, 1981).

The influence of DTC to increase lymphoproliferations induced by the mitogens, PHA, Con A and pokeweed (PWM) was tested on 16–18 week-old female BALB/c and C3H/He mice,

1 hour, 1 day, 2 days and 7 days after a treatment with 25 mg/kg DTC, or pyrogen-free saline in controls.

The results (Renoux and Renoux, 1981) indicate that DTC exerts an inhibitory influence on the lymphocyte population responsive to PWM, and increases the responses to PHA and Con A. However, identical numbers of spleen cells of BALB/c or C3H female mice assayed on the same days exhibit a different pattern of responses. Cells of BALB/c mice evidence a depressed early responses to T cell mitogens, followed at day 7 by significantly increased responses. In contrast, splenocytes of C3H mice respond within 1 hour after treatment by a sharp rise in [^{3}H] thymidine uptake, which was followed by responses depressed, or not significantly different from controls.

These data suggest a genetic regulation of lymphocyte stimulation by DTC might exist. They also question the use of mitogens as *in vitro* probes to mimic the abilities of lymphocytes to divide in the presence of specific antigens, as the stimulation by DTC of the response to SRBC was found almost identical in female mice of the same age, in both strains.

Current studies shows that DTC induces also increased lymphoproliferative responses to allogeneic antigens (Renoux *et al.*, 1984).

A single treatment with DTC, at the time of immunization, elicits in mice immunized with SRBC higher and longer sustained levels of DTH than in controls (Renoux and Renoux, 1979b).

The data evidence that DTC affects the macrophage and T-cell induced DTH response to SRBC. It is of interest for further studies and correlation with clinical assay, to lay stress on the finding that a high dose of DTC, 25 mg/kg, positivates the response when an excess of antigen (10^8 SRBC) was present, whereas a low dose of the agent, 2.5 mg/kg increases already positive DTH response to a suboptimal dose (10^5 SRBC). Interesting also is the finding that DTC can impair the immediate antibody-mediated hypersensitivity to DNP and enhance the DTH to BGG in guinea pigs immunized with BGG-DNP (Neveu, 1978).

In all assays, including the chronic administration of 25 mg/kg for one month (Renoux and Renoux, 1980a), DTC has elicited increased T-cell associated responses, in contrast with the immunodepression afforded by long-term administration, or large doses, of other immunomodulating agents.

Thus, administration of DTC increases either the proliferative responses to T-cell mitogens and alloantigens, the antibody responses against a complex antigen (SRBC) or delayed-type-hypersensitivities. The results correlate with the efficacy of DTC to recruit Thy-1^+ cells from precommitted precursor spleen cells in *nu/nu* mice, without apparent changes in the number of B (Fc receptor-positive) cells (section 7.1). These effects were not accompanied with an influence of DTC on the B-cell mitogen, PWM, nor with polyclonal activation.

6.2. Influences of DTC on NK and ADCC of Female C3H/He Mice

Natural killer activity (NK) and antibody-dependent cell-mediated cytotoxicity (ADCC), were measured in a 4-hour ^{51}Cr release assay (Bardos *et al.*, 1981).

A treatment with 25 mg/kg DTC, 4 days before test, significantly ($P<0.01$) increases the NK activity of female C3H mice at E/T ratios from 1:25 to 1:100, whereas this treatment is unable to modify ADCC to CRBC. The data are to be confirmed by other experiments including variable time- and dose-schedules of treatment, and other mouse strains of different genetic level of NK activity. If confirmed, the specific stimulating effect of DTC on NK reactivity and its inefficacy to trigger an increased ADCC on erythrocytes, will provide a mean to further delineate the cell subsets active in the resistance to tumors.

6.3. Influence of DTC on Mice Immunosuppressed by Chemotherapeutic Agents

In view of its potential use in cancer therapy, DTC was chronically administered (25 mg/kg three times a week for 4 weeks) to BALB/c mice treated for 4 weeks with therapeutic-like doses of cyclophosphamide (CY), azathioprine (AZA) or cortisone acetate HC (Renoux and Renoux, 1980a).

Immune responses were evaluated by mitogen-induced lymphocyte proliferation and by *in vivo* primary antibody responses to SRBC. One-half of the mice were sacrificed for lymphoproliferative assays, and the second half were immunized with 10^8 SRBC, 4 days after the end of treatment to minimize the role of residual drug activity or of stress on lymphocyte responsiveness. The administration of DTC alone, even for 1 month, stimulated the host to increased T-cell associated responses. Chronic treatments with the chemotherapeutic agents impaired, or inhibited, mitogen-induced lymphoproliferations and antibody responses. DTC, administered simultaneously to AZA or HC, increased these responses above that of untreated controls, at levels comparable to those of mice treated with DTC alone, and partially restored the responses abrogated by CY. The results raise the possibility of developing a rational chemoimmunotherapy using DTC in association with a compatible cytoreductive drug.

7. MECHANISMS OF ACTION OF DTC

DTC is inactive *in vitro*. It is not a polyclonal activator and it does not induce granuloma or increase in organ weight. DTC acts by enhancing, or inducing, the synthesis of hormone-like factors specific for the T-cell lineage.

7.1. DTC as a Trigger of Hormone-like Factors

Administered to congenitally thymusless mice, DTC induces the *in vivo* acquisition of specific T-cell markers by precommitted and undifferentiated precursor spleen cells, and concomitantly, functional immune activation (Renoux and Renoux, 1977b; Renoux *et al.*, 1977b, 1979b; Renoux and Renoux, 1980b).

The serum of DTC-treated *nu/nu* mice transfers, like the serum of treated thymus-bearing mice, the *in vivo* activities and allows precursor spleen cells of *nu/nu* mice to differentiate *in vitro* into Thy-1^+ cells. As low as 0.01 ml of serum, sampled on *nu/nu* mice 4 days after a treatment with 25 mg/kg DTC, induces the appearance of about 20% Thy-1^+ cells in a 3.5-hour induction assay on *nu/nu* spleen cells, whereas even a 18-hour incubation was unable to modify the percentage of B (Fc receptor-positive) cells.

At present, DTC (and DTC-induced serum factor) is the only known agent able to induce in thymusless mice the *in vivo* acquisition of specific T-cell markers by undifferentiated precursor lymphoid cells, following a single administration of the agent.

7.2. Activity Across Species Barrier of the DTC-induced Serum Factor

Mouse serum was obtained 24-hours after a s.c. injection of 25 mg/kg of DTC to female BALB/c mice. Its effect to induce HTLA$^+$ cells or Fc receptor-positive (B) cells was tested on a mixture of peripheral blood lymphocytes deprived of mature T cells by repeated depletion of E rosettes on density gradient. After 4-hours incubation at 37°C in a humidified atmosphere of 5% CO_2 in the presence of mouse serum, the cells with surface T-lymphocyte differentiation antigens (HTLA$^+$ cells) were identified in a microcytotoxicity assay, and B (Fc receptor-positive) cells were enumerated, after 6 or 18 hours of incubation (Renoux *et al.*, 1980b).

The studied populations include 54–57% CR$^+$ cells, before and after 18 hours *in vitro* incubation, evidencing the absence of effect on the B-cell lineage of DTC-treated mouse serum. Between 2–6% of cells with the HTLA phenotype remain after elimination of the E-rosette forming cells. A 4-hour incubation of E$^-$ human lymphocytes with as low as 10 μl of serum of DTC-treated BALB/c mice was sufficient to convert an additional 7–12% HTLA$^-$ cells into HTLA$^+$ cells, at a level comparable to the effect of calf thymus extract. The serum of DTC-treated mice is also capable of increasing functional activities of human peripheral blood lymphocytes, as measured by enhancement of Con A-induced proliferation. In addition, blast cells induced by Con A or by the serum of DTC-treated mice suppressed equally the proliferative response in MLC, in contrast to the blasts induced by calf thymus extract, which did not display a significant suppressor activity (Renoux *et al.*, 1980b).

In conclusion, DTC appears to promote or to stimulate the *in vivo* synthesis of a potent inducer of prothymocyte maturation and acquisition of functional activities. This inducer is active across species barrier.

7.3. Influences of Brain Neocortex

Partial ablation of the left neocortex caused an inhibition of the hormone(s) active on T cells and inhibited both NK activity and the response to allogeneic antigens, while similar lesions of the right neocortex did not modify these responses (Renoux *et al.*, 1980a, c; Renoux, 1980c, 1981; Bizière *et al.*, 1981; Bardos *et al.*, 1981) In contrast, administration of DTC to left decorticated animals resulted in a complete reconstitution of immune activities, whereas a treatment with DTC of right decorticates was unable to modify these responses. The number and activities of B cells were unchanged (Renoux *et al.*, 1984).

The data show that a role of the left neocortex in maintaining body integrity in response to environment is displayed through the control of the T-cell lineage and suggest that an intact right cortex would control the effects of DTC.

8. INFLUENCES OF DTC ON IMMUNE PARAMETERS IN MAN

The effects of DTC were evaluated on the informed-consent volunteers of the Phase I studies (section 5.5) by the following tests: serum levels of IgA, IgG and IgM, total hemolytic complement (CH50), and C4 and C3; T cells (E rosettes) and B cells (Ig-bearing cells, by immunofluorescence); response to PHA and Con A. Tests were performed before administering DTC (day 0) and at day +1, +2 and +7 after each injection.

In a first series of assays, low doses of DTC (0.5 to 2.2 mg/kg per i.v. injection) were administered to cancer patients, prior to surgery. In all cases but one (a 70-year-old woman severely affected by a recurrent breast cancer and extensive radio-dermitis on the thorax), the responses to T-cell mitogens were restored at normal levels, even above. Thus, low doses of DTC prevent the well known immunodepression associated with surgery and anesthesia, in patients whose immune responses were already altered by cancer (Renoux *et al.*, 1980d)

A second series was made up of male patients affected with chronic pulmonary infections. They were treated with 5 mg/kg DTC (Renoux *et al.*, 1980d; Renoux and Renoux, 1981). A single administration of DTC increased at normal values the responses to PHA or Con A, that were impaired prior to treatment (day 0). The percentage of T cells returned to normal values, either when the figure was abnormally high or low at day 0 before treatment. The following tests were not affected by the treatment: percent of B (sIg^+) cells, levels of IgA, IgG, IgM, or complement activity in the serum. The percent of autologous rosette-forming cells was lowered ($\overline{m}$ 15.35) in all patients, and not affected by the treatment with DTC.

In man, as in animals, DTC was not a polyclonal activator. The mean values of background responses (cpm ± SE in the absence of mitogens) were: 638 ± 504 at day 0, 737 ± 541 at day +1, 482 ± 343 at day +2, and 554 ± 400 at day +7.

These preliminary results confirm in man the unique, and specific influence of DTC to regulate the activities of the T-cell lineage, without apparent, direct effect on B cells.

Although analysis is far from complete, the findings suggest a unique influence of DTC on the immune system.

DTC is a non-toxic agent devoid of untoward pharmacological effects, at least at the doses effective on the immune system.

DTC has no direct influence on B cells, nor polyclonal activities or *in vitro* enhancing effects. DTC did not act directly to differentiate T cells but, through stimulation of the Central Nervous System network, influences the endocrinological network and, at the example of thymusless mice, might correct a genetically determined immunodeficiency disease.

DTC induces through the increased synthesis of selective hormone-like factors, the recruitment and the regulation of cells of the T-cell lineage. These actions are put forth in the absence of events initiated by other triggering influences, and contrast with those of other immunostimulants known to act as promoters to increase an already evoked immune event or as adjuvants to augment the responses to an antigen. Since DTC is a non-toxic agent, the data suggest it would be a drug effective to treat syndromes and diseases where the underlying immune defect is a T-cell deficiency or dysfunction, such as cancers, viral or bacterial diseases, some autoimmune diseases and the immunological effects of aging.

9. GENERAL CONCLUSIONS

Levamisole, a synthetic low molecular weight compound, was the first member of a new class of drugs to augment the immune response. In addition to their clinical usefulness, sulfur compounds may well serve as tools to unravel the complexities of immunological activation.

Levamisole increases the functions of cellular immunity in normal, healthy man and animal, as evidenced by increased vaccinal protection, accelerated isogenic graft rejection, enhanced levels of delayed hypersensitivity and augmented proliferative responses to antigens or mitogens.

Available findings bear evidence to a direct effect on macrophage function, recruitment of T-cells from committed precursors and activation of T-cells for an increased immune response. The potention of levamisole as an immunological stimulant is dictated by a complex relationship between dose of the drug, the degree of antigenic challenge and the capacity of the treated man or animal to produce a hormone-like product. Indeed, levamisole promotes, particularly in the presence of antigen, the production of a soluble factor that combines with cell-membranes of precursor cells in the thymus and also activates T-cells.

The modulation of the immune response in the immunodeficient, the immunodepressed, or the cancer bearing patient accounts for the encouraging results already obtained in clinical trials. Therapeutic effectiveness of levamisole constantly parallels improvement in tests of cellular immunity. Genetic and environmental factors, sex, age, nutrition and associated therapies are important factors to modulate the effectiveness of levamisole. Unlike antibiotics specific for the bacteria, the activity of immunomodulators, or immunopotentiators, is strongly host-dependent.

The ambivalence in effects of levamisole, warranted by inconsistencies in both experimental results and clinical testings, has been related to imidazole's cholinergic-like action. It induced the search for a sulfur compound devoid of imidazole yet still active.

Table 6 summarizes the main differences we have found thus far between levamisole and DTC.

TABLE 6. *Differences between LMS and DTC*

Test	Responses	
	LMS	DTC
Mouse LD_{50} i.v. route (mg/kg)	28	>1000
Range of activity	narrow and variable	large
Evidence for nonresponders	yes	no
In vitro activities	yes	no
Suppression of endotoxin-induced emaciation	no	yes
Antibiotic-like effects	no	yes

Range of activity, evidence for nonresponders, were evaluated in both the hemolytic plaque assay response to sheep erythrocytes (PFC) and the survival of leukemic AKR mice. Synergy with theophylline or imidazole was assayed in the PFC test. *Brucella* fractions were employed to evaluate the effects of levamisole (LMS) or sodium diethyldithiocarbamate (DTC) on endotoxin-induced cachexia (Renoux *et al.*, 1976b). *In vitro* blastogenesis was measured by ^{3}H-thymidine uptake. *In vitro* increase of Ig excretion is described in Renoux *et al.*, (1977b).

DTC has proven to be a T-cell recruiting and regulating agent through the production of a hormone specific for the T-cell lineage. At present, this hormone of maturation and differentiation of T cells is the only known selective inducer of prothymocyte maturation *in vivo* not affecting B cells.

The presence of a thymus is not a prerequisite for the elaboration of the inducer. Our results are compatible with a function of the thymus which is the release of a signal to trigger in another cellular system the synthesis of the hormone active on T cells, and control of its production by a feedback regulation. Furthermore, DTC has led to studies strongly suggesting interrelationships between the Central Nervous System and the Immune System to maintain internal homeostasis and control the responses to environmental factors, through the control of the T-cell lineage by the neocortex.

The unique properties of DTC on T cells are associated with the absence of polyclonal activities. Also, DTC does not evidence time- or dose-dependent characteristics to enhance or inhibit immune responses, a feature which clearly distinguishes DTC from other adjuvants or immunomodulators. In addition, DTC does not create the granulomatous disease evoked by adjuvants of bacterial origin.

These properties are all the most interesting that at immunostimulant doses (0.5–25 mg/kg) purified DTC appears to be completely devoid of toxic and side effects.

In man, a treatment with DTC increases for about 1 week the response of peripheral blood lymphocytes to T-cell mitogens, in such a way that it prevents in aged cancer patients the immunodepression created by surgical trauma, in spite of the existing impairment associated with cancer.

DTC might, therefore, be employed in the preoperative management of cancer patients to lessen, or suppress, the immune impairment provoked by surgical and anesthetic trauma, thus reducing the risk of disseminating micro-metastases. The use of DTC after radical surgery may, hopefully, prevent recurrences or metastases, in as much as the development of neoplasic cells be controlled by the immune system. Similarly, a treatment with DTC during ionizing radiation therapy could protect against the detrimental influence of radiations on the immune system. DTC might also be the basis for an improved chemoimmunotherapy. Its unique influence on the T cell lineage and its antibiotic-like effects may well deserve further studies to determine the usefulness of DTC in the treatment of viral and bacterial diseases.

In conclusion, DTC satisfies all criteria required for a non-toxic agent devoid of untoward side effects for the restoration of deficient or impaired cellular immunity in cancer and likely in a variety of diseases or syndromes associated with dysfunction of T cells.

REFERENCES

ABANONI, S. E., POPP, J. A., CHANG, S. K., HARRINGTON, G. W., LOTLIKAR, P. D., HADJIOLOV, D., LEVITT, M., RAJALAKOHIMI, S. and SARMA, D. R. S. (1977) Inhibition of dimethylnitrosamine-induced strand breaks in liver DNA and liver cell necrosis by diethyldithiocarbamate. *J. Natn. Cancer Inst.* **58:** 263–271.

ALBERT, A. (1973) Metal-binding substances. In: *Selective Toxicity,* 5th ed. pp. 334–391. Chapman and Hall, London.

AL-IBRAHIM, M. S., HOLZMAN, R. S. and LAWRENCE, H. S. (1975) Stimulation of human macrophages *in vitro* by levamisole. *Clin. Res.* **23:** 286A.

ANDERSON, R., GLOVER, A., KOORNHOF, H. J. and RABSON, A. R. (1976) *In vitro* stimulation of neutrophil mobility by levamisole: maintenance of cGMP levels in chemotactically stimulated levamisole-treated neutrophils. *J. Immun.* **117:** 428–432.

BARDOS, P., DEGENNE, D., LEBRANCHU, Y., BIZIÈRE, K. and RENOUX, G. (1981) Neocortical lateralization of NK activity in mice. *Scand. J. Immunol.* **13:** 609–613.

BETEL, I and MARTIJNSE, J. (1976) Drugs that disrupt microtubuli do not inhibit lymphocyte activation. *Nature* **261:** 318–319.

BIZIÈRE, K., RENOUX, G., RENOUX, M., GYENES, L., DEGENNE, D., GUILLAUMIN, J. M., BARDOS, P. and LEBRANCHU, Y. (1981) Effects of the ablation of the left cerebral cortex on T-cell number and cell-mediated responses in the mouse. *Neurosciences Abst.* **6:** 31.

BORCH, R. F. and PLEASANT, M. E. (1979) Inhibition of *cis*-platinum nephtotoxicity by diethyldithiocarbamate rescue in rats. *Proc. Natl. Acad. Sci. USA* **76:** 6611–6614.

BORCH, R. F., KATZ, J. C., LIEDER, P. M. and PLEASANT, M. E. (1980) Effect of diethyldithiocarbamate rescue on tumor response to *cis*-platinum in a rat model. *Proc. Natl. Acad. Sci. USA* **77:** 5441–5444.

BRULEY-ROSSET, M., FLORENTIN, I., KIGER, N., DAVIGNY, M. and MATHÉ, G. (1978) Effects of Bacillus Calmette-Guérin and Levamisole on immune responses in young adult and age-immunodepressed mice. *Cancer Treat. Rep.* **62:** 1641–1650.

CHAN, S. H. and SIMONS, M. J. (1975) Levamisole and lymphocyte responsiveness. *Lancet* **ii:** 1246–1247.

CHANG, P., WIERNIK, P. H., RICHTENFELD, J. L. and SCHIFFER, C. A. (1978) Levamisole (L), cytosine arabinose (Ara-C) and daunorubicin (DNR) induction therapy of adult acute non-lymphocytic leukemia (ANLL). *Proc. Am. Assoc. Cancer Res. Am. Soc. Clin. Oncol.* **19:** 370–374.

CHIRIGOS, M. A., PEARSON, J. W. and PRYOR, J. (1973) Augmentation of chemotherapeutically induced remission of a murine leukemia by a chemical immunoadjuvant. *Cancer Res.* **33:** 2615–2619.

COLPAERT, F. C., LENAERTS, F. M., NIEMEGEERS, C. J. E. and JANSSEN, P. A. J. (1975) A critical study on RO-4-1284 antagonism in mice. *Archs Int. Pharmacodyn. Ther.* **215:** 40–44.

DE BRABANDER, M., AERTS, F., GEUENS, G., VAN DE VEIRE, R. and VAN BELLE, H. (1978) O.M.P.I. A sulfhydryl metabolite of levamisole that interacts with microtubules. *Chem. Biol. Interactions* **28:** 45–49.

DE DIEGO, A. I., CARRILLO, C. G., SUADROME, A. and CASTRO, H. W. R. (1974) Influencia de los antiparasitarios sistemicos sobre las aglutininas. I. Aglutininas producidas por vacuna. *Gac. Vet.* **36:** 164–170. II. Aglutininas de vacas enfermas. *Gac. Vet.* **36:** 584–588.

DESOWITZ, R. S. (1975) Plasmodium berghei: immunogenic enhancement of antigen by adjuvant addition. *Exptl. Parasit.* **38:** 6–13.

DOUGLAS, S. D., SCHMIDT, M. E. and DAUGHADAY, C. C. (1976) Effects of levamisole on monocyte-macrophage immunoprotein receptors and *in vitro* function. *Fedn. Proc.* **35:** 335.

DURAND, P., BEGUET, M., HORRENBERGER, R. and RENOUX, G. (1942) Recherche du pouvoir neutralisant du sérum des vaccinés contre le typhus exanthématique. *Bull. Acad. Med.* **126:** 410–415.

FIALA, E. S., BOBOTAS, G., KULAKIS, C., WATTENBERG, L. W. and WEISBERGER, I. H. (1977a) Effects of disulfuram and related compounds on the metabolism *in vivo* of the colon carcinogen, 1,2-dimethylhydrazine. *Biochem. Pharmacol.* **26:** 1763–1768.

FIALA, E. S., FIALA, E. A. and KELLER, R. W. (1977b) Activation of β-glutamyl transferase in rat liver by disulfuram and its effects on the first stage of azo-dye induced carcinogenesis. *Fed. Proceed.* **36:** 349.

FISCHER, G. W., PODGORE, J. K., BASS, J. W., KELLEY, J. L. and KOBAYASHI, G. Y. (1975) Enhanced host defense mechanisms with levamisole in suckling rats. *J. Infect. Dis.* **132:** 578–581.

FORBES, L. S. (1972) Toxicological and pharmacological relations between levamisole, pyrantel and diethylcarbamazine and their significance in helminth chemotherapy. *Southeast Asian J. Trop. Med. Pub. Health* **3:** 235–241.

GORDON, B. L. and YANAGIHARA, R. (1977) Treatment of systemic lupus erythematosus with the T-cell immunopotentiator, levamisole: a follow-up report of 16 patients under treatment for a minimum period of four months. *Ann. Allergy* **39:** 227–236.

GRAZIANI, G. and DE MARTIN, G. L. (1977) Pharmacokinetic studies on levamisole: on the pharmacokinetics and relative bioavailability of levamisole in man. *Drug. Exp. and Clin. Res.* **2:** 235–239.

HADDEN, J. W., COFFEY, R. G., HADDEN, E. M., LOPEZ-CORRALES, E. and SUNSHINE, G. H. (1975) Effects of levamisole and imidazole on lymphocyte proliferation and cyclic nucleotide levels. *Cellular Immun.* **20:** 98–103.

HADDEN, J. W., LOPEZ, C., O'REILLY, R. J. and HADDEN, E. M. (1976) Levamisole and inosiplex: antiviral agents with immunopotentiating action. *Ann. N.Y. Acad. Sci.* **284:** 139–152.

HADDEN, J. W. (1977) Cyclic nucleotides in lymphocyte proliferation and differentiation. In: *Immunopharmacology*, pp. 1–28. HADDEN, COFFEY and SPREAFICO (eds.). Plenum Medical Book Co., New York, London.

HOEBEKE, J. and FRANCHI, G. (1973) Influence of Tetramisole and its optical isomers on the mononuclear phagocytic system. Effect on carbon clearance in mice. *J. Reticuloendothelial. Soc.* **14:** 317–323.

IRWIN, M. R. and KNIGHT, H. D. (1975) Enhanced resistance to *Corynebacterium pseudotuberculosis* infections associated with reduced serum immunoglobulin levels in levamisole-treated mice. *Infect. Immun.* **12:** 1098–1103.

KULKARNI, V. B., MULBAGAL, A. N., PARANJAPE, V. L., KHOT, J. B. and MANDA, A. V. (1973) Immunostimulating effect of tetramisole on antibody formation against Newcastle disease virus in chicks. *Indian Vet. J.* **50:** 225–227.

LEHTINEN, M., AHRENBERG, P., HÄNNINEN, A., IKKALA, E., LEVANTO, A., PALVA, I., RAJAMÄKI, A., ROSENGARD, S., SAARNI, M., SELROOS, O., TIMONEN, T., WARIS, E., WASASTJERNA, C. and VUPPIO, P. (1978) Levamisole as immunotherapy in acute non-lymphocytic leukemia. *Abstracts (I) XVII Cong. Internat. Soc. Hematol., Paris,* pp. 469.

LICHTENFELD, J. L., DESNER, M., MARDINEY, M. R. and WIERNIK, P. H. (1974) Amplification of immunologically induced lymphocyte ^{3}H thymidine incorporation by levamisole. *Fedn. Proc.* **33:** 790.

LIMA, A. O., JAVIERRE, M. Q., DA SILVA, W. D. and CAMARA, D. S. (1974) Immunological phagocytosis: effect of drugs on phosphodiesterase activity. *Experienta* **30:** 945–946.

LUTZ, L. M., GLENDE, E. A. and RECKNAGEL, R. O. (1973) Protection by diethyldithiocarbamate against carbon tetrachloride lethality in rats and against carbon tetrachloride-induced lipid peroxidation *in vitro. Biochem. Pharmacol.* **22:** 1729–1734.

MERLUZZI, V. J., BADGER, A. M., KAISER, C. W. and COOPERBAND, S. R. (1975b) *In vitro* stimulation of murine lymphoid cell cultures by levamisole. *Clin. Exp. Immun.* **22:** 486–492.

MERLUZZI, V. J., KAISER, C. W. and COOPERBAND, S. R. (1976) Differential effects of levamisole on murine lymphoid tissues. *Fedn. Proc.* **35:** 334.

NATIONAL CANCER INSTITUTE (1979) Bioassay of sodium diethyldithiocarbamate for possible carcinogenesis. *Techn. Rep. Series* No. 172.

NEVEU, P. J. (1978) The effect of thiol moiety of levamisole on both cellular and humoral immunity during the early response to a hapten-carrier complex. *Clin. Exp. Immunol.* **32:** 419–422.

NICKEL, (1975) Committee on medical and biological effects of environmental pollutants. *Proc. Nat. Acad. Sci. USA,* pp. 113–123.

PABST, H. F. and CRAWFORD, J. A. (1974) Enhancement of *in vitro* cellular immune response by L-tetramisole. *Pediatr. Res.* **8:** 416.

PAVLOSKY, S., GARAY, G., GIRAUDO, C., SACKMANN, F., HAYES, A., and SVARCH, E. (1978) Chemoimmunotherapy with levamisole in acute lymphocytic leukemia. *6th Ann. Meet. Am. Assoc. Cancer Research.*

PASTAN, I. H., JOHNSON, G. S. and ANDERSON, W. B. (1975) Role of cyclic nucleotides in growth control. *Ann. Rev. Biochem.* **44:** 491–507.

PERK, K., CHIRIGOS, M. A., FUHRMAN, F. and PETTIGREW, H. (1975) Some aspects of host response to levamisole after chemotherapy in a murine leukemia. *J. Natn. Cancer Inst.* **54:** 253.

PLOMMET, M., RENOUX, G., PHILIPPON, A., LORENTZ, C. and GESTIN, J. (1970) Brucellose bovine expérimentale. I. Comparaison de l'efficacité des vaccins B19 et H38. *Ann. Rech. Vet.* **1:** 189–201.

PROVOST, A., TACHER, G. et BORREDON, C. (1974) Recherche de l'activité immunostimulante de trois dérivés à action antihelminthique de l'imidazole sur les immunogénèses bovipestique, péripneumonique et charbonneuse. *Revue Elev. Mêd. Vêt. Pays Trop.* **27:** 39–52.

RENOUX, G. (1951) Traitement de la brucellose *(B. melitensis)* expérimentale du cobaye par le BAL (2,3 dimercaptopropanol ou dithioglycerol) seul ou associé au chloramphenicol ou à l'auréomycine. *Ann. Inst. Pasteur* **81:** 541–549.

RENOUX, G. (1969) Interférences chez la souris de l'infection par *Coxiella burneti* avec la résistance ou l'immunité contre l'épreuve par *Brucella abortus*. *C.R. Acad. Sci.* **269:** 1467–1469.

RENOUX, G. (1978) Modulation of immunity by levamisole. *Pharm. Ther. A.* **2:** 397–423.

RENOUX, G. (1980a) Trends in immunopotentiation. *Int. J. Immunopharmacol.* **2:** 1–6.

RENOUX, G. (1980b) The general immunopharmacology of levamisole. *Drugs* **19:** 89–99.

RENOUX, G. (1980c) Differentiation of the T-cell lineage by sodium diethyldithiocarbamate (DTC). Influence of the neocortex. In: *New Trends in Human Immunology and Cancer Immunotherapy*, pp. 986–994. B. SERROU and C. ROSENFELD (eds.). Doin, Paris.

RENOUX, G. (1982) Immunopharmacologie et pharmacologie du diethyldithiocarbamate de sodium, DTC. *J. Pharmacol. (Paris)* **13:** 95–134.

RENOUX, G. and RENOUX, M. (1971) Effet immunostimulant d'un imidothiazole dans l'immunisation des souris contre l'infection par *Brucella abortus*. *C.R. Acad. Sci.* **272D:** 349–350.

RENOUX, G. and RENOUX, M. (1972a) Action immunostimulante de dérivés du phenylimidothiazole sur les cellules spléniques formatrices d'anticorps. *C.R. Acad. Sci.* **274D:** 756–757.

RENOUX, G. and RENOUX, M. (1972b) Restauration par le phenylimidothiazole de la réponse immunologique des souris âgées. *C.R. Acad. Sci.* **274D:** 3034.

RENOUX, G. and RENOUX, M. (1972c) Action du phenylimidothiazole (tetramisole) sur la réaction du greffon contre l'hôte. Rôle des macrophages. *C.R. Acad. Sci.* **274D:** 3320.

RENOUX, G. and RENOUX, M. (1972d) Antigenic competition and nonspecific immunity after a rickettsial infection in mice: restoration of anti-bacterial immunity by phenyl-imidothiazole treatment. *J. Immun.* **109:** 761.

RENOUX, G. and RENOUX, M. (1973a) Liens entre les événements immunologiques et le contrôle génétique de l'activité enzymatique des macrophages et des lymphocytes. *C.R. Acad. Sci.* **276D:** 861.

RENOUX, G. and RENOUX, M. (1973b) Stimulation of anti-*Brucella* vaccination in mice by tetramisole, a phenylimidothiazole salt. *Infect. Immunity* **8:** 544–548.

RENOUX, G. and RENOUX, M. (1974a) Immunopotentiation par les thiols et disulfures. *C.R. Acad. Sci.* **278D:** 1139–1141.

RENOUX, G. and RENOUX, M. (1974b) Modulation of immune reactivity by phenyl-imidothiazole salts in mice immunized by sheep red blood cells. *J. Immun.* **113:** 779–790.

RENOUX, G. and RENOUX, M. (1975) Influences du lévamisole sur l'induction immunologique des lymphocytes. T. *Ann. Immun.* **126C:** 91.

RENOUX, G. and RENOUX, M. (1977a) Roles of the imidazole or thiol moiety on the immunostimulant action of levamisole. In: *Control of Neoplasia by Modulation of the Immune System*, pp. 67–80. CHIRIGOS, M. A. (ed.). Raven Press, New York.

RENOUX, G. and RENOUX, M. (1977b) Thymus-like activities of sulphur derivatives on T-cell differentiation. *J. Exp. Med.* **145:** 466–471.

RENOUX, G. and RENOUX, M. (1977c) Influence du lévamisole sur la production d'anticorps. *Ann. Immun.* **128C:** 273–274.

RENOUX, G. and RENOUX, M. (1977d) Mécanismes d'action du lévamisole, stimulant des réponses d'immunité cellulaire. *Ann. Immun.* **128C:** 275–277.

RENOUX, G. and RENOUX, M. (1979a) Immunodépression par le lévamisole. *Nouv. Presse Méd.* **8:** 1427.

RENOUX, G. and RENOUX, M. (1979b) Immunopotentiation and anabolism induced by sodium diethyldithiocarbamate. *J. Immunopharmacol.* **1:** 247–267.

RENOUX, G. and RENOUX, M. (1980a) The effects of sodium diethyldithiocarbamate, azathioprine, cyclophosphamide or hydrocortisone acetate administered alone or in association for 4 weeks on the immune responses of BALB/c mice. *Clin. Immunol. Immunopath.* **15:** 21–32.

RENOUX, G. and RENOUX, M. (1980b) Administration of DTC evidences a role of the thymus in the control and regulation of factors inducing thymocyte differentiation in the mouse. *Thymus* **2:** 139–146.

RENOUX, G. and RENOUX, M. (1981) Immunologic activity of DTC: potential for cancer therapy. In: *Augmenting Agents in Cancer Therapy: Current Status and Future Prospects*, pp. 427–440. E. M. HERSH, M. A. CHIRIGOS and M. J. MASTRANGELO (eds.). Raven Press, New York.

RENOUX, G., RENOUX, M., BIZIERE, K., GUILLAUMIN, J. M., BARDOS, P. and DEGENNE, D. (1984). Involvement of Brain Neocortex and Liver in the regulation of T cells: the mode of action of sodium diethyldithiocarbamate (imuthiol). *Immunopharmacology*, **7:** 89–100.

RENOUX, G., RENOUX, M., GUILLAUMIN, J. M., KASSEL, R. L. and FIORE, N. (1975) L'action antitumorale du lévamisole (LMS) dans la leucémie spontanée AKR et sa stimulation des réponses aux erythrocytes sont médiatisées par des facteurs sériques. *Ann. Immun.* **126C:** 99.

RENOUX, G., RENOUX, M. and AYCARDI, D. (1976a) Levamisole promotes the killing of *Listeria monocytogenes* by macrophages. *Fedn. Proc.* **3:** 336.

RENOUX, G., RENOUX, M. and GUILLAUMIN, J. M. (1976b) Cachexie des souris induite par une fraction de *B. melitensis*. Ses modifications par le lévamisole ou par le diethyldithiocarbamate de sodium. *Internat. Symp. Brucellosis (II). Develop. Biol. Standard., Karger, Basel.* **31:** 110–114.

RENOUX, G., RENOUX, M., TELLER, M. N., MCMAHON, S. and GUILLAUMIN, J. M. (1976c) Potentiation of T-cell mediated immunity by levamisole. *Clin. Exp. Immunol.* **25:** 288–296.

RENOUX, G., RENOUX, M. and GUILLAUMIN, J. M. (1977a) Effets de la prednisone, de la pénicillamine et du lévamisole sur quelques paramètres immunologiques. *La Nouv. Presse Méd.* **6:** 3863.

RENOUX, G., KASSEL, R. L., RENOUX, M., FIORE, N. C., GUILLAUMIN, J. M. and PALAT, A. (1977b) Immunomodulation by levamisole in normal and leukemic mice. Evidence for a serum transfer. In: *Moduation of Host Immune Resistance in the Prevention or Treatment of Induced Neoplasias*, pp. 77–79. I. M. A. CHIRIGOS (ed.). Fogarty Internat. Center Proc. No. 28; US Government Printing Office, Washington.

RENOUX, G., RENOUX, M. and GUILLAUMIN, J. M. (1977c) Le diethyldithiocarbamate de soude est un stimulant de l'immunité. *C.R. Soc. Biol.* **171:** 313–318.

RENOUX, G., RENOUX, M. and GUILLAUMIN, J. M. (1979a) Genetic and epigenetic control of levamisole-induced immunostimulation. *Internat. J. Immunopharmacol.* **1:** 43–48.

RENOUX, G., RENOUX, M., GUILLAUMIN, J. M. and GOUZIEN, C. (1979b) Differentiation and regulation of lymphocyte populations: evidence for immunopotentiator-induced T cell recruitment. *J. Immunopharamacol.* **1:** 415–422.

RENOUX, G., BIZIÈRE, K., RENOUX, M. and GUILLAUMIN, J. M. (1980a) Le cortex cérébral règle les réponses immunes des souris. *C.R. Acad. Sci. (Paris)* **290D:** 719–722.
RENOUX, G., TOURAINE, J. L. and RENOUX, M. (1980b) Induction of differentiation of human null cells into T lymphocytes by the serum of mice treated with sodium diethyldithiocarbamate. *J. Immunopharmacol.* **2:** 49–59.
RENOUX, G., BIZIÈRE, K., RENOUX, M., GYENES, L., DEGENNE, D., GUILLAUMIN, J. M., BARDOS, P. and LEBRANCHU, Y. (1980c) Effects of the ablation of the left cerebral cortex on T-cell number and cell-mediated responses in the mouse. *Internat. J. Immunopharmacol.* **2:** 156.
RENOUX, G., RENOUX, M., GRECO, J., BAUDOIN, J., LAVANDIER, M. and LEMARIÉ, D. (1980d) Phase I–II studies of sodium diethyldithiocarbamate, DTC. In: *New Trends in Human Immunology and Cancer Immunotherapy,* pp. 974–995. B. SERROU and C. ROSENFELD (eds.). Doin, Paris.
RENOUX, G., RENOUX, M., GYENES, L. and GUILLAUMIN, J. M. (1980e) A comparison of the *in vivo* T-cell recruiting capacity of DTC, serum of DTC-treated mice, and two synthetic 'Thymic Hormones'. *Internat. J. Immunopharmacol.* **2:** 167.
SARMA, D. S. R., RAJALAKSHISNI, S. and HADJIOLOV, D. (1974) Effect of diethyldithiocarbamate (DEDTC) and aminoacetylnitrile (AAN) on the induction of strand breaks in rat liver DNA by chemical carcinogens *in vivo. Fed. Proceed.* **33:** 395.
SCHEID, M. P., GOLDSTEIN, G. and BOYSE, E. A. (1978) The generation and regulation of lymphocyte populations. Evidence for differentiative induction systems *in vitro. J. Exp. Med.* **147:** 1727–1743.
SCHMIDT, M. E. and DOUGLAS, S. D. (1976) Effects of levamisole on human monocyte function and immunoprotein receptors. *Clin. Immun. Immunopath.* **6:** 279–288.
SCHMIED, L. M. and ROSENBUSCH, C. (1973) Effectors del levamisole sobre et indice de sueroprotection en primo vaccination antiaftosa. *Rev. Med. Vet.* **54:** 467–471.
SCHREIBER, A. D., PARSONS, J. and COOPER, R. A. (1975) Effect of levamisole on the human monocyte IgG receptor. *Blood* **46:** 1018.
SHEPPARD, J. R. (1972) Difference in the cyclic adenosine 3′5′-monophosphate levels in normal and transformed cells. *Nature New Biol.* **236:** 14–16.
STECHER, V. J., LIAUW, L. and CHINEA, G. (1976) Effect of levamisole on adherence and chemotaxis of leukocytes. *Fedn. Proc.* **35:** 531.
STOS, G. (1978) Modification du métabolisme oxydatif du polynucléaire chez les cancéreux. Thèse Médecine Tours, p. 207.
STROM, T. B., HIRSH, M. S., BLACK, P. H., CARPENTER, C. B. and MERRIL, J. P. (1973) Modulation of lymphocyte blast transformation by cyclic monocleotides. *J. Clin. Invest.* **52:** 83.
STROMME, J. H. and ELDJARN, L. (1966) Distribution and chemical forms of diethyldithiocarbamate and tetraethylthiuram disulphide (disulfuram) in mice in relation to radioprotection. *Biochem. Pharmacol.* **15:** 287–297.
SUNDERMAN, P. W. (1979) Efficacy of sodium diethyldithiocarbamate (Dithiocarb) in acute nickel carbonyl poisoning. *Ann. Clin. Lab. Sci.* **9:** 1–10.
SUNSHINE, G., LOPEZ-CORRALES, E., HADDEN, E. M., COFFEY, R. G., WANEBO, H., HADDEN, J. W. and ROJAS, A. (1977) Levamisole and Imidazole: *in vitro* effects in mouse and man and their possible mediation by cyclic nucleotides. In: *Modulation of Host Immune Resistance in the Prevention or Treatment of Induced Neoplasias',* pp. 31–37. M. A. CHIRIGOS (ed.). Fogarty Internat. Center Proc. No. 28, US Government Printing Office, Washington.
SUNSHINE, G., BASCH, R. S., COFFEY, R. G., COHEN, K. W., GOLDSTEIN, G. and HADDEN, J. W. (1978) Thymopoietin enhances the allogeneic response and cyclic GMP levels of mouse peripheral, thymoderived lymphocytes. *J. Immunol.* **120:** 1594–1599.
THIENPONT, D., VANPARIJS, O. F. J., RAEYMAEKERS, A. H. M., VANDERBERK, J., DEMOEN, P. J. A., ALLEWIJN, F. T. N., MARSBOOM, R. P. H., NIEMEGEERS, C. J. E., SCHELLEKENS, K. H. L. and JANSSEN, P. A. J. (1966) Tetramisole (R8299), a new, potent broad spectrum anthelmintic. *Nature* **209:** 1084–1086.
THORLING, K., BRINCKER, H. and BJÖRN JENSEN, K. (1978) Chemoimmunotherapy of acute myeloid leukaemia with levamisole and nine cytostatic. (Abstracts I) *XVII Cong. Internat. Soc. Hematol., Paris,* p. 471.
TURK, J. L. and PARKER, D. (1979) Sensitization of guinea pigs to levamisole. *Internat. Archs. Aller. and Appl. Immunol.* **58:** 237–240.
VAN BELLE, H. (1972) Kinetics and inhibition of alkaline phosphatases from canine tissues. *Biochim. Biophy. Acta* **289:** 158–168.
VAN BELLE, H. (1976) Alkaline phosphatase. I. Kinetics and inhibition by levamisole of purified isoenzymes from humans. *Clin. Chem.* **22:** 972.
VAN DEN BOSSCHE, H. (1972) Biochemical effects of Tetramisole. In: *Comparative Biochemistry of Parasites,* pp. 117–125. Academic Press, New York, London.
VAN NUETEN, J. M. (1972) Pharmacological aspects of Tetramisole. In: *Comparative Biochemistry of Parasites,* pp. 101–115. Academic Press, New York, London.
VERSIJP, G., VAN ZWET, T. L. and VAN FURTH, R. (1975) Levamisole and functions of peritoneal macrophages. *Lancet* **i:** 798.
VITETTA, E. S. and UHR, J. W. (1975) Immunoglobulin-receptors revisited. *Science* **189:** 964–968.
WATSON, J. (1975) The influence of intracellular levels of cyclic nucleotides on cell proliferation and the induction of antibody synthesis. *J. Exp. Med.* **141:** 97–111.
WATTENBERG, L. W. (1974) Inhibition of carcinogenic and toxic effects of polycyclic hydrocarbons by several sulfur-containing compounds. *J. Natl. Cancer Inst.* **52:** 1583–1587.
WATTENBERG, L. W. (1975) Inhibition of dimethylhydrazine-induced neoplasia of the large intestine by disulfuram. *J. Natl. Cancer Inst.* **54:** 1005–1006.
WATTENBERG, L. W. and FIALA, E. S. (1978) Inhibition of 1, 2-dimethylhydrazine-induced neoplasia of the large intestine in female CP_1 mice by carbon disulfide: brief communication. *J. Natl. Cancer Inst.* **60:** 1515—1517.
WERNER, G. H. (1979) Immunopotentiating substances with antiviral activity. *Pharmac. Ther.* **6:** 235–273.
WOODS, W. A., FLIEGELMAN, M. J. and CHIRIGOS, M. A. (1975) Effect of levamisole (NSC-177023) on DNA synthesis by lymphocytes from immunosuppressed C57BL mice. *Cancer Chemother. Rep.* **59:** 531–536.

CHAPTER 12

THE INFLUENCE OF SYNTHETIC HOMORIBOPOLYNUCLEOTIDE COMPLEXES ON THE IMMUNE RESPONSE

ROBERT E. CONE

Department of Pathology
University of Connecticut School of Medicine, Farmington, Connecticut, 06030, USA

1. INTRODUCTION

The response of an individual to antigenic challenge consists of multiple events which lead to either the production of specifically activated effector cells and/or humoral products; or to the specific inactivation of responding clones to further challenge (tolerance). As with most complex systems, the Immune System functions under strict regulatory controls, exerted in part by the system itself. Thus, interacting subsets of responding cells as well as their products modify the nature, time course, intensity and quality of an immune response. Adjuvants can be interposed on a 'natural' immune response to alter normal regulatory balances. Such agents permit weakly immunogenic substances to stimulate an immune response, and can decrease the induction period and increase the intensity and duration of an immune response. Adjuvants can thus be used as an agent to provide a stronger immune response both experimentally and clinically and additionally to magnify and provide insight into what Johnson has called 'subliminal events' in the immune response (Johnson *et al.*, 1971).

A host of agents have been used experimentally to amplify the immune system (Waksman, 1978). However untoward side effects of many of these agents do not permit their use in a clinical setting. In this respect homoribopolynucleotide complexes of polyadenylic and polyuridylic acids (poly A:U) offer promise because of their low toxicity in animal systems (Han *et al.*, 1973). Moreover, since poly (A:U) is chemically well defined, analysis of its cellular target(s) and mode of action as an adjuvant are feasible.

2. HISTORICAL

That exogenous nucleic acids might influence an immune response was demonstrated first by the observation that administration of nucleic acids would restore immunocompetence to animals in which the immune response was suppressed by drugs (Merritt and Johnson, 1965) or X-irradiation (Jaroslow and Taliaferro, 1956). These findings suggested a possible mechanism for the immunoenhancing effects of endotoxin or other cytotoxic agents. Endotoxin was shown to cause an *in vivo* destruction of small lymphocytes located perifollicularly to antibody forming cells (Ward *et al.*, 1959). Since endotoxin

ABBREVIATIONS

poly (A:U), polyadenylic–polyuridylic acid complex; FUDR, 5-fluorodeoxyuridine; DNA, deoxyribonucleic acid; poly (I:C), polyinosinic–polycytidylic acid complex; PFC, plaque-forming cell; RFC, rosette-forming cell; SRBC, sheep red blood cells; VLB, vinblastine; T lymphocyte, thymus-influenced lymphocyte; DNP-POL, dinitrophenol-polymerized flagellin; CMI, cell-mediated immunity; DH, delayed type hypersensitivity; poly A, polyadenylic acid; poly U, polyuridylic acid; poly C, polycytidylic acid; EAE, experimental autoimmune encephalomyelitis; PHA, phytohemagglutinin; B lymphocyte, bone marrow-derived lymphocyte; RNA, ribonucleic acid; IgM, immunoglobulin M; IgG, immunoglobulin G; IgE, immunoglobulin E; AUSF, poly A:U-induced supernatant factor; HGG, human gamma globulin; cyclic AMP, 3′,5′ cyclic adenosine monophosphate; BGG, bovine gamma globulin; BSA, bovine serum albumin; PPD, purified protein derivative.

partially restored the immune response of sub-lethally irradiated rabbits (Kind and Johnson, 1959) and could partially overcome the immunosuppressive effects of FUDR in mice (Merritt and Johnson, 1963), it was suggested that endotoxin restored immunocompetence to irradiated rabbits by causing the release of nucleic acids necessary for the repair of cells damaged, but not killed by irradiation. Similarly, the ability of endotoxin to overcome FUDR-induced immunosuppression was thought to be due to a release of an endogenous supply of nucleic acid precursors which would circumvent the inhibition of DNA synthesis caused by FUDR (Merritt and Johnson, 1963). Subsequent studies demonstrated that nucleic acids and low molecular weight oligonucleotides had a potent adjuvant effect on antibody formation to soluble (Merritt and Johnson, 1965) or particulate (Braun and Nakano, 1967) antigens in normal animals.

Analysis of the adjuvant properties of nucleic acids has been facilitated greatly by the availability of chemically defined synthetic homoribopolynucleotides. Helical complexes of polyadenylic (poly A) and polyuridylic (poly A:U) or polyinosinic and polycytidylic acids (poly I:C) are readily formed when mixed in the presence of sodium ion. Administration of the polynucleotide complexes with antigen was shown to have adjuvant effects identical to those observed previously with crude preparations of nucleic acids (Braun *et al.*, 1968; Johnson *et al.*, 1968).

3. AUGMENTATION OF HUMORAL IMMUNE RESPONSE

3.1. *In Vivo*

As shown in Table 1, poly (A:U) and poly (I:C) both augment the *in vivo* production of antibody to soluble and particulate antigens. The essential manifestations of the adjuvant properties of poly (A:U) and poly (I:C) are similar are are outlined in Table 2. However, because of the relative toxicity of poly (I:C) (Stinebring and Absher, 1971; Philips *et al.*, 1971) the adjuvant properties of poly (A:U) have been studied more extensively. Administration of homoribopolynucleotide complexes will augment serum IgM, IgG and IgE antibody levels in the primary response, characteristically with a shortened time required to detect specific antibody and prolonged maintenance of high levels of circulating antibody (Schmidtke and Johnson, 1971; Mota and Ferini, 1975, Johnson, 1976). In general antigen does not enhance the anamnestic response (Schmidtke

TABLE 1. *Adjuvant Effects of Polynucleotide Complexes on the* In Vivo *Humoral Immune Response*

Antigen	Effect	Author
SRBC	Increased rate of appearance of antibody-secreting cells	Braun *et al.*, 1968 Braun and Nakano, 1967
SRBC	Increased number of antibody-secreting cells in splenic hemolytic foci. No increase in number of foci	Braun *et al.*, 1968 Campbell and Kind, 1971
SRBC	Accelerated increase in antigen-binding T and B cells	Cone and Wilson, 1973
BGG	Increase in IgM, IgG antibodies Increased priming	Schmidtke and Johnson, 1971
BSA	Increased priming	*ibid*
HGG	Increased priming	*ibid*
Ferritin	Increased priming	*ibid*
Vi antigen	Increased priming	*ibid*
Seminal antigens	Increased antibody	Menge, 1970
DNA	Increased antibody	Okuhara *et al.*, 1976
Foot and mouth disease (vaccine)	Increased antibody	
Swine influenza	Increased antibody	Stephen *et al.*, 1977
Venezuelan equine encephalomyelitis virus	Increased antibody	Houston *et al.*, 1976
BGG	Inhibition of tolerance induction	Kong and Capanna, 1974

TABLE 2. *Adjuvant Properties of Polynucleotide Complexes in Humoral Immunity*

1. Decreased induction period for detectable antibody-forming cells
2. No affect on burst size
3. Augmentation of levels of IgM, IgG, IgE antibodies
4. Augmentation of primary (and sometimes) secondary antibody response
5. Augmented priming for secondary response
6. Abrogation of tolerance induction

and Johnson, 1971). However administration of poly (A:U) in the primary response will augment markedly priming for the secondary response (Schmidtke and Johnson, 1971).

The amplifying effect of homoribopolynucleotide complexes on events in the humoral immune response which occur earlier than when serum antibodies can be detected may be demonstrated when antibody secreting cells (plaque forming cells, PFC) or antigen binding cells (rosette forming cells, RFC) are enumerated in the response to sheep erythrocytes). Anti-SRBC PFC or RFC are detected 24–48 hrs earlier in the spleens of mice receiving poly (A:U) (Braun *et al.*, 1968; Braun and Nakano, 1967; Cone and Johnson, 1972; Marchalonis *et al.*, 1973). However, in most cases the maximum number of antibody-forming cells generated in poly (A:U) and non-poly (A:U) treated animals is the same (Braun *et al.*, 1968; Marchalonis *et al.*, 1973). In short, poly (A:U) or poly (I:C) appear to shorten the induction period required for the generation of antibody producing cells. The actual rate of increase in antibody forming cells and the final numbers obtained however are not influenced by these adjuvants. In some cases, however, elevated levels of antibody secreting cells are maintained longer in poly (A:U) treated animals (Braun *et al.*, 1968). The earlier appearance and prolonged maintenance of antibody secreting cells is thus responsible for the augmented serum antibody levels in animals receiving poly (A:U). Interestingly, when numbers of antibody-forming precursor cells (or inductive units, see below) were measured, poly (A:U) was found to have no effect on numbers of precursors or inductive units but rather enhanced the number of antibody-forming cells per inductive unit (Braun *et al.*, 1968; Campbell and Kind, 1971). These observations support further the contention that poly (A:U) does not amplify the number of cells responding to antigen but rather the rate at which they begin to respond. One of the most striking examples of the effect of poly (A:U) on the induction period is the influence of the polynucleotide complexes on the time at which the immune response becomes susceptible to the immunosuppressive action of vinblastine (VLB). Since this vincaalkaloid kills cells entering metaphase the time at which it suppresses the immune response has been taken as a measure of when responding cells are entering division (Perkins *et al.*, 1969). VLB inhibits the humoral response of mice to sheep erythrocytes when given 24 hr after immunization. However, when vinblastine is given within 6 hr after mice receive antigen and poly (A:U) the immune response to that antigen is inhibited (Cone and Johnson, 1972).

The ability of poly (A:U) to shorten so drastically the time between injection of antigen and the first evidence of division of responding cells suggests that the adjuvant action of poly (A:U) is most likely exerted at the very earliest stages of the immune response. In support of this view is the observation that poly (A:U) will prevent the induction of tolerance to soluble antigens (Kong and Capanna, 1974). Moreover, the influence of antigen dose and the timing of administration of poly (A:U) relative to antigen (*vide infra*) also indicate that the influence of poly (A:U) may be during the initial interaction of immunocompetent cells with antigen.

3.2. *In Vitro* HUMORAL IMMUNE RESPONSE

The limited (if any) toxicity and chemical homogeneity of poly (A:U) has facilitated analysis of its adjuvant properties on the humoral and cell-mediated (*vide infra*) response *in vitro*. The adjuvant effect of poly (A:U) *in vitro* is generally similar to those observed *in vivo*; namely, a much more rapid (by 24–48 hr) appearance and peak production of antibody-forming cells (Cone and Marchalonis, 1973; Braun and Ishizuka, 1971; Jaroslow and Ortiz-Ortiz, 1972). However, *in vitro* the effective dose of poly (A:U) is far lower than that used *in vivo* and dosage requirements are considerably more stringent. Dose requirements have varied considerably and have ranged from 0.0001–10 mg/ml. It is clear however, that high doses of poly (A:U) can suppress the immune response *in vitro* (Cone and Marchalonis, 1973; Braun and Ishizuka, 1971). The variation in dosage probably depends on the culture system employed and the antigen dose. Thus when suboptimal amounts of SRBC are added to spleen cell cultures, the dose of poly (A:U) required to achieve maximum adjuvant activity is dependent on the day at which the immune response is assayed. When the response is assayed on day 2, 10 μg of poly (A:U)/culture is required, and 0.1 μg culture shows little if any adjuvant activity. However, there is no further increase in PFC in the presence of 10 μg/ml and by day 4 there are fewer PFC than control cultures. On day 3, cultures containing 1 μg poly (A:U) exhibit a further increase in PFC but the response is similarly 'shut down' after 3 days. At 3 days 0.1 μg poly (A:U) gives maximum adjuvant activity with further increases in PFC on day 4. The dose of poly (A:U) required for maximum adjuvant activity *in vitro* is also dependent on antigen dose. Thus on day 3 if 0.01–0.1 μg poly (A:U) provides maximum adjuvant activity for 10^5 SRBC, 0.1–1 μg is required for 10^4 SRBC. Higher doses than these become suppressive. That the inhibitory influence of poly (A:U) on the *in vitro* immune response is not due to a non-specific toxic effect on the cultured cells is evidenced by experiments in which spleen cells were cultured with SRBC and dinitrophenylated polymerized flagellin (DNP-POL). This antigen stimulates antibody formation in the absence of thymus-influenced (T) lymphocytes and macrophages while the antibody formation to the former antigen requires T cells and macrophages (see below). Poly (A:U) had no amplifying or suppressive activity for the PFC response to DNP-POL while these effects were evident in the response to SRBC in the same culture (Cone and Feldman, unpublished results). It is thus more likely that the suppressive effect of poly (A:U) is mediated through the influence of suppressor T cells (see below).

4. CELL MEDIATED IMMUNITY

4.1. *In Vivo*

Homoribopolynucleotide complexes of poly (A:U) or poly (I:C) can also exert a strong adjuvant effect on cell-mediated immune responses (Table 3). Cell-mediated reactions (CMI) are effected by T lymphocytes (which provide specificity) and macrophages and monocytes which may act as auxilliary cells under the influence of T cells. Production of humoral antibody does not necessarily play a role in CMI. Demonstration of an adjuvant effect may be somewhat more difficult in CMI because the antigen dose requirements are often quite different (and much lower) than required to stimulate humoral responses (Askenase *et al.*, 1975). Thus poly (A:U) has little effect on the rejection time of skin grafts across a strong H-2 allogeneic 'barrier' in mice (Cone and Johnson, 1971), unless the mice receiving the graft have been made immunodeficient by neonated thymectomy (see below). However when the antigenic stimulus is weak, as is the case when male skin (H–Y) is grafted to syngeneic female mice graft rejection is accelerated by the administration of poly (I:C) (Turner *et al.*, 1970). Similarly, poly (A:U) administered to mice with doses of SRBC which are suboptimal for the induction of delayed hypersensitivity (DH) augments the DH reaction (measured by swelling after subsequent challenge with antigen) (Askenase and Cone, unpublished observations). In this regard DH is augmented without concomitant production of antibody. Poly (A:U) administered with doses of SRBC optimal for DH will suppress DH, but augment antibody production. This latter observation is consistent with the finding that doses of antigen which lead to antibody formation tend to suppress DH in the mouse (Askenase *et al.*, 1975; LaGrange, *et al.*, 1974). Thus administration of poly (A:U) results in a shift to the left in the antigen dose response curve for DH and antibody formation. Other manifestations of *in vivo*

TABLE 3. *Adjuvant Effects of Polynucleotide Complexes on Cell-mediated Immunity*

Antigen	Adjuvant	Assay	Author
		In Vivo	
H-2	Poly (A:U)	Skin grafts in neonatally thymectomized (adult) mice	Cone and Johnson, 1971
H-2	Poly (A:U)	Graft vs Host reaction	Cantor *et al.*, 1970
H-Y	Poly (I:C)	Skin grafts	Turner *et al.*, 1970
PPD	Poly (A:U) Poly (U)	Dermal reactions assay for Migration Inhibitory Factor (MIF)	Casavant and Youmans, 1975
Myelin basic protein	Poly (A:U)	Experimental autoimmune encephalomyelitis (EAE)	Gumbiner *et al.*, 1973
Spinal cord homogenate	Poly (A:U) Poly (U) Poly (C)	EAE	Patterson and Drobish, 1974
		In Vitro	
PPD	Poly (A:U)	Blast transformation DNA synthesis	Friedman *et al.*, 1969
Tetanus toxoid	Poly (A:U)	Blast transformation DNA synthesis	Chess *et al.*, 1972
Allogeneic cells	Poly (A:U)	DNA synthesis	Chess *et al.*, 1972
H-2	Poly (A:U)	Generation of cytotoxic T cells	Wagner and Cone, 1974
H-2	Poly (A:U)	Generation of cytotoxic T cells	Bick and Moller, 1977

CMI such as the graft vs host reaction (Cantor *et al.*, 1970) and induction of autoimmune disease (Gumbiner *et al.*, 1973; Patterson and Drobish, 1974) are also augmented by polynucleotide complexes. Interestingly non-complexed homopolymers of poly A, poly U or poly C have been shown to augment experimental autoimmune encephalomyelitis (EAE) induced in response to immunization with nerve tissue (Patterson and Drobish, 1974). In most cases (see below) single stranded homopolymers are without significant adjuvant activity.

4.2. *In Vitro*

In vitro correlates of cell-mediated immunity include blast transformation and DNA synthesis in response to antigen and the production of cytotoxic T cells capable of killing target cells bearing surface antigens to which the T cells have been stimulated. Poly (A:U) has been shown to enhance blast transformation and DNA synthesis by T cells in response to suboptimal amounts of soluble antigens (Friedman *et al.*, 1969; Chess *et al.*, 1972) or allogeneic cells. However, in some cases no enhanced stimulation of DNA synthesis in T cells in response to allogeneic cells have been observed (J. Schmidtke, personal communication). Quite possibly this is due to antigen dose effects. An earlier increase and attainment of maximum numbers of cytotoxic T cells under the influence of poly (A:U) has been observed when responding T cells are co-cultivated with allogeneic lymphocytes (Wagner and Cone, 1974) or syngeneic tumor cells bearing tumor specific transplantation antigens (Wagner and Cone, unpublished observations). The effective adjuvant dose in this system was at least 2–3 orders of magnitude lower than that required for *in vitro* simplification of antibody-forming cells to SRBC. In fact, amounts of poly (A:U) which were optimal *in vitro* for augmentation of humoral immunity suppressed the development of cytotoxic T cells. However, recent observations in this regard have shown that very high concentrations of poly (A:U) (100 μg/ml) *in vitro* will induce the appearance of cytotoxic T cells to allogeneic cells, within 2 hr of culture and in the absence of antigen (Bick and Moller, 1977). The homoribopolynucleotide complexes did not induce DNA synthesis in the T cells to achieve this effect. The relationship between the 'polyclonal activation' of T cells achieved with high doses of poly (A:U) and the antigen specific amplification of the response of T cells to allogeneic cells by 1×10^{-5}-fold less poly (A:U) is uncertain. Perhaps small amounts of poly (A:U) in concert with an antigenic stimulus to several clones has the same effect as high doses of poly (A:U) to many clones. Lectins such as phytohemogglutinin (PHA) will also induce the polyclonal activation of T cells into cytotoxic cells. However, this occurs only after a round of DNA synthesis. Interestingly poly (A:U) suppresses the mitotic activity induced by PHA (Friedman *et al.*, 1969; Johnson *et al.*, 1968).

5. IMMUNE DEFENSE

5.1. Viruses and Microorganisms

From the preceding it is apparent that homoribonucleotide complexes can exert potent adjuvant effects on both humoral and cell-mediated immunity. Since both of these 'arms' of the immune system are operant in resistance to infection it might be expected that polynucleotide adjuvants facilitate immunologic defense against infectious micro-organisms. However, at this juncture it should be stressed that in some instances the effect of the polynucleotides is not as dramatic or complete as when these adjuvants are tested for augmentation of single facets of an immune response to a non-living antigen. As shown in Table 4, poly (A:U) and poly (I:C) enhance resistance to a wide range of infectious agents. Increased antibody responses and resistance to challenge to a number of viruses has been observed when virus vaccines were administered concomitantly with poly (A:U) or poly (I:C). With regard to poly (I:C), increased resistance may also be due to the greater ability of poly (I:C) as compared to poly (A:U) to induce interferon production (Hilleman *et al.*, 1971; Colby *et al.*, 1971). Administration of poly (A:U) together with attenuated *Brucella abortus* reduced the number of microorganisms in spleen or liver of mice 1000-fold as compared to mice receiving *B. abortus* alone (Cheers and Cone, 1974). However the residual microorganisms in the spleen were able to proliferate such that 30 days later they reached levels (which were maintained) in mice

TABLE 4. *Effect of Polynucleotide Complexes on Response to Infectious Agents*

Agent	Adjuvant	Effect	Authors
Viruses			
Murine pneumonia (PVM)	Poly (I:C)	Enhanced resistance	Hilleman *et al.*, 1971
Vaccinia	Poly (I:C)	Enhanced resistance	
Columbia SK	Poly (I:C)	Enhanced resistance	
Sendai	Poly (I:C)	Enhanced resistance	
Influenza	Poly (A:U) Poly (I:C)	Increased antibody	Woodhour *et al.*, 1969
Rabies	Poly (I:C)	Enhanced resistance	Fenge and Postic, 1970
Foot and mouth disease virus	Poly (A:U) Poly (I:C)	Enhanced resistance	Cunliffe *et al.*, 1977
Bacteria			
Brucella	Poly (A:U)	Enhanced protection by vaccine	Renoux *et al.*, 1972
Brucella abortus	Poly (A:U)	Inhibition of primary infection	Cheers and Cone, 1974
Listeria monocytogenes	Poly (A:U)	Inhibition of primary infection	Fauve, 1971 Remington and Merigan, 1970
Parasites			
Toxoplasma gondii	Poly (A:U) Poly (I:C)	Enhanced protection	Araujo and Remington, 1974
Plasmodium berghei	Poly (I:C)	Enhanced protection	Desowitz, 1975

infected without poly (A:U). Moreover, poly (A:U) had no appreciable effect on chronically infected mice. Again it appeared that poly (A:U) exerted its adjuvant effect at or near the time of initial immune stimulus only. Since protection against *B. abortus* is thought to be effected through cell-mediated immunity it was felt that poly (A:U) exerted its adjuvant effect through T lymphocytes (see below). Accordingly the ability of poly (A:U) to reduce the primary infection to *B. abortus* was tested in congenitally athymic mice. In contrast to expectations poly (A:U) reduced the primary infection in these mice to the same extent as normal mice. Since poly (A:U) has been shown to have little or no direct effect on B lymphocytes (see below) it was postulated that the major influence of poly (A:U) on the primary defence against *B. abortus* was exerted through the macrophage. However, other studies (Renoux *et al.*, 1972) have shown that poly (A:U) can reduce the effective immunogenic dose of a *B. abortus* vaccine by 3 $\log_{10}$ when protection was tested by subsequent challenge with *B. abortus.* In this report no antibody was found in protected animals so that selective stimulation of cell-mediated immunity (and therefore T cells) seemed likely. It would thus appear that poly (A:U) can be used to amplify (and dissect) both the macrophage and T lymphocyte facets of the immune response to *Brucella*. A similar effect of poly (A:U) on protection against *L. monocytogenes* infection (Fauve, 1971) may also be due to action of the polynucleotide complexes on macrophages. However, the possibility that poly (A:U) enhanced the activity of T lymphocytes which in turn activated macrophages cannot be ruled out.

6. TUMOR IMMUNITY

The possibility that the immune system might be used as a therapeutic adjunct in the treatment of neoplasms has received considerable attention in recent years (Smith and Landy, 1975). Homoribopolynucleotide complexes would seem to be useful candidates for enhancement of anti-tumor immunotherapy because of their low toxicity [particularly poly (A:U)] and their well-defined chemistry. However, it should be stressed that as the case with infectious agents, the relationship between the tumor and the immune system is highly complex. Thus an immune response to the tumor might destroy the tumor but alternatively can facilitate its spread. Introduction of polynucleotide adjuvants into this relationship may thus be a 'double-edged sword'. Timing, antigen dose effects and the nature of the potentiated immune response are critical. Moreover it is conceivable that the polynucleotides could have a direct effect on the tumor cell which may enhance the means by which a neoplastic cell escaped attack by the immune system.

The results of studies on the ability of polynucleotide complexes to potentiate an immunoprotective response against neoplasms have been somewhat disappointing (Table 5). In general it can be said that when a positive (protective) effect of polynucleotides was observed it was of a temporary and moderate nature. Part of the difficulty in evaluating the effects of poly (A:U) or poly (I:C) on tumor immunity is the wide variations in experimental protocols. If an immune response to the tumor has already been induced prior to administration of the adjuvant the polynucleotides are likely to have no effect. If no immune response has occurred previously, the enhanced immune response generated by polynucleotide treatment could eventually result in a response which serves to protect the tumor. Alternatively, polynucleotide treatment may result in the direct opposite of the desired effect. Thus, administration of poly (A:U) to C58 mice 1 hr to 7 days after injection with viable line Ib leukemia cells did not increase survival time.* When poly (A:U) was administered 24 hr before injection of viable line Ib cells or concurrently with X-irradiated cells enhanced lethality by the tumor cells resulted. Spleen cells from such animals were unable to transfer immunity to non-poly (A:U)-treated recipients whereas such cells from non-poly (A:U)-treated donors conferred immunity on recipient mice. As will be discussed below the net effect of poly (A:U) in these experiments is probably due to an activation of suppressor T cells.

*Maryanski *et al.*, Immune mechanisms in leukemia: Suppressive effect of polyadenylic-polyuridylic acid on the active and adoptive immune response of C58 mice to line Ib cells, submitted for publication.

TABLE 5. *Effects of Homoribopolynucleotide Complexes on Immunity to Neoplasms*

Homoribopoly-nucleotide	Neoplasm	Effect	Author
Poly (I:C)	Murine reticulum cell; Sarcoma	Reduced tumor size, increased survival	Levy *et al.*, 1971
Poly (A:U) Poly (I:C)	Murine L1210 Leukemia	25–40 per cent increase in survival time	Zeleznick and Bhuyan, 1969
Poly (I:C)	SV40 tumor tumor transplant (hamsters)	None	Larson *et al.*, 1970
Poly (I:C)	Transplanted methylcholanthrene induced fibrosarcoma and murine polyoma (mice)	Temporary inhibition of growth rate	Fisher *et al.*, 1972
Poly (A:U)	Mammary adenocarcinoma (hamsters)	Increased median survival time after surgical removal of tumor	Lacour *et al.*, 1972
Poly (A:U)	Murine WEHI-3B myelomonocytic leukemia	Increased survival	Maryanski *et al.**
Poly (A:U)	Murine line Ib leukemia	Increased lethality	Maryanski *et al.**

*Immune mechanisms in leukemia: Suppressive effect of polyadenylic–polyuridylic acid on the active and adoptive immune response of C58 mice to line Ib cells, submitted for publication.

7. IMMUNOSUPPRESSIVE EFFECTS OF POLYNUCLEOTIDE ADJUVANTS

The immune system consists of a multicomponent network of interacting cell subsets. The system is delicately regulated by the interacting cells and by antibody. As with any interacting network, perturbation of one facet will likely lead to effects on another. As discussed above, the amplifying effect of polynucleotides on humoral and cell-mediated responses is critically dependent on the dose of antigen and the timing of the administration of the adjuvant in relation to antigen encounter. When poly (A:U) is administered concurrently with antigen the result is usually an amplified response. However, *in vivo* poly (A:U) has no effect on an immune response elicited by high doses of antigen. *In vitro* high doses of poly (A:U) and antigen either suppress the response (Braun and Ishizuka, 1971) or result in an aborted response after an accelerated induction (Cone and Marchalonis, 1973). When poly (A:U) is given *in vivo* 24 hr before antigen suppression is often observed (Schmidtke and Johnson, 1971). Interestingly, the suppressive effects of poly (A:U) pre-treatment can be reversed if a second injection of poly (A:U) is given with antigen. At least part of the suppressive effect of poly (A:U) pre-treatment is mediated through macrophages. When macrophages obtained from mice treated 24 hr previously with poly (A:U) were incubated with BGG they were unable to induce an immune response upon transfer into naive animals (Johnson and Johnson, 1971). However, incubation of these macrophages with antigen and poly (A:U) reversed the suppressive effect of poly (A:U) pre-treatment. The *in vivo* humoral response of mice to sheep erythrocytes is generally not affected by poly (A:U) pre-treatment however profound suppressive effects by poly (A:U) pre-treatment have been observed when delayed hypersensitivity responses were studied (Askenase and Cone, unpublished). Administration of poly (A:U) with low doses of antigen potentiated the delayed sensitivity response while pre-treatment completely suppressed the response. When the polynucleotides were given with moderate doses of antigen antibody production was enhanced and delayed sensitivity was suppressed. However, the suppressive effect of poly (A:U) could be prevented when mice were also given cytoxan before immunization with low or moderate doses of antigen. These results have been interpreted to suggest that poly (A:U) may be amplifying the activity of a cytoxan-sensitive suppressor T cell (Askenase *et al.*, 1975). More direct evidence for this notion has been obtained by Morris and Johnson (1978). Spleen cells obtained from mice treated with poly (A:U) 24 hr prior to cell culture with sheep erythrocytes fail to produce antibody-forming cell response to SRBC. Removal of nylon-adherent splenic T cells from the spleen cell population will permit the remaining cells to respond to SRBC. In fact it was shown that poly (A:U) pre-treatment had amplified the activity of helper T cells in the spleen. These results indicate that poly (A:U) pre-treatment had amplified the activity of both suppressor and helper T cell subsets. The suppressor T cells were able to prevent the activity of helper T cells required in an anti-SRBC response. Since administration of poly (A:U) concurrently with antigen appears to amplify helper T cell activity (see below) the results of Morris and Johnson suggest further that a longer time is required before the amplifying influence of poly (A:U) on suppressor T cells is manifested. Conceivably the activation of suppressor T cells was the direct result of prior activation of helper T cells (Eardley *et al.*, 1978a).

Although administration of poly (A:U) prior to antigenic stimulation can result in suppression of an immune response to the antigen the homoribopolynucleotide complex can prevent the induction of tolerance to antigens when given 0–12 hr *after* injection of tolerizing antigen doses (Kong and Capanna, 1974). Cortisone-resistant T cells appeared to be the target for the poly (A:U) effect in these studies (Capanna and Kong, 1975).

8. CELLULAR SITES OF ACTION OF POLYNUCLEOTIDE ADJUVANTS

The temporal relationship between administration of poly (A:U) and antigen suggests that polynucleotide adjuvants influence the early phases of an immune response. Stem cells, macrophages and/or immunocompetent T or B cells could be affected. Thus, these adjuvants might increase the number of cells responding to antigen by activation of the differentiation of stem cells or recruitment of immunocompetent cells. Alternatively the rate of proliferation or the functional efficiency of responding cells might be amplified without increasing the frequency of responding units.

In vitro and *in vivo* poly (A:U) has been shown to increase the number of hematopoietic colony-forming units (McNeill, 1971; McNeill and Killen, 1971). Whether this is a direct effect of the polynucleotides on stem cells, or the result of enhanced secretion of colony stimulating factor is not known. Additionally, poly (A:U) has been shown *in vitro* to cause the expression of differentiation antigens on precursor cells (Scheid *et al.*, 1973). These results support the contention that polynucleotide adjuvants might exert an adjuvant effect by increasing the number of cells which might respond to an antigenic stimulus. However, as discussed previously poly (A:U) does not, in many cases, increase the maximum number of cells responding to antigen but rather increases the rate at which they respond.

Poly (A:U) has been shown to have marked effects on macrophage function. Incubation of macrophages with antigen *in vitro* and subsequent transfer of antigen-pulsed macrophages to naive animals results in an enhanced immune response to the antigen (Johnson and Johnson, 1971). When macrophages are cultured with antigen and poly (A:U) the ability of the antigen-pulsed macrophages to induce an immune response was amplified (Johnson and Johnson, 1971). Moreover, incubation of macrophages with polynucleotides can result in a non-specific activation of these cells into cytotoxic cells (Alexander and Evans, 1971; Johnson, 1976). Both RNA and protein synthesis is required for the polynucleotide-induced activation (Johnson and Johnson, 1971) of macrophages.

Poly (A:U)-induced suppression may also be mediated in part through macrophages. Macrophages obtained from mice treated with poly (A:U) 24 hr before culture with antigen will not transfer an enhanced immune response after antigen pulsing. Incubation of such cells with antigen and poly (A:U) will however override the poly (A:U)-induced suppression (Johnson and Johnson, 1971). The ability of poly (A:U) to provide partial protection against experimental *Brucella* infection in mice (Cheers and Cone, 1974) appears to be due to non-specific activation of macrophages (Madraso and Cheers, 1978). In these studies poly (A:U) failed to enhance T cell-mediated responses to the organism, adoptive transfer of immunity or the production of IgG or IgM antibodies to *Brucella*. Macrophage spreading, an indicator of activation was enhanced *in vivo* after administration of poly (A:U) and *B. abortus*. Similar activation of macrophages after *in vitro* culture with poly (A:U), in the absence of T cells was also observed. These observations, taken together with the finding that poly (A:U) was able to enhance protection against *B. abortus* infection in congenitally athymic mice (Cheers and Cone, 1974) suggest that the enhanced activation of macrophages by poly (A:U) was completely responsible for the adjuvant effects of the polynucleotides in this system.

Given the central role of the macrophage in the immune response it would appear that a significant part of the adjuvant effects of polynucleotides is mediated through these cells. However, there is a large body of evidence to indicate that another major locus of action of poly (A:U) is the T (thymus-derived) lymphocyte. Early studies in this regard demonstrated that poly (A:U) when injected with antigen into adult mice thymectomized at birth, restored the antibody response to sheep erythrocytes as effectively as administration of thymocytes (Cone and Johnson, 1971). The effect of poly (A:U) was shown to be due to amplification of small numbers of T cells present in the thymectomized mice. Thus treatment of such mice with anti-thymocyte serum to further reduce T cell numbers reduced or abrogated the poly (A:U) effect. Moreover, injection of poly (A:U) restored the ability of thymectomized mice to reject allogeneic skin grafts. If the mice were fully depleted of T cells restoration of graft rejection would be impossible.

The influence of poly (A:U) on T lymphocytes was subsequently defined more precisely with the aid of lethally-irradiated mouse model systems reconstituted with thymocytes and bone marrow cells. It was shown that *in vivo* administration of poly (A:U) with bone marrow cells and thymocytes permitted an immune response with 200-fold less thymocytes than normally required (Cone and Johnson, 1972). Moreover, a potentiating effect of poly (A:U) on the activity of thymocytes was observed if these cells were incubated with poly (A:U) and antigen *in vitro* for 90 min prior to injection. These studies provided evidence for a direct effect of poly (A:U) on T cells. No direct amplification of B cell activity was observed (Cone and Johnson, 1972). Similar results were obtained when poly (A:U) was employed to amplify *in vitro* immune responses to sheep erythrocytes (Cone and Marchalonis, 1973) or the *in vitro* generation of cytotoxic T cells by alloantigens (Wagner and Cone, 1974). More recent studies have shown that *in vitro* incubation of T cells with poly (A:U) can induce, in the absence of macrophages or antigen, the polyclonal activation of T cells into cytotoxic cells (Bick and Moller, 1977). In other *in vivo* studies it was found that injection of poly (A:U) and sheep erythrocytes resulted in a three-fold enhancement in the number of B cells forming rosettes (RFC) with SRBC and a ten-fold increase in the number of T-RFC (Cone and Wilson, 1973). In an adoptive transfer system it was shown further that poly (A:U)-induced enhancement of an immune response to hapten-carrier conjugates was due to amplification of the activity of carrier-primed T cells (Hamaoka and Katz, 1973; Yamashita and Kitazawa, 1974).

The immunosuppressive effects of poly (A:U) are also manifested in part through an influence on T cells. Spleen cells obtained from mice injected with poly (A:U) 24 hr before cultivation of the cells *in vitro* with sheep erythrocytes will not produce an immune response to SRBC. Similar immunosuppression can be obtained by *in vitro* culture of spleen cells with poly (A:U) for 24 hr before addition of antigen (Morris and Johnson, 1978). Removal of a nylon adherent T cell population from the poly (A:U)-treated cell population will permit an immune response to take place. Moreover, the helper T cell population in such spleens exhibits amplified activity. It appears that exposure to poly (A:U) causes a rapid amplification of suppressor T cells. If antigen is present the system is driven towards amplified help while in the absence of antigen suppressor activity apparently overrides the helper activity. The temporal sequence of events suggests that the amplified helper activity may be responsible for activation of suppressor cells (feedback suppression, Eardley *et al.*, 1978a). Alternatively, it could be a direct effect of poly (A:U) on suppressor cells simply takes more time to be manifested.

From the preceding it is clear that the amplifying effects of polynucleotide complexes are to a large extent mediated through macrophages and T lymphocytes. Since the activities of these cells are often interdependent in many cases it is difficult to determine whether the polynucleotide complexes directly influence the activity on one cell type with a resulting indirect effect on the other. Since both macrophages and T cells can influence the activity of B lymphocytes the net effect of poly (A:U) on the humoral immune response will be an indirect amplification of B cell activity. Because of this fact direct influences of the polynucleotide complexes on B cells are difficult to demonstrate. No effect of poly (A:U) on B lymphocytes has been observed when these cells are incubated with poly (A:U) and antigen prior to transfer into irradiated mice (Cone and Johnson, 1972) or *in vitro* culture (Cone and Marchalonis, 1973). The number of plasma cells secreting antibody in hemolytic foci is increased by poly (A:U) (Campbell and Kind, 1971) however this could be due to an influence on macrophage and/or T cells. In addition poly (A:U) has no effect on the *in vitro* immune response of murine spleen cells to polymerized flagellin, a thymus independent antigen (Feldman and Cone, unpublished observations).

Poly (A:U) and poly (I:C) have been shown to be mitogenic *in vitro* for B lymphocytes when the polynucleotide complexes are added in high concentration (Diamanstein *et al.*, 1971a,b; Diamanstein and Blittstein-Willinger, 1975; Scher *et al.*, 1973). T cells do not appear to be required for the mitogenic effect (Scher *et al.*, 1973). Whether the observed mitogenicity is related to the adjuvant effects of poly (A:U) is uncertain. However, amounts of poly (A:U) which are mitogenic *in vitro* generally suppress the immune response (Cone and Marchalonis, 1973). *In vitro* synthesis and secretion of immunoglobulin by peripheral blood lymphocytes from normal human donors is enhanced 2–6-fold by poly (A:U) suggesting a polyclonal activation of human B cells*. However, an indirect stimulation of B cells via activation of T cells was not ruled out in these experiments. Poly (A:U) had significant effects on immunoglobulin secretion by peripheral blood lymphocytes from patients with acquired hypogammaglobulinemia. B cells from such individuals are capable of synthesizing and secreting immunoglobulin but either lack a required T cell helper signal or are inhibited by suppressor T cells (Waldman *et al.*, 1975). Poly (A:U) may substitute for, or provide this T cell helper signal†.

9. MODE OF ACTION OF POLYNUCLEOTIDE ADJUVANTS

Despite the fact that polynucleotide adjuvants are well defined chemically information on the relationship between structure and adjuvant activity is limited. At present, the most important requirements for effective adjuvanticity by polynucleotide complexes are helix formation and molecular size. Poly A or poly U alone do not exhibit adjuvant properties while the helical complex of poly A:poly U is a potent adjuvant (Schmidtke and Johnson, 1971). It has been suggested that poly A is the active principle of the complex since poly A complexed to methylated bovine albumin can function as an adjuvant (Braun and Nakano, 1967), however triple stranded complexes of two parts poly A to one part poly U are no more effective than poly (A:U) (Johnson *et al.*, 1971). Moreover, purine and/or pyrimidine mono or oligonucleotides do not show adjuvant effects (Johnson *et al.*, 1971). Heat treatment (100°C) or disruption of hydrogen bonding of the polynucleotide complex will destory or diminish adjuvant activity supporting further the contention the helix formation between poly A and poly U or poly I and poly C is a strict requirement for adjuvanticity (Schmidtke and Johnson, 1971).

Helix formation might be required for the polynucleotide complexes to assume a conformation which permits binding to cell membranes (see below) and to protect the polynucleotides from serum nucleases. The effects of thermal activation on the ability of

*Lederman, H. M., Johnson, A. G. and Tubergen, D. G., Regulation of the immune system by synthetic polynucleotides—VII. Enhancement of IgG synthesis by human peripheral blood leukocytes *in vitro*, submitted for publication.

†Lederman *et al.*, submitted for publication.

poly (A:U) to stimulate interferon production are illuminating in this regard. When poly (A:U) is heated for 5 min at 37°C the concentration required to induce interferon production by fibroblasts was reduced 6 orders of magnitude (Merigan *et al.*, 1971; De Clercq *et al.*, 1970). It was postulated that this treatment (a) altered the conformation of poly (A:U) which then resulted in an increased rate of binding to cells and resistance to nuclease attack at the cell surface and (b) decreased the susceptibility of poly (A:U) to endonucleases. The effects of thermal activation on the adjuvant activity of poly (A:U) have not however been tested.

The effect of poly (A:U) on immunocompetent cells is manifested quickly. Incubation of lymphoctyes with poly (A:U) *in vitro* for 10 min and subsequent removal of the polynucleotides will potentiate the *in vivo* or *in vitro* activity of the cells as effectively as injection of poly (A:U) *in vivo* (Cone and Johnson, 1972) or inclusion of poly (A:U) throughout *in vitro* culture (Wagner and Cone, 1974). Moreover, incubation of poly (A:U) *in vitro* with normal mouse serum will destroy the adjuvant activity of the polynucleotides suggesting rapid degradation by serum nucleases (Schmidtke and Johnson, 1971). Consequently the *in vivo* activity of poly (A:U) must be accomplished quickly.

The fact that poly (A:U) appears to act rapidly suggests that the polynucleotide complexes must be absorbed by the affected cell. Polynucleotide complexes are indeed absorbed by a variety of cell types (Johnson, 1976) however the ultimate fate of poly (A:U) and poly (I:C) differs. Poly (A:U) is taken up be Ehrlich ascites tumor cells as an intact complex while the strands of poly (I:C) are separated at the cell surface (Schell and Muller, 1971). Poly I only enters the cell. Adsorbtion of polynucleotides by cells probably depends in part on charge since pretreatment of cells with poly L-lysine enhances the adsorption of poly (A:U) (Schell, 1971). Since most cells bear a net negative surface charge, alteration of surface charge by polycations would be expected to increase the binding of negatively charged polynucleotides. However aggregation of polynucleotide complexes in the absence of any change in the charge of the polynucleotide also results in increased binding to cells (Noronha-Blob and Pitha, 1978). Increased aggregation of poly I:poly vinyl C correlates directly with increased antiviral activity of this compound. On the other hand increased aggregation of poly (I:C) does not improve upon the very effective antiviral activity of this polynucleotide (Noronha-Blob and Pitha, 1978). It has been suggested that this difference between poly (I:C) and poly I:poly vinyl C is due to the fact that poly (I:C) is a highly ordered double stranded complex (Noronha-Blob and Pitha, 1978). Conformation of the polynucleotide complexes is thus important for both binding to the cell and resistance to serum or cell associated nucleases. It is not known, however, whether the adjuvant effect of polynucleotides requires membrane binding only, or subsequent internalization of the bound complexes.

The adjuvant effects of polynucleotide complexes could be manifested at several levels. Binding to target cells might initiate cell division, expanding reactive cell populations in a polyclonal fashion. Cell metabolism might increase such that cells responding to antigen function more efficiently or differentiate more rapidly. On the other hand the polynucleotide complexes might have more selective effects on secretory and/or membrane mediated-events. Poly (A:U) has been shown to be weakly mitogenic for splenic T cells in culture (Han and Johnson, 1976) in the absence of antigen and a somewhat stronger mitogen for B cells (Ruhl *et al.*, 1974; Scher *et al.*, 1973). However, the amount of poly (A:U) required to demonstrate a mitogenic effect was far in excess of that needed to demonstrate adjuvant activity *in vitro* (see above). In fact such doses would generally suppress an *in vitro* immune response. Polynucleotides have also been shown to induce *in vitro* some differentiative functions in T cells (Bick and Moller, 1977) and the expression of differentiation antigens by immature B cells (Scher *et al.*, 1973). Again the doses of poly (A:U) required were in excess of those needed to demonstrate adjuvant activity.

When considering the mode of action of polynucleotide adjuvants it should be kept in mind that these agents exert an immunopotentiating effect only when given with or near the time that antigen is presented. It is therefore unlikely that these agents greatly expand the number of responding clones by mitogenic effects or induction of differentiation.

Limiting dilution studies of poly (A:U)-treated T cells (Cone and Johnson, 1972) support this contention. It is thus more probable that poly (A:U) accelerates the rate at which the immune system responds to antigen. Indeed, the *in vivo* doubling time of T cells responding to antigen and the time required for responding cells to enter mitosis (Cone and Johnson, 1972) is halved by poly (A:U) treatment. These effects could be due to (a) increases in cellular metabolism, (b) amplification of recognition of antigen and/or triggering signals induced by antigen-receptor interactions, (c) increased efficiency of cell collaboration, (d) enhanced antigen processing and presentation by macrophages.

9.1. Effects on Macrophage Activity

Poly (A:U) and poly (I:C) both stimulate macrophage metabolism in whole cell and cell-free systems (Morrell, 1971). RNA and protein synthesis are affected including the activity of DNA-dependent RNA polymerase. An increase in RNA synthesis was also noted by Johnson and Johnson (1971) when poly (A:U) was added to macrophages incubated with bovine gamma globulin. Synthesis of messenger RNA may have been involved since the enhanced synthesis was blocked by actinomycin D. This enhanced RNA synthesis was correlated with an increased ability of the antigen-pulsed macrophages to induce an immune response in naive animals. It would seem likely that the enhancement of protein synthesis and RNA metabolism in macrophages by poly (A:U) may result in increased or more efficient antigen processing and presentation by these cells. Conceivably the production of macrophage factors which activate T lymphocytes (Waksman, 1978) was enhanced by the polynucleotide adjuvant.

9.2. Effects on T Cell Activity

As discussed above, the major effect of polynucleotide adjuvants on T cell activity appears to be an acceleration in the rate at which T cells respond to antigen and an increase in the functional activity of individual cells (Cone and Johnson, 1972). Some of these effects may be due to amplification of macrophage activity which in turn results in amplification in T cell activation. Although detailed studies on the effects of polynucleotides on T cell metabolism have not been performed the studies of Bick and Johnson (1977) indicate that the ability of T cells to release a soluble helper factor is enhanced or activated by poly (A:U). Thus murine thymocytes incubated with poly (A:U) for 1.5 hr are induced to release a soluble factor (AUSF) which potentiates the *in vitro* humoral immune of normal spleen cells to erythrocytes. Untreated thymocytes also released 'helper factors' but incubation with poly (A:U) shortened by 3–4-fold the time required for production of the factor. AUSF has also been shown to prevent the induction of tolerance in much the same fashion as polynucleotide adjuvants (Fessia *et al.*, 1977). Another similarity between the immunopotentiating effect of AUSF and poly (A:U) is the observation that the activity of AUSF requires the presence of T cells (Bick and Johnson, 1977). These results suggest that the cells producing AUSF [and one of the targets of poly (A:U)] may be amplifier cells of the Lyt 1, 2, 3 phenotype (Eardley *et al.*, 1978b). These cells may amplify the activity of Lyt 1^+, 2, 3^- helper cells and induce suppressor cells (feedback suppression). Poly (A:U)-induced suppression (see above) might thus be explained by activation of Lyt 1^+, 2^+, 3^+ amplifier cells. It may well be, as suggested by Johnson (1976) that a major portion of the adjuvant activity of poly (A:U) is due to the stimulation of T cells to secrete immunoregulatory factors.

9.3. Effects on B Lymphocytes

There is scant evidence for a direct adjuvant effect of polynucleotide complexes on B lymphocytes (see above). This is not to say, however, that polynucleotides do not influence B cell activity. It is possible that the effects of polynucleotides on B cells, while not being relevant in terms of direct adjuvant effects on B cells nevertheless provide insight as regards adjuvant activity on T cells and/or macrophages.

When murine spleen cells obtained from mice primed 6 weeks previously to human gamma globulin (HGG) were incubated *in vitro* for 1 hr with poly (A:U) and HGG a 4–8-fold increase in antigen binding cells was observed (Stout and Johnson, 1972). Similar results were obtained if the primed mice were injected with poly (A:U) in the absence of antigen. *In vivo* the rise in antigen-binding cells occurred within 48 hr after injection and then rapidly fell to background levels. Functional and serological assays suggested that these cells belonged to a memory B cell pool. Moreover, incubation of these cells with poly (A:U) for 1 hr in the absence of antigen *prior* to the antigen binding assay resulted in a loss in the ability of the cells to bind antigen. Removal of the poly (A:U) and subsequent culture of the cells for 6 hr resulted in a recovery of the ability of the cells to bind antigen when cultured again with poly (A:U) and antigen. Although the initial induction of antigen-binding cells by poly (A:U) did not require *de novo* protein synthesis, re-expression of antigen binding ability was sensitive to inhibitors of protein synthesis. It was suggested that poly (A:U) induced a rapid expression of cryptic membrane receptors for HGG in the primed cell population which were rapidly turned over in the presence of polynucleotides. If no antigen were present the loss of receptors occurred faster than resynthesis such that cells incubated with poly (A:U) in the absence of antigen were 'stripped' of their receptors. In these experiments it cannot be said with certainty whether the induction of receptors represented poly (A:U)-induced increased in immunoglobulin synthesis and secretion or expression of membrane immunoglobulins. It is also possible that this apparent direct effect on memory B cells occurred through a poly (A:U)-induced release of T cell factors.

Poly (A:U)-induced changes in B cell surface membrane topology and physiology have been explored further by Stout and Coons (1973). Poly (A:U) was shown to inhibit antigen binding by non-primed cells in a fashion similar to that described above. Moreover analysis of the shedding of membrane proteins by surface labelling techniques indicated that the polynucleotide complexes caused an accelerated shedding of membrane proteins. Other studies (Cone, R. E., unpublished observations) indicated that the shedding of membrane receptor immunoglobulins was accelerated by poly (A:U). These effects of poly (A:U) appeared to medicited by elevation in the levels of cyclic AMP (Stout and Coons, 1973). It is significant in this regard that the adjuvant effects of poly (A:U) are enhanced by agents which stabilize intracellular levels of cyclic AMP (Ishizuka *et al.*, 1970). These results suggest that the action of poly (A:U) on lymphocytes may be mediated via a direct membrane activating signal which results in an accelerated release of pharmacologically active membrane proteins or secretion of lymphokines and monokines.

10. FUTURE PROSPECTS

In the ten years following the discovery that homoribopolynucleotide complexes can amplify the immune response considerable information has been obtained which illuminate the nature and mode of action of these agents. It is likely that the primary targets for immunopotentiation by polynucleotides are the T lymphocyte and the macrophage. Within the T lymphocyte pool it remains to be determined whether all or certain subsets of T cells are stimulated by polynucleotides. The precise mode of adjuvant action is still unclear, however, available evidence suggests that polynucleotides can stimulate secretion and/or shedding of pharmacologically active lymphocyte and macrophage products. This stimulation may involve a membrane activating event. These adjuvants may thus be useful tools for the production of such factors such that the factors may be characterized and their mode of action elucidated.

The limited toxicity of poly (A:U) suggests a potential use of this agent for proplylactic immunization, particularly when the immunizing antigen is weak or tolerogenic. Conversely, the immunosuppressive activity of these adjuvants might be exploited in situations such as organ transplantation. Quite possibly regimens may be found for the use of polynucleotides to amplify *specific* tolerance induction. Moreover, the ability of polynucleotide adjuvants to amplify the activity of small numbers of T cells holds promise for the use of these agents in immunodeficiency diseases where T cell function is minimal but not absent.

REFERENCES

ALEXANDER, P. and EVANS, R. (1971) Endotoxin and double-stranded RNA render macrophages cytotoxic. *Nat. New Biol.* **232**: 76–78.

ARAUJO, F. G. and REMINGTON, J. S. (1974) Protection against *Toxoplasma gondii* in mice immunized with *Toxoplasma* cell fractions, RNA and synthetic polynucleotides. *Immunology* **27**: 711–721.

ASKENASE, P., HAYDEN, B. J. and GERSHON, R. K. (1975) Augmentation of delayed type hypersensitivity by doses of cyclophosphamide which do not affect antibody responses. *J. Exp. Med.* **141**: 697–702.

BICK, P. and JOHNSON, A. G. (1977) Homoribopolynucleotide-induced secretion of immunocompetent cell enhancing factors from mouse thymocytes. *Scand. J. Immunol.* **6**: 1133–1144.

BICK, P. and MOLLER, G. (1977) Cytotoxic T cell activation by polyribonucleotides: DNA synthesis is not required. *J. Exp. Med.* **144**: 844–856.

BRAUN, W. and NAKANO, M. (1967) Antibody formation: Stimulation by polyadenylic and polyuridylic acids. *Science* **157**: 819–821.

BRAUN, W., NAKANO, M., JARASKOVA, L., YAJIMA, Y. and JIMENEX, L. (1968) Stimulation of antibody-forming cells by oligonucleotides of known composition. In *Nucleic Acids in Immunology*, pp. 347–363, PLESCIA, O. J. and BRAUN, W. (eds). Springer-Verlag, N.Y.

BRAUN, W. and ISHIZUKA, M. (1971) Antibody formation: Reduced responses after administration of excessive amounts of nonspecific stimulators. *Proc. Nat. Acad. Sci. U.S.A.* **68**: 1114–1116.

CAMPBELL, P. A. and KIND, P. (1971) Bone marrow-derived cells as targets for polynucleotide adjuvants. *J. Immunol.* **107**: 1419–1423.

CANTOR, H., ASOFSKY, R. and LEVY, H. B. (1970) The effect of polyinosinic-poly-cytidylic acid upon graft versus host activity in Balb/c mice. *J. Immunol.* **104**: 1035–1038.

CAPANNA, S. L. and KONG, Y. M. (1975) Further studies on the prevention of tolerance induction by poly (A:U). *Immunology* **27**: 647–653.

CASAVANT, C. H. and YOUMANS, G. P. (1975) The adjuvant activity mycobacterial RNA preparations and synthetic polynucleotides for induction of delayed hypersensitivity to purified protein derivative in guinea pigs. *Immunol.* **114**: 1014–1022.

CHEERS, C. and CONE, R. E. (1974) Effect of polyadeninine:polyuridine on brucellosis in conventional and congenitally athymic mice. *J. Immunol.* **112**: 1535–1539.

CHESS, L., LEVY, C., SCHMUKLER, M., SMITH, K. and MARDINEY, M. R. JR. (1972) The effect of synthetic polynucleotides on immunologically-induced tritiated thymidine incorporation. *Transplantation* **14**: 748–755.

COLBY, C., CHAMBERLIN, M. J., DUESBERG, P. H. and SIMON, M. T. (1971) The specificity of interferon production. In *Biological Effects of Polynucleotides*, p. 79, BEERS, R. F. and BRAUN, W. (eds). Springer-Verlag, N.Y.

CONE, R. E. and JOHNSON, A. G. (1971) Regulation of the immune system by synthetic polynucleotides—II. Action on antigen-reactive cells of thymic origin. *J. Exp. Med.* **133**: 665–679.

CONE, R. E. and JOHNSON, A. G. (1972) Regulation of the Immune System by synthetic polynucleotides—IV. Amplification of proliferation of thymus-influenced lymphocytes. *Cell Immunol.* **3**: 283–291.

CONE, R. E. and MARCHALONIS, J. J. (1973) Adjuvant action of poly (A:U) on T cells during the primary immune response *in vitro*. *Aust. J. Exp. Biol. Med. Sci.* **50**: 69–81.

CONE, R. E. and WILSON, J. D. (1973) Adjuvant action of poly (A:U) on T and B rosette-forming cells in SRBC-immunized mice. Analysis by two rosette assay methods. *Int. Arch. Allergy and Appl. Immunol.* **43**: 123–130.

CUNLIFFE, H. R., RICHMOND, J. Y. and CAMPBELL, C. H. (1977) Interferon inducers and foot and mouth disease vaccines: influence of two synthetic polynucleotides on antibody response and immunity in guinea pigs and swine. *Can. J. Comp. Med.* **41**: 117–121.

DECLERQ, E. WELLS, R. D. and MERIGAN, T. C. (1970) Increase in antiviral activity of polynucleotides by thermal activation. *Nature* **226**: 364–366.

DESOWITZ, R. S. (1975) *Plasmodium bergheii*: immunologic enhancement of antigen by adjuvant addition. *Exp. Parasitol.* **38**: 6–13.

DIAMANSTEIN, T., WAGNER, B., BAYSE, I., ODENWALD, M. V. and SCHULZ, G. (1971a) Stimulation of humoral antibody formation by polyanions—I. Effect of polyacrylic acid on the primary immune response of mice immunized with SRBC. *Eur. J. Immunol.* **1**: 335–341.

DIAMANSTEIN, T., WAGNER, B., BAYSE, I., ODENWALD, M. V. and SCHULZ, G. (1971b) Stimulation of the humoral antibody formation by polyanions—II. The influence of sulfate esters of polymers on the immune response in mice. *Eur. J. Immunol.* **1**: 341–351.

DIAMANSTEIN, T. and BLITTSTEIN-WILLENGER, E. (1975) Relationship between biological activities of polymers—I. Immunogenicity, C3 activation, mitogenicity for B cells and adjuvant properties. *Immunology* **29**: 1087–1092.

EARDLEY, D. D., HUGENBERGER, J., MCVAY-BOUDREAU, L., SHEN, F. W., GERSHON, R. K. and CANTOR, H. (1978a) Immunoregulatory circuits among T cell sets—I. T-helper cells induce other T cell sets to exert feedback inhibition. *J. Exp. Med.* **147**: 1106–1115.

EARDLEY, D. D., SHEN, F. W., CONE, R. E. and GERSHON, R. K. (1978b) Antigen-binding T cells: Dose response and kinetic studies on the development of different subsets. *J. Immunol.*: In Press.

FAUVE, R. M. (1971) Influence of synthetic polynucleotides on the bacteriocidal power of mouse macrophages against *Listeria monocytogenes*. In *Biological Effects of Polynucleotides*, p. 215, BEERS, R. F. and BRAUN, W. (eds). Springer-Verlag, N.Y.

FENGE, P. and POSTIC, B. (1970) Protection of rabbits against experimental rabies by poly (I:C). *Nature* **226**: 171–172.

FESSIA, S. L., KONG, Y.-C., BICK, P. H. and JOHNSON, A. G. (1977) Prevention of tolerance induction to a thymus-dependent antigen by poly (A:U)-induced thymocyte fluid. *Eur. J. Immunol.* **8**: 508–510.

FISHER, J. C., COOPERBAND, S. R. and MANNICK, J. A. (1972) The effect of polyinosinic–polycytidylic acid on the immune response of mice to antigenically distinct tumors. *Cancer Res.* **32**: 889–892.

FRIEDMAN, H. M., JOHNSON, A. G. and PAN, P. (1969) Stimulatory effect of polynucleotides on short-term leukocyte cultures. *Proc. Soc. Exp. Biol. Med. Sci.* **132**: 916–920.

GUMBINER, C., PATERSON, P. Y., YOUMANS, G. R. and YOUMANS, A. S. (1973) Adjuvanticity of mycobacterial RNA and poly (A:U) for induction of experimental allergic encephalomyelitis in guinea-pigs. *J. Immunol.* **110**: 309–312.

HAMAOKA, T. and KATZ, D. H. (1973) Mechanism of adjuvant activity of poly (A:U) on antibody responses to hapten-carrier conjugates. *Cell Immunol.* **7**: 246–260.

HAN, I. H., JOHNSON, A. G., COOK, J. and HAN, S. S. (1973) Comparative biological activity of endotoxin and synthetic polyribonucleotides. *J. Infec. Dis.* **128**: 5232.

HAN, I. H. and JOHNSON, A. G. (1976) Regulation of the immune system by synthetic polynucleotides—VI. Amplification of the immune response in young and aging mice. *J. Immunol.* **117**: 423–427.

HILLEMAN, M. R., LAMPSON, G. P., TYTELL, A. A., FIELD, A. K., NEMES, M. M., KRAKOFF, I. H. and YOUNG, C. W. (1971) Double stranded RNAs in relation to interferon induction and adjuvant activity. In *Biological Effects of Polynucleotides*, pp. 27–44, BEERS, R. F. and BRAUN, W. (eds). Springer-Verlag, N.Y.

HOUSTON, W. E., CRABBS, C. L., STEPHEN, E. L. and LEVY, H. B. (1976) Modified polyriboinosinic–polyribocytidylic acid, and immunological adjuvant. *Infect. Immun.* **14**: 318–319.

ISHIZUKA, M., GAFNI, M. and BRAUN, W. (1970) Cyclic AMP effects on antibody formation and their similarities to hormone-mediated events. *Proc. Soc. Exp. Biol. Med.* **134**: 963–968.

JAROSLOW, B. and TALIAFERRO, W. (1956) Restoration of hemolysin-forming capacity in X-irradiated rabbits by tissue and yeast preparations. *J. Infect. Dis.* **98**: 75–81.

JAROSLOW, B. N. and ORTIZ-ORTIZ, L. (1972) Influence of poly A–poly U on early events in the immune response *in vitro*. *Cell Immunol.* **3**: 123–132.

JOHNSON, A. G. (1976) The adjuvant action of synthetic polynucleotides on the immune response. In *Immune RNA*, pp. 17–27, COHEN E. P. (ed.).

JOHNSON, A. G., SCHMIDTKE, J., MERRITT, K. and HAN, I. (1968) Enhancement of antibody formation by nucleic acids and their derivatives. In *Nucleic Acids in Immunology*, pp. 347–363, PLESCIA, O. J. and BRAUN, W. (eds). Springer-Verlag, N.Y.

JOHNSON, A. G., CONE, R. E., FRIEDMAN, H. M., HAN, I. H., JOHNSON, H. G., SCHMIDTKE, J. R. and STOUT, R. D. (1971) Stimulation of the immune system by homoribopolynucleotides. In *Biological Effects of Polynucleotides*, pp. 157–178, BEERS, R. F. JR. and BRAUN, W. (eds). Springer-Verlag, N.Y.

JOHNSON, H. G. and JOHNSON, A. G. (1971) Regulation of the immune system by synthetic polynucleotides—II. Action on peritoneal exudate cells. *J. Exp. Med.* **133**: 649–664.

KIND, P. and JOHNSON, A. G. (1959) Studies on the adjuvant action of bacterial endotoxins on antibody formation—I. Time limitation of enhancing effect and restoration of antibody formation in X-irradiated rabbits. *J. Immunol.* **82**: 415–427.

KONG, Y. and CAPANNA, S. L. (1974) Interference with tolerance induction in mice by poly (A:U). *Cell Immunol.* **11**: 488–492.

LACOUR, F., SPIRA, A., LACOUR, J. and PRADE, M. (1972) Polyadenylic–polyuridylic acid, and adjunct to surgery in the treatment of spontaneous mammary tumors in C_3H-He mice and transplantable melanoma in the hamster. *Cancer Res.* **32**: 648–649.

LAGRANGE, P. H., MACKANESO, G. B. and MILLER, T. E. (1974) Influence of dose and route of antigen injection on the immunological induction of T cells. *J. Exp. Med.* **139**: 528.

LARSON, V. M., PANTELAKIS, P. N. and HILLEMAN, M. K. (1970) Influence of synthetic double stranded RNA (poly I:C) on SV_{40} viral oncogenesis and transplant tumor in hamsters. *Proc. Soc. Exp. Biol. Med.* **133**: 14–17.

LEVY, H. B., ADAMSON, R., CARVONE, P., DEVITA, V., GAZDAR, A., RHIM, J., WEINSTEIN, A. and RILEY, F. (1971) Studies on the anti-tumor action of poly I:poly C. In *Biological Effects of Polynucleotides*, pp. 55–66, BEERS, R. F. and BRAUN, W. (eds). Springer-Verlag, N.Y.

MADRASO, E. D. and CHEERS, C. (1978) Polyadenylic–polyuridylic acid poly (A:U) and experimental murine brucellosis—II. Macrophages as target cells of poly (A:U) in experimental brucellosis. *Immunology* **35**: 69–78.

MARCHALONIS, J. J., CONE, R. E. and ROLLEY, R. T. (1973) Amplification of thymus-influenced lymphocytes by poly (A:U): Inhibition of antigen binding by antiserum to immunoglobulin light chain. *J. Immunol.* **110**: 561–566.

MCNEILL, T. A. (1971) The effect of synthetic double stranded polyribonucleotides on haemopoietic cloony forming cells *in vitro*. *Immunology* **21**: 741–750.

MCNEILL, T. A. and KILLEN, M. (1971) The effect of synthetic double stranded polyribonucleotides on haemopoietic colony forming cells *in vivo*. *Immunology* **21**: 751–759.

MENGE, A. C. (1970) Use of polynucleotides with seminal antigens to induce isoantibodies and infertility in rabbits. *Proc. Soc. Exp. Biol. Med.* **135**: 108–112.

MERIGAN, T. C., DECLERQ, E., ECKSTEIN, F. and WELLS, R. D. (1971) Molecular requirements for synthetic RNA to act in interferon stimulation. In *Biological Effects of Polynucleotides*, pp. 67–78, BEERS, R. F. JR. and BRAUN, W. (eds). Springer-Verlag, N.Y.

MERRITT, K. and JOHNSON, A. G. (1963) Studies on the adjuvant action of bacterial endotoxins on antibody formation—V. The influence of endotoxin and 5-fluoro-2-deoxyuridine on the primary antibody response of the Balb mouse to a purified protein antigen. *J. Immunol.* **91**: 266–272.

MERRITT, K. and JOHNSON, A. G. (1965) Studies on the adjuvant action of bacterial endotoxin on antibody formation—IV. Enhancement of antibody formation by nucleic acids. *J. Immunol.* **94**: 416–422.

MORRELL, R. M. (1971) Effect of polynucleotides (poly I:C and poly A:U) on protein, RNA and polysomal synthesis in rabbit and human lung and rat and human lung peritoneal macrophages. In *Biological Effects of Polynucleotides*, pp. 179–196, BEERS, R. F. JR. and BRAUN, W. (eds). Springer-Verlag, N.Y.

MORRIS, C. K. and JOHNSON, A. G. (1978) Regulation of the immune system by synthetic polynucleotides—VII. Suppressor cells induced by pre-treatment with poly (A:U). *Cell. Immunol.* **39**: 345–354.

MOTA, I. and FERINI, A. (1975) The effect of a synthetic double stranded RNA on IgG_1 and IgE production by guinea pigs. A comparative study with lipopolysaccharide. *Immunology* **29**: 319–326.

NORONHA-BLOB, L. and PITHA, J. (1978) Binding of polynucleotides to fibroblasts. Effects of complex formation with vinyl analogs of nucleic acids. *Biochim. Biophys. Acta* **519**: 285–290.

OKUHARA, E., IGARASHI, J. and MATSUMOTO, T. (1976) An adjuvant effect of poly A–poly U production of antibodies to DNA in rabbits. *J. Immunol. Methods* **10**: 177–182.

PATTERSON, P. Y. and DROBISH, D. G. (1974) Adjuvanticity of synthetic polynucleotides for induction of experimental allergic encephalomyelitis in guinea pigs. *J. Immunol.* **113**: 1942–1946.

PERKINS, E. H., SADO, T. and MAKINODAN, T. (1969) Recruitment and proliferation of immunocompetent cells during the long phase of the primary antibody response. *J. Immunol.* **103**: 668–678.

PHILIPS, F. S., FLEISHER, M., HAMILTON, L. D., SCHWARTZ, M. K. and STERNBERG, S. S. (1971) Polyinosenic–polycytidylic acid toxicity. In *Biological Effects of Polynucleotides*, pp. 259–274, BEERS, R. F. JR. and BRAUN, W. (eds). Springer-Verlag, N.Y.

REMINGTON, J. S. and MERIGAN, T. C. (1970) Synthetic polyanions protect mice against intracellular bacterial infections. *Nature* **226**: 361–363.

RENOUX, G., RENOUX, M. and BRANCHE, R. (1972) Stimulation of antibacterial vaccination in mice by poly-adenylic acid:polyuridylic acid. *Infect. Immun.* **6**: 699–702.

RUHL, H., VOGT, W., BOCHERT, G. and DIAMANSTEIN, T. (1974) Stimulation of B cells by poly A:poly U and poly I:poly C *in vitro*. *Immunology* **26**: 937–941.

SCHEID, M. P., HOFFMAN, M. K., KOMURO, K., HAMMERLING, V., ABBOTT, J., BOYSE, E. A., COHEN, G. H., HOOPER, J. A., SCHULOF, R. S. and GOLDSTEIN, A. L. (1973) Differentiation of T cells induced by preparations from thymus and by non-thymic agents. *J. Exp. Med.* **138**: 1027–1032.

SCHELL, P. L. and MULLER, W. (1971) Uptake of polynucleotides by intact mammalian cells—XII. Stimulation of the uptake of rabopolynucleotides by deoxyribonuclease. *Biochim. Biophys. Acta* **247**: 502–505.

SCHELL, P. L. (1971) Uptake of polynucleotides by intact mammalian cells—XI. pH dependent permeability changes for synthetic ribopolymers. *Biochim. Biophys. Acta* **262**: 467–475.

SCHER, I., STRONG, D. M., AHMED, A., KNUDSEN, R. C. and SELL, K. W. (1973) Specific murine B cell activation by synthetic single- and double-stranded polynucleotides. *J. Exp. Med.* **138**: 1545–1563.

SCHMIDTKE, J. R. and JOHNSON, A. G. (1971) Regulation of the immune system by synthetic polynucleotides—I. Characterization of adjuvant action on antibody synthesis. *J. Immunol.* **106**: 1191–1200.

SMITH, R. T. and LANDY, M. (1975) In *Immunobiology of the Tumor-Host Relationship*, SMITH, R. T. and LANDY, M. (eds). Academic Press, N.Y.

STEPHEN, E. L., HILMAS, D. E., MANGIAFICO, J. H. and LEVY, H. B. (1977) Sevine influenza virus vaccine: potentiation of antibody responses in Rhesus monkeys. *Science* **197**: 1289–1290.

STINEBRING, W. R. and ABSHER, M. (1971) The double-bitted axe: A study of toxicity of interferon releasers. In *Biological Effects of Polynucleotides*, pp. 249–258, BEERS, R. F. JR. and BRAUN, W. (eds). Springer-Verlag, N.Y.

STOUT, R. D. and JOHNSON, A. G. (1972) Regulation of the immune system by synthetic polynucleotides—V. Effect on cell-associated immune globulin receptors and immunological memory. *J. Exp. Med.* **135**: 45–60.

STOUT, R. D. and COONS, A. H. (1973) Studies on membrane bound receptors for antigen. Preparation of populations of receptor-depleted lymphocytes. *J. Exp. Med.* **138**: 875–886.

TURNER, W., CHAN, S. P. and CHIRIGOS, M. A. (1970) Stimulation of humoral and cellular antibody formation in mice by poly Ir:Cr. *Proc. Soc. Exp. Biol. Med.* **133**: 334–337.

WAGNER, H. and CONE, R. E. (1974) Adjuvant effect of poly (A:U) upon T cell-mediated *in vitro* cytotoxic allograft responses. *Cell Immunol.* **10**: 394–403.

WAKSMAN, B. H. (1978) Modulation of Immunity by soluble mediators. *Pharmacology and Therapeutics* **2**: 623–672.

WALDMAN, T. A., BRODER, S., BLAESE, R. M., DUNN, M., BLACKMAN, M. and STROBER, W. (1975) Role of suppressor T cells in pathogenesis of common variable hypogammaglobulinemia. *Lancet* **ii**: 609.

WARD, P. A., JOHNSON, A. G. and ABELL, M. R. (1959) Studies on the adjuvant action of bacterial endotoxins on antibody formation—I. Time limitation of enhancing effect and restoration of antibody formation in X-irradiated rabbits. *J. Exp. Med.* **109**: 463–474.

WOODHOUR, A. F., FRIEDMAN, A., TYTELL, A. A. and HILLEMAN, M. R. (1969) Hyperpotentiation by synthetic double stranded RNA of antibody responses to influenza virus vaccine in adjuvant 65. *Proc. Soc. Exp. Biol. Med.* **226**: 171–175.

YAMASHITA, U. and KITAZAWA, M. (1974) Enhancing activity of synthetic polynucleotides on the induction of anti-hapten response. *Immunology* **26**: 925–936.

ZELEZNICK, L. D. and BHUYAN, B. K. (1969) Treatment of leukemia (L1210) mice with double stranded polynucleotides. *Proc. Soc. Exp. Biol. Med.* **130**: 126–128.

CHAPTER 13

THE BIOLOGICAL ACTIVITY OF THE SYNTHETIC POLYANION, PYRAN COPOLYMER (DIVEEMA, MVE, 46015) AND THE HETEROCYCLIC BIS DEAE FLUORENONE DERIVATIVE, TILORONE AND CONGENERS: CLINICAL AND LABORATORY EFFECTS OF THESE AGENTS AS MODULATORS OF HOST RESISTANCE

WILLIAM REGELSON

Medical College of Virginia, Virginia Commonwealth University, Richmond, Virginia 23298, U.S.A.

1. INTRODUCTION

This paper will discuss two diverse series of chemical compounds: the synthetic polyanions as represented by pyran copolymer (divinyl ether maleic anhydride copolymer, NSC 46015, diveema) now called 'MVE' and related synthetic polyanions, and the carbazol derivative tilorone (bis DEAE fluorenone) and its analogs (Fig. 1a, b).

This review is clinically pertinent as synthetic polyanions of fixed molecular weight uniformity are in clinical trial. These are MVE 2 from Hercules and NED from 137 from Monsanto (Hersh *et al.*, 1981; Powell *et al.*, 1981; Falk *et al.*, 1979, 1980).

Alternative uses for polyanions, their combination with polynucleotides (Waschke *et al.*, 1979) or as carriers of chemotherapy (i.e. 5-FU, methotrexate) or as enzyme inhibitors have been discussed elsewhere (Przybylski *et al.*, 1978; Regelson, 1979; Butler, 1980), as has the biologic role of naturally derived polysaccharides or synthetically derived polynucleotides which have related activity to the synthetic polyanionic polymers described here.

The effective anti-viral or anti-tumor action of 'interferon inducers' may not relate to interferon levels both *in vitro* and *in vivo* indicating possible alternative effects on lymphokines or cell metabolism (Breinig *et al.*, 1980).

Physico-chemically, pyran (MVE) and the synthetic polyanions resemble polynucleotides and differ strikingly from tilorone and the related carbazol fluorenone series of compounds, which are heterocyclic ring structures. Pyran is only active parenterally in contrast to tilorone and its derivatives. Despite differences in structure, charge, molecular weight and mode of administration, these agents have much in common.

The role of pyran, tilorone and their cogeners as nonspecific protective agents and adjuvants against a variety of infections and tumors has been shown. In the main protection against bacterial, protozoal, fungal and viral infection has been seen. The difference in effect depends on the tumor or pathogen studied, the agent used and the route of administration.

The main clinical anti-tumor emphasis for new, uniform low (m.w. $\leqslant$ 15,000) molecular weight polyanions is that they may be useful as adjuvants post-surgically (Kaplan *et al.*, 1974; Kaplan, 1980) with radiation (Collins and Song, 1977) or post chemotherapeutically when tumor burden is minimal (Pearson *et al.*, 1974; Mohr *et al.*, 1975; Mohr and Chirigos, 1978). This is where one can expect the best clinical results with newer, uniform low molecular weight MVE or NED 137 polyanions. Although, for pyran, if molecular weight is too low, immunologic stimulating effects may not be seen.

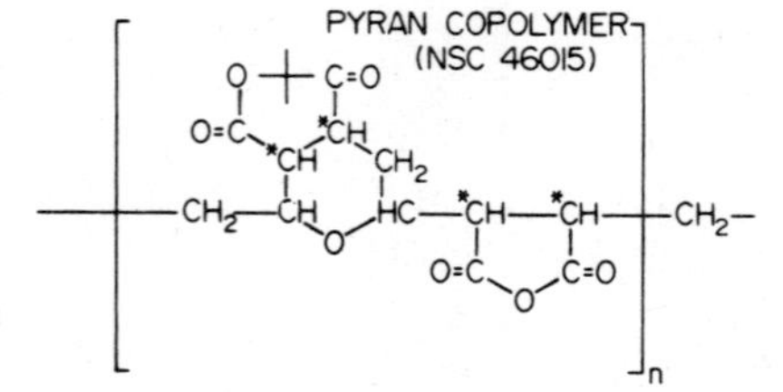

FIG. 1a. Pyran copolymer, Diveema, NSC 46015, MVE 2. This compound hydrolyzes to form polycarboxylates. The asterisks indicate where ^{14}C-tagging has been placed to study its biological distribution.

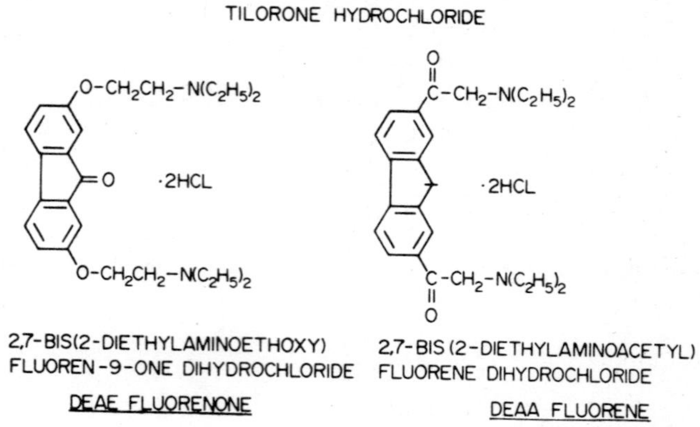

FIG. 1b. Tilorone, DEAE fluorenone and DEAA fluorene (RMI 11002DA) are the two known derivatives clinically tested.

With the older, molecular weight mixed fractions of pyran series, clinical dosage were limited by pyrexia, vascular collapse and thrombocytopenia. In Phase I study, it appears that the uniform MVE 2 (Hercules) clinical fraction is free of these symptoms (Powell *et al.*, 1981) as is true for the amide/acid maleic anhydride NED 137 derivative (Falk *et al.*, 1979, 1980) of Monsanto.

Tilorone and DEAA fluorene toxicity does not relate to marrow suppressing action but to CNS, retinal damage or corneal and epithelial inclusion effects (Weiss *et al.*, 1980a,b).

This paper reviews the diverse and related features of these interesting agents whose clinical exploration, despite past disappointment, is quite active. Current knowledge and the availability of pure molecular weight fractions for pyran, MVE 2, and NED 137, and better understanding of tilorone action should lead to more effective anti-tumor drugs or vaccine adjuvants developed alone or in combination from these agents.

2. SYNTHETIC POLYANIONS

The biologic action of synthetic polyanions with major emphasis on anti-viral, anti-tumor and immunologic effects has been presented in a number of reviews (Anaclerio *et al.*, 1978; Breslow *et al.*, 1973, 1976; Kaplan and Morahan, 1976a,b,c; Merigan, 1967a,b; Merigan and Finklestein, 1968; Niblack, 1971; Ottenbrite *et al.*, 1978; Ottenbrite and Regelson, 1976; Regelson, 1968a,b,c; 1973a,b; 1974, 1976, 1979, 1980; Regelson *et al.*, 1970a,b,c,d; 1974, 1975, 1978; Regelson and Munson, 1970; Pucetti and Giampietri, 1978).

A new review of polyanions has been published in *Polymers in Biology*, (edited by Donaruma *et al.*, 1980) which includes an extensive review of the anti-tumor, anti-viral and immunologic effects of pyran and related compounds (Breinig *et al.*, 1980; Kaplan, 1980; Baird and Kaplan, 1980; Regelson, 1980) as well as metabolic polyanion effects (Pitha, 1980; Barnes, 1980), and effects on cation and nuclear relationships (Fiel, 1980).

Of increasing interest is their possible role in governing the physical and physiologic state of the nucleus with resultant effects on protein synthesis (Coffey *et al.*, 1973; Fiel *et al.*, 1976a, 1980; Miller *et al.*, 1971, 1972; Tunis and Regelson, 1965) or on cell differentiation (Ekblom *et al.*, 1978). In this regard, polyanions and the synthetic polynucleotides resemble one another (Adamson *et al.*, 1970).

Other activities for polyanions include enzyme inhibition and activation (Regelson, 1968b,c, 1973, 1979), anti-coagulant action (Regelson, 1968a; Roberts *et al.*, 1973a; Shamash and Alexander, 1969), diuretic effects (Regelson, 1968b), inhibition of adrenocortical function, and effects on the iso-electric point of proteins, blood viscosity and oxygen diffusion (Regelson, 1968b) and mobilization of lymphocytes (Ormai *et al.*, 1973).

Pyran has been linked to 5-FU (Butler, 1980) and to methotrexate or polynucleotides with results that indicate the feasibility of combined action but with equivocal success in the models studied (Przybylski *et al.*, 1978).

The most striking recent interest in these agents has developed from efforts to define their anti-tumor activity which appears to involve activation of macrophages as effector cells which can distinguish the tumor cell's surface from that of normal cells. This results in selective tumor cell killing, sparing normal cells, when these polyanions activated macrophages are in contact with the tumor cell surface (Harmel and Zbar, 1975; Baird and Kaplan, 1975; Kaplan, 1980; Baird, 1976; Baird *et al.*, 1974; Kaplan *et al.*, 1977b; Kaplan and Morahan, 1976a,b; Morahan, 1977; Regelson *et al.*, 1974). Current work from Kaplan's laboratory suggests that this could be mediated by reduction division (Kaplan *et al.*, 1978a,b; 1980) and/or free radical formation.

Most recently, in preparation for clinical trial of MVE 2, a series of papers discussing the development of these pure molecular weight fractions of pyran has been presented (Chirigos and Stylos, 1980; Donaruma *et al.*, 1980; Dean *et al.*, 1978; Pavilidis *et al.*, 1978; Stylos *et al.*, 1978; Morahan *et al.*, 1978; Breinig *et al.*, 1980; Stolfi and Martin, 1978). MVE 2 (m.w. 15,000), which differs from past clinical fractions of pyran (NSC 46015) by being of uniform fixed molecular weight, has entered into clinical trials under NCI contracts (Powell *et al.*, 1981).

Most recently, Monsanto has entered into clinical study of one of their maleic anhydride copolymer fractions. Work with these polymers was extensively reviewed by Regelson *et al.* in the 1960's (Regelson, 1968a,b) and one, NED 137, was selected for clinical trial. Falk's group in Toronto has reported on this polyanion which has a molecular weight of less than 1000 and shows no evident toxicity at anti-tumor levels. Data suggest that this maleic anhydride polymer is a B-cell stimulator with IgM long term antibody stimulation but with no interferon or macrophage stimulating or anti-coagulant activity (Falk *et al.*, 1979, 1980). Preliminary data suggests a beneficial clinical effect of NED 137 in preventing post-surgical tumor recurrences (Falk *et al.*, 1980).

2.1. Pyran

Pyran copolymer (divinyl ether maleic anhydride copolymer, NSC 46015, diveema, MVE) (Fig. 1a) is parenterally active against a variety of transplanted, virus and carcinogen induced tumors. These have included CA 755, Lewis lung carcinoma (Kaplan *et al.*, 1976a,b; Kaplan and Morahan, 1976a; Little, 1964; Morahan *et al.*, 1974; Morahan and Kaplan, 1976a,b; Ottenbrite and Regelson, 1976; Ottenbrite *et al.*, 1978); B_{16} melanoma (Morahan *et al.*, 1974); Ehrlich carcinoma (Little, 1964); Friend leukemia (Little, 1964; Regelson, 1967, (Regelson *et al.*, 1967, 1970b; Regelson and Munson, 1970; Schuller *et al.*, 1975); Rauscher leukemias (Hirsch *et al.*, 1974; Little, 1964; Pearson *et al.*, 1970); the Dunning ascites leukemia (Little, 1964); L1210 leukemia (Mohr, 1976; Mohr and Chirigos, 1977; Mohr *et al.*, 1975; Sandberg and Goldin, 1971); C3H mammary tumor transplants (Sandberg and Goldin, 1971); methylcholanthrene derived transplants (Kopila *et al.*, 1971) and dimethylbenzanthracene (DMBA) induced tumors (Elzay and Regelson, 1977); the LSTRA sarcoma (Pearson *et al.*, 1970); Madison lung carcinoma

(Papamatheakis, 1976); prostatic adenocarcinoma in the rat (Coffey, 1976); and the Murine (M2) fibrosarcoma (Collins and Song, 1977).

This has been confirmed for the newer MVE fractions against an established autochthonous murine mammary tumor (Stolfi & Martin, 1978), Lewis lung carcinoma, P 815 mastocytoma (Morahan *et al.*, 1978) and as an adjuvant with BCNU in the LSTRA murine leukemia (Dean *et al.*, 1978).

Pyran prevents polyoma induced tumors and Rauscher leukemia in thymectomized mice (Hirsch *et al.*, 1972). In contrast to MVE–BCNU effects on inhibition of the LSTRA murine leukemia, methyl CCNU and radiation showed no potentiation of MVE action as an adjuvant against Lewis lung carcinoma (Morahan *et al.*, 1978), but this was not true for radiation in the C3H/He fibrosarcoma (Collins and Song, 1977).

Both MVE pure molecular weight fractions and pyran NSC 46015 (Papamatheakis *et al.*, 1978a) inhibited pulmonary metastases of the M109 tumor when given before or on day 0 of tumor innoculation. Of interest, MVE polymers of the lowest molecular weight were the most active (Pavilidis *et al.*, 1978). Kaplan (1980) and Kaplan *et al.* (1978a,b) showed similar effects for Lewis lung carcinoma.

Pyran induces interferon in both man and mouse (Merigan, 1967a,b; Merigan and Finklestein, 1968; Merigan and Regelson, 1967; Regelson, 1967) but anti-tumor and anti-viral activity do not correlate with interferon induction (Gresser, 1976; Regelson, 1970); Regelson *et al.*, 1970c).

Of interest, pyran can both stimulate and inhibit the immune response (Baird and Kaplan, 1975, 1977a,b,c; 1978, 1980; Baird, 1976; Braun *et al.*, 1970; Kapusta and Mendelson, 1969; Regelson, 1970), and alter *in vitro* lymphoblastic response to lipopolysaccharide (LPS) or phytohemagglutinin (PHA) (Baird and Kaplan, 1975; 1977a,b,c; 1980; Baird, 1976).

The mechanism of action for pyran is mediated through direct effects on both B and T cell function and also through macrophage activation. Stimulation of 'suppressor' macrophages appears responsible for inhibition of lymphocyte blastogenesis.

In our laboratory, in conjunction with Upjohn (White, 1976) we showed that pyran inhibits the early cation dependent steps of complement activity which was confirmed by Colsky *et al.* (1976) and can activate the C3 alternative pathway. Pyran can prevent adjuvant induced arthritis (Kapusta and Mendelson, 1969), but its effects on skin graft survival are controversial.

Toxicologically, the clinically tested pyran fraction (NSC 46015) interferes with liver microsomal enzyme hydrolysis (Munson *et al.*, 1972b; Munson and Wooles, 1969; Wooles and Munson, 1971; Barnes, 1980), causes hepato-splenomegaly (Regelson, 1970; Regelson *et al.*, 1970), anemia, weight loss, leukopenia, increases sensitivity to endotoxin lethality (Munson and Regelson, 1971) and prevents fibrin formation (Dennis *et al.*, 1969; Roberts *et al.*, 1973a; Shamash and Alexander, 1969).

This toxicity and the anti-viral and immune modulating effects of pyran relate to its molecular weight. Higher molecular weights ($>15{,}000$) are more toxic and inhibit macrophage function, while lower molecular weights ($<15{,}000$) stimulate phagocytosis and have absent or decreased anti-viral or immunostimulating effects.

The role of molecular weight of pyran fractions have been reviewed in numerous articles (Breslow, 1976; Breslow *et al.*, 1973; Morahan *et al.*, 1972a,b, 1971; Ottenbrite *et al.*, 1976, 1980; Ottenbrite and Regelson, 1976; Regelson, 1968b, 1970, 1979; Regelson *et al.*, 1974, 1975, 1976). Pertinent to clinical development of the MVE 2 fraction, all molecular weight fractions have anti-tumor effects.

Pyran also accelerates the removal of plutonium bound to liver in animal models (Guilmette and Linderbaum, 1975) and this apparently requires molecular weights greater than 15,000. In current reviews, Regelson (1979) and Ottenbrite (1980) discuss the chelating or cation binding capacity of biologically active copolymers which have affinities for Me, Fe and Ca (Fiel *et al.*, 1980). In this regard, the administration of metal complexed polyanions might be explored. MVE 2 has no clinical effects on calcium levels although this was looked for in Phase I studies (Powell *et al.*, 1981).

Pyran's anti-tumor action can be related to macrophage activation (Baird and Kaplan, 1975, 1978; Baird, 1976; Kaplan *et al.*, 1974, 1977b; Kaplan and Morahan, 1976a; Mobraaten *et al.*, 1973; Morahan *et al.*, 1974; Morahan and Kaplan, 1976a,b; Regelson, 1974; Regelson *et al.*, 1974, 1975; Schultz *et al.*, 1976, 1978) in mice and anti-viral action may be based on similar mechanisms (Kaplan and Morahan, 1976b; Morahan, 1977). Anti-tumor effects may relate to the number of carboxylic groups and if analogies can be made to polyacrylics may reflect magnesium ion binding capacity (Hodnett *et al.*, 1978).

Clinical samples of pyran (NSC 46015) initially inhibit phagocytic clearance of colloidal particulates followed by a later stimulation (Morahan *et al.*, 1972a,b; Morahan and Kaplan, 1976b; Munson *et al.*, 1970; Ottenbrite *et al.*, 1978; Ottenbrite and Regelson, 1976; Regelson, 1968b; 1970; 1973a,b; Regelson *et al.*, 1970c,d; 1974, 1975; Regelson and Munson, 1970). However, it was found that low molecular weight fractions ($<12{,}000$) stimulate phagocytosis while higher molecular weight fractions ($>12{,}000$) inhibit.

Pyran enhances resistance to infection (Kartasheva, 1977), particularly to staphylococcal, pneumococcal, and cryptococcal infection (Munson *et al.*, 1970; Regelson, 1970; Regelson and Munson, 1970; Regelson *et al.*, 1970d). Resistance to cryptococcal lethality does not relate to phagocytic stimulation while anti-bacterial resistance is only seen during the period of increased phagocytosis.

Of potential clinical importance is the adjuvant action of pyran copolymer in enhancing anti-viral vaccine activity (Campbell and Richmond, 1973; Richmond and Campbell, 1973). Pyran also produces prolonged adjuvant anti-tumor activity at non-toxic concentrations following chemotherapeutic response (Mohr, 1976; Mohr and Chirigos, 1977); Mohr *et al.*, 1971, 1975; Dean *et al.*, 1978), or the injection of irradiated tumor cells (Mohr and Chirigos, 1977; Mohr *et al.*, 1975; Chirigos and Stylos, 1980).

Clinical study with pyran began in 1966 but was delayed several times because of problems related to providing similar samples of the same average molecular weight and evidence of increased toxicity of the sterile hydrolyzed lyophilized salt after storage. A new formulation of pyran as the acid hydrolysate, containing up to 15 per cent of the anhydride, was tested in 1971 but proved too toxic for continued clinical trial.

Of interest, the NED 137 ethylene maleic anhydride copolymer of Monsanto was derived from a fraction which on greater than 10 years of shelf storage showed a decrease in toxicity. In contrast, increased toxicity for pyran has been found on prolonged shelf storage.

NED 137, whose structure has not yet been released, but is said to be an amide/acid ethylene maleic anhydride copolymer, is a low molecular weight compound ($<1{,}000$) and in contrast to pyran shows no anticoagulant activity, platelet or renal toxicity, or T-cell, macrophage or interferon inducing effects, but may stimulate IgM production (Falk *et al.*, 1980).

2.2. Chemistry and Toxicology

Pyran copolymer (NSC 46015), pyran-3,4-dicarboxylic anhydride, tetrahydro-2-methyl-6-(tetrahydro-2,5-dixo,3-furyl)-polymer (Fig. 1a) was originally provided by Hercules, Inc., (Wilmington, Delaware) through the Cancer Chemotherapy National Service Center.

Pyran copolymer is a typical anhydride which in the presence of water, becomes hydrolyzed to the corresponding carboxylic acid. The active tumor inhibitory agent is the polycarboxylic material and in this, it resembles other anionic poly-electrolytes which have shown anti-tumor, anti-viral and enzyme inhibitory activity (Breslow, 1976; Breslow *et al.*, 1973; Niblack, 1971; Ottenbrite *et al.*, 1978; Ottenbrite and Regelson, 1976; Butler, 1980; Ottenbrite, 1980). It's activity is similar to those Monsanto compounds reported on by Regelson (1968a,b), but is apparently different from that reported for NED 137 (Falk *et al.*, 1979, 1980).

The initial clinical and all the animal toxicity studies were done with the lyophilized hydrolysate of pyran; the animal toxicity studies with material of an average molecular weight (m.w.) of 30,000, while the clinical studies (NSC 46015) were done with pyran of an average m.w. of 18,000 or 23,000. Toxicity in dogs and monkeys was characterized by severe liver, parenchymal and renal tubular injury at dosages as low as 4 mg kg^{-1} day^{-1} which was not observed in man.

Studies of ^{14}C-labelled pyran, similar to NSC 46015 showed that the highest concentration of pyran was present in liver and spleen within 24 hr, with persistance of up to 25 per cent of the drug at 5 weeks (Regelson *et al.*, 1970c). This has been confirmed by Papametheakis *et al.* (1978a,b).

The clinical use of the acid hydrolysate, which contained 15 per cent anhydride, was quite toxic. Apart from its low pH of 2.4, which was probably responsible for sclerosing veins, it showed less activity as an anti-viral or immune stimulating agent than the earlier clinical material; the sodium salt hydrolysate which was given at pH 7.5 or 7.7.

For all pyran preparations, the anti-viral and immune stimulating activity do not appear to be necessary for anti-tumor action (Regelson *et al.*, 1974) and this has been a factor in the selection of the MVE 2 fraction for clinical study.

2.3. Clinical Studies

In the initial Phase I study, pyran copolymer (NSC 46015) was given to advanced cancer patients no longer responsive to other treatment modalities. The detailed clinical experience with pyran has been published elsewhere and we will only summarize it here. (Regelson *et al.*, 1978).

Pyran copolymer was given initially for 36 courses to 29 patients and the consistent limiting toxicity of pyran was transient thrombocytopenia. However, leukopenia could accompany thrombocytopenia but was a less constant, although an equally reversible finding. Cytoplasmic inclusions were seen in circulating leukocytes, nucleated marrow cells and phagocytic cells of liver and spleen after pyran administration. Pyrexia, although not dose limiting, was seen in 50% of patients despite the absence of pyrogen on rabbit test. In addition, fever frequently developed in the absence of shaking chills.

In an independent pediatric study of pyran's anti-viral action against Dawson's encephalitis, hemolysis, helmet cell (schizontocyte) formation and reversible renal failure were seen (Leavitt *et al.*, 1971). Two of three patients in this study also developed transient maculopapular eruptions following single injection, which was not seen in our more extensive study.

In our clinical study, hypotension, seizure activity, transient blindness and one death were unpredictable side effects, particularly when pyran was given too rapidly as an intravenous push. This toxicity appeared to be a consistent consequence of utilization of the acid hydrolysate rather than the earlier lyophilized hydrolyzed formulation previously used. Immediate anticoagulant effects were seen but hemorrhage was not a limiting factor in drug administration.

In contrast to pediatric experience in single dosage trial, pyran as the hydrolyzed salt was given to four adults at 18 mg/kg without toxicity despite potent anticoagulant action (Dennis *et al.*, 1969; Ottenbrite and Regelson, 1977).

In phase I study, significant anti-tumor action lasting three months was seen in one patient with ovarian cancer who received drug at 12 mg/kg biw, but evaluation of any single tumor type was inadequate. In Phase II study, a total of 33 patients were given pyran at the starting dose of 12 mg kg^{-1} day^{-1}. This program included patients with measurable disease but based on survival data, only pre-terminal patients were studied (Regelson *et al.*, 1978).

In both Phase I and II studies, 39 patients received more than two doses of pyran at 12 mg/kg. The largest number included 11 epidermoid carcinomas of the lung and 8 head and neck epidermoid tumors. The rest were a variety of sarcomas and carcinomas.

For all pyran, NSC 46015, preparations, basophilic cytoplasmic inclusions were found within two weeks of drug administration in the peripheral white blood cells of all patients receiving 8 mg kg^{-1} day^{-1} or more.

One patient with acute myeloblastic leukemia also had intranuclear inclusions in her myeloblasts following one dose of pyran. Of interest, these intranuclear inclusions are similar to what has been seen in astrocytes following heat trauma to the skull during tilorone administration (Levine *et al.*, 1974). It will be of interest to see if similar cytoplasmic and nuclear findings are seen in the MVE 2 clinical study.

Increased histiocytic activity was noted in the bone marrow of patients receiving pyran and large amounts of reddish-purple basophilic or metachromatically appearing material is seen in the cytoplasm of all nucleated marrow elements. These cytoplasmic inclusions were spherical or lobular in form and could show Feulgen positivity (Regelson, 1967, 1976).

As mentioned earlier, pyran was found to interfere with all three stages of blood coagulation including the formation of thromboplastin, the activation of thrombin and the interaction of thrombin and fibrinogen to form fibrin. Significant thrombocytopenia ($<50\%$ of initial platelet level) was noted during three rapid serial determinations but no clinical bleeding was encountered with pyran administration despite a mild increase in bleeding time (Dennis *et al.*, 1972).

Based on clotting studies in dogs and man, it was estimated that 0.2 mg/ml of pyran can be present in blood with doubling of clotting time after 2 hr of pyran infusion at 12 mg/kg. It should be stressed that *in vivo* anticoagulant effects in dogs, mice and man were strikingly different, with man the most sensitive to anticoagulant effects. Despite this, no clinical bleeding problems developed. Of additional interest, there was a distinct 2–3-fold decrease in sedimentation rate in dogs following pyran. This latter observation was, unfortunately, not studied in man (Regelson *et al.*, 1974, 1978).

MVE 2 effects on blood clotting have not been seen, nor fever and cytoplasmic inclusions in Phase I study (Powell *et al.*, 1981), and Falk has seen no anticoagulant activity for his low molecular weight Monsanto NED 137 maleic anhydride copolymer (Falk *et al.*, 1980).

3. PYRAN DISCUSSION

Apart from thrombocytopenia and fever, the major limiting toxicity for clinical studies with pyran NSC 46015 has been associated with the unpredictable development of hypotension in six cases (mottled cyanosis in one of these), seizure in two patients and impairment of vision in three with complete loss of vision in one case, who expired in shock, of 62 patients treated. Vision fully returned in 2 hr to 2 days in the other two patients. Occasional, but significant toxic side effects have included facial edema, onset of angina with myocardial infarction in another and confusion and somnolence in three patients.

Our experience with pyran copolymer is not surprising in view of our past clinical trial with polyethylene sulfonate (PES) (Regelson and Holland, 1962). This 'heparinoid' of average molecular weight 13,000 which possessed both lipolytic and anticoagulant activity was given to 49 cancer patients, and in similar fashion to pyran, intravenous injection was associated with unpredictable hypotension in seven. However, unlike pyran, pain in the tumor or peripheral extremities was seen in 16 of the 49 patients, and fever and chills was a rarity. This was in contrast to pyran where chills and fever was a constant feature at high dosage (>8 mg/kg). Pyran, like PES, produced thrombocytopenia but unlike PES produced leukopenia in occasional patients.

The platelet and vascular toxicity of heparin and heparinoids has been discussed in a past review (Regelson, 1968a). In brief, polydisperse polyanions produce what has been defined as a 'macromolecular syndrome' (Regelson, 1968a) resembling anaphylactic or anaphylactoid responses. Vascular, as well as pyrogenic effects have also been produced by synthetic polynucleotides (Black *et al.*, 1973; Morahan *et al.*, 1972a; Philips *et al.*, 1971; Phillips *et al.*, 1971) and similar toxicity has been observed clinically from the nuclease-resistant polynucleotides or glucan polysaccharides (DiLuzio, 1978).

Pyran caused thrombocytopenia similar in fashion to the polysulfonate PES (Regelson and Holland, 1962). *In vitro* thrombocytopenia for pyran may resemble that induced by collagen but is not seen consistently. Clinically, unlike PES, pyran did not cause a rise in acid phosphatase which in the case of PES correlated with clinical platelet fall (Regelson and Holland, 1962).

In regard to the above, it may be that intravascular platelet aggregation could account for some of the clinical hypotensive effects seen as thrombocytopenia occurred concomitantly with blood pressure fall. Alternatively, pyran, as a polyanion and polycarboxylate, can cause changes in the isoelectric point of blood proteins similar in fashion to heparin (Regelson, 1968a,b,c; 1975a,b) to produce changes in blood viscosity (Regelson, 1968a; Regelson *et al.*, 1978), which could alter blood pressure. A decrease of 2–3-fold in sedimentation rate, which was seen in dogs with pyran, may be an example of the above. It should be remembered that polyanions, like heparin, alter globulin stability with precipitation at low temperatures and similar effects have been seen for dextrans (Berezney and Coffey, 1976; Regelson, 1968a). Alternatively, platelet destruction can release vasoactive agents, but other possible explanations for vascular effects can range from the aldosterone blocking action of polyanion to diamine oxidase inhibition (Regelson, 1968b, 1973a,b).

Pyran, like heparin or heparinoids, can activate lipases (Regelson, 1968b,c) or change the distribution of lipoproteins (Regelson, 1968b,c). This is of current importance in view of the observation that low density lipoproteins can inhibit immune response (Curtiss *et al.*, 1977).

One can postulate that pyran with its physiologic and polyanionic relationships to heparinoids which block the physiological action of aldosterone (Regelson, 1968b), may also interfere with steroid maintenance and/or regeneration of the adrenal cortex which is responsible for aldosterone production (Chremos *et al.*, 1969). This is suggested by the fact that pyran sensitizes to both heat, stress and endotoxic shock (Munson and Regelson, 1971) which may also relate to effects on the P-450 microsomal hydrolases which are present in both the liver and adrenal cortex (Barnes, 1981).

Pyran as a pyrogen superficially behaves like an endotoxin but is not pyrogenic in the rabbit (Gander and Goodale, 1973). Polynucleotides, given systemically, have similar toxicity to the synthetic polyanions (De Clercq *et al.*, 1973; Black *et al.*, 1973; Morahan *et al.*, 1971, 1972a) and resemble endotoxins in their toxicity. Among the toxicities of poly I:C are prothrombin time prolongation (Philips *et al.*, 1971; Phillips *et al.*, 1971) and endotoxin pyrogenic and leukopenic side effects as well as Schwartzman-like reactions which may explain some examples of polyanion related tumor necrosis. However, synthetic polynucleotides in the rabbit produce pyrogens that are not granulocyte dependent (Gander and Goodale, 1973) while pyran is apparently only pyrogenic in man. These actions, like those of the polynucleotides, vary with higher molecular weight fractions being the most toxic. In addition, pyran and polynucleotides are both toxic to the liver, causing central necrosis in dogs, and interference with drug metabolizing enzymes (Little, 1964; Munson *et al.*, 1970, 1972b; Wooles and Munson, 1971; Barnes, 1981). Again, molecular weight is critical as low m.w. fractions ($<30{,}000$) of pyran and the MVE series do not appear to have liver damaging effects.

Anemia as well as leukopenia is characteristic of pyran's effect in mouse toxicology studies (Breslow, 1976; Breslow *et al.*, 1973; Regelson *et al.*, 1974) where lower molecular weight fractions ($<15{,}000$) do not do this. This is not an uncommon finding for polymeric substances including branched and unbranched polysaccharides (Regelson, 1968a) as well as uncharged polymers such as polyvinyl pyrrolidone (PVP), (Ohbuchi, 1968).

Clinical pyran (NSC 46015) sensitizes to gram negative bacterial endotoxin lethality in mice which is another possible explanation for its clinical hypotensive action (Breslow, 1976; Breslow *et al.*, 1973; Munson and Regelson, 1971; Regelson *et al.*, 1974), although sepsis was not an apparent factor in clinical study (Regelson *et al.*, 1978). Although pyran, in most studies, increases resistance to bacterial infection, there are exceptions which may relate to the molecular weight fractions studied (Kartasheva *et al.*, 1977).

The binding of polyanions to endothelial surfaces (as is seen with heparin) can produce changes in vascular physiology (Regelson, 1968a,b, 1974). Indeed, the evidence that high dosage pyran causes anemia (Breslow, 1976; Breslow *et al.*, 1973; Regelson *et al.*, 1974, 1975) and destruction of red blood cells (Schizontocyte formation) (Leavitt *et al.*, 1971) suggests the possibility that pyran's destruction of red cells is similar to that seen with plastic heart valve prosthesis. Again, this has not been seen for MVE2 (Powell *et al.*, 1981).

3.1. Anticoagulant Effects

As mentioned previously, pyran (NSC 46015) is a potent anticoagulant which differs in its action from heparin and PES (Dennis *et al.*, 1969; Regelson *et al.*, 1976, 1978; Roberts *et al.*, 1973a; Shamash and Alexander, 1969). Pyran complexes with fibrinogen to prevent its polymerization by thrombin (Regelson *et al.*, 1976, 1978; Shamash and Alexander, 1969). However, despite its potent thrombocytopenic and dose-related anticoagulant activity in man, no clinical hemorrhage has been seen (Regelson *et al.*, 1978).

Inhibitory effects of pyran upon the clotting system suggest similarities with the effects of dextran (Spector *et al.*, 1975) i.e. reduced thromboplastin activity, reduced Factor V and increased anti-thrombin activity, and interference with normal platelet function and platelet Factor III activity (Regelson, 1968a). These effects were noted at all levels of pyran copolymer administration, but increased with increasing dosage (Dennis *et al.*, 1969; Regelson *et al.*, 1978).

Anticoagulant effects could be explained by pyran's physical-chemical alteration of fibrinogen which prevents its polymerization to fibrin by thrombin (Roberts *et al.*, 1973a; Shamash and Alexander, 1969) and *in vitro* studies from our laboratory show that pyran can substitute for heparin in all laboratory determinations (i.e. blood gases).

It should be stressed that pyran shows striking species differences in relation to effects on clotting as is seen in the variations found in mice, dog and man. The former two species, are less susceptible to anticoagulant effects. MVE 2 and NED 137 do not appear to have anticoagulant activity at clinically projected dosage.

The route of pyran injection is important as i.v. pyran reduces benzoyl-L-arginine methyl ester (BAME) and *p*-toluenosulfonyl-L-arginine methyl ester (TAME) esterase in the liver whereas the i.p. drug increases the level of this fibronolytic enzyme. It is of unexplained interest that increases in BAME, TAME esterase activity correlates with increased mouse strain resistance to virus infection (Roberts and Regelson, 1977).

In another area, the native polyanion, heparin, has been reported to increase the oxygen tension of tumors thus making squamous cell carcinoma in a mouse model more vulnerable to radiation. This has been discussed by Regelson (1979) with an emphasis on radiation sensitization related to described effects on deoxyribonucleoprotein displacement and nuclear morphology (Matyasova *et al.*, 1974). Certainly pyran, which apparently alters sedimentation constants in the dog can also alter the partition of blood proteins which could effect blood flow or oxygen diffusion.

In relation to the intravascular biologic action of pyran, Ormai *et al.* (1973) have shown that polymethacrylic acid (PMAA) has potent lymphocyte mobilizing capacity. Lymphocytosis has been reported for heparin administration (Regelson, 1968b) and in one case it has been observed by us clinically for pyran (Regelson *et al.*, 1978).

The synthetic polyanion, PMAA, has been used by Van Bekkum's group (Ormai *et al.*, 1973) as a lymphocyte mobilizing adjuvant for extra-corporeal radiotherapy for the treatment of acute leukemia. However, in mice, pyran causes the loss of lymphocytes from spleen and lymph node germinal centers (Snodgrass *et al.*, 1975, 1976) which is similar to what has been seen for the non charged polyvinyl pyrrolidone (Ohbuchi, 1968). Pertinent to this, some of the pyran related polycarboxylate ethylene maleic anhydride copolymers of Monsanto produced a striking leukemoid reaction in dogs along with hemolysis and changes in blood viscosity (Mihich *et al.*, 1960).

As discussed previously, clinical pyran (NSC 46015) in mice caused hepatosplenomegaly, anemia, leukopenia, sensitized to gram negative endotoxin and interfered with drug metabolizing hepatic enzymes. Depending on the fraction studied, with falling molecular weight, anti-viral and immunological stimulating capacity was lost (Breslow, 1976; Breslow *et al.*, 1973; Ottenbrite *et al.*, 1978; Ottenbrite, 1980; Ottenbrite and Regelson, 1976; Regelson *et al.*, 1974). One can only speculate that molecular weights below 15,000 can be more rapidly excreted, interact with proteins differently, or possess a different distribution pattern to effect host responses differently. The clinical material which contains high molecular weight fractions up to 200,000 or higher can remain for long periods (30% at 5 weeks) in liver and spleen (Regelson *et al.*, 1970d, 1974; Papamatheakis *et al.*, 1978), which may explain the differences between fractions studied.

Pyran induced splenomegaly does not correlate with anti-tumor activity which is in contrast to the work of Kaplan *et al.* (1978a,b) which showed that anti-tumor activity for strains of cornyebacteria correlated with their capacity to induce splenomegaly.

It should be stressed that for pyran or MVE 2, man as the test system, is unique and this requires empiric clinical testing. For example, no pyran induced liver toxicity was seen clinically for NSC 46015 despite the marked sensitivity of the dog to hepatotoxicity for this pyran sample. In contrast, man is apparently more sensitive to anticoagulant and thrombocytopenic effects. The dog is also more sensitive to renal toxicity as renal damage, with the exception of the high dose pediatric study (Leavitt *et al.*, 1971) was not seen in man. In our adult clinical studies, no renal toxicity was seen following pyran administration despite significant hypotension in several patients at doses as high as 18 mg/kg.

The route of administration is critical as intravenous pyran in the mouse reduces resistance to Friend leukemia while the i.p. drug increases resistance (Schuller *et al.*, 1975). Differences can be seen regarding pyran's effects on macrophage and esterase and immune response with i.p. vs i.v. dosage (Roberts and Regelson, 1977; Schuller *et al.*, 1975).

3.2. NUCLEAR AND CYTOPLASMIC EFFECTS

The presence of basophilic inclusions in the cytoplasm of histiocytes and white blood cells of bone marrow and peripheral blood of patients, and in the liver and spleen of phagocytes in mice are characteristic for both pyran copolymer, polyethylene sulfonate and, as will be discussed later, tilorone. In an excellent review, Pitha (1980) has recently reviewed the action of nucleic acids and polyanions on nuclear and cellular function.

The mechanism for both formation of these basophilic inclusions is not clear, but both pyran and PES cause swelling of the nucleus with extrusion of DNA and histone (Berezney and Coffey, 1976; Coffey *et al.*, 1973; Miller *et al.*, 1971, 1972; Regelson, 1968b,c; Tunis and Regelson, 1965) and nucleic acids exert similar effects (Pitha, 1980). This is seen to be associated with an increase in nucleolar size and the turning on of RNA and protein synthesis in resting cells (Berezney and Coffey, 1976; Miller *et al.*, 1971). *In vitro* pyran and related polyanions cause tremendous swelling of cell surface in tissue culture which is particularly true of the macrophage (Goodell *et al.*, 1976; Snodgrass *et al.*, 1976).

On exposure of washed cells to polyanions in phosphate buffered saline; initially, there is a change in heterochromatin to euchromatin ratios in the nucleus followed by increased nuclear RNA and protein synthesis (Arnold *et al.*, 1972; Miller *et al.*, 1971, 1972). With increased *in vitro* concentrations of pyran or increased exposure time, this results in increased nucleolar definition and the expansion followed by contraction and collapse of the nucleus with extrusion of nuclear contents (Arnold *et al.*, 1972; Berezney and Coffey, 1976; Coffey *et al.*, 1973; Tunis and Regelson, 1965).

We have shown that high concentrations of pyran in the tissue culture medium (>1 mg/ml) induce abnormally appearing cytoplasmic microtubules but the nuclear membrane is largely intact. These nuclear effects are associated with a characteristic blebbing of the cell surface and eventually major portions of the cytoplasm break loose as large membrane contained vacuoles which drift away into the medium (Arnold *et al.*, 1972; Regelson, 1968b; Tunis and Regelson, 1965). Of interest, this is similar to what is seen on tumor cell death produced by activated macrophages (Snodgrass *et al.*, 1976).

The idea that pyran effects might be a model for physiologic effects produced by nuclear acidic proteins which function to alter regulation of gene activity through alteration of affinities of histone or deoxyribonucleoproteins has been suggested by Regelson (1967) and the work of Miller *et al.* (1971, 1972) which has been expanded by Fiel *et al.*, (1976a,b).

Pyran's actions on cells or nuclei may reflect on the development of divalent cation complexes with pyran which form nuclear microspheres which exert lysomotrophic action within narrow intracellular pH ranges. In non-nucleated cells, Fiel's group has found red blood cell hemolysis as a pyran effect which can be blocked by Ca^{2+} ions or by the presence of serum. The latter is similar to what has been seen for nuclear lysis induced by pyran and other polyanions.

The cytoplasmic blebs released from cells by pyran and other polyanions contain DNA and histone along with RNA and protein derived from the cytoplasm. The nucleus left behind following pyran lysis resembles that seen with residual nuclear protein matrix following DNA extraction with high salt and phospholipase *in vitro* (Berezney and Coffey, 1976). These effects are similar to that seen with fusion of prophase cells with cells in metaphase where chromosomal pulverisation occurs (Obara *et al.*, 1975).

Cytoplasmic inclusions produced by polyanions are similar to what has been seen for tilorone and related congeners as well as atabrine and other small molecular weight interferon inducers which, like tilorone, can also induce interferon (Glaz and Talas, 1975; Levine *et al.*, 1975; Rehovsky *et al.*, 1970; Siminoff *et al.*, 1973; Wampler *et al.*, 1973). These effects are different than those produced by glucan (Mansell *et al.*, 1978) as all of these compounds which induce these characteristic cytoplasmic inclusions have anti-viral activity and in similar fashion to pyran copolymer, tilorone and related compounds inhibit both DNA polymerase and reverse transcriptase (Papas *et al.*, 1974a,b; Pitha, 1980). This will be discussed in detail in the section on tilorone. However, despite anti-viral activity, paradoxically, these interferon inducers and anti-tumor agents can stimulate the formation of C-type virus particles in similar fashion to what one sees in host graft rejection (Dennis *et al.*, 1969; Gazdar, 1972). Because of this, one has to ask if RNA and DNA polymerase induced by these agents play some role vital to viral production which can result in paradoxic RNA virus formation which somehow may relate to the cytoplasmic inclusions. Alternatively, cytoplasmic inclusion can be the result of DNA or DNA-template restriction as has been seen for acid polymers including synthetic polyribonucleotides, pyran and polysulfonates or simply the inclusion of polyanionic complexes in lysosomes.

While it is possible that basophilic inclusions seen in the cytoplasm indicate lysosomal presence, they are morphologically and time distinct from those inclusions produced by glucan (Mansell *et al.*, 1978). For this reason, it is our feeling that they derive from the nucleus and indeed nuclear inclusions have been seen, as well as budding of nuclear surface in association with pyran and PES administration. However, it must be remembered that pyran is significantly concentrated for long periods in the cytoplasm of Kupffer and parenchymal cells of liver and spleen (Regelson *et al.*, 1970d; Papamatheakis *et al.*, 1978) and thus it could also reflect on lysosomal interactions of the polymer or polymer complexes as well.

The importance of the above to molecular weight differences in polyanions is critical as it may relate to their ability to displace deoxyribonucleoprotein (DNP) from its binding position in the nucleus. It should be remembered that DNA itself can be lethal to tumor cells (Glick, 1967, 1968) and apparently, radiated tissue is more vulnerable to DNP displacement by polyanions. One area of projected clinical investigation for pyran is whether it can act as a synergist for radiation or radiomimetic induced tumor injury (Matyasova *et al.*, 1974).

Fiel *et al.* (1976a,b, 1980) have established that pyran's action on isolated nuclei relates to complexing with Mg^{2+}. Depending on concentration of pyran copolymer present, one gets nuclear disruption with soluble complexes forming with DNP or the formation of stable microspheres with DNP which might account for cytoplasmic inclusions. In Fiel's studies, pyran did not cause nuclear swelling in contrast to other polyanions unless Mg^{2+} concentrations was held below a certain threshold. With Mg^{2+} concentrations above 5 mM, nuclear swelling is reversed and microsphere formation occurs. Nuclear swelling or microspherole production can also be induced by polynucleotides (Fiel *et al.*, 1976a,b) or the chelator EDTA.

In regard to Fiel's work (Fiel *et al.*, 1976a,b; Fiel, 1980), which suggests that nuclear interaction with polyanions may relate to effects on divalent cations. It has been known for many years that polyanions interact with divalent calcium with pyran being the most effective chelator. In fact, the capacity for cationic binding by heparinoids was used as a screening method for anti-tumor selection of both synthetic and naturally derived heparinoids (Regelson, 1968b,c). This harks back to the work of Victor Heilbrun in the 1930's who suggested that cytoplasmic calcium ion shifts were responsible for sol–gel alterations in the cytoplasm resulting in cell division.

Calcium effects may involve pyran's action as an inhibitor of DNA polymerase of RNA tumor viruses (Papas *et al.*, 1974). Most recently, Di Cioccio and Sahai Srivastava (1978) have found that pyran fractions can inhibit DNA polymerases of the simian sarcoma virus which they felt was a consequence of bivalent cation binding. The inhibitory action for pyran varied for different polymerases and bivalent cations present.

Work by Carchman with P388D1 macrophages in tissue culture has shown that macrophage activation produced by pyran and polymethacrylic acid copolymers is associated with dramatic shifts in ionic calcium. This is concomitant with increases in macrophage volume and increased lethality for target tumor cells (Goodell *et al.*, 1976; Kaplan and Morahan, 1976b). In similar fashion, Hodnett *et al.* (1978) have reported a correlation between anti-tumor activity and magnesium binding for low molecular weight polyanions.

In regard to the above, it must be stressed that the effect of pyran on the nucleus of cells is best seen in the absence of tissue culture media or serum, and in the presence of phosphate buffer (Arnold *et al.*, 1972; Tunis and Regelson, 1965). Recent work has shown that differences in buffers may reflect on the presence or absence of iron salts as a contaminant of the buffers used.

It is an educated guess that synthetic polyanions will be found to alter the stabilization of chromatin by poly ADP-ribosylation. This system effects transcription of nucleosomes associated DNA, and is dependent on NAD, NADH, spermine and specific histone loci all of which could be effected by charged polyanions (Smulson and Sugimura, 1980).

In regard to effects on cell nuclei, recent evidence suggests that macrophage killing of tumor cells is associated with an amitotic division of nuclear fragmentation followed by cell division (Kaplan *et al.*, 1978a,b; Kaplan, 1980). Current work by this group suggests that free radical formation and/or adenosine deaminase effects might be involved (Gerrard *et al.*, 1981).

3.3. Anti-Inflammatory and Anti-Complement Activities

Synthetic polyanions have anti-inflammatory and thrombolytic activity on topical application: this has included polyethylene sulfonate (polyvinyl sulfonate, Peson), (Farbwerke Hoechst, 1963) and polyphloretin phosphate (Regelson, 1968b,c) both of which have anti-tumor activity.

Pyran inhibits serum complement; in a study by Upjohn Laboratories, the capacity of pyran copolymer to inhibit serum complement was related to molecular weight. The system used was that of Wasserman and Levine (1961) (semi-micro) and utilized sheep erythrocytes, sensitized with rabbit heolysin, and dilute guinea-pig serum as a source of complement.

On closer examination with various erythrocyte intermediates, it was observed that only the early components of the complement cascade, the cation dependent stages, were inhibited. Indeed, if one increased the concentrations of calcium and magnesium in the incubation mixture, the inhibition of hemolysis by the copolymers was reversed. Of interest to polyanion effects on cell growth, spermine would also reverse their action. It was concluded that the biological activity of the copolymers on complement was, in large part, due to charge distribution and chelator potential. Of interest to the above, in preliminary studies, clinical pyran (NSC 46015) can activate the C3 alternative pathway. In this regard, Majeski and Stinnet (1977) have shown that the chemoattractant properties of *Corynebacterium parvum* and pyran were complement mediated.

4. PYRAN: ADJUVANT ACTION

To recapitulate, as mentioned in our introduction, pyran has been shown to be an effective anti-tumor agent in a number of allogeneic, syngeneic, carcinogen induced and virally induced tumor systems.

Of major clinical importance, Chirigos and colleagues have found that mice could be cured of a syngeneic leukemia or lymphosarcoma when pyran was given after treatment with the chemotherapeutic agent (BCNU) which reduced, but did not eliminate the tumor burden (Pearson *et al.*, 1970, 1974; Dean *et al.*, 1978). Similarly, pyran acts as an immunoadjuvant with radiated L1210 leukemia cells (Mohr, 1976; Mohr and Chirigos, 1977, 1978; Mohr *et al.*, 1975) and with radiation against a fibrosarcoma (Collins and Song, 1977). Pyran decreases metastases and recurrence after surgical excision (Kaplan, 1980). Similar results have been seen for the MVE series of pure molecular weight fractions (Chirigos and Stylos, 1980).

In addition, Campbell and Richmond (1973) (see also Richmond and Campbell, 1973) have found that pyran given with an otherwise ineffective vaccine induced good protection against foot and mouth disease virus in mice.

Pyran has been shown on prophylactic local or systemic administration to diminish local lip or vaginal herpes type I and II infection without aborting latent herpes type I trigeminal ganglionic involvement. Pyran aborts systemic herpes type II infection but no studies of its adjuvant action with a herpes virus vaccine have been reported (Morahan *et al.*, 1979).

The bulk of anti-viral activity is thought to be mediated by activated macrophages (McCord *et al.*, 1976) but the exact role of activated macrophages in viral adjuvant action for pyran has not been explained as an interferon or immunostimulating effect (Breinig *et al.*, 1980).

Adjuvant anti-tumor and anti-viral effects occur for pyran at concentrations far below the clinically tolerated dose. This suggests that MVE 2 should be used clinically in patients after surgery, radiation, or successful chemotherapy where the tumor burden is small. We should, however, remember that depending on the timing of the agent relative to induction of tumor, pyran can stimulate as well as inhibit tumor growth (Gazdar, 1972; Gazdar *et al.*, 1972; Schuller *et al.*, 1975; Schultz, 1976; Schultz *et al.*, 1976, 1977a; Kripke and Borsos, 1974). The action of MVE 2 clinically has shown significant but minimal immunostimulating activity in Phase I clinical trial (Hersh *et al.*, 1981; Powell *et al.*, 1981).

4.1. Macrophage Activation, NK Cell Activation and Immunologic Effects

The major mechanism of pyran's action against tumor is its effect on activation of macrophages. It must be stressed that pyran is effective against viral tumor induction in immunosuppressed mice (Hirsch *et al.*, 1972) and its effect is independent of interferon levels (Gresser, 1976; Regelson, 1967; Regelson *et al.*, 1970c). Most recently, Gresser has shown that a globulin anti-interferon blocked poly I:C and statolon action against tumor growth (Gresser *et al.*, 1978) but could not block pyran's anti-tumor action.

The evidence indicates that pyran's action may be due to macrophage activation and enhanced phagocytosis (Baird and Kaplan, 1975; Baird, 1976; Baird *et al.*, 1974a; Kaplan *et al.*, 1976a,b, 1978a,b; Kaplan and Morahan, 1976a,b; Morahan *et al.*, 1974; Morahan and Kaplan, 1976a,b, 1977; Morahan, 1977; Regelson *et al.*, 1974; Stinnett and Majeski, 1980).

Killing by activated macrophages may be the mechanism by which pyran can exert its anti-tumor activity since histopathologically, tumors from pyran-treated mice show a markedly increased histiocytic infiltration (Morahan and Kaplan, 1976b; Snodgrass *et al.*, 1976). Based on this, clinical testing of pyran intratumorally, subcutaneously or intradermally into primary or metastatic tumors, as with *C. parvum*, BCG or glucan, has shown local anti-tumor action (Kaplan, 1980).

Macrophage activation is seen in intraperitoneal injection as measured by the *in vitro* tumor killing response of peritoneal exudate cells. Again, it should be stressed that the route of pyran administration may be critical since pyran given intraperitoneally inhibits Friend leukemia in contrast to the intravenous route where paradoxic stimulation of the splenomegaly due to Friend leukemia is seen (Schuller *et al.*, 1975).

The role of interferon as the unifying feature in macrophage activation has been suggested by Schultz *et al.* (1977a,b,c,d). This has been extended by them to *in vitro* studies of macrophage interferon stimulation (Schultz *et al.*, 1978a,b), which Chirigos and Stylos (1980) suggests may be a prostaglandin mediated effect.

Most recently, Stinnett and Majeski (1980) have found pyran to induce macrophage responses independent of T-cell relationships in nude mice. Nude mice respond with greater macrophage mobilization when pyran is given i.p. as compared to normal mice. This effect was independent of splenomegaly or granuloma formation.

The action of pyran activated macrophages in producing a nuclear fragmentation or reduction division has been reported earlier (Kaplan *et al.*, 1978a,b, 1980).

In summary:

(1) Peritoneal macrophages taken from mice treated with pyran intraperitoneally were cytotoxic to tumor cells while non pyran stimulated macrophages had no effect (Morahan, 1977; Morahan and Kaplan, 1976a,b; Kaplan and Morahan, 1976a,b; Kaplan *et al.*, 1977a,b, 1974).

(2) Systemic treatment with pyran increases infiltration of tumors by histiocytes (Snodgrass, *et al.*, 1975).

(3) Pyran activated peritoneal exudate cells mixed with tumor cells and transferred to untreated recepients show tumor inhibition (Kaplan & Morahan, 1976a,b; Morahan and Kaplan, 1976a,b).

(4) Pyran activated macrophages respond cytotrophically to soluble by products of neoplastic cells (Snodgrass *et al.*, 1978).

(5) Amitotic reduction division is seen within 24–48 hours following exposure of tumor target cells to pyran activated macrophages (Kaplan *et al.*, 1978a,b, 1980).

(6) Recent work by Kaplan's group has shown that pyran activated macrophages show free radical singlet oxygen and peroxide formation as well as adenosine deaminase induction which may be pertinent to their anti-tumor effects (Gerrard *et al.*, 1981).

Interferon and interferon inducers stimulate NK cell activity and pyran has been found to enhance NK cell activity as well as stimulate splenic effector cell antibody-dependent cell mediated cytotoxicity (Tagliabue *et al.*, 1977). As NK cells have nonspecific anti-tumor action, their action alone or in conjunction with macrophages may be the clue to their anti-tumor action. A similar case will be made for tilorone's effect on NK cells in the neighboring section of this paper.

The immunologic response data has been reviewed by Baird and Kaplan (1977a,b, 1978, 1980). Pyran's effects which are both T- and B-cell mediated are related in complex fashion to inhibition of blastogenesis by pyran stimulated macrophages. Pyran can prolong allograft survival (Mohr *et al.*, 1971) which is similar to what has been reported for other interferon inducers (Mobraaten *et al.*, 1973).

In whole body radiated tumor bearing mice, T-cell response is aided by pyran (Stylos *et al.*, 1978). The bulk of pyrans's immunostimulation is seen in B-cell mediated responses and its action on T-cell function are varied.

Data are not yet available as to whether immunological adjuvancy to augment anti-viral vaccines (Ottenbrite *et al.*, 1978); Ottenbrite and Regelson, 1976) can be obtained by newer MVE low molecular weight fractions of pyran or the NED 137 in clinical use. Anti-tumor vaccine adjuvancy has been seen for pyran copolymer MVE fractions (Chirigos and Stylos, 1980). Similar data is necessary to see if newer low molecular weight fractions for pyran or related compounds can be useful in removing plutonium from the liver. Here, higher molecular weight fractions may be necessary (Guilmette and Lindenbaum, 1975; Lindenbaum *et al.*, 1975).

MVE 2, clinically given i.v. at doses $>200\,mg/m^2$ increases the level of adherent monocyte-macrophages in peripheral blood, increase antibody dependent cellular toxicity to chicken and human RBC's and a human leukemia cell line, and increase NK cell activity (Powell *et al.*, 1981), as well as increase circulating 'progenator' cells from the bone marrow.

Macrophage activation produced by pyran is associated with new antigenic markers at the macrophage cell surface (Waldrep *et al.*, 1981a,b; Kaplan and Mohanakuma, 1977) and with an apparent increase in adenosine deaminase activity (Gerrard *et al.*, 1981). The relationship of this to the mechanism of macrophage induced tumor cell killing is under study.

Phagocytosis is a different process than pinocytosis as macrophage mediated events. Pratten *et al.* (1981) have recently demonstrated that pyran and fixed molecular weight MVE derivatives had no effect on stimulating pinocytic uptake of peritoneal macrophages or rat embryonic yolk sac cells. The uptake of pyran fractions by peritoneal macrophages is attributed to a receptor mediated process related to an adsorptive process which they feel may be of chemotherapeutic advantage when methotrexate is linked to pyran (Diveema) fractions.

5. PYRAN: SUMMARY AND CONCLUSION

The following can be said for past clinical experience with pyran copolymer and the possible clinical role of the MVE 2 derivative.

(1) The older clinical formulations (the lyophilized hydrolyzed salt and the acid hydrolysate of pyran copolymer (m.w. average 18–23,000) NSC 46015) were too toxic for continued intravenous trial.

(2) Pyran has dose related *in vitro* and *in vivo* anticoagulant effects but prolonged anticoagulant activity (block to fibrin formation) was not associated with clinical hemorrhage for NSC 46015. Mice and dogs do not show the same sensitivity to the anticoagulant action of pyran as does man. Pyran is a useful substitute for heparin as an *in vitro* anticoagulant. The effect of MVE 2 on blood clotting has not been reported.

(3) In view of laboratory animal evidence of improved therapeutic anti-tumor index of lower molecular weight ($<15,000$) pyran the MVE 2 fraction is now in clinical trial. However, although the lower molecular weight fractions stimulate macrophage function, it loses anti-viral and immunologic stimulating activity. MVE effects on NK cell and the immune response are clinically significant and dose related (Powell *et al.*, 1981).

(4) Basophilic cytoplasmic inclusions and occasional PAS positive intranuclear inclusions are found in leukocytes with clinical pyran, but not MVE 2. The mechanism for inclusion formation has not been ascertained.

(5) It must be stressed that polyanions apparently have unique species related toxicity. NSC 46015 pyran in mice and dogs, in pre-clinical toxicity, produces liver and renal damage and inhibits drug metabolizing enzymes. This was not a clinical problem at the dosage studied for pyran and MVE 2.

(6) Intravenous pyran NSC 46015, reduces BAME and TAME splenic esterase activity, which in contrast with administration i.p. correlates with resistance to Friend leukemia and mouse strain viral susceptibility. Thus, the route of pyran administration is critical to its biologic action, but this has not been ascertained for the lower, uniform m.w. MVE 2.

(7) In view of pyran's action in mobilizing polutonium from liver binding (Guilemette and Lindenbaum, 1974; Lindenbaum *et al.*, 1975), its clinical use with chelators could be warranted by plutonium poisoning. This deserves exploration with newer available lower molecular weight MVE fractions of pyran copolymer.

(8) The clinical MVE 2 or NED 137 (Monsanto) studies should keep in mind complications developing from polyanionic antibiotic complexing properties as with polymixins or aminoglycoside antibiotics (Edberg *et al.*, 1976).

(9) The clinical MVE 2 and other MVE fractions should be examined for anti-complement or complement activating activity in view of pyran's *in vitro* inhibiting effects and similarities to endotoxin action.

(10) Significant anti-tumor activity of NSC 46015 pyran with objective and subjective improvement was seen in one patient with a myxomatous ovarian cancer. However, a sufficient number of patients were not treated in any tumor category and almost all patients in Phase II study were in the pre-terminal phases of their disease with treatment limited to a median of 9–14 days. Studies of MVE 2 in advanced cancer should pave the way for clinical adjuvant programs in patients with minimal disease, regardless of study outcome in advanced cancer patients.

(11) MVE 2 and NED 137 should be looked at for vaccine adjuvant action and for trypanocidal activity both for their immunostimulating activity and their physico-chemical resemblance to the anionic trypanocidal dye suramin (Regelson, 1968b,c).

(12) As has been seen for pyran, MVE 2 should be looked at for effects on homograft and allograft survival (Mobraaten *et al.*, 1973; Mohr *et al.*, 1971) and effects in blocking arthritis (Kapusta and Mendelson, 1969).

6. TILORONE AND ITS ANALOGS

Tilorone, 2,7-bis-{2-(diethyl amino) ethoxy} fluoren-9-one (Fig. 1b), is an effective *in vivo* interferon inducer which has been tested clinically for anti-viral and anti-cancer activity. In the search for anti-viral agents of this series, approximately 800 compounds related to the parent compound have been synthesized. These have been examined for anti-viral, anti-tumor, immunologic and anti-inflammatory properties. In summary, a few generalizations can be made concerning structural activity anti-viral relationships (Albrecht, 1974; Albrecht *et al.*, 1972; Fleming *et al.*, 1971; Witkowski *et al.*, 1979; Veckenstedt *et al.*, 1979).

(1) Monobasic derivatives do not yield potent anti-viral agents but induce interferon when compared to the corresponding bis basic derivatives.

(2) Removal of the amine terminal results in the loss of anti-viral activity.

(3) Maximum activity is observed with no less than three rings in the central aromatic or heteroaromatic nucleus.

The structure activity effects may relate to the capacity of fluorenone derivatives to intercalate with DNA (Witkowski *et al.*, 1979).

In relation to drug distribution, over 50% of tilorone is present in mice after 72 hr but ketone derivatives disappear more rapidly with 10–15% of the compound present at 72 hr.

The anti-viral activity for tilorone.HCl and related congeners has been established for a wide range of viruses (Fornosi *et al.*, 1971; Krueger and Mayer, 1970; Krueger *et al.*, 1970, 1971; Mayer and Krueger, 1970a,b; Portnoy and Merigan, 1971; Schiff *et al.*, 1973; Stringfellow, 1973; Stringfellow *et al.*, 1974). This activity relates to interferon production, but interferon levels do not necessarily correlate with anti-viral activity seen (DeClercq, 1972; DeClercq and Merigan, 1971; Giron *et al.*, 1972a,b; Niblack, 1971).

Tissue levels of interferon produced by tilorone are similar to what has been seen for poly I:C with the exception of the thymus where tilorone induces higher levels than poly I:C (DeClercq, 1972; DeClercq and Merigan, 1970).

The route of administration is critical to the effect seen; e.g. in mice, against Semliki Forest virus, tilorone was not effective intravenously but was effective by all other routes. In contrast, tilorone is effective when given intravenously in the rat (Krueger *et al.*, 1970). However, tilorone has been found to be protective against influenza A virus and equine and tick encephalitis virus when given intranasally to mice (Balezina *et al.*, 1976).

Tilorone, in drinking water, can induce continuous levels of interferon (Glaz and Talas, 1973) and show anti-tumor activity Wampler *et al.*, 1972). In this regard, it should be remembered that the presence of infection makes mice hyporeactive to interferon inducers such as tilorone and poly I:C (Stringfellow and Glasgow, 1972a,b).

Exposure of cells to cyclohexamide after tilorone or pyran administration increases the level of interferon produced during the late period when interferon levels are ordinarily falling. In contrast, it blocks production of interferon during the early phase of induction. This is similar to what has been seen for the polynucleotides (Black *et al.*, 1973; DeClercq, 1972; DeClercq and Merigan, 1970).

Again, the anti-viral action for tilorone has been shown to be independent of circulating interferon levels (Giron *et al.*, 1972a,b). This is demonstrated in that protection of mice from virus infection can be seen at levels as low as 0.5 and 1.5 mg/kg whereas interferon at significant levels appears at 160 mg/kg. Similar absence of correlation has been found for other interferon inducers including pyran.

Poly I:C can enhance tilorone's capacity to generate *in vitro* interferon in L 929 cells (Groelke *et al.*, 1975). As is true for polyanions and poly rI:rC, DEAE dextran with tilorone can enhance *in vitro* interferon induction, but this has not been pursued *in vivo* (Groelke *et al.*, 1975). The stabilizing action of DEAE dextran against ribonucleases, raises the question that tilorone's action may be mediated through some secondary effect involving the stabilization of polynucleotides. Alternatively, effects on cyclic nucleotides have been reported to be a factor, perhaps related to lymphokine induction in tilorone action (Romer and Zschiesche, 1979).

6.1. Drug Metabolizing Effects

An interesting feature of tilorone is the depression of the cytochrome P-450 monooxygenase system (Leeson *et al.*, 1976; Renton and Mannering, 1976a,b) in similar fashion to pyran. Rats lose hepatic microsomal ethylmorphine N-dimethylase, benzopyran hydroxylase and analinehydroxylase activities. Cytochrome P-450 shows reduction to significant levels and similar effects are seen on prolongation of hexabarbitol and zoxazolamine metabolism and aminopyrine demethylase (Barnes, 1980).

Tilorone is among a wide range of interferon inducers such as mengo virus, statolon, poly I:C, pyran and endotoxin which inhibit the cytochrome P-450 drug metabolizing enzymes (Munson *et al.*, 1972; Mannering *et al.*, 1976; Renton and Mannering, 1976a,b; El Azhary and Mannering, 1979; Zerkle *et al.*, 1980). In some way, interferon inducers may dissociate heme proteins from the P-450 system to depress drug metabolism and amino-levulinic acid synthetase with changes in tryptophane 2,3-dioxygenase and stimulation of heme oxygenase. Other heme dependent systems are effected, which include depression of catalase activity. The effects and timing vary with the cell system and interferon inducer evaluated in that liver P-450 is more vulnerable than that found in intestinal epithelium. The long-term action of tilorone or other interferon inducers on mitochondrial cytochrome pigments has not been ascertained. Zerkle *et al.* (1980) have shown that drug metabolism changes are not associated with changes in heme relationships in contrast to poly I:C.

Ascorbate synthesis is blocked by tilorone as is the action of phenobarbital or methylcholanthrene or benzopyrene which stimulate ascorbate formation (Renton *et al.*, 1979; El Azhary and Mannering, 1979). The importance of this in relation to interferon action is not known, but it raises an alternative clinical action for interferon and interferon inducers as agents potentially useful in the prevention of carcinogen activation.

Tilorone may act in promoting hepatic protein kinase activity which may be a general interferon effect, blocking hemin inhibition of protein kinase at a competitive site (Pierre and Loeb, 1977). This result in restoration of phosphorylation of phosphopolypeptides which can be blocked by hemin action on liver microsome. Quinacrine and tilorone behave similarly in prevention of casein kinase inhibition by heme while both agents block protein synthesis (Bogdanovsky and Pierre, 1979).

Of interest, along with chloroquine, quinacrine, imipramine and a wide range of phenothiazines and antihistamines which are capable of ionic binding to phosphate groups of DNA, tilorone is capable of stimulating phenylalanine ammonia lyase activity in plant tissue (Hadwiger, 1972). The mechanism of action is associated with the formation of pisatin, an isoflavanoid that increases plant resistance to fungal pathogens. Other compounds which induce pisatin interreact with DNA and these have included alkylating agents, polyamines, cationic polypeptides, ethidium bromide, actinomycin D and nogalamycin.

It is this author's speculation that the final common pathway for the effect of interferon inducers on drug metabolizing enzymes will relate to effects on NAD/NADH ratios which also involve the activity of poly ADP ribosylation (Smulson and Sugimura, 1980) or the 2′,5′-isoadenylate trimer or its synthetase which can block erythro-differentiation of Friend leukemia and are mediators of interferon effects (Gazitt, 1981).

6.2. Nucleic Acid Complexing

Tilorone has been shown to form molecular complexes with DNA (Chandra et al., 1972a,c). Tilorone intercalates with DNA (Chandra, 1974; Chandra *et al.*, 1974; Chandra and Wiltersdorf, 1974, 1976) and this explains tilorone's block to DNA and RNA polymerase activity (Chandra, 1974; Chandra and Woltersdorf, 1974; Chandra *et al.*, 1972a,b,c; Green and Gerard, 1974; Green *et al.*, 1974, 1975; Smith and Gallo, 1974; Witkowski *et al.*, 1979).

Tilorone's *in vitro* effect as an inhibitor of RNA virus directed DNA polymerase is due to its specific binding to dAT sites of double stranded DNA (Chandra *et al.*, 1974; Chandra and Woltersdorf, 1976), and the closest distance between bound tilorone is four base pairs. This binding affinity for tilorone is structurally related to side chain positions in the tilorone molecule and holds for related congeners such as dibenzofuran, fluorene, and dibenzothiophene, bis basic substituted polycyclic aromatics (Chandra *et al.*, 1974; Chandra and Woltersdorf, 1976; Green *et al.*, 1975). Tilorone's effect on the super-coiling of DNA or the action of the gyrase has not yet been reported.

Other agents such as the pyrolle-amidine antibiotic distamycin (Zimmer *et al.*, 1971) and netropsin have been reported to bind poly (dA–dT) in similar fashion to tilorone (Chandra, 1974). Chandra and Woltersdorf (1976), have discussed this at great length and have compared the action of distamycin, daunomycin, tilorone and thiolated derivatives of polynucleotides on RNA virus directed DNA polymerase in relation to mechanisms involving intercalation or interaction with DNA templates. Similar effects have been reported for neutral pentazulene dyes derived from plants such as azoanthoxanthin (Quadrifoglio *et al.*, 1975).

Witkowski *et al.* (1979) explain fluorenone analog anti-viral effects as related to intercalating action with DNA.

6.3. RNA and DNA Polymerase Inhibition

Tilorone is a specific inhibitor of DNA polymerases for RNA tumor viruses from the FLV and MSV (Moloney) mammalian RNA tumor viruses (Chandra *et al.*, 1972b). While these effects may be significant to the anti-viral action of tilorone and/or polyanions independent of their interferon inducing capacity, this has not been pursued. Unfortunately, studies which utilize inhibition of DNA polymerases for primary anti-tumor screening by a variety of agents have failed to lead to effective anti-tumor agents (Waalkes *et al.*, 1974).

Based on the RNA directed DNA polymerase of the oncorna viruses, rational screening for anti-tumor agents was made in the hope that RNA tumor virus directed DNA polymerases might be critical to control of tumor growth and malignant transformation (Chandra, 1974; Schafer *et al.*, 1974; Vilcek and Ng, 1971; Rana *et al.*, 1975). A broad spectrum of anti-tumor and DNA intercalating agents have been looked at in this system which included tilorone and related structures (anthraquinine, fluorene, xanthenone, dibenzfuran and fluroanthene derivatives) as well as actinomycin D, ethidium bromide, daunomycin, distamycin and analogs, chromamycin A_3 and olivomycin. Other inhibitors have included congo red, heparin, bleomycin, thiosemicarbazones and selected cations. This work should be reevaluated with respect to possible alteration of poly ADP-ribosylation which is so important to nucleosome formation, DNA repair and translational activity (Smulson and Sugimura, 1980).

The mechanisms of action for tilorone and pyran's stimulation of interferon has been thought by Cahn and Lubin (1973) to be due to inhibition of protein synthesis. Similar effects have been found for polynucleotide action (Cordell-Stewart and Taylor, 1973), and for tilorone and pyran utilizing reticulocyte lysates.

The observation that inhibitors of protein synthesis can induce interferon has been shown for kanamycin (Lukas and Hruskova, 1968), cyclohexamine (De Clercq, 1972; De Clercq and Merigan, 1970, 1971) and polynucleotides (Black *et al.*, 1973; De Clercq, 1972).

The rifamycin antibiotics were the most active as compounds which possess a naphthoquinone chromophore. Ansamycins are another series of compounds, which are the streptovaracins, of similar action to tilorone. These compounds inhibit MSV and RSV focus formation at levels blow those which inhibit cell proliferation.

Of interest, all the above agents behave similarly to synthetic polynucleotides and pyran, which block polymerase activity. This has been discussed in detail by Green and Gerard (1974), Green *et al.* (1975) and others (Vilcek and Ng, 1971; Schafer *et al.*, 1974; Smith and Gallo, 1974; Pitha, 1980).

A common relationship to tilorone and polyanions should be looked for in that ethidium bromide which intercalates with DNA, also acts to block the exogenous incorporation of purines into DNA. Similar action is also seen for nine alkyl substituted purines and these latter compounds have been found to be potent immunostimulating agents with anti-tumor action on pretreatment of mice (Van deVoorde, 1970).

As mentioned previously, tilorone fluoranthene derivatives inhibit the viral reverse transcriptase by combining with the template primer, poly (dA–dT). Low levels of fluoranthene compounds also inhibit activated calf thymus DNA and 70S RNA as well as poly I:C templates. Amine side chains or tilorone and its analogs (Chandra, 1974; Chandra *et al.*, 1974, 1972a,b; Chandra and Woltersdorf, 1974, 1976; Schafer *et al.*, 1974), influence the binding to template with resultant DNA polymerase inhibition which was associated with a block to MSV viral transformation on preincubation of cells.

Excess nucleic acid template can reverse the above inhibition (Green *et al.*, 1975). This may be important to the role of tilorone on lymphocytes (i.e. inhibiting T-cells) as work indicates that lymphocytes leak DNA into the medium without effecting their viability (Boldt *et al.*, 1976; Cordell-Stewart and Taylor, 1973). In addition, lymphocytes contain the reverse transcriptase inhibited by these compounds. This is more than theoretical consideration if both pyran and/or tilorone can increase the leak of DNA polynucleotides from cells. DNA itself can be toxic to cells which is an effect which can be blocked by cyclohexamide (Glick, 1967, 1968).

Of interest to nucleic acid effects on drug distribution studies, tilorone is subcellularly concentrated in the nucleus. The highest levels are found in the liver and spleen, (Gaur and Chandra, 1973; Wacker *et al.*, 1972).

6.4. TOPICAL AND *IN VITRO* EFFECTS

Tilorone acts topically against herpes virus (Adamson, *et al.*, 1972; Lieberman *et al.*, 1973; Yochimura *et al.*, 1973) and has been successfully administered internasally as an anti-viral agent in mice (Balezina *et al.*, 1976). Tilorone *in vitro* can inactivate viruses (Camyre *et al.*, 1973), and tilorone has been reported to inhibit mitosis at 3 μg/mg in kangaroo rat cell lines with evidence of chromosomal abnormalities (Green and West, 1971).

Studies of tilorone cytotoxicity *in vitro* against the L5178Y, Walker 256 and Novikoff hepatoma showed toxicity at concentrations in tissue culture of 4 and 1.2 μg/ml. We found similar effects (Adamson, 1971a,b,c; Morahan *et al.*, 1974) at somwhat higher concentration against Lewis lung and B16 melanoma cells. In contrast, tilorone was stimulatory *in vitro* to rat myeloma lines with stimulation of cell growth and IgE synthesis (Eber and Gavin, 1978).

Cytotoxicity has also been seen at 10 μg/ml when exposed to human skin fibroblasts (De Clercq and Merigan, 1971). This cytotoxic action of tilorone contrasts with that of pyran or the polynucleotides which are relatively non-toxic *in vitro* (Morahan *et al.*, 1974) while in contrast to pyran tilorone is well tolorated *in vivo* at dosages up to 50 mg kg^{-1} day^{-1} and higher.

Tilorone *in vitro* resembles pyran and endotoxin which have minimal interferon inducing capacity in culture, but tilorone differs from endotoxin and pyran in being a more potent *in vitro* cytocidal agent. In view of increased *in vivo* toxicity for interferon inducers such as the polyribonucleotides, in the presence of virus infection (De Clercq *et al.*, 1973; Niblick, 1971) a relationship to endogenous virus infection in tissue culture should be looked for when there are high *in vitro* interferon yields to tilorone or enhanced *in vitro* toxicity. In support of this possibility, a direct relationship has been reported between increased interferon release and the degree of toxicity to normal and leukemic human lymphocyte cells grown in culture (Dennis *et al.*, 1972).

Tilorone has formed complexes with bacterial plasmids and may be of major importance for potential antibacterial action or block to bacterial resistance as tilorone has been shown to inhibit bacterial plasmid survival and transfer (Hahn and Ciak, 1977).

6.5. CYTOKINE AND INTERFERON INDUCTION

The interferon inducing capacity and anti-viral activity for the fluoronone derivatives is based on their route of administration (Glaz and Talas, 1973; Krueger *et al.*, 1970; Wampler and Regelson, 1974). This is of clinical significance but tilorone has only been tested in man by the topical or oral route.

Tilorone blocks the migration of leukocytes into subcutaneous implanted sponges (Ford-Hutchinson *et al.*, 1976) which led Clark and Robins (1978) to test tilorone for antipyretic activity. Antipyretic effects were seen for tilorone against leukocyte pyrogen, arachnidonic acid and endotoxin. Larger doses of systemic tilorone produced hypothermia, tachypnea, mydriasis and vocalization in cats.

Tilorone has no antagonistic action to prostaglandins despite evident antipyretic and anti-inflammatory effects. The absence of any antiprostaglandin activity for tilorone is of interest in view of the fact that prostaglandins can enhance interferon action and it has been postulated that prostaglandin stimulation may be a mechanism by which macrophage activation is thought to be stimulated by pyran and other interferon inducers (Schultz *et al.*, 1977b).

As mentioned previously, not all tilorone derivatives produce cytoplasmic inclusions nor do all tilorone derivatives produce significant interferon levels despite significant antiviral action. In fact, it should be stressed that significant levels of circulating interferon titers do not necessarily correlate with viral inhibition produced by these agents. A potent anti-viral agent of this series which does not increase circulating interferon is DEAP fluroanthene (Fleming *et al.*, 1971; Krueger *et al.*, 1971).

Most recently, Zschiesche *et al.* (1978) have shown that tilorone, in addition to interferon, can induce macrophage migration inhibitory factor (MIF) from lymphocytes in mice, as well as a macrophage derived bacterial inhibiting factor in the serum. This effect is related to stimulation of cyclic nucleotides in lymphocytes (Romer and Zschiesche, 1979). Thus, cytokine induction is an effect of tilorone. Tilorone aborts lymphocyte MIF induced by endotoxin (Jirillo *et al.*, 1977) and a factor is induced by tilorone which changes polymorpholeukocyte electrophoretic migration (Jirillo *et al.*, 1977b). Similar effects have been seen by Fahlbusch *et al.* (1977) on MIF production by interferon.

As with interferon itself and other interferon inducers, tilorone induces an NK cell response, which correlates with the degree of interferon induction in the mouse strain studied, and to the response of these mice to tumor growth (Gidlund *et al.*, 1979, 1980; Orn *et al.*, 1979).

6.6. Teratogenesis and Virus Induction

Tilorone is not teratogenic but increases embryonic resorption (32%) in rodents as compared to controls at 50 mg/kg on day 6–8 of pregnancy. Poly I:C has similar action and pyran copolymer has not been studied in this regard (Sieber and Adamson, 1972).

In view of reports that interferon inducers such as tilorone and poly I:C can increase C-particle virus induction in tumor (Fiel *et al.*, 1976a, b; Fitzwilliam and Griffith, 1976) and the evidence of increased C-particle formation in embryonic or growing tissue, it would be of interest to see if C-particle virus formation in developing embryos is effected by tilorone administration.

6.7. Host Resistance

In addition to anti-viral activity, interferon inducers such as pyran, statolon and endotoxin can protect mice from klebsiella pneumonia (Pindak, 1970). Similar effects for pyran and endotoxin have been seen against *Pasteurella tularansis* whereas poly I:C, tilorone and exogenous interferon have no effect and statolon increases mortality. In the case of *D. pneumoniae*, poly I:C, pyran and endotoxin reduce mortality and increase survival time while tilorone and exogenous interferon have no effect and statolon decreased acute mortality (Giron *et al.*, 1972a; Glick, 1968).

Tilorone decreases resistance to Listeria monocytogenes unless the innoculum was extremely small but had no effect on staphylococcal infection (Gruenewald and Levine, 1976). Why this difference between response to various infecting organisms following administration of these agents which effect the reticuloendothelial system is not known.

In the case of the structurally unrelated polyanions, we have seen pyran protection against *D. pneumoniae*, staphylococcus, cryptococcosis and trypansomiasis (Munson *et al.*, 1970; Regelson, 1973a,b, 1970; Regelson *et al.*, 1974; 1970c,d; Regelson and Munson, 1970) in addition to its anti-tumor and anti-viral action. In that regard, while tilorone is not as effective as pyran, the anthraquinone analog has shown profound protective activity against lethal staphylococcal infection (Munson *et al.*, 1972a). In contrast, in pathogen free mice, oral tilorone can increase lethality and the growth of intravenously administered mycobacteria and salmonella (Collins, 1975).

The reason for these above differences is not clear, but must be studied as it relates to the effect of these agents on macrophage function. Tilorone and its analogs can stimulate phagocytic function in liver and spleen (Munson *et al.*, 1972a; Regelson *et al.*, 1970a) which correlates with resistance to staphylococcal infection.

Tilorone, given orally, enhances liver sinusoidal phagocytic activity (Munson *et al.*, 1972a,b). Tilorone can enhance sheep RBC erthyrophagocytosis of mouse peritoneal exudate cells, an effect that is abrogated by an anti-interferon globulin. This has been used as evidence that interferon is a stimulus to phagocytosis (Rabinovitch and Manejias, 1974). Tilorone, by itself, does not stimulate bone marrow macrophage stem cell numbers except in tumor bearing animals (Fisher and Gebhardt, 1978).

If interferon induction or NK cell response is the common mechanism for tilorone or pyran increased resistance to a variety of infections, then one must take into account the hyporeactive state immediately after interferon is induced (Stringfellow and Glasgow, 1972a,b; Stringfellow, 1973; Stringfellow *et al.*, 1974). In regard to the above, in infection, both pyran and tilorone can sensitize to the lethal action of endotoxin (Munson and Regelson, 1971; Rose *et al.*, 1971). This resembles lead acetate effects which can significantly enhance the toxicity of mice to the intravenous injection of polynucleotides (Black *et al.*, 1973). This group found that polynucleotide toxicity and anti-viral potency were inversly related and are also similar to what we have seen with poly I:C complexes (Morahan *et al.*, 1972a,b, 1971).

A factor in host resistance to tilorone effects may relate to the character of monocyte/phagocyte mobilized by the infection and its response to tilorone. This is seen in experimental allergic encephalomyelitis where tilorone enhanced patterns of injury by stimulating increased levels of macrophage derived cathepsin C in the rat (Marks *et al.*, 1977).

6.8. Eye Lesions

Rehovsky *et al.* (1970) showed that tilorone can produce cytoplasmic inclusions in leukocytes and phagocytic cells of liver and spleen. Kaufman *et al.* (1971) gave tilorone topically to the eye in man at very high concentration (200 mg/ml) for up to 9 days in 10 subjects and reported the presence of epithelial inclusions in the cornea which he attributed to drug localization. Fortunately, this was reversible at 2 months. Similar corneal inclusions have been seen in patients in our clinical study receiving oral tilorone for sustained periods. This is a dose related effect and reversible. It is of interest in studies of drug distribution in the rat that the longest storage period of tilorone is found in the eye (Gaur and Chandra, 1973).

We now know that tilorone induced corneal inclusions are clinically reversible and can level off and maintain an equilibrium without worsening of symptoms. In a patient who was on tilorone for more than 31 months (totaling 189 gm) at 8.8 mg/kg biw, corneal inclusions were seen as the visible symptoms of cytoplasmic inclusion and were also found clinically in conjunctiva as well as white blood cells (Weiss *et al.*, 1980a,b; Blanke *et al.*, 1979). Unfortunately, this patient now has evidence of retinopathy.

In a second patient who received a total of 152 gm of tilorone in 16 months, similar findings to that produced by atabrine with retinopathy have been found. Therefore, systemic tilorone produces not only corneal lesions but retinal lesions as well. This should be studied as a photoactivating effect (Weiss *et al.*, 1980) in view of tilorone's fluorescent action at visible blue light frequencies.

7. ANTI-TUMOR ACTIVITY

Anti-tumor activity for tilorone was first found against Walker 256 in rats and reticulum A-RCS in mice (Adamson 1971a,c; Adamson *et al.*, 1972) on i.p. or s.c. administration. The rationale for Adamson's testing of tilorone was based on evidence of anti-tumor activity for pyran and the polynucleotides, both of which possess interferon inducing capacity.

Based on a concept of parallelism between anti-viral and anti-tumor activity, Adamson compared rifampacin, tilorone and poly I:C and found them all to be active against the Walker 256 in the rat (Adamson, 1971b,c). This was done at a time before it was known that these agents could inhibit virus related RNA controlled DNA polymerase (reverse transcriptase).

Oral tilorone has been shown to inhibit Friend leukemia and these effects occurred long after interferon titers had fallen, which suggested an alternative (i.e. immune) or direct metabolic effect on tumor growth for the anti-tumor action of this agent (Barker *et al.*, 1971).

Anti-tumor activity has been seen for tilorone and related compounds. These include activity against Friend leukemia, Ehrlich and Lewis lung carcinomas, B16 melanoma, L1210 leukemia (Adamson, 1971a,c; Adamson *et al.*, 1972; Morahan *et al.*, 1974; Munson *et al.*, 1972a; Rheins *et al.*, 1971; Rana *et al.*, 1975) and methycholanthrene induced tumors (Barker *et al.*, 1971) in mice. Inhibition of Morris hepatomas, in addition to the transplanted Walker 256 carcinoma (Rheins *et al.*, 1971; Rhoads *et al.*, 1971) and spontaneous tumors in the rat (Baslet *et al.*, 1978).

In a broad study of the activity of tilorone and its analogs, we found anti-tumor activity against Friend Leukemia and Ehrlich carcinoma (Munson *et al.*, 1972a). In addition, as mentioned previously, increased resistance to *Staphylococcus aureus* was found depending on the structure of the compound studied.

Those tilorone related compounds which can significantly stimulate phagocytosis, as determined by carbon or sheep red blood cell clearance in liver and spleen were most effective in increasing resistance to bacterial infection as well as inhibiting tumor growth (Munson *et al.*, 1972a; Regelson *et al.*, 1970a). Enhanced Jerne plaquing to sheep red blood cells was seen and the anti-tumor activity could relate to enhanced B-cell mediated immune responses or alternatively, to activation of macrophages (Munson *et al.*, 1972a; Regelson *et al.*, 1970a).

Of interest, tolerance to tilorone was seriously compromised with the presence of Friend leukemia virus infection. This is similar to what others have seen for polynucleotide toxicity (Niblack, 1971; De Clercq *et al.*, 1973). The most active anti-Friend leukemia compounds tested in this series were DEAA fluroene and DMAE fluoranone. Tilorone, while effective against other tumors when given subcutaneously, did not inhibit the allogeneic Ehrlich tumor but four other congeners were active which included DEAP fluoranthrene and DEAA fluorene which inhibited both Friend leukemia and the Ehrlich carcinoma.

Although L1210 was not inhibited by tilorone or its congeners when given subcutaneously in the above experiments, putting it in drinking water produced minimal but significant L1210 and P388 leukemia inhibition (Wampler *et al.*, 1972; Wampler & Regelson, 1974). Tilorone DMEA-xanthone and DEAA fluorene are also effective inhibitors of the Lewis lung tumor by this route (Wampler and Regelson, 1974).

Tilorone, put into drinking water, also inhibits induction by methylcholanthrene of tumors in C57BL mice. Administration of tilorone at a daily dose of 50 mg/kg for a year, significantly retarded the appearance of tumors when the mice were treated in this way. Again, the route of administration is critical as tilorone is a potent stimulator of phagocytosis when given orally (Regelson, *et al.*, 1974). In addition, it has been shown to maintain levels of circulating interferon when given in this way.

When tilorone is given subcutaneously, it is not as effective as a phagocytic stimulator in contrast to the DBAP anthraquinone analog. The anthraquinone derivative when given subcutaneously (Morahan *et al.*, 1972b) could increase resistance to lethal staphylococcal infection at 0 time or 24 hr post i.p. bacterial injection (Munson *et al.*, 1972a).

Others have also found tilorone to be active against Friend leukemia (Rheins *et al.*, 1971). In DBA/2 mice with established Friend leukemia, tilorone given seven days post inoculation at seven day intervals increased mean survival time (Rheins *et al.*, 1971). In this system, there was a decrease of Friend leukemia virus titer as well as electron microscopic evidence of decrease in C-type particles seen in the spleen. This is in contrast to Gazdar *et al.* (1972), who showed that the *in vivo* growth rate of several transplanted tumors was enhanced by pretreatment of syngeneic animals with single dosage of interferon inducers such as tilorone, poly I:C and Newcastle disease virus. In Gazdar's study, his tumors all released infectious C-type virus despite tilorone pretreatment of the mice prior to tumor inoculation.

In similar fashion to pyran (Hirsch *et al.*, 1972) for polyoma virus, a delay was found in lymphoma formation in immunosuppressed NZB M2W mice treated with tilorone (Walker and Anver, 1974). These animals, while showing increased survival, showed a higher incidence of glomerularnephritis related to DNA antibody complex localization in the nephron. The latter phenomena is not at all dissimilar to what has been seen for tilorone's effect in blocking acute lethality from allergic encephalopathy (EAE) in rats. Where, while death following hyperimmune encephalitis is delayed, necrotic myelopathy involving the cord is increased (Levine and Sowinski, 1976a,b).

Tilorone, given orally at weekly intervals to rats, was effective against Walker 256 carcinosarcoma and Morris hepatomas 777 and 3924A. This inhibition did not relate to interferon levels (Walker and Anver, 1974).

Herpes samiri, which is a potent lymphoma inducing agent in monkeys, showed *in vitro* inhibition of virus titration following administration of tilorone to the tissue culture medium at 10 μg/ml (Katz *et al.*, 1976). In view of the association of herpes virus with tumor induction and growth, the anti-herpetic action of tilorone with local and systemic use is of importance (Lieberman *et al.*, 1973; Regelson, 1976; Tokumaru, 1975; Yoschimura *et al.*, 1973).

In a study of an acute lymphocytic leukemia arising in BALB/cXDBA2F1 mice, Yancey and Bleyer (1974) found that tilorone was effective against a murine leukemia which was resistant to alkylating agents and less resistant to vincristine and prednisolone. This tumor was sensitive to 5-FU and hycanthone as well as tilorone with an increase of 67–68% in survival time. The increase in the resistance to this tumor is of interest in that there are some suggestions that it may be of T-cell origin. In contrast to the effects of tilorone on increasing resistance to the acute lymphocytic leukemia of Yancey and Bleyer (1974), Frei *et al.* (1974) found that tilorone had no effect on the development of leukemia in the spontaneous AKR mouse.

8. EFFECTS ON IMMUNE AND INFLAMMATORY RESPONSE

Tilorone stimulates the antibody response (Diamantstein, 1973; Hoffman *et al.*, 1972; Megel *et al.*, 1974a,b; Munson *et al.*, 1972a; Regelson, 1976; Regelson *et al.*, 1970a). In contrast, prolongation of allograft survival in mice by inducers of interferon has been shown by Mobraaten *et al.* (1973). Three different agents were used which included Newcastle's disease virus, statolon and tilorone. Tilorone was the best agent for prolonging graft survival when given in drinking water.

Tilorone, and other agents, when combined with cytoxan do no better than *C. parvum* in producing additional antitumor activity against the C3H mammary tumor (Fisher *et al.*, 1978). Tilorone, like zymosan, can restore liver phagocytic function in rabbits with the Brown–Pearce carcinoma (Veksler *et al.*, 1979).

Tilorone prolonged skin grafts, from rats of Fischer (AgB^1) strain, with survival increases of from 9.9 ± 1.1 days to 13.7 ± 2.3 days in the tilorone treated recipients. In contrast, steroids, when combined with tilorone, increased the survival of skin only 6.7 ± 2.6 days. Similar tilorone effects were found with heart allografts from Fischer and Brown–Norway rats given to Lewis rats. Allograft heart survival was prolonged from 14.7 ± 1.0 days to 31.0 ± 3.8 days in the Brown–Norway to Lewis rat combination.

The theory behind the above relates to T-cell depression in the recipient animals but also may represent increased production of interferon which can inhibit bone marrow cellular proliferation and also diminish cellular immune response (Mobraaten *et al.*, 1973; Wildstein *et al.*, 1975). However, the timed interval and the pattern of tilorone administration suggests that interferon levels were not the answer to the effect. Of interest, cytotoxic antibody of the IgG type to the donors lymphocytes were present at higher levels one week after tilorone administration (Wildstein *et al.*, 1975, 1976) despite sustained graft survival.

Tilorone causes severe lymphopenia in rats with depletion of small lymphocytes from lymph follicles in the spleen (Levine *et al.*, 1974). As discussed previously, this is associated with the appearance of vacuoles and basophilic granules in the cytoplasm. Granules are also found in the cytoplasm of granulocytes. Following the administration of pyran, within 12 hr, 80% of the lymphocytes have disappeared, whereas there is a relative increase in granulocyte levels. There is a decrease in neutrophilic granulocyte levels and both neutrophil and eosinophilic promyelocytes contain extensive coarse basophilic granulation as well as small vacuoles (Zbinden and Emch, 1972). Tilorone also induces nuclear inclusions in astrocytes following heat damage to the brain of rats (Levine *et al.*, 1975).

Apart from morphologic changes in leukocytes, the evidence for the action of tilorone hydrochloride as a modulator of host immune responsiveness has been presented in a large series of papers: Tilorone stimulates antibody production involving IgM, IgG, and IgE in mice and rats (Diamantstein, 1973; Hoffman *et al.*, 1972; Megel *et al.*, 1974a,b,c; 1976).

Tilorone is a potent inhibitor of a variety of cell mediated immune responses in rats. As mentioned previously, it inhibits paralysis in experimental allergic encephalomyelitis (EAE) (Megel *et al.*, 1974a) but in contrast, while it delays the encephalomyelitis, it can enhance onset and extent of paralysis depending upon the dose timing of its administration (Levine and Sowinski, 1976a). In the latter case, while interfering with the onset of lymphocytic infiltration of neural tissue, it can accelerate the penetration of monocytes into the spinal cord with the resultant malacia. Pertinent to this enhancement of hyperimmune disease has been seen in the NZB/NZW mouse unless cytoxan is added (Walker, 1977; Walker and Anver, 1978).

Tilorone suppresses the tuberculin skin reaction (Megel *et al.*, 1974a) and suppresses the local graft vs host (GVH) response in Lewis and Brown–Norway hybrids (Megel *et al.*, 1976), and the paw edema of adjuvant induced arthritis (Chang and Hoffman, 1975; Megel *et al.*, 1974a; Chang, 1977). In Chang's study (1977), there was no correlation between the inhibition of adjuvant induced arthritis and immune response.

Of significant interest to clinical transplantation, the suppression of the local graft vs host response in Lewis and Brown–Norway hybrids is seen in pretreatment of the donor animal. There is also some evidence that pretreatment of donor animals, i.e. dogs prior to renal homografting, increases the degree of take of the transplanted kidney (Cawein *et al.*, 1975).

Zschiesche *et al.* (1977) have found a block to graft vs host when tilorone was given at day 0–2 post graft in mice, but when given day -4 or -2, it enhanced graft vs host disease. Tilorone effects on graft vs host in chickens has been obscurred by its toxicity (Donahoe *et al.*, 1977).

The mechanism of action for tilorone as an immune inhibitor has developed from the observation of Zbinden and Emch (1972) as well as others who have shown that tilorone produces a transient lymphopenia (Megel, 1977; Megel *et al.*, 1974a,b,; 1976). While this effect is transient, in that continued administration results in the return of peripheral lymphocytes to control levels, the effect is associated with a significant depletion of lymphocytes in the T-cell areas of lymph nodes, spleen, and Peyer's patches. Raychaudhuri and Megel (1977) and Megel *et al.* (1977, 1978) have shown that peripheral lymphocytic recovery following daily tilorone administration is of B-lymphocytes which have replaced the T-lymphocyte population.

Continued daily administration of tilorone increased the weight of spleens and this increase in splenic weight was due to a significant increase in the percentage of splenic B-lymphocytes. These changes, showing replacement of T-lymphocytes with B-lymphocytes, obviously explain the mechanism by which tilorone can interfere with graft vs host reactivity while stimulating antibody production.

Further evidence for the specificity of tilorone as a T-cell suppressing agent, is the fact that athymic mice treated with tilorone did not show a fall in their leukocyte count while in contrast, normal mice showed a significant transient depletion of lymphocytes. There was also no difference between interferon induction in the normal control mice and the athymic mice and interferon induction occurred despite the absence of T-cells in the athymic animals (Gibson *et al.*, 1976).

The T-lymphocyte depletion in normal mice following tilorone treatment occurs more or less simultaneously with the appearance of anti-viral activity which reaches a maximum in 24 hr. T-lymphocytes are obviously not necessary for significant interferon induction and tilorone's action is similar to what has also been shown for anti-lymphocyte serum (Gibson *et al.*, 1976).

Tilorone's action as an immunoadjuvant or T-cell inhibitor may be mediated via its stimulation of macrophage function (Munson *et al.*, 1972a; Regelson, 1976; Regelson *et al.*, 1970a). Pyran works by similar action (Regelson *et al.*, 1974), and Friedlaender *et al.* (1974) have found that cell-mediated immunity during tilorone administration can be enhanced if one removes adherent cells (i.e. macrophages or perhaps adherent B-cells) from the medium which is similar to what has been found for pyran. In the case of pyran, removal of activated macrophages results in enhancement of blastogenesis (Baird and Kaplan, 1977a,b,c; 1975; Baird, 1976; Kaplan and Morahan, 1976a,b).

As discussed previously, apart from delay in paralysis for the hyperimmune encephalomyelitis (EAE) model in the rats (Megel *et al.*, 1974a, 1976) and prolongation of skin and heart graft in rats (Wildstein *et al.*, 1975, 1976), there is also evidence that tilorone can cause significant reduction of tuberculin skin reaction (Megel, 1977; Megel *et al.*, 1974b; Argentieri *et al.*, 1978).

As mentioned previously, tilorone enhances autoimmune glomerular nephritis in the young NZB/NEW mice (Walker, 1977). But when it is combined with cytoxan, survival is enhanced and tumor induction and glomerular nephritis are decreased (Walker and Anver, 1978).

In addition to effects on tuberculin skin sensitivity, tilorone can prevent cell-mediated immune adjuvant arthritis (Chang and Hoffman, 1975). This again is in the rat using subplantar injection of *Mycobacterium tuberculosis.* Tilorone not only inhibits the secondary immunologically induced inflammatory response, but also the primary inflammatory response showing that tilorone possesses anti-inflammatory properties as well.

Tilorone p.o. decreased *M. leprae* reactive infection in mouse foot pads, but it enhanced the infectivity of *M. marinum* and *M. lepraemurium* under the same circumstances. Suggesting an anti-inflammatory effect for *M. leprae* that balances out the decreased resistance to infection seen with enhanced sensitivity to *M. marinum* and *lepraemurium* (Levy *et al.*, 1978).

Tilorone is equal to hydrocortisone in its effects on blocking tuberculin reactions when given prophylactically (Megel, 1977; Megel *et al.*, 1974b). When given therapeutically, following the administration of the tuberculin, tilorone inhibited inflammation but hydrocortisone appears to be more effective in reducing edema (Megel, 1977; Megel *et al.*, 1974b).

In addition to the effects of tilorone in decreasing immunologic inflammation, carageenan paw edema in adult female Sprague-Dawley rats can also be modified by tilorone. This effect is independent of adrenalectomy and tilorone has to be given 24 hr prior to the carageenan injection for the effect to be seen. In contrast, phenylbutazone was most effective when given at the time of injection of the inflammatory agent.

In Megel's (1977) study of direct passive Arthus reaction, female Sprague Dawley rats were injected with antiserum produced in rabbits against bovine serum albumin. Cobra venom factor, a complement depleting agent, aspirin and tilorone significantly inhibited the Arthus reaction when these agents were administered 24 or 1.5 hr before sensitization. Tilorone was effective at 24 hr before, but when given 30 min prior to sensitization, was inactive. This is similar to what has been seen for its effects on carageenan reaction.

Attempts have been made to distinguish B- and T-subpopulations of lymphocytes using fluoroscein conjugated anti-mouse IgG antiserum (Raychaudhuri and Megel 1977; Megel *et al.*, 1977, 1978). Tilorone caused a marked reduction in total white blood count 24 hr after the first dose with depression at 3 days which returned to control levels at 9 days. There was a striking increase in the per cent of B-lymphocytes in the peripheral blood of the tilorone-treated mice compared with the controls. Although tilorone caused a slight but statistically significant depletion of B-cells 24 hr after the first dose, highly significant increases in B-cells were noted on the 3rd and 9th days equivalent to a 1.3 and

2.5-fold increase over control levels. T-cells remained significantly depressed during the 9 day study period although there may have been some mild recovery.

During this same period of tilorone administration, there was a 2–3-fold increase in serum hemolytic complement levels over that of control. This is of interest in view of the fact that while tilorone behaved in similar fashion to cobra venom in preventing Arthus paw edema, cobra venom produces a striking depletion of complement 30 min after administration which persists for 24 hr while tilorone, after a single oral dose, elevates complement levels for periods as long as 96 hr. In contrast, *in vivo* in the NAB/NZY young mouse along with accelerated immune complex disease, C_3 complement is depleted with tilorone administration (Walker, 1977). The above is of interest in view of recent observations that interferon titers are inversely related to serum complement levels (Koliskova *et al.*, 1979).

As is to be expected, the guinea-pig behaves differently under the influence of tilorone as compared to rats and mice. Using rosette forming cells in experimental tests for T-lymphocytes, tilorone along with cytoxan and cortisone increased and percentage of rosette-forming cells. Of interest, *in vitro* incubation of guinea-pig lymphocytes with cytoxan, azathioprine and tilorone, induced similar increases in the percentage of rosette-forming cells (Johansen *et al.*, 1974). In contrast to mice and rats, tilorone caused no change in spleen weight, number of mononuclear cells or T-cell percentage in guinea-pigs treated with tilorone for 2 days. When treated for 2 weeks there was a slight increase in splenic weight and the number of mononuclear cells as well as an increase in rosette cell percentage in both spleen and thymus.

Why this species difference is seen has not been explained. There is also no note by Johansen of cytoplasmic inclusions found in the leukocytes of the guinea-pig. This indicates that the guinea-pig is quite different and that there is an obvious species specificity for the action of tilorone.

Although not seen clinically, tilorone has produced renal lesions particularly of distal tubules in rats. This was associated with vacuoles containing myelin (lamellar) bodies of acid phosphastase positivity which were also contained in the ascending limb of Henle (Thelmo and Levine, 1978). Similar changes have been reported for K^+ depletion, chlorphentermine, chloroquin, and psychotropic drugs of the phenothiazine type where such lesions are primarily found in the liver and related to endoplasmic reticulum changes (Lullman *et al.*, 1973). Again, no renal functional abnormalities of this kind were noted in man.

9. CLINICAL ANTI-TUMOR STUDIES

Based on the animal model anti-tumor data, tilorone was entered into Phase I and Phase II clinical trial (Kuperminc and Gelber, 1976; Richter *et al.*, 1975a,b; Wampler *et al.*, 1973).

While the number of responding patients has been small, and the effects of minimal value, anti-tumor activity has been seen. The problem relates to the development of optimal schedules versus the presence of side-effects which are different from the usual cytotoxic agents. These include bizarre dreams, seborrheic dermatitis, transient corneal inclusions and retinopathy; the latter two side-effects are seen on prolonged administration. The CNS effects are not surprising in view of animal evidence of drug concentration similar to that found in the spleen and present in the eye. (Gaur and Chandra, 1973, Wacker *et al.*, 1972).

Nausea and vomiting and diarrhea are also limiting side-effects, while tilorone has no suppressing effect on the bone marrow and may actually increase the platelet count. Up to 15 mg/kg weekly, single doses and 6 mg/kg daily doses have been tolerated.

Following Phase I study in 15 patients in our clinic, Phase II study was undertaken in 66 patients. Patients studied were beyond hope of surgical or radiotherapy cure, and in most cases had failed on other chemotherapy.

In our Phase II study, 45 patients were evaluable (Richter *et al.*, 1975a). Partial transient responses were noted in single breast and renal cancer patients. Although 13 melanomas were treated, unlike Phase I study where benefit was obtained in 2 of 3 melanomas, no significant response was seen.

The major limiting toxicity of tilorone were reversible corneal inclusions at high cumulative dose which was found when drug was given on a daily basis (Kuperminc and Gelber, 1976; Richter *et al.*, 1975a; Weiss *et al.*, 1980a,b). In our Phase II study, 3 patients of 32 who received tilorone at total doses of 310–463 mg/kg of drug, from 62–105 days, showed corneal inclusions. No inclusions were seen in a comparable group receiving an average of 226 mg/kg for a mean of 29 days (range 2–80 days) (Richter *et al.*, 1975a).

Our Phase II study compared 2 dosage levels of 6 mg/kg q.d. × 7 weeks versus 10 mg/kg g.d. × 14 days, but the latter dose schedule was too toxic for patient acceptance beyond a single cycle.

If one adds up our Phase I and Phase II studies, then two significant clinical responses were seen in 16 patients with melanoma. The next largest series of patients studied included 7 lung (4 squamous, 3 adeno) and 4 breast cases with no more than 2 or 3 patients in other tumor categories. A total of 16 adenocarcinomas from different sites were evaluated, 10 squamous cell carcinomas, 3 lymphomas and one each of acute lymphocytic leukemia, ovarian teratocarcinoma and seminoma. This was not an adequate Phase II evaluation, with the exception of our melanoma experience (Richter *et al.*, 1975a).

Basophilic cytoplasmic inclusions have always been seen in the cytoplasm of leukocytes of patients receiving drug for one week or more. The relation of this to corneal inclusions is suggestive (Weiss *et al.*, 1980a,b; Blanke *et al.*, 1979). The inclusions seen in leukocytes are similar to those produced by atabrine, which also induces interferon and produces basophilic inclusions in leukocyte cytoplasm (Glaz *et al.*, 1973; Glaz and Talas, 1975). These compounds can induce similar corneal or retinal changes to tilorone (Hobbs *et al.*, 1961; Von Sallmann and Bernstein, 1963 Weiss *et al.*, 1980a,b).

Based on our experience, we feel that the use of tilorone in advanced cancer patients is not warranted. For example, a randomized study in 25 previously treated advanced breast cancer patients at 340 mg m^{-2} day^{-1} showed that the tilorone treated patients had a median decrease in survival of 7 weeks in contrast to 24 weeks in patients receiving ARA-C and FUDR chemotherapy (Kuperminc and Gelber, 1976).

However, Edelstein and Israel (1974) and Israel *et al.* (1977) gave tilorone at weekly intervals of 1500 mg and this group reported arrest of tumor growth in 6 of 11 patients with measurable metastases from a variety of tumors but have subsequently abandoned its study.

Up to now, 120 cancer patients have received oral tilorone, but its role in advanced cancer and leukemia is limited (Cawein *et al.*, 1975). However, tilorone's clinical potential may reside in the treatment of T-cell related leukemia, mycosis fungoides or Sezeryi's disease where responses for 6 months or more have been seen. Alternatively, tilorone should be used as an adjuvant in post operative or radiotherapy patients with minimal disease. Cawein *et al.* (1975) have recently reported on a trial of tilorone in acute leukemia with changes in B-cell:T-cell relationships secondary to tilorone administration.

In an oral study with a tilorone congener, we have completed a Phase I study of RMI 11,002DA (DEAA fluorene, 2,7-bis(2-diethyamino) acetylfluorene dihydrochloride) a congener of tilorone.HCL which has similar biologic activity (Richter *et al.*, 1975b) (Fig. 1).

Prior experience in animals indicated better tolerance of RMI 11,002DA. The latter was found by Merrell–National investigators to have a shorter half life (in mice) 1.3 days vs 3.8 days for tilorone. As an acetylcholinesterase inhibitor, RMI 11,002DA is five times less potent than its tilorone congener. Monkeys tolerated up to 75 mg kg^{-1} day^{-1} but neurological abnormalities were reported in 15% receiving the high dosages. Inclusion bodies were reported in rodent and monkey macrophages and lymphocytes in similar fashion to what has been seen for tilorone, but this was not seen clinically.

No tumor regression or stabilization of disease process was observed in the 32 patients treated in our Phase I study (Richter *et al.*, 1975b). Side effects were similar to tilorone with the exeption of the absence of leukocyte cytoplasmic inclusions, seborrheic keratitis and corneal inclusions. Maximum tolerated dose appears to be at the 22 mg kg^{-1} day^{-1} level and the acceptable dose will be 10 or 12 mg kg^{-1} day^{-1}. Single weekly administration for DEAA fluorene would be 14–16 mg/kg with dosage limited to that level by its psychedelic action.

Toxicity was principally manifested by nausea, sleep disturbances, bizarre dreams, and three cases of an acute allergic dermatitis which responded promptly to drug withdrawal. RMI 11,002DA (DEAA fluorene) should be placed in Phase II study in view of its greater potency against the Friend virus tumor, Lewis lung and B16 melanoma tumors in mice.

In support of the adjuvant use for tilorone or RMI 11,002DA (DEAA fluorene), the most exciting laboratory utilization of tilorone has been with combined drug administration. Utilizing the syngeneic murine lymphoid leukemia (MCAS-10 following treatment with 1,3-bis(2-chloroethyl)-1-nitrosourea (BCNU) at a dose which significantly suppressed the disease, the administration of tilorone post chemotherapy significantly prolonged survival in similar fashion to pyran. These effects again do not correlate with interferon induction (Pearson *et al.*, 1974). In contrast, pyran has been reported to be effective against the spontaneous transplantable prostatic adenocarcinoma in Lobund Wistar rats (Coffey, 1976) but tilorone has not been shown to be effective against this tumor (Burleson and Pollard, 1976).

10. MISCELLANEOUS ACTION

Apart from cancer studies in a therapeutic double-blind placebo-controlled study, tilorone was given to 8 patients with amyotrophic lateral sclerosis of whom 6 could be evaluated and no difference was seen to a comparable placebo control group. Eye problems were identical to that seen in the tumor population and those described by Weiss *et al.*, (1980), (Olson *et al.*, 1978).

In other areas, tilorone has also been used in the treatment of Herpes type I, subacute sclerosing panmyeloencephalopathy (Cawein *et al.*, 1975) with questionable benefit.

We have given tilorone and prednisone to a renal transplant patient with panleukoencephalopathy. She functionally improved for two years with no sign of host–graft rejection, despite two previous episodes of threatened rejection on immuran and cytoxan. Drug was discontinued at two years because of asymptomatic corneal and retinal lesions and she is maintaining her renal graft on prednisone alone two years post tilorone (Selhorst *et al.*, 1978).

The optimal oral dose for tilorone will prove to be 10 mg/kg biw which the above patient received. Based on the T-cell inhibiting action of tilorone and our experience in this one patient, the use for this agent may best be seen in the prevention of host graft rejection in organ transplantation provided one is alert for conjunctival and retinal changes and limits dosage accordingly.

Tilorone's cytoplasmic inclusions are found in conjunctiva, buccal mucosa and leukocytes on clinical administration. We postulate that these inclusions will be found in all nucleated cells on sufficient dose and length of administration. It suggests that similar inclusions reported in the cornea or retinal lesions on atabrine administration may relate to similar cellular entry which also may account for the cutaneous pigmentation of atabrine administration. Of interest, NZB/NZW mice and guinea-pigs do not show cytoplasmic leukocyte inclusions on prolonged tilorone treatment suggesting that there is a species difference that governs this effect.

Other facts of interest in relation to tilorone's activity are reports; that i.v. tilorone lowers body temperature (Glaz and Talas, 1973), and that tilorone acts as an *in vitro* photoactive inhibitor of platelet aggregation (Mackenzie and Schatzman, 1975). In addition, tilorone and related congeners can photoinactivate viruses in vitro (Camyre *et al.*, 1973). These photoinactivating effects were similar to what has been seen for acridine, and the neutral red phenazine dye.

Tilorone and many of its congeners possess cholinesterase inhibiting activity (Albrecht, 1974; Albrecht *et al.*, 1972) and in view of cholinergic receptors on lymphocytes, this could be critical to its effects on lymphocyte response. There are also similarities between the anti-parasitic agents hycanthone and lucanthone, which have similar structural and central nervous system action and which have been reported to have effects on radiation, repair and sensitivity of tumors to radiotherapy.

Tilorone has activity in eliminating plutonium from liver binding, but it is less active than pyran or glucan (Guilmette and Lindenbaum, 1975; Lindenbaum *et al.*, 1975).

Tilorone has anticoagulant activity *in vitro* with slight acceleratory effects on the hydrolysis of TAME (*p*-toluensulfonyl-L-arginine methyl ester) by thrombin but is a strong accelerator of the hydrolysis of TAME by thrombokinase (activated Factor X), where even 4×10^{-4} M compound produced rates that are 140% of controls. The hydrolysis of BAME (Benzoyl-L-arginine methyl ester), however, by either thrombin or thrombokinase is very weakly inhibited by tilorone.

The activation of plasminogen by streptokinase is inhibited by 0.01 M tilorone, but the hydrolysis of TAME by plasmin is only weakly inhibited. The thrombin–plasmin reaction is slightly accelerated by low concentrations, but is strongly inhibited by 0.01 M tilorone and this concentration of tilorone inhibits both modified one-stage prothrombin and recalcification tests (Roberts *et al.*, 1973b).

Electron micrographs of rat liver show the presence of many branched structures of the endoplasmic reticulum in the form of whorls (myelin bodies). Tilorone also decreases albumin levels by 15% which are synthesized by the endoplasmic reticulum (Leeson *et al.*, 1976).

Other interferon inducers are also reported to do this which include poly I:C, CP20961, quinacrine and statolon (Renton and Mannering, 1976). Pyran does this as well and it appears to relate to molecular weight, as fractions of pyran less than 15,000 m.w. do not do this (Breslow, 1976; Breslow *et al.*, 1973; Munson *et al.*, 1972b; Munson and Wooles, 1969; Ottenbrite *et al.*, 1978; Ottenbrite and Regelson, 1976; Regelson, 1973; Regelson *et al.*, 1974; Wooles and Munson, 1971; Barnes, 1980).

Tilorone has been reported to protect mice from whole body radiation when it is given 30 min before radiation (Chertkov *et al.*, 1978), which is important, as radiation protection has also been seen for interferon.

11. RELATED COMPOUNDS

In relation to the action of tilorone, it should be remembered that there are other small molecular weight interferon inducers and that tilorone behaves similarly to acridine drugs (Glaz *et al.*, 1973; Glaz and Talas, 1975). Acranil produces levels of mouse interferon equivalent to that of tilorone where atabrine (mepacrine) is not as effective. These tricyclic compounds with dialkyl amino aklyl side chains behave similarly to tilorone in relation to their effect as metabolic inhibitors and their effect as interferon inducers, Of interest, both tilorone and mepacrine can produce latent antiviral activity as long as 14 days after administration and acranil can block tilorone's interferon inducing capacity. Both atabrine and acranil induce cytoplasmic inclusions and atabrine also produces corneal and retinal lesions in similar fashion to tilorone (Hobbs *et al.*, 1961; Von Sallmann and Bernstein, 1963; Blanke *et al.*, 1979; Weiss *et al.*, 1980a,b). Both tilorone and quinacrine block the action of hemin on reticulocyte lysates which involves interaction with a protein kinase (Bogdanovsky and Pierre, 1979).

Compounds which can induce interferon include bis-piperidinylacetyl dibenzofuran hydrochloride (MA 56) (Soehner *et al.*, 1974) and BL-20803 which is 4-(3-dimethyl aminopropylamino)-1,3-dimethyl-1H-pyrazolo-(3,4-b)-quinoline dihydrochloride. This compound, like tilorone, induces basophilic inclusions. Most recently, Veckenstedt *et al.*

(1979a,b) have synthesized a series of fluorenones with similar antiviral activity to tilorone.

12. CONCLUSION: TILORONE AND ANALOGS

In conclusion, tilorone and DEAA fluorene, like pyran copolymer, requires further clinical trial with appropriate caution in regard to ocular toxicity. Tilorone and its congeners have had only minimal clinical exploration and their most effective use might be in:

(1) The treatment of acute and chronic virus infection (i.e. subacute sclerosing panmyelopathy).

(2) There should be clinical study for possible inhibition of bacterial transformation and resistance based on observations indicating that tilorone can interfere with plasmid transfer.

(3) Their adjuvant use in the treatment of cancer patients when minimal tumor is present.

(4) Their use in prolongation of organ transplants and skin grafts.

(5) Their use in the treatment of arthritis, lupus and other manifestations of hyperimmune disease alone or in combination with cytotoxic immune suppressors.

(6) Their use in study of plutonium decorporation or drug binding and metabolism in liver parenchyma.

(7) Their study as radiation protective agents.

(8) Their use as pharmacologic agents to distinguish T-cells from B-cells.

They represent a series of compounds with ocular toxicity that can be reversible and dose related. Tilorone apparently has no major suppressing effects on bone marrow reserve and while it interferes with T-cell function, does not seriously compromise host resistance to most bacterial infections.

13. FINAL SUMMARY: PYRAN, TILORONE AND THEIR DERIVATIVES

Pyran and polyanions and the fluorenone derivatives, i.e. tilorone, and its congeners (DEAA fluorene) (Fig. 1) have the following activities in common: interferon induction, anti-tumor activity and anti-viral activity.

They inhibit reverse transcriptase and modulate resistance to bacterial, fungal and protozoal infection. Both series of compounds produce basophilic cytoplasmic inclusions in phagocytic cells or leukocytes. However, in the case of tilorone derivatives, the presence of these inclusions does not necessarily relate to interferon induction or anti-viral activity.

Pyran copolymer produces nuclear alteration with euchromatization of the nucleus and depression of nuclear function (Arnold *et al.*, 1973; Berezney and Coffey, 1976; Coffey *et al.*, 1973; Miller *et al.*, 1971, 1972). Both series of compounds produce macrophage activation (Baird and Kaplan, 1980, 1977a,b,c; 1975; Baird, 1976; Baird *et al.*, 1974; Kaplan *et al.*, 1976a,b; Kaplan and Morahan, 1976a,b; Morahan, 1977; Munson *et al.*, 1972a; Regelson *et al.*, 1974, 1970a) and B-cell stimulation (Diamantstein, 1973; Hoffman *et al.*, 1972; Megel *et al.*, 1974; 1976; Munson *et al.*, 1972a; Regelson, 1976; Regelson *et al.*, 1970a).

Tilorone and related congeners inhibit cellular immune response (Chang and Hoffman, 1975; Megel *et al.*, 1974a, 1976; Mobraaten *et al.*, 1973; Wildstein *et al.*, 1975, 1976) while this has not been clearly defined for pyran except with inhibition of adjuvant induced arthritis (Kapusta & Mendelson, 1969) and suggestive effects on skin graft survival. This may be secondary to phagocytic effects as the presence of activated macrophages interferes with phytohemagglutinin and lipolysaccharide induced blastogenic response (Baird and Kaplan, 1975, 1977a,b,c; 1980; Baird, 1976; (Baird *et al.*, 1974; Friedlaender *et al.*,

1974). Tilorone depletes T-cells (Levine *et al.*, 1974; Megel, 1977; Megel *et al.*, 1974a,b; 1976; Raychaudhuri and Megel, 1977; Zbinden and Emch, 1972) and both compounds can produce hepatosplenomegaly with this being dependent on molecular weight for pyran copolymer (Breslow, 1976; Breslow *et al.*, 1973; Ottenbrite *et al.*, 1978; Ottenbrite and Regelson, 1976; Regelson *et al.*, 1974, 1975).

In the case of pyran copolymer, germinal center morphology is destroyed and monocytic activity is increased in the spleens of treated mice (Regelson, 1967; Regelson and Munson, 1970; Regelson *et al.*, 1970c). Depletion of Peyers patches and changes in splenic morphology has been reported for tilorone (Mobraaten *et al.*, 1973; Wildstein *et al.*, 1975).

Both compounds can sensitize to the lethal action of endotoxin (Breslow, 1976; Breslow *et al.*, 1973; Munson and Regelson, 1971; Regelson *et al.*, 1974, 1975; Rose *et al.*, 1971) and both inhibit drug metabolizing enzymes (Munson *et al.*, 1972b; Munson and Wooles, 1969) with alterations in hepatic endoplasmic reticulum and P-450, 448 response, which is characteristic of interferon inducers (Mannering *et al.*, 1976; Renton *et al.*, 1979; Zerkle *et al.*, 1980; Barnes, 1980).

Both agents have complement effects with pyran inhibiting serum complement or activating the C3 alternative pathway. In the case of tilorone (Raychaudhuri and Megel, 1977; Megel *et al.*, 1978) serum complement levels are increased along with anti-inflammatory activity and block to secondary immune response. This deserves special interest in view of inverse relationships between complement and interferon induction (Koliskova *et al.*, 1979).

Pyran is a potent anticoagulant which acts through interference with fibrin formation (Dennis *et al.*, 1969; Regelson *et al.*, 1975, 1978; Roberts *et al.*, 1973a; Shamash and Alexander, 1969), while tilorone has *in vitro* effects through activation of BAME or TAME esterase activity (Roberts *et al.*, 1973b). Interperitoneal pyran stimulates BAME and TAME splenic esterase activity while i.v. pyran inhibits. This correlates with virus susceptibility (Roberts and Regelson, 1977).

Pyran is a thrombocytopenic agent, both *in vivo* and *in vitro* whereas tilorone may actually increase blood platelet levels on clinical trial and *in vitro* exerts its anti-platelet effect through a photoactivation process (MacKenzie and Schatzman, 1975).

Pyran is pyrogenic clinically in man, whereas tilorone has no effect on clinical temperature regulation but does cause hypothermia in mice (Glaz and Talas, 1975).

Tilorone produces bizarre dreams, corneal inclusions and retinopathy and seborrheic keratitis (Wampler *et al.*, 1973; Richter *et al.*, 1975a,b); Weiss *et al.*, 1980a,b), while pyran, as the polydispease polymer can produce vascular collapse and transient blindness (Regelson *et al.*, 1978). In contrast, MVE 2, a pyran copolymer of fixed molecular weight, is apparently free of vascular toxicity or pyrogenecity (Powell *et al.*, 1981).

Both pyran and tilorone can mobilize (decorporate) plutonium from liver with pyran being the more active agent (Guilmette and Lindenbaum, 1975; Lindenbaum *et al.*, 1975). Both can produce *in vitro* viral neutralization but in the case of tilorone (Camyre *et al.*, 1973), this is a photoactivation process. Tilorone blocks plasmid capability in bacterial transformation studies (Hahn and Ciak, 1977).

Pyran can inhibit aldosterone activity (Chremos *et al.*, 1969; Regelson, 1968b, 1973), and can increase calcium flux in the activation of macrophages *in vitro* while this has not been tested for tilorone.

Tilorone activates plant phenylalanine ammonia lyase (Hadwiger, 1972) and hepatic phosphoprotein kinase (Pierre and Loeb, 1977) while pyran and synthetic polyanions inhibit or activate a wide range of enzymes (Regelson, 1968b,c, 1973, 1974).

Tilorone has radiation protection activation (Chertkov *et al.*, 1978) in similar fashion to interferon while pyran, theoretically, may be sensitizing (Matyasova *et al.*, 1974) to radiation effects because of polyanionic histone displacement.

It would be of interest to study combinations of the fixed lower molecular weight pyran, MVE 2 and the Monsanto NED 137 in combination with tilorone or other immune modulators in view of the absence of clinical toxicity for these newer polyanions.

In conclusion, both pyran and tilorone, their congeners and pure molecular weight pyran fractions require further basic and clinical studies for elaboration of mechanism and clinical usefulness which, fortunately, is under continued study at this time.

One must ask what common mechanisms are present that link such two diverse series of compounds in such striking similarity in relation to functional activity?

Acknowledgements—This research was supported by U.S.P.H.S. and N.C.I., Eastern Cooperative oncology Group Programs CA 10572, CA 02824, CA 02822 and CA 06594; The Hercules Company, Wilmington, Delaware; the Merrill-National Company, Cincinnati, Ohio; the Harvey Marler Fund and the MCV/VCU Cancer Center. We wish to thank Eva Gross, Bea Wiggins and Lynn Baird, Ph.D., for editorial assistance.

REFERENCES

ADAMSON, R. H. (1971a) Antitumor activity of tilorone hydrochloride against some rodent tumors: preliminary report. *J. natn Cancer Inst.* **46**: 431–434.

ADAMSON, R. H. (1971) Evaluation of the antitumor activity of rifamycin SV. *Archs Int. Pharmacodyn.* **192**: 61–65.

ADAMSON, R. H. (1971) Antitumour activity of two antiviral drugs—rifampicin and tilorone. *Lancet* **1**: 398.

ADAMSON, R. H., ABLASHI, D. V., ARMSTRONG, G. R. and ELLMORE, N. W. (1972) Effect of cytosine arabinoside, adenine arabinoside, tilorone, and rifamycin SV on multiplication of herpes virus Saimiri *in vitro*. *Antimicrob. Agents Chemother.* **1**: 82–83.

ADAMSON, R. H., FABRO, S., HOMAN, E. R., O'GARA, R. W. and ZENDZIAN, R. P. (1970) Pharmacology of polyriboinosinic: polyribocytidylic acid a new antiviral and antitumor agent. *Antimicrob. Agents Chemother.* **9**: 148–152.

ALBRECHT, W. L. (1974) In: *Progress in Chemotherapy (Antibacterial, Antiviral and Antineoplastic)*, Vol. 2, pp. 865–880, DAIKOS, G. K. (Ed). Proceeding of the 8th International Congress of Chemotherapy, Athens 1973, Hellenic Society for Chemotherapy, Athens.

ALBRECHT, W. L., ANDREWS, E. R., CARR, A. A., FLEMING, R. W., GRISAN, J. M., HORGAN, S. W., SILL, A. D., SWEET, F. W. and WENSTRUP, D. L. (1972) Antiviral and interferon inducing bis-basic substituted polycyclic aromatic and heteroaromatic compounds. *Med. Chem. Sympos.* Iowa City 18–22 June (13th Mtg.).

ANACLERIO, A., CONTI, G., MORAS, J. L., MACONI, A. and SPREAFICO, F. (1978) Effect of immunomopolymers on thymocyte suppressive activity in mice. **00**, 000–000.

ARGENTIEGRI, D. C., MEZZATESTA, J. R. and CARLSON, R. P. (1978) Effects of standard immunological agents on (foot pad) hypersensitivity reactions in tuberculin sensitive guinea-pigs. *Fed. Proc.* **37**: 604.

ARNOLD, E. A., YAWN, D. H., FROWN, D. G., WILLIE, R. C. and COFFEY, D. S. (1972) Structural alteration in isolated rat liver nuclei after removal of template restriction by polyanions. *J. Cell Biol.* **53**: 737–757.

BAIRD, L. G. (1976) The mechanisms of immunoadjuvant activity of pyran copolymer. Ph.D. Thesis, Dept. of Microbiology, Medical College of Virginia, Virginia Commonwealth University, Richmond, Virginia 23298.

BAIRD, L. G., KAPLAN, A. M. and LUCAS, D. O. (1974) *Regulatory Mechanisms in Lymphocytic Activation.* Academic Press, New York, p. 794.

BAIRD, L. G. and KAPLAN, A. M. (1975) Immunoadjuvant activity of pyran copolymer—I. Evidence for direct stimulation of T-lymphocytes and macrophages. *Cell Immunol.* **20**: 167–176.

BAIRD, L. G. and KAPLAN, A. M. (1977a) Macrophage regulation of mitogen induced blastogenesis—I. Demonstration of inhibitory cells in the spleens and peritoneal exudates of mice. *Cell Immunol.* **28**, 22–35.

BAIRD, L. G. and KAPLAN, A. M. (1977b) Macrophage regulation of mitogen induced blastogenesis—II. Mechanisms of inhibition. *Cell Immunol.* **28**: 36–50.

BAIRD, L. G. and KAPLAN, A. M. (1977c) Macrophage regulation of mitogen induced blastogenesis—III. Demonstration of inhibitory cells in the spleens and peritoneal exudates of mice. *Cell Immunol.* **28**: 22–35.

BAIRD, L. G. and KAPLAN, A. M. (1978) Immunoregulatory macrophages frrm pyran treated mice. In *Immune Modulation and Control of Neoplasia by Adjuvant Therapy*, CHIRIGOS, H. A. (Ed). *Prog. Cancer Res. Therapy.* **7**: 435–445. Raven Press, New York.

BAIRD, L. G. and KAPLAN, A. M. (1980) Effects of polyanion immunomodulators on the immune system. In *Anionic Polymeric Drugs*, (Polymers in Biology and Medicine Series), pp. 105–121, DONARUMA, L. G., OTTENBRITE, R. M. and VOGL, O. (Eds). John Wiley, New York.

BALEZINA, T. I., FADEEVA, L. L., ZEMSKOV, V. M., KORNEEVA, L. E., LOIDINA, G. I., NIKOLAEVA, O. V. and ERMOLIEVA, Z. V. (1976) Interferonogenic and antiviral activity of tobacco mosaic virus, tilorone and sodium nucleinate. *Antibiotiki* **21**: 250–254.

BLANKE, R. V., SAADY, J. J., DRUMMOND, D. C. and WEISS, J. N. (1979) Tilorone determination in a corneal biopsy. *J. analyt. Toxicol.* **00**, 206–208.

BARKER, A. D., RHEINS, M. S. and WILSON, H. E. (1971) Amelioration of Friend virus leukemia by sequential administration of viral and non viral interferon inducers. *Proc. Soc. exp. Biol. Med.* **137**: 981–987.

BARNES, D. W. (1980) Effects of anionic polymeric drugs and other immunoactive agents on hepatic microsomal mixed function oxidases. In *Anionic Polymeric Drugs* (Polymers in Biology and Medicine Series), pp. 255–275, DONARUMA, L. G., OTTENBRITE, R. M. and VOGL, O. (Eds). John Wiley, New York.

BASLET, W. A., GRENGER, J. A., REES, R. C. and BALDWIN, R. W. (1978) Therapy of metatasizing rat tumors of spontaneous origin. *Br. J. Cancer* **38**: 176.

BEREZNEY, R. and COFFEY, D. S. (1976) The nuclear protein matrix: isolation, structure and function. In *Advances in Enzyme Regulation*, Vol. 14, pp. 63–100, WEBER, G. (Ed.). Pergamon Press, Oxford.

BLACK, D. R., ECKSTEIN, F., DECLERCQ, E. and MERIGAN, T. C. (1973) Studies on the toxicity and antiviral activity of various polynucleotides. *Antimicrob. Agents Chemother.* **3**: 198–206.

BOGDANOVSKY, D. and PIERRE, M. (1979) Effect of tilorone and quinacrine on translation in reticulocyte lysates. *Biochem. Pharmac.* **28**: 3683–3685.

BOLDT, D., MACDERMOTT, R., SPECKART, S. and NASH, G. (1976) DNA excretion by purified lymphocyte populations. 11th Leukocyte Culture Conference Sept. 12–23, Tucson, Arizona. **ABS 60**: 37.

BRAUN, W., REGELSON, W., YAJIMA, Y. and ISHIZUKA, M. (1970) Stimulation of antibody formation by pyran copolymer. *Proc. Soc. exp. Biol. Med.* **133**: 171–175.

BREINIG, M. C., MUNSON, A. E. and MORAHAN, P. S. (1980) Antiviral activity of synthetic polymers. In *Anionic Polymeric drugs*, pp. 211–226, DONARUMA, L. G., OTTENBRITE, R. M. and VOGL O. (Eds). John Wiley, New York.

BRESLOW, D. S. (1976) Biologically active synthetic polymers. *Pure appl. Chem.* **46**: 103–110.

BRESLOW, D. S., EDWARDS, E. I. and NEWBURG, N. R. (1973) Divinyl ether–maleic anhydride (pyran) copolymer used to demonstrate the effect of molecular weight on biological activity. *Nature* **246**: 160–162.

BUTLER, G. B. (1980) Synthesis, characterization and biological activity of pyran copolymers. In *Anionic Polymeric Drugs*, pp. 49–141, DONARUMA, L. G., OTTENBRITE, R. M. and VOGL, O. (Eds). John Wiley, New York.

BURLESON, G. R. and POLLARD, M. (1976) Chemotherapy of spontaneous transplantable prostatic adenocarcinomas in Lobund Wistar rats. *Fed. Proc.* **35**, Pt. I: 624.

CAHN, F. and LUBIN, M. (1973) Antiviral drugs and protein synthesis in reticulocyte lysates. *Intervirology* **I**: 376–385.

CAMPBELL, C. H. and RICHMOND, J. Y. (1973) Enhancement by two carboxylic acid interferon inducers of resistance stimulated in mice by foot and mouth disease vaccine. *Infect. Immun.* **7**: 199–204.

CAMYRE, K. P., GROELKE, J. W. and ALBRECHT, W. L. (1973) Viral photoinactivation—a property of some tilorone related compounds. 73rd Mtg. Amer. Soc. Microbiol., Miami Beach, March 6–11.

CAWEIN, M., LAMPKIN, B. C., TSUKIMOTO, I., REGELSON, W. and SCHIFF, G. (1975) Clinical studies with tilorone. *Symp. Proc. on Antivirals with Clinical Potential.* Stanford University, Aug. 26–29.

CHANDRA, P. (1974) Molecular approaches for designing antiviral and antitumor compounds. In *Topics in Current Chemistry*, Vol. 52, pp. 99–139, Springer-Verlag, Berlin.

CHANDRA, P., WILL, G., GERICKE, D. and GOTZ, A. (1974) Inhibition of DNA polymerases from RNA tumor viruses by tilorone and congeners: site of action. *Biochem. Pharmac.* **23**: 3259–3265.

CHANDRA, P. and WOLTERSDORF, M. (1974) Influence of tilorone and congeners on the secondary structure and template activity of DNA. *FEBS Lett.* **41**: 169–173.

CHANDRA, P. and WOLTERSDORF, M. (1976) Tilorone hydrochloride. A specific probe for A–T regions of duplex deoxyribonucleic acid. *Biochem. Pharmac.* **25**: 877–880.

CHANDRA, P., ZUNINO, F., GAUR, V. P., ZACCARA, A., WOLTERSDORF, M., LUONI, G. and GOTZ, A. (1972a) Mode of tilorone hydrochloride interaction to DNA and polydeoxyribonucleotides. *FEBS Lett.* **28**: 5–9.

CHANDRA, P., ZUNINO, F. and GOTZ, A. (1972b) Bis-deae-fluorenone: a specific inhibitor of DNA polymerases from RNA tumor viruses. *FEBS Lett.* **22**: 161–164.

CHANDRA, P., ZUNINO, F., ZACCARA, A., WACKER, A. and GOTZ, A. (1972c) Influence of tilorone hydrochloride on the secondary structure and template activity of DNA. *FEBS Lett.* **23**: 145–148.

CHANG, Y. H. and HOFFMAN, W. W. (1975) Suppression of adjuvant-induced arthritis by tilorone: lack of association with alterations of immune response, possibly mediated through interferon. *Pharmacologist* **17**: 226.

CHANG, Y. H. (1977) Adjuvant polyartheritis—II. Suppression by tilorone. *J. Pharmac. exp. Ther.* **203**: 156–161.

CHERTKOV, K. S., TALOSH, M., MOSINA, Z. M. and PREOBRAZHENSKIJ, T. T. (1978) Radioprotective effectiveness of tylorone. *Radiobiology* **19**: 455–458.

CHIRIGOS, M. A. and STYLOS, W. A. (1980) Immunomodulatory effect of various molecular weight maleic anhydride divinyl ethers and other agents *in vivo*. *Cancer Res.* **40**: 1967–1972.

CHREMOS, A. N., LAIDLAW, J. C. and RUSE, J. L. (1969) Effect of sulfated mucopolysaccharide (R01-8307) on the zona glomerulosa of regenerating rat adrenal glands and intact glands in sodium deprived rats. *Endocrinology* **85**: 337–341.

CLARK, W. G. and ROBINS, J. A. (1978) The antipyretic effect of tilorone HCl in the cat. *Br. J. Pharmac.* **62**: 281–287.

COFFEY, D. S.; BARRACK, E. R. and HESTON, W. D. (1973) The regulation of nuclear DNA template restrictions by acidic polymers. *Brady Research Monograph II*. Johns Hopkins University School of Medicine. Baltimore, Maryland.

COFFEY, D. S. (1976) Response of a prostatic adenocarcinoma to combined chemotherapy and pyran. 3rd Conf. on Modulation of host immune Resistance in the Prevention or Treatment of Induced Neoplasias. Virus Cancer Program. N. C. I., J. E. Fogarty Int. Ctr., Dec. 13–15.

COLLINS, A. L. T. and SONG, C. W. (1977) Studies on combined radiotherapy and immunotherapy using pyran copolymer on experimental tumors. *Radiat. Res.* **70**: 688.

COLLINS, F. M. (1975) Effect of tilorone treatment on intracellular microbial infections in specific-pathogen-free mice. *Antimicrob. Agents Chemother.* **7**: 447–452.

COLSKY, J., MCKENZIE, D. and HETTRICK, D. L. (1976) Complement reactivity of cancer patients measurements by immune lysis and immune adherents. *Cancer Res.* **27**: 2386–2394.

CORDELL-STEWART, B. and TAYLOR, M. W. (1973) Effect of viral double-stranded RNA on protein synthesis in intact cells. *J. Virol.* **11**: 232–237.

CURTISS, L. K., DEHEER, D. H. and EDGINGTON, T. S. (1977) *In vivo* suppression of the primary immune response by a species of low density serum lipoprotein. *J. Immunol.* **118**: 648–652.

DEAN, J. H., PADARATHSINGH, B. L. and KEYS, L. (1978) Response of murine leukemia to combined BCNU maleic anhydride vinyl ether (MVE) adjuvant therapy and correlation with macrophage activation by MVE in the *in vitro* growth inhibition assay. *Cancer Treat. Rep.* **62**: 1807–1816.

De Clercq, E. (1972) Future possibilities of interferon and interferon inducers in human medicine. *Tijdschp. Geneesk* **28**: 307–318.
De Clercq, E. and Merigan, T. C. (1970) Stimulation or inhibition of interferon production depending on time of cyclohexamide administration. *Virology* **42**: 799–802.
De Clercq, E. and Merigan, T. C. (1971) Bis-deae-fluorenone: mechanism of antiviral protection and stimulation of interferon production in the mouse. *J. infect. Dis.* **123**: 190–199.
De Clercq, E., Stewart, W. E. II, and De Somer, P. (1973) Increased toxicity of double-stranded ribonucleic acid in virus infected animals. *Infect. Immun.* **7**: 167–172.
Dennis, A. J., Wilson, H. E., Barker, A. D. and Rheins, M. S. (1972) Interferon induction in normal and leukemia human leukocyte cultures by tilorone hydrochloride. *Proc. Soc. exp. Biol. Med.* **141**: 782–785.
Dennis, L. H., Angeles, A., Baig, M. and Shnider, B. I. (1969) The effect of pyran polymer on the hemostatic mechanism. In *Proc. Soc. clin. Pharmacol.*
Diamantstein, T. (1973) Stimulation of humoral immune response by tilorone hydrochloride. *Immunology* **24**: 771.
Di Cioccio, R. A. and Sahai Srivastava, B. I. (1978) Inhibition of deoxyribonucleic acid polymerases from human cells and from simian sarcoma virus by pyran. *Biochem. J.* **175**: 519–524.
Di Luzio, N. R., Cook, J. A., Cohen, C., Rodregue, J., Kakoshis, P. and McNamee, R. B. (1978) Enhancement of the inhibitory effect of cyclophosphamide on experimental acute myelogenous leukemia by glucan immunopotentiators and response of serum lysosome in immune modulation and control of neoplasia by adjuvant therapy. Chirigos, M. A. (Ed). *Prog. Cancer Res. Ther.* **7**: 171–182.
Donahoe, J. P., Giambrone, J., Fletcher, O. J. and Kleven, S. H. (1977) *In vivo* function tests of the effect of tilorone and niridazole on cell-mediated immunity in chickens. *Am. J. vet. Res.* **38**: 2013–2017.
Donaruma, G., Ottenbrite, R. and Vogl, O. (1980) Eds. *Anionic Polymeric Drugs* (Polymers in Biology and Medicine Series) John Wiley, New York.
Edelstein, R. and Israel, L. (1974) Presented at Conference on Modulation of Host Immune Resistance in the Prevention or Treatment of Induced Neoplasias. N. I. H., N. C. I. Dec. 9th.
Eber, K. W. and Gavin, J. (1978) Drug modulation of *in vitro* immunoglobulin G synthesis. *Fed. Proc.* **37**: 838.
Edberg, S. C., Bottenbley, C. J. and Gam, K. (1976) Use of Sodium polyanethol sulfonate to selectively inhibit amino glycoside and polymixin antibiotics in a rapid blood level antibiotic assay. *Antimicrob. Agents Chemother.* **9**: 414–417.
Ekblom, P., Nordling, S. and Saxen, L. (1978) Inhibition of kidney tubule induction by charged polymers. *Cell Differentiation* **7**: 345–353.
El Azhary, R. and Mannering, G. J. (1979) Effects of interferon inducing agents (polyriboinosinic acid, polyribocytidylic acid, tilorone) on hepatic hemoproteins (cytochrome P450 catalase, tryptophane, 2,3-dioxygenase, mitochondrial cytochromes) heme metabolism and cytochrome P450 linked monoxygenase systems. *Molec. Pharmac.* **15**: 698–707.
Elzay, R. and Regelson, W. (1977) Effect of pyran copolymer on DMBA experimental oral carcinogenesis with golden Syrian hamster. *Research Annotation. J. D. Res.* **55**, No. 6: 1138.
Fahlbusch, B., Zschiesche, W., Schumann, I. and Tonew, E. (1977) Induction of lymphokines by tilorone. *Archs Immunol. Ther. Ex.*, **25**: 702–705.
Falk, R. E., Makowka, L., Nossal, N., Falk, J. A., Fields, J. E. and Asculai, S. S. (1979) Modulation of the immune response and control of tumor spread by a new synthetic compound. *Br. J. Surg.* **66**: 861–863.
Falk, R. E., Makowka, L., Nossal, N. A., Falk, J., Rotstein, L. E., Fields, J. E. and Asculai, S. S. (1980) Mechanism of increased antitumor immunity by a synthetic polymer. *J. Surg. Res.* **28**: 485–491.
Farbwerke Hoechst, A. G., (1963) Investigators Brochure: LB-504, Peson creme, Frankfurt, Germany.
Fiel, R. J., Mark, E. J. and Levine, H. I. (1976a) Polyanion induced nuclear swelling and microsphere formation. *J. Colloid Interface Sci.* **55**: 133–142.
Fiel, R. J., Mark, G. H. and Levine, H. I. (1976b) Divalent cation binding specificities and microsphere formation of pyran copolymer and related polycarbocylates. 172nd Am. Chem. Soc. Mtg. San Francisco, Calif. Aug. 29–Sept. 3.
Fiel, R. J., Mark G. H. and Levine, H. I. (1980) Physico-chemical characteristics and molecular pharmacology of pyran copolymer. In *Anionic Polymeric Drugs*, pp. 143–183, Donaruma, L. G., Ottenbrite, R. M. and Vogl, O. (Eds). John Wiley, New York.
Fisher, B. and Gebhardt, M. (1978) Comparative effects of *Corynebacterium parvum, Brucella abortus* extract, *Bacillus calmette–guerin*, glucan, levamisole and tilorone with or without cyclophosphamide on tumor growth, macrophage production and macrophage cytotoxicity in a murine mammary tumor model. *Cancer Treat. Rep.* **62**: 1919–1930.
Fisher, B., Linta, J., Hanlon, J. and Saffer, E. (1978) Further observations on the inhibition of tumor growth by *Corynebacterium parvum* with cyclophosphamide—V. Comparison of the effects of tilorone HCl, Levamisole, methanol-soluble fraction of *Mycobacterium butyricum*, BCG, and a nonviable aqueous extract of brucella *abortus* in treatment of mice with tumors. *J. natn. Cancer Inst.* **60**: 391–399.
Fitzwilliam, J. F. and Griffiths, J. F. (1976) Experimental encephalitis caused by herpes simplex virus: comparison of treatment with tilorone hydrochloride and phosphonoacetic acid. *J. infect. Dis.* **133** (Suppl.): A221–225.
Fleming, R. W., Albrecht, W. L., Andrews, E. R., Grisar, J. M., Horgan, S. W., Sill, A. D., Sweet, F. W. and Wenstrup, O. L. (1971) Some bis-basic substituted polycyclic aromatic compounds: a new class of antiviral interferon inducers. Int. Colloq. on Interferon and Interferon Inducers, Leuven, Belgium, Sept. 13–16.
Ford-Hutchinson, A. W., Bolms, J. P. and Walker, S. R. (1976) Tilorone HCl, a non-steroidal anti-inflammatory agent devoid of prostaglandin synthetase inhibitory activity. *J. Pharm. Pharmac.* **28**: 790–791.
Fornosi, F., Weiszfeiler, G. and Talas, M. (1971) Effect of tilorone hydrochloride on the experimental rabies of mice. *Acta microbiol. hung.* **18**: 327–331.

FREI, W. III, SCHABEL, F. M., Jr. and GOLDIN, A. (1974) Comparative chemotherapy of AKR lymphoma and human hematological neoplasia. *Cancer Res.* **34**: 184–193.

FRIEDLAENDER, G. E., MITCHELL, M. S. and MOSHER, M. R. (1974) Effect of 2,7-Bis{2-(diethylamino)ethoxy} fluoren-9-one dihydrochloride (tilorone) upon cell-mediated immunity in mice. *Cancer Res.* **34**: 304–307.

Gander, G. W. and GOODALE, F. (1973) Studies on the endogenous pyrogen released in response to poly I:poly C. The Pharmacology of Thermoregulation Symp., San Francisco, 1972, pp. 255–263, Karger, Basel.

GAUR, V. and CHANDRA, P. (1973) Subcellular distribution of ^{14}C-tilorone hydrochloride in tissues of mice and rats. *Naturwissenschaften* **60**: 1–3.

Gazdar, A. F. (1972) Brief communication: enhancement of tumor growth rate by interferon inducers. *J. natn. Cancer Inst.* **49**: 1435–1438.

GAZDAR, A. F., STEINBERG, A. D., SPAHN, G. F. and BARON, S. (1972) Interferon inducers: enhancement of viral oncogenesis in mice and rats. *Proc. Soc. exp. Biol. Med.* **139**: 1132–1137.

GAZITT, Y. (1981) Inhibition of induced L-ornithine decarboxylase stimulation and erythrodifferentiation in Friend erythroleukemia cells by 2',5'-isoadenylate trimer core. *Cancer Res.* **41**: 2959–2961.

GERRARD, T. L., AULTMAN, M. D. and KAPLAN, A. M. (1981) Role of adenosine deaminase in human monocyte differentiation. I. effects of EHNA on monocyte mediated tumor cell cytotoxicity and monocyte-mediated antibody dependent cytotoxicity. *J. Immunol.* In Press.

GIBSON, J. P., MEGEL, H., CAMYRE, K. P. and MICHAEL, J. G. (1976) Effect of tilorone on the lymphoid and interferon responses of athymic mice. *Proc. Soc. exp. Biol. Med.* **151**: 264–266.

GIDLUND, M., ORN, A., WIGZELL, H., SENIK, A. and GRESSER, I. (1979) Enhanced NK cell activity in mice injected with interferon and interferon inducers. *Nature.* **273**: 759–761.

GIDLUND, M., OJO, E. A., ANDERS, O., WIGZELL, H. and MURGITA, R. A. (1980) B-cells are of no importance for the maturation of natural killer cells in mice. *Scand. J. Immunol.* In Press.

GIRON, D. J., BALL, R. J., SCHMIDT, J. P. and PINDAK, F. F. (1972a) Effect of interferon on bacterial infections. *Antimicrob. Agents Chemother.* **1**: 90–81.

GIRON, D. J., PINDAK, F. F. and SCHMIDT, J. P. (1972b) Tilorone hydrochloride: Lack of correlation between interferon induction and viral protection. *Antimicrob. Agents Chemother.* **1**: 78–79.

GLAZ, E. T., STOGER, I., SZOLGAY, E. and TALAS, M. (1973) Antiviral activity and induction of interferon-like substance by quinacrine and acranil. *Antimicrob. Agents Chemother.* **3**: 537–541.

GLAZ, E. T. and TALAS, M. (1973) Continual serum interferon induced by prolonged drinking of tilorone solution. *Acta. virol.* **17**: 168.

GLAZ, E. T. and TALAS, M. (1975) Comparison of the activity of small molecular interferon inducers: tilorone and acridine drugs. *Archs Virol.* **48**: 375–384.

GLICK, J. L. (1967) The specificity of inhibition of tumor cell viability by DNA. *Cancer Res.* **27**: 2338–2341.

GLICK, J. L. (1968) Induction of an allogeneic-like inhibition by means of DNA obtained from untreated cells. In *Nucleic Aids in Immunology* pp. 414–436, PLESCIA, O. J. and BRAUN, W. (Eds). Springer-Verlag, New York.

GOODELL, E. M., MUNSON, A. E. and CARCHMAN, R. A. (1976) Growth and phagocytosis characteristics of P388Di cells in tissue culture. *Proc. 13th Natn. Mtg. Reticuloendothelial Soc.* Dec. 15–18, New Orleans, La.

GREEN, M. and GERARD, G. F. (1974) Inhibitors of oncornavirus RNA directed DNA polymerase and animal cell DNA polymerases. In *Progress in nucleic acid research and molecular biology*. Vol. 14, pp. 255–75, 322–34, COHN, W. E. (Ed). Academic Press, New York.

GREEN, M. and GERARD, G. F. (1974) Inhibitor of oncornavirus RNA directed DNA polymerase and animal cell DNA polymerases. In *Progress in nucleic acid research and molecular biology*. Vol. 14, pp. 255–75, 322–34, COHN, W. E. (ed). Academic Press, New York.

GREEN, M., RANKIN, A., GERARD, G. F., GRANDGENETT, D. P. and GREEN, M. R. (1975) Inhibition of purified DNA polymerase of RNA tumor viruses by fluoranthene derivatives and analogues of tilorone hydrochloride. *J. natn. Cancer Inst.* **55**: 433–442.

GREEN, S. and WEST, W. L. (1971) *In vitro* cytogenetic effects of tilorone HCl. *Pharmacologist* **13**: 260 (Abs).

GREEN, M., GRANOGENETT, D. P., RANKIN, A. M., CASSELL, D. M., GERARD, G. F., GURGO, C. and GREEN, M. R. (1974) Biochemical suppression of tumor virus activity. *Cancer* **34**: 1427–1438.

GRESSER, I. (1976) Antitumor Effect of Interferon. In *Cancer: A Comprehensive Treatise*, BECKER, F. (Ed). Plenum Press, New York.

GRESSER, I., MAYRY, C., BANDY, B. T., TOVER, B. and MAVNORY, M. T. (1978) Role of endogenous interferon in the anti-tumor effect of poly I:C and statolon as demonstrated by the use of antimouse interferon serum. *Int. J. Cancer* **21**: 72–77.

GROELKE, J. W., CAMYRE, K. P. and MAYER, G. O. (1975) Enhancement of interferon production *in vitro*: a property of tiloronepoly rI:rC/DEAE-dextran. *Proc. Soc. exp. Biol. Med.* **148**: 1044–1047.

GRUENEWALD, R. and LEVINE, S. (1976) Effect of Tilorone on susceptibility of mice to primary and secondary infection with Listeria monocytogenes. *Infect. Immun.* **13**: 1613–1618.

GUILMETTE, R. A. and LINDENBAUM, A. (1975) Progress in the use of pyran copolymers for decorporation of polymeric plutonium. *Proc. of the Workshop on the Biological Effects and Toxicity of Pu-239 and Ra-226*, Sun Valley, Idaho, October, In press.

HADWIGER, L. A. (1972) Increased levels of pisatin and phenylalanine ammonia lyase activity in *Pisum sativum* treated with antihistaminic, antiviral, antimalarial, tranquilizing and other drugs. *Biochem. Biophys. Res. Commun.* 46: 71–79.

HAHN, F. E. and CIAK, J. (1977) Bactericidal effects of combinations of Ampicillin with anti-plasmid compounds on *Salmonella typhimurium* Rt. *Antimicrob. Agents Chemother.* **11**: 176–177.

HAMILTON, L. (1972) Brookhaven, National Laboratories. Personal communication.

HARMEL, R. P. and ZBAR, B. (1975) Tumor suppression by pyran-copolymer: correlation with production of cytotoxic macrophages. *J. natn. Cancer Inst.* **54**: 989–988.

HERSH, E. M., GUTTERMAN, J. Y., ALEXANIAN, R., LOTZOVA, E. and MURPHY, S. G. (1981) A seven parameter host defense assay system for evaluating biological response modifiers (BRM) therapy of human cancer. *ABS American Soc. Clinical Oncology*. **22**: C156, 372.

HIRSH, M. S., BLOCK, P. H., WOOD, M. L. and MONACO, A. P. (1972) Effects of pyran copolymer on oncogeneic virus infections in immunosuppressed hosts. *J. Immunol.* **108**: No. 5: 1312–1318.

HOBBS, H. E., EADIE, S. P. and SOMERVILLE, F. (1961) Ocular lesions after treatment with chloroquine. *Br. J. Ophthal.* **45**: 284–297.

HODNETT, E., AMIRMOAZZAMI, J. and TIEN HAI TAI, J. (1978) Anionic polymers and biological activities; effects of some new polycarboxylic acids on the ascites sarcoma 180 of mice. *J. med. Chem.* **21**: 652–657.

HOFFMAN, P. F., RITTER, H. W. and KRUEGER, R. F. (1972) Tilorone hydrochloride stimulation of the primary immune response of mice. In *Advances in Antimicrobial and Antineoplastic Chemotherapy*. p. 217, HEJZLAR, M., SEMONSKY, M. and MOSAK, S., (Eds). Urban & Schwarzenberg, Munich.

ISRAEL, L., MILLER, P. and EDELSTEIN, R. (1977) Antitumor activity of tilorone in man: a preliminary report. 1st Conference on Modulation of Host Immune Resistance in the Prevention and Treatment of Induced Neoplasias. N.I.H., Bethesda, Md., pp. 145–152, CHIRIGOS, M. A. (Ed). U.S. Government Printing Office, Washington D.C.

JIRILLO, E., MONNO, R., MUNNO, I. and DE SANTIS, A. (1977a) Effects of Supernatants of Lymphocyte cultures stimulated with tilorone, on the electrophoretic mobility of human leukocytes. *Annali Sclavo* **19**: 1102–1108.

JIRILLO, E., MONO, R., MUNO, I., DE SANTIS, A. and FUMAROLA, D. (1977b) Effects of tilorone HCl on cellular immunity (leukocyte inhibiting factor production from human lymphocyte stimulated by E-coli lipopoly saccharide. *Boll. Ist. Sieroterapico Milan.* **56**: 299–302.

JOHANSEN, K. S., TALMAGE, D. W. and JOHANSEN, T. S. (1974) T-cell rosette formation in primates, pigs and guinea-pigs. The influence of immunosuppressive agents. *J. Allergy clin. Immunol.* **54**: 86–93.

KAPLAN, A. M., MORAHAN, P. S. and REGELSON, W. (1974) Induction of macrophage-mediated tumor-cell cytotoxicity by pyran copolymer. *J. natn. Cancer Inst.* **52**: 1919–1921.

KAPLAN, A. M. and MORAHAN, P. S. (1976a) Macrophage mediated tumor cell cytotoxicity. *Ann. N. Y. Acad. Sci.* **276**: 134–145.

KAPLAN, A. M. and MORAHAN, P. S. (1976b) Macrophage activity against viruses and tumor cells and in regulation of lymphoproliferation. *Proc. 13th Natn. Meeting of Reticuloendothelial Society*, Dec. 15–18, p. 60.

KAPLAN, A. M. and MORAHAN, P. S. (1976c) Macrophage mediated tumor cell cytotoxicity. *Ann. N.Y. Acad. Sci.* **776**: 134–145.

KAPLAN, A. M., BAIRD, L. G. and MORAHAN, P. S. (1977a) Macrophage regulation of tumor cell growth and mitogen induced blastogenesis. In *Control of Neoplasia by Modulation of the Immune System*, (Prog. Cancer Res. Ther. series, Vol. 2), pp. 461–468, CHIRIGOS, M. A. (Ed). Raven Press, New York.

KAPLAN, A. M., WALKER, P. L. and MORAHAN, P. S. (1977b) Tumor cell cytotoxicity versus cytostasis of pyran activated macrophages. 1st Conf. on Modulation of Host Immune Resistance in the Prevention or Treatment of Induced Neoplasias. *Fogarty Int. Center Proc.* No. **28**, pp. 277–286, U.S. Government Printing Office, Washington, D.C.

KAPLAN, A. M. and MOHANA KUMAR, U. (1977) Expression of a "new" cell surface antigen on activated murine macrophages. *J. exp. Med.* **146**: 1461–1466.

KAPLAN, A. M., BROWN, J., COLLINS, J. M., MORAHAN, P. S. and SNODGRASS, M. J. (1978a) Mechanisms of macrophage-mediated tumor cell cytotoxicity. *J. Immunol.* **121**: 1781.

KAPLAN, A. M., COLLINS, J. M., MORAHAN, P. S. and SNODGRASS, M. J. (1978b) Potential mechanisms of macrophage mediated tumor cell toxicity. *Cancer Treat. Rep.* **62**: 1823–1829.

KAPLAN, A., CONNOLY, K. and REGELSON, W. (1980) Induction of aberrant tumor cell division using 5-FU or activated macrophages. In *proceedings on the host-invader interplay*. pp. 429–483, VAN DEN BOSSCHE, H. (Ed). Elsevier/North Holland, Netherlands.

KAPLAN, A. M. (1980) Antitumor activity of synthetic polymers. In *Anionic polymeric drugs*. (Polymers in Biology and Medicine series), pp. 227–253, DONNARUMA, L. G., OTTENBRITE, R. M. and VOGL, O. (Eds). John Wiley, New York.

KAPUSTA, M. A. and MENDELSON, J. (1969) The inhibition of adjuvant disease in rats by interferon inducing agent pyran copolymer. *Arthr. Rheum.* **12**, No. 5: 463–471.

Kartasheva, A. L., *et al.* (1977) Nature of animal sensitization to Y Pestis EV induced by pyran copolymer. *J. Microbiol. Epidemiol. Immunobiol.* (Russ.) **11**: 143–144.

KATZ, E., MARGALITH, E. and WINER, B. (1976) The effect of tilorone hydrochloride on the growth of several animal viruses in tissue cultures. *J. gen. Virol.* **31**: 125–129.

KAUFMAN, H. E., CENTRIFANTO, Y. M., ELLISON, E. D. and BROWN, D. C. (1971) Tilorone hydrochloride: human toxicity and interferon stimulation. *Proc. Soc. exp. Biol. Med.* **137**: 357–360.

KOLISKOVA, D., BORECKY, L. and ORAVEC, C. (1979) The effect of interferon induction on complement level in rats. *Acta. biol. med. germ.* **38**: 837–841.

KOPILA, K., SMITH, C. and RUBIN, A. A. (1971) Methylcholanthrene transplants. *J. reticuloendol. Soc.* **9**: 447–450.

KRIPKE, M. L. and BORSUS, T. (1974) Accelerated development of benzapyrene-induced skin tumors in mice treated with pyran copolymer *J. natn. Cancer Inst.* **53**: 1409–1410.

KRUEGER, R. F. and MAYER, G. D. (1970) Tilorone hydrochloride: an orally active antiviral agent. *Science* **169**: 1213–1214.

KRUEGER, R. F., MAYER, G. O., YOSHIMURA, S. and LUDWIG, K. A. (1970) *In vivo* evaluations of tilorone hydrochloride against Semliki forest virus. *Antimicrob. Agents Chemother.* 486–490.

KRUEGER, R. F., MAYER, G. D., CAMYRE, K. P. and YOSHIMURA, S. (1971) Comparative interferon and antiviral responses of tilorone hydrochloride and other bis-basic substituted polycyclic aromatic compounds. Int. Colloq. on Interferon and Interferon Inducers, Leuven, Belgium, Sept. 13–16.

KUPERMINC, M. and GELBER, R. (1976) Tilorone: a phase II trial for advanced breast carcinoma. *Proc. Am. Assoc. Cancer Res.* **17**: 260 (Abs.).
LEAVITT, T. J., MERIGAN, T. C. and FREEMAN, J. M. (1971) Hemolytic–uremic-like syndrome following polycarboxylate interferon induction. Treatment of Dawson's inclusion-body encephalitis. *Am. J. Dis. Child.* **121**: 43–47.
LEESON, G. A., BIEDENBACH S. A., CHAN, K. Y., GIBSON, J. P. and WRIGHT, G. J. (1976) Decrease in the activity of the drug-metabolizing enzymes of rat liver following the administration of tilorone hydrochloride. *Drug. metab. Dispos.* **4**: 232–238.
LEVINE, S., GIBSON, J. P. and MEGEL, H. (1974) Selective depletion of thymus dependent areas in lymphoid tissue hy tilorone. *Proc. Soc. exp. Biol. Med.* **146**: 245–248.
LEVINE, S. and SOWINSKI, R. (1976a) Necrotic myelopathy myelomalacia) in rats with allergic encephalomyelitis treated with tilorone. *Am. J. Pathol.* **82**: 381–392.
LEVINE, S. and SOWINSKI, R. (1976b) Endotoxin toxicity in rats is enhanced by tilorone. *Proc. Soc. exp. Biol. Med.* **151**: 329–332.
LEVINE, S., SOWINSKI, R. and HOENIG, E. M. (1975) Nuclear bodies produced in astrocytes by tilorone. *Am. J. Pathol.* **78**: 319–332.
LEVY, L., AIZER, F., NG, H. and WELCH, T. Y. (1978) The effects of tilorone on bacterial infections of mice. *Lepr. Rev.* **49**: 215–222.
LIEBERMAN, M., SCHAFER, T. W. and CAME, P. E. (1973) Chemotherapy of cutaneous herpes virus infection of hairless mice. *J. invest. Derm.* **60**: 203–206.
LINDENBAUM, A., ROSENTHAL, M. W. and GUILMETTE, R. A. (1975) Retention of polymeric plutonium in mouse tissues as affected by antiviral compounds and their analogs. *Proc. of I.A.E.A. Symp. on diagnosis and treatment of internally deposited radionucleotides.* Vienna, Austria, Dec. IAEA-SR-6/22.
LITTLE, A. P. (1964) Preclinical toxicology of NSC 46015 hydrolysate report to Cancer Chemotherapy National Service Center, March 5, 1964, Contract No. SA-43-ph-3789. Arthur D. Little, Inc. Boston, Mass.
LUKAS, R. and HRUSKOVA, J. (1968) *In vivo* induction of an interferon-like inhibitor by kannamycin. *Acta virol. Prague* **12**: 263–267.
LULLMAN, H., LULLMAN-RAUCH, R. and WASSERMAN, D. (1973) Drug induced lipidosis. *Ger. Med.* **3**: 128–135.
MACKENZIE, R. D. and SCHATZMAN, G. L. (1975) The *in vitro* and *in vivo* evaluation of tilorone hydrochloride as a platelet aggregation inhibitor. *Scand. J. Haematol.* **15**: 58–62.
MAJESKI, J. A. and STINNETT, J. D. (1977) Chemoattractant properties of *Corynebacterium parvum* and pyran copolymer for human monocytes and neutrophils. *J. natn. Cancer Inst.* **58**: 781–783.
MANNERING G. J., EL-AZHARY, R. and RENJON, K. W. (1976) Depression of the hepatic cytochrome p450 monoxygenase system by administering interferon inducing agents. Microsomes and Drug Oxidations IIIrd Int. Symp. **357**: 1039–1040.
MANSELL, P. W. A., ROWDEN, G. and HAMMER, C. (1978) Clinical experiences with the use of glucan. In *Immune Modulation and Control of Neoplasia by Adjuvant Therapy.* (Prog. Cancer Res. Ther. series, Vol. 7) pp. 255–280, CHIRIGOS, M. A. (Ed). Raven Press, New York.
MARKS, N., GRYNBAUM, A. and LEVINE, S. (1977) Proteolytic enzymes in ordinary, hyperacute, monocytic and passive transfer forms of experimental allergic encephalomyelitis. *Brain Res.* **123**: 147–157.
MATHÉ, G. (1973) Personal communication.
MATYASOVA, J., SKALKA, M. and CEJKOVA, M. (1974) The importance of molecular weight of inorganic polyphosphates for their interaction with deoxyribonucleoprotein of animal tissue. *Folia biol.* (*Praha*) **20**: 193–204.
MAYER, G. D. and KRUEGER, R. F. (1970a) Tilorone hydrochloride: A new antiviral agent and interferon inducer. *Proc. Int. Congr. infect. Dis.*, Vienna, Aug. 31–Sept. 5., pp. 245–255.
MAYER, G. D. and KRUEGER, R. F. (1970b) Tilorone hydrochloride: Mode of action. *Science* **169**: 1214–1215.
MCCORD, R. S., BREINIG, M. K. and MORAHAN, P. S. (1976) Antiviral effects of pyran against systemic infection of mice with herpes simplex virus type II. *Antimicrob. Agents Chemother.* **10**: 28–33.
MEGEL, H., RAYCHAUDHURI, A., GOLDSTEIN, S., KINSOLVING, C. R., SHEMANO, I. and MICHAEL, J. G. (1974a) Tilorone: its selective effects on humoral and cell-mediated immunity. *Proc. Soc. exp. Biol. Med.* **145**: 513–518.
MEGEL, H., RAYCHAUDHURI, A., SHEMANO, I. and GIBSON, J. P. (1974b) Immunological responses with tilorone. In *Proc. Fogarty Int. Center* Dec. 9–11, 1974. U.S. Government Printing Office, Washington, D.C.
MEGEL, H., RAYCHAUDHURI, A., SHEMANO, I., THOMAS, L. L. and BEAVER, T. H. (1974c) Tilorone hydrochloride as an anti-inflammatory agent. *Fed. Proc.* **33**: 558.
MEGEL, H., RAYCHAUDHURI, A. and THOMAS, L. (1976) The effect of tilorone on the local graft-versus-host reaction in rats. *Transplantation* **21**: 81–83.
MEGEL, H. (1977) The immunologic and anti-inflammatory properties of tilorone hydrochloride in animals. Int. Symp. New Anti-Inflammatory Drugs, June 11–12, Pisa, Italy.
MEGEL, H., RAYCHAUDHURI, A., SHEMANO, I. and GIBSON, J. P. (1977) Immunological responses with tilorone—update. Conference on modulation of host immune resistance in the prevention or treatment of induced neoplasias. N.I.H., Bethesda, Md. pp. 103–111 CHIRIGOS, M. A. (Ed). U.S. Government Printing Office, Washington, D.C.
MEGEL, H., RAYCHAUDHURI, A., BAKER, M. and BEAVER, T. H. (1978) The Immunopharmacologic and anti-inflammatory properties of RMI 9563 with special reference to its effect on the complement system agents in its actions 8/3: pp. 218–228, Birkau Ser Verlag, Basel.
MERIGAN, T. C. (1967a) Induction of circulating interferon by synthetic anionic polymers of known composition. *Nature* (*London*) **214**: 416–417.
MERIGAN, T. C. (1967b) Discussion, Ciba Foundation Symposium on Interferon. pp. 50–60, WOLSTENHOLME, G. E. W. and O'CONNOR, M. (Eds). J. A. Churchill Ltd., London.
MERIGAN, T. C. and FINKELSTEIN, M. S. (1968) Interferon-stimulating and *in vivo* antiviral effects of various synthetic anionic polymers. *Virology* **35**: 363–374.

MERIGAN, T. C. and REGELSON, W. (1967) Interferon induction in man by a synthetic polyanion of defined composition. *New Engl. J. Med.* **277**: 1283–1287.
MIHICH, E., SIMPSON, C. L., REGELSON, W. and MULHERN, P. I. (1960) Pharmacological study of ammoniated ethylene maleic polymer, m.w. 20,000–30,000 (AEMA 20–30) *Fed. Proc.* **19**: A 142.
MILLER, G., BERLOWITZ, L. and REGELSON, W. (1971) Chromatin and histones in mealy bug cell explants: Activation and decondensation of facultative heterochromatin by a synthetic polyanion. *Chromasoma* **32**: 251–261.
MILLER, G. J., BERLOWITZ, L. and REGELSON, W. (1972) Chromatin and histones in hen erythrocyte nuclei: Morphologic change induced by selective binding of histones with a synthetic polyanion. *Exp. Cell. Res.* **71**: 409–421.
MOBRAATEN, L. E., DE MAEYER, E. and DE MAEYER-GUIGNARD, L. (1973) Prolongation of allograft survival in mice by inducers of interferon. *Transplantation* **16**: 415–420.
MOHR, S. J., CHIRIGOS, M. A. and FUHRMAN, F. S. (1971) Enhancement of a tumor allograft in BALB/C × DBA/2F, mice by pyran copolymer. *Cancer Res.* **36**: 1315–1319.
MOHR, S. J., CHIRIGOS, M. A., FUHRMAN, F. S. and PRYOR, J. W. (1975) Pyran copolymer found to be effective adjuvant to chemotherapy against a murine leukemia and solid tumor. *Cancer Res.* **35**: 3750–3754.
Mohr, S. J. (1976) Potentiation of L1210 vaccine with pyran adjuvant. In *3rd Conf. on Modulation of Host Immune Resistance in the Prevention or Treatment of Induced Neoplasias.* Virus Cancer Program. N.C.I., J. E. Fogarty Int. Center, Dec. 13–15.
MOHR, S. J. and CHIRIGOS, M. A. (1977) Potentiation of a tumor cell vaccine by pyran copolymer. In *Control of Neoplasia by Modulation of the Immune System.* (Prog. Cancer Res. Ther. series, Vol. 2) pp. 421–435, CHIRIGOS, M. A. (Ed). Raven Press, New York.
MOHR, S. J. and CHIRIGOS, M. A. (1978) Immunopotentiation against the L1210 leukemia by pyran copolymer and crude tumor antigen. In *Immune Modulation and Control of Neoplasia by Adjuvant Therapy.* (Prog. Cancer Res. Ther. series, Vol. 7) pp. 415–426, CHIRIGOS, M. A. (Ed). Raven Press, New York.
MORAHAN, P. S., MUNSON, A. E., REGELSON, W. and HAMILTON, L. D. (1971) Pyran and polynucleotides: comparison of biologic activities. Int. Colloq. on Interferon and Interferon Inducers. Leuven, Belgium, Sept.
MORAHAN, P. S., MUNSON, A. E., REGELSON, W., COMMERFORD, S. L. and HAMILTON, L. D. (1972a) Antiviral activity and side effects of polyriboinosinic cytidylic acid complexes as effected by molecular size. *Proc. natn. Acad. Sci. U.S.A.* **69**: 842–846.
MORAHAN, P. S., REGELSON, W. and MUNSON, A. E. (1972) Pyran and polyribonucleotides: Differences in biological activities. *Antimicrobial. Agents Chemother.* **2**: 16–22.
MORAHAN, P. S., MUNSON, J. A., BAIRD, L. G., KAPLAN, A. M. and REGELSON, W. (1974) Antitumor action of pyran copolymer and tilorone against Lewis lung Carcinoma and B-16 melanoma. *Cancer Res.* **34**: 506–511.
MORAHAN, P. S. and KAPLAN A. M. (1976a) Host cells associated with Lewis lung carcinoma. *Proc. 13th natn. Mtg. reticuloendothl. Soc.*, Dec. 15–18, p. 71.
MORAHAN, P. S., KAPLAN, A. (1976b) Macrophage activation and antitumor activity of biologic and synthetic agents. *Int. J. Cancer* **17**: 82–89.
MORAHAN, P. S. (1977) Antitumor and antiviral function of activated macrophages. In *3rd Conference on Modulation of Host Immune Resistance in the Prevention or Treatment of Induced Neoplasias.* Virus Cancer Program, N.C.I., J. E. Fogarty Center, Dec. 13–15.
MORAHAN, P. S. and KAPLAN, A. (1977) Macrophage mediated tumor resistance. In *Control of Neoplasia by Modulation of the Immune System.* (Prog. Cancer Res. Ther., Vol. 2) pp. 449–459, CHIRIGOS, M. A. (Ed). Raven Press, New York.
MORAHAN, P. S., BARNES, D. W. and MUNSON, A. E. (1978) Relationship of molecular weight to antiviral and antitumor activities and toxic effects of maleic anhydride divinyl ether (MVE) polyanions. *Cancer Treat. Rep.* **62**: 1797–1805.
MORAHAN, P. S., CLINE, P. F., BREINIG, M. C. and MURRAY, B. K. (1979) Effect of pyran on latency after herpes simplex virus infections. *Antimicrob. Agents Chemother.* **15**: 547–553.
MUNSON, A. E. and WOOLES, W. R. (1969) The relationship between hexobarbital metabolism and reticuloendothelial (RE) activity *Pharmacologist* **11**: 174, 261.
MUNSON, A. E., REGELSON, W., LAWRENCE, W., JR and WOOLES, W. R. (1970) The biphasic response of the reticuloendothelial system (RES) produced by pyran copolymer and its relation to immunologic response. *J. reticuloendothl. Soc.* **7**: 375–385.
MUNSON, A. E. and REGELSON, W. (1971) Sensitization to endotoxin by pyran copolymer. *Proc. Soc. exp. Biol. and Med.* **137** (2): 553–557.
MUNSON, A. E., MUNSON, J. A., REGELSON, W. and WAMPLER, G. L. (1972a) Effect of tilorone hydrochloride and congeners on reticuloendothelial system, tumors, and the immune response. *Cancer Res.* **32**: 1397–1403.
MUNSON, A. E., REGELSON, W. and MUNSON, J. A. (1972b) Effect of four antiviral agents on hepatic micrisomal mixed functional oxidase enzymes. *Toxic. appl. Pharmac.* **22**: 299–300.
NIBLACK, J. F. (1971) Interferon inducers in antiviral research. 23rd Int. Congr. Pure and Applied Chem. Special Lectures, Boston, July 25–30, Vol. III, pp. 111–131.
OBARA, Y., WEINFIELD, H. and SANDBERG, A. A. (1975) Detection by means of cell fusion of macromolecular synthesis involved in the reconstruction of the nuclear envelope in mitosis. *J. Cell Biol.* **64**: 378–388.
OHBUCHI, S. (1968) Suppression of antibody formation by the reticuloendothelial (RES) blockade. I. Effects of the RES-blockade with macromolecular polyvinyl pyrrolidone. *Acta med. okayama* **22**: 37–49.
OLSON, W. H., SIMONS, J. A. and HALLAAS, G. (1978) Therapeutic trial of tilorone in ALS: Lack of benefit in a double-blind, placebo controlled study. *Neurology* **28**: 1293–1295.
ORMAI, S., HAGENBEEK, A., PAKLOVITS, M. and VAN BEKKUM, D. W. (1973) Changes of lymphocyte kinetics in the normal rat induced by the lymphocyte mobilizing agent polymethacrylic acid. *Cell Tiss. Kinet.* **6**: 407–423.

Orn, A., Gidlund, M. and Wigzell, H. (1979) Genetics of interferon induced increased NK activity. *Abs. 9th Scand. Soc. Immunol.* p. 156.

Ottenbrite, R. M. and Regelson, W. (1976) Biological activity of water soluble polymers. In *Encyclopedia of Polymer Sciences and Technology*, Suppl. Vol. 2, Bikales, H. M. (Ed). Interscience Publishers.

Ottenbrite, R. M., Regelson, W., Kaplan, A. M., Carchman, R., Morahan, P. S. and Munson, A. E. (1978) Biological activity of polycarboxamic acid polymers. In *Polymeric Drugs*, pp. 263, Donaruma, L. G. and Vogl, O. (Eds). Academic Press, New York.

Ottenbrite, R. M., Enright, N., Munson, A. and Kaplan, A. M. (1979) Biologic activity of a new micyclic-ether polyanion. *Polymer Preprints* **20**: 600–604.

Ottenbrite, R. M. (1980) Structure and Biological Activities of Some Polyanionic Polymers. In *Anionic Polymeric Drugs*. (Polymers in Biology and Medicine series) pp. 21–48, Donaruma, L. G., Ottenbrite, R. M. and Vogl, O. (Eds). John Wiley, New York.

Papamatheakis, J. D., Chirigos, M. A. and Schultz, R. M. (1978a) Effect of dose, route and timing of pyran copolymer therapy against Madison lung carcinoma. In *Immune Modulation and Control of Neoplasia by Adjuvant Therapy*. (Prog. Cancer Res. Ther. series, Vol. 7) pp. 427–438, Chirigos, M. A. (Ed). Raven Press, New York.

Papamatheakis, J. D., Schultz, R. M., Chirigos, M. A. and Massicot, J. G. (1978b) Cell and tissue distribution of ^{14}C-labelled pyran copolymer. *Cancer Treat. Rep.* **62**: 1845–1851.

Papas, T. S., Woods, W. A. and Chirigos, M. A. (1974a) Active site probes and the selective inhibition of RNA tumor viral DNA polymerase, In *1st Conf. on Modulation of Host Immune Resistance in the Prevention or Treatment of Induced Neoplasias. Fogarth Int. Center Proc.* U.S. Govt. Printing Office, Bethesda, Md. Dec. 9–11.

Papas, T. S., Pry, T. W. and Chirigos, M. A. (1974b) Inhibition of RNA-dependent DNA polymerase of avian myeloblastosis virus by pyran copolymer. *Proc. natn. Acad. Sci. USA* **7**: 367–370.

Pavilidis, N. A., Schultz, R. M., Chirigos, M. A. and Luetzeler, J. (1978) Effect of maleic anhydride-divinyl ether copolymers on experimental M109 metastases and macrophage tumoricidal function. *Cancer Treat. Rep.* **62**: 1817–1822.

Pearson, J. W., Chirigos, M. A., Chaparas, S. D. and Sher, N. A. (1974) Combined drug and immunostimulation therapy against a syngeneic murine leukemia. *J. natn. Cancer Inst.* **52**: 463–468.

Pearson, J. W., Gibson, W. T. and Chirigos, M. A. (1970) Use of a murine sarcoma virus in an *in vivo* assay for anti-viral and anti-tumor agents. *Cancer Res.* **30**: 2024–2028.

Philips, F. S., Fleisher, M., Hamilton, L. D., Schwartz, M. K. and Sternberg, S. S. (1971) Polyinosinic–polycytidylic acid toxicity. In *Biological Effects of Polynucleotides*, pp. 259–273, Beers, R. F. and Braun, W. (Eds). Springer-Verlag, New York.

Phillips, B. M., Hartnagel, R. E., Kraus, P. J., Tamako R. P. Fronesca, E. C. and Kowlaski, R. L. (1971) Systemic toxicity of polyinosinic acid: Polycytidylic acid in rodents and dogs. *Toxicol. appl. Pharmac.* **18**: 220–239.

Pindak, F. F. (1970) Protection of mice against bacterial infection by interferon inducers. *Infect. Immun.* **1**: 271–273.

Pierre, M. and Loeb, J. E. (1977) Regulation of a microsomal protein Kinase from mouse liver by hemin and the interferon inducer tilorone. *Biochem. Biophys. Res. Commun.* **77**: 481–488.

Pitha, A. J. (1980) Nucleic acids and sulfate and phosphate polymers. In *Anionic Polymeric Drugs* (Polymers in Biology and Medicine series) pp. 000–000, Donaruma, L. G., Ottenbrite, R. M. and Vogl, O. (Eds). John Wiley, New York.

Portnoy, J. and Merigan, T. C. (1971) The effect of interferon and interferon inducers on avian influenza. *J. infect. Dis.* **124**: 545–552.

Powell, M. L., Hersh, E. M., Gutterman, J. U., Zander, A. R., Granati, L., Alexanian, G., Hortobagyi, G. and Murphy, S. G. (1981) Phase I study of MVE-2 therapy in human cancer. *Abs Am. Ass. Cancer Res.* **22**: 750, p. 189.

Pratten, M. K., Duncan, R., Cable, A. Z., Schnee, R., Ringsdorf, H. and Lloyd, J. B. (1981) Pinocytic uptake of divinyl ether maleic anhydride (pyran copolymer) and its failure to stimulate pinocytosis. *Chem-Biol. Interact.* **35**: 319–330.

Przybylski, M., Zaharko, D. S., Chirigos, M. A., Adamson, R. H., Schultz, R. M. and Ringsdorf, H. (1978) Divema-methotrexrate immune-adjuvant role of polymeric carriers linked to antitumor agents. *Cancer Treat. Rep.* **62**: 1837–1843.

Pucetti, P. and Giampietri, A. (1978) Immunopharmacology of pyran copolymer. *Pharm. Res. Commun.* **10**: 489–501.

Quadrifoglio, P., Crescenzi, V., Prota, G., Capiello, L., Di Marco, A. and Zunino, F. (1975) The interaction of natural tetraazacyclopentazulene dyes with DNA and their effects on the DNA

Raychaudhuri, A. and Megel, H. (1977) The effect of tilorone on immunoglobulin-bearing lymphocytes (B-cells) in peripheral blood and spleen of mice. *J. reticuloendothl. Soc.* **20**: 127–134.

Rabinovitch, M. and Manejias, R. C. (1974) Anti-interferon globulin inhibits macrophage phagocytic enhancement *in vivo* by tilorone on Newcastles disease virus. *Cell Immunol.* **39**: 402–406.

Rana, M. W., Pinkerton, H. and Rankin, A. (1975) Effect of rifamycin and tilorone derivatives of Friend virus leukemia in mice. *Proc. Soc. exp. Biol. Med.* **150**: 32–35.

Regelson, W. and Holland, J. F. (1962) The effect of an anionic polyelectrolyte (polyethylene sulfonate) in patients with cancer. The clinical pharmacology of a macromolecule. *Clin. Pharmac. Ther.* **3**: 730–749.

Regelson, W., Munson, A. E. and Merigan, T. C. (1967) The control of susceptibility to leukemia virus infection and tumor induction by synthetic polyanions and other compounds which induce or block interferon production: their possible relation to the reticuloendothelial system. *Abs. Vth Int. Cong. on Chemotherapy, V. Weiner Med. Akad.* 407.

Regelson, W. (1967) Prevention and treatment of Friend leukemia virus infection by interferon inducing synthetic polyanions. The reticuloendothelial system and artherosclerosis. *Adv. exp. Med. Biol.* **1**: 315–332.

REGELSON, W. (1968a) Thrombocytopenic and related physiologic effects of heparin and heparinoids: a macromolecular-induced syndrome? *Hematol. Rev.* **1**: 193–227.

REGELSON, W. (1968b) The growth regulating activity of polyanions. *Adv. Cancer Res.* **11**: 223–287.

REGELSON, W. (1968c) Anionic polyelectrolytes as antimitotic agents. *Adv. Chemother.* **3**: 303–371.

REGELSON, W. (1970) Part I: The biologic activity of polyanions: A brief review of antitumor, antiviral antibacterial action and some theories in regard to mechanism. *L'Interferon* **6**: 353–379.

REGELSON, W., MUNSON, A. E. (1970) The reticuloendothelial effects of interferon inducers: Polyanionic and non-polyanionic phylaxis against microorganisms. *Ann. N.Y. Acad. Sci.* **173**: 831–841.

REGELSON, W., MUNSON, A. E., MUNSON, J. A., MAYER, G. D. and KRUEGER, R. F. (1970a) The phagocytic stimulating activity of a new oral interferon inducer: tilorone hydrochloride. *Proc. Int. Mtg. Ret. Soc.* Freiburg, Germany, July 29–Aug. 1 (6th Mtg.) (Abs).

REGELSON, W., MUNSON, A. E. and the Eastern Oncology Study Group (1970b) Polyanions as antitumor agents: the biologic activity and reticuloendothelial activity of pyran copolymer and poly: inosinic and cytidylic acid (poly rI:rC). Xth Int. Cancer Cong., Houston, Texas.

REGELSON, W., MUNSON, A. E., WOOLES, W. R., LAWRENCE, W., JR. and LEVY, H. (1970c): Part II: Reticuloendothelial action of interferon inducers: the biphasic action of pyran copolymer and polynucleotides on phagocytic and immunologic response. *L'interferon* **6**: 381–395.

REGELSON, W., MUNSON, A. E. and WOOLES, W. (1970d) The biologic activity of synthetic polymers: Interferon inducers and reticuloendothelial response: polyanions. *Interferon Symp. Series Immunobiol. Standard* **14**: 227–236.

REGELSON, W. (1973a) Host modulation of resistance to infection and neoplasia. *Medicinal Chemistry* 8, **17**: 160–172.

REGELSON, W. (1973b) The biologic activity of water-soluble polymers. In *Water Soluble Polymers II*, pp. 161–177, BIKALES, N. M. (Ed). Plenum Press, New York.

REGELSON, W., MORAHAN, P. S., KAPLAN, A. M., BAIRD, L. G. and MUNSON, J. A. (1974) Synthetic polyanions: molecular weight, macrophage activation and immunologic response. In *Activation of Macrophages*, pp. 98–110, WAGNER, W. H. and HAHN, H. (Eds). Excerpta Medica, Elsevier, New York.

REGELSON, W. (1974) The antimitotic activity of polyanions: Heparin and heparinoids. *J. Med.* **5**: 50–68.

REGELSON, W., MORAHAN, P. and KAPLAN, A. M. (1975) The role of molecular weight in pharmacologic and biologic activity of synthetic polyanions. In *Polyelectrolytes and their application*, pp. 131–144, REMBAUM, A. and SELIGNY, E. (Eds). Reidel Publ., Dordrecht-Holland.

REGELSON, W. (1976) Clinical immunoadjuvant studies with tilorone DEAA fluorene (RMI 11,002), corynebacterium parvum and some observations on the role of host resistance and herpes-like lesions on tumor growth. *Ann. N.Y. Acad. Sci.* **277**: 269–287.

REGELSON, W., SHNIDER, B. I., COLSKY, J., OLSON, K. B., HOLLAND, J. F., JOHNSTON, JR., C. L. and DENNIS, L. H. (1978) Clinical study of the synthetic polyanion pyran copolymer (NSC 46015) diveema and its role in future clinical trials. In *Immune Modulation and Control of Neoplasia by Adjuvant Therapy*, pp. 469–490, CHIRIGOS, M. A. (Ed). Raven Press, New York.

REGELSON, W. (1978) Future direction of synthetic polyanions (pyran copolymer) *Cancer Treat. Rep.* **62**: 1853–1856.

REGELSON, W. (1979) The biologic activity of polyanions: past history and new prospectives. In *Microsymposium Volume of J. Polymer Science, Symposium* **66**: 483–538, SEDLACEK, B. (Ed).

REGELSON, W. (1980) Clinical and Research concepts regrading polyanions and starch microspheres. In *Antionic Polymeric Drugs*. (Polymers in Biology and Medicine Series), pp. 303–325, DONARUMA, L. G., OTTENBRITE, R. M. and VOGL, O. (Eds). John Wiley, New York.

REHOVSKY, M. W., NEWBERNE, J. W. and GIBSON, J. P. (1970) Effects of an oral interferon-inducer on the hematopoietic and reticuloendothelial system. *Toxicol. appl. Pharmac.* **17**: 556–558.

RENTON, K. W., KEYLER, D. E. and MANNERING, G. J. (1979) Depression of inductive effects of phenobarbital and 3-methycholanthrene on ascorbic acid synthesis and hepatic cytochrome P-450 linked monooxygenase systems by the interferon inducer, poly I:C and tilorone. *Biochem. Biophys. Res. Commun.* **88**: 1017–1023.

RENTON, K. W. and MANNERING, G. J. (1976a) Depression of the hematopoietic cytochrome P-450 monooxygenase system by administered tilorone. *Drug Metab. Dispos.* **4**: 223–231.

RENTON, K. W. and MANNERING, G. J. (1976b) Depression of hepatic cytochrome P-450 dependent monooxygenase systems with administered interferon inducing agents. *Biochem. Biophys. Res. Commun.* **73**: 343–348.

RHEINS, M. S., BARKER, A. D. and WILSON, H. E. (1971) Therapeutic effects of a series of non-viral interferon inducers on a viral-induced leukemia. *Can. J. Microbiol.* **17**: 1257–1265.

RHOADS, A., ROYE, D., WEST, W. and MORRIS, H. P. (1971) The effect of tilorone on the growth rate of Morris hepatomas 777, 392A, and Walker 256 carcinosarcoma. *Am. chem. Soc.* Washington, D.C. Sept. 13–16. (162nd Mtg.).

RHOADS, A. R., WEST, W. L. and MORRIS, H. P. (1973) Interferon induction and suppression of solid tumor growth in rats by tilorone hydrochloride. *Res. Commun. chem. Pathol. Pharmac.* **6**: 741–750.

RICHMOND, J. Y. and CAMPBELL, C. H. (1973) Foot and mouth disease virus: protection induced in infected mice by two orally administered interferon inducers. *Arch. Gesamte Virusforsch* **42**: 102–105.

RICHTER, P., WAMPLER, G., KUPERMINC, M. and REGELSON, W. (1975a) Tilorone: Phase II study. In *1st Conference on Modulation of Host Immune Resistence in the Prevention of Induced Neoplasia. Fogarty Int. Center Proc.* No. **28**, pp. 141–143, CHIRIGOS, M. A. (Ed) N.I.H. 77–893, U.S. Government Printing Office, Washington, D.C.

RICHTER, P., WAMPLER, G., KUPERMINC, M. and REGELSON, W. (1975b) Phase I study of RMI 11,002DA (DEAA-fluorene). *Ibid.* p. 139.

ROBERTS, P. S., REGELSON, W. and KINGSBURY, B. (1973a) Determination of fibrinogenin normal plasma in the presence and absence of anticoagulants. *J. Lab. clin. Med.* **2**: 822–828.

ROBERTS, P. S., REGELSON, W. and KUPERMINC, M. (1973b) The effects of tilorone on clotting reactions and enzymes. 3rd Mediterranean Congress on Thromboembolism. *Israel J. med. Sci.* **9**: 12 (Abs.).

ROBERTS, P. S. and REGELSON, W. (1977) Splenic proteolytic enzymes and resistance to viral infections. In *Control of Neoplasia by Modulation of the Immune System.* (Prog. Cancer Res. Ther. series, Vol. 2), pp. 549–562, CHIRIGOS, M. A. (Ed). Raven Press, New York.

RÖMER, W. and ZSCHIESCHE, W. (1979) Cyclic nucleotide metabolism in the mouse spleen after treatment with tilorone hydrochloride *Acta. biol. med. germ.* **38**: 791–794.

ROSE, W. C., BRADLEY, S. G. and LEE, I. P. (1971) Enhanced toxicity for mice of combinations of antitumor drugs with *Salmonella typhosa* endotoxin. *Pharmacologist* **13**: 289 (Abs.).

SANDBERG, J. and GOLDIN, A. (1971) Use of first generation transplants of a slow growing solid tumor for the evaluation of new cancer chemotherapeutic agents. *Cancer Chemother. Rep.* **55(1)**: 233–238.

SCHAFER, M. P., CHIRIGOS, M. A. and PAPAS, T. S. (1974) Inhibition of Rauscher leukemia virus and avian myeloblastosis virus DNA polymerases by tilorone (NSC-143969) and its analogs. *Cancer Chemother. Rep.* **58(1)**: 821–827.

SCHIFF, G. M., LINNEMANN, C. C., ROTTE, T., MAYER, G. and TRIMBLE, S. (1973) Effect of tilorone HCl against rubella virus challenge in humans. *Clin. Res.* **21**: 882.

SCHULLER, G. B., MORAHAN, P. S. and SNODGRASS, M. (1975) Inhibition and enhancement of Friend leukemia virus by pyran copolymer. *Cancer Res.* **35**: 1915–1920.

SCHULTZ, R. (1976) Correlation between anti-tumor activity and macrophage activation by polyanions. In *3rd Conference on Modulation of Host Immune Resistance in the Prevention or Treatment of Induced Neoplasias.* Fogarty Int. Center. Proc., Virus Cancer Program, N.C.I.

SCHULTZ, R. M., PAPAMATHEAKIS, J. D. and CHIRIGOS, M. A. (1976) Correlation between polyanion induced macrophage activation and anti-tumor activity. *Proc. 13th natn Mtg. of Reticuloendothl. Soc.* Dec. 15–18, p. 71.

SCHULTZ, R. M., PAPAMATHEAKIS, J. D., WETZELER, J. and CHIRIGOS, M. A. (1977a) Association of macrophage activation with antitumor activity by synthetic and biological agents. *Cancer Res.* **37**: 3338–3343.

SCHULTZ, R. M., PAPAMATHEAKIS, J. D. and CHIRIGOS, M. A. (1977b) Interferon: an inducer of macrophage activation by polyanions. *Science* **197**: 674–676.

SCHULTZ, R. M., PAPAMATHEAKIS, J. D., LUETZELER, J. RUIZ, P. and CHIRIGOS, M. A. (1977c) Macrophage involvement in the protective effect of pyran copolymer against the Madison lung carcinoma (M109), *Cancer Res.* **37**: 358–364.

SCHULTZ, R. M., PAPAMATHEAKIS, J. D. and CHIRIGOS, M. A. (1977d) Direct activation *in vitro* of mice peritoneal macrophages by pyran copolymer (NSC 46015). *Cell Immunol.* **29**: 403–409.

SCHULTZ, R. M., CHIRIGOS, M. A. and HEINE, V. I. (1978a) Functional and morphological characteristics of interferon-treated macrophages. *Cell Immunol.* **35**: 84–91.

SCHULTZ, R. M., PAPAMATHEAKIS, J. D. and CHIRIGOS, M. A. (1978b) Correlation between antitumor activity and macrophage activation by polymers. In *Immune Modulation and Control of Neoplasia by Adjuvant Therapy.* (Prog. Cancer Res Ther. Series, Vol. 7) pp. 459–467, CHIRIGOS, M. A. (Ed). Raven Press, New York.

SELHORST, J. B., DUFEY, K. F., THOMAS, J. M. and REGELSON, W. (1978) PML: Remission and immunologic reversals. *Neurology* **28**: 337.

SHAMASH, J. and ALEXANDER, B. (1969) Coagulation studies with linear copolymers of aliphatic hydrocarbons and maleic acid: new ideas of anticoagulants. *Biochem. Biophys. Acta.* **194**: 449–461.

SIEBER, S. M. and ADAMSON, R. H. (1972) Embryotoxic activity of interferon and tilorone, and synthetic interferon inducer in mice. *5th Int. Congr. Pharmac.*, San Francisco, 23–28 July p. 231.

SIMINOFF, P., BERNARD, A. M., HURSKY, V. S. and PRICE, K. E. (1973) BL-20803 a new low molecular weight interferon inducer. *Antimicrob. Agents Chemother.* **3**: 742–743.

SMITHE, R. G. and GALLO, R. C. (1974) Agents which inhibit reverse transcriptases. *Life Sci.* **15**: 1711–1730.

SMULSON, M. E. and SUGIMURA, T. (1980) *Novel ADP. Ribosylations of regulatory enzymes and proteins.* Elsevier/North Holland, New York.

SNODGRASS, G. J., HARRIS, T. G. and KAPLAN, A. M. (1978) Chemokinetic response of activated macrophages to soluble products of neoplastic cells. *Cancer Res.* **78**: 2925–2929.

SNODGRASS, M. J. and KAPLAN, A. M. (1977) The *in vitro* response of non-specifically activated macrophages to carcinoma cells and their soluble by products. *Anat. Rec.* **187**: 718.

SNODGRASS, M. J., KAPLAN, A. M. and HARRIS, T. M. (1976) Macrophage mobility in response to carcinoma cells and their soluble by-products. *Proc. 13th natn Mtg. reticuloendothl. Soc.*, Dec. 15–18, p. 113.

SNODGRASS, M. J., MORAHAN, P. S. and KAPLAN, A. M. (1975) Histopathology of the host response to Lewis lung carcinoma: Modulation by pyran. *J. natn. Cancer Inst.* **55**: 455.

SOEHNER, R. L., GAMBARDELLA, M. M. and HOU, E. F. (1974) Oral induction of interferon by a low-molecular-weight compound. *Proc. Soc. exp. Biol. Med.* **145**: 1114–1119.

SPECTOR, J. I., LANG, E. and CROSBY, W. H. (1975) Coagulation changes in baboons during acute experimental hemoglobinemia and dextran infusion. *Am. J. Pathol.* **78(3)**: 469–476.

STINNETT, J. D. and MAJESKI, J. A. (1980) Macrophage activation and mobilization in nude mice by corynebacterium parvum and pyran. A functional histiologic study *J. Surg. Oncol.* **14**: 327–332.

STOLFI, R. L., MARTIN, D. S. (1978) Therapeutic activity of maleic anhydride-vinyl ether copolymers against spontaneous autochthonous murine mammary tumors. *Cancer Treat. Rep.* **62**: 1791–1796.

STRINGFELLOW, D. and GLASGOW, L. A. (1972a) Hyporeactivity of infection: potential limitation to therapeutic use of interferon-inducing agents. *Infect. Immun.* **6**: 743–747.

STRINGFELLOW, D. A. and GLASGOW, L. A. (1972b) Tilorone hydrochloride: an oral interferon-inducing agent. *Antimicrob. Agents Chemother.* **2**: 73–78.

STRINGFELLOW, D. A. (1973) Interferon inducers as antiviral agents. *Diss. Abstr. Intern. B* **33(7)**: 3219–3220.

STRINGFELLOW, D. A., OVERALL, J. C., JR and GLASGOW, L. A. (1974) Interferon inducers in therapy of infection with encephalomycarditis virus in mice. 1. Effect of single doses of polyriboinosinic–polyribocytidylic acid and tilorone hydrochloride on viral pathogenesis. *J. infect. Dis.* **130**: 470–480.

STYLOS, W. A., CHIRIGOS, M. A., LENGEL, C. R. and WEISS, J. F. (1978) T and B lymphocytes of irradiated, tumor-bearing mice treated with an immunostimulator, pyran. *Cell. Immunol.* **40**: 437–444.

TAGLIABUE, A., MANTOVANI, A., POLENTARVITI, N., VECCHI, A. and SPREAFICO, F. (1977) Effect of immunomodulators on effector cells involved in antibody-dependent cellular cytotoxicity. *J. natn. Cancer Inst.* **59**: 1019.

THELMO, W. L. and LEVINE, S. (1978) Renal lesions induced by tilorone and an analog. *Am. J. Pathol.* **91**: 355–360.

TOKUMARU, T. (1975) The mode of inhibition of herpes simplex and vesicular stomatitis ocular viral infections in the rabbit and hamster by an interferon inducer tilorone dihydrochloride. *Res. Commun. Chem. Pathol. Pharmac.* **11**: 289–301.

TUNIS, M. and REGELSON, W. (1965) The interaction of nucleated cells with anionic polyelectrolytes and inhibition of the interaction by pancreatic deoxyribonuclease. *Exp. Cell Res.* **40**: 383–395.

VAN DE VOORDE, J. (1970) Concomitant immunosuppressive effect of azaserine and thiopurine on AD-755 tumors in mice. 7th natn. Mtg. Reticuloendothl. Soc., Dec. 2–5, Augusta, Ga.

VECKENSTEDT, A., WITKOWSKI, W. and HOFFMANN, S. (1979a) Antiviral properties in mice of bis-basic fluorenone base-pair analogs. *Acta biol. med. Germ.* **38**: 745–749.

VECKENSTEDT, A., WITKOWSKI, W. and HOFFMAN, S. (1979b) Comparison of antiviral properties in mice of bis-pyrrolidino acetamino-fluorenone (MLV-B75), Bis-dipropylamino acetamido-fluorenone (MLV-B76), and tilorone hydrochloride. *Acta virol.* **23**: 153–158.

VILCEK, J. and NG, M. H. (1971) Post transcriptional control of interferon synthesis. *J. Virol.* **7**: 588–594.

VON SALLMANN, L. and BERSTEIN, H. N. (1963) Adverse effects on chloroquine and related antimalarial drugs on ocular structures. *Bull. rheum. Dis.* **15**: 327–330.

VEKSLER, I. G., RYABUKHA, U. N. and ANANENKO, U. P. (1979) Radiometric determination of the functional state of liver cells following the experimental use of certain stimulants of immunity. *Fitziol. Zh. SSSR.* **25**: 710–714.

WAALKES, T. P., SANDERS, K., SMITH, R. G. and ADAMSON, R. H. (1974) DNA polymerases of Walker 256 carcinosarcoma. *Cancer Res.* **34**: 385–391.

WACKER, A., LODEMANN, E., GAUR, V. and DIEDERICH, J. (1972) Distribution of ^{14}C-tilorone in mice. *Naturwissenschaften* **59**: 520.

WALKER, S. E. and ANVER, M. R. (1974) Delayed lymphoma formation in immunosuppressed NZB/NZW mice treated with tilorone HCl. *Clin. Res.* **22**: 612A.

WALKER, S. E. (1977) Accelerated mortality in young NZB/NZW mice treated with the interferon inducer tilorone hydrochloride. *Clin. Immunol. Immunopath.* **8**: 204–212.

WALKER, S. E. and ANVER, M. R. (1978) Stimulated autoantibody response and increased longevity in NZB/NZW mice treated with cyclophosphamide and tilorone. *Clin. exp. Immunol.* **33**: 453–462.

WALDREP, J. G., KAPLAN, A. M. and MOHANA KUMAR, T. (1981). Differentiation antigens of the human mononuclear phagocyte system I identification and characterization. *Cell Immunol.* In Press.

WALDREP, J. G., MOHANA KUMAR, T. and KAPLAN, A. M. (1981). Human mononuclear phagocyte associated antigens II lymphokine inducible antigens on the macrophage cell line, U 937. *Cell Immunol.* In Press.

WAMPLER, G. L., MUNSON, A. E. and REGELSON, W. (1972) Tilorone and congeners: new antitumor agents with stimulating effects on host defense mechanisms. *Proc. Am. Ass. Cancer Res.* **13**: 120.

WAMPLER, G. L., KUPERMINC, M. and REGELSON, W. (1973) Phase I study of tilorone, a non-marrow depressing antitumor agent. *Cancer Chemother. Rep.* **57**: 209–217.

WAMPLER, G. L. and REGELSON, W. (1974) Antitumor activity of tilorone and congeners in murine screening tumor systems. In *1st Conf. on Modulation of Host Immune Resistance in the Prevention or Treatment of Induced Neoplasiasl Fogarty Int. Center Proc.* No. **28**, pp. 123–129 CHIRIGOS, M. A. (Ed). U.S. Government Printing Office, Washington, D.C., (N.I.H. 77-893).

WASCHKE, K., WASEHKE, S.-R., HOFFMAN, S. and WITKOWSKI, W. (1979) Interferon induction in human lymphocytes by complexes of vinyl copolymers with polynucleotides. *Acta. biol. med. germ.* **38**: 739–744.

WASSERMAN, E. and LEVINE, L. (1961) Quantitative microcomplement fixation and its use in the study of antigenic structure by specific antigen-antibody inhibition. *J. Immunol.* **87**: 290–295.

WEISS, J. N., OCHS, A., ABEDI, S. and SELLHORST, J. (1980a) Retinopathy after tilorone HCl. *Am. J. Opthal.* **XX**: 846–853.

WEISS, J. N., WEINBERG, R. S. and REGELSON, W. (1980b) Kerathopathy after oral administration of tilorone HCl. *Am. J. Ophthal.* **89**: 46.

WILDSTEIN, A., STEVENS, L. E. and HASHIM, G. (1976) Skin and heart allograft prolongation in tilorone-treated rats. *Transplantation* **21**: 129–132.

WILDSTEIN, A., STEVENS, L. E. and HASHIM, G. (1975) Allograft prolongation by tilorone, an inducer of interferon. *Clin. Res.* **23**: 229A.

WITKOWSKI, W., HOFFMAN, S., VECKENSTEDT, A., SKOLZIGER, R., LUCK, G. and ZIMMER, C. H. (1979) Structure activity relationships of antiviral bis-basic fluorenone base-pair analogs. *Acta biol. med. germ.* **38,** 733–737. 733–737.

WOOLES, W. and MUNSON, A. E. (1971) The effect of stimulants and depressants of reticuloendothelial activity on drug metabolism. *J. reticuloendothl. Soc.* **9**: 108–119.

YANCEY, S. T. and BLEYER, W. A. (1974) Characteristics and response to certain cancer chemotherapeutic agents of an acute lymphocytic leukemia arising in a BALB/c X DBA/2F1 mouse. *Cancer Res.* **34**: 1866–1869.

YOSHIMURA, S., CHRISTIAN, R. T., CAMYRE, K. P. and KREUGER, P. F. (1973) Herpes virus hominis, type 1 and 2, infections in mice and rats. *8th Int. Congr. Chemother.* Athens, Greece, Sept.

ZBINDEN, G. and EMCH, E. (1972) Effect of tilorone HCl, an oral interferon-inducer, on leukopoiesis in rats. *Acta haemat.* **47**: 49–58.

ZERKLE, T. B., WADE, A. E. and RAGLAND, W. L. (1980) Selective depression of hepatic cytochrome P-450 hemoprotein by interferon inducers. *Biochem. Biophys. Res. Commun.* **96**: 121–127.

ZIMMER, C., BEINERT, K. E., LUCK, G., WAHNERT, U., LOBER, G. and THRUM, H. (1971) Interaction of the oligopeptide antibiotics netropsin and distamycin A with nucleic acids. *J. mol. Biol.* **58**: 329–348.
ZSCHIESCHE, W., SLAVINA, E. and LEIPUNSKARA (1977) The interferonogenic agent tilorone as a modulator of GvH reaction in mice. *Arch. Immunol. Ther. Experimentalis* **25**: 725–730.
ZSCHIESCHE, W., FAHLBUSCH, B., SCHUMANN, I. and TONEW, E. (1978) Induction of cytokines by tilorone hydrochloride *Agents Actions* **8**: 515–522.

INDEX

Acquired cellular immunity 243
Actinomycin D 361, 367, 373, 378, 379, 382, 383
Adriamycin 363, 372, 382
AFP 164, 167, 185
Alkylating agents 360, 366
Allograft rejection 258
Allotype suppression 119
Anaerobic coryneform bacteria 339–40
Anaphalactic antibody 133
Antibodies
derived from immunoglobulin 108
Fc portions of 89–95, 124–5
immunity modulation by 81–158
Antibody-dependent cell-mediated cytotoxicity (ADCC) assay 116–17, 167, 213, 381, 382, 383, 403
Antibody-feedback 104–6, 112, 113, 116–18
mediated by T cells 120–2
Antibody forming cells (AFC) 41, 42, 48, 64
Antibody responses 82–6
generation *in vitro* 41
Antibody synthesis 3
effect of BCG 278
T cell facilitation of 7–10
Antigen-antibody complexes 81–158
Antigen-binding vs antigen-masking 103–8
Antigen binding capacity (ABC) 346
Antigen-masking vs antigen-binding 103–8
Antigen presentation by macrophages
effects on B cells 50–1
effects on T cells 47–50
Antigen processing 46–7
Antigen-receptors 114, 138
Antigens
immunity modulation by 81–158
MHC 95–102
Antilymphocytes serum (ALS) 5
Anti-thymocyte serum (ATS) 327
Ara-C. *See* Cystosine arabinoside
Asparaginase 364, 376
Assay systems 55
Autoanatiidiotypic antibodies 122
Avian viruses 218, 222–3
Azathioprine 360, 363, 381, 383, 403–4
Azobenzenearsonate (ABA) 15

B cell inactivation model 112–13
B cell maturation 83
B cells 4–5, 7–10, 12
and BCG 282, 283
and *C parvum* 340, 351–2
and chemotherapy 359, 362–8, 373–6, 379, 380
and immunity modulation by antigens, antibodies and antigen-antibody complexes 83–6, 89, 102, 112, 113, 117–23, 128–38
and immunity modulation by levamisole 406
and immunity modulation by soluble mediators 183
and macrophage effects 35, 42, 50–1, 69
and methanol extraction residue (MER) 303, 323, 328–9
and synthetic homoribopolynucleotide complexes 421
and viruses and the immune response 213, 214, 217, 219, 224
effects of polynucleotide complexes 423–4
in tilorone treatment 454
inactivation of 113
Babesia 282
Babesia microti 261
Bacillus Calmette-Guérin (BCG)
and chemotherapy 370, 381
and immunity modulation by macrophages 37, 54, 57, 69, 70
and methanol extraction residue (MER) 304, 305, 319, 322, 324, 329
and micro-organisms 244, 245, 249, 251, 253, 254, 255, 262, 263, 266
antagonism of immunosuppression by 280–1
as adjuvant to specific antigen 295
clinical immunotherapy with 291–4
hazards and toxicity 294
therapeutic trials 291–2
effects of specific types of lymphoid cell 281–6
effects on antibody synthesis 278–9
effects on cell-mediated immunity 279–80
effects on interferon, colony-stimulating factor and pyrogens 287–8
effects on lymphocytes 286–91
effects on T cells 286–7
fractions of 288–91
immunity modulation by 275–301
immunological effects in man 292–4
lipid contribution to therapeutic effects 288
stimulation of afferent macrophages 284
suppressor adherent cells 284–6
BCG. *See* Bacillus Calmette-Guérin
BCNU (1,3-bis(2-chloroethyl)-1-nitrosourea) 363, 366, 457
Benzoyl-L-arginine methyl ester (BAME) 437, 460
Benzyl-penicilloyl (BPO) 105
Besnoitia infection 259–60
Besnoitia jellisoni 241, 246, 247
BGG 347
bis DEAE fluorenone. *See* Tilorone
Bleomycin 361, 364
Bordetella pertussis 245, 343
Brown-Pearce carcinoma 452
Brucella 393–4
Brucella abortus 40, 218, 243, 281, 342, 416–17, 420
Brucella melitensis 244
Burro red blood cells (BRBC) 47
Busulfan 373

cAMP 398
Cancer 66
Candida 282, 318
Candida albicans 252, 261, 343
Carminomycin 361, 367
Cell-mediated immunity 3, 86–9, 220, 277, 283, 293, 303, 414–16
effect of BCG 279–80
effect of MER 308–9
effect of MER *in vitro* 310
Cell-mediated lymphocytotoxicity 45, 53–5, 59, 67, 167
Cell-mediated lympholysis 42, 129
Cellular mechanisms in immune responses 82–102
cGMP 398

Chemotherapy 359–92
Clone elimination or inactivation 127–33
Cloning inhibition factor 165
Colchinine 361, 380–3
Colony stimulating factor 287–8
Complement-dependent cellular cytotoxicity (CDCC) 381
Complement-independent cellular cytotoxicity 381
Complement-independent phagocytosis 381
Complement-receptor lymphocytes (CRL) 95
Complete Freund's adjuvant (CFA) 44, 247, 248, 249, 262, 281, 304, 377
Concanavalin A (Con A) 42, 43, 262
Cortisone acetate 361, 382, 403–4
Corynebacterium diphtheriae 352
Corynebacterium granulosum 249
Corynebacterium parvum 53, 54, 57, 62, 63, 70, 245, 249, 255, 262, 287, 308, 322, 339–58, 381, 382, 441, 452
  adjuvant effect of 348
  antitumour activity 343–5
  antitumor effects in man 345–6
  clinical applications 354
  delayed hypersensitivity (DH) 347
  effects on antibody responses to T cell dependent antigen 346–7
  effects on antibody responses to T-independent antigens 347
  effects on B cells 351–2
  effects on macrophages 348–51
  effects on NK cell activity 354
  effects on primary and memory cytotoxicity 353
  effects on T cells 352–3
  mechanism of action 348
  modulation of immune response 346–7
  modulation of RES 342
  morphologic alterations following 340–2
  resistance to infectious agents 342–3
  reticulostimulant 354
Coxiella burneti 393
Cryptococcus neoformans 243
Cyclic nucleotides 398
Cyclohexamide 445
Cycloheximide 383
Cyclophosphamide 280–1, 362–9, 372–83, 403–4
Cyclosporin A 364, 372, 379
Cytochalasin A 361, 382, 383
Cytochalasin B 361, 365, 381–3
Cytochalasin D 361
Cytochalasin E 361
Cytokines 159, 448–9
  action on target cell functions 180–6
  biological role 163–5
  classification of 159–63
  in vitro observations in relation to *in vivo* events 165–8
  purification and characterization of 169–72
Cytomegalovirus infection 261
Cytosine arabinoside (Ara-C) 363, 364, 366, 378
Cytotoxic effector cells 330
Cytotoxic effector functions 381
Cytotoxic immune responses 353
Cytotoxic peritoneal exudate macrophages 283
Cytotoxic T cells 378, 379, 381
Cytotoxic T lymphocytes (CLT) 4, 11, 17, 87

Dacarbazine (DTIC) 318–19
Daunomycin 382
Daunorubicin 364, 372
Delayed hypersensitivity 10, 21, 48, 347, 414, 418
Delipidated mycobacterial cells (DMC) 278, 288
Deoxyribonucleoprotein (DNP) 41–2, 105, 110, 439
Dimethyl benzene anthracene (DMBA) 312
Dinitrochlorobenzene (DNCB) 68, 166, 293, 307, 378
Dinitrofluorobenzene (DNFB) 306–7, 368, 377
Dinitrophenylated Ficoll 262
Diplococcus pneumoniae 449
Direct allogeneic anaphylactic degranulation (DAAD) 117, 118
DNA polymerase 439, 440, 446, 450
DMA precursors 87
DNA synthesis 55, 64, 134, 184, 185, 265, 278, 281, 360, 363, 365–79, 381, 415, 416
DNA viruses 218–19, 234
DNase 55
Drugs effects
  on afferent immune responses 359–65
  on central immune responses 365–79
  on efferent immune response 379–83
DTC (sodium diethyldithiocarbamate) 394
  absence of carcinogenicity 401
  activity across species barrier 404
  anabolic effect 401
  anti-cancer effects 401
  anti-toxic effects 402
  as trigger of hormone-like factors 404
  chemistry, metabolism and pharmacology of 400–2
  comparison with levamisole 406
  experimental immunomodulation studies 402–4
  general remarks on 406–7
  influences of brain neocortex 405
  influences of immune parameters in man 405
  influences on mice immunosuppressed by chemotherapeutic agents 403–4
  influences on mouse spleen weight or lymphocyte numbers 402
  influences on NK and ADCC 403
  mechanisms of action 404–5
  potentiation of T–cell activities by 402–3
  ratio-protective properties 401
  toxico-pharmacology in man 402

Echinococcus 282
Effector B cells 373–6, 379
Effector cells, differentiation of 373–9
Effector functions, mature non T cell-non B cell 381–3
Effector T cells 376–81
Encephalomyelitis (EAE) 454
Escherichia coli 163, 219, 282, 287
Extracellular proliferation 241
Eye lesions 450

Fc-dependent antibody-feedback 112–13
Fc-dependent feedback suppression 116–20
Fc-portion binding to Fc receptors 113–16
Fc portion on immunoregulatory antibody 110–12
Fc-receptors 89–95, 102, 107, 113–17, 121, 124, 126
5-Fluorodeoxyuracil 375, 412
5-Fluorouracil 361, 363, 378
Francisella tularensis 241
Freund's complete adjuvant (FCA) 44, 247, 248, 249, 262, 281, 304, 377
Freund's incomplete adjuvant 247, 248, 347
Friend leukemia virus 220–21
Friend virus 212, 215–17

Genetic control of T cell interactions 19–23
L-Glutamic acid-L-alanine-L-tyrosine (GAT) 14

Graft-versus-host (GVH) reactions 4, 10, 15, 63, 65, 87, 108, 264
Granulocyte-macrophage colony forming units 285
Granulomatous hepatitis 294
Gross leukemia virus 218

Hanks balanced salt solution (HBSS) 247, 248
Haptens 8
Helper cells, differentiation of 372–3
Hemophilus influenzae 241
Hepatitis virus 219
High density lipoprotein (HDL) 266
Histoplasma capsulatum 241
Hodgkin's disease 67
Homoribopolynucleotide complexes 411–27
  adjuvant effects on cell mediated immunity 415
  adjuvant effects on *in vivo* humoral immune response 412
  adjuvant properties in humoral immunity 413
  augmentation of humoral immune response 412–14
  cellular sites of action of 419–21
  effects of B lymphocytes 423–4
  effects on cell-mediated immune responses 414
  effects on macrophage activity 423
  effects on response to infectious agents 416
  effects on T cell activity 423
  future prospects 424–5
  immune defense effects 416–17
  immunosuppressive effects of 419–20
  in vitro correlates of cell-mediated immunity 415–16
  in vivo humoral immune response 413–14
  mode of action of 421–4
  tumor immunity effects 417
Horse red blood cells (HRBC) 64
Host response
  modulation by micro-organisms 241–73
  to intracellular infection 245–9
  to intracellular infection and suppressed response to specific immunologic stimuli 256–62
  to intracellular micro-organisms 242–3
Human gammaglobulin (HGG) 105, 424
Human serum albumin (HSA) 40, 110
Hydrocortisone 367, 370, 372, 376, 381, 383, 454
Hydrocortisone succinate 382
Hydroxyurea 360, 378

IDS-mediated suppression of DNA synthesis 184, 185
Immune responses 3–7
  cellular mechanisms in 82–102
  effects of macrophages on. *See* Macrophages
  modulation by T lymphocytes 22–3
  negative cell regulation of 12–19
  T cell regulation 7–12
Immunocomponent cells, inactivation of 116–20
Immunoglobulin binding factor (IBF) 102
Immunoglobulins
  Fc portions of 89
  IgA 84, 123
  IgD 82, 91
  IgE 118, 127, 368
  IgG 84, 89, 90, 93–5, 98, 99, 102, 108–24, 127, 131–7, 217, 303, 368, 374, 375, 378, 395, 454
  IgM 82, 84, 89–95, 98, 108, 120–2, 131–3, 135, 217, 303, 368, 374, 375, 378, 395, 433
Immunomodulation effect 303
Immunomodulators, action of 321–3
Incomplete Freunds adjuvant (ICFA) 247, 248, 347
Influenza infection 261

Initiator T lymphocytes (ITL) 86
Interferon 287, 382, 429, 442, 444, 448–9
Interleukin 1 (IL-1) 51
Intermediate density lipoprotein (IDL) 266
Intracellular proliferation 241
Irreversible tolerance 127–33

K-cells 167, 213
Keyhold limpet hemocyanin (KLH) 14, 39–42
Klebsiella infection 290
Klebseilla pneumoniae 256, 257

Lactic dehydrogenase (LDH) 219, 223
Lepromatous leprosy 66, 68
Leukopenia 363
Levamisole 393–410
  chemistry, pharmacology and metabolism of 394–5
  clinical use of 399–400
  comparison with DTC 406
  effect on cyclic nucleotides 398
  effects on immune system 399
  experimental immunomodulation studies 395–9
  general remarks on 406
  genetic and epigenetic control effects 397–8
  in animal cancer therapy 397
  influence on antibody response to various antigens 396
  in vivo effectiveness 396
  mechanisms of action of 397–9
  mediation through serum factors induced by sulphur moiety 398–9
  potentiation of functions of polymorphonuclears by 397
  potentiation of macrophage activities 396–7
  potentiation of T-cell activity 395–6
  protective influence of metabolites 398
  time- and dose-dependent regulatory characteristics 398
Lipid contribution to therapeutic effects of BCG 288
Lipopolysaccharide (LPS) 44, 61, 62, 113, 352, 432
Lipoproteins 266
Listeria 282, 325, 397
Listeria monocytogenes 57, 58, 59, 241, 244, 247, 256, 257, 264, 281, 343, 417
Low density lipoprotein (LDL) 266
Lymph node cell immunocompetence 365
Lymphocyte-activating factor (LAF) 45, 51, 177, 284, 324–5
Lymphocyte components 361–4
Lymphocyte homing patterns 361
Lymphocyte immunocompetence 365
Lymphocytes, effects of BCG on 289–91
Lymphocytic choriomeningitis cirus (LCM) 219
Lymphoid cells, effects of BCG on 281–6
Lymphoid hyperplasia 340
Lymphoid-RES 324
Lymphokines (LK) 159, 263–4, 382
  biological role 163–5
  classification of 159–63
  identity of cells producing 175–6
  in vitro observations in relation to *in vivo* events 165–8
  mechanism of production and release 177–80
  purification and characterization of 169–72
Lysosomal enzyme activity 325

Macrophage-activating agent 62
Macrophage activating factor (MAF) 166, 181, 187, 252–4, 263

Macrophage-derived suppressor factor (MØSF) 59
Macrophage-induced suppression, metabolic requirements for 55–6
Macrophages 5
activation 52
activation as result of interaction with exogenous agents or with lymphocytes and their mediators 57–8
activation by pyran 441
activation induced by soluble lymphocyte products 263–4
and nonspecific resistance to neoplastic cells 249–56
BCG-activated 282
categories of 37
central role of 168–9
cytotoxicity of 349
differential effect on normal versus neoplastic cells 68–9
distinction between activated and resting 54
effect of *C. parvum* 348–51
effect of MER 324
effect of polynucleotide complexes 423
effect of viruses on 224–32
effect on B cells, antigen presentation 50–1
effect on T cells, antigen presentation by 47–50
effector cell in expression of increased nonspecific resistance to intracellular micro-organisms 243–5
enhancement of immune response by 38–51
enhancement of immune response *in vitro* 41–6
enhancement of immune response *in vivo* 39–41
from single tissue source 38
from various sources 37–8
immunity modulation by 35–79
methods used for harvesting 38
OVA-pulsed 49
peritoneal, cytotoxic effects 254
potentiation by levamisole 396–7
requirement for generation of antibody-producing cells *in vitro* 41
requirement for production of lymphokines *in vitro* 44–6
requirement for T cell responses *in vitro* 42–6
role in immunosuppression associated with cancer and other pathological conditions 66–8
role in immunosuppression associated with graft host disease 65
stimulation of afferent 284
subpopulations of 38
suppression of immune responses by 51–71
suppression of immune responses *in vivo* 59–69
suppression of immunologic responses 262–3
suppressor effects mediated by soluble factors 56–7
suppressor role in antigenic competition 63–5
tumoricidal effect by activated 263
Major histocompatibility gene complex (MHC) 4, 11–15, 20–2, 46–50, 69, 84–90, 95–102, 106, 107, 130, 137, 159
Mammary tumor virus 222, 261
MCF 165, 166, 167
MDP 290
Melphalan 373
Mengo virus 343
2-Mercaptoethanol (2–ME) 45
6–Mercaptopurine 360, 363, 365, 367, 372, 373, 375, 378, 380
Mesocestoides coiti 261
Methanol extraction residue (MER) 278, 279, 281, 284, 303–37
and chemotherapy 330
antigenic stimulation by 323
antimicrobial activity 305–6
antitumor activity in experimental systems 310–15
clinical trials on effectiveness of 315, 318
clinical trials summary 320
effect in solid tumors 318–21
effect on antibody-forming cells 307
effect on antibody response 325
effect on antibody response *in vitro* 309–10
effect on B cells 328–9
effect on circulating antibodies 307–8
effect on CMI 308–10
effect on immunologic responsiveness to particulate and soluble antigens 306–10
effect on immunotherapy in man 315–21
effect on LAF production 324–5
effect on lysosomal enzyme activities 325
effect on macrophages 324
effect on morphology and function of lymphoid-RES 324
effect of oral administration of 316
effect on phagocytic, bacteriostatic and bactericidal activity 325
effect on spontaneous tumor development 312–13
effect on states of resistance and immunological reactivity 305–21
effect on T cell function 308–9, 326–8
effect on tumor cells 325–6
effect on tumor challenge 311–12
heterogeneity of test groups 316
immunomodulatory effect of 329
immunotherapeutic studies 313–15
in acute myelocytic leukemia (AML) 317–18
in vitro systems 309–10, 326
in vivo systems 307–9, 324–6
mode of action studies 321–30
occurrence of side effects 316
optimal experimental conditions for 317
preparation, properties and activities of 305
properties 323–4
role of shared antigens 329
safety of use 316
tumor enhancement by 316
tumor relationships 317
unexpected discontinuation of treatment 317
use of combined treatments 316–17
Methotrexate 360, 363, 365, 366, 371, 372, 375, 378
Methyl-CCNU 363
Methylprednisolone 383
Microbial agents, immunosuppression mechanisms 265–6
Micro-organisms
effects of homoribonucleotide complexes 416
intracellular
and neoplasia resistance 245–9
host response to 242–3
macrophage in increased nonspecific assistance to 243–5
modulation of immunity and host resistance by 241–73
Migration inhibition factor (MIF) 44, 58, 59, 70, 164–6, 175, 181, 186–8, 220, 221, 263, 449
Miliary tuberculosis 66
Mineral oil induced plasmcytoma (MOPC) 285
Mitoclomine 373
Mixed leukocyte culture 42, 45, 49, 54, 56, 57, 59, 66, 67
Mixed leukocyte reaction (MLR) 15–17

Mixed lymphocyte culture 96, 106, 107, 118
Mixed lymphocyte-tumor interaction (MLTI) 53, 55
Moloney sarcoma virus (MSV) 52, 62, 222, 264, 280
Monocyte/macrophage components 360–1
Monocyte-mediated antibody-dependent cell-mediated cytotoxicity (MMADCC) 43
Monokines (MK) 159
  biological role 163–5
  classification of 159–63
  in vitro observations in relation to *in vivo* events 165–8
  purification and characterization of 169–72
Mononuclear phagocytes 241
Multicellular cell pathway 16
Murine leukemia viruses 215–18
Murine sarcoma virus (MSV) 53, 67
Murine tumor viruses 222
MVE-2 429–35, 438, 443, 444, 460
Mycobacterium bovis 241, 275, 304
Mycobacterium butryicum 245–7
Mycobacterium leprae 68, 454
Mycobacterium lepraemurium 454
Mycobacterium marinum 454
Mycobacterium tuberculosis 57, 241, 243, 244, 281, 304, 454

Natural killer (NK) cells 53, 69, 213, 221, 283, 323, 354, 403, 442
NED-137 429–31, 433, 435, 443, 444, 460
Negative cell regulation of immune responses 12–19
Neocortex, influence of DTC 405
Neoplasia, effect of intracellular infection 245–9
Neuraminidase galactose oxidase 43
Neutrophils 36, 397
Newcastle disease (NDV) virus 223
Nippostrongylus brasilienis 249
Nitrogen mustard 363, 373
Non-oncogenic viruses 219–20, 223–4
Nonspecific factors 160
Nucleic acid complexing 446

OMPI 398
Oncogenic viruses 215–24
Osteoclast-activating factor (OAF) 45
Ovalbumin (OVA) 44, 64
OVA pulsed macrophages 49

Pactamycin 382
Pasteurella tularansis 449
Periodate oxidation 342
Peripheral blood leukocytes (PBL) 37, 42–5, 53, 66, 67
Peritoneal exudate cells (PEC) 36, 53, 54, 69
Peritoneal lymph nodes 254
Peritoneal macrophages 349, 350
Phosphodiesterase 397
Phytoemagglutinin (PHA) 5, 42–6, 52, 62, 99, 223, 262, 264, 416, 432
Plaque forming cells (PFCs) 56, 215, 346, 395
Plasmodium 282
Plasmodium berghei 262, 343
Pokeweed mitogen (PWM) 43, 56, 66
Polio virus vaccine 261
Polyethylene sulfonate (PES) 435–6, 438–40
Polymethacrylic acid (PMAA) 437
Polymorphonuclear leukocytes (PMNs) 241
Polynucleotide complexes. *See* Homoribopolynucleotide complexes
Polyphoretin phosphate 440
Polyvinyl pyrrolidone (PVP) 436
Precursor T cells 381
Prednisolone 382
Prednisone 373
Procarbazine 371
Prostaglandins 265
Protein synthesis 134, 361, 376, 423, 438
Protozoan infection 256
Pseudomonas aeruginosa 261
Purified protein derivative of tuberculin (PPD) 44–6
Puromycin 361, 382, 383
Puromycin aminonucleoside 371
Pyran copolymer 429
  adjuvant action 441–3
  anticoagulant effects 437–8
  antitumor effects 275–8, 433
  chemistry and toxicology 433–4
  clinical studies 434–5
  cytoplasmic effects 438–40
  discussion 435–41
  final summary 459–61
  general remarks on 431–3
  immunologic effects 441–3
  macrophage activation 441–3
  molecular weight 460
  NK cell activation 441–3
  nuclear effects 438–40
  past clinical experience and possible clinical role 443
  resistance to infection 433
  role of molecular weight 432
  serum complement inhibition 440
  toxicity 432
Pyrogenic substances 288

Rapamycin 375
Rauscher leukemia virus (RLV) 217, 313
Recruited T Lymphocytes (RTL) 86–7
Reticuloendothelial system (RES) 52, 57, 60, 63, 69, 70, 304
  lymphoid 324
  modulation of 342
  stimulation of 321–2, 342
Reversible tolerance, active suppression 133–5
Rifamycin 447
RNA polymerase 446
RNA synthesis 134, 361, 376, 423, 438
RNA viruses 234
RNase 55
Rowson Parr virus (RPB) 217
Rubidomycin 364
Rubomycin 367

Salmonella enteritidis 243, 245, 282, 342
Salmonella typhimurium 216, 244, 264
Sarcoidosis 66
Schistosoma mansoni 243, 262
Serologically-defined antigens 88
Serum antibody 133
Sheep red blood cell (SRBC) 56, 61, 64, 65, 215, 217, 259–66, 278–80, 305–10, 324, 328, 346
Sheep red blood cell (SRBC) glycophorin specific TsF 23
Shigella paradysentheria 40
SIRS (soluble immune response suppressor) 15, 17, 59, 64, 263
Skin grafts 258, 279, 452
Small cell carcinoma of the lung (SCC) 320
Sodium diethyldithiocarbamate. *See* DTC
Sodium periodate 43

Soluble immune response suppressor (SIRS) 15, 17, 59, 64, 263
Soluble mediators
identity of cells producing 175–6
mechanisms of production and release 177–80
modulation of 159–208
nonspecific 160–62
restricted by MHC 160
unrestricted by MHC 161–2
specific 159
specificity for 172–5
Specific factors 159
Spleen cells 284
Staphylococcus 325
Staphylococcus aureus 261, 343
Stem cells 3–4
Steroid hormones 361, 367, 376
Streptococcus pneumoniae 241, 256, 257
Streptococcus pyogenes 241
Streptozotocin 364
Suppressor adherent cells 284–6
Suppressor cell differentiation 367–71
Suppressor T cells 118, 420
Susulfan *See* also Busulfan
Synthetic polyanions 429-35
anti-complement activity 440–1
anti-inflammatory activity 440–1
biologic action 431–2

T cell-derived suppressor products 16
T cell facilitation
of antibody synthesis 7–10
of cell-mediated immune responses 10–11
of macrophage effector functions 11–12
T cell interactions, genetic control of 19–23
T cell replacing factor (TRF) 9, 102, 121
T cell suppressor dysfunction and disease 17–19
T cell suppressor factor (TsF) 14, 16, 17, 23
T cells 4–5, 7–10, 13–17, 21–2
and BCG 279, 283, 284, 286
and *C. parvum* 340–2, 352–3, 359
and chemotherapy 362–8, 374, 376–80
and immunity modulation by antigens, antibodies and antigen-antibody complexes 82–6, 89–102, 106, 108, 112, 119, 122, 124, 128–38
and immunity modulation by levamisole 395–6, 402–3, 406, 407
and immunity modulation by soluble mediators 167, 184
and macrophage effects 35, 42–4, 47–50, 59–60, 69, 70
and methanol extraction residue (MER) 303, 322–3, 326–8
and synthetic homoribopolynucleotide complexes 415, 416, 421
and viruses and the immune response 213, 214, 217, 219, 220, 221, 224
antibody-feedback mediated by 120–2
effects of polynucleotide complexes 423
in tilorone treatment 454–5
mechanism of modulation of immune responses by 22–3
T lymphocytes 84
TAME (*p*-toluensulfonyl-L-arginine methyl ester) 437, 458, 460
Target cell functions 180–6
Target cell receptors 172–5
Tetanus toxoid 259
Tetramisole 394
6-TG 365, 375
Thymus cells 364
Thymus-derived lymphocytes 3–34
Tilorone 371, 429, 444–50
anti-tumor activity 450–2
as immune inhibitor 453
capacity to generate *in vitro* interferon 445
clinical anti-tumor studies 455–7
conclusions from clinical trial 459
cytokine induction 448–9
DNA polymerase inhibition 446–7
drug metabolizing effects 445–6
effects on immune and inflammatory response 452–5
eye lesions 450
final summary 459–61
host resistance 449–50
interferon induction 448–9
miscellaneous action 457–8
nucleic acid complexing 446
related compounds 458
RNA polymerase inhibition 446–7
route of administration 445
teratogenesis 449
tissue levels of interferon produced by 445
topical and *in vitro* effects 448
virus induction 449
Tolerance-breaking immunogen 128
Tolerance-breaking protein 127
Tolerance classification 130
Tolerance induction 130, 134
p-Toluenosulfonyl-L-arginine methyl ester (TAME) 437, 458, 460
Toxoplasma gondii 241, 246, 281, 343
Toxoplasma infection 257–61
Transfer of delayed hypersensitivity (DTN) 48
Treponema pallidum 282
Trichinella spiralis 262, 379
Trinitrophenol (TNP) 129
Trypanosoma brucei 261, 263
Trypanosoma congolense 261
Trypanosoma cruzi 241
Tuberculosis 261
Tumor cells 62–3
Tumor necrosis factor (TNF) 287
Tumor-specific immunity 293

Very low density lipoprotein (VLDL) 266
Vesicular stomitis virus (VSV) 223
Vibrio cholerae 216
Vinblastine 361, 364, 375, 381, 382
Vincristine 364, 375
Viruses
and immune response 211–40
current concept of 212–14
effect of homoribonucleotide complexes 416
effect on macrophage functions 224–32
historical background 211–12
implications of 212
mechanisms of 214–15
modulation of immunoresponsiveness by 225

Wax D 304

YAC-1 target cells 221
Yersinia tularensis 282